CONTENTS

Foundations of
Maternal-Newborn
and Women's
Health Nursing

EIGHTH EDITION

Sharon Murray,
MSN, RN

Professor Emerita, Health Professions, Golden West College, Huntington Beach, California

Emily McKinney,
MSN, RN, C (deceased)

Nurse Educator and Consultant, Dallas, Texas

Karen S. Holub,
MS, RNC-OB

Assistant Clinical Professor, Baylor University, Louise Herrington School of Nursing, Dallas, Texas

Reneé Jones,
DNP, RNC-OB, WHNP-BC

Clinical Associate Professor, Baylor University, Louise Herrington School of Nursing, Dallas, Texas

Kristin L. Scheffer,
MSN, RNC-OB, C-EFM

Nursing Professional Development Specialist, Baylor University Medical Center; Adjunct Faculty, Louise Herrington School of Nursing, Baylor University, Dallas, Texas

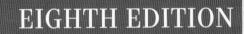

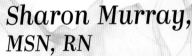

ELSEVIER

Elsevier
3251 Riverport Lane
St. Louis, Missouri 63043

> **Notice**
>
> Practitioners and researchers must always rely on their own experience and knowledge in evaluating and
> using any information, methods, compounds or experiments described herein. Because of rapid advances
> in the medical sciences, in particular, independent verification of diagnoses and drug dosages should be
> made. To the fullest extent of the law, no responsibility is assumed by Elsevier, authors, editors or contrib-
> utors for any injury and/or damage to persons or property as a matter of products liability, negligence or
> otherwise, or from any use or operation of any methods, products, instructions, or ideas contained in the
> material herein.

Previous editions copyrighted 2019, 2014, 2010, 2006, 2002, 1998, 1994.

Senior Content Strategist: Sandy Clark
Director, Content Development: Laurie Gower
Senior Content Development Specialist: Betsy McCormac
Publishing Services Manager: Deena Burgess
Senior Project Manager: Julie Taylor
Design Direction: Amy Buxton

Printed in India

Last digit is the print number: 9 8 7 6 5 4 3 2 1

Working together
to grow libraries in
developing countries

www.elsevier.com • www.bookaid.org

Susan A. Angelicola, MSN, RNC, APRN, WHNP-BC
Women's Health Nurse Practitioner
Department of Obstetrics & Gynecology
Summit Health, New Providence
New Jersey
United States

Suzanne McMurtry Baird, DNP, RN
Nursing Director
Clinical Concepts in Obstetrics, LLC
Brentwood, Tennessee
United States;
Adjunct Assistant Professor of Nursing
Vanderbilt University School of Nursing
Nashville, Tennessee
United States

Lynn Clark Callister, PhD, RN, FAAN
Professor Emerita
College of Nursing
Brigham Young University
Provo, Utah
United States

Jane Lin Chien, MS, CRNA, APRN, CCRN
Labor and Delivery
Medical City of Dallas
Dallas, Texas
United States

Rebecca L. Cypher, MSN, PNNP, RNC-OB, C-EFM
Perinatal Consultant and President
Cypher Maternal-Fetal Solutions, LLC
Washington
United States

Kristine DeButy, MSN, RNC-OB, NE-BC
Director of Nursing
Women & Children's Services
Baylor University Medical Center
part of Baylor Scott and White Health
Dallas, Texas
United States

Emily Drake, PhD, RN
Professor
Department of Family, Community and
    Mental Health Systems
University of Virginia
Charlottesville, Virginia
United States

Melissa R. Espey-Mueller, LCCE, CD, CLE, GTA
Director of Prenatal Education
Women's and Children's Services
Baylor University Medical Center
Baylor Scott and White Health
Dallas, Texas
United States

Heather S. Hendrikson, RDN, CSP, LD
Clinical Dietitian
Women's Services/NICU
Baylor University Medical Center
part of Baylor Scott and White Health
Dallas, Texas

Karen S. Holub, MS, RNC-OB
Assistant Clinical Professor
Louise Herrington School of Nursing
Baylor University
Dallas, Texas
United States

Reneé Jones, DNP, RNC-OB, WHNP-BC
Clinical Associate Professor
Louise Herrington School of Nursing
Baylor University
Dallas, Texas,
United States

Nan Ketcham, PhD (c), RN, CNE
Clinical Associate Professor
Louise Herrington School of Nursing
Baylor University
Dallas, Texas
United States

Courtney M. Kujansuu, MSN, RNC-OB, RNC-IAP, C-EFM, C-ONQS
Clinical Professional Development
    Educator
HCA Center for Clinical
    Advancement-Mountain Division
Alaska Regional Hospital
Anchorage, Alaska
United States

Sharla McDaniel, MSN, RN
Staff Nurse
Labor and Delivery
Baylor University Medical Center
part of Baylor Scott and White
Dallas, Texas
United States

Jessica L. McNeil-Santiel, DNP, APRN, CNM, RNC-OB, C-EFM
Certified Nurse Midwife
WISH
Parkland Health and Hospital System
Dallas, Texas
United States;
Adjunct Clinical Faculty
Louise Herrington School of Nursing
Baylor University
Dallas, Texas
United States

Cathy L. Miller, PhD, RN
Professor
College of Nursing and Health Sciences
University of Texas at Tyler
Tyler, Texas
United States

Dawn Piacenza, MSN, APRN, RNC-OB, C-EFM
NICU Data Coordinator
Women's and Infant's Services
Wesley Medical Center
Wichita, Kansas
United States

Emily Roberts, MSN, AGCNS-BC, RNC-OB, C-EFM
Clinical Nurse Specialist
Women's Services
Roper St. Francis Healthcare
Charleston, South Carolina
United States

Jennifer Rodriguez, DNP, RN
Professor of Nursing
Kellogg Community College
Battle Creek, Michigan
United States

Cheryl K. Roth, PhD, WHNP-BC, RNC-OB, RNFA
Nurse Practitioner
Labor & Delivery/Couplet Care
HonorHealth
Scottsdale Shea/Osborn Medical Centers
Scottsdale, Arizona
United States

Kristin L. Scheffer, MSN, RNC-OB, C-EFM
Nursing Professional Development Specialist
Baylor University Medical Center
part of Baylor Scott and White Health
Dallas, Texas
United States;
Adjunct Faculty
Louise Herrington School of Nursing
Baylor University
Dallas, Texas
United States

Allison L. Scott, DNP, PCPNP-BC, IBCLC
Associate Professor
Eleanor Mann School of Nursing
University of Arkansas
Fayetteville, Arkansas
United States

Lisa Wallace, DNP, RNC-OB, NE-BC
Assistant Professor
Department of Nursing
Morehead State University
Morehead, Kentucky
United States

Suzanne White, DNP, RN, PHCNS-BC
Associate Professor of Nursing
Morehead State University
Morehead, Kentucky

Della Wrightson, MSN, APRN, RNC-NIC
Levine Children's Hospital
Atrium Health
Charlotte, North Carolina
United States

INSTRUCTOR AND STUDENT RESOURCES

Kimberly Amos, PhD, MSN, RN, CNE
Director
Foothills Nursing Consortium
Isothermal Community College
Rutherfordton
North Carolina
United States

INSTRUCTOR RESOURCES

Tiffany Jakubowski, MS, RN, AGCNS-BC, CMSRN, ONC
Nursing Instructor
Front Range Community College
Westminster
Colorado
United States

Katherine McDannel, MSN, RN
Assistant Professor,
Nursing,
Lewis University College of Nursing and
    Health Sciences,
Romeoville, Illinois

Rita J. Nutt, DNP, RN
Assistant Professor,
School of Nursing,
Salisbury University,
Salisbury, Maryland

Courtney Orelup-Fitzgerald,
    MSN, RN, CPN
Instructor,
School of Nursing,
Salem State University,
Salem, Massachusetts

Tina Rorick, DNP, MSN, RN, CPN
Maternal Child Health Content Expert,
Professor,
Nursing,
College of the Canyons,
Santa Clarita, California

Dr. Sheilena Sanders, DNP, MSN, MBA/
    HCM, RN
Nursing Professor,
Nursing,
Augusta Technical College/Augusta Uni-
    versity,
Augusta, Georgia

To our families: Bill and Jill Holub, Grant and Amanda Pearson, Jamie, Hannah and Cole Jones; Bobby, Cole, and Cade Scheffer and Julie Odom for the sacrifices you made for this book and for your love and support every day.

To all nurses and nursing students, past, present, and future. You embody the best of all of us as you offer your knowledge, skill, and compassion to heal, support, and comfort others. Stay strong.

One of our challenges as educators and providers of nursing care in many settings is to keep up with the rapid changes in health care while preparing students to stay focused on the *care* of nursing. Nursing faculty teach the student ways to use critical thinking, the nursing process, and clinical judgment along with advances in pharmaceuticals and technology while imparting the values of client-centered care. Our text tries to help the student learn to balance "high-touch" care with "high-tech" care in different settings.

An effective textbook must present comprehensive content that can be read with ease because nursing students differ in learning styles, experience, and primary language. Our objective for the eighth edition of *Foundations of Maternal-Newborn and Women's Health Nursing* continues to be presenting complex material as simply and clearly as possible. We provide instruction in assessments and interventions so students can function quickly in the clinical area at a beginning level. To this end, proven learning aids, such as summaries, illustrations, and tables, are used generously throughout the book.

CONTENT

The five elements we consider most important are (1) a scientific base of information; (2) critical thinking, the nursing process, and clinical judgment; (3) communication; (4) client and family teaching; and (5) diversity and inclusion.

Scientific Base

Effective nursing care depends on having a sound understanding of the basis for medical treatments and nursing actions. Although anatomy and physiology courses are part of every curriculum, students often need a review, particularly of the specific content related to childbearing and women's health. Because of this, we have incorporated principles of physiology and pathophysiology throughout the book. We have presented these scientific concepts in a clear and understandable manner so that the reader can comprehend the forces underlying both health and dysfunction.

Critical Thinking, The Nursing Process, and Clinical Judgment

Nurses must learn critical thinking skills to overcome habits or impulses that can lead to poor clinical decisions. Chapter 1 discusses critical thinking and describes how critical thinking is used in each step of the nursing process.

The nursing process is a five-step process of clinical decision making that forms the foundation of holistic client-centered nursing care. It is used to plan and provide nursing care and evaluate the client's response. To demonstrate the application of this process in childbearing and newborn and women's health nursing, many of the chapters have an "Application of the Nursing Process" section, which leads the reader through the five steps of the nursing process as it applies to a specific client condition or need. Basic information about the condition is presented, and general nursing care follows, organized by the steps of the nursing process. Interventions are general rather than client-specific and are explained by rationales.

Although clinical judgment is part of the nursing process, research has demonstrated that entry-level nurses lack clinical judgment ability. Driven by this research and an increased focus on client safety, the National Council of State Boards of Nursing (NCSBN) developed the NCSBN Clinical Judgment Measurement Model (NCJMM) as an "evidence-based framework for measuring whether nurse licensure candidates demonstrate at least minimal competence with respect to clinical judgment and decision making" (NCSBN, n.d., "Does the NCSBN Clinical Judgment Measurement Model (NCJMM) replace the need for the nursing process?" section). The model is not intended to replace the nursing process, but rather it is a specific framework for testing (NCSBN, n.d., "How is the NCSBN defining Clinical Judgement for purposes of a Next Generation NCLEX® (NGN)" section). The Next Generation Nursing (NGN) style questions associated with this model are different than the traditional NCLEX® question style students and faculty are accustomed to on examinations. To facilitate student confidence with these question styles, we have added a series of NGN-style questions throughout the book. Chapter 1 discusses critical thinking, clinical judgment, and the nursing process.

Communication

Although they seldom are included as core content in childbearing and women's health nursing texts, communication skills are essential to providing adequate care for a childbearing family. Throughout the text, we reinforce the student's previous learning and give practical examples of ways in which communication skills can be used in childbearing and women's health settings.

Teaching

While health care delivery has changed dramatically, with greater emphasis on outcome management, the family's need for education and support has increased. Nurses have responded to families' needs by developing alternative means of education that use every possible moment before admission and during their stay in the health care facility. Childbearing families are entitled to comprehensive information about how to achieve the best pregnancy outcome and how to best care for the postpartum client and the baby after birth. Clients of all ages need current information about maintaining their health. Nurses may be their primary instructors in many areas of childbearing and newborn and women's health nursing.

We present client teaching in two ways:
- Chapters are organized to highlight key content so the student can gather information and translate it into teaching

that is individualized for the person or group of people. For example, Chapter 23, Infant Feeding, lays a foundation of basic information, discusses some common problems, identifies relevant assessments, and presents nursing interventions devoted to teaching parents ways to feed their infant successfully.

- Teaching guidelines are highlighted in Client Teaching features, which give ideas on ways to answer the most common questions on a topic. These features are constructed to show students ways to present information in everyday language rather than in professional language so the family will better understand the teaching. For instance, the feature "When to Go to the Hospital or Birth Center" (Chapter 15) addresses the concern of many expectant parents that they will not recognize the onset of labor.

The internet is often used by lay people and professionals alike as a source of health information. We provide the addresses for many websites throughout our text that contain reliable, current information relevant to childbearing and newborn and women's health nursing. Examples of these sites are the March of Dimes, Centers for Disease Control and Prevention, National Institutes of Health, and American Cancer Society. Websites for professional associations and other reliable sources are included when appropriate.

Diversity, Equity, and Inclusion

Cultural values are among the most significant factors influencing a family's perception of childbirth, and effective nursing care must be culture specific. This requires nurses to consider their own cultural values and implicit biases in order to examine how these values may create conflict with those whose values are different. Chapter 2 offers an overview of Western cultural values and identifies some areas such as communication and health beliefs that may be sources of conflict. Because many different cultural groups exist in the United States, emphasis is placed on ways to do a cultural assessment. Understanding a family's culture helps nurses provide care that shows respect for cultural differences and traditional healing practices while providing the necessary education and support.

In the last several years, there has been a growing awareness of the marginalization of gender diverse persons and the effects of this marginalization, including inequities in health care. In this edition of our textbook, we identified the need for gender inclusiveness. A significant challenge for us has been one of gender-neutral terminology in the obstetric and gynecologic specialties. There is a wide variety of individual differences in gender identification, expression, and preferred terminology. When working with clients and their families, nurses should demonstrate respect for the individual by asking about preferred names, pronouns, and parent titles (mother, father, parent). However, this is not a solution when writing a text. We have tried to be consistent with the use of "sex," "male," and "female" to describe the chromosomes and genitalia present at birth. Identifying concise, gender-neutral terms for "maternal," "mother," "father," and "women's health"

has been more difficult. Where possible, we have used the term "client" to identify the pregnant or postpartum person and "partner" for the nonchildbearing parent, and we have reserved "mother" and "father" as role descriptors rather than biological identifiers in the childbearing chapters. We have removed the gender-specific pronouns as much as possible. Like many others, we struggle to find an inclusive term for "women's health" that still communicates respect for the person as more than a vessel of organs. For this edition, we have retained "women's health" to refer to the health care of persons with ovaries, a uterus, and breasts. We hope that we will have better terminology identified in the literature before our next edition of this text. Chapter 2 introduces some of the issues of gender-diverse clients and families, especially in the childbearing environment. We acknowledge the need for, and support research in the area of, the childbearing experience and women's health issues for these families.

ORGANIZATION

The eighth edition of *Foundations of Maternal-Newborn and Women's Health Nursing* is divided into five parts. Part 1, Foundations for Nursing Care of Childbearing Families, presents an overview of contemporary nursing care of the family, including, social, cultural, and ethical aspects. A review of reproductive anatomy and physiology and the hereditary and environmental factors that affect care are also presented.

Part 2, The Family Before Birth, begins with conception and prenatal development. These chapters also cover the physiologic and psychosocial adaptations to pregnancy and include a thorough explanation of recommended nutrition during pregnancy and after childbirth. A chapter addressing antepartum fetal assessments and their purpose and two chapters covering families with special needs and antepartum complications are included in Part 2.

Part 3, The Family During Birth, addresses the physiologic processes of birth, nursing care during labor, and birth and intrapartum complications. These chapters include intrapartum fetal monitoring, pain management, and obstetric procedures such as cesarean birth.

Part 4, The Family Following Birth, describes care of the new parent and infant, as well as infant feeding and postpartum and neonatal complications. Chapter 19 is a new chapter that addresses obstetric critical care, a growing subspecialty of obstetric nursing due to the increased maternal morbidity and mortality in the United States. It is also included in Part 4, as many of the critical conditions span the antepartum, intrapartum, and postpartum periods.

Part 5, Women's Health Care, focuses on family planning, care of the infertile couple, and women's health care.

FEATURES

- *Visual Appeal.* The book is visually appealing, with numerous up-to-date, full-color illustrations and photographs that clarify concepts and reinforce learning.

- *Objectives.* Each chapter begins with a list of objectives that spell out the purposes of the chapter.
- *Glossary.* A glossary at the back of the book contains key terms and their definitions from all chapters and other terms related to this course.
- *Knowledge Check.* Questions to help students monitor their understanding of the material presented are placed at intervals throughout each chapter. Answers to questions are placed in Appendix A so that students can have immediate feedback.
- *Critical to Remember* and *Safety Checks.* Condensed summaries of the essential facts to remember are boxed and set apart to reinforce critical information.
- *Client Teaching.* This feature can be used by students who must begin client teaching very early in their clinical rotations. These include answers to the most common questions asked by parents, often phrased in lay terms or as the nurse would actually answer a client.
- *Procedures.* Illustrated procedures that are specific to childbearing and newborn and women's health nursing, such as assessment of the uterine fundus, are presented in a step-by-step format.
- *Drug Guides.* Guides for medications often administered in childbearing and newborn and women's health care are available in appropriate chapters.
- *Complementary and Alternative Therapies.* We have included content about these therapies when appropriate throughout the text.
- *Summary Concepts.* A concise review of content is provided at the end of each chapter. In addition, tables, flow charts, and diagrams are used to summarize complex material.
- *Next-Generation NCLEX® (NGN)-Style Questions.* Samples of NGN questions are included at the end of most of the chapters throughout the book, and answers are found in Appendix B.

ANCILLARIES

Materials that complement *Foundations of Maternal-Newborn and Women's Health Nursing* include:

For Students

- ***Evolve:*** Evolve is an innovative website providing a wealth of content, resources, and state-of-the-art information on childbearing and women's health nursing. Learning resources for students include Audio Glossary, Printable Key Points, and NCLEX®-Style Review Questions and Next Generation NCLEX®-(NGN)-Style Cases

For Instructors

Evolve includes these teaching resources for instructors:
- ***Electronic Test Bank in ExamView format*** contains more than 900 NCLEX®-style test items, including alternative-format questions. Additional Next-Generation NCLEX® (NGN)-Style Cases (and Answers) for Maternity Nursing are also included.
- ***TEACH for Nurses*** includes teaching strategies; in-class case studies; and links to animations, nursing skills, and nursing curriculum standards such as QSEN concepts and BSN Essentials.
- ***Electronic Image Collection,*** containing more than 350 full-color illustrations and photographs from the text, helps instructors develop presentations and explain key concepts.
- ***PowerPoint Slides,*** with lecture notes for each chapter of the text, assist in presenting materials in the classroom. ***Case Studies*** and ***Audience Response Questions*** for i-clicker are included.

REFERENCE

National Council of State Boards of Nursing. (n.d.). *NGN FAQs for educators.* https://www.ncsbn.org/11447.htm.

ACKNOWLEDGMENTS

Many people made the eighth edition of *Foundations of Maternal-Newborn and Women's Health Nursing* a reality. Thank you to the Elsevier team who brought us together, kept us focused, and assisted throughout the publication process: Sandy Clark, Content Strategist; Betsy McCormac, Content Development Specialist; Julie Taylor, Project Manager; and Amy Buxton, Designer.

Thank you to the chapter contributors who shared their passion. Their clinical expertise and commitment to the future of nursing are deeply appreciated.

We also want to thank our photographer, Dianna Rich, RN, a labor and delivery nurse with a talent for photography who contributed the much-needed new photographs.

We will be forever grateful to Sharon Murray and Emily McKinney, whose vision and endless work brought us the previous editions of this book and whose love for nursing and nursing students will live on in future editions.

Karen Holub, Reneé Jones, and Kristin Scheffer

CONTENTS

Clinical Judgment and the Nursing Process

Kristin L. Scheffer, Karen S. Holub

OBJECTIVES

After studying this chapter, you should be able to:

1. Discuss the need for heightened awareness on safety and quality in women's health.
2. Describe programs that address safety and quality within women's health.
3. Explain choices in childbearing.
4. Define family-centered care.
5. Discuss current trends that affect women's health nursing, such as Healthy People 2030, focus on safety and quality,

cost containment, community-based care, advances in technology, and increased use of complementary and alternative medicine.

6. Describe the influence of regulatory and professional organizations on the development of standards within women's health nursing.
7. Discuss how nurses use critical thinking, clinical judgment, and the nursing process.

Major changes in maternity and women's health care occurred throughout the twentieth century. Explosive increases in knowledge, including technological advances; government funding, oversight and regulations; cost containment efforts; and the desire of consumers to be active participants and decision makers in their care led to increasing complexity of care. Despite advancements, comparison of current maternal and neonatal outcomes in the United States to those of other countries demonstrates the need for continued improvement. Health care professionals continually focus on patient safety and quality of care. Nursing skills of critical thinking, clinical judgment, and the nursing process combined with standards, guidelines, and evidence position the professional nurse as a critical member of the health care team in this environment.

SAFETY AND QUALITY WITHIN WOMEN'S HEALTH

High rates of maternal and infant mortality have become a major focus for many nations, including the United States. Although improvements in health care and government funding have resulted in a significant decline in maternal and infant mortality, statistics show a wide disparity between outcomes based on a variety of client characteristics. Proportionately more adverse outcomes are seen in rural areas compared with outcomes in urban areas (American College of Obstetricians and Gynecologists [ACOG], 2021a). Racial and ethnic disparities fueled by social determinants, implicit bias, racism,

and other inequities create increased morbidity and mortality in women's health (ACOG, 2021b; Association of Women's Health, Obstetric and Neonatal Nurses [AWHONN], 2021b; Centers for Disease Control and Prevention [CDC], 2019; Nurse Practitioners in Women's Health, 2020).

While safety and quality standardization has been implemented throughout obstetric care, the CDC (2021) reported maternal mortality rates increased from 17.4 deaths per 100,000 births in 2018 to 20.1 in 2019. Currently, programs to improve women's health safety and quality include The Joint Commission, Interprofessional Collaboration and Education, Alliance for Innovation on Maternal Health, and Women's Health and Perinatal Nursing Care Quality Measures.

The Joint Commission

The Joint Commission (TJC) is an independent organization that accredits health care organizations. It focuses on continual quality improvement and standardization of practices creating safe and effective care. Accredited organizations report their performance with the Perinatal Care Measures for best practice annually. The four perinatal care measures are decrease the rate of elective deliveries, decrease the rate of primary cesarean births, decrease the rate of newborns with unexpected complications, and increase the rate of exclusive breastfeeding (TJC, 2021). In January 2021, TJC also issued standards in the provision of care, treatment, and services in relation to maternal safety. These two standards focus on reducing the likelihood of harm related to maternal hemorrhage and severe hypertension/preeclampsia.

Interprofessional Collaboration and Education

Interprofessional collaborative practice has been identified as a key to safe, high-quality, accessible, patient-centered care (Interprofessional Education Collaborative [IPEC], 2021). To promote team-based patient care and improve outcomes, IPEC has encouraged health professional schools to incorporate learning experiences and defined core competencies into their curricula for interprofessional collaborative practice. Studies have shown interprofessional interactions enhance communication, increase appreciation for other disciplines, and delineate the contribution to the whole when providing care in practice (Wei et al., 2019; Zechariah et al., 2019).

Alliance for Innovation on Maternal Health

The Alliance for Innovation on Maternal Health (AIM) is a quality improvement alliance of professional organizations, patient representatives, and a health industry informational forum (AIM, 2020). AIM has developed patient safety bundles for maternal care representing best practices and is supported by multidisciplinary professional organizations (ACOG, 2018).

Patient Safety Bundles

A bundle is a set of evidence-based practices performed together to improve patient outcomes (AIM, 2020). Maternal safety bundles have been developed for mental health: depression and anxiety, obstetric hemorrhage, severe hypertension in pregnancy, venous thromboembolism, safe reduction of primary cesarean birth, reduction of peripartum racial/ethnic disparities, support after a severe maternal event, opioid use disorder, cardiac conditions in obstetric care, postpartum discharge transition, pregnant/postpartum care of substance use disorder, prevention of surgical site infections after gynecologic surgery, and enhanced recovery after surgery (AIM, 2020). (See https://www.safehealthcareforeverywoman.org.)

Women's Health and Perinatal Nursing Care Quality Measures

Nurses' actions have a significant impact on client outcomes. To help guide those actions, AWHONN has developed practice standards to provide standardization and a means to measure the quality of nursing care. These standards address multiple aspects of care including educational preparation of nurses, access to health care, risk-based screenings, care of specific client populations (incarcerated, substance users, analgesia/anesthesia, etc.), gender bias, fetal monitoring, cardiovascular health, and many others (AWHONN, 2021a). Practice briefs are quick-reference guides providing standardized techniques and the evidence-based rationale behind the interventions incorporated. A few of the topics addressed include quantification of blood loss, prevention of newborn falls, and venous thromboembolism (AWHONN, 2021c).

Standards of care support consistency in safety and quality of care for all clients. However, as a consumer, the client can choose different health care settings and providers, as well as what interventions are implemented or withheld.

CHOICES IN CHILDBIRTH

In the early 1950s, consumers began to insist on their right to be involved in their own health care. Childbearing families wanted to be active decision makers in the extraordinary time of pregnancy and childbirth. Health care professionals such as Dr. Grantly Dick-Read, Dr. Fernand Lamaze, and Dr. Robert Bradley responded with programs that included client and family education to support them. Most families now recognize they have choices in the childbirth experience. These choices include provider, birth setting, support persons for labor and birth, and education.

Health Care Provider

Clients contemplating pregnancy and birth may choose a physician, either an obstetrician or family practice doctor; a nurse practitioner (NP); a certified nurse midwife (CNM), or a direct-entry midwife to be their health care provider. Direct entry midwives include certified midwife (CM), certified professional midwife (CPM), or traditional midwife. Clients and their families need to know what to expect from each of these practitioners.

Midwives care for clients at low risk for complications and refer them to a backup physician if problems develop. A CNM is trained in nursing and midwifery and licensed by the state as an advanced practice registered nurse, where a direct-entry midwife is trained to provide the midwife model of care, performing prenatal and delivery care out of the hospital setting, without receiving a nursing degree or license. CMs complete training much like CNMs, including graduation from a master's level training program, adhere to the same standards as CNMs but do not have a degree or license in nursing. CPMs and traditional midwives train in community, out of hospital settings; however, CPMs pursue certification where traditional midwives do not (Midwives Alliance of North America, 2020).

CNMs, NPs, and physicians treat clients during pregnancy and the postpartum period, but NPs do not perform deliveries. NPs usually work in a physician's office or clinic and see clients for routine prenatal care, but the delivery is performed by the physician. A CNM, NP, or family practice physician also may care for the newborn; an obstetrician only cares for the pregnant and postpartum client; and a pediatrician cares for the baby.

Some couples visit several different care providers before choosing the one they think is best for them. They may ask about the provider's usual practices and beliefs regarding medications, episiotomies, or aspects of infant care.

Birth Setting

Hospitals

The majority of births in the United States occur in the hospital settings, most of which provide family-centered care. *Family-centered care* describes safe, high-quality care that recognizes and adapts to both the physical and psychosocial needs of the family, including the newborn. The goal is to foster family unity while maintaining physical safety.

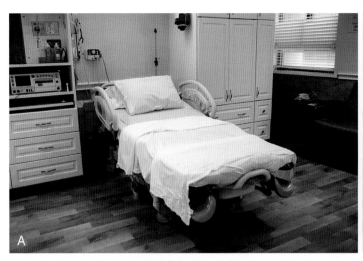
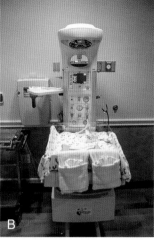

FIG. 1.1 Typical labor, delivery, and recovery room.

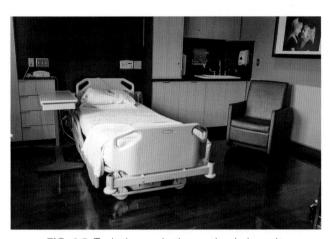

FIG. 1.2 Typical room in the mother-baby unit.

Labor, Delivery, and Recovery Rooms. Today, the most common location for vaginal birth in a hospital is the labor, delivery, and recovery (LDR) room. In an LDR room, normal labor, birth, and recovery from birth take place in one setting (Fig. 1.1A–B).

During labor, the client's significant others can remain at the bedside. These people may include relatives, friends, and other children, depending on the policies of the facility and the client's desires. After birth, the client and newborn typically remain in the LDR room for up to 2 hours, then they are transferred to the mother-baby unit for the remainder of the hospital stay (Fig. 1.2). Upon transfer to the mother-baby unit, the infant may be taken to the nursery for more extensive assessment or may remain with the client in the postpartum room while being assessed.

Labor, Delivery, Recovery, and Postpartum Rooms. Some hospitals offer rooms like LDR rooms in layout and function, with the exception that the client is not transferred to a postpartum or mother-baby unit after recovery. The couplet remains in the labor, delivery, recovery, and postpartum (LDRP) room until discharge. The primary support person is encouraged to stay with the client and infant, and sleeping facilities for that person may be provided.

Birth Centers

Freestanding birth centers are designed to provide maternity care for low-risk clients outside a hospital setting. Many centers also provide gynecologic services such as annual well-woman examinations and contraceptive counseling. The client usually attends classes at the birth center or elsewhere to prepare for childbirth, breastfeeding, and infant care. Both the client and the infant continue to receive follow-up care during the first 6 weeks after birth. This may include help for breastfeeding problems, a postpartum examination at 4 to 6 weeks, family planning information, and examination of the newborn.

Birth centers are less expensive compared with traditional hospitals, which provide advanced technology that may be unnecessary for low-risk clients. Clients who want a safe birth in a familiar, home-like setting often express satisfaction with birth centers.

The main disadvantage is most independent birth centers are not equipped for major obstetric emergencies. If unforeseen difficulties develop during labor, the client should be transferred to a hospital for continued care provided by a physician. Although procedures have been designed for these situations, a sudden transfer is frightening for the family.

Home Births

In the United States only a small number of clients give birth at home. Many CNMs have moved their practices to hospitals or birth centers and may be in practice with physicians. Clients who once sought home births have found they can have many of the advantages of family-centered care in the hospital or birth center and yet retain the nurse–midwife's care and low-intervention approach they prefer.

Home birth provides the advantage of keeping the family together in its own familiar environment throughout the childbirth experience. When all goes well, birth at home can be a growth-enhancing experience for every family member. Bonding with the infant is unimpeded by hospital routines, and breastfeeding is highly encouraged and supported.

Clients who have their babies at home maintain a feeling of control because they actively plan and prepare for each detail of the birth.

Giving birth at home also has disadvantages. Clients who plan a home birth should be screened carefully to make sure they are low risk for complications. If transfer to a nearby hospital becomes necessary, the time required may be an issue. Other problems associated with home birth include the need for the parents to provide a setting and adequate supplies for the birth. The client must provide care for themselves and their infant without the immediate help typically provided in a hospital or birth center setting.

Support Person

Inclusion of the client's support system is paramount during labor. Evidence demonstrates continuous labor support results in higher client satisfaction, shorter duration of labors with a higher rate of vaginal birth, and decreased incidence of operative vaginal delivery and low 5-minute Apgar scores (Bohren et al., 2017). The support person can be a partner, relative, friend, or nursing personnel. For hospital births, only one or two people may be permitted to be present where other settings may allow more support people.

Some clients hire a **doula** to provide support during labor. A doula is a trained labor support person who provides physical and emotional support throughout labor and sometimes during the postpartum period. Many doulas are certified childbirth educators and certified lactation consultants. They are able to provide family teaching and support throughout the pregnancy and postpartum/newborn period.

Siblings

Many viewpoints exist regarding the presence of children at birth. Some think children become closer to their new siblings when they are present at birth. Others think the sights of the birth process, blood, and the client in pain may be too frightening for children.

Children who participate in the birth of a sibling may attend all or part of the labor and birth or may join the parents just after the birth to participate in the immediate celebration. An adult support person is necessary to stay with the child throughout the experience. The support person should have no role other than attending to the child. This role includes gauging the child's response, providing explanations and reassurance, and taking the child out of the room as needed.

Education

Perinatal education is important to help couples learn about pregnancy, birth, and parenting. Many programs not only focus on preparation for childbirth but also include information formerly received during the birth facility stay. There are options for perinatal education. New families make their choices based on the program (online or in-person), costs, and types of information they need. Small classes are ideal but may be too expensive or unavailable (see Chapter 7).

CURRENT FACTORS AFFECTING PERINATAL AND WOMEN'S HEALTH CARE

In addition to the focus on safety and quality, current factors affecting women's health include Healthy People 2030, cost containment, community-based perinatal nursing, advances in technology, and complementary medicine.

Healthy People 2030

Healthy People 2030 is a set of 10-year objectives for improving the health of the people of the United States. The overarching goals are as follows (U.S. Department of Health and Human Services, 2020):

- Attain high-quality, longer lives free of preventable disease, disability, injury, and premature death.
- Achieve health equity, eliminate disparities, and improve health literacy contributing to an increase in the health of all groups.
- Create social, physical, and economic environments that promote good health for all.
- Promote quality of life, healthy development, and healthy behaviors across all life stages.
- Engage leaders to take action and design policies impacting the health of all.

Cost Containment

Government, insurance companies, health care facilities, and providers have made a concerted effort to control the increasing cost of health care in the United States. Cost containment efforts have had major effects on maternity care, primarily regarding length of stay (LOS). Clients who have a normal vaginal birth are typically discharged with their newborns from the hospital at 24 to 48 hours, and those who give birth by cesarean section leave at 72 to 96 hours. This is a short time to accomplish the teaching needed before discharge, particularly when the client is tired and uncomfortable from the birth.

Community-Based Perinatal and Women's Health Nursing

Community-based care has increased in perinatal and women's health nursing due to the increased cost associated with the acute care setting. Advances in portable technology and wireless transmission allow nurses in many practice areas to perform procedures in the home once limited to the hospital. Documentation and data retrieval are available by secure wireless internet connections. Additionally, clients and their families are taught to manage less severe problems at home under the supervision of a nurse, entering the hospital only for possible worsening of the problem. Consumers often prefer home care because of decreased stress on the family when a client or newborn is not separated from the family support system for hospitalization.

Public health agencies have existed for many years, and many clients obtain all antepartum, postpartum, and neonatal care in these clinics. Other community facilities such as neighborhood health centers, shelters for women and children, school-age mothers' programs, and nurse-managed postpartum centers also provide care to a variety of clients.

Nurses need a broad array of skills to function effectively in community-based care, whether that care takes place in individuals' homes or in large clinics. They should understand the communities in which they practice and the diversity within those communities.

In addition to the perinatal services provided by CNMs and NPs, the role of the perinatal registered nurse (RN) encompasses antepartum, postpartum, and neonatal care in the community setting. Care may be given in an environment physically separate from acute care settings; therefore nurses should be able to function independently and have superior clinical and critical thinking skills. They should be proficient in interviewing, counseling, and teaching. They assume a leadership role in the coordination of the services a family may require in a complex case, and they frequently supervise the work of other care providers.

Advances in Technology

Technological advances are changing the way that health care is delivered; perinatal care should keep pace with these changes. Health care professionals and clients have online access to information from a variety of databases. Nurses have an important responsibility to help childbearing families verify the source of information and interpret the information appropriately. Telemedicine is used for consultation between professionals and may provide access to care for people in underserved areas. As we have seen in recent years, the use of telemedicine has continued to evolve and is utilized by many more providers. Fetal monitoring data may be stored on electronic media rather than on paper. Video and digital imaging methods are used to preserve and recall crisp images and allow image overlay and computerized comparison, often at distant locations. Electronic medical records are standard in health care facilities. Electronic devices can be used to support nurses with medication information, send and receive wireless email, maintain contacts, and download journal articles from publications such as the *Journal of Obstetric, Gynecologic, and Neonatal Nursing* and *Nursing for Women's Health*. Maintaining security is essential to ensure appropriate privacy for personal and professional information.

Complementary and Alternative Medicine

Complementary and alternative medicine (CAM) is common. CAM refers to health care approaches that differ from conventional Western medicine. When these practices are integrated with conventional treatments, they are complementary; when used in place of the mainstream practices, they are "alternative." Integrative medicine refers to the coordinated use of conventional and complementary approaches to health care (National Center for Complementary and Integrative Health, 2020). Table 1.1 gives examples of therapies for complementary or alternative care.

Safety is a major concern with the use of CAM. Many people who use these techniques or substances are self-referred. They may delay seeking necessary care from a conventional provider, or the client may ingest herbal remedies or other harmful substances during pregnancy or lactation. Some CAM therapies are harmful if combined with conventional medications or when taken in excess. Because herbs and vitamins are classified as foods rather than medications, they are not strictly regulated. Therefore people may consume variable amounts of active ingredients from these substances. Herbal therapies may be used for infertility, premenstrual syndrome, dysmenorrhea, menopausal

TABLE 1.1 Complementary and Alternative Medicine Categories

Category	Examples
Mind–body interventions: behavioral, psychological, social, and spiritual approaches to health	Yoga, relaxation response techniques, meditation, tai chi, hypnotherapy, music therapy, spirituality, and biofeedback; some such as support groups and cognitive–behavioral therapy are now mainstream
Manipulative and body-based methods: based on manipulation or movement of one or more parts of the body	Chiropractic or osteopathic manipulation; massage
Alternative medical systems: systems developed outside the Western biomedical approach or that evolved apart from the early conventional medical approach in the United States	Examples of systems developed within Western cultures include homeopathy, naturopathic, and chiropractic medicine; non-Western approaches include traditional Chinese medicine, Ayurveda, Native American medicine, and acupuncture
Biologically based therapies: use of substances found in nature such as herbs, foods, and vitamins	Dietary supplements, herbal products, or medicinal plants such as ginkgo biloba, ginseng, echinacea, saw palmetto, witch hazel, bilberry, aloe vera, feverfew, and green tea; aromatherapy
Energy therapies: two types involve the energy fields	
Biofield therapies: presumed to affect energy fields that surround the body	Biofield therapies have not been scientifically proved; examples include qi gong, Reiki, and therapeutic touch
Bioelectromagnetic-based therapies: unconventional use of electromagnetic fields	Examples of bioelectromagnetic-based therapies include pulsed fields, magnetic fields, and alternating-current or direct-current fields

symptoms, pregnancy and perineal discomforts, and lactation support. Also, many people may not consider some therapies as alternative because they are considered mainstream in their cultures. Assessment for the use of CAM therapies is becoming more common for many client assessment tools in medicine, nursing, pharmacy, and other health care specialties.

Nurses may find their professional values are consistent with many of the CAM therapies. As a profession, nursing supports a self-care and preventive approach to health care, in which individuals bear much of the responsibility for their health. Nursing practice has traditionally emphasized a holistic, or body–mind–spirit, model of health that fits with CAM. Nurses may already practice some CAM therapies such as therapeutic touch. The rising interest in CAM provides opportunities for nurses to participate in research related to the legitimacy of these treatment modalities.

STANDARDS OF PRACTICE FOR PERINATAL AND WOMEN'S HEALTH NURSING

Standards are statements of responsibility or duty established by an authority (American Nurses Association [ANA], 2021) such as the government, the state board of nursing, accrediting organizations, the professional organization or the agency. "Practice guidelines are systematically developed statements to assist practitioner and patient decisions about appropriate health care for specific clinical circumstances" (Institute of Medicine, 1990). Both community-based and acute care services should meet standards and guidelines for practice established by the agency itself, appropriate specialty practice organizations, and accrediting agencies.

Agency Standards

Health care agencies are required to have policies, procedures, and protocols to define and guide elements of care. These standards, which should comply with established national standards, should be kept current and accessible to the nursing personnel. Manuals for these agency standards are often available online within the agency for easier access. Updates and periodic reviews are required to maintain validity.

Professional Organizational Standards

Professional organizational standards provide broader guidelines that are nationally recognized. AWHONN is recognized as the national professional organization for perinatal, neonatal and women's health nursing services, publishing standards, education guides, monographs, professional issues, and nursing practice guidelines. Standards set by other professional organizations, such as the ACOG, the American Academy of Pediatrics (AAP), and the National Association of Home Care and Hospice, may influence standards for perinatal and women's health nurses.

Legal Standards

Nurses who practice in any health care delivery system should understand the definition of nursing practice and the rules and regulations that govern its practice in their work settings. Nurses also should be aware of their scope of practice in varying locations as defined by state nurse practice acts.

Other regulatory bodies, such as the Occupational Safety and Health Administration (OSHA), the U.S. Food and Drug Administration (FDA), and the CDC, also provide guidelines for practice in those areas. Accrediting agencies such as TJC and the Community Health Accreditation Program (CHAP) give their approval after visiting facilities and observing whether standards are being met in practice. Approval from these accrediting agencies affects reimbursement and funding decisions as well.

Evidence-Based Practice

Clinically based nursing research is increasing rapidly as nurse researchers strive to develop an independent body of knowledge demonstrating the value of nursing interventions. This is achieved through evidence-based practice. Evidence-based practice utilizes continual critical analysis of current literature (scientific knowledge) and available data (clinical expertise) to develop policy and practice standards improving the outcomes of consumers. This approach promotes high-quality care through evaluation of practice for measurable, defined outcomes and continual reevaluation for future improvements (Agency for Healthcare Research and Quality [AHRQ], n.d.; National Institute of Corrections, n.d.).

AWHONN has an ongoing commitment to develop and disseminate evidence-based practice guidelines. Implementation of evidence-based guidelines promotes application of the best available scientific evidence for nursing care rather than care based on tradition alone.

The AHRQ, a branch of the U.S. Public Health Service, actively sponsors research in health issues facing mothers and children. From research generated through this and other agencies, high-quality evidence can be accumulated to guide the best and lowest-cost clinical practices. Clinical practice guidelines are an important tool in developing parameters for safe, effective, and evidence-based care to mothers, infants, children, and families. Many professional and regulatory organizations have developed guidelines related to adult and pediatric care. Safety and quality improvements, enhanced primary care, access to high-quality care, and specific illnesses are addressed in available practice guidelines. AHRQ's guidelines are available at https://www.guidelines.gov.

ESSENTIAL SKILLS FOR PROFESSIONAL NURSING

Critical thinking, clinical judgment, and the nursing process are critical skills that nurses use in daily practice. These skills are interrelated and complementary.

Critical Thinking

Critical thinking is a disciplined and systemic way of forming judgments and making decisions. It has a cognitive (skills) and affective (disposition) aspect (Facione, 1990). In nursing, the skills include information seeking, analyzing, discriminating, applying standards, logical reasoning, and predicting and transforming knowledge. The affective habits of the mind in nursing include inquisitiveness, intellectual integrity, contextual perspective, intuition, confidence, creativity, open-mindedness, flexibility, perseverance, and reflection (Scheffer & Rubenfeld, 2000). Critical thinking requires the nurse to examine how judgments and decisions are made including what data is collected, how it is analyzed, what biases (personal, institutional, cultural, etc.) and assumptions may influence decisions, what alternative decisions are considered, and what are the likely consequences of the decision or judgment.

Critical thinking is based on reason rather than preference or prejudice. It also seeks to examine feelings to understand how emotions affect thinking. Finally, critical thinking requires the suspension of **judgment** (opinion) until evidence is adequate to support **inferences** or drawing conclusions.

Clinical Judgment

The purpose of critical thinking is to help nurses make the best clinical judgments. Clinical judgment involves an iterative process which begins when nurses realize accumulating knowledge from texts and lectures is not enough. They attempt to apply this knowledge to specific clinical situations, prioritize client concerns, and reach conclusions providing the most effective care in each situation.

To improve the evaluation of the clinical judgment skills of entry level nurses, the National Council of State Boards of Nursing (NCSBN) developed the Clinical Judgment Measurement Model (CJMM) and Next-Generation NCLEX examination-style questions. The CJMM is a framework for measuring minimal competence in clinical judgment and decision making (National Council of State Boards of Nursing, 2021).

Knowledge checks and a series of Next-Generation Nursing (NGN) questions are presented throughout the book to help students develop skills in critical thinking and application of knowledge in possible real-life situations.

The Nursing Process

The Nursing Process is "the essential core of practice for the registered nurse" (ANA, n.d.). It is a "scientific clinical reasoning approach to client care that includes assessment, analysis, planning, implementation, and evaluation" (NCSBN, 2018). The nursing process requires the professional nurse to use nursing judgment, a competency that includes critical thinking, clinical judgment, and integration of evidence-based practice (National League for Nursing, 2010). See Table 1.2 for a comparison of the nursing process, critical thinking, and clinical judgment. In maternal-newborn and women's health nursing, the nursing process applies to a population that is often healthy and experiencing a life event that holds the potential for both growth and problems. Nursing activity in these settings is often devoted to the assessment and diagnosis of client strengths and healthy functioning to achieve a higher or more satisfying level of wellness. This focus often differs from that of providing care for adults or children who are ill when the nurse encounters them.

TABLE 1.2 Use of the Nursing Process, Critical Thinking, and Clinical Judgment		
Nursing Process	Critical Thinking Skills	Clinical Judgment
Assessment	Collecting complete data, validating data	Recognize cues
	Clustering data (normal versus abnormal, important versus unimportant, relevant versus irrelevant)	
	Identifying emotions	
Analysis	Identifying cues and making inferences	Analyze cues
	Reflecting and suspending judgment	
	Examining thought processes for biases and assumptions	
	Identifying alternatives	
	Determining priorities	Prioritize hypotheses
Planning	Identifying expected client outcomes	Generate solutions
	Planning evidence-based actions	
	Validating plan with client and/ or coworker	
	Communicating plan	
	Acknowledging defensive behavior	
Implementation	Applying knowledge/ prioritizing actions	Take action
	Testing plan	
	Carrying out plan	
Evaluation	Comparing actual outcomes to expected outcomes	
	Examining insights gained	
	Recognizing new ways of thinking or acting	
	Examining options and criteria for action	
	Appraising self and others in the situation	

The nursing process is written in the text as a linear, step-by-step process. However, with knowledge and experience, the nurse applies the nursing process in the clinical setting dynamically. For example, the nurse may discover the client has a full bladder early in a postpartum assessment. The nurse skips to an intervention and helps the client to the restroom to urinate before completing the assessment. This action is taken by the nurse to prevent discomfort and possible excessive bleeding caused by a full bladder.

Assessment

Nursing assessment should be accomplished systematically and deliberately and include objective and subjective data related to physiologic, psychological, social, and cultural status of the client. Although the client or infant may be the primary patient, nurses should assess the belief systems, available support, perceptions, and plans of other family members to provide the best nursing care. Two levels of nursing assessment are used to collect comprehensive data: screening assessments and focus assessments.

Screening Assessment. The screening, or database, assessment is usually performed at the first contact with the person. Its purpose is to gather information about all aspects of the person's health. This information, called **baseline data**, describes the health status before interventions begin. It forms the basis for the identification of both strengths and problems.

Focused Assessment. A focused assessment is used to gather information specifically related to an actual health problem or a problem that the woman or family is at risk for acquiring. A focused assessment is often performed at the beginning of a shift and centers on areas immediately relevant. For instance, in care of the mother and infant after birth, the nurse should assess the breasts and nipples because clients are at risk for problems if they do not have adequate information about breastfeeding or care of the nipples. A focused assessment also may reveal strengths that nursing care will enhance.

Analysis: Identification of Client Problems

The data gathered during assessment should be analyzed to identify existing or potential strengths or problems and their causes. Data are validated and grouped in a process of critical thinking to recognize cues and inferences. The problems identified may be actual, or an increased risk for a problem or the nurse may identify wellness opportunities (Table 1.3).

Health needs for which nurses can provide **independent nursing interventions** and for which they are legally accountable are termed *nursing diagnoses*. At present, more than 200 nursing diagnoses have been identified by the North American Nursing Diagnosis Association International (NANDA-I) (https://www.nanda.org).

Planning

The third step in the nursing process involves planning care for the problems identified. During this step, nurses set priorities, develop goals or outcomes, and plan interventions to accomplish these goals.

Setting Priorities. Setting priorities includes (1) determining which problems need immediate attention (life-threatening problems) and taking action; (2) determining whether potential problems call for a provider's order for diagnosis, monitoring, or treatment; and (3) discriminating actual problems that take precedence over an increased risk.

Establishing Goals and Expected Outcomes. Although the terms *goals* and *expected outcomes* are sometimes used interchangeably, they are different. Broad goals should be linked with specific and measurable outcome criteria. For example, if the goal is for the parents to demonstrate effective parenting by discharge, then the expected outcomes might include prompt, consistent responses to infant signals and competence in bathing, feeding, and comforting the infant.

The following rules apply to written expected outcomes:
- Outcomes should be stated in client-oriented terms, identifying who is expected to achieve the goal.
- Measurable verbs should be used. For example, *identify, demonstrate, express, walk, relate,* and *list* are observable and measurable verbs. Examples of verbs that are difficult to measure are *understand, appreciate, feel, accept, know,* and *experience.*
- A time frame is necessary. When is the person expected to perform the action?
- Goals and expected outcomes should be realistic and attainable.
- Goals and expected outcomes are collaborated with the client and family to ensure their participation in the plan of care.

TABLE 1.3	**Examples of Actual and Increased Risk for Client Problems and Wellness Opportunities**	
ACTUAL CLIENT PROBLEMS		
Problem	**Etiology**	**Signs and Symptoms**
Inadequate nutrition	Lack of knowledge about nutritional needs during lactation	Weight loss of 5 kg and daily caloric intake <1500 calories
Inadequate breastfeeding	Nipple trauma	Cracked nipples and reports of discomfort during nursing
INCREASED RISK FOR A CLIENT PROBLEM		
Problem	**Risk Factors**	
Risk for inadequate nutrition	Lack of knowledge of nutritional needs during lactation issue	
Risk for inadequate breastfeeding	Lack of knowledge of correct positioning of infant and appropriate breast care	
WELLNESS OPPORTUNITIES		
Topic	**Selected Defining Characteristics**	
Opportunity for improved self-care	Expressed or observed desire to seek information for health promotion	
Opportunity for improved nutrition	Follows an appropriate standard for food intake such as MyPlate or American Diabetic Association guidelines	

Nursing Interventions

After the goals and expected outcomes are developed, nurses write nursing interventions to help the client meet the established outcomes.

Interventions for Actual Client Problems. Nursing interventions for actual client problems are aimed at reducing or eliminating the causes or related factors. For instance, if the problem is ineffective attachment between the parents and the newborn resulting from separation from the infant because of illness, the desired outcome might include the parents demonstrating progressive attachment behaviors such as touching, palming, eye contact, and participation in infant care within 1 week. Nursing interventions focus on role modeling attachment behaviors and increasing contact between parents and their baby.

Interventions for Risk for Client Problems. Interventions are aimed at (1) monitoring for onset of the problem, (2) minimizing risk factors, and (3) preventing the problem. For example, if baby Sam is at an increased risk for skin breakdown because of frequent, loose stools, the planned outcome is the skin remains intact. Nursing interventions include monitoring the condition of the skin at prescribed intervals for signs of skin impairment and initiating measures to keep the skin clean and dry to reduce the risk for skin impairment.

Wellness Interventions. Interventions also focus on opportunities for health enhancement. Nursing care seeks to promote client success through the teaching of self-care measures. Examples of wellness interventions include teaching related to weight reduction, exercise to lower chronic hypertension, or reconditioning the body after birth.

Implementing Interventions. Implementing nursing interventions may be a problem if written interventions are not specific. Nursing interventions should be as specific as provider's orders. If a physician orders hydrocodone with acetaminophen, 5 mg/500 mg, 1 tablet PO (orally) every 6 hours as needed for pain, the order specifies the combination drug to be given, the dose to be given, the route of administration, the time, and the reason. A well-written nursing intervention is equally specific: "Teach client not to break, chew, or crush the medication tablet."

Conversely, poorly written interventions such as "Assist with breastfeeding" provide generalizations rather than specific interventions. Specific methods the nurse should use to assist breastfeeding are more effective. For example, "Demonstrate correct positioning in cradle and football hold at first attempt to breastfeed. Teach client to elicit rooting reflex by stroking infant's lips with nipple. Demonstrate how to latch infant to nipple, and request a return demonstration before client and baby are discharged."

Evaluation

The evaluation determines the effectiveness of the plan and its goals or expected outcomes. The nurse should assess the status of the client and compare the current status with the goals or outcome criteria developed during the planning step. The nurse then judges the progression toward goal achievement and makes a decision: Should the plan be continued? Modified? Abandoned? Are the problems resolved or the causes diminished? Is a different problem more relevant?

The nursing process is dynamic, and evaluation frequently results in expanded assessment and additional or modified client problems and interventions. Nurses are cautioned not to view lack of goal achievement as a failure but as a signal to reassess and begin the process anew.

Individualized Nursing Care Plans

Nurses are responsible for documenting the client problem or nursing diagnosis, expected outcomes, interventions, and evaluation of actual outcomes for each problem. This information is often communicated to colleagues through a written plan of care. Many institutions have standards of care for groups of clients such as those who have had normal spontaneous vaginal births. However, individual nursing care plans may be necessary based on needs or problems identified during the assessment step of the nursing process. When nurses write individualized plans of care, they implement the plans through interventions that direct the care (Box 1.1). Some client situations end with a single office visit, whereas others progress over time such as normal or complicated birth. Specific planned nursing care may be documented by office, clinic, or hospital computer systems, and the systems may be linked to improve continuity.

KNOWLEDGE CHECK

5. What is the purpose of critical thinking?
6. How do "actual" client problems differ from "risk of" client problems?
7. How should goals and expected outcome criteria be stated?
8. Why are interventions sometimes difficult to implement? How can this difficulty be overcome?

SUMMARY CONCEPTS

- Programs to improve patient safety and quality of care include The Joint Commission, Interprofessional Collaboration and Education, Alliance for Innovation on Maternal Health, and Women's Health and Perinatal Nursing Care Quality Measures.
- Families must make many decisions about childbirth, including choosing a birth attendant, a birth setting, a support person for labor, and the type of educational classes to attend.
- Family-centered maternity care, which is based on the principle that families can make decisions about health

BOX 1.1 Developing Individualized Nursing Care through the Nursing Process

Although the nursing process is the foundation for nursing, initially it is a challenging process to apply in the clinical area. It requires proficiency in focused assessments of the new mother and infant and the ability to analyze data and plan nursing care for individual patients and families. Asking questions at each step of the nursing process may be helpful.

Assessment

1. Did some data not fit within normal limits or expected parameters? For example, the client states, "I feel dizzy when I try to walk," or the postmenopausal client describes vaginal bleeding at an annual well-woman examination.
2. If so, what else should be assessed? (What else should I evaluate? What might be related to this symptom? How do my assessments compare with previous assessments?) For example, what are the blood pressure, pulse rate, skin color, temperature, and amount of lochia if the client feels dizzy? Is my assessment similar to earlier ones, or has there been a change?
3. Did the assessment identify the cause of the abnormal data? What are the hemoglobin and hematocrit laboratory values? What was the blood loss at childbirth? Was blood loss excessive during the hours and days after birth?
4. Are other factors present? What medication was given during labor? Was an anesthetic for labor pain administered? When? What medication is being administered now? How long has it been since the last oral intake? Is the environment a related factor (crowded, warm, unfamiliar)? Is the client reluctant to ask for assistance?

Analysis: Identification of Client Problems

1. Are adequate data available to reach a conclusion? What else is needed? (What do you wish you had assessed? What would you look for next time?)
2. What is the major concern? (On the basis of the data, what are your concerns?) The client who is dizzy may fall when ambulating to the bathroom, particularly if unassisted. The client with postmenopausal vaginal bleeding will need evaluation by a provider for possible cancer.
3. What might happen if no action is taken? (What might happen to the person if you do nothing?) Will injury or a complication occur?
4. Is there a NANDA-I–approved diagnostic category that reflects your major concern? How is it defined? Suppose during analysis you decide the major concern is injury if the

patient falls. What diagnostic category most closely reflects this concern?
5. Does this diagnostic category "fit" this client? Is this problem a greater risk for this client than others in a similar situation? Why? What are the additional risk factors?
6. Is this a problem that nurses can manage independently? Are medical interventions also necessary?
7. If the problem can be managed by nurses, is it an actual problem (defining characteristics present) or a risk problem (risk factors present)?

Planning

1. What expected outcomes are desired? The client will remain free of injury during the hospital stay? The client will demonstrate position changes reducing the episodes of vertigo?
2. Would the outcomes be clear, specific, and measurable to anyone reading them?
3. What nursing interventions should be initiated and carried out to accomplish these goals or outcomes?
4. Are your written interventions specific and clear? Are action verbs used (*assess, teach, assist*)? After you have written the interventions, examine them. Do they define exactly what is to be done (when, what, how far, how often)? Will they prevent the client from suffering an injury?
5. Are the interventions based on sound rationale? For instance, dehydration possible during labor causes weakness resulting in falls; loss of blood during delivery may exceed 500 mL, which results in hypotension when the client stands suddenly. A client who has recently delivered after receiving an epidural may have lingering effects from this form of labor pain relief.

Implementing Nursing Interventions

1. What are the expected effects of the planned intervention? Are adverse effects possible? What are they?
2. Are the interventions acceptable to the client and family?
3. Are the interventions clearly written so they can be carefully followed?

Evaluation

1. What is the status of the client at this time?
2. What were the goals and outcomes? Were they specific and measurable or should they be clarified?
3. Compare the current status of the client with the stated goals and outcomes.
4. What should be done now?

NANDA-I, North American Nursing Diagnosis Association International.

care if they have adequate information, has greatly enhanced the role of nurses.
- Technologic advances, increasing knowledge, government involvement, cost containment efforts, and consumer demands have changed maternity care in the United States.
- Reduced lengths of stay make it more difficult for the nurse to provide information regarding self-care and infant care to the client who is recovering from the fatigue and discomfort of birth.
- Nurses provide care based on standards, guidelines and evidence using the skills of critical thinking, clinical judgment, and the nursing process.

REFERENCES

Agency for Healthcare Research and Quality (AHRQ). (n.d.). Evidence-based practice. https://www.ahrq.gov/topics/evidence-based-practice.html.

Alliance for Innovation on Maternal Health (AIM). (2020). Patient safety bundles. https://safehealthcareforeverywoman.org/aim/patient-safety-bundles/.

American Nurses Association (ANA). (2021). Nursing: Scope and standards of practice (4th ed., pp. 73).

American Nurses Association (ANA). (n.d.). The nursing process. https://www.nursingworld.org/practice-policy/workforce/what-is-nursing/the-nursing-process/.

American College of Obstetricians and Gynecologists (ACOG). (2018). *AIM program awarded millions to expand efforts to reduce maternal mortality and morbidity.* https://www.acog.org/news/news-releases/2018/08/aim-program-awarded-millions-to-expand-efforts-to-reduce-maternal-mortality-and-morbidity.

American College of Obstetricians and Gynecologists (ACOG). (2021a). *Health disparities in rural women.* ACOG Committee Opinion 586. Published 2014, reaffirmed 2021.

American College of Obstetricians and Gynecologists (ACOG). (2021b). *Importance of social determinants of health and cultural awareness in the delivery of reproductive health care.* ACOG Committee Opinion 729. Published 2018, reaffirmed 2021.

Association of Women's Health, Obstetric and Neonatal Nurses (AWHONN). (2021a). *AWHONN position and consensus statements.* https://www.awhonn.org/news-advocacy-and-publications/awhonn-position-statements/.

Association of Women's Health, Obstetric and Neonatal Nurses (AWHONN). (2021b). AWHONN position statement: Racism and bias in maternity care settings. *Journal of Obstetric, Gynecologic and Neonatal Nurses, 50*(5), e6–e8. https://doi.org/10.1016/j.jogn.2021.06.004.

Association of Women's Health, Obstetric and Neonatal Nurses (AWHONN). (2021c). *AWHONN practice briefs.* https://www.awhonn.org/practice-briefs/.

Bohren, M. A., Hofmeyr, G. J., Sakala, C., Fukuzawa, R. K., & Cuthbert, A. (2017). Continuous support for women during childbirth. *Cochrane Database of Systematic Reviews, 2017*(7), CD003766. https://doi.org/10.1002/14651858.CD003766.pub6.

Centers for Disease Control and Prevention (CDC). (2019). *Social Determinants and Eliminating Disparities in Teen Pregnancy.* Centers for Disease Control and Prevention. Retrieved from https://www.cdc.gov/teenpregnancy/about/social-determinants-disparities-teen-pregnancy.htm#action.

Centers for Disease Control and Prevention (CDC). (2021). *Maternal mortality rates in the United States, 2019.* https://www.cdc.gov/nchs/data/hestat/maternal-mortality-2021/maternal-mortality-2021.htm.

Facione, P. A. (1990). *Critical thinking: A statement of expert consensus for purposes of educational assessment and instruction.* Millbrae, CA: The California Academic Press (ERIC ED 315423).

Institute of Medicine (US). (1990). In M. J. Field, & K. N. Lohr (Eds.), *Committee to advise the public health service on clinical practice guidelines clinical practice guidelines: directions for a new program* (p. 38). National Academies Press (US).

Interprofessional Education Collaborative. (2021). *What is interprofessional education (IPE)?* https://www.ipecollaborative.org/about-us.

Midwives Alliance of North America. (2020). *Types of midwives.* https://mana.org/about-midwives/types-of-midwife.

National Center for Complementary and Integrative Health (NCCIH). (2020). *Be an informed consumer.* https://www.nccih.nih.gov/health/be-an-informed-consumer.

National Institute of Corrections. (n.d.). Evidence-based practices. https://nicic.gov/projects/evidence-based-practices-ebp.

National Council of State Boards of Nursing. (2018). *NCLEX-RN® Examination: Test plan for the National Council Licensure Examination for Registered Nurses* (p. 5).

National Council of State Boards of Nursing. (2021). *NGN FAQs for educators* (p.5). Retrieved from https://www.ncsbn.org/11447.htm.

National League for Nursing (NLN). (2010). *Outcomes and competencies for graduates of practical/vocational, diploma, associated degree, baccalaureate, master's, practice doctorate, and research doctorate programs in nursing* (p. 34).

Nurse Practitioners in Women's Health. (2020). *Structural racism and implicit bias in women's healthcare.* https://www.npwomenshealthcare.com/structural-racism-and-implicit-bias-in-womens-healthcare/.

Scheffer, B. K., & Rubenfeld, M. G. (2000). A consensus statement of critical thinking in nursing. *Journal of Nursing Education, 39*(8), 352–359.

The Joint Commission (TJC). (2021). *Perinatal care measures.* https://www.jointcommission.org/measurement/measures/perinatal-care/.

U.S. Department of Health and Human Services. (2020). *Healthy People 2030.* https://health.gov/healthypeople.

Wei, H., Corbett, R. W., Ray, J., & Wei, T. L. (2019). A culture of caring: The essence of healthcare interprofessional collaboration. *Journal of Interprofessional Care, 34*(3), 324–332. https://doi.org/10.1080/13561820.2019.1641476.

Zechariah, S., Ansa, B. E., Johnson, S. W., Gates, A. M., & De Leo, G. (2019). Interprofessional education and collaboration in healthcare: An exploratory study of the perspectives of medical students in the United States. *Healthcare, 7*(4), 117. https://doi.org/10.3390/healthcare7040117.

2

Social, Cultural, and Ethical Issues

Lynn Clark Callister, Cathy L. Miller, Sharla McDaniel, Reneé Jones

OBJECTIVES

After studying this chapter, you should be able to:

1. Explain family structure.
2. Describe characteristics of functional families and factors that interfere with family functioning.
3. Give examples of high-risk families.
4. Compare Western cultural values with those of differing cultural, racial, and ethnic groups.
5. Explain cultural negotiation.
6. Relate how social determinants of health, including socioeconomic status, poverty, homelessness, adverse childhood events, racism/discrimination, immigrant/refugee status, transportation, geographic variability, disparity in health care, implicit bias, and LGBTQ status, affect maternal-newborn and women's health nursing.
7. Describe the role of the nurse in assessment, prevention, and intervention of intimate partner violence.
8. Define human trafficking, also known as trafficking in persons.
9. Identify possible indicators ("red flags") of human trafficking.
10. Apply theories and principles of ethics to managing ethical dilemmas.
11. Describe how the steps of the nursing process can be applied to ethical decision-making.
12. Discuss ethical conflicts related to reproductive issues such as elective pregnancy termination, forced contraception, and infertility therapy.
13. Discuss the maintenance of client, institutional, and colleague confidentiality when using electronic communication.
14. Describe the legal basis for nursing practice.
15. Identify measures to prevent or defend malpractice claims.

The family forms the foundation of society. It is the first social institution a person knows in which one learns values, norms, and expected behaviors. The family exists within a "culture." The culture affects the values, beliefs, and traditions of the family. The individual and family are part of a society. The American society is faced with social and ethical dilemmas affecting individuals and families for whom nurses provide care. Some ethical and social issues result in flaws regulating reproductive practice. The nurse should understand the legal basis for their scope of practice.

THE FAMILY

Family Structures

There are multiple family structures, including the most common nuclear or conjugal family with a husband, wife, and children. Extended family includes the nuclear family with grandparents, aunts, uncles, or cousins living together. One adult who is divorced, separated, or widowed living with a child or children is a single-parent family. Adolescent mothers constitute a type of family formation regardless of whether the mother is single or coupled, what her developmental age is, and whether she is living with her parents or living alone. These mothers may have difficulty constructing their maternal identity. A blended or reconstituted family is one in which one or more parents bring into the union children from a previous relationship. Couples living without the legal bonds of marriage with or without children are in a cohabitative relationship. A communal family is a group of unrelated people who choose to live together, with the children becoming the responsibility of the group. Foster or adoptive families are those who take responsibility for children who were not born to them. This may include foster or adoptive children from another country or of another cultural, ethnic, or racial group. Same gender families include two adults of the same sex living together, some with children. New family formations are emerging, including those who identify as LGBTQ+ orientation (Griggs et al., 2021; Simpson 2021a; Sundus et al., 2021).

Differing family patterns of functioning are defined by how members of the family relate to each other. These include authoritarian or autocratic, authoritative or democratic, permissive or laissez-faire, or uninvolved. In an authoritarian family, the parents make the decisions and enforce rules. In democratic families, choices and responsibility are balanced in an atmosphere of respect for all family members. In the permissive family, there is freedom with little accountability. Families are also functional (healthy) or nonfunctional (unhealthy). Functional families exhibit characteristics which are helpful for a nurse to use to assess the way a specific family is functioning, including:

- Open communication, with family members expressing their needs and concerns
- Flexibility in role assignments, with family members working together to assist and support each other
- Agreement of adults on the basic principles of parenting with minimal discord
- Resiliency and adaptability

Factors that may interfere with healthy family functioning include lack of financial resources, absence of adequate family support, birth of an infant who has special needs, presence of unhealthy habits such as substance abuse or impaired anger management, and the inability to make mature decisions necessary to provide care to an infant.

High-risk families include those who live below the poverty level, those who live with chronic food insecurity, those headed by a single adolescent parent, and those with unanticipated stressors such as a preterm or ill newborn or a newborn with special needs. Families with lifestyle problems such as alcoholism, substance abuse, and family violence are considered at high risk for problems in providing adequate care for the infant. It is the responsibility of nurses to refer these families to social services agencies for financial assistance, crisis intervention, home visits, substance abuse rehabilitation, and anger management programs.

There are stages of families across the life span, from the beginning couple stage through the childbearing stage, the grown-child stage, and the older family stage. The childbearing phase creates some of the most powerful changes in a family as the relationship between the adults changes to include the care of a dependent infant. Family dynamics change when children must learn to share their parents' attention with a new sibling.

Cultural beliefs and practices influence what is considered normal or abnormal in family structure and relationships. Cultural patterns of behavior are transmitted from generation to generation. There are multiple cultural beliefs, practices, and behaviors, and these are dynamic and evolving beyond traditional cultural, racial, and/or ethnic groups. This includes socially disadvantaged families, refugees/immigrants, and multiple other "cultures" as well as variations related to assimilation and acculturation or identification with varying gender orientation (Callister, 2021b).

> **❓ KNOWLEDGE CHECK**
>
> 1. What are characteristics of a functional family?
> 2. What factors may interfere with family functioning?

Family Demographics in the United States

In 2020 non-Hispanic Whites constituted 72.0% of the population of the United States (U.S.) and Hispanics/Latinos (H/L) were 18.4%. African American/Black (AA/B) alone were

12.8%, American Indian/Alaska Natives (AI/AN) were 0.9%, Asians were 5.7%, and Native Hawaiians/Pacific Islanders (NH/PI) were 10.2%. Some other races alone constituted 5% of the population, and two or more races 3.4% (United States Census Bureau [USCB], 2020).

According to the census, those who are foreign-born constitute 13.7% of the population. Over 21% of those over 5 years of age live in households where a language other than English is spoken in the home (USCB, 2020). Languages spoken at home include: English 78%, Spanish 13.5%, other Indo-European languages 3.7%, Asian and Pacific Islander languages 3.6%, and other 1.2%. (USCB, 2020).

The poverty rate is 12.3%, and 9.2% of the population is without health insurance; moreover, 16.8% of children under 18 years of age are living in poverty. Also, 12.7% of people have a disability. Nearly 90% of adults are educated at a high school level or higher, and the employment rate is 62% (USCB, 2020).

The U.S. fertility rate in 2019 was 58.3 births per 1000 women 15 to 44 years of age, with H/L women having the highest fertility rate (65.3 births per 1000 women aged 15–44 years of age). The 2019 birth rates ranged from 9.8 per 1000 population in non-Hispanic (non-H/L) Whites to 11.9 in AI/AN, 13 in Asians, 13.4 in AA/B, 14.6 in H/L, and the highest birth rates (17.0) in NH/PIs (Martin et al., 2020; Martin et al., 2021).

The percentage of mothers who had early prenatal care in 2019 was 82.8% in non-Hispanic Whites and 72.1% in the H/L population. Slightly over 67% of the non-H/L AA/B women had early prenatal care (Martin et al., 2020; Martin et al., 2021).

There were 3,747,540 registered births in the U.S. in 2019 (Martin et al., 2020; Martin et al., 2021). Infant mortality rates (IMR) declined 1.17 from 2018. There are racial and ethnic differences in the IMR, with rates of 4.6 in non-Hispanic Whites, 4.9 in H/Ls, and 10.8 in AA/B per 1000 live births (Martin et al., 2020; Martin et al., 2021).

The 2019 preterm birth rate (prior to 37 weeks' gestation) was 9.26% of live births in non-H/L Whites, 9.97% for H/Ls, and 14.39% for non-H/L AA/Bs and was lowest among births to non-H/L and Asian mothers at 8.72% (Martin et al., 2020; Martin et al., 2021). For maternal mortality rates, see Chapter 19.

CULTURE AND CHILDBEARING FAMILIES

Culture is the sum of beliefs and values that are learned, shared, and transmitted from generation to generation in a specific group of people. Cultural values guide the thinking, decisions, and actions of a group, particularly during pivotal life events such as childbirth and child-rearing. Ethnic characteristics are religious, racial, national, or cultural group characteristics, such as speech patterns, social customs, and physical characteristics. Ethnicity is the condition of a group of people who share race, specific languages and dialects, religious faiths, traditions, values, and symbols. Ethnocentrism is when people think their cultural beliefs and practices are superior to those of others, and it forms the basis for interpersonal conflicts. Transcultural nursing is concerned with the provision of nursing care with sensitivity for and respect of the needs of individuals, families, and groups of people (Callister 2021b; Douglas et al., 2014; Giger & Haddad, 2021; Lauderdale, 2020; Purnell, 2019).

Cultural Considerations
Cultural Values

Dominant Western cultural values that may influence the thinking and action of the majority of nurses in the U.S. but may not be shared by culturally diverse childbearing clients and their families include the following:

- Democracy is a cultural value that may not be shared by families who think decisions should be made by the family, religious figures, or higher authorities in their cultural group. Fatalism, or the belief that events and results are predestined, also may affect health care decisions.
- Individualism conflicts with the values of many cultural groups.
- Cleanliness is considered by some groups to be an American "obsession."
- Preoccupation with time is a major source of conflict with those who mark time by different standards.
- Reliance on technology may be intimidating.
- The belief that optimal health is a right is in direct conflict with beliefs in many cultures in which health care is not a major expected right.
- Admiration for self-sufficiency and financial success may conflict with beliefs of other societies that place less value on wealth and more value on less tangible factors such as spirituality.

Differing cultures and lack of understanding of cultures (between the nurse and the childbearing family) may create communication difficulties related to communication style, decision-making, touch, spirituality and religiosity, and time orientation.

Communication Style

Styles in communication differ among cultures. For example, among Asians, nodding and smiling may mean, "Yes, I hear you," but may not indicate agreement or even understanding. When presenting information, the nurse should validate understanding by asking the client to repeat the information, saying: "Tell me what you understood" or "Show me what you learned."

Knowing communication principles helps nurses avoid making errors in communication. For example, Hispanics are traditionally diplomatic and tactful. They frequently engage in "small talk" before introducing questions about their care. Nurses should remember that small talk is a valuable use of time. It establishes rapport and helps accomplish the goals of care. It helps create an atmosphere of trust *(confianza)* in the relationship and helps the client feel comfortable. Another example is that AI/ANs often converse in a low tone that may be difficult to hear. They may consider note-taking taboo and expect the caregiver to remember what was said.

Decision-Making

It is important to determine who makes decisions for the family. Is it the individual client, the partner, other family members, or traditional authority figures? If decisions are collectively made or may be beyond the client's control, such as whether prenatal care is accessed and at what time during the pregnancy, the decision makers should be included in the conversation.

Eye Contact

Many Whites and African Americans consider eye contact important to communication. Eye-contact avoidance sometimes frustrates health care personnel, who believe eye contact denotes honesty. In some cultures, such as AI/AN cultures, avoiding eye contact is a sign of respect. Eye-contact behavior is also an important consideration when nurses deal with Latino infants and children. *Mal ojo* (evil eye) is a sudden unexplained illness when an individual with special powers admires a child too openly. Eye contact between a woman and man may be considered seductive by those from Middle Eastern cultures.

Touch

Touch is also an important component of communication. In some cultures, such as those espousing Hinduism or the Islamic faith, touch by a woman other than the wife may be offensive to men. Hispanics are more likely to appreciate touch, which is viewed as a sign of sincerity. Nurses should remain sensitive to the response of the client being touched and should refrain from touching if the client indicates it is not welcomed.

Spirituality and Religiosity

Many culturally diverse clients may espouse deeply held religious and spiritual practices and beliefs (Callister & Khalaf, 2010; Crowther et al., 2020) and may be reluctant to share these with their nurses. For example, Thai clients describe the adherence to practices and rituals associated with their beliefs about three essences: the body, mind–heart, and energy.

Time Orientation

Time orientation can create conflict between health care professionals and culturally diverse childbearing clients. AI/ANs, Middle Easterners, and H/Ls tend to emphasize the present moment rather than the future. If clients do not place the same importance on keeping appointments, they may encounter anger and frustration in the health care setting that leaves them bewildered, ashamed, and unlikely to return for care. See **Nursing Care Plan: Language Barriers During Pregnancy** for an example of the issue of communication difficulties.

Culture and Health Beliefs in Childbearing

Childbirth is viewed by most clients as a meaningful, life-changing event (Callister, 2020; 2021b; Lauderdale, 2020). It is important to note "childbirth is a time of transition and social celebration in all cultures. Giving birth has the potential to be a rich and cultural spiritual experience facilitated by

◎ NURSING CARE PLAN

Language Barrier During Pregnancy

Assessment

Diep T., a young Vietnamese primigravida at 16 weeks of gestation, speaks very little English. She listens quietly to the nurse's health care instructions, and although she appears confused, she asked no questions. Her husband, Bao N., nods and smiles frequently and speaks more English than his wife but has difficulty responding to questions about his wife's health.

Critical Thinking

Why should additional assessments be made before client problems can be formulated? **Answer:** Nodding and smiling do not always mean that persons from another culture understand health teaching. Instead, such actions simply may indicate the information has been heard or perhaps Mr. N. is being polite and does not want the nurse to feel inadequate. Before assuming Mr. N. can translate health care teaching for his wife, the nurse should validate his learning by asking Mr. N. to explain what he has learned.

Client Problem

Ineffective communication resulting from language barriers.

Planning: Expected Outcomes

Throughout the pregnancy the family will demonstrate adequate understanding of instructions by (1) keeping scheduled appointments, (2) following health care instructions, and (3) verbalizing basic needs and concerns at each prenatal visit.

Interventions and Rationales

- Assess the couple's ability to speak, read, and write in English and determine whether they are fluent in other languages. *People who are not fluent in speaking a language may be more adept at reading it.*
- Obtain the assistance of a fluent interpreter, preferably of the same gender.
- Establish a list of bilingual staff who are willing to interpret and understand the importance of confidentiality and exactness. Ensure staff are knowledgeable about the phone interpreter services used by the clinical agency. Use a translator to develop written material in languages most commonly encountered in the facility. Develop communication aids about common teaching topics in various languages. Use communication cards with questions and answers printed in Vietnamese with Diep and her husband.
- Use posters, pictures, and models to demonstrate anatomy, birth, or other concepts clearly.

- *A fluent interpreter is essential because people do not always reveal they do not understand instructions. This hinders follow-up questions. Printed materials help elicit basic information, reinforce information given verbally, and may answer unasked questions. Written materials and communication cards in the client's language convey interest in communicating and provide a means of eliciting basic information. Pictures or models make information more understandable* (Callister, 2021a; Koh et al., 2014; Lau et al., 2021; Kynoe & Hanssen, 2020; Lor et al., 2021).
- Face Diep and her husband rather than the interpreter when talking. Use quiet tones. Use the same interpreter whenever possible. Watch facial expressions for a clue to clients' understanding. *Talking directly to the client while facing her shows respect and concern. Soft speech protects the client's privacy and modesty. A natural response when people do not understand is to raise the voice. This may convey impatience or anger. A consistent interpreter enhances communication. Facial expressions may show confusion if the client does not understand.*
- Ask the interpreter to explain exactly what the nurse says as much as possible instead of paraphrasing. *If the interpreter paraphrases the nurse's words, important information may be lost.*
- Consider nonverbal factors when communicating. Speak slowly and smile when appropriate. Keep an open posture. Do not cross the arms over the chest or turn away from the family. Listen carefully to what the family says. Nod, lean forward, or encourage continued talk with frequent "uh-huhs." Avoid fidgeting or watching a clock.
- Determine Diep's response to a light touch on the arm, and use or avoid touch depending on her response.
- Do not expect prolonged eye contact.
- *Even subtle body language can indicate interest and empathy or impatience, annoyance, or hurry. Touch and eye contact are sensitive cultural variables, and nurses should be aware they are not always welcomed.*
- Use phone interpreter services, which are provided in some clinical agencies, ensuring both the nurse and the client receive accurate information.

Evaluation

Diep keeps each prenatal appointment. She follows all recommendations and gradually asks appropriate questions more often at each visit.

---

a culturally competent nurse" (Callister, 1995, p. 33; Wehbe-Alamah et al., 2021).

There are more than 100 ethnocultural groups in the United States with traditional health beliefs, but it is important to recognize "culture" defined broadly means more than ethnocultural characteristics. "Culture" may include childbearing clients who have been sexually abused as children, or others who have definite ideas about not using birth technologies but prefer traditional means of managing labor and birth that may even include having a home birth. "Culture"

may include clients living in poverty, clients struggling with low health literacy, clients who have experienced female genital cutting, clients with a disability, or clients dealing with anxiety and depression.

There is a growing number of those who identify as LGBTQ+ for whom perinatal nurses provide care across the childbearing years (Everett et al., 2019; Griggs et al., 2021).

There are multiple cultures. You may not know exactly what to expect when you walk into a client's room in the clinic or the birthing unit, but being creative, flexible, and resilient in your approach to caring will bring many satisfying cultural experiences (Callister, 2016).

Take the opportunity to learn about the uniqueness of each person you care for and about their cultural beliefs and practices surrounding childbirth. For example, Asians may believe health is the balance between "yin" and "yang." Those of Haitian origin may define health as "harmony with nature." Hispanics often consider health as a balance between "hot" and "cold."

Traditional methods to prevent illness are related to cultural beliefs such as the "evil eye," which causes injury, illness, or misfortune. Others are phenomena, such as soul loss because of jealousy, environmental factors, such as bad air, and natural events, such as solar eclipses. Practices to prevent illness developed from beliefs regarding the cause of illness. This includes protective or religious objects such as amulets with magic powers or consecrated religious objects (such as talismans) frequently worn or carried to prevent illness. Orthodox Jewish people make major decisions only after conferring with their rabbi (Candelaria et al., 2019).

Health Maintenance

The predominant culture in the U.S. may treat pregnancy as high-risk, with frequent prenatal visits and multiple tests, hospitalization for giving birth, and significant use of technology, including epidural analgesia/anesthesia and induced labor. On the other hand, many cultures view pregnancy as a normal physiologic condition with little or no need for health care because the childbearing person is not ill and birth is considered low-risk.

Traditional practices may be used to maintain health during pregnancy and birth. For example, Mexican clients may keep active to ensure a small newborn and easy birth and may continue sexual intercourse to lubricate the birth canal. East Indians maintain a balance between "hot" (eggs, nuts, chili, garlic, mango, ginger) and "cold" foods (fresh fruit, yogurt, buttermilk). Prenatal care may not begin for Indonesians until the second trimester, when the soul is believed to enter the unborn child. Korean childbearing clients may practice Qi during pregnancy, which consists of physical postures, breathing techniques, and meditation. In many cultures, including Korean, immigrant postpartum rituals are practiced, including seclusion and hot/cold-related prohibitions (Han et al., 2020). Native Americans may not tie knots or make braids during pregnancy to prevent complications involving the umbilical cord. Some groups believe unclean things and strong emotions such as anger cause harm to the fetus or can precipitate a difficult childbirth.

Immigrants and refugees may have particular challenges as they describe the experience of living between two cultures (Pangas et al., 2019). They may feel the vulnerability of being marginalized, struggling with low socioeconomic status, and experiencing lack of access to social resources, including prenatal care. The establishment of a trusting relationship between the nurse and the immigrant is critical (Kyno & Hanssen, 2021).

Somali immigrants have described the limitations of support because of separation from their families, which highlights the importance of cultural and religious beliefs. Some clients develop distinct birth cultural practices that combine their traditional beliefs with Western childbirth practices to promote positive outcomes. Hispanic childbearing clients may desire *(el anhelo)* to learn and understand more but without sacrificing their ethnic and cultural identity *(la identidad)*.

Belief in Fate

Some cultures believe in fate determining outcomes. This includes adverse events over which they have no personal control. This may mean in some instances they do not take personal responsibility for what happens when they bear a child.

Preventing Illness

Childbearing clients may think they can ensure positive outcomes by observing cultural taboos. Advance preparation for the newborn may also be avoided in some cultures. Arabic Muslim clients believe preparing for the baby defies the will of Allah. Navajo families do not choose a name for their unborn child until after birth because they fear it will harm the infant if identified earlier. Russian clients may not buy clothes or baby equipment until the fetus is born healthy. Clients in many cultures eat raw garlic or onion or adhere to food taboos and prescribed combinations of foods.

Strict adherence to religious codes and moral conduct is also believed to prevent illness. The nurse should ask, "What do pregnant clients take to protect themselves and the baby?" and "What special foods and drinks are important?"

Use of Complementary and Other Therapies

Natural substances such as herbs and plants may be used to promote wellness and treat illness. Tongan clients use *vaikita* made from orange peels and mango leaves to prevent postpartum illness *(kita)*. Dermabrasion, which is the rubbing or irritation of the skin to relieve discomfort, is a common health practice in Southeast Asia. This includes coining, in which an area is covered with an ointment and the edges of a coin rubbed over the area. These methods leave marks resembling bruises or burns on the skin, often mistaken for signs of physical abuse.

Clients may use religious charms, holy words, prescribed acts, and traditional healers before seeking other health advice. AA/B clients and others may seek the provision of information from wise women (Devido et al., 2020). Hispanics may consult *curanderas* for illness or a *partera* for care during pregnancy. Some Africans and Haitians may rely on folk medicine, including witchcraft, voodoo, or magic.

Modesty

Fear, modesty, and a desire to avoid examination by men may keep some clients from seeking health care during pregnancy. In many cultures (such as Muslim, Hindu, Hispanic), exposure of the genitals to men is considered demeaning. In these cultures, the reputations of women depend on their demonstrated modesty. If possible, female health care providers should perform examinations. If this is not possible, the client should be carefully draped with all areas of the body covered except those that must be exposed for examination. A female nurse should remain with these clients at all times. Obtaining permission from the male partner may be necessary before any examination or treatment can be performed. In addition, the client's partner or support person should be allowed to be present during examinations.

Clients who have experienced female genital cutting may be fearful and anxious about modesty issues, and nurses should be respectful and nonjudgmental (Johnson-Aghakwu et al., 2019).

KNOWLEDGE CHECK

3. How can differences in Western and traditional cultural values be reconciled?
4. How can nurses show respect for traditional cultural practices that are harmless?

Culturally Competent Care

Nursing standards emphasize the importance of providing culturally competent care. The American Nurses Association (ANA) standards for professional nurses include culturally competent care: "The registered nurse practices in a manner that is congruent with cultural diversity and inclusion principles" (ANA, 2021). The U.S. Department of Health and Human Services (DHHS) released the enhanced National Standards for Culturally and Linguistically Appropriate Services (CLAS) in Health and Health Care (Koh et al., 2014). Standards of the Association of Women's Health, Obstetric, and Neonatal Nurses (AWHONN) also emphasize the importance of culturally competent care for childbearing clients and their families (AWHONN, 2019).

Childbearing experiences are enriched through quality interactions with health care providers. Outcomes of culturally competent care include enhanced relationships between clients and their providers, reduced complications, adherence to health care provider recommendations, improved quality of life, increased trust, and an appreciation of cultural diversity by providers. Assessing, developing, and using culturally appropriate health education for childbearing clients is essential for the culturally competent nurse to improve client outcomes (Callister, 2021a).

Culturally competent nursing care requires an awareness of, sensitivity to, and respect for the diversity of the clients served. It involves assessment of the family's culture and cultural negotiation when necessary. Barriers to health care may include linguistic and sociocultural differences; socioeconomic barriers, including lack of health insurance; a lack of health knowledge; a reluctance to question a health care provider; and the biomedical health care environment (Callister, 2021a). For example, Muslim clients with higher levels of modesty and religiosity may be more likely to delay seeking prenatal care (Wehbe-Almah et al., 2021).

Cultural Assessment

The following questions might be considered when performing a cultural assessment, which should be used to develop plans for care that respect cultural differences and traditional health practices (Callister, 2021a; Giger et al., 2021; Lauderdale, 2020; Purnell, 2019):

- What is the family's ethnic affiliation?
- Is childbearing viewed as a normal physiologic process, a time of vulnerability and risk, or a state of illness?
- What are the prescribed practices, customs, and rituals related to diet, activity, and behavior during pregnancy and childbirth?
- How is childbirth pain managed, and what maternal and paternal behaviors are appropriate?
- What maternal restrictions or precautions are considered necessary during childbearing? Are any religious expectations required to be met after birth?
- Who provides support during pregnancy, childbirth, and beyond?
- What are the prescribed practices and restrictions related to care of the newborn?
- Who in the family hierarchy makes health care decisions?
- What are the views of life and death, including predestination and fatalism?
- Do you need help understanding health care information?
- How can health care professionals be most helpful?

Cultural Negotiation

Cultural negotiation involves providing information but also acknowledging the client may hold views different from those of the nurse. A client may not follow health care advice because of cultural beliefs. If the client or their family indicates that information is not helpful or is harmful in their opinion, the conflict should be acknowledged openly and clarified. "I sense that you are unsure about this. Tell me your concerns." After allowing the client and the family to express their beliefs, the nurse explains why the recommendation was made and works with them to find a compromise satisfactory to all.

Cultural negotiation also involves sensitivity to specific concerns. For example, nurses should be aware of Islamic laws governing modesty when caring for Muslims. Some Muslim women must cover their hair, body, arms to the wrist, and legs to the ankles at all times when in the presence of men. A Muslim woman may be prohibited from being alone in the presence of a man other than her husband or a male relative.

"Perinatal nurses should seek a health care encounter with childbearing women that respects the sociocultural and spiritual context of life and moves beyond the superficial to understand the deeper meaning of childbearing. Perinatal nurses should never lose sight of the fact that a woman's childbirth experience is not only about making a baby but also about creating a mother—a mother who is strong and competent and who trusts her own capacities because she has been cared for by a culturally competent nurse" (Callister, 2006a, 2006b, p.214; 2020; Lauderdale, 2020; Morton & Simkin, 2019; Oladapo et al., 2018; Simpson, 2019; Vedam et al., 2019).

❓ KNOWLEDGE CHECK

5. Why is it important for nurses to examine their own cultural beliefs and values?
6. What is meant by the term "cultural negotiation?"

SOCIAL ISSUES

Nurses caring for clients and families must assess social determinants of health that influence health care, including socioeconomic status, poverty, homelessness, and disparity in health care.

Socioeconomic Status

The socioeconomic status of the family has significant influence on childbearing practices. The term *socioeconomic status* refers to the resources available for the family to meet the needs for food, shelter, and health care. Socioeconomic status can be divided into the affluent, the middle class, the working poor, and the new poor (Table 2.1).

The Affluent

Affluent families have resources to provide for their needs and purchase health care. They have a good income, secure shelter in a safe neighborhood, and the education and reserves to protect themselves from economic fluctuations. They can pay for health care through either private means or insurance.

Affluent families think they deserve the best in health care and respect from health care providers. They are future-oriented and therefore value preventive care. In general, they seek early regular antepartum care and comply with recommendations of the health care providers.

The Middle Class

The middle class constitutes the largest group of families in the U.S. They usually are able to rent or own homes in relatively safe neighborhoods. They have adequate food and either education or skills that assist them to obtain and keep jobs for long periods.

Middle-class families rely on group insurance, obtained as a benefit of employment, to shield themselves from exorbitant health care costs. A major concern is loss of a job, which results in loss of health insurance. They are future-oriented and usually seek health care early in pregnancy.

The Working Poor and Unemployed

The working poor and unemployed include unskilled or unemployed workers. They work for low wages and are often the last-hired and the first-fired. They may live below the poverty level and have barely enough to survive. Some have difficulty meeting their basic needs for food and shelter, and some become homeless.

Because of economic uncertainty, these families place more emphasis on meeting present needs and less value on preventive (future-oriented) care. This often causes them to postpone prenatal care until the second or even the third trimester.

The New Poor

The new poor constitute a group of individuals and families who were previously self-sufficient but are now without resources because of circumstances such as loss of a job or health care insurance. They must find their way in an unfamiliar and complicated health care system.

TABLE 2.1	Impact of Socioeconomic Factors on the Family's Response to Pregnancy		
Affluent	**Middle Class**	**Working Poor and Unemployed**	**New Poor**
Resources			
Is confident of ability; has financial reserves to protect from economic fluctuations; owns or rents home in a safe neighborhood; has health insurance or can pay for health care; is able to provide enriched environment	Has relative security but fewer reserves and more debt; owns or rents home in relatively safe neighborhood; depends on employment for health insurance	Lacks skills and bargaining power; is most vulnerable to economic fluctuations; struggles to meet basic needs	Was previously self-sufficient but has lost prior resources; may have recently lost job and insurance; unused to public assistance
Value Placed on Health Care			
Values preventive care	Values health care but must rely on health insurance related to employment	May value health care but often does not see a way to improve situation	Values health care but may no longer have finances to access it
Time Orientation			
Is future-oriented and seeks prenatal care early; expects best possible care and education for children	Is future-oriented and seeks early prenatal care; makes plans to provide best possible care and education for children	Priority is to meet needs of present; often seeks prenatal care late; has an uncertain future	Has middle-class time orientation but must meet present needs; may begin prenatal care late

NURSING CARE PLAN

Socioeconomic Problems During Pregnancy

Assessment

Theresa, a 19-year-old primigravida, is seen for initial prenatal care at 24 weeks of gestation. She took the day off from work without pay in a factory and rode the bus to the clinic. She is currently living with her sister and brother-in-law, who receive Temporary Assistance for Needy Families. During the interview, Theresa states she will not be able to keep clinic appointments because she cannot afford to take more time off until the baby comes. She is unmarried and says the father of the baby is "gone." Physical assessment shows Theresa and her fetus are healthy. She declares she does not need further prenatal care and only needs to find someone to support her during labor and birth.

Identification of Client Problems

Potential for inadequate prenatal care because of lack of knowledge of the importance of prenatal care and lack of resources.

Planning: Expected Outcomes

During the first prenatal visit, Theresa will do the following:
1. Describe the benefits of prenatal care.
2. Verbalize a plan for obtaining regular prenatal care.

Interventions and Rationales

1. Use active listening to show concern and empathy with Theresa's difficulties in obtaining prenatal care. *Expressing interest in Theresa's situation may make her more likely to listen to health teaching.*
2. Emphasize why regular prenatal care is essential:
   a. To monitor the growth and development of the baby
   b. To evaluate Theresa's health, which directly affects the health of the fetus

   c. To detect problems and intervene before they become severe

   Preventive care often is not a priority when the client has conflicting needs for food and shelter. Many clients are unaware that complications such as preeclampsia or gestational diabetes, which may be identified and treated with routine care, are serious hazards if they remain undetected.
3. Assist Theresa in devising a plan to obtain regular prenatal care.
   a. Provide her with a list of prenatal clinics near her home or place of work and the hours they are open.
   b. Discuss transportation services and determine whether family or friends can help her keep prenatal appointments.
   c. Explore dates, times, and alternatives until she finds a schedule that works for her.
   d. Obtain a list of phone numbers (e.g., friends, family, employer) at which she can be reached for follow-up.

   Some clinics are open on weekends and evenings to accommodate those who work. Unreliable transportation is a major reason for failure to keep scheduled appointments, and clinic schedules that allow some flexibility are helpful. Interest in a client's individual situation is highly motivating for her to find a way to continue prenatal care.

Evaluation

Theresa is attentive as the nurse talks about the importance of health care. She shows interest in finding a way to have regular prenatal care and makes an appointment for the next visit. If she misses scheduled appointments, follow-up phone calls to arrange alternative appointments may be necessary.

The values of the new poor are those of the middle class: they demonstrate self-sufficiency, hard work, and pride in the ability to succeed. Seeking public assistance is very difficult for this group. These families are devastated when they encounter the lack of respect that may occur when some health care workers interact with families unable to pay for health care.

Poverty

Poverty remains an underlying factor in problems such as homelessness and inadequate access to health care. Poverty in the U.S. was projected to be 9.2% in 2020, which means there were 29.3 million people living in poverty (USCB, 2020). Because of adverse living conditions, poor health care, and poor nutrition, infants born to people in low-income groups are more likely to begin life with problems such as low birth weight (LBW).

Poverty often breeds poverty. In poor families, children may leave the educational system early, making them less likely to learn skills necessary to obtain good jobs. Childbearing at an early age is common and further interferes with education and the ability to work. The cycle of poverty may continue from one generation to the next as a result of hopelessness and apathy (Fig. 2.1).

As health care costs have risen, the ability to pay for employer-sponsored health insurance has become more difficult for low- and middle-income workers. The working poor have jobs but receive wages barely adequate to meet their day-to-day needs or may work just under the full-time hours required to qualify them for employer insurance and other benefits. These jobs may not offer health insurance at all, or high premiums may be the only option. The working poor have little opportunity to save for emergencies such as serious illness.

Preliminary data indicates 8.8% (28.2 million) of Americans do not have health insurance (USCB, 2020). Millions of other people have limited insurance and would not be able to survive financially in the event of serious illness. People without insurance seek care only when absolutely necessary. Health maintenance and illness prevention may seem costly and unnecessary to them. Some receive no health care during pregnancy until they arrive at the hospital for birth.

Homelessness

At least 567,715 people in the U.S. were homeless on a given night in January 2019. Seventy percent were individuals, and 30% were people in families with children. This included all parts of the country, with the highest counts being in California,

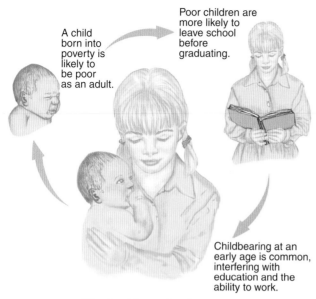

A child born into poverty is likely to be poor as an adult.

Poor children are more likely to leave school before graduating.

Childbearing at an early age is common, interfering with education and the ability to work.

Fig. 2.1 The cycle of poverty.

> ## BOX 2.1   Social, Economic, and Environmental Determinants of Health
>
> - Income, poverty
> - Employment status
> - Access to and use of health care and preventive services
> - Age (adolescents, aging)
> - Racial, ethnic, cultural minority
> - Geographic (rural, inner city, urban/suburban, between states)
> - Marital status
> - Education
> - Linguistic (inability to speak English)
> - Immigration status
> - Transportation
> - Housing
> - Public safety
> - Behavioral risk factors
> - Available social support

Florida, New York, and Texas. The homeless include those with varied family status, genders, and racial/ethnic groups. One in two of the homeless were unsheltered, and 60% were male. NH/PIs and AI/AN were most likely to be homeless. AA/B or multiracial individuals and H/L were more likely than White Americans to be homeless (National Alliance to End Homelessness, 2020). Homeless people may wait until health concerns are severe because of shame related to being homeless and an inability to pay for the care needed. Health care may be delayed until the homeless person enters the emergency department, and needed care is far more costly than the preventive care the homeless person could not afford.

The pregnant homeless client is less likely to seek prenatal care that might identify complications such as maternal hypertension, diabetes, substance abuse, or inadequate maternal weight gain, which adds to the risk for prematurity and LBW infants (March of Dimes, 2020). Pregnancy may interfere with one's ability to work and may reduce income to the point that housing is unattainable.

Disparity in Health Care

Health disparities exist in a population when different groups of people have differences in health outcomes. These disparities may be perceived by culturally diverse groups of clients as influencing birth outcomes (morbidity and mortality) in a variety of ways (Dove-Meadows et al., 2020). These include social, economic, and environmental determinants of health (Callister, 2021c). Disparities considered to be determinants of health are listed in Box 2.1.

The MMR has decreased in many countries but has increased in the U.S. despite expenditures on childbirth being higher than any other country in the world (National Academies of Sciences, Engineering & Medicine, 2020). Racial/ethnic variation is significant, with AA/B and AI/AN people being the most impacted by the maternal health crisis (Hoyert & Minino, 2020). White clients experience 13.0 deaths per 100,000 births compared with 42.8 deaths per 100,000 births in AA/B clients. Implicit bias may contribute to racial/ethnic disparities to MMR (Saluja & Bryant, 2021).

Racial and ethnic variation in the rates of sexually transmitted infections and diseases may be influenced by issues such as access to health care and the ability to pay for such services (Sutton et al., 2021). AA/B clients are more likely to die of cancer than White clients, even though they have a lower incidence of being diagnosed with a malignancy (American Cancer Society, 2021).

The IMR among non-H/L AA/B infants is twice the rate of White infants (10.8 vs. 4.8 per 1000 live births; Burris & Parker, 2021). There are also racial and ethnic disparities in fetal deaths, with AA/B clients having three times the rate of fetal deaths associated with maternal complications (Pruitt et al., 2020).

Prenatal care is widely accepted as an important element in a good pregnancy outcome. Late or no prenatal care is associated with increased risks for maternal and infant morbidity and mortality. Use of prenatal care varies by race/ethnicity. First trimester prenatal care is 82.5% for non-H/L White clients, 72.1% for H/L clients, 67.1% for AA/B clients, and 62.6% for AI/AN clients. H/L and AA/B clients are more likely to receive late or no prenatal care compared with Asian or NH/PI clients and White clients (Johnson, 2020; Martin et al., 2021). Adolescent clients are the most likely to receive late or no prenatal care. The younger the client, the less likely it is that the client will receive prenatal care: late or no care is highest for adolescent clients under 15 years of age (25.7%) and is approximately 11% for adolescent clients aged 15 to 19 years (National Vital Statistics Report, 2018).

Factors limiting access to care should be addressed to increase the use of preconception and prenatal care. There are multiple overlapping and contributing factors that interfere with access to care during childbearing.

Barriers to Prenatal Care

Access to prenatal care is limited by financial, systemic, and attitudinal barriers. Financial barriers are among the most important factors limiting prenatal care. The 2018 U.S. poverty rate was 10.5%, with 8% of the population (26.1 million people) having no health insurance (Semega et al., 2020). Many childbearing families have no insurance or insufficient insurance to cover care during pregnancy and birth. Although Medicaid finances prenatal care for indigent persons, the enrollment process is burdensome and lengthy. Some clients do not know how to access this resource or do not qualify. Immigrant and refugee expectant clients may be at risk for delayed or inadequate prenatal care (Oerther et al., 2020; Olukorun et al., 2020) and should be targeted for interventions to improve both maternal and infant outcomes (Sinclair et al., 2020).

Systemic barriers include institutional practices that interfere with consistent care. Prenatal visits are usually scheduled during daytime hours that conflict with working clients' schedules. Taking time off from work often means loss of wages and may put the client's job in jeopardy. In addition, child care is rarely available at sites of care, and some clients are unable to find affordable care. Lack of transportation may keep clients from getting prenatal care. In addition, interpreters may not be available for clients who do not speak English well.

An important barrier to health care results from the unsympathetic attitude of some health care workers toward those who are unable to pay for prenatal care. Poor families may experience long waits to access their first prenatal visit, long delays, hurried examinations, rudeness, and arrogance from some members of the health care team. Staff may be overworked and frustrated with the workloads they carry. Clients may wait hours for an examination that lasts only a few minutes. Many never see the same health care provider more than once. These clients may not keep clinic appointments because they do not see the importance of the hurried examinations.

Nurses should treat all childbearing families with respect and consideration and eliminate racism and inequities in care delivery (Butler et al., 2019; Callister, 2020; Declerq et al., 2020; Killion, 2021; McGowan et al., 2019; Shorey et al., 2021; Simpson, 2021b). Nurses can work to determine which barriers apply to the clients and find ways to meet the needs of the specific population being served. Scheduling prenatal visits in the evening or on weekends, setting aside times for walk-in prenatal visits, and offering other services such as applications for Medicaid and Women, Infants, and Children (WIC) programs may increase use of prenatal services. Decreasing waiting time before appointments as much as possible is important. Cultural sensitivity is important for all caregivers (Callister, 2012b).

Some clients do not obtain early prenatal care because they do not realize they are pregnant, do not want the pregnancy confirmed, do not want anyone to know about the pregnancy, or are considering an abortion. A client with an unintended pregnancy may be too depressed to begin prenatal care early. Many clients rely on advice from family and friends during pregnancy, and some believe prenatal care is unimportant, especially when they are healthy and have no obvious problems with the pregnancy.

Allocation of Health Care Resources

In addition to the social factors involved in health disparities, how the available health care money is spent is an issue to be addressed. In 2020 the U.S. spent $4 trillion on health care (NIH, 2021). Expenditures for health care continue to rise. Areas to be addressed include ways to provide care for indigent persons, the uninsured or underinsured, and those with long-term care needs. Distribution of the limited funds available for health care among all these areas is a major concern.

Care Versus Cure

Another issue is whether the focus of health care should be on preventive and caring measures or cures for diseases. In the past, health care has focused more on treatment and cure rather than on prevention and care, but prevention avoids suffering and is less expensive than treating diseases after diagnosis.

The focus on cure has resulted in technologic advances that enable some people to live longer, healthier lives. Nevertheless, the costs of technology should be balanced against the benefits obtained and by the number of people who benefit.

Although LBW infants constitute a small percentage of all newborns, they require a large percentage of total hospital expenditures. The expenses of one preterm infant for a single day in an intensive care nursery are more than enough to pay for the care of the mother throughout her pregnancy and birth, and if the mother had received prenatal care early and regularly, the infant might have avoided intensive care.

Quality-of-life issues are important with regard to technology. Neonatal nurseries are able to keep very-low-birth-weight (VLBW) babies alive because of advances in high neonatal technology for this group. Some of these infants go on to lead normal or near-normal lives. Others gain time but not quality of life. Families and health care professionals face difficult decisions about when to treat, when to end treatment, and how to recognize when the suffering outweighs the benefits.

KNOWLEDGE CHECK

7. Why do many low-income clients delay seeking health care until the second or third trimester?
8. How do the attitudes of health care workers affect the care of poor families?

Solutions

Addressing social determinants of health (Lathrop, 2020) is essential to move toward health equity. The use of screening tools for social determinants of health include PRAPARE (National Association for Community Health Centers); the American Academy of Family Physicians Social Needs Screening Tool; and the Health Leads Toolkit (Lathrop, 2020).

One way a nurse can personally address social determinants of health is by providing a disadvantaged childbearing client with a list of food assistance resources and the nearest WIC office.

Government Programs for Health Care. Government programs for health care are intended as a safety net for vulnerable populations such as women and children with low socioeconomic status. Pre- and postpartum home visits as part of health care for AI/AN childbearing persons may be helpful as part of Indian Health Services (Johnson, 2020).

Medicare, Medicaid, and Children's Health Insurance Program. Medicare provides health insurance for people over 65 years of age, with disabilities, or with end-stage renal disease. Medicare is federally funded and administered by the Centers for Medicare and Medicaid Services (CMS), a division of the DHHS. Medicaid provides health care for indigent persons, older adults, and persons with disabilities. Pregnant women and young children are especially targeted. Medicaid is funded by both the federal and individual state governments. The states administer the program and determine which services are offered. Although the qualifying level of poverty varies across states, all women with an income less than 133% of the current federal poverty level are eligible for perinatal care. The Children's Health Insurance Program provides health care for children up to age 19 years through Medicaid and other programs. Like Medicaid, it is funded by both the federal and state governments and administered by the state.

Public Clinics. Clients who do not have private insurance or Medicaid may receive prenatal care at public clinics, which typically base their fees on the family's income. Nevertheless, barriers to care such as limited staff, hours of operation, lack of transportation, and lack of childcare for other children may affect the feasibility of such care.

Temporary Assistance to Needy Families. Temporary Assistance to Needy Families (TANF) provides financial assistance for basic living costs for pregnant persons and families with one or more dependent children. Eligibility requirements, income limits, allowances for homelessness, and time limitations vary across states. Group prenatal care such as the Centering Pregnancy model at low-resource health clinics is proving to be effective for culturally diverse childbearing persons, including Somali refugees (Banke-Thomas et al., 2019; Madeira et al., 2019).

Shelters and Health Care for the Homeless. Federal funding has assisted homeless people with shelter and health care. Nevertheless, the homeless have additional difficulties in obtaining health care because of lack of transportation, inconvenient hours, and poor continuity of care.

Quality and quantity of care in clinics may be poor because of inadequate funding. Nurses have been instrumental in opening shelters, clinics, and outreach services for the homeless, with nurse practitioners and certified nurse midwives often playing a major role. Clinics headed by nurse practitioners, advanced care nurses, are often opened in underserved rural and inner city areas. Nurses also help inform the public and legislatures about the needs of the homeless and others with few health care options (Sutton et al., 2021).

Innovative Programs. Innovative programs to ensure all clients receive good prenatal care are necessary to improve pregnancy outcomes. Some outreach programs are designed to improve health in clients who traditionally do not seek prenatal care. Bilingual health care workers and bilingual educational classes are included in some programs. Programs may be located in schools, shopping centers, churches, workplaces, and neighborhoods that are easily accessible to people. Mobile vans outfitted with basic equipment bring prenatal care to clients who are unable or unwilling to attend care at fixed locations or in more distant neighborhoods. The number of such neighborhood programs is insufficient to make adequate health care for clients a reality.

> ### KNOWLEDGE CHECK
> 9. How do poverty and inadequate prenatal care affect infant mortality and morbidity?
> 10. What is the effect of health care disparities in the United States?

LGBTQ Families

According to a Gallop poll in 2021, 5.6% of adults in the United States identify as lesbian, gay, bisexual, transgender, or queer (LGBTQ; Jones, 2021). The number of LGTBQ-identifying adults is especially increasing in younger populations such as Gen Z (born 1997–2002: 15.9%) and Millennials (born 1981–1996: 9.1%; Jones, 2021). Although research regarding LGBTQ families is sparse, LGBTQ families are becoming more common in the pregnant and childbearing population. One goal of Healthy People 2030 is to improve the health, safety, and well-being of lesbian, gay, bisexual, and transgender people (National Institutes of Health [NIH], 2021). In this segment, we will discuss appropriate terms for and issues specific to the LGBTQ population during childbearing (Box 2.2).

Appropriate Terms

Traditionally, the person giving birth is called the "mother" and the male partner is called the "father." Although these words have defined meanings, both are gendered terms and have many implications regarding roles and gender identity. Although no particular terms have been defined for LGBTQ families, birth parent and parent (or non-birth giving partner) are without gender implications. It is always appropriate to ask the client what they would like to be called or to call them by their chosen name. These preferences to names and pronouns should be noted in their chart to ensure the entire care team is aware of the client's choice. Until the client's preference is known, avoid using gendered terms like "here comes your baby, mama," or "do you want to take pictures, dad?" and instead use gender neutral terms or the client's name like "push, Ryan," and "here's how you put on a diaper, Support Person." Regardless of sexual orientation or gender

BOX 2.2 Gender-Inclusive Terms

- **Asexual:** The lack of a sexual attraction or desire for other people.
- **Cisgender:** A term for someone who identifies as the sex that they were assigned at birth.
- **Gender expression:** External appearance of one's gender identity, usually expressed through behavior, clothing, haircut, or voice, and which may or may not conform to socially defined behaviors and characteristics typically associated with being either masculine or feminine.
- **Gender Identity:** One's innermost concept of self as male, female, a blend of both, or neither—how individuals perceive themselves and what they call themselves. One's gender identity can be the same or different from their sex assigned at birth.
- **Heterosexual:** Being sexually attracted to members of the opposite sex.
- **Nonbinary:** An adjective describing a person who does not identify exclusively as a man or a woman. Nonbinary people may identify as being both a man and a woman, somewhere in between, or as falling completely outside these categories. Although many also identify as transgender, not all nonbinary people do. Nonbinary can also be used as an umbrella term encompassing identities such as agender, bigender, genderqueer, or gender-fluid.
- **Queer:** A term sometimes used to describe a fluid gender identity. In the past, this was a negative term for people who are gay. Now, however, queer is used by some people to describe themselves, their community, or both in a positive way. Typically used when self-identifying or quoting someone who self-identifies as queer.

- **Bisexual:** Being attracted to people of more than one gender.
- **Gay:** A person who is emotionally, romantically or sexually attracted to members of the same gender. Men, women, and nonbinary people may use this term to describe themselves.
- **Gender fluid:** A person who does not identify with a single fixed gender or has a fluid or unfixed gender identity.
- **Gender incongruence:** Clinically significant distress caused when a person's assigned birth gender is not the same as the one with which they identify.
- **Lesbian:** A woman who is sexually attracted to other women.
- **Pansexual:** Describes someone who has the potential for emotional, romantic or sexual attraction to people of any gender though not necessarily simultaneously, in the same way or to the same degree. Sometimes used interchangeably with bisexual.
- **Sexual orientation:** An inherent or immutable enduring emotional, romantic or sexual attraction to other people.
- **Transgender:** A person whose gender identity differs from the sex they were assigned at birth.

identity, use gender-inclusive language with all clients such as "partner" or "significant other" rather than "boyfriend" or "husband" when the client's partner status is unknown. Ask what preferences the client may have regarding pronouns and parent names. Use gender-neutral terms or chosen names if unable to ask preferences.

Many issues related to LGBTQ families occur before childbirth and therefore will not be a part of the care given during the intrapartum and postpartum period, but it is important to recognize barriers these families have had to overcome and disparities faced in their journey to parenthood.

LGBTQ individuals face a number of health disparities including:
- LGBTQ youth are two to three times more likely to attempt suicide.
- LGBTQ youth are more likely to be homeless.
- Lesbians are less likely to get preventive services for cancer.
- Gay men are at higher risk for human immunodeficiency virus (HIV) and other sexually transmitted infections (STIs), especially among communities of color.
- Lesbians and bisexual females are more likely to be overweight or obese.

- Transgender individuals have a high prevalence of HIV/STIs, victimization, mental health issues, and suicide and are less likely to have health insurance than heterosexual or LGB individuals.
- LGBTQ populations have the highest rates of tobacco, alcohol, and other drug use.

Before Pregnancy

Regardless of the genetic sex or gender identity of the parents, LGBTQ families have to consider how to start a family. This decision to start a family will involve considering all options from adoption to surrogacy to in-vitro fertilization. Family planning must be considered early in the process of transitioning of transgender clients, before hormone therapy or gender-affirming surgery. It is important to remember pregnancy is still possible after transitioning, and contraceptive counseling is crucial to preventing unwanted pregnancies. To have parental rights, non-birth parents may have to pay substantial legal fees to adopt the child, even if the non-birth giving parent's genetic material was used. LGBTQ couples may have faced barriers in finding an inclusive provider and may have faced discrimination in health care. As with any other parents, LGBTQ parents bring the problems, disparities, discriminations, and fears that they had before pregnancy into pregnancy with them, which can put them at higher risk for poor outcomes.

Pregnancy and Postpartum

Very few studies investigate needs of the LGBTQ client during pregnancy and the postpartum period. Pregnancy can be a stressful event for any person, but LGBTQ clients can experience discrimination and stigma that can increase stress levels. LGBTQ clients are more likely to report stillbirths and miscarriage compared with heterosexual clients and also have a comparatively higher percentage of LBW infants and very preterm births (Everett et al., 2019). These risks have been correlated to systemic exposure to discrimination and to high-risk behaviors, such as smoking and drinking during pregnancy, that are more prevalent in pregnancies of sexual minorities. Finally, mental health issues, such as depression and anxiety, are more pervasive in the LGBTQ population, leading to poor outcomes in neonatal morbidity and a higher rate of postpartum mood disorders.

Issues regarding the transgender male client and pregnancy must be considered. Prenatal care is one of the most important influencers of positive pregnancy outcomes. The pregnant transgender man has several barriers to overcome to receiving prenatal care, including:

- How to present as pregnant: As a pregnant man, as a cisgender woman, as a nonpregnant man
- The client–provider relationship: Finding supportive care, presenting to a "women's clinic" as a transgender man
- The "othering" of the client experience: How uniqueness makes the client feel like their experience is inferior
- Discomfort at the possible lack of provider/facility experience with trans pregnancy and delivery
- Social isolation and limited resources
- Mental health and self-perception: Some men view pregnancy as a parasite and experience gender dysmorphia, whereas others view it as the body's purpose and it brings feelings of peace.
- Loss of control and bodily autonomy
- Childbirth: Minimal information is available, which can increase sense of unknown and fear

Researchers are only starting to look into the LGBTQ community and ask questions regarding their experiences in pregnancy and family attainment. It is important that all health care providers be sensitive to this population and adopt policies and habits that are inclusive of all parents and reproductive humans.

Implicit Bias

Implicit bias is defined as "thoughts and feelings that exist outside of conscious awareness and subsequently affect human understanding, actions, and decisions unknowingly" (Saluja & Bryant, 2021, p.271). These attitudes can be positive or negative, developed as humans have evolved to assist in making quick decisions, and many times go unrecognized in the individual. Explicit bias, alternatively, is based on one's discriminatory beliefs and values and can be targeted in nature. Implicit bias has been shown to be correlated with a lower quality of care and is seen in times of overload or stress when the unconscious belief is activated (Saluja & Bryant, 2021). This affects health care decisions toward treatment and health outcomes.

Mitigating Implicit Bias

The first step in addressing implicit bias is recognizing it exists. The implicit association test (IAT) is a test developed in 1998 by scientists wanting to measure the strength of "associations between concepts (e.g., black people, gay people) and evaluations (e.g., good, bad) or stereotypes (e.g., athletic, clumsy)" (Project Implicit, 2011). Results of over 4.5 million completed IAT found: (1) implicit bias is pervasive; (2) people are often unaware of their biases; (3) implicit biases predict behavior; and (4) people differ in levels of implicit bias.

Being aware of cultural humility is a life-long commitment to self-evaluation to advocate for others. Cultural humility promotes empathy and respects client's individuality instead of assuming expertise on a client's race, culture, or ethnicity (Saluja & Bryant, 2021). Additionally, mindfulness has been shown to be effective to decrease implicit bias (Saluja & Bryant, 2021). Additional strategies to mitigate implicit bias are listed in Box 2.3.

Once implicit bias has been acknowledged, mitigating its effects requires a multifaceted approach. Organizational systems must include diverse populations and must evaluate whether policies include biases toward particular groups of people. Additionally, to decrease the effect implicit bias has on health care outcomes, the use of symptom-specific checklists to aid in standardized decision-making is a key recommendation. Personal reflection can help individuals recognize biases and correct them before interactions. Take the IAT test at http://implicit.harvard.edu/implicit/takeatest.html.

Intimate Partner Violence

Intimate partner violence (IPV) is defined as abuse by a current or former partner or spouse. It includes physical, sexual, and emotional abuse (e.g., threatening a partner's loved ones or possessions or harming a partner's self-worth). It is estimated that a third of adolescents and adult women in the U.S. have experienced physical violence by an intimate

---

BOX 2.3 Strategies to Combat Implicit Bias

Have a basic understanding of the cultures your patients come from.

Don't stereotype your patients; individuate them.

Understand and respect the tremendous power of unconscious bias.

Recognize situations that magnify stereotyping and bias.

Know the National Culturally and Linguistically Appropriate Services (CLAS) Standards.

Perform a "Teach Back." Teach Back is a method to confirm patient understanding of health care instructions that is associated with improved adherence, quality, and patient safety.

partner or have been raped by their partner or have experienced other forms of sexual violence from their partner (Ramaswamy et al., 2019). This is a major health concern, with an estimated 1.47 million rape-related physical assaults occurring in women in the U.S. annually (American College of Obstetrics and Gynecology [ACOG], 2019b). Although some studies show an increased incidence of IPV in culturally diverse women, IPV is seen at all socioeconomic levels (Ali et al., 2020).

Physical abuse may involve threats, slapping, and pushing. It may escalate to punching, kicking, and beating resulting in internal injury, wounds from weapons, or death. Sexual abuse, including rape, often is part of physical abuse, with many abused women reporting being forced into sex by their male partner (Ramaswamy et al., 2019).

Physical violence occurs within the context of continuous emotional abuse, threats, and coercion, and the abuser blames the victim for causing the abuse. As a result, victims feel shame, loss of self-respect, and powerlessness. They are often isolated from friends and family. Abused women often report reproductive coercion, attempts by the abuser to interfere with contraception use, and pregnancy. Although IPV spans all demographic categories, some factors associated with an increased risk include low self-esteem, low income, heavy alcohol and drug use, depression, and history of abuse (Grace et al., 2020).

Effects of Intimate Partner Violence During Pregnancy

Violence may start or escalate in frequency and severity during pregnancy with the risk for abuse continuing into the postpartum period. Childbearing adds more stress to the relationship. The partner may feel trapped in the relationship and under increased pressure to provide emotional and financial support for the client and the infant. Up to 20% of clients may be physically abused during pregnancy. Abuse occurs more often during pregnancy than any other commonly screened medical complication, with the possible exception of pregnancy-induced hypertension (ACOG, 2020; Grace et al., 2020).

Abuse during pregnancy is correlated with maternal/child complications. Abused clients are more likely than nonabused clients to start prenatal care late. They have an increased risk for uterine rupture, placental abruption, preterm birth, LBW infants, and maternal and fetal death. They may have increased risk for sexually transmitted infections (STIs) and perinatal depression.

Physical abuse of the client may be an indication of what life holds for the unborn child. Some abusers who batter women also batter children, and some women who are victims of violence abuse their children. Children who witness violence in the home may have psychological, social, emotional, and behavioral problems.

Factors That Promote Violence

Family violence occurs in families in which roles are gender-based and little value is placed on the woman's role. Men hold the power, and women are viewed as less worthy of respect.

There are gender differences in the wage market, and some women may remain in unhealthy relationships because they are financially dependent on their partners.

The woman's role in her own culture is important. For example, in many cultures, women think they should be submissive and sacrifice for their families because it is their duty to keep the family together. They may not have the education to be able to access help or obtain employment to provide a means of support if they should leave their partners. If the woman is an illegal immigrant, she is less likely to seek help from authorities for fear of being deported.

Stereotyping males as powerful and females as weak and without value has a profound effect on the self-esteem of women. Many women internalize these messages and may believe they are less worthy than their partners and they are the cause of their own punishment.

The woman may come to accept her partner's statements indicating she is the cause of the violence. She may minimize the abuse or indicate to others that it is rare. Women often feel a need to help the abuser and hope the partner will change and the abuse will end. As the relationship becomes increasingly abusive, the woman may begin to look for help.

Although alcohol is often stated as a cause of violence against women, chemical dependence and IPV are two separate problems. Chemical dependence is a disease of addiction, but abuse is a learned behavior. Nevertheless, violence may become more severe or bizarre when alcohol or drugs are involved. Table 2.2 summarizes the myths and realities of violence against women.

Characteristics of the Abuser

Physical abuse is about power, and it is only one of multiple tactics abusive partners use to control their partners. Other tactics include isolation, intimidation, and threats. Extreme jealousy and possessiveness are typical of the abuser. An abuser often attempts to control every aspect of the woman's life, such as where she goes, to whom she speaks, and what she wears. They control access to money and transportation and may force the woman to account for every moment spent away from them.

The abuser often has a low tolerance for frustration and poor impulse control who does not perceive the violent behavior as a problem and often denies responsibility for the violence by blaming the woman. Most abusers come from homes in which they witnessed the abuse of their mothers or were themselves abused as children.

Cycle of Violence

Although IPV may appear to be random, there is often a pattern. The violence occurs in a cycle consisting of three phases: (1) a tension-building phase, (2) a battering incident, and (3) a "honeymoon" or "calm phase." Being aware of the behaviors associated with each phase will enable the nurse to provide counseling (Fig. 2.2).

Nurse's Role in Prevention of Abuse

Nurses can do a great deal to prevent physical and sexual abuse in intimate relationships. First, they should examine

TABLE 2.2	**Myths and Realities of Violence Against Women**
Myths	**Realities**
The battered woman syndrome affects only a small percentage of the population.	Battering is a major cause of injury to women. Approximately 25% of women have experienced severe violence from IPV.
Violence against women occurs only in lower socioeconomic classes and minority groups.	Violence occurs in families from all social, economic, educational, racial, and religious backgrounds.
The problem is really "partner abuse," couples who assault each other.	Women experience IPV more often than men. Violence against women is about control and power.
Alcohol and drugs cause abusive behavior.	Substance abuse and violence against women are two separate problems. Substance abuse is a disease, but violence is a learned behavior and can be unlearned.
The abuser is "out of control."	He is not out of control. Instead, he is making a decision because he chooses who, when, and where he abuses.
The woman "got what she deserved."	No one deserves to be beaten. No one has the right to beat another person. Violent behavior is the responsibility of the violent person.
Women "like it," or they would leave.	Women are threatened with severe punishment or death if they attempt to leave. Many have no resources and are isolated, and they and their children are dependent on the abuser.
Couples' counseling is a good recommendation for abusive relationships.	Couples' counseling not only is ineffective for the couple but also can be dangerous for the abused woman.

IPV, Intimate partner violence.

their own beliefs to determine whether they accept the attitude that blames the victim: "Why were they wearing that?" "They shouldn't have flirted with someone else." "Why do they stay within the relationship?" Second, nurses can consciously practice empowerment of women. They should make it clear that the client owns their body and has the right to decide how it should be treated. Nurses should use language that indicates the client is an active partner in their care, such as: "You understand your body; what do you think?"

During examinations, nurses can introduce aspects of care to increase the client's control over the situation and help them feel supported (Kirkner et al., 2021). For example, make sure when the client first meets the health care provider who is to examine them, they are seated and clothed instead of being unclothed and in a lithotomy position.

School nurses are in an excellent position to influence how teenagers define gender roles: "Real men don't beat up women." "Girls don't have to put up with verbal or physical abuse from anyone." "Use a condom; it's not cool to give STIs or an unwanted pregnancy to someone you care about." Gaining understanding of cyberbullying abuse and strategies to manage it is important for nurses caring for adolescent clients who may be at risk for this kind of abuse (Van Ouytsel et al., 2020).

Nurses should be familiar with resources designed to provide health care workers with technical assistance, training materials, posters, bibliographies, and relevant articles. The National Domestic Violence Hotline offers information on crisis assistance throughout the United States. They have interpreters for 170 different languages and are available 24 hours a day. The other sources listed here provide information but are not crisis lines.

- National Domestic Violence Hotline: 800-799-SAFE and TTY 1-800-787-3224
- National Coalition against Domestic Violence: 303-839-1852
- National Resource Center on Domestic Violence: 1-800-787-3224 or TTY 1-800-799-7233
- StrongHearts Native Helpline: 1-844-762-8483
- Love is Respect National Teen Dating Abuse Helpline: 1-866-331-9474 or TTY 1-866-331-8453
- Rape, Abuse & Incest National Network (RAINN) National Sexual Assault Hotline: 1-800-656-HOPE (4673) to be connected with a trained staff member from a sexual assault service provider in your area

People who are being abused should be warned not to use their home computers to access the internet for sources of information about abuse because their partners may be able to find out about recently used internet sites.

KNOWLEDGE CHECK

11. What is the effect of pregnancy on battering behavior?
12. How can nurses alter their practice to help prevent violence against clients?

Human Trafficking

Human trafficking is the recruitment, harboring, transportation, provision, or obtaining of a person for labor, commercial sex, or domestic services, through the use of force, fraud, or coercion for the purpose of subjection to involuntary servitude, peonage, debt bondage, or slavery (The United States Department of Justice [DOJ], 2021). Trafficking in persons (TIP) takes many forms; however, the most commonly reported is sexual exploitation (United Nations Office on Drugs and Crime [UNODC], 2020).

Although it is commonly recognized there is no sound methodology for accurately generating the U.S. and global incidence of TIP, the U.S. Department of State (DOS) (2021) estimates approximately 24.9 million persons are trafficked

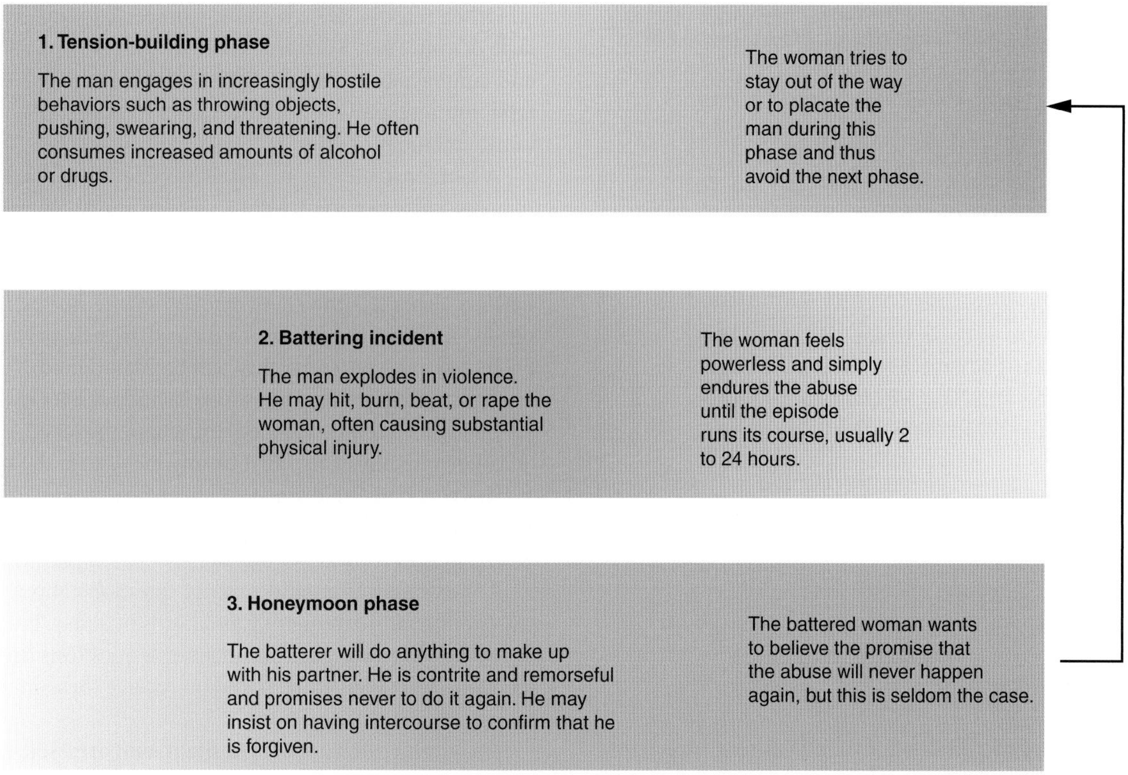

1. Tension-building phase

The man engages in increasingly hostile behaviors such as throwing objects, pushing, swearing, and threatening. He often consumes increased amounts of alcohol or drugs.

The woman tries to stay out of the way or to placate the man during this phase and thus avoid the next phase.

2. Battering incident

The man explodes in violence. He may hit, burn, beat, or rape the woman, often causing substantial physical injury.

The woman feels powerless and simply endures the abuse until the episode runs its course, usually 2 to 24 hours.

3. Honeymoon phase

The batterer will do anything to make up with his partner. He is contrite and remorseful and promises never to do it again. He may insist on having intercourse to confirm that he is forgiven.

The battered woman wants to believe the promise that the abuse will never happen again, but this is seldom the case.

Fig. 2.2 Types of behaviors that are evident in each step of the cycle of violence.

annually globally. This number is staggering considering estimates of only 1 in 100 victimizations are actually identified. The lack of scholarly evidence, especially as it pertains to pregnant clients that are victims of TIP, accurate estimations of victimization, and lack of evidence-based and trauma-informed best practices, is commonly attributed in part to a lack of identification and reporting by health care providers (Stoklosa et al., 2019). De Chesnay (2013) recognized sex trafficking as a global pandemic.

Women and children of childbearing age make up the majority of reported TIP cases (UNODC, 2020), with the average age of entry into sex trafficking reported to be women and girls in their childbearing years. Victims of TIP are subjected to an extensive myriad of abuses, including but not limited to sexual abuse, physical abuse, torture, psychological abuse, and the denial of basic human needs such as food and shelter (Chisolm-Straker et al., 2019). Further complicating the provision of care to this population is the isolation from support networks such as friends, family, and spiritual services.

Considering the abuses sustained by victims while under control of the trafficker and the inherently secretive nature of human trafficking, it is important to recognize that victims of TIP typically do not receive routine health care, much less prenatal care and education. Subsequently, mental and physical health outcomes seen in this population include but are not limited to increased incidence of HIV infection, pelvic inflammatory disease, botched home abortions, retained products of conception, damage to reproductive organs, precipitous deliveries, anxiety, depression, suicidal ideation, and self-harm attempts. Concurrent experiences such as violence,

stress, and a myriad of complex social factors further put victims at high risk for adverse pregnancy outcomes (Collins & Skarparis, 2020).

Although the scope and magnitude of providing evidence-based, survivor informed, and trauma-informed care (TIC) to this population is beyond the scope of this chapter, it is important for nurses caring for clients of childbearing age to be aware and to recognize cues or client "red flags" of TIP exploitation, recognizing that victims of TIP rarely self-identify (Stoklosa et al., 2019). A list of possible cues and "red flags" the nurse may recognize in client encounters with victims of TIP is provided in Box 2.4. Although one red flag may not be indicative of the client being a victim of TIP, the nurse should be assessing for patterns of red flags and analyzing the cues to inform their care priorities. For instance, a client who is not English-speaking would not necessarily raise suspicion, but a non-English-speaking minor client who does not know their address, presents with a history of multiple abortions, and is accompanied by an older person who will not let the client speak should raise the nurse's index of suspicion. Maternal-newborn nurses are in a unique position to recognize victimized clients and begin the critical chain of recognition, analysis, and intervention for this most vulnerable population (Miller, 2013).

Application of the Nursing Process: The Battered Woman

Assessment

During pregnancy, a woman is likely to have more frequent contact with health care providers than at any other time in

---

BOX 2.4 Human Trafficking Red Flags

- A person who is accompanied by an individual who insists on answering your questions
- Reluctance or inability of the victim to reveal the true situation
- Signs and symptoms of physical and mental abuse
- Evidence of being controlled
- Fearful
- Submissive
- Fear of authority figures
- Lack of identification documents
- Cannot relate their physical address
- Inconsistent stories and/or histories
- Foreign/non-English-speaking
- Homeless
- Previous and/or current prostitution charges
- History of sexual abuse
- Possession of expensive electronics, jewelry, and other luxury items
- History of substance abuse
- Markings on the body that appear to be branding
- High number of sexual partners relative to age

---

her life. Because of the prevalence of IPV during pregnancy, women should be asked about IPV at each prenatal visit, on admission to the birthing center, and again at the postpartum checkup. After pregnancy, visits to the pediatrician usually occur frequently during the infant's first year and provide other opportunities for further screening.

Unfortunately, few clients identify themselves as victims of IPV, and many remain unrecognized. When they are first approached, they may deny abuse has occurred. They may feel judged and stigmatized because they do not want to leave the relationship and fear their children will be taken away if they reveal the situation. The client who is not ready to seek help when they are first asked may be ready at a later time. Asking in a nonjudgmental way, and especially asking more than once, may lead the client to seek help at a later time.

Written information about abuse should be placed in places such as restrooms, where it will not be seen by the partner. This implies discussion of violence is encouraged and safe.

Many nurses are unsure about how to approach the issue of suspected abuse. Clients often seek care during the "honeymoon phase" of the violence cycle. During this phase, the abuser is often overly solicitous ("hovering husband syndrome") and eager to explain any injuries exhibited. The abuser often answers questions directed at the victim.

Introducing the subject of violence in the presence of the abuser who may be responsible for it places the victim in danger. It is absolutely essential to separate the victim from the abuser for the discussion of violence. No other family members should be present during the interview. Even children may reveal the discussion of abuse to the partner or family members.

A common concern about discussing IPV is having time with the victim without their partner. Sometimes the partner can be sent to another area to give insurance information or to eat a meal.

Other reasons nurses cite for not discussing IPV include lack of time, not knowing what to do if IPV is discovered, and language barriers. If language barriers are present, a professional interpreter should be used to translate and never a family member or friend.

When a private, secure place has been found, explain that many women experience abuse. For example, "Because abuse is very common and can affect the woman's health, it is the policy at this hospital to ask every woman about abuse situations." This lets the client know they are not being singled out for questioning. Reassure them that their privacy will be protected and confidentiality will be maintained.

Common screening questions include the following:
- Have you been threatened, hit, slapped, kicked, choked, or otherwise physically hurt by anyone within the last year?
- Has this happened since you have been pregnant?
- Has anyone forced you to have sexual activities?
- Are you ever afraid of anyone?

A "yes" answer should prompt questions about who hurt the client and the frequency and kinds of abuse. If a client has old or new signs of possible abuse, ask questions such as "Did someone hurt you?" and "Did you receive these injuries from being hit?"

The victim often appears hesitant, embarrassed, or evasive. They may speak in a low tone of voice, be unable to look the nurse in the eye, and appear guilty, ashamed, jumpy, or frightened. They may have a flat affect (absence of facial response) or one inappropriate for the situation.

Evaluate and document all signs of injury, both past and present. This includes areas of welts, bruising, swelling, lacerations, burns, and scars. Injuries are most commonly noted on the face, breasts, abdomen, and genitalia. Many victims have new or old fractures of the face, nose, ribs, or arms. A photograph or a drawing may be used to record areas of injury. These may be important for future legal action.

If sexual abuse has occurred, a gynecologic examination is necessary because trauma to the labia, vagina, cervix, or anus often is present. Types of forced sex may include vaginal/anal intercourse and insertion of foreign objects into the vagina and anus.

CRITICAL TO REMEMBER

Cues Indicating Violence Against Women

Nonverbal—Facial grimacing, slow and unsteady gait, vomiting, abdominal tenderness, absence of facial response

Injuries—Welts, swelling, burns, vaginal or rectal bleeding; bruises or lacerations in various stages of healing; evidence of old or new fractures of the nose, face, ribs, or arms; injuries to the face, breasts, abdomen, or genitals

Vague somatic complaints—Anxiety, depression, panic attacks, sleeplessness, anorexia

Discrepancy between history and type of injuries—Wounds that do not match the victim's story; multiple bruises in various stages of healing; bruising on the arms (which may have been raised as a form of self-protection); old, untreated wounds

Be particularly alert for nonverbal cues indicating abuse has occurred. Facial grimacing or a slow, unsteady gait may indicate pain. Vomiting or abdominal tenderness may indicate internal injury. A flat affect is indicative of victims who emotionally withdraw from the situation to protect themselves from the horror and humiliation they experience. Keep in mind the victim may fear for their life because abusive episodes tend to escalate. Open-ended questions help prompt full disclosure and the expression of feelings. Record direct quotes of what the victim says about the abusive experience.

Identification of Client Problems

A variety of client problems may be applicable, depending on assessment data. The most meaningful may be fearfulness secondary to the potential for injury to self or children.

Planning: Expected Outcomes

The victim may have difficulty developing a long-term plan of care without a great deal of specialized assistance. They often are unwilling to leave the abusive situation, and nurses should focus on working with the victim to make short-term plans to protect them from future injury. The expected outcomes are that the victim will:
1. Acknowledge the physical assaults.
2. Develop a specific plan of action for when the abusive cycle begins.
3. Identify community resources that can provide protection for the victim and their children.

Interventions

Listening. Use therapeutic communication techniques to listen and encourage the victim to share feelings. Assure them you understand their situation is a difficult one and they have been surviving as well as they can. Praise even small positive steps they have taken to ensure safety for themselves and their children. The victim should make their own decisions about whether to continue the relationship and should not feel coerced to end it.

Developing a Personal Safety Plan. Ask the victim what is done to decrease or avoid violence from the abuser. Help the victim make concrete plans to protect their safety and the safety of their children. For example, if the abused client insists on returning to the shared home, describe the cycle of behavior that culminates in physical abuse and factors such as drug or alcohol use that precipitate a violent episode. Discuss behaviors indicating the level of frustration and anger is increasing to the point at which the danger is escalating.

Assist them to do the following:
- Locate the nearest shelter, safe house, or another safe place and make specific plans to go there once the cycle of violence begins.
- Identify the safest, quickest routes out of the home.
- Hide extra keys to the car and house, money, personal information (social security numbers, birth certificates, insurance policy information, driver's license, bank account numbers, passport), medications, some clothes for themselves and their children, and personal necessities.

They should not hide them in the house but find another place such as the house of a friend or relative.
- Devise a code word and prearrange with someone to call the police when the word is used.
- Memorize the telephone number of the shelter or hotline because time is often a crucial element in the decision to leave. An easy number to remember is the one for the National Domestic Violence Hotline (1-800-799-SAFE), which provides immediate crisis assistance in the caller's community.
- Review the safety plan frequently because leaving the partner is one of the most dangerous times. Victims are more likely to be injured or killed when they are leaving than at any other time.

Affirming They Are Not to Blame. The victim often believes they are responsible for the abuse. Let them know no one deserves to be hurt for any reason. The one who hurt them is the person responsible. They did not provoke it or cause it and could not have prevented it. Nurses are often responsible for teaching basic family processes, such as the following:
- Violence is not normal.
- Violence usually is repeated and escalates.
- Battering is against the law.
- Those being abused have alternatives.

They also need nonjudgmental acceptance and recognition of the difficulties involved in making changes in their situation. Praise them for any actions they take, even if they are only minor steps toward making their life safer. Reassure them that they are doing the right thing for themselves and their children when they seek help and make plans for escape.

Providing Education. The childbearing client is likely to worry about the effect of abuse on their pregnancy. Discuss the increased incidence of preterm labor with them and explain the signs. If they are using substances, explain the effects of smoking and of the use of alcohol and other substances and help them make plans to decrease or stop their use. Help them identify stressors and explore ways to reduce them wherever possible.

Providing Referrals. When contact with the victim is a short-term one, many interventions are outside the scope of nursing practice. Refer the family to community agencies such as the police department, legal services, community shelters, counseling services, and social service agencies, as needed. Include mental health referrals, if necessary, for treatment of depression or for counseling. Document that referrals were made and whether the client accepted them.

It is essential to accept the decisions of the battered client and acknowledge they are on their own timetable. They may not take any actions at the time they are recommended. Listening to them, believing them, and providing information about resources may be the only help the nurse can provide until the client is ready to do more.

Do not become negative or pass judgment on the abuser. The one being abused is often tied to the abuser by both economic and emotional bonds and may become defensive if the partner is criticized. Tell them resources are available for the abuser, but the abuser must first admit abuse and seek assistance before help can be offered. *Initiating referrals for the partner before they ask for help will increase the danger to the abused if they think they have been betrayed.*

Evaluation

The plan of care can be deemed successful if the client acknowledges the violent episodes in the home, makes concrete plans to protect themselves and their children from future injury, and makes plans to use the community resources available to them.

> ### ? KNOWLEDGE CHECK
>
> 13. What major cues indicate a client has been physically abused?
> 14. How can nurses intervene to help those being abused protect their safety if they choose to remain in a home situation with a partner who physically abuses them?
> 15. What are possible indicators that a client is a victim of human trafficking?

ETHICS AND BIOETHICS

Ethics involves determining the best course of action in a certain situation. Ethical reasoning is the analysis of what is morally right and reasonable. **Bioethics** is the application of ethics to health care. Ethical behavior for nurses is discussed in codes such as the ANA *Code of Ethics for Nurses with Interpretive Statements* (ANA, 2015). Ethical issues have become more complex as technology has created more options in health care. These issues are controversial because agreement over what is right or best does not exist and because moral support is possible for more than one course of action.

Ethical Dilemmas

An **ethical dilemma** is a situation in which no solution is completely satisfactory. Opposing courses of action may seem equally desirable, or all possible solutions may seem undesirable. Ethical dilemmas are among the most difficult situations in nursing practice. To find solutions, nurses and other health care personnel should apply ethical theories and principles and determine the burdens and benefits of any course of action.

Ethical Theories

Three models guide ethical decision-making: deontologic, utilitarian, and human rights. Few people use one decision-making model exclusively. Instead, they make decisions by examining models and determining which is most appropriate for the circumstances.

Deontologic Model. The **deontologic model** determines what is right by applying ethical principles and moral rules. It does not vary the solution according to individual situations. One example is the rule, "Life must be maintained at all costs and in all circumstances." Strictly used, the deontologic model would not consider the quality of life or weigh the use of scarce resources against the likelihood that the life maintained would be near-normal.

Utilitarian Model. The **utilitarian model** approaches ethical dilemmas by analyzing the benefits and burdens of any course of action to find one that will result in the greatest amount of good. Appropriate actions may vary with the situation when using the utilitarian model. The utilitarian approach is concerned more with the consequences of actions than the actions themselves. In its simplest form, the utilitarian approach is "The end justifies the means." If the outcome is positive, the method of arriving at that outcome is less important.

Human Rights Model. The belief that each person has human rights is the basis for the **human rights model** to making ethical decisions. The nurse may find personal difficulty in the right of a person to refuse care that the nurse and possibly other care providers believe is best. A nurse's goal is usually to save lives, but what if the person's life is intolerable or care is refused?

Ethical Principles

Ethical principles or rules are also important for solving ethical dilemmas. Four of the most important principles are beneficence, nonmaleficence, respect for autonomy, and justice. Other important ethical principles such as accountability, confidentiality, truth, and keeping promises are derived from these four basic principles (Box 2.5). These principles guide decision-making, but in some situations, the application of one principle conflicts with another. In such cases, one principle may outweigh another in importance.

Treatments designed to do good also may cause harm. For example, a cesarean birth may prevent permanent harm to a fetus in jeopardy. Nevertheless, the surgery that saves the fetus also has effects on the mother, causing pain, temporary disability, possible complications, and increased financial expenses. Both the mother and the health care providers may decide the principle of beneficence outweighs the principle of nonmaleficence. If the client does not want surgery, the principles of autonomy and justice also should be considered. Is the client's right to determine what happens to their body more or less important than the right of the fetus to fair and equal treatment?

Solving Dilemmas in Daily Professional Practice

Nurses are often involved in supporting parents when tragedy strikes during a birth. They should be knowledgeable regarding the disease process and the appropriate nursing care in these situations and also be able to support family's needs when ethical dilemmas arise. Ethical challenges also may arise, however, during day-to-day professional practice. Nurses and other professionals should learn to analyze and resolve these dilemmas. Personal values and cultural and language differences are some of the issues that have an impact on the solving of ethical dilemmas.

Ethical dilemmas, a situation in which no solution seems completely satisfactory, also may have legal ramifications. For example, although the American Medical Association (AMA) has stated anencephalic organ donation is ethically permissible, it may be illegal. In many states, the legal criteria for death

BOX 2.5 Ethical Principles in Health Care

- Autonomy—People have the right to self-determination. This includes the right to respect, privacy, and information necessary to make decisions based on their personal values and beliefs.
- Beneficence—Make a decision that produces the greatest good or the least harm.
- Nonmaleficence—Avoid risking or causing harm to others.
- Justice—All people should be treated equally and fairly regardless of disease or social or economic status.
- Fidelity—Keep promises and do not make promises that cannot be kept.
- Truth (veracity)—Tell the truth.
- Confidentiality—Keep information private.
- Accountability—Accept responsibility for actions as a health care professional.

Applying the Nursing Process to Solve Ethical Dilemmas
- Assessment—Gather data to clearly identify the problem and the decisions necessary. Obtain viewpoints from all who will be affected by the decision and applicable legal, agency policy, and common practice standards.
- Analysis—Decide whether an ethical dilemma exists. Analyze the situation using ethical theories and principles. Determine whether and how these conflict.
- Planning—Identify as many options as possible, determine their advantages and disadvantages, and conclude which options are most realistic. Predict what is likely to happen if each option is followed. Include the option of doing nothing. Choose the solution.
- Implementation—Carry out the solution. Determine who will implement the solution and how. Identify all interventions necessary and what support is needed.
- Evaluation—Analyze the results. Determine whether further interventions are necessary.

From Alfaro-LeFevre, R. (2021). *Critical thinking, clinical reasoning, and clinical judgment* (8th ed). Elsevier.
Arnold, E.C. & Boggs, K.N. (2019). Clinical judgment and ethical decision making. In *Interpersonal relationships: Professional communication skills for nurses* (8th ed). Elsevier.

include cardiopulmonary and brain death. Therefore, donor organs from the baby with anencephaly are likely unusable for transplantation because of lengthy anoxia.

Greater understanding about conflicts and misunderstandings that may arise from the differences among people helps nurses find better solutions to ethical dilemmas and other problems common to daily life. Many approaches can be used to solve ethical dilemmas in nursing practice. No single approach guarantees a right decision, but it provides a logical, systematic method for decision-making. Because the nursing process is also a method of problem solving, nurses can use a similar approach when faced with ethical dilemmas.

Decision-making in ethical dilemmas may seem straightforward, but it rarely results in answers acceptable to everyone. Health care agencies often have bioethics committees to formulate policies for ethical situations, provide education, and help make decisions in specific

cases. The committees include a variety of professionals such as nurses, physicians, social workers, ethicists, and clergy members. The family members most closely affected by the decision also participate, if possible. A satisfactory solution to ethical dilemmas is more likely to occur when people work together.

KNOWLEDGE CHECK

16. What is the difference between ethics and bioethics?
17. How do the deontologic, utilitarian, and human rights models differ within ethical theories?
18. When might two ethical principles conflict?
19. How do the steps of the nursing process relate to ethical decision-making?

Ethical Issues in Reproduction

Many issues cross the boundary between ethics and legality and apply to all caregivers. These issues apply to many fields of care, including reproduction and women's health. Respectful care for childbearing clients and their families is a human right. "One hopes the memory [of giving birth] will be cherished as one of the peak experiences of their lives, perhaps challenging but one in which they felt safe and received dignified, compassionate care" (Morton & Simkin, 2019, p. 395).

Reproduction issues often involve conflicts in which a client's behaviors may cause harm to the fetus or be disliked by some or most members of society. Conflicts between a mother and fetus occur when the mother's needs, behavior, or wishes may injure the fetus. The most obvious instances involve abortion, substance abuse, and a mother's refusal to follow the advice of caregivers. Health care workers and society may respond to such a client with anger rather than support. Nevertheless, the rights of both mother and fetus should be examined.

Elective Pregnancy Termination

Abortion, or elective termination of pregnancy, was a volatile legal, social, and political issue even before the *Roe v. Wade* decision by the U.S. Supreme Court in 1973. Before then, states could outlaw abortion within their boundaries. In *Roe v. Wade,* the Supreme Court stated abortion was legal in the U.S. and existing state laws prohibiting abortion were unconstitutional because they interfered with the mother's constitutional right to privacy. This landmark decision was overruled in 2022 by *Dobbs v. Jackson Women's Health Organization* which returned the rights to regulate abortion back to individual states (Britannica, 2022). At the time of this publication, the changes to state laws involving abortion access and limitations is still uncertain.

Some people believe abortion should be illegal at any time because it deprives the fetus of life. In contrast, others believe women have the right to control their reproductive functions and political discussion of reproductive rights is an invasion of a woman's most private decisions.

For many people the woman's constitutional right to privacy conflicts with the right to life of the fetus; however, the Supreme Court did not rule on when life begins. This omission provokes debate between those who think life begins at conception and those who think life begins when the fetus is viable, or capable of living outside the uterus. Those who think life begins at conception may be opposed to abortion at any time during pregnancy. Those who think life begins when the fetus is viable (22 to 24 weeks of gestation) may oppose abortion after that time. Nurses need to understand abortion laws and the conflicting beliefs that divide society on this issue.

Implications for Nurses. Nurses' responsibilities in the conflict about abortion cannot be ignored. First, they should be informed about the complexity of the abortion issue from legal and ethical standpoints and know the regulations and laws in their state. Second, they should realize that for many people, abortion is an ethical dilemma resulting in confusion, ambivalence, and personal distress. Next, they should also recognize that for many others, the issue is not a dilemma but a fundamental violation of the personal or religious views that give meaning to their lives. Finally, nurses should acknowledge the sincere convictions and strong emotions of those on all sides of the issue, including themselves.

Professional Obligations. Nurses have no obligation to support a position with which they disagree. The nursing practice acts of many states allow nurses to refuse to assist with the procedure if it violates their ethical, moral, or religious beliefs. Nevertheless, nurses are obligated to disclose this information before they are employed in an institution where abortions are performed. It is unethical for a nurse to withhold this information until assigned to care for a woman having an abortion and then refuse to provide care. As always, nurses should respect the decisions of women who look to nurses for care. If nurses think they are not able to provide compassionate care because of personal convictions, they should inform a supervisor so appropriate care can be arranged.

> ### ❓ KNOWLEDGE CHECK
> 20. What are the major conflicting beliefs about abortion?

Mandated Contraception

The availability of contraception that does not require taking a regular oral dose, such as using a hormone-releasing patch or having hormone injections or an intrauterine device (IUD), has led to speculation about whether certain people should be forced to use this method of birth control. Requiring contraception has been used as a condition of probation, allowing women accused of child abuse to avoid incarceration.

Some people think mandated contraception is a reasonable way to prevent additional births in the case of women who are considered unsuitable parents and to reduce government expenses for dependent children. A punitive approach to social problems does not provide long-term solutions. Requiring poor women to use contraception to limit the money spent on supporting them is legally and ethically questionable and does not address the obligations of the children's father. Such a practice interferes with a woman's constitutional rights to privacy, reproduction, refusal of medical treatment, and freedom from cruel and unusual punishment. In addition, medication may pose health risks to the woman. Surgical sterilization (tubal ligation) also carries risks and should be considered permanent. Access to free or low-cost information on family planning would be more appropriate and ethical.

Fetal Injury

If a mother's actions cause injury to the fetus, the question of whether they should be restrained or prosecuted has legal and ethical implications. In some instances, courts have issued jail sentences to women who have caused or who may cause injury to the fetus. This response punishes the woman and places them in a situation in which they cannot further harm the fetus. In other cases, women have been forced to undergo cesarean births against their will when providers have testified such a procedure was necessary to prevent injury to the fetus.

The state has an interest in protecting children, and the U.S. Supreme Court has ruled a child has the right to begin life with a sound mind and body. Many state laws require evidence of prenatal drug exposure be reported. Women have been charged with negligence, involuntary manslaughter, delivery of drugs to a minor, and child endangerment.

Nevertheless, forcing women to behave in a certain way because they are pregnant violates the principles of autonomy, self-determination of competent adults, bodily integrity, and personal freedom. Because of fear of prosecution, this practice could impede, not advance, health care during pregnancy.

The punitive approach to fetal injury also raises the question of how much control the government should have over a pregnant woman. Laws could be passed to mandate maternal HIV testing with no right to refuse, fetal testing, intrauterine surgery, or even the foods the woman eats during pregnancy. The decision with regard to just how much control should be allowed in the interests of fetal safety is difficult.

Fetal Therapy

Fetal therapy is becoming more common as techniques improve and knowledge grows. Although intrauterine blood transfusions are relatively standard practice in some areas, fetal surgery is still relatively uncommon.

The risks and benefits of surgery for major fetal anomalies should be considered in every case. Even when surgery is successful, the fetus may not survive, may have other serious problems, or may be born severely preterm. The mother may require weeks of bed rest and a cesarean birth. Nevertheless, despite the risks, successful fetal surgery may result in birth of an infant who could not otherwise have survived.

Parents need help balancing the potential risks to the mother and the best interests of the fetus. They might feel pressured to have surgery or other fetal treatment they do not understand. As with any situation involving informed consent, women need adequate information before making a decision. They should understand if procedures are still experimental, the known chances of a procedure's success, and if any alternative treatments are available and their chances of success.

Issues in Infertility

Infertility Treatment. Perinatal technology has found multiple ways for some previously infertile couples to bear children. Many techniques are more successful, but ethical concerns include the high cost and overall low success of some infertility treatments. Because many of these costs are not insured, their use is limited to the affluent. Techniques may benefit only a small percentage of infertile couples. Despite treatment, many couples never give birth, regardless of the costs or invasiveness of therapy. Successful treatment may lead to multiple gestations and complications related to maternal age.

Other ethical concerns focus on the fate of unused embryos. Should they be frozen for later use by the woman or someone else or used in genetic research? What if the parents divorce or die? Who should make these decisions? In multiple pregnancies with more fetuses than can be expected to survive intact, reduction surgery may be used to destroy one or more fetuses for the benefit of those remaining. The ethical and long-term psychological implications of this procedure are also controversial.

Assisted reproductive technologies (ART) now allow postmenopausal women to become pregnant. What are the ethical implications of conceiving and giving birth to children whose mother is several decades older than their friends' mothers and is more likely to die when the children are relatively young? Should the age and health of the parents be a factor in determining whether this treatment is offered? Should a consideration be the risk these women face for complications that might result in unhealthy infants? Should average life expectancy enter the decision?

Surrogate Parenting. In surrogate parenting, a woman agrees to bear an infant for another woman. Conception may take place outside the body using ova and sperm from the couple who wish to become parents. These embryos are then implanted into the surrogate mother, or the surrogate mother may be inseminated artificially with sperm from the intended father. Donated embryos also may be implanted into a surrogate mother. Sensitive and respectful care should be provided for the biologic parents and the gestational surrogate or carrier (Palmer & Cullen, 2019).

Cases in which the surrogate mother has wanted to keep the child have created controversy. No standard regulations govern these cases, which are decided individually. Ethical concerns involve who should be a surrogate mother, what her role should be after birth, and who should make these decisions. Screening of parents and surrogates is necessary to determine whether they are suited for their roles. Who should perform the screening? Should it be left to the private interests of those involved, or should government become involved?

An issue closely related to surrogate parenting is the use of donor gametes or unused embryos from another infertile couple. Will the use of donor gametes or embryos violate the religious or moral beliefs of the parents? Does the child thus conceived have a right to know the identity of the biologic parents? What are the rights of the biologic parents?

Privacy Issues

Many people are concerned about the possible misuse of their health information. They may fear that health information in the wrong hands, whether that information is accurate or not, may cost them a job, promotion, loan, or something equally valuable. Privacy concerns and fear of health care or other insurance loss may cause a person to withhold genetic or other medical history information from a provider. Quality of genetic counseling may be impaired if family members refuse to release their medical records.

Government Regulations

The 1996 Health Insurance Portability and Accountability Act (HIPAA) was designed to reduce fraud in the insurance industry and make it easier for people to remain insured if they move from one job to another. Within HIPAA's provisions was the mandate for Congress to pass a law to protect the privacy of personal medical information by August 1999. Congress failed to do so, and the Secretary of the DHHS proposed interim regulations in October 1999 to protect personal medical privacy as required by HIPAA. The DHHS regulations provide consumers with significant new power over their records, including the right to see and correct their records, the application of civil and criminal penalties for violations of privacy standards, and protection against deliberate or inadvertent misuse or disclosure.

Electronic Communications. A person's health data are generally maintained in various computerized formats. Although this allows nearly instantaneous exchange of data among providers, it also may carry the potential for greater violation of privacy than data maintained on paper. Terminals may be placed in hallways or client rooms to facilitate quick entry and retrieval of information for staff. The nurse should remember this information also may be easily accessed by a computer-literate person despite the use of passcodes and other security measures. Nurses should take care to avoid violating client confidentiality by promptly logging off terminals when finished and following facility protocols for protection of security pass codes.

Social media sites allow nurses to exchange information and nursing care tips that can improve practice. These forums also have the potential to allow lapses of client or institutional confidentiality because their communications cannot be considered private. When participating in discussion lists or using e-mail, nurses should respect the confidentiality of clients, colleagues, and institutions. Institutional documents such as chart forms, policies, and procedures should not be shared without the facility's approval. A personal message should not be forwarded without the original sender's permission. The ANA and National Council for State Boards of Nursing provide resources for nursing regarding appropriate use of social media.

LEGAL ISSUES

The legal foundation for the practice of nursing provides safeguards for clients and sets standards by which nurses can be evaluated. Nurses need to understand how the law applies specifically to them. When nurses do not meet the standards expected, they may be held legally accountable.

Safeguards for Health Care

Three categories of safeguards determine the law's view of nursing practice: (1) nurse practice acts, (2) standards of care set by professional organizations, and (3) rules and policies set by the institution employing the nurse. Clinical judgment should guide ethical and legal decision-making (Boggs, 2019).

Nurse Practice Acts

The nurse practice act of each state determines the scope of practice of registered nurses in that state. Nurse practice acts define what the nurse is allowed to do when caring for clients. The acts also specify what the nurse is expected to do when providing care. Some parts of the law may be very specific. Others are stated broadly to allow flexible interpretation of the role of nurses. Nurse practice acts vary across states, and nurses should understand these laws wherever they practice. Nurses should have a copy of the nurse practice act for their state and refer to it for questions about their scope of practice. Most state nurse practice acts are available on the internet. The website of the National Council of State Boards of Nursing (NCSBN) has information on nurse practice acts for all states, all territories, and the District of Columbia, as well as other information related to licensing and practice.

Laws relating to nursing practice also delineate methods, called standard procedures or *protocols,* by which nurses may assume certain duties commonly considered part of medical practice. The procedures are written by committees of nurses, physicians, and administrators. They specify the nursing qualifications required for practicing the procedures, define the appropriate situations, and state the education required. Standard procedures allow the role of the nurse to change to meet the needs of the community and expanding knowledge.

Standards of Care

Court decisions have generally held that nurses should practice according to established standards and health agency policies in addition to nurse practice acts. Standards of care are set by professional associations and describe the level of care that can be expected from practitioners. For example, perinatal nurses are held to the national standards published by AWHONN, which are based on research and the agreement of experts. AWHONN also publishes practice resources, position statements, and other guidelines for nurses. Nurses should be familiar with the latest standards of care that cover their own practices in the provision of safe, quality, and respectful care (Simpson, 2021b).

Agency Policies

Each health care agency sets specific policies, procedures, and protocols governing nursing care. Nurses are frequently involved in writing and revising nursing policies and procedures. Policies and procedures increase staff adherence to professional, legal, and regulatory standards, statutes, and accreditation requirements, decrease variation in practice, and provide a reference for staff, decreasing dependence on memory, which can be a major source of human errors or oversights. In the event of a malpractice claim, the applicable policy, procedure, or protocol is likely to be used as evidence. The case of the professionals is strengthened if all agency policies are followed properly. These policies should be revised and updated regularly.

Malpractice: Limiting Loss

Negligence is the failure to perform as a reasonable, prudent person of similar background would act in a similar situation. Negligence may consist of doing something that should not be done or failing to do something that should be done.

Malpractice is negligence by professionals such as nurses and other health care providers in the performance of their duties. Nurses may be accused of malpractice if they do not perform according to established standards of care and in the manner of a reasonable, prudent nurse with similar education and experience in a similar situation. Four elements must be present to prove negligence: duty, breach of duty, damage, and proximate cause.

> ### CRITICAL TO REMEMBER
> #### Elements of Negligence
>
> **Duty**—The nurse must have a duty to act or give care to the client. It must be part of the nurse's responsibility. Emerging ethical dilemmas were engendered by the COVID-19 global pandemic in which issues arose such as the obligation to provide care regardless of client diagnosis and the dilemma of protecting self from a highly contagious life-threatening disease versus providing clinical care (Alayi et al., 2021; Barbosa-Leiker, et al. 2021).
> **Breach of duty**—A violation of that duty must occur. The nurse fails to conform to established standards in performing that duty.
> **Damage**—An actual injury or harm to the client as a result of the nurse's breach of duty must occur.
> **Proximate cause**—The nurse's breach of duty must be proved to be the cause of harm to the client.

Malpractice claims continue to be a major cost in health care. As a result of awards from such claims, the cost of malpractice insurance has risen for all health care workers. More health care workers practice defensively and accumulate evidence that their actions are in the client's best interests.

Many reasons exist for perinatal malpractice claims. Complications are usually unexpected because parents view pregnancy and birth as normal. The birth of a compromised child is a tragic shock, and parents may look for someone to blame. Although very small preterm infants may survive, some have long-term disabilities and require expensive care. Statutes of limitations vary across states, but plaintiffs often have more than 20 years to file lawsuits involving a newborn. Therefore the period during which a malpractice suit may be filed is longer.

Health care agencies and individual nurses should work together to prevent malpractice claims. Nurses are responsible and accountable for their own actions. Therefore they should be aware of the limits of their knowledge and scope of practice, and they should practice within those limits.

Prevention of claims is sometimes referred to as *risk management* or *quality assurance*. Although prevention of all malpractice claims is impossible, nurses can prevent malpractice judgments against themselves by following guidelines for informed consent, refusal of care, and documentation; acting as a client advocate; and maintaining their levels of expertise.

Informed Consent

When clients receive adequate information, they are less likely to file malpractice suits. Informed consent is an ethical concept that has been enacted into law. Clients have the right to decide whether to accept or reject treatment options as part of their right to function autonomously. To make wise decisions, they need full information about treatments offered.

CRITICAL TO REMEMBER

Requirements of Informed Consent

Patient's competence to consent
Full disclosure of information needed
Patient's understanding of information
Patient's voluntary consent

Competence. Certain requirements should be met before consent is considered informed. First, the client should be competent or able to think through a situation and make rational decisions. Infants, children, and adult clients who are comatose or severely cognitively impaired are incapable of making such decisions. A client who has received drugs that impair the ability to think is temporarily incompetent. In these cases, another person is appointed to make decisions for the client.

In most states, the age of majority (the age at which a person can give consent to health care) is 18 years. In some states, however, younger adolescents can consent independently to some treatments, such as those for mental illness, abortions, contraceptives, drug abuse, and STIs/STDs. An emancipated minor is younger than the age of majority, usually 18 years, and considered medically competent to make some medical decisions independent of a parent or guardian. Pregnant adolescents may be considered emancipated minors in some states. Nurses should be familiar with laws governing age of consent in their practice area.

Another exception to the usual requirement of informed consent is in emergency circumstances; in such situations, consent is considered implied. Treatment may proceed if there is no evidence the client does not want the treatment. *Emergency* may be specifically defined by state law and is usually restricted to unforeseen conditions that, if uncorrected, would result in severe disability or death. Emergency consent applies only for the emergency condition and does not extend to any other nonemergency problem that coexists with the emergency condition.

Patient information about advance directives such as a living will, durable power of attorney for health care, and an alternative decision maker for the client should be assessed on admission to the health care facility. Often, hospitals are required to inform clients about advance directives during the nursing admission assessment. The person who has not made advance directives should be offered the opportunity to make these choices.

Full Disclosure. The second requirement is full disclosure of information, including details of what the treatment entails, the expected results, and the meaning of those results. The risks, side effects, benefits, and other treatment options should be explained to clients. The person also should be informed about the consequences if no treatment is chosen.

Understanding of Information. The third requirement is that the person should comprehend information about proposed treatment. Health care professionals should explain the facts in terms the person can understand. If a client does not speak English, an interpreter is required. A client with hearing impairment should have a sign-language interpreter of the appropriate level to sign all explanations before consent is given. Interpreters should not be family or friends because these people may interpret selectively rather than objectively. Additionally, client confidentiality is compromised when nonprofessional interpreters are used for sensitive information. Nurses should be advocates for the client when they find the client does not fully understand or has questions about a treatment. If it is a minor point, the nurse may be able to explain it. Otherwise, the nurse should inform the physician or other health care provider of the need for clarification.

Voluntary Consent. The fourth requirement is that the client should be allowed to make choices voluntarily without undue influence or coercion from others. Although others may give information, the client alone makes the decision. Clients should not feel pressured to choose in a certain way, and they should not think their future care depends on their decision.

Refusal of Care. Occasionally, some persons decline treatment offered by health care workers. Clients refuse treatment when they think the benefits of treatment are insufficient to balance the burdens of the treatment or their quality of life after treatment. Clients have the right to refuse care, and they can withdraw agreement to treatment at any time. When a person makes this decision, a number of steps should be taken (Simpson, 2021b).

If the provider is unaware of the client's decision, the nurse should notify that provider and document the notification accordingly. There should be verification that the client understands the treatment and consequences of refusal. Opinions by other providers may be offered to the client. A description of the treatment refused should be documented in the client's chart, as well as the explanations given to the client and their refusal.

Every effort should be made to obtain a written refusal from the client indicating they have been informed of the risks and benefits of the treatment and the refusal of the treatment. The nurse should refer to the facility's procedure for client refusal of treatment for other requirements. If no ethical dilemma exists, the client's decision stands.

In cases of an ethical dilemma, a referral may be made to the hospital ethics committee. In rare situations, the physician may seek a court ruling to force treatment. For example, when a childbearing client refuses a cesarean birth, their decision may gravely harm the unborn child. This situation is the only legal instance in which a person is forced to undergo surgery for the health of another. Nevertheless, court action is avoided, if possible, because it places the client and their caregiver in adversarial positions. In addition, it invades the client's privacy and interferes with their autonomy and right to informed consent. If legally mandated surgery were to become widespread and cause persons to avoid health care during pregnancy, the resulting harm would affect more clients and infants than those who would be protected by the surgery.

Coercion is illegal and unethical in obtaining consent. Even though the nurse may strongly think a client should receive the treatment, they should not feel forced to submit to unwanted procedures. Nurses should not allow personal feelings to adversely affect the quality of their care. People have the right to good nursing care, regardless of their decisions to accept or reject treatment.

Documentation

Nurses are expected to meet the **standard of care**, or the level of care expected of a professional as determined by laws, professional organizations, and health care agencies (Alfaro-LeFevre, 2021; ANA, 2021). Documentation is essential for collaborative client care and is also the best evidence that a standard of care has been maintained. It includes nurses' notes, fetal monitoring strips, electronic data, flow sheets, care paths, consent forms, and any other data recorded on paper, recorded electronically, or both. In many instances, notations in hospital records are the only proof care has been given. When documentation is not present, juries may assume that care was not given.

Documentation should demonstrate thorough initial and ongoing assessments, identification of problems, interventions used, and evaluation of their effectiveness, as well as information reported to other members of the health care team.

Documenting Discharge Teaching. Discharge teaching is important to ensure clients know how to take care of themselves and their infants after they leave the facility. To prevent or defend against lawsuits, nurses should document the teaching they perform and the client's understanding of that teaching. Various documentation forms verify teaching and the degree of understanding about important topics. The nurse also should note the need for reinforcement and the method of providing reinforcement.

Documenting Incidents. Another form of documentation used in risk management is the incident report, sometimes called a *quality assurance report* or *variance report.* The nurse completes a report when something occurs that might result in legal action—for example, injury to a client, visitor, or staff member. The report alerts the agency's legal department that a problem may exist. It also identifies situations that might endanger clients in the future. Incident reports are not a part of the client's chart and should not be referred to on the chart. When an incident occurs, documentation on the chart should include the same type of factual information about the client's condition that would be recorded in any other situation.

Late entries in documentation may be necessary after an emergency in which the nurse should provide client care quickly. Late entries should be accurate and objective rather than defensive, especially if the outcome was negative.

The Nurse as Client Advocate

Nurses are ethically and legally bound to act as the client's advocate. When nurses think the client's best interests are not being served, they are obligated to seek help from appropriate sources. This usually involves relaying the problem through the facility's chain of command. The nurse consults a supervisor and the client's physician or other health care provider. If the results are not satisfactory, the nurse continues through administrative channels to the director of nurses, hospital administrator, and chief of the medical staff, if necessary. All nurses should know the chain-of-command process for their workplaces.

Nurses should document their efforts to seek help for clients. For example, when postpartum clients are experiencing excessive bleeding, nurses document the methods used to control the bleeding. They also document each time they call the physician, the information given to the physician, and the response received. When nurses cannot contact the physician or do not receive adequate instructions, they should document their efforts to seek instruction from others such as the supervisor. Nurses should continue their efforts until the client receives the care needed (Simpson, 2021b).

Maintaining Expertise

The nurse also can reduce malpractice liability by maintaining expertise. To ensure nurses maintain their expertise in provision of safe care, states require proof of continuing education for renewal of nursing licenses. Nursing knowledge grows and changes rapidly, and all nurses should keep current. New information from classes, conferences, and professional publications can help nurses perform as would a reasonably prudent peer. Nurses should analyze research articles to determine whether changes in client care are indicated by the research evidence. Nurses should demonstrate evidence-based clinical practice.

Employers often provide continuing education classes for their nurses through conferences, satellite television systems, computer networks, and other means. Membership in professional organizations such as state branches of the ANA or in specialty organizations such as AWHONN provides nurses access to new information through publications, nursing conferences, podcasts, and other educational offerings. Continuing nursing education is also widely available electronically.

Expertise is a concern when nurses are "floated," or required to work with clients whose needs differ from those of the nurses' usual clients. A nurse may be floated from one maternal-newborn setting to another or to a nonmaternity setting. In these situations, nurses need cross-training, which includes orientation and education to perform care safely in new areas. The employer should provide appropriate cross-training for nurses who float. Nurses who work outside their usual area of expertise should assess their own skills and avoid performing tasks or taking responsibilities in areas until they have been educated to be competent in those areas.

KNOWLEDGE CHECK

24. How do state boards of nursing safeguard clients?
25. How do standards of care and agency policies influence judgments about malpractice?
26. How can standards of care be used to help defend malpractice claims against nurses?

COST CONTAINMENT AND DOWNSIZING

Measures to lower health care costs continue to directly and indirectly affect nurses' work. Two measures of special concern are the use of unlicensed assistive personnel (UAP) and brief length of stay (LOS) for clients.

Delegation to Unlicensed Assistive Personnel

Delegation of care to an UAP may allow the nurse to focus on greater needs within their group of clients. Orientation and education of UAP should be completed and is competency based in both initial training and ongoing evaluations. UAP should be identified to the client as a nonlicensed person (ANA, 2012).

Nurses should be aware that they remain legally responsible for client assessments and make the critical judgments necessary to ensure client safety when delegating tasks to UAP. Nurses should know the capabilities of each UAP who is caring for clients and supervise them sufficiently to ensure competence (ANA, 2012; AWHONN, 2016).

Early Discharge

Regardless of the client's diagnosis, the time from admission to discharge is as short as possible to keep costs in check and to reduce chances for hospital-acquired infections. Because birth is considered a wellness experience that does not require a long LOS, care of new mothers and infants requires teaching from the earliest encounters. In 1996 federal legislation was passed to require insurance companies allow the option of a 48-hour hospital LOS after vaginal birth and a 4-day LOS after cesarean birth. Discharge may be earlier, if deemed appropriate, after discussion between the physician or nurse midwife and the client. Although it is not required by federal law, many states mandate prompt follow-up for early discharge in the client's home, an office, or a clinic. Some third-party payers voluntarily cover home visits for mothers who opt for earlier discharge because of the lower total cost for the home visit plus a short hospital LOS.

Concerns About Early Discharge

Although advantages of early discharge include prompt ambulation and reduced risk for hospital-acquired infection, concerns exist for new mothers and their families. Clients may be exhausted from a long labor or complicated birth and unable to absorb all the information nurses attempt to teach before discharge. Once home, many new mothers also must care for other children. Nurses may detect early signs of maternal or infant complications that may not be evident to parents while in the health care facility. Parents at home may not recognize the development of a serious maternal or neonatal infection or jaundice, and care may be delayed until the illness has become severe.

There may be cultural traditions that influence the expectations the mother may have for her postpartum course that the nurse should be aware of (Heck, 2021). The mother may experience postpartum depression, which may compromise her ability to recover from birth in a timely manner and care for her infant and family (Park et al., 2019). The ethical and legal implications of sending mothers home before they are able to adequately care for themselves and their newborns are very real concerns for nurses who should balance cost constraints with client needs.

Similar problems may occur in older people who must care for themselves after an inpatient or outpatient procedure. Sedating drugs given for a procedure may have prolonged effects, especially on older adults. Although the older person may appear to understand all instructions and sign papers indicating their understanding, they may not remember what was taught after returning home. It is ideal for a trusted friend or family member to be taught with the client and for printed or online instructions in simple language to be provided. Follow-up phone calls or visits are often scheduled to reevaluate the healing process after a procedure.

Methods to Deal with Short Lengths of Stay

Teaching begins at admission. Self-care during pregnancy or in women's health begins at first encounter. More teaching should occur during pregnancy when the mother's physical needs do not interfere with her ability to comprehend the new knowledge. In the facility, careful documentation and notification of the primary care provider are essential so clients are not discharged inappropriately if abnormal findings develop. Self-care and infant-care discharge instructions should be explained to the client and their support person. A printed form, signed by both the client and the nurse, is placed in the chart, with a copy given to the client for later reference in self-care and care of the baby. Other methods for follow-up such as home visits, phone calls, and return visits to the birth facility for nursing assessments after discharge may identify complications early, when they can be addressed most effectively.

Nursing follow-up by phone calls (telehealth) is the least expensive of postdischarge methods. Nevertheless, the nurse does not see or physically examine the client or the infant, and specific protocols and procedures should be in place for nursing actions that should be taken if a potential problem is identified during the call. Documentation should be kept for follow-up phone calls. Any instructions given to the client (recommended actions if problems arise, if a minor problem does not improve, or if a problem worsens) during the phone call should be documented (Jokinen et al., 2021; Simpson, 2021b).

? KNOWLEDGE CHECK

27. What concerns do nurses have about unlicensed assistive personnel?
28. Why is early discharge a concern for nurses?
29. What are the important points in follow-up phone call?

SUMMARY CONCEPTS

- Families vary in their structures and patterns of functioning.
- Functional families are characterized by open communication, flexibility in role assignments, and adult agreement on basic principles of parenting, resiliency, and adaptability.
- Culture is the sum of beliefs and values that are learned, shared, and transmitted from generation to generation in a specific group of people.
- Dominant Western cultural values may influence the thinking and action of nurses in the U.S. but may not be shared by culturally diverse childbearing clients and their families.
- Professional nurses are expected to provide culturally competent care, which requires an awareness of, sensitivity to, and respect for the diversity of clients served.
- Health care disparity is a major social issue that underlies adequacy of health care resources, access to prenatal care, government programs to increase health care to indigent persons and children, and health care rationing.
- Multiple factors are associated with intimate partner violence, which is deliberate, severe, and generally repeated in a predictable cycle that often causes severe physical harm (or death) to the client.
- Perinatal nurses should screen for intimate partner violence and provide appropriate education and resources.
- Human trafficking, also called trafficking of persons, is the recruitment and movement of individuals for the purpose of exploitation. Sex and labor trafficking are the most common forms.
- Persons and children of childbearing age make up the majority of reported cases of human trafficking, with the average age of entry into sex trafficking reported to be between 12 to 14 years of age.
- Ethical dilemmas are a difficult area of practice and are best solved by applying common ethical methods and principles and the steps of the nursing process.
- When ethical principles of beneficence, nonmaleficence, autonomy, and justice result in ethical dilemmas, the nursing process may be used to guide ethical decision-making.
- Punitive approaches to ethical and social problems may prevent clients from seeking adequate prenatal care.
- Nurses are expected to perform in accordance with nurse practice acts, standards of care, and agency policies.
- Nurses can help defend malpractice claims by following guidelines for informed consent, refusal of care, and documentation and by maintaining their levels of expertise.
- Complete and timely documentation is the best evidence that the standard of care received by a client was met.
- Continuing pressures on optimal nursing practice include unlicensed assistive personnel and short lengths of stay.

REFERENCES & READINGS

Alayi, K. V., Harvey, I. S., Panjwani, S., Uwak, I., Garney, W., & Page, R.L. (2021). Narrative analysis of childbearing experiences during the Covid-19 pandemic. *MCN: The American Journal of Maternal Child Nursing, 46*(5), 10–18.

Alchu-Allouban, A., Khater, W., Zaheya, L., & Almonani, M. (2021). Nursing ethics in the care of patients during the COVID-19 pandemic. *Frontiers of Medicine, 8,* 1–7.

Alfaro-LeFevre, R. (2021). In *Critical thinking, clinical reasoning and clinical judgment* (8th ed., pp. 121–142). Elsevier.

Ali, B., Mittal, M., Schroder, A., Ishman, N., Quinton, S., & Boekeloo, B. (2020). Psychological violence and sexual risk behavior among predominantly African American women. *Journal of Interpersonal Violence, 35*(23–24), S574–S5588.

American Academy of Pediatrics (AAP) & American College of Obstetricians and Gynecologists (ACOG). (2018). In *Guidelines for perinatal care* (8th ed.).

American Cancer Society. (2021). *Cancer facts and figures for African Americans 2019–2021.*

American College of Obstetricians and Gynecologists (ACOG). (2019a). *Human trafficking. ACOG committee opinion 787.*

American College of Obstetricians and Gynecologists (ACOG). (2019b). *Sexual assault. ACOG committee opinion 777.*

American College of Obstetricians and Gynecologists (ACOG). (2020). *Reproductive and sexual coercion. ACOG committee opinion 796.*

American College of Obstetricians and Gynecologists (ACOG). (2021). *Health care for transgender and gender diverse individuals. ACOG Committee Opinion, No. 823.*

American Nurses Association (ANA). (2012). *Principles for delegation by registered nurses to unlicensed assistive personnel (UAP)*.

American Nurses Association (ANA). (2015). *Code of ethics for nurses with interpretive statements*.

American Nurses Association (ANA). (2021). In *Nursing scope and standards of practice* (4th ed.).

Association of Women's Health, Obstetric & Neonatal Nurses (AWHONN). (2019). In *Standards for professional nursing practice in the care of women and newborns* (8th ed.).

AWHONN. (2016). The role of UAP in the care of women and newborns. Position paper. *Journal of Obstetric, Gynecologic, and Neonatal Nursing, 45*(1), 137–139.

Banke-Thomas, A., Agebemenu, K., & Johnson-Agbakwu, C. (2019). Factors associated with access to maternal and reproductive health care among Somali women resettled in Ohio. *Journal of Immigrant and Minority Health, 21*, 946–953.

Barbosa-Leiker, C., Smith, C. L., & Drespi, E. J. (2021). Stressors, coping, and resources needed during the COVID-19 pandemic in a sample of perinatal women. *BMC Pregnancy and Childbirth, 171*(21), 1–13. https://doi.org/10.1186/s12884-021-03665-0.

Boggs, K. U. (2019). Clinical judgment and ethical decision making. In E. C. Arnold, & K. U. Boggs (Eds.), *Interpersonal relationships: Professional communication skills for nurses* (8th ed., pp. 40–56). Elsevier.

Britannica. (2022). *Dobbs v. Jackson Women's Health Organization*. https://www.britannica.com/topic/Dobbs-v-Jackson-Womens-Health-Organization.

Burris, H. H., & Parker, M. G. (2021). Racial and ethnic disparities in preterm birth outcomes. *Journal of Perinatology, 41*, 365–366.

Butler, M. M., Fullerton, J., & Aman, C. (2019). Competencies for respectful maternity care. *Birth, 47*, 346–356.

Callister, L. C. (1995). Cultural meanings of childbirth. *Journal of Obstetric, Gynecologic, and Neonatal Nursing, 24*(4), 327–334.

Callister, L. C. (2006a). Culturally competent care of women and newborns: Knowledge, attitude, and skills. *Journal of Obstetric, Gynecologic, and Neonatal Nursing, 30*(2), 209–2015. https://doi:10.111/j.1552-6909.z001.tb01537.x.

Callister, L. C. (2006b). The meaning of giving birth and mastery of the experience. *International Journal of Childbirth Education, 21*(3), 7–8.

Callister, L. C. (2016). What do the childbearing women in your practice look like? *Nursing for Women's Health, 20*(1), 9–11.

Callister, L. C. (2020). Surviving and having a healthy baby are low bars for childbirth: Women have the right to expect much more. Global health and nursing column. *MCN: The American Journal of Maternal/Child Nursing, 45*(2), 127.

Callister, L. C. (2021a). *Developing and assessing culturally appropriate health education for childbearing women*. Arlington, VA: March of Dimes Foundation.

Callister, L. C. (2021b). Integrating cultural beliefs and practices when caring for childbearing women and families. In K. F. Simpson, P. A. Creehan, N. O'Brien-Abel, C. K. Roth, & A. J. Rohan (Eds.), *Perinatal nursing* (5th ed., pp. 18–47). Lippincott Williams & Wilkins.

Callister, L. C. (2021c). Reducing racial and ethnic disparities in the care of women and newborns. Global health and nursing column. *MCN: The American Journal of Maternal/Child Nursing, 46*(6), 302.

Callister, L. C., & Khalaf, I. (2010). Spirituality in childbearing women. *The Journal of Perinatal Education, 19*(2), 16–24.

Candlelaria, M., Bressler, T., & Spatz, D. L. (2019). Breastfeeding guidance of Orthodox Jewish families when newborns require special care and continued hospitalization. *MCN: The American Journal of Maternal/Child Nursing, 44*(2), 80–85.

Centers for Disease Control and Prevention. (2020). *First data released on maternal mortality in over a decade*. https://www.cdc.gov/nchs/maternal-mortality/index.htm.

Chisolm-Straker, M., Miller, C. L., Duke, G., & Stoklosa, H. (2019). A framework for the development of healthcare provider education programs on human trafficking part two: Survivors. *Journal of Human Trafficking*. https://doi.org/DOI:10.1080/23322705.2019.1635333.

Cohn, T., & Harrison, C. V. (2022). A systematic review exploring racial diparities, social determinants of health, and sexually transmitted infections in Black women. *Nursing for Women's Health, 25*. Advanced online publication. https://doi.org/10.1016/j.nwh.2022.01.006.

Collins, C., & Skarparis, K. (2020). The impact of human trafficking in relation to maternity care: A literature review. *Midwifery*, 1–13. https://doi.org/10.1016/j.midw.2020.102645. Epub 2020 Jan 23. 32035342.

Crowther, S., & Hall, J. (2020). Association of psychosocial-spiritual experiences around childbirth and subsequent perinatal mental health outcomes. *Journal of Reproductive and Infant Psychology, 38*(1), 50–84.

De Chesnay, M. (2013). *Sex trafficking: A clinical guide for nurses*. New York: Springer.

Declerq, E., Sakala, C., & Belanoff, C. (2020). Women's experience of agency and respect in maternity care by type of insurance in California. *PLoS One, 15*(7), e235–262.

Devido, J., Appelt, C. J., & Szalla, N. (2020). Wise women's provision of maternal child information and support for urban African American women. *Journal of Transcultural Nursing, 31*(5), 554–564.

Douglas, M. K., Rosenkoetter, M., Pacquiao, D., Callister, L. C., Callister, L. C., Hattar-Pollara, M., Lauderdale, J., Milstead, J., Nardi, D., & Purnell, L. (2014). Guidelines for implementing culturally competent care. *Journal of Transcultural Nursing, 25*(2), 109–121.

Dove-Meadows, W., Deriemacker, A., Dailey, R., Nolan, D. S., Vamaugh, K., & Giurgescu, C. (2020). Pregnant African American women's perceptions of neighborhood, racial discrimination, and psychological distress as influences on birth outcomes. *MCN: The American Journal of Maternal/Child Nursing, 45*(1), 49–55.

Ely, D., & Driscoll, A. K. (2020). Infant mortality in the United States, 2018: Data from the period linked birth/infant death file. *National Vital Statistics Reports, 69*(7), 1–18.

Everett, B. G., Kominiarek, M. A., Mollborn, S., Adkins, D. E., & Hughes, T. L. (2019). Sexual orientation disparities in pregnancy and infant outcomes. *Maternal and Child Health Journal, 23*(1), 72–81.

Giger, J. N., & Haddad, L. (2021). In *Transcultural nursing: Assessment and interventions* (8th ed.). Elsevier.

Grace, K. T., Decker, M. R., Alexander, K. A., Campbell, J., Miller, E., Perrin, N., & Glass, N. (2020). Reproductive coercion intimate partner violence, and unintended pregnancy among Latina women. *Journal of Interpersonal Violence, 32*(21), 3302–3320.

Griggs, K. M., Waddill, C. B., Bive, A., & Ward, N. (2021). Care during pregnancy, childbirth, postpartum, and human milk feeding for individuals who identify as LGBTQ+. *MCN: The American Journal of Maternal/Child Nursing, 46*(1), 43–53.

Han, M., Goyal, D., Lee, J., & Kim, A. (2020). Korean immigrant women's postpartum experiences in the United States. *MCN: The American Journal of Maternal/Child Nursing, 45*(1), 42–48.

Heck, J. L. (2021). Postpartum depression in American Indian/Alaska native women: A scoping review. *MCN: The American Journal of Maternal/Child Nursing, 46*(1), 6–13.

Hoyert, D. L., & Minino, A. M. (2020). Maternal mortality in the United States. *National Vital Statistics Reports, 69*(2), 1–18.

Johnson, M. B. (2020). Prenatal care for American Indian women. *MCN: The American Journal of Maternal/Child Nursing, 45*(4), 221–227.

Johnson-Aghakwu, C. E., Warren, N., Budhatoki, C., & Cole, F. (2019). Female genital cutting (FGC): Clinical knowledge, attitudes, and practices from a provider survey in the US. *Journal of Immigrant and Minority Health, 21*, 954–964.

Jokinen, A., Stolt, M., & Suhonen, R. (2021). Ethical issues related to eHealth: An integrative review. *Nursing Ethics, 28*(2), 254–271.

Jones, J. M. (2021). *LGBT identification rises to 5.6% in latest U.S. estimate.* The Gallup Poll. https://www.optumhealtheducation.com/sites/default/files/LGBT%20Identification%20Rises%20to%205.6%25%20in%20Latest%20U.S.%20Estimate.pdf.

Karp, C., Wood, S. N., Galadanci, H., Kibira, S. P. S., Makumbi, F., Omoluabi, E., Shiferaw, S., Seme, A., Tsui, A., & Moreau, C. (2020). I am the master key that opens and unlocks. *Social Science & Medicine, 258.* https://doi.org/10.1016/j.socscimed.2020.113086.

Killion, M. M. (2021). Improving maternity care by eliminating racism and inequities. *MCN: The American Journal of Maternal/Child Nursing, 46*(2), 123.

Kirkner, A., Lorenz, K., & Ulman, S. E. (2021). Recommendations for responding to survivors of sexual assault: A qualitative study of survivors and support providers. *Journal of Interpersonal Violence, 36*(3–4), 1005–1028.

Koh, H. K., Gracia, J. N., & Alvarez, M. E. (2014). Culturally and linguistically appropriate service: Advancing with class. *The New England Journal of Medicine, 37*(3), 198–201.

Kyne, N. M., & Hanssen, I. (2021). *Establishing a trusting nurse-immigrant mother relationship in the neonatal unit.* Nursing Ethics. https://doi.org/10.1177/09697330211003258.

Kynoe, M., Fugelseth, D., & Hanssen, I. (2020). When a common language is missing: Nurse-mother communication in the NICU. *Journal of Clinical Nursing, 29*(13–14), 2221–2230.

Lane, J., Johnson-Agbakwu, C. E., Warren, N., Budhatoki, C., & Cole, E. C. (2019). Female genital cutting (FGC): Clinical knowledge, attitudes, and practices from a provider survey in the US. *Journal of Immigrant and Minority Health, 21*, 954–964.

Lathtrop, B. (2020). Moving toward health equity by addressing social determinants of health. *Nursing for Women's Health, 24*(1), 36–44. https://doi.org/10.1016/j.nwh.2019.11.003.

Lauderdale, J. (2020). Transcultural perspectives in childbearing. In M. M. Andrews, & J. S. Boyle (Eds.), *Transcultural concepts in nursing care* (8th ed.). Wolters & Kluwer.

Lau, J. D., Zhu, Y., & Vora, S. (2021). An evaluation of a perinatal education and support program to increase breastfeeding in a Chinese American community. *Maternal and Child Health Journal, 25*, 214–220. https://doi.org/10.1007/s10995-020-03016-z.

Logan, R. G., Daley, E. M., Vamos, C. A., Louis-Jacques, A., & Marhefka, S. L. (2021). *When is health care actually going to be care?" the lived experience of family planning care among young black women.* Qualitative Health Research, 1–14. https://doi.org/10.1177/1049732321993094.

Lor, M., Badenoch, N., & Yang, J. (2021). Technical meets traditional: Language, culture, and the challenges faced by Hmong medical interpreters. *Journal of Transcultural Nursing.* https://doi.org/10.1177/10436596211039553.

Madeira, A. D., Rangen, C. M., & Avery, M. D. (2019). Design and implementation of a group prenatal care model for Somali women at a low-resource health clinic. *Nursing for Women's Health, 23*(3), 224–233.

March of Dimes. (2020). *Nowhere to go:" Maternity care deserts across the US: 2020 report.*

Martin, J. A., Hamilton, B. E., & Osterman, M. J. K. (2020). *Births in the United States, 2019. NCHS brief 287.* National Center for Health Statistics.

Martin, J. A., Hamilton, B. E., Osterman, M. J. K., & Driscoll, A. K. (2021). Births: Final data for 2019. *National Vital Statistics Reports, 70*(2), 1–51.

McGowan, E. C., Abdulla, L. S., Hawes, K. K., Tucker, R., & Vohr, B. R. (2019). Maternal immigrant status and readiness to transition to home from the NICU. *Pediatrics, 143*(5).

Miller, C. L. (2013). Child sex trafficking in the emergency department: Opportunities and challenges. *Journal of Emergency Nursing, 39*(5), 477–478.

Morton, C. H., & Simkin, P. (2019). Can respectful maternity care save and improve lives? *Birth, 46*(3), 391–395.

National Academies of Sciences, Engineering and Medicine. (2020). *Birth settings in America: Outcomes, quality, access, and choice.* The National Academies Press.

National Alliance to End Homelessness. (2020). *Snapshot of homelessness.*

National Institutes of Health (NIH). (2021). *Strategic plan to advance research on the health and well-being of sexual & gender minorities 2021–2025.*

National Vital Statistics Reports. (2018). Timing and adequacy of prenatal care in the United States. 67(3), 1–14.

Oerther, S., Lah, H. W., & Oerther, C. (2020). Immigrant women's experiences as mothers in the United States. *MCN: The American Journal of Maternal/Child Nursing, 45*(1), 1–16.

Oladapo, O. T., Tuncalp, O., Bonet, M., Lawrie, T. A., Portela, A., Downe, S., Gulmezoglu, A. M. (2018). WHO model of intrapartum care for a positive birth experience: Transforming care of women and babies for improved health and well being. *British Journal of Obstetrics and Gynecology, 125*, 918–922.

Olukorun, O., Kako, P., Dressel, A., & Mkandawire-Valhmu, L. (2020). A qualitative exploration of undocumented African immigrant women in the health care delivery system. *Nursing Outlook, 68*, 242–251.

Palmer, C. A., & Cullen, M. (2019). Nursing care birth plan for the surrogate family. *Journal of Obstetric, Gynecologic, and Neonatal Nursing, 48*(3), S30.

Pangas, J., Ogunsiji, O., Elmir, R., Raman, S., Liamputtong, P., Burns, E., Dahlen, H.G., & Schmied, V. (2019). Refugee women's experiences negotiating motherhood and maternity care in a new country. *International Journal of Nursing Studies, 90*, 31–45.

Park, V. M. T., Goyal, D., Suen, J., Win, N., & Tsoh, J. Y. (2019). Chinese American women's experiences with postpartum depression symptoms and mental health seeking behaviors. *MCN: The American Journal of Maternal/Child Nursing, 44*(3), 144–149.

Project Implicit (2011). https://implicit.harvard.edu/implicit/takeatest.html.

Pruitt, S. M., Hoyert, D. L., Anderson, K. N., Martin, J., Waddell, L., Duke, C., Honein, M. A., & Reefhuis, J. (2020). Racial and ethnic disparities in fetal deaths. *Morbidity and Mortality Weekly Report, 69*(37), 1277–2182.

Purnell, L. (2019). Update: The Purnell theory and model for culturally competent health care. *Journal of Transcultural Nursing, 30*(2), 98–105.

Ramaswamy, U. R., Ranji, U., & Salganicoff, A. (2019). *Intimate partner violence (IPV) screening and counseling services in clinical settings. Issue brief.* Kaiser Family Foundation.

Saluja, B., & Bryant, Z. B. (2021). How implicit bias contributes to racial disparities in maternal morbidity and mortality in the United States. *Journal of Women's Health, 30*(2), 270–273.

Semega, J., Kollar, M., Shrider, E. A., & Creamer, J. (2020). *Income and poverty in the United States: 2019. Current population reports P60-270.* U.S. Government Printing Office.

Shorey, S., Ng, E. D., & Downe, S. (2021). Cultural competence and experiences of maternity health care providers on care for migrant women: A qualitative meta-synthesis. *Birth, 48*(4), 458–469.

Simpson, K. R. (2019). Listening to women, treating them with respect, and honoring their wishes during childbirth are critical aspects of safe, high-quality maternity care. *MCN: The American Journal of Maternal/Child Nursing, 44*(6), 168.

Simpson, K. R. (2021a). A new report on understanding the well-being of LGBTQI+ population. *MCN: The American Journal of Maternal/Child Nursing, 46*(2), 68.

Simpson, K. R. (2021b). Perinatal safety and quality. In K. R. Simpson, P. A. Breehan, N. O'Brien-Abel, C. K. Roth, & A. J. Rohan (Eds.), *Perinatal nursing* (5th ed., pp. 1–17). Wolters Kluwer.

Sinclair, I., St-Pierre, M., Vaillancourt, C., Gagnon, S., & Dancause, K. N. (2020). Variations in relations between perceived stress and birth outcomes by immigration status. *Maternal and Child Health Journal, 24*(12), 1–11.

Stoklosa, H., Miller, C. L., Duke, G., & Chisolm-Straker, M. (2019). A framework for the development of healthcare provider education programs on human trafficking part one: Experts. *Journal of Human Trafficking, 1*(22).

Sundus, A., Shahzad, S., & Younas, A. (2021). Ethical and culturally competent care of transgender patients. *Nursing Ethics, 28*, 1–20.

Sutton, M., Anachebe, N. F., & Lee, R. (2021). Racial and ethnic disparities in reproductive health services and outcomes. *Obstetrics & Gynecology, 37*(2), 225–233.

United Nations Office on Drugs and Crime. (2020). *Trafficking in persons.*

United States Census Bureau. (2020). *Poverty: 2018 and 2019. report # ACSBR/20-04.* U.S. Government Printing Office.

United States Department of Justice. (2021). *Human Trafficking.* https://www.justice.gov/humantrafficking.

United States Department of State. (2021). *About human trafficking.* https://www.state.gov/humantrafficking-about-human-trafficking/.

Van Ouytsel, J., Ponnet, K., & Walrave, M. (2020). Cyber dating abuse: Investigating digital monitoring behaviors among adolescents. *Journal of Interpersonal Violence, 35*(23–24), S157–S178.

Vedam, S., Stoll, K., Taiwo, T. K., Rubashkin, N., Cheyney, M., Stauss, N., McLemore, M., Cadena, M., Nethery, E., Rushton, E., Schummers, L., Declercq, E., & GVtM-US Steering Council. (2019). The giving voice to mothers study: Inequity and mistreatment during pregnancy and childbirth in the United States. *Reproductive Health, 16*(1), 77.

Wehbe-Alamah, H., Hammonds, L. C., & Stanley, D. (2021). Culturally congruent care from the perspectives of Judaism, Christianity, and Islam. *Journal of Transcultural Nursing, 32*(2), 119–128.

Reproductive Anatomy and Physiology

Jennifer Rodriguez

An understanding of the structure and function of the reproductive organs is necessary for the effective nursing care of clients during and after their reproductive years and for couples who require family planning or infertility care. This chapter reviews basic prenatal development, sexual maturation, and the structure and function of the female and male reproductive systems. Because of its emphasis in this book, the female reproductive system is discussed most extensively.

SEXUAL DEVELOPMENT

Sexual development begins at conception when the **genetic sex** is determined by the union of an ovum and a sperm. During childhood, the sex organs are inactive and then become active during puberty.

Prenatal Development

The ovum carries a single X chromosome. Spermatozoa carry either an X chromosome or a Y chromosome. If an X-bearing spermatozoon fertilizes the ovum, the offspring's genetic sex is female. If a Y-bearing spermatozoon fertilizes the ovum, a genetic male offspring results.

Although genetic sex is determined at conception, the reproductive systems of males and females are similar, or sexually undifferentiated, for the first 6 weeks of prenatal life. During the seventh week, differences between males and females appear in the internal structures. The external genitalia continue to look similar until the ninth week, when these outer structures begin to change. Differentiation of the external sexual organs is complete at approximately 12 weeks of gestational age.

During fetal life, both ovaries and testes secrete their primary hormones, which are estrogen and testosterone, respectively. Testosterone causes development of male sex organs and external genitalia, and its absence results in development of female sex characteristics. Although estrogen is secreted by the fetal ovary, the hormone is not required to initiate development of female sex structures.

Childhood

The sex glands are inactive during infancy and childhood. At sexual maturity the hypothalamus stimulates the anterior pituitary gland to produce hormones that, in turn, stimulate sex hormone production by the **gonads**, the reproductive (sex) glands.

Sexual Maturation

Puberty refers to the time during which the reproductive organs become fully functional. It is not a single event but a series of changes occurring over several years during late childhood and early adolescence. Primary sex characteristics relate to the maturation of the organs directly responsible for reproduction. Examples of primary sex characteristics are maturation of ova in the ovaries and production of sperm in the testes. **Secondary sex characteristics** are changes in other systems that differentiate females and males but do not directly relate to reproduction. Examples of secondary sex characteristics in the female include breast development; selective distribution of fat in breasts, buttocks, and thighs; pubic and axillary hair; and higher pitched voice. Secondary sex characteristics in the male include increased muscle mass, growth of hair on the face and body, growth of pubic and axillary hair, and development of a deeper voice.

Initiation of Sexual Maturation

Changes of puberty occur in an orderly sequence in the **somatic cells** (body cells other than the gametes). Not all factors involved in the initiation of sexual maturation are known. Secretions of the hypothalamus, anterior pituitary, and gonads all play a role. The hypothalamus can secrete gonadotropin-releasing hormone (GnRH) to initiate puberty during infancy and early childhood, but it does not do so in significant amounts until late childhood. Production of even tiny quantities of sex hormones by the young child's ovaries or testes inhibits secretions of the hypothalamus, preventing premature onset of puberty. Maturation of another brain area, as yet unknown, probably triggers the hypothalamus to initiate puberty (Hall, 2021).

The maturing child's hypothalamus gradually increases production of GnRH beginning at age 9 to 12 years (Blackburn, 2018; Hall, 2021). The level of GnRH increases slowly until it reaches a level adequate to stimulate the anterior pituitary to increase its production of follicle-stimulating hormone (FSH) and luteinizing hormone (LH). The ovaries and testes increase production of sex hormones and begin maturing **gametes** (reproductive cells, an ovum in females and a sperm in males) in response to higher levels of FSH and LH. Sex hormones also induce development of secondary sex characteristics. Table 3.1 lists the major hormones that play a role in reproduction.

Puberty varies among individuals; these variances include the age puberty begins and the time required to complete these changes. Hormonal changes of puberty begin approximately 6 months to 1 year earlier in females than in males. The growth spurt associated with puberty also begins earlier for females than for males. The obvious changes of puberty in females, such as breast development and height increase, begin an average of 2 years before changes in males. Changes of puberty occur in an orderly sequence in both males and females. Increases in height and weight are dramatic during puberty but slow after puberty until mature heights and weights are attained. Research has identified a link between early onset of puberty and obesity in females (Li et al., 2017).

Female Puberty Changes

As females mature, the anterior pituitary gland secretes increasing amounts of FSH and LH in response to the hypothalamic secretion of GnRH. These two pituitary secretions stimulate secretion of estrogens and progesterone by the ovary, resulting in maturation of the reproductive organs and breasts and development of secondary sex characteristics. The first noticeable change of puberty in females, development of the breasts, begins at approximately 8 to 13 years of age. Menstruation occurs about 2 to 2.5 years after breast development, with an average age range of 9 to 16 years.

Breast changes. Initially, the nipple enlarges and protrudes. The areola surrounding the nipple also enlarges and becomes somewhat protuberant. These changes are followed by growth of the glandular and ductal tissue. Fat is deposited in the breasts to give them the characteristic rounded female appearance. During puberty, a female's breasts often develop at different rates, resulting in a lopsided appearance until one breast catches up with the other.

Body contours. The pelvis widens and assumes a rounded, basin-like shape that favors passage of the fetus during childbirth. Fat is deposited selectively in the hips, giving them a rounder appearance than those of the male.

Body hair. Pubic hair first appears downy and becomes thicker as puberty progresses. Axillary hair appears near the time of menarche. The texture and quantity of pubic and axillary hair vary among females and ethnic groups. Females of African descent usually have body hair that is coarser and curlier than that of White females. Asian females often have sparser body hair compared with females of other racial groups.

Skeletal growth. Females grow taller for several years during early puberty in response to estrogen stimulation. The growth spurt begins approximately 1 year after breast development begins. Estrogen also causes the epiphyses (growth areas of the bone) to unite with the shafts of the bones, which eventually stops growth in height.

Reproductive organs. The female's external genitalia enlarge as fat is deposited in the mons pubis, labia majora, and labia minora. The vagina, uterus, fallopian tubes, and ovaries grow larger. In addition, the vaginal mucosa changes, becoming more resistant to trauma and infection in preparation for sexual activity. Cyclic changes in the reproductive organs occur during each female reproductive cycle.

Menarche. Approximately 2 to 2.5 years after the beginning of breast development, females experience their **menarche**, or first menstrual period. Early menstrual periods are often irregular and scant. These early menstrual cycles are not usually fertile because ovulation occurs inconsistently. Fertile reproductive cycles require preparation of the uterine lining precisely timed with ovulation. Nevertheless, ovulation may occur during any female reproductive cycle, including the first. The sexually active female can conceive even before her first menstrual period.

Delayed onset of menstruation is called *primary* **amenorrhea** if the female's periods have not begun within 2 years after the onset of breast development or by 16 years of age or if the female is more than 1 year older than their mother or sisters were when their menarche occurred. *Secondary amenorrhea* describes absence of menstruation for at least three cycles after regular cycles have been established or for 6 months. Both primary and secondary amenorrhea are more common in females who are thin. Females who are competitive athletes or dancers or who suffer from eating disorders (e.g., anorexia nervosa or bulimia) may have too little fat to produce enough sex hormones to stimulate ovulation and menstruation. Pregnancy is also a common cause of secondary amenorrhea. Both primary and secondary amenorrhea may result from inadequate pituitary stimulation of the ovary or failure of the ovary to respond to pituitary stimulation. Amenorrhea also may be caused by excessive androgenic hormones from the adrenal glands, which have a masculinizing effect.

Male Puberty Changes

Secretion of GnRH by the hypothalamus stimulates secretion of LH and FSH from the anterior pituitary. LH and FSH then stimulate secretion of testosterone and eventually cause **spermatogenesis**, or formation of male gametes, or sperm, in the maturing adolescent. Testosterone stimulates development of a male's reproductive organs and secondary sex characteristics. The first outward sign of male puberty is growth of the

TABLE 3.1   Major Hormones in Reproduction

Produced By	Target Organs	Action in Female	Action in Male
Gonadotropin-Releasing Hormone			
Hypothalamus	Anterior pituitary	• Stimulates release of FSH and LH, initiating puberty and sustaining female reproductive cycles; release is pulsatile.	Stimulates release of FSH and LH, initiating puberty; release is pulsatile.
Follicle-Stimulating Hormone			
Anterior pituitary	Ovaries (female) Testes (male)	• Stimulates final maturation of follicle. • Stimulates growth and maturation of graafian follicles before ovulation.	Stimulates Leydig cells of testes to secrete testosterone.
Luteinizing Hormone			
Anterior pituitary	Ovaries (female) Testes (male)	• Stimulates final maturation of follicle. • Surge of LH approximately 14 days before next menstrual period causes ovulation. • Stimulates transformation of graafian follicle into corpus luteum, which continues secretion of estrogens and progesterone for about 12 days if ovum is not fertilized. If fertilization occurs, placenta gradually assumes this function.	Stimulates Leydig cells of testes to secrete testosterone.
Estrogens			
• Ovaries and corpus luteum (female) • Placenta (pregnancy) • Formed in small quantities from testosterone in Sertoli cells of testes (male); other tissues, especially liver, produce estrogen in male	• Internal and external reproductive organs • Breasts (female) • Testes (male)	• Reproductive organs: maturation at puberty; stimulation of endometrium before ovulation • Breasts: Induce growth of glandular and ductal tissue; initiate deposition of fat at puberty; stimulate growth of long bones but cause closure of epiphyses, limiting mature height. • Pregnancy: Stimulates growth of uterus, breast tissue; inhibits active milk production; relaxes pelvic ligaments.	Necessary for normal sperm formation.
Progesterone			
Ovary, corpus luteum, placenta	Uterus, female breasts	• Stimulates secretion of endometrial glands; causes endometrial vessels to become dilated and tortuous in preparation for possible embryo implantation. • Pregnancy: Induces growth of cells of fallopian tubes and uterine lining to nourish embryo; decreases contractions of uterus; prepares breasts for lactation but inhibits prolactin secretion.	Not applicable.
Prolactin			
Anterior pituitary	Female breasts	• Stimulates secretion of milk (lactogenesis); estrogen and progesterone from placenta have an inhibiting effect on milk production until after placenta is expelled at birth; suckling of newborn stimulates prolactin secretion to maintain milk production.	Not applicable.
Oxytocin			
Posterior pituitary	Uterus, female breasts	• Uterus: Stimulates contractions during birth and stimulates postpartum contractions to compress uterine vessels and control bleeding. • Stimulates let-down, or milk-ejection reflex, during breastfeeding.	Not applicable.

TABLE 3.1 **Major Hormones in Reproduction—cont'd**			
Produced By	**Target Organs**	**Action in Female**	**Action in Male**
Testosterone			
• Leydig cells of the testes (male) • Adrenal glands (female) • Ovaries (female)	• Sexual organs (male) • Male body conformation after puberty	• Small quantities of androgenic (masculinizing) hormones from adrenal glands cause growth of pubic and axillary hair at puberty; most androgens, such as testosterone, are converted to estrogen.	• Induces development of male sex organs in fetus. • Induces growth and division of cells that mature sperm. • Induces development of male secondary sex characteristics.

FSH, Follicle-stimulating hormone; *GnRH,* gonadotropin-releasing hormone; *LH,* luteinizing hormone.

testes, which may begin as early as 9.5 years of age. Penile growth begins approximately 1 year later as the circumference and length of the penis increase. The skin of the scrotum thins and darkens as the sexual organs mature. Final male sexual maturation is complete at approximately 17 years of age (Blackburn, 2018).

Nocturnal emissions. Often called *wet dreams,* nocturnal emissions commonly occur during the teenage years. The male experiences a spontaneous ejaculation of seminal fluid during sleep, often accompanied by dreams with sexual content. Males should be prepared for this normal occurrence so they do not feel abnormal or ashamed or fear they have an infection or other problem.

Body hair. Pubic hair growth begins at the base of the penis. Gradually, the hair coarsens and grows upward and in the midline of the abdomen. Approximately 2 years later, axillary hair appears. Facial hair begins as a fine, downy mustache and progresses to the characteristic beard of the adult male. In most males, chest hair develops, and some males have hair on their upper backs. The amount and character of body hair vary among males of different racial groups, with Asian and Native American males often having less than White males or males of African descent. The quantity and character of body hair among males of the same racial group also vary.

Body composition. Because of the influence of testosterone, males develop a greater average muscle mass than females. At maturity a male's muscle mass exceeds the female's by an average of 50% (Hall, 2021), explaining the biologic advantage of males in tasks requiring muscle strength.

Skeletal growth. Testosterone causes males to undergo a rapid growth spurt, especially in height. The linear growth of males begins approximately 1 year later than in females and may continue into their 20s. Testosterone eventually causes union of the epiphysis with the shaft of long bones, as estrogen does in females. The height-limiting effect of testosterone is not as strong as that of estrogen in females, with the result that males grow in stature for several years longer than females. The male's greater average height at maturity is the combined result of beginning the growth spurt at a slightly later age and continuing it for a longer time.

The shoulders of males broaden as their height increases. Their pelvis assumes a more upright shape, with narrower diameters and heavier composition than the female pelvis. A male's pelvis is structurally suited for tasks requiring load bearing.

Voice changes. Hypertrophy of the laryngeal mucosa and enlargement of the larynx cause the male's voice to deepen. Before reaching their lower tones at maturity, many males experience embarrassing "cracking" or "squeaking" of their voices when they speak.

Decline in Fertility

The **climacteric** is a transitional period that starts as female fertility declines and extends through menopause and the postmenopausal period. In most females, the climacteric occurs between ages 40 and 50 years. Maturation of ova and production of ovarian hormones gradually decline. The external and internal reproductive organs atrophy somewhat as well. **Menopause** is the term used to describe the final menstrual period; however, *menopause* (permanent cessation of menstruation) and *climacteric* are often used interchangeably to describe the entire gradual process of change. Perimenopause is the time from the onset of changes associated with the climacteric, continuing for approximately 2 to 5 years after the last menstrual period (Blackburn, 2018). (See Chapter 28 for more information about the female's needs during this phase of life.)

Males do not experience a distinct marker event like menopause. Production of testosterone and sperm gradually declines, and sexual function decreases in the late 40s and 50s.

❓ KNOWLEDGE CHECK

1. What are the first noticeable changes of puberty in females and males?
2. What are basic differences between the mature male and female pelvis?
3. Why do males generally attain greater mature height than females?
4. What are common male and female secondary sex characteristics?

TABLE 3.2 Functions of Female Reproductive and Accessory Organs

Organ	Function
Vagina	• Passageway for menstrual flow • Female organ for coitus; receives male penis during coitus • Passageway for fetus during birth
Uterus	• Houses and nourishes fetus to sufficient maturity to function outside mother's body; propels fetus to outside
Fallopian tube	• Passageway for ovum as it travels from ovary to uterus • Site of fertilization
Ovaries	• Secrete estrogens and progesterone • Contain ova within follicles for maturation during female's reproductive life
Breasts Alveoli	• Secrete milk after childbirth (acinar cells within alveoli)
Lactiferous ducts	• Collect milk from alveoli and conduct it to outside

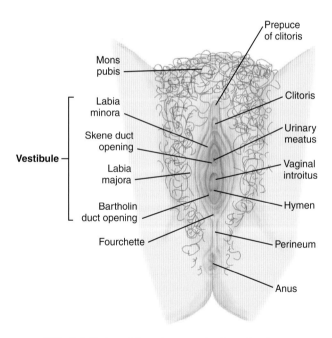

FIG. 3.1 External female reproductive structures.

FEMALE REPRODUCTIVE ANATOMY

The nurse needs a basic knowledge of the structure and function of the external and internal reproductive organs to understand their roles in pregnancy and childbirth (Table 3.2).

External Female Reproductive Organs

Collectively, the external female reproductive organs are called the *vulva*. These structures include the mons pubis, labia majora and minora, clitoris, structures of the vestibule, and perineum (Fig. 3.1).

Mons Pubis

The mons pubis is the rounded, fleshy prominence over the symphysis pubis that forms the anterior border of the external reproductive organs. It is covered with varying amounts of pubic hair.

Labia Majora and Minora

The labia majora are two rounded, fleshy folds of tissue that extend from the mons pubis to the perineum. They have a slightly deeper pigmentation than surrounding skin and are covered with pubic hair. The labia majora protect the more fragile tissues of the external genitalia.

The labia minora run parallel to and within the labia majora. The labia minora extend from the clitoris anteriorly and merge posteriorly to form the fourchette, which is the posterior rim of the vaginal introitus, or vaginal opening. The labia minora do not have pubic hair. They are highly vascular and respond to stimulation by becoming engorged with blood.

Clitoris

The clitoris is a small projection at the anterior junction of the two labia minora. This structure is composed of highly sensitive erectile tissue similar to that of the penis. The labia majora merge to form a prepuce over the clitoris.

Vestibule

The *vestibule* refers to structures enclosed by the labia minora. The urinary meatus, vaginal introitus, and ducts of Skene and Bartholin glands lie within the vestibule. Skene, or periurethral, glands provide lubrication for the urethra. Bartholin glands provide lubrication for the vaginal introitus, particularly during sexual arousal.

The vaginal introitus is surrounded by erectile tissue. During sexual stimulation, blood flows into the erectile tissue, allowing the introitus to tighten around the penis. This adds a massaging feeling that heightens the male's sexual sensations and encourages ejaculation.

The hymen is a thin fold of mucosa partially separating the vagina and the vestibule. The intactness, or lack thereof, of the hymen is not a criterion of virginity. The hymen may be broken by injury, tampon use, intercourse, or childbirth.

Perineum

The perineum is the most posterior part of the external female reproductive organs. The perineum extends from the fourchette anteriorly to the anus posteriorly. It is composed of fibrous and muscular tissues that provide support for pelvic structures.

Internal Female Reproductive Organs

The internal reproductive structures are the vagina, uterus, fallopian tubes, and ovaries (Figs. 3.2 and 3.3). These organs are supported and contained within the bony pelvis.

Vagina

The vagina is a tube of muscular and membranous tissue approximately 8 to 10 cm long between the bladder anteriorly

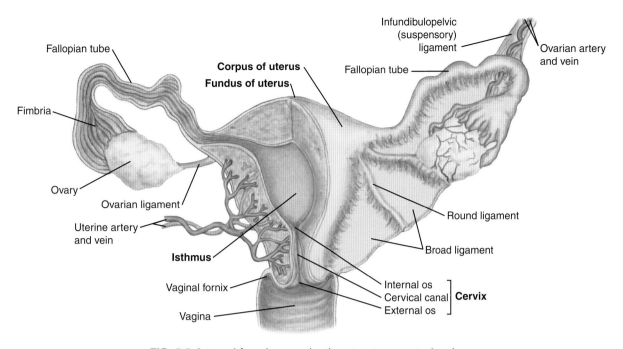

FIG. 3.2 Internal female reproductive structures, anterior view.

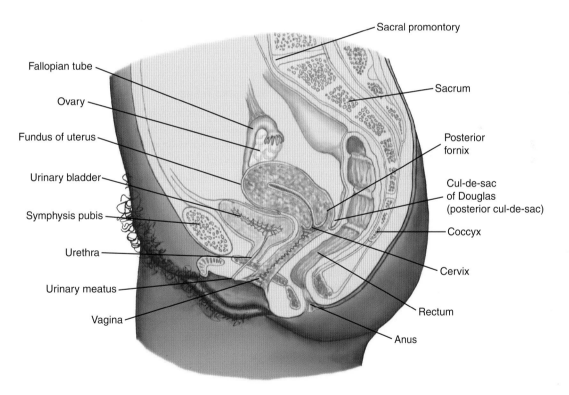

FIG. 3.3 Internal female reproductive structures, midsagittal view.

and the rectum posteriorly. The vagina connects the uterus above with the vestibule below. The vaginal lining has multiple folds, or **rugae**, and a muscular layer capable of marked distention during childbirth. The vagina is lubricated by secretions of the cervix (the lowermost part of the uterus) and Bartholin glands.

The vagina does not end abruptly at the uterine opening but arches to form a pouch-like structure called the *vaginal* **fornix**. Each fornix is described by its location: anterior, posterior, and lateral.

The vagina has three major functions: (1) it allows discharge of the menstrual flow; (2) it is the female organ of

coitus (male–female sexual union); and (3) it allows passage of the fetus from the uterus to outside the mother's body during childbirth.

Uterus

The uterus is a hollow, thick-walled, muscular organ shaped like a flat, upside-down pear. The uterus houses and nourishes the fetus until birth and then contracts rhythmically during labor to expel the fetus. Each month the uterus is prepared for a pregnancy, regardless of whether conception occurs.

The uterus measures approximately 7.5 × 5 × 2.5 cm and is larger in females who have borne children. It is suspended above the bladder and is anterior to the rectum. Its normal position is anteverted (rotated forward over the bladder) and slightly anteflexed (flexed forward).

Divisions of the uterus. The uterus has three divisions: the corpus, the isthmus, and the cervix.

Corpus. The corpus, or body, is the upper division of the uterus. The uppermost part of the uterine corpus, above the area where the fallopian tubes enter the uterus, is the fundus of the uterus.

Isthmus. A narrower transition zone, the isthmus, is located between the corpus of the uterus and the cervix. During late pregnancy the isthmus elongates and is known as the *lower uterine segment.*

Cervix. The cervix is the tubular "neck" of the lower uterus and is approximately 2 to 3 cm in length. During labor, the cervix effaces (thins) and dilates (opens) to allow passage of the fetus. The os is the opening in the cervix between the uterus and vagina. The upper cervix and lower cervix are marked by the internal os and external os, respectively. The external os of a childless female is round and smooth. After vaginal birth the external os has an irregular, slit-like shape and may have tags of scar tissue.

Layers of the uterus. The uterus has three layers: the perimetrium, the myometrium, and the endometrium.

Perimetrium. The perimetrium is the outer peritoneal layer of serous membrane that covers most of the uterus. Laterally the perimetrium is continuous with the broad ligaments on both sides of the uterus.

Myometrium. The myometrium is the middle layer of thick muscle. Most muscle fibers are concentrated in the upper uterus, and their number diminishes progressively toward the cervix. The myometrium contains three types of smooth muscle fiber, each suited to specific functions in childbearing (Fig. 3.4):
- Longitudinal fibers are found mostly in the fundus and are designed to expel the fetus efficiently toward the pelvic outlet during birth.
- Interlacing figure-8 fibers constitute the middle layer. These fibers contract after birth to compress blood vessels that pass between them to limit blood loss.
- Circular fibers form constrictions where the fallopian tubes enter the uterus and surround the internal cervical os. Circular fibers prevent reflux of menstrual blood and tissue into the fallopian tubes, promote normal implantation of the fertilized ovum by controlling its entry into the uterus, and retain the fetus until the appropriate time of birth.

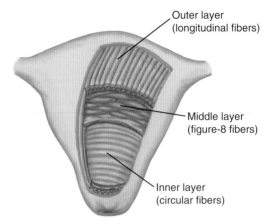

FIG. 3.4 Layers of the myometrium showing the three types of smooth muscle fiber.

Endometrium. The endometrium is the inner layer of the uterus. It responds to the cyclic variations of estrogen and progesterone during the female reproductive cycle (Fig. 3.7) The endometrium has two layers:
- The basal layer is the area nearest the myometrium that regenerates the functional layer of the endometrium after each menstrual period and after childbirth.
- The functional layer lies above the basal layer. Endometrial arteries, veins, and glands extend into the functional layer and are shed during each menstrual period and after childbirth in the lochia, the vaginal drainage after childbirth.

Fallopian Tubes

The fallopian tubes, also called *oviducts,* are 8 to 14 cm long and quite narrow (2 to 3 mm at their narrowest and 5 to 8 mm at their widest). They form a pathway for the ovum between the ovary and uterus. Fertilization occurs in the fallopian tubes. Each fallopian tube enters the upper uterus at the cornu, or horn, of the uterus.

The fallopian tubes are lined with folded epithelium containing hairlike processes called **cilia** that beat rhythmically toward the uterine cavity to propel the ovum through the tube. The rough, folded surface of its lining and small diameter make the fallopian tube vulnerable to blockage from infection or scar tissue. Tubal blockage may result in sterility or a tubal (ectopic) pregnancy because the fertilized ovum cannot enter the uterus for proper implantation.

The fallopian tubes have four divisions:
- The interstitial portion runs into the uterine cavity and lies within the uterine wall.
- The isthmus is the narrow part adjacent to the uterus.
- The ampulla is the wider area of the tube lateral to the isthmus, where fertilization occurs.
- The infundibulum is the wide, funnel-shaped terminal end of the tube. Fimbriae are fingerlike processes that surround the infundibulum.

The fallopian tubes are not directly connected to the ovary. The ovum is expelled into the abdominal cavity near the fimbriae at ovulation. Wavelike motions of the fimbriae draw the ovum into the tube. Nevertheless, the tubal isthmus remains

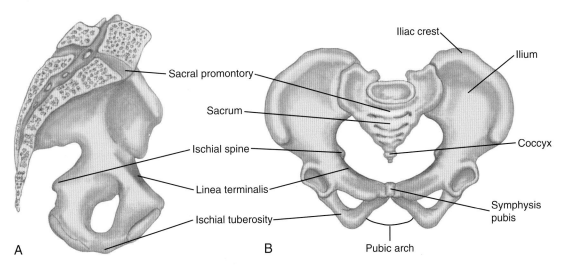

FIG. 3.5 Structures of the bony pelvis, shown in lateral (A) and anterior (B) views.

contracted until 3 days after conception to allow the fertilized ovum to develop within the tube. Initial growth of the fertilized ovum within the fallopian tube promotes its normal implantation in the upper uterus.

Ovaries

The ovaries are the female gonads, or sex glands. There are two functions of the ovary: (1) sex hormone production and (2) maturation of an ovum during each reproductive cycle.

The ovaries secrete estrogen and progesterone in varying amounts during a female's reproductive cycle to prepare the uterine lining for pregnancy. Ovarian hormone secretion gradually declines to very low levels during the climacteric.

At birth, the ovary contains all the ova it will ever have. Approximately two million immature ova are present at birth. Many of these degenerate during childhood, and at puberty approximately 200,000 to 400,000 viable ova remain. Many ova begin the maturation process during each reproductive cycle, but most never reach maturity. During a female's reproductive life, only about 400 of the ova ever mature enough to be released and fertilized. By the time a female reaches the climacteric, almost all the ova have been released during ovulation or have regressed. The few remaining ova are unresponsive to stimulating hormones and do not mature (Blackburn, 2018; Moore et al., 2020).

Support Structures

The bony pelvis supports and protects the lower abdominal and internal reproductive organs. Muscles and ligaments provide added support for the internal organs of the pelvis against the downward force of gravity and increases in intraabdominal pressure.

Pelvis

The bony pelvis is a basin-shaped structure at the lower end of the spine (Fig. 3.5). Its posterior wall is formed by the sacrum. The side and anterior pelvic walls are composed of three fused bones: the ilium, ischium, and pubis.

The linea terminalis, also called the *pelvic brim* or *iliopectineal line*, is an imaginary line dividing the upper, or false, pelvis from the lower, or true, pelvis. The false pelvis provides support for the internal organs and the upper part of the body. The true pelvis is most important during childbirth (see Chapter 12).

Muscles

Paired muscles enclose the lower pelvis and provide support for internal reproductive, urinary, and bowel structures (Fig. 3.6). In addition, a fibromuscular sheet, the pelvic fascia, provides support for the pelvic organs. Vaginal and urethral openings are located in the pelvic fascia.

The levator ani is a collection of three pairs of muscles: the pubococcygeus, which is also called the *pubovaginal muscle* in the female; the puborectal; and the iliococcygeus. These muscles support internal pelvic structures and resist increases in the intraabdominal pressure.

The ischiocavernosus muscle extends from the clitoris to the ischial tuberosities on each side of the lower bony pelvis. The two transverse perineal muscles extend from fibrous tissue of the perineum to the two ischial tuberosities, stabilizing the center of the perineum.

Ligaments

Seven pairs of ligaments maintain the internal reproductive organs and their nerve and blood supplies in their proper positions within the pelvis (see Fig. 3.2).

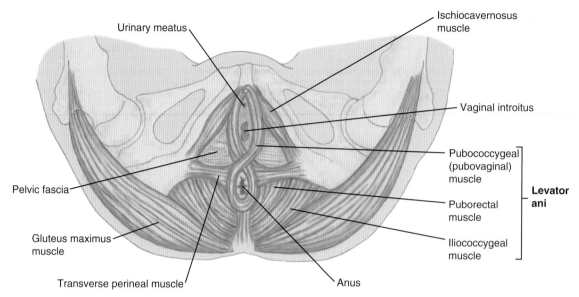

FIG. 3.6 Muscles of the female pelvic floor.

Lateral support. Paired ligaments stabilize the uterus and ovaries laterally and keep them in the midline of the pelvis. The broad ligament is a sheet of tissue extending from each side of the uterus to the lateral pelvic wall. The round ligament and fallopian tube mark the upper border of the broad ligament, and the lower edge is bounded by the uterine blood vessels. Within the two broad ligaments are the ovarian ligaments, blood vessels, and lymphatics.

The right and left cardinal ligaments provide support to the lower uterus and vagina. They extend from the lateral walls of the cervix and vagina to the side walls of the pelvis.

The two ovarian ligaments connect the ovaries to the lateral uterine walls. The infundibulopelvic (suspensory) ligaments connect the lateral ovary and distal fallopian tubes to the pelvic side walls. The infundibulopelvic ligament also carries the blood vessel and nerve supply for the ovary.

Anterior support. Two pairs of ligaments provide anterior support for the internal reproductive organs. The round ligaments connect the upper uterus to the connective tissue of the labia majora. These ligaments maintain the uterus in its normal anteflexed position and help direct the fetal-presenting part against the cervix during labor.

The pubocervical ligaments support the cervix anteriorly. They connect the cervix and interior surface of the symphysis pubis.

Posterior support. The uterosacral ligaments provide posterior support, extending from the lower posterior uterus to the sacrum. These ligaments also contain the sympathetic and parasympathetic nerves of the autonomic nervous system.

Blood Supply

The uterine blood supply is carried by the uterine arteries, which are branches of the internal iliac artery. These vessels enter the uterus at the lower border of the broad ligament near the isthmus of the uterus. The vessels branch downward to supply the cervix and vagina and upward to supply the uterus. The upper branch also supplies the ovaries and fallopian tubes. The vessels are coiled to allow for elongation as the uterus enlarges and rises from the pelvis during pregnancy. Blood drains into the uterine veins and from there into the internal iliac veins.

Additional ovarian and tubal blood supply is carried by the ovarian artery, which arises from the abdominal aorta. The ovarian blood supply drains into the two ovarian veins. The left ovarian vein drains into the left renal vein, and the right ovarian vein drains directly into the inferior vena cava.

Nerve Supply

Most functions of the reproductive system are under involuntary, or unconscious, control. Nerves of the autonomic nervous system from the uterovaginal plexus and inferior hypogastric plexus control automatic functions of the reproductive system.

Sensory and motor nerves that innervate the reproductive organs enter the spinal cord at the T12 through L2 levels. These nerves are important for pain management during childbearing (see Chapter 13).

> ### ❓ KNOWLEDGE CHECK
>
> 10. Where is the true pelvis located?
> 11. What are the purposes of the muscles of the pelvis? What are the purposes of the ligaments?

FEMALE REPRODUCTIVE CYCLE

The term *female reproductive cycle* refers to the regular and recurrent changes in the anterior pituitary secretions, ovaries, and uterine endometrium designed to prepare the body for pregnancy (Fig. 3.7). Associated changes in the cervical mucus promote fertilization during each cycle. The female reproductive cycle is often called the *menstrual cycle* because menstruation provides a marker for each cycle's beginning and end if pregnancy does not occur.

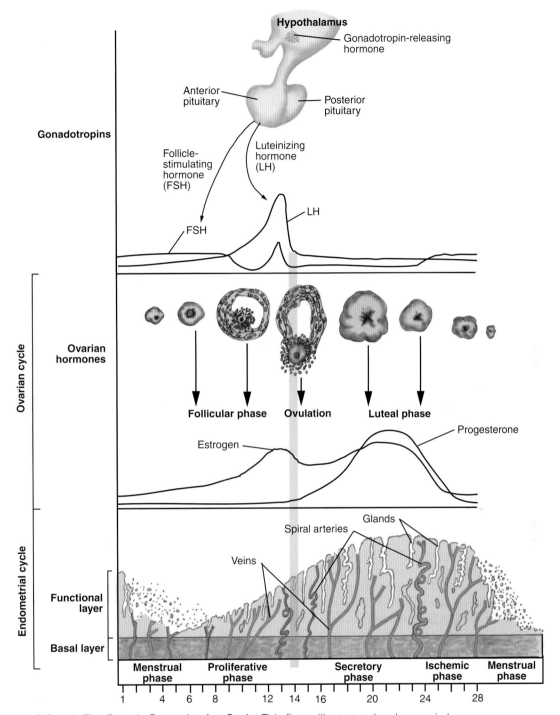

FIG. 3.7 The Female Reproductive Cycle. This figure illustrates the changes in hormone secretion from the anterior pituitary and interrelated changes in the ovary and uterine endometrium.

The female reproductive cycle is driven by a feedback loop between the anterior pituitary and ovaries. A feedback loop is a change in the level of one secretion in response to a change in the level of another secretion. The feedback loop may be positive, in which rising levels of one secretion cause another to rise, or negative, in which rising levels of one secretion cause another to fall.

The duration of the cycle is approximately 28 days, although it may range from 20 to 45 days (Hall, 2021). Significant deviations from the 28-day cycle are associated with reduced fertility. The first day of the menstrual period is counted as day 1 of the female's cycle. The female reproductive cycle is further divided into two cycles reflecting changes in the ovaries and uterine endometrium.

Ovarian Cycle

In response to GnRH from the female's hypothalamus, the anterior pituitary secretes FSH and LH. These secretions stimulate the ovaries to mature and release an ovum and secrete additional hormones to prepare the endometrium for implantation of a fertilized ovum. The ovarian cycle consists of three phases: follicular, ovulatory, and luteal.

Follicular Phase

The follicular phase is the period during which an ovum matures. It begins with the first day of menstruation and ends approximately 14 days later in a 28-day cycle. The length of this phase varies more among different females than do the lengths of the other two phases. The fall in estrogen and progesterone secretion by the ovary just before menstruation stimulates secretion of FSH and LH by the anterior pituitary. As the FSH and LH levels rise slightly, 6 to 12 **graafian follicles** (sacs within the ovary), each containing an immature ovum, begin to grow. Each follicle secretes fluid containing high levels of estrogen, which accelerates maturation by making the follicle more sensitive to the effects of FSH. Eventually, one follicle outgrows the others to reach maturity. The mature follicle secretes large amounts of estrogen, which depresses FSH secretion. The dip in FSH secretion just before ovulation blocks further maturation of the less-developed follicles. Occasionally, more than one follicle matures and releases its ovum, which can lead to a multifetal pregnancy. Females who take fertility drugs may release multiple mature ova that are used for assisted reproductive techniques (see Chapter 27).

Ovulatory Phase

Near the middle of a 28-day reproductive cycle and about 2 days before ovulation, LH secretion rises markedly. Secretion of FSH also rises but to a lesser extent than that of LH. These surges in LH and FSH levels cause a slight fall in follicular estrogen production and a rise in progesterone secretion, which stimulates final maturation of a single follicle and release of its ovum. Ovulation marks the beginning of the luteal phase of the female reproductive cycle and occurs 14 days before the next menstrual period.

The mature follicle is a mass of cells with a fluid-filled chamber. A smaller mass of cells houses the ovum within this chamber. At ovulation, a blister-like projection called a *stigma* forms on the wall of the follicle, the follicle ruptures, and the ovum with its surrounding cells is released from the surface of the ovary, where it is picked up by the fimbriated end of the fallopian tube for transport to the uterus.

Luteal Phase

After ovulation and under the influence of LH, the remaining cells of the old follicle persist for approximately 12 days as a corpus luteum. The corpus luteum secretes estrogen and large amounts of progesterone to prepare the endometrium for a fertilized ovum. During this phase, levels of FSH and LH decrease in response to higher levels of estrogen and progesterone. If the ovum is fertilized, it secretes a hormone (chorionic gonadotropin) that causes persistence of the corpus luteum to maintain an early pregnancy. If the ovum is not fertilized, FSH and LH fall to low levels, and the corpus luteum regresses. Decline of estrogen and progesterone levels, along with corpus luteum regression, results in menstruation as the uterine lining breaks down.

The loss of estrogen and progesterone from the corpus luteum at the end of one cycle stimulates the anterior pituitary to again secrete more FSH and LH, initiating a new female reproductive cycle. The old corpus luteum is replaced by fibrous tissue called the *corpus albicans.*

Endometrial Cycle

The uterine endometrium responds to ovarian hormone stimulation with cyclic changes. Four phases mark the changes in the endometrium: proliferative, secretory, ischemic, and menstrual.

Proliferative Phase

The proliferative phase occurs as the ovum matures and is released during the first half of the ovarian cycle. After completion of a menstrual period, the endometrium is very thin. The basal layer of endometrial cells remains after menstruation. These cells multiply to form new endometrial epithelium and endometrial glands under the stimulation of estrogen secreted by the maturing ovarian follicles. Endometrial spiral arteries and endometrial veins elongate to accompany thickening of the functional endometrial layer and nourish the proliferating cells. As ovulation approaches, the endometrial glands secrete thin, stringy mucus that aids entry of sperm into the uterus.

Secretory Phase

The secretory phase occurs during the last half of the ovarian cycle as the uterus is prepared to receive a fertilized ovum. The endometrium continues to thicken under the influence of estrogen and progesterone from the corpus luteum, reaching its maximum thickness of 5 to 6 mm. The blood vessels and endometrial glands become twisted and dilated.

Progesterone from the corpus luteum causes the thick endometrium to secrete substances to nourish a fertilized ovum. Large quantities of glycogen, proteins, lipids, and minerals are stored within the endometrium, awaiting arrival of the ovum.

Ischemic and Menstrual Phases

If fertilization does not occur, the corpus luteum regresses, and its production of estrogen and progesterone falls. About 2 days before the onset of menstruation, vasospasm of the endometrial blood vessels causes the endometrium to become ischemic and necrotic. The necrotic areas of endometrium separate from the basal layers, resulting in the menstrual flow. The durations of the menstrual phase, from the first day of flow to the last is approximately 5 days.

During a menstrual period, females lose approximately 40 mL of blood. Because of the recurrent loss of blood, many females are mildly anemic during their reproductive years, especially if their diets are low in iron.

Changes in Cervical Mucus

During most of the female reproductive cycle, the mucus of the cervix is scant, thick, and sticky. Just before ovulation, cervical mucus becomes thin, clear, and elastic to promote passage of sperm into the uterus and fallopian tube, where they can fertilize the ovum. **Spinnbarkeit** refers to the elasticity of cervical mucus. Females may assess the elasticity of their cervical mucus to either avoid or promote conception (see Chapter 26).

(see Chapter 26).

KNOWLEDGE CHECK

12. Which ovarian structures secrete estrogen and progesterone during the female reproductive cycle?
13. What three ovarian phases occur during each female reproductive cycle?
14. How does the uterine endometrium change during a female's reproductive cycle?
15. Why does the cervical mucus become thin, clear, and elastic around the time of ovulation?

THE FEMALE BREAST

Structure

The breasts, or mammary glands, are not directly functional in reproduction, but they secrete milk after childbirth to nourish the infant. The small, raised nipple is located at the center of each breast (Fig. 3.8). The nipple is composed of sensitive erectile tissue and may respond to sexual stimulation. A larger circular areola surrounds the nipple. Both the nipple and areola are darker than surrounding skin. Montgomery's tubercles are sebaceous glands in the areola. They are inactive and not obvious except during pregnancy and lactation, when they enlarge and secrete a substance that keeps the nipple soft.

Within each breast, lobes of glandular tissue secrete milk. These lobes are arranged in a pattern similar to spokes of a wheel around the hub. Between 15 and 20 of these lobes are arranged around and behind the nipple and areola. Fibrous tissue and fat in the breast support the glandular tissue, blood vessels, lymphatics, and nerves.

Alveoli are small sacs containing acinar cells to secrete milk. The acinar cells extract the necessary substances from the mammary blood supply to manufacture milk when the breasts are properly stimulated by the anterior pituitary gland. Myoepithelial cells surround the alveoli to contract and eject the milk into the ductal system when signaled by secretion of the hormone oxytocin from the posterior pituitary gland. The alveoli drain into lactiferous ducts, which connect at the nipple to drain milk from all areas of the breast.

Function

The breasts are inactive until puberty, when rising estrogen levels stimulate growth of the glandular tissue. In addition, fat is deposited in the breasts, resulting in the mature female contour. The amount of fat is the major determinant of breast size; the amount of glandular tissue is similar for all mature females. Therefore breast size is unrelated to the amount of milk a female can produce during lactation.

During pregnancy, high levels of estrogen and progesterone produced by the placenta stimulate growth of the alveoli and ductal system to prepare them for lactation. Prolactin secretion by the anterior pituitary gland stimulates milk production during pregnancy, but this effect is inhibited by estrogen and progesterone produced by the placenta. Inhibiting effects of estrogen and progesterone stop when the placenta is expelled after birth, and active milk production occurs in response to the infant's suckling while breastfeeding.

KNOWLEDGE CHECK

16. What is the function of Montgomery's tubercles?
17. How is breast size related to the amount of milk that can be produced?
18. Why is milk not actively secreted during pregnancy?

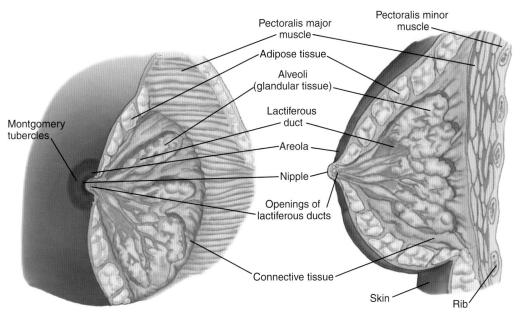

FIG. 3.8 Structures of the female breast.

MALE REPRODUCTIVE ANATOMY AND PHYSIOLOGY

External Male Reproductive Organs

The male has two external organs of reproduction: the penis and scrotum (Fig. 3.9).

Penis

The penis has two functions. As part of the urinary tract, it carries urine from the bladder to the exterior during urination. As a reproductive organ, the penis deposits semen into the female vagina during coitus.

The penis is composed mostly of erectile tissue, which is spongy tissue with many small spaces inside. The three areas of erectile tissue are the corpus spongiosum, which surrounds the urethra, and two columns of the corpus cavernosum on each side of the penis.

The penis is flaccid most of the time because the small spaces within the erectile tissue are collapsed. During sexual stimulation, arteries within the penis dilate and veins are partly occluded, trapping blood in the spongy tissue. Entrapment of blood within the penis causes erection and enables penetration of the vagina during sexual intercourse.

The glans is the distal end of the penis. The urinary meatus is centered in the end of the glans. The loose skin of the prepuce, or foreskin, covers the glans. The prepuce may be removed during circumcision, a surgical procedure usually performed during the newborn period, although it may be performed later. The glans is very sensitive to tactile stimulation, which adds to the male's sensation during coitus.

Scrotum

The scrotum is a pouch of thin skin and muscle suspended behind the penis. The skin of the scrotum is somewhat darker than the surrounding skin and is covered with small ridges called *rugae*. The scrotum is divided internally by a septum. One of the male gonads (testicle) is contained within each pocket of the scrotum.

The scrotum's main purpose is to keep the testes cooler than the core body temperature. Formation of normal male sperm requires that the testes not be too warm. A cremaster muscle is attached to each testicle. Contraction of the cremaster muscles draws the testicles closer to the body for warming, and relaxation of these muscles allows the testicles to move away from the body for cooling.

Internal Male Reproductive Organs

The functions of the male external and internal reproductive organs are summarized in Table 3.3.

Testes

The male gonads, or testes, have two functions: they serve as endocrine glands, and they produce male gametes, or sperm, also called *spermatozoa*. Androgens (male sex hormones) are the primary endocrine secretions of the testes. Androgens are produced by Leydig cells of the testes. The primary androgen produced by the testes is testosterone.

Unlike females, who experience a cyclic pattern of hormone secretion, males secrete testosterone in a relatively even pattern. A feedback loop with the hypothalamus and anterior pituitary stabilizes testosterone levels. A small amount of

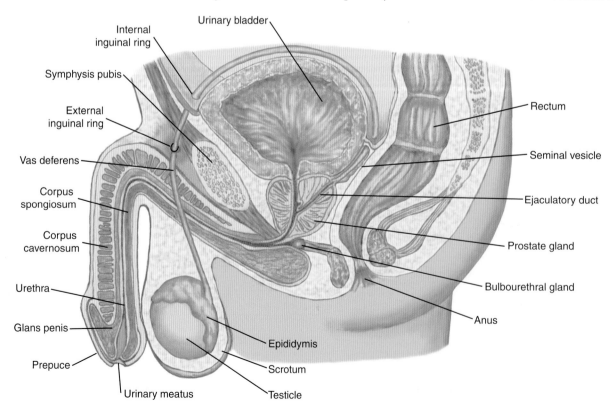

FIG. 3.9 Structures of the male reproductive system, midsagittal view.

TABLE 3.3 Functions of Male Reproductive and Accessory Organs

Organ	Function
Penis	• Conduit for urine from bladder • Male organ of sexual intercourse
Scrotum	• Housing of testes and maintenance of their temperature at a level cooler than trunk of the body, thus promoting normal sperm formation
Testes	• Endocrine glands that secrete primary male hormone (testosterone) • Sperm formation
Seminiferous tubules	• Location of spermatogenesis within testes
Epididymis	• Storage of some sperm • Final sperm maturation • Location where sperm develop ability to be motile
Vas deferens	• Storage of sperm • Conduction of sperm from epididymis to urethra

Seminal vesicles, prostate, and bulbourethral glands	• Secretion of seminal fluids that carry sperm and provide the following:
	  • Nourishment of sperm
	  • Protection of sperm from hostile acidic environment of vagina
	  • Enhancement of motility of sperm
	  • Washing of all sperm from urethra

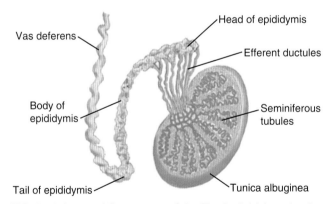

FIG. 3.10 **Internal Structures of the Testis.** Initial production of sperm begins within the tiny, coiled seminiferous tubules. Immature sperm pass from the seminiferous tubules to the epididymis and then to the vas deferens. During their passage through these structures, sperm mature and acquire the ability to propel themselves after ejaculation.

testosterone is converted to estrogen in males and is necessary for sperm formation.

Spermatogenesis occurs within tiny coiled tubes, the seminiferous tubules of the testes (Fig. 3.10). Leydig cells are interstitial cells supporting the seminiferous tubules and secrete testosterone, which is necessary to form new cells that will mature into sperm. Sertoli cells within the seminiferous tubules respond to FSH secretion by nourishing and supporting sperm as they mature. Unlike females, who have a lifetime supply of ova in their gonads at birth, males do not begin producing sperm until puberty. Normal males produce new sperm throughout life, although production declines with age.

At ejaculation, approximately 35 to 200 million sperm are deposited in the vagina (Blackburn, 2018; Hall, 2021). This large number is needed for normal fertility, although a single sperm fertilizes the ovum. Only a few sperm ever reach the fallopian tube, where an ovum may be available for fertilization. When the first sperm penetrates the ovum, changes within the ovum prevent other sperm from also fertilizing it (see Chapter 5).

Accessory Ducts and Glands

From the seminiferous tubules, sperm pass into the epididymis within the scrotum for storage and final maturation. In the epididymis, sperm develop the ability to be motile, although secretions within the epididymis inhibit actual motility until ejaculation occurs.

The epididymis empties into the vas deferens, where larger numbers of sperm are stored. The vas deferens leads upward into the pelvis and then downward toward the penis through the internal and external inguinal rings. Within the pelvis the vas deferens joins the ejaculatory duct before connecting to the urethra.

Three glands—the seminal vesicles, the prostate, and the bulbourethral gland—secrete seminal fluids that carry sperm into the vagina during intercourse. The seminal fluid has four functions: (1) nourishing the sperm, (2) protecting the sperm from the hostile pH (acidic) environment of the vagina, (3) enhancing the motility of the sperm, and (4) washing the sperm from the urethra to maximize the number deposited in the vagina.

? KNOWLEDGE CHECK

19. What are the two functions of the penis?
20. What two types of erectile tissue are in the penis? What is their function?
21. Why is it important for the testes to be contained within the scrotum?
22. What are the two functions of the testes?

SUMMARY CONCEPTS

• Initial prenatal development of the reproductive organs is similar for both males and females. If a critical part of the Y chromosome is not present at conception, female reproductive structures will develop.
• During puberty the reproductive organs become fully functional, and secondary sex characteristics develop.

• Puberty begins approximately 6 months to 1 year earlier in females than in males, although the early growth spurt in females makes it seem like they begin puberty much earlier than males.
• Females are generally shorter than males at the completion of puberty because they begin their growth spurt at an earlier age and complete it more quickly than males.

- Females often do not ovulate in early menstrual cycles, although they can ovulate even before the first cycle. Therefore, a sexually active female can become pregnant before the first menstrual period.
- The onset of puberty is more subtle in males than in females, beginning with growth of the testes and penis.
- Males may have nocturnal emissions of seminal fluid, which may be distressing if the male has not been educated that these events are normal and expected.
- All of the female's ova are present at birth. New ova are not formed after birth; most are depleted when the female reaches the climacteric.
- The female reproductive cycle is often called the *menstrual cycle*. It includes changes in the anterior pituitary gland, ovaries, and uterine endometrium to prepare for a fertilized ovum. The character of cervical mucus also changes during the cycle to encourage fertilization.
- Breast size is unrelated to glandular tissue or the quantity or quality of milk a female can produce for an infant after birth. Breast size is primarily related to the amount of fat present.
- For normal sperm formation, the testes of males must be cooler than their core body temperature.
- Seminal fluids secreted by the seminal vesicles, the prostate, and the bulbourethral glands nourish and protect the sperm, enhance their motility, and ensure most sperm are deposited in the vagina during sexual intercourse.

REFERENCES

Blackburn, S. T. (2018). *Maternal, fetal, and neonatal physiology: A clinical perspective* (5th ed.). Elsevier.

Hall, J. C. (2021). *Guyton and Hall textbook of medical physiology* (14th ed.). Elsevier.

Li, W., Liu, Q., Deng, X., Chen, Y., Liu, S., & Story, M. (2017). Association between obesity and puberty timing: A systematic review and meta-analysis. *International Journal of Environmental Research and Public Health, 14*(10), 1266.

Moore, K. L., Persaud, T. V. N., & Torchia, M. G. (2020). *Before we are born: Essentials of embryology and birth defects* (10th ed.). Elsevier.

Hereditary and Environmental Influences on Childbearing

Suzanne White

OBJECTIVES

After studying this chapter, you should be able to:

1. Describe the structure and function of normal human genes and chromosomes.
2. Give examples of ways to study genes and chromosomes.
3. Explain benefits and ethical implications of the Human Genome Project.
4. Describe the characteristics of single gene traits and their transmission from parent to child.
5. Relate chromosomal abnormalities to spontaneous abortion and birth defects in the infant.
6. Explain characteristics of multifactorial birth defects.
7. Identify environmental factors that can interfere with prenatal development and ways to prevent or reduce their negative effects.
8. Describe genetic counseling.
9. Explain the role of the nurse in caring for individuals or families with concerns about birth defects.

Hereditary and environmental forces shape a person's development from before conception until death. The nurse needs a basic knowledge of these forces to better understand disorders evident at birth (**congenital**) and those developing later in life. This chapter reviews the basics of hereditary influences on development and the impact of environmental factors in causing **birth defects**. The nursing role in relation to genetic knowledge is also discussed.

HEREDITARY INFLUENCES

Hereditary, or **genetic**, influences pertain to the results of development directing cellular functions provided by genes that constitute the 46 chromosomes in every somatic cell. Disorders can result if too much or too little genetic material is present in the cells and if one or more genes are abnormal and provide incorrect directions.

Structure of Genes and Chromosomes

A review of the structure of genes and chromosomes aids in understanding the reasons for the occurrence of disorders. Chromosomes are composed of genes that in turn are composed of deoxyribonucleic acid (DNA) (Fig. 4.1).

Deoxyribonucleic Acid

DNA is the building block of genes and chromosomes. It is made up of three units: (1) a sugar (deoxyribose), (2) a phosphate group, and (3) one of four nitrogen bases (adenine, thymine, guanine, and cytosine).

DNA resembles a spiral ladder, with a sugar and a phosphate group forming each side of the ladder and a pair of nitrogen bases forming each rung of the ladder. The four bases of the DNA molecule pair in a fixed way, allowing the DNA to be accurately duplicated during each cell division.

- Adenine pairs with thymine.
- Guanine pairs with cytosine.

The DNA directs the manufacture of proteins needed for cell function. The sequence of bases within the DNA determines which amino acids will be assembled to form a protein and the order in which they will be assembled for cell processes. Some proteins form the structure of body cells, whereas others are enzymes that control metabolic processes within the cell. If the sequence of nitrogen bases in the DNA is incorrect or some bases are missing or added in critical places, a defect in body structure or function may result.

Bases are arranged in groups of three called *codons* for translation into a specific amino acid in the cell. For example, a triplet base codon may consist of the bases GCC (guanine, cytosine, cytosine), which tells the cell to produce the amino acid alanine. Other codons, known as *stop codons*, signal the end of a gene sequence.

Genes

A **gene** is a segment of DNA that directs the production of a specific product needed for body structure or function. Humans have 23,000 genes arranged on their chromosomes. Only a portion of the long strand of DNA that forms a chromosome makes a single gene. Some genes are active only during prenatal life, and others become functional at various times after birth. Gene regulation is the process of turning genes on and off. During early development, cells begin to

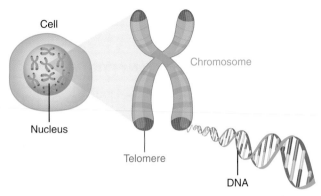

Fig. 4.1 DNA helix is the building block of genes and chromosomes. (From iStock: 961320764_FancyTapis)

take on specific functions. Gene regulation ensures the appropriate genes are expressed at the proper times. Gene regulation also helps an organism respond to its environment. Gene regulation is accomplished by a variety of mechanisms, including chemical modification of genes and the use of regulatory proteins to turn genes on or off (National Human Genome Research Institute [NHGRI], 2021a).

Genes that code for the same trait often have two or more alternative forms, or **alleles**. Familiar examples of alleles are the ABO blood types. Normal alleles provide genetic variation and sometimes a biologic advantage. If an allele occurs at least 1% of the time in the population, it is called a **polymorphism**.

Some changed gene forms, or **mutations**, may be harmless, but many are harmful, such as those that cause the production of abnormal hemoglobin in sickle cell disease. Mutations may cause harm by the following actions:

- Substituting incorrect bases for the normal bases
- Interrupting the normal gene sequence or stopping it prematurely
- Duplicating some bases or entire gene sequences
- Adding or subtracting some bases within those making up a gene's sequence of bases, which will alter the amino acids it causes to be assembled

A mutation may occur in **gametes** (reproductive or germ cells) or **somatic cells** (other body cells). If the mutation occurs in a gamete, the mutation can be transmitted from one generation to the next. Mutations occurring in somatic cells are often associated with malignant change, but they are not transmitted from generation to generation.

Genes are too small to be seen under a microscope, but they can be studied in the following ways:

- By measuring the products they direct cells to produce, such as an enzyme or other substance
- By directly studying the gene's DNA
- By analyzing the gene's close association (linkage) with another gene that can be studied in one of the previous two ways

The tissue used for study of a gene depends on where the gene product is present in the body and the available technology. These tissues may include blood, skin cells, hair follicles, and fetal cells from the amniotic fluid or chorionic villi.

Genes can be identified by direct analysis of DNA and can be studied in any cells containing a nucleus, even if the gene product is not present in that tissue. Although not always used, DNA analysis of the blastomere (eight-cell stage of prenatal development) can be used to select embryos to be implanted in the uterus after in-vitro fertilization. This prevents implantation of embryos with a specific gene defect or common chromosome defects.

The National Human Genome Research Institute is part of the National Institutes of Health. The Human Genome Project is an international effort started in 1990 to identify all genes contained in the human body. Benefits of greater knowledge about specific human genes include the following:

- Performing genetic testing to determine the risk for a disorder or the actual or probable presence of the disorder
- Basing reproductive decisions on more accurate and specific information than has previously been available
- Identifying genetic susceptibility to a disorder so interventions to reduce risk can be instituted
- Using gene therapy to modify a defective gene
- Modifying therapy such as medication based on an individual's genetic code or the genetic makeup of tumor cells
- Individualizing treatment or medications for a specific person

The explosion of knowledge about the genetic basis for many diseases raises many legal and ethical issues for which we do not yet have answers (Box 4.1). As our knowledge base grows, new issues are likely to emerge:

- Genetic information has implications for others in the person's family, raising privacy issues.
- Knowledge about a genetic disorder often precedes knowledge about treatment of the disorder.
- Identification of genetic problems could lead to poor self-esteem, guilt, and excessive caution, or, conversely, a reckless lifestyle.
- Presymptomatic identification of genetically influenced illness would be a source of long-term anxiety.
- Genetic knowledge could affect one's choice of a partner.

Concern about employment or insurance coverage related to genetic tests was addressed in the United States in 2008 with the enactment of the Genetic Information Nondiscrimination Act (GINA). Insurance companies and employers are prohibited from discriminating on the basis of information from genetic tests. Insurance companies are prohibited from discriminating in ways such as canceling, denying, refusing to renew, or changing the terms or premiums based solely on a genetic predisposition toward a specific disease. Employers are prohibited from using genetic information when making employment decisions. A genetic test cannot be demanded by an employer or insurance company. The GINA document further clarified genetic information as part of an individual's health information, and this rule was implemented in 2013 (NHGRI, 2020).

Chromosomes

Genes are organized in 46 paired **chromosomes** in the nucleus of somatic cells. A gene can be likened to a single

BOX 4.1 Ethical Issues Created by Greater Genetic Knowledge

- Should testing be offered for a genetic disease for which no treatment is available? What if the disease is fatal? Should testing be required if a person may carry a diagnosable disorder that might be passed on to the children, even if the person does not want the test?
- Huntington's disease is an example of a genetic disease that can be diagnosed. It has serious effects, with a fatal outcome during midlife. Should testing be offered? Should it be required before the person is allowed to reproduce?
- Who should own and control genetic information? Does an insurer have the right to a person's genetic information to assess risk and therefore set more accurate rates? Or is this information private? Should this information be disregarded for everyone when insurance rates are set? Geneticists may have the ability to identify conditions that a person will develop in the future even if the problem is not present. Examples include hypertension, diabetes, and heart disease. If an insurance company knows the person will develop this disorder, rates would be higher or coverage would be denied. If an employer has this information, the person might not be hired, to avoid raising insurance costs for the company. Yet the reverse could be true. Genetic testing might prove a person *would not* develop a disorder, thereby gaining them lower rates. If genetic testing before being insured is not permitted, is it right that all persons insured by a company subsidize those who develop disorders that could have been determined before being insured by paying higher rates?
- How should issues of racial or ethnic identification be handled? What if a person's parentage is not what he or she has always believed? Discoveries in the process of genetic analysis may determine that a person is not of the racial identity previously thought, or a person might discover a parent is not the biologic parent. What should be done if information of this nature is uncovered? What are possible implications for self-image and identity? How might other members of the family be involved in the unexpected discovery?

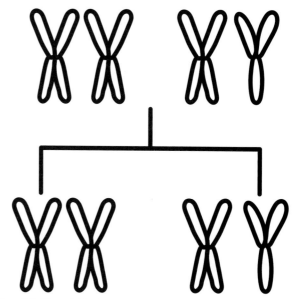

Fig. 4.2 X and Y chromosome sex determination system. (From iStock: 1299322282_Azam Ishaq)

Unlike genes, chromosomes can be seen under the microscope but only during cell division for a full chromosome analysis. Specimens should be obtained and preserved carefully to provide enough living cells for chromosomal analysis. Temperature extremes, blood clotting, and the addition of improper preservatives can kill the cells and render them useless for analysis.

Chromosomes look jumbled before they are arranged into a karyotype. A systematic study is possible using imaging of prepared chromosomes and then arranging them into a karyotype. In a karyotype, autosomal pairs are arranged from largest to smallest. Letters describe groups of similar size and appearance. Sex chromosomes are arranged in a separate group.

A person's karyotype is abbreviated by a combination of numbers and letters. The number describes the total number of chromosomes, followed by either an XX to indicate the sex chromosomes are female or an XY to indicate they are male. Therefore the chromosome complement is abbreviated as 46,XX for a normal female and as 46,XY for a normal male (Fig. 4.2). If the chromosome number or structure is abnormal, as in Down's syndrome (trisomy 21), which has an extra 21 chromosome, an added abbreviation indicates the abnormality: 47 (total number of chromosomes), XY (male), + 21 (the number of the extra chromosome). Other abbreviations describe karyotypes with missing or structurally altered chromosomes.

Finer chromosome analysis uses fluorescent-labeled DNA probes that attach to specific chromosomes. This technique is called fluorescence in-situ hybridization (FISH) and permits testing for added, missing, or rearranged chromosome material that otherwise may not be visible microscopically. FISH analysis can be done rapidly because stimulation of cells to divide is not required as in other types of chromosome analysis. More specific chromosome analysis is the comparative

bead; a chromosome is like a string of beads. Each chromosome is composed of varying numbers of genes. A total of 22 chromosome pairs are **autosomes** (non-sex chromosomes), and the 23rd pair is composed of the **sex chromosomes**, XX (female) or XY (male). Added, missing, and structurally abnormal chromosomes are usually harmful. **Homologous** chromosomes carry matching genetic information; that is, they have the same genes in the same sequence.

Mature gametes have half the chromosomes (23) of other body cells. One chromosome from each pair is distributed randomly in the gametes, allowing variation of genetic traits among people. When the ovum and sperm unite at conception, the total is restored to 46 paired chromosomes.

Cells for full chromosome analysis must have a nucleus and be living. Chromosomes can be studied by using any of several types of cells: white blood cells, skin fibroblasts, bone marrow cells, and fetal cells from the chorionic villi of the placenta or suspended in amniotic fluid.

genomic hybridization used to identify losses or duplications of specific chromosome regions, which often occur in tumor cells.

KNOWLEDGE CHECK

1. What is the relationship among DNA, genes, and chromosomes?
2. Can genes be studied by examining them under a microscope? Why or why not? What methods are used to study them?
3. Why do cell specimens for chromosomal analysis have to be alive, regardless of the tissue used?
4. What do each of these abbreviations mean: 46, XY and 46, XX? How are chromosome abnormalities described?

Transmission of Traits by Single Genes

Inherited characteristics are passed from parent to child by the genes in each chromosome. These traits are classified according to whether they are **dominant** (strong) or **recessive** (weak) and whether the gene is located on one of the autosome pairs or on the sex chromosomes. Both normal and abnormal hereditary characteristics are transmitted by these mechanisms.

Because humans have pairs of matched chromosomes, except for the sex chromosomes in the male, they have one allele for a gene at the same location on each member of the chromosome pair. The paired alleles may be identical (**homozygous**) or different (**heterozygous**).

Some genes, both normal and abnormal, occur more frequently in certain groups than in the population as a whole. For example, the gene causing Tay-Sachs disease on chromosome 15 is carried by approximately 1 of every 30 Jews in the United States. This rate is also similar in persons of French–Canadian ancestry and members of the Cajun population in Louisiana and is approximately 100 times its occurrence in the general population (National Tay-Sachs and Allied Diseases Association [NTSAD], 2021). Because the abnormal gene occurs more frequently in these groups, their incidence of Tay-Sachs disease is also higher. Other disorders that are more common in certain ethnic groups are cystic fibrosis, which occurs primarily in White people of northern European descent, and sickle cell disease, which occurs more frequently in people of African descent.

Dominance

Dominance describes the way a person's **genotype** (genetic composition) is translated into the **phenotype**, or observable characteristics. In the case of a dominant gene, one copy is enough to cause the trait to be expressed. For example, in the ABO blood system, genes for types A and B are dominant. Therefore, a single copy of either of these genes is enough for it to be expressed in the person's blood type.

Two identical copies of a recessive gene are required for the trait to be expressed. The gene for blood type O is recessive. Laboratory testing identifies a person's blood type as O only if that person receives a gene for blood type O from both parents. If the person receives a gene for type O from one parent and type A from the other parent, blood type A is expressed in laboratory blood typing.

On the basis of dominant and recessive forms of a gene, a person with type A blood can have one of the following two possible combinations of gene alleles:

- Two type A alleles
- One type A allele and one type O allele

Other alleles are equally dominant. The person who receives a gene for blood type A from one parent and type B from the other will have type AB blood because both alleles are equally dominant and expressed in blood typing.

Dominance and recessiveness are relative qualities for many genes. Some people with a single copy of an abnormal recessive gene (carriers) may have a lower than normal level of the gene product (e.g., an enzyme) that can be detected by biochemical methods. These people often do not have overt disease because the normal copy of the gene produces enough of the required product to allow normal or near-normal function.

Chromosome Location

Genes located on autosomes are either autosomal dominant or autosomal recessive, depending on the number of identical copies of the gene needed to produce the trait. However, genes located on the X chromosome are paired only in females because males have one X chromosome and one Y chromosome.

A female with an abnormal recessive gene on one of her X chromosomes usually has a normal gene on the other X chromosome that compensates and maintains relatively normal function. However, the male is at a disadvantage if his lone X chromosome has an abnormal gene. The male has no compensating normal gene because his other sex chromosome is a Y. The abnormal gene is expressed in the male because it is unopposed by a normal gene.

Patterns of Single Gene Inheritance

Three major patterns of single gene inheritance are autosomal dominant, autosomal recessive, and X-linked (Box 4.2). Few genes are found on the Y chromosome, primarily the one that causes the embryo to differentiate into a male (NHGRI, 2021b). Because few Y-linked traits have been identified, these will not be discussed.

Although the word **pedigree** is widely used among genetic professionals, the nurse may need to interpret it for the client. Be cautious when referring to the illustration of a family's genetic history as a *pedigree* because some associate the word only with animals. For example, when taking a genetic family history, the nurse might say, "I'm going to use several symbols to depict your family tree and its members' health histories. This diagram is called a *genogram,* but it's also often called a *pedigree.*"

Single gene traits have mathematically predictable and fixed rates of occurrence. For example, if a couple has a child with an autosomal recessive disorder, the risk that future children will have the same disorder is 1 in 4 (25%) at every conception. The risk is the same at every conception, regardless of how many of a couple's children have been affected.

BOX 4.2 Single Gene Traits

Genogram (Pedigree) Symbols

A genogram symbolically represents a family's medical history and the relationships of its members to one another. It helps identify patterns of inheritance that may help distinguish one type of disorder from another.

- ☐ Male
- ◯ Female
- ◇ Sex not specified (number indicates the number of persons represented by the symbol)
- ■ ● Affected
- ◪ ◑ Carriers (heterozygous) for an autosomal recessive trait
- ⊙ Female carrier of an X-linked recessive trait
- ⊘ Deceased
- ☐—◯ Mating/marriage
- ☐=◯ Consanguineous mating/marriage
- I Roman numerals indicate generations

Autosomal Recessive

Characteristics

Two autosomal recessive genes are required to produce the trait.

Males and females are equally likely to have the trait.

There is often no prior family history of the disorder before the first affected child.

If more than one family member is affected, they are usually full siblings.

Consanguinity (close blood relationship) of the parents increases the risk for the disorder.

Disorders are more likely to occur in groups isolated by geography, culture, religion, or other factors.

Some autosomal recessive disorders are more common in specific ethnic groups.

Transmission of Trait from Parent to Child

Unaffected parents are carriers of the abnormal autosomal recessive trait.

Children of carriers have a 25% (1 in 4) chance for receiving both copies of the defective gene and thus having the disorder.

Children of carriers have a 50% (1 in 2) chance of receiving one copy of the gene and being carriers like the parents.

Children of carriers have a 25% (1 in 4) chance of receiving both copies of the normal gene. They are neither carriers nor affected.

Examples

Normal traits: Blood group O, Rh-negative blood factor.

Abnormal traits: Tay-Sachs disease, sickle cell disease, cystic fibrosis.

Genogram

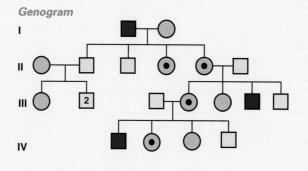

Autosomal Dominant

Characteristics

A single copy of the gene is enough to produce the trait.

Males and females are equally likely to have the trait.

Often appears in every generation of a family, although family members having the trait may have widely varying manifestations of it.

May have multiple and seemingly unrelated effects on body structure and function.

Transmission of Trait from Parent to Child

A parent with the trait has a 50% (1 in 2) chance of passing the trait to the child.

The trait may arise as a new mutation from an unaffected parent. The child who receives the mutated gene can then transmit it to future generations.

Examples

Normal traits: Blood groups A and B, Rh-positive blood factor.

Abnormal traits: Huntington's disease, neurofibromatosis.

Genogram

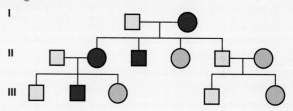

X-Linked Recessive

Characteristics

Although recessive, only one copy of the gene is needed to cause the disorder in males, who do not have a compensating X without the trait.

Males are affected, with rare exceptions.

Females are carriers of the trait but not usually adversely affected.

Affected males are related to one another through carrier females.

Affected males do not transmit the trait to their sons.

Transmission of Trait from Parent to Child

Males who have the disorder transmit the gene to 100% of their daughters and none of their sons.

Sons of carrier females have a 50% (1 in 2) chance of being affected. They also have a 50% chance of being unaffected.

Daughters of carrier females have a 50% (1 in 2) chance of being carriers like their mothers. They also have a 50% chance of being neither affected nor carriers.

A new X-linked recessive gene also may arise by mutation.

Examples

Colorblindness, Duchenne muscular dystrophy, hemophilia A.

Genogram

Autosomal Dominant Traits

An autosomal dominant trait is produced by a dominant gene on a non-sex chromosome. The expression of abnormal autosomal dominant genes may result in multiple and seemingly unrelated effects in the person. The gene's effects also may vary substantially in severity, leading a family to believe incorrectly that a trait skips a generation. A careful physical examination may reveal subtle evidence of the trait in each generation. In other cases, some people may carry the dominant gene but have no apparent expression of it in their physical makeup.

In some autosomal dominant disorders, such as Huntington's disease, those with the gene will always have the disease if they live to the age at which the disorder becomes apparent. In other disorders, only a portion of those carrying the gene ever exhibit the disease.

New mutations account for the introduction of abnormal autosomal dominant traits into a family with no history of the disorder. In this case parents of the child are not affected because their body cells do not have the altered gene.

The person who is affected by an autosomal dominant disorder is usually heterozygous for the gene; that is, the person has a normal gene on one chromosome and an abnormal gene on the other chromosome of the pair. Occasionally, a person receives two copies of the same abnormal autosomal dominant gene. Such an individual is usually much more severely affected than someone with only one copy (NHGRI, 2021c).

Autosomal Recessive Traits

An autosomal recessive trait occurs if a person receives two copies of a recessive gene carried on an autosome. Everyone is estimated to carry abnormal autosomal recessive genes without manifesting the disorder because everyone has a compensating normal gene. Because of the low probability of two unrelated people sharing even one of the same abnormal genes, the incidence of autosomal recessive diseases is relatively low in the general population.

Situations increasing the likelihood of two parents sharing the same abnormal autosomal recessive gene are as follows:
- Consanguinity (blood relationship of the parents): Blood relatives have more genes in common, including abnormal ones.
- Groups isolated by culture, geography, religion, or other factors: The isolation allows abnormal genes to become concentrated over the years and occur at a greater frequency than in more diverse groups.

Many autosomal recessive disorders are severe, and affected persons may not live long enough to reproduce. Two notable exceptions are phenylketonuria (PKU) and cystic fibrosis. Improved care of people with these disorders has allowed them to live into their reproductive years. If one member of the couple has the autosomal recessive disorder, all their children will be carriers. Their child's risk for having similarly affected children is also higher, depending on the prevalence of the abnormal gene in the general population and the likelihood their mate is a carrier (American College of Obstetricians and Gynecologists [ACOG], 2020).

> ### CRITICAL TO REMEMBER
> #### Single Gene Abnormalities
> - A person affected with an autosomal dominant disorder has a 50% chance of transmitting the disorder to each biologic child.
> - Two healthy parents who carry the same abnormal autosomal recessive gene have a 25% chance of having a child affected with the disorder caused by this gene.
> - Parental consanguinity increases the risk for having a child with an autosomal recessive disorder.
> - One copy of an abnormal X-linked recessive gene is enough to produce the disorder in a male.
> - Abnormal genes can arise as new mutations. If these mutations are in the gametes, they are transmitted to future generations.

X-Linked Traits

X-linked recessive traits are more common than X-linked dominant traits and are the only X-linked pattern discussed in this chapter. Sex differences in the occurrence of X-linked recessive traits and the relationship of affected males to one another are important factors distinguishing these disorders from autosomal dominant and recessive disorders. In general, males are the only ones to show full effects of an X-linked recessive disorder because their only X chromosome has the abnormal gene on it. One of the two X chromosomes is inactivated randomly in a normal female embryo. The active X chromosome in cells usually provides adequate cell function, although one of the two X chromosomes is inactivated. Barr bodies seen in female cells indicate the inactive X, and they are not seen in normal male tissue samples. Females can show the full disorder in the following two uncommon circumstances:
- If a female has a single X chromosome (Turner syndrome)
- If a female child is born to an affected father and a carrier mother

X-linked recessive disorders can be relatively mild (e.g., colorblindness), or they may be severe (e.g., hemophilia). In addition, those having the disorder may be affected with varying degrees of severity.

> ### KNOWLEDGE CHECK
> 5. If a parent has an autosomal dominant disorder, what are the chances the child will have the same disorder?
> 6. Why would parents who are first cousins be more likely to have a child with an autosomal recessive disorder?
> 7. If each member of a couple carries the gene for an autosomal recessive disorder, what are the chances the children will have the disorder? What are the chances the children will be carriers? What are the chances the children will not receive the abnormal gene from either parent?
> 8. Why are males more often affected by X-linked recessive disorders? If a female carries an X-linked recessive disorder such as hemophilia, what are the chances her sons will have the disorder? What are the chances her daughters will be carriers?

Chromosomal Abnormalities

Chromosomal abnormalities can be numerical or structural. They are quite common (≥50%) in the embryo or fetus spontaneously aborted (miscarried). Chromosomal abnormalities often cause major defects because they involve deletion or duplication of many genes. The normal number of chromosomes in body cells other than reproductive cells is 46, referred to as **diploid**.

Numerical Abnormalities

Numerical chromosomal abnormalities involve added or missing single chromosomes or multiple sets of chromosomes. **Trisomy** and **monosomy** are numerical abnormalities of single chromosomes. The term **polyploidy** refers to abnormalities involving full sets of chromosomes.

Trisomy. A trisomy exists when each body cell contains an extra copy of one chromosome, bringing the total number to 47. Each chromosome is normal, but too many are present in each somatic cell. The most common trisomy is Down's syndrome, or trisomy 21, in which three copies of chromosome 21 are in each somatic cell. Trisomies of chromosomes 13 and 18 are less common and have more severe effects. The incidence of bearing children with trisomies increases with maternal age, so most clients who are 35 years or older and become pregnant are offered prenatal diagnostic screening to determine whether the fetus has Down's syndrome or another trisomy.

Infants with Down's syndrome have characteristic features usually noticed at birth. Chromosomal analysis is performed during the neonatal period to confirm the diagnosis and determine whether Down's syndrome is caused by trisomy 21 or a rarer chromosomal anomaly involving a structural rather than a numerical abnormality of chromosome 21.

Children with Down's syndrome reach developmental milestones more slowly than unaffected children. Their intellectual development is delayed, although the severity varies, just as intelligence varies in the general population. Early intervention programs and regular medical care help these children reach their full ability and manage the physical issues associated with Down's syndrome.

Klinefelter syndrome is a trisomy of the sex chromosomes. Klinefelter syndrome (KS), 47,XXY, occurs in 150 per 100,000 live-born males. In addition to possessing one or more extra X chromosomes, affected males typically exhibit phenotypical traits that include hypergonadotropic hypogonadism, testosterone deficiency, and infertility (Gravholt et al., 2018).

Monosomy. A monosomy exists when each body cell has a missing chromosome, with a total number of 45. The only monosomy compatible with postnatal life is Turner syndrome, or monosomy X. The person with Turner syndrome has a single X chromosome and is always born with female genitalia.

Prenatal ultrasound of a baby with Turner syndrome may reveal a large fluid collection on the back of the neck or other abnormal fluid collections (edema), heart abnormalities, or abnormal kidneys. Symptoms noticed at birth or during infancy may include a wide or webbed neck, broad,

shield-like chest with widely spaced nipples, low-set ears, swelling of the hands and feet, and slightly less than average length. The most common signs in children, adolescents, and adults are short stature and ovarian insufficiency. This includes a lack of growth spurts at expected times during childhood, short adult stature compared to other females in the family, puberty which is delayed or which stalls during the teen years, reduced fertility and an early end to menstrual cycles not due to pregnancy. Treatment with estrogen at the age of puberty promotes development of secondary sexual characteristics. Continuing estrogen throughout life reduces development of osteoporosis (Mayo Clinic, 2017).

CRITICAL TO REMEMBER
Chromosome Abnormalities

Chromosome abnormalities are either numerical or structural.

Numerical	**Structural**
Entire single chromosome added (trisomy)	Part of a chromosome missing or added
Entire single chromosome missing (monosomy)	Rearrangements of material within chromosome(s)
One or more added sets of chromosomes, resulting in cells containing 69 (triploidy) or 92 (tetraploidy) chromosomes	Two chromosomes that adhere to each other
	Fragility of a specific site, such as on the X chromosome ("fragile X syndrome")

Polyploidy. Polyploidy may occur when gametes do not halve their chromosome number during meiosis and retain both members of each pair or when two sperm fertilize an ovum simultaneously. The result is an embryo with one or more extra sets of chromosomes. The total number of chromosomes is a multiple of the **haploid** number of 23 (69 or 92 total chromosomes). Polyploidy usually results in an early spontaneous abortion but may occasionally be seen in a live-born infant. This abnormality may be found in chorionic villus sampling (see Chapter 9) and may reflect an abnormality of the chorionic villi rather than of the fetus.

Structural Abnormalities

Chromosomal abnormalities may involve the structure of one or more chromosomes. Part of a chromosome may be missing or added, or DNA within the chromosome may be rearranged. Some of these rearrangements are common, harmless variations. Others are harmful because important genetic material is lost or duplicated in the structural abnormality or the position of the genes in relation to other genes is altered so that their normal function is not possible.

Another structural abnormality occurs when all or part of a chromosome is attached to another (**translocation**) (Fig. 4.3). Many people with a translocation chromosomal abnormality are clinically normal because the total of their genetic material is normal or balanced. If a parent has a balanced translocation, the offspring, like the parent, may have completely normal chromosomes or a balanced translocation.

CHROMOSOMAL TRANSLOCATION

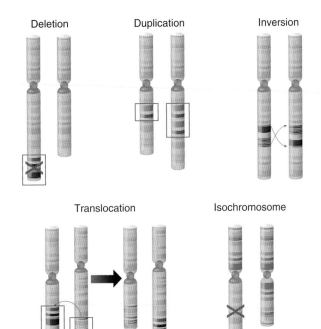

Fig. 4.3 Illustration of a translocation of chromosome material. (From iStock: 509313346_ttsz)

However, the offspring may receive too much or too little chromosomal material and be spontaneously aborted or have birth defects.

Balanced translocations are often discovered when amniocentesis reveals a translocation in the fetus or during infertility evaluations if a history of recurrent spontaneous abortions is reported. Either balanced or unbalanced chromosomal translocations may occur spontaneously in the offspring of parents who have no translocation.

Fragile X syndrome is an X-linked chromosomal abnormality. The syndrome was so named because a site on the X chromosome demonstrates breaks and gaps when the cells are grown in a medium deficient in folic acid. The syndrome is now usually diagnosed by molecular DNA studies. As in other X-linked traits, males are more severely affected than females, who have a compensating X chromosome that is usually normal. Fragile X syndrome is the most common inherited form of male intellectual disability (NHGRI, 2021d).

？ KNOWLEDGE CHECK

9. What is a chromosomal trisomy? Describe a common trisomy.
10. What is a chromosomal monosomy? Which monosomy is compatible with life?
11. Why are structural chromosomal abnormalities often harmful?
12. What are the possible outcomes of the offspring of a parent who has a balanced chromosomal translocation?

MULTIFACTORIAL DISORDERS

Multifactorial disorders result from an interaction of genetic and environmental factors. The genetic tendency toward the disorder is modified by the environment. These interactions may either positively or negatively influence prenatal and postnatal development. For example, two embryos may have an equal genetic susceptibility for the development of a disorder such as spina bifida (open spine). However, the disorder will not occur unless an environment that favors its development, for example, deficient maternal intake of folic acid, also exists.

Characteristics

Multifactorial birth defects are typically present and detectable at birth and isolated defects rather than defects which occur with unrelated abnormalities. However, a multifactorial defect may cause a secondary defect. For example, infants with spina bifida often have hydrocephalus (abnormal collection of spinal fluid within the brain) as well. The hydrocephalus is not a separate defect but one that occurs because the primary defect—abnormal development of the spine and spinal cord—disrupts spinal fluid circulation, allowing the fluid to accumulate within the brain's ventricular system.

However, the infant who has defects other than those known to be associated with spina bifida probably does not have a multifactorial disorder. In this case the spina bifida is more likely to be part of a syndrome such as a chromosome defect, which may pose a different risk for recurrence in a future child.

Multifactorial disorders are some of the most common birth defects encountered. Examples include the following (Driscoll & Simpson, 2021):
- Heart defects
- Neural tube defects such as anencephaly (absence of most of the brain and skull), spina bifida, and encephalocele
- Cleft lip and cleft palate
- Pyloric stenosis

Risk for Occurrence

Unlike single gene traits, multifactorial disorders do not follow mathematical probabilities but do tend to recur in families. Unaffected parents of an affected child have a 1% to 5% risk of parenting another child with the disorder (Driscoll & Simpson, 2021). Factors which influence the risk include:
1. Number of affected close relatives—Risk increases as the number of affected close relatives (parent, full sibling, or child) increases.
2. Severity of the disorder in affected family members—For example, bilateral cleft lip is associated with a higher risk for recurrence in a close relative than is a unilateral cleft lip on one side of the upper lip.
3. Sex of the affected person(s)—For example, pyloric stenosis occurs five times as often in males as in females. The couple who has a daughter with pyloric stenosis faces a higher risk for recurrence with future children because the genetic influence for development of the defect is greater if a female develops it.

4. Geographic location—The risk for some disorders, such as neural tube defects, is more prevalent in one population than another. Because a group at greater risk often lives near others with the same risk, occurrence of the disorder may be more frequent in that area.

CRITICAL TO REMEMBER

Multifactorial Birth Defects

- Multifactorial defects are some of the most common birth defects encountered in maternity and pediatric nursing practice.
- They are a result of interaction between a person's genetic susceptibility and environmental factors during prenatal development.
- These are usually single, isolated defects, although the primary defect may cause secondary defects.
- Some occur more often in certain geographic areas and among more closely related population groups.
- A greater risk for occurrence exists with the following:
  - Several close relatives have the defect, whether mild or severe.
  - One close relative has a severe form of the defect.
  - The defect occurs in a child of the less frequently affected sex.
  - Infants who have several major or minor defects that are not directly related probably do not have a multifactorial defect but have another syndrome such as a chromosomal abnormality.

If multifactorial disorders had no environmental component, the risk for occurrence and recurrence would be a precise percentage rather than a range. However, if no genetic component exists (if the disorder were totally related to environment), the ability to predict the risk for occurrence or recurrence would be minimal.

ENVIRONMENTAL INFLUENCES

Environment, for example, good nutrition that supplies all necessary raw materials for fetal growth and adequate folic acid intake before conception, may positively influence prenatal development. However, some environmental influences such as *teratogens* (environmental agents) or mechanical forces that can cause defects as the baby develops are harmful.

Environmental influences on childbearing are those not known to have a genetic component. At one time, the placenta was thought to be a shield against harmful agents. Now it is recognized that most agents can cross the placenta and affect the developing fetus.

Teratogens

Teratogens are agents in the fetal environment that either cause or increase the likelihood that a birth defect will occur. Some drugs have been established as safe or harmful. With most agents, however, their potential for harming the fetus is not clear. Several factors make it difficult to establish the teratogenic potential of an agent:

1. Retrospective study—Investigators must rely on the mother's memory about substances she ingested or was exposed to during pregnancy. The conclusion that a specific agent is harmful and the ways in which it harms the fetus is possible only when many cases are collected in which the exposure history is similar and the birth defects are also similar.
2. Timing of exposure—Agents may be harmful at one stage of prenatal development but not at another. Exposure may be harmful but may vary with the prenatal development stage.
3. Different susceptibility of organ systems—Some agents affect only one fetal organ system, or they affect one system at one stage of development and another at a different stage of development.
4. Uncontrolled fetal exposure—Exposures cannot be controlled to eliminate extraneous agents or ensure a consistent dose. Interactions with other agents may reduce or compound the fetal effects. An agent toxic at one dose may have no apparent effect at another.
5. Placental transfer—Agents vary in their ability to cross the placenta.
6. Individual variations—Fetuses show varying susceptibility to harmful agents.
7. Nontransferability of animal studies—Results of animal studies cannot always be applied to humans. Agents that do not harm animal fetuses may damage the human embryo or fetus.
8. Risk for damage from an uncontrolled maternal disorder—Some maternal disorders, such as epilepsy or hypertension, may cause fetal damage if not controlled. A poorly controlled maternal disorder raises a question of whether the disorder itself or the medication used to control the disorder harms the fetus.

Teratogens typically cause more than one defect, which distinguishes teratogenic defects from multifactorial disorders. However, children affected by single gene and chromosome defects are also likely to have multiple defects. Therefore, clinicians consider single gene disorders, chromosomal abnormalities, and effects of teratogenic agents when trying to diagnose an infant born with multiple anomalies.

Hundreds of individual agents are either known or suspected teratogens (Box 4.3). Types of teratogens include the following:

- Maternal infectious agents (e.g., viruses, bacteria) that cross the placenta
- Drugs and other substances used by the client (e.g., therapeutic agents, illicit drugs, tobacco, alcohol)
- Pollutants, chemicals, and other substances to which the client is exposed in daily life
- Ionizing radiation
- Maternal hyperthermia
- Effects of maternal disorders such as diabetes mellitus and PKU

Preventing Fetal Exposure

Ideally, prevention of exposure to harmful influences begins before conception because all major organ systems develop

BOX 4.3   Selected Environmental Substances Known or Thought to Harm the Fetus

The nurse should adhere to new information about adverse fetal effects from these or other drugs given during pregnancy.

- Alcohol
- Aminoglycosides
- Anticonvulsant agents
- Antihyperlipidemic agents (statins)
- Antineoplastic agents
- Antithyroid drugs
- Cocaine
- Diethylstilbestrol (DES)
- Folic acid antagonists
- Infections
- Cytomegalovirus
- Herpes simplex virus
- Human immunodeficiency virus
- Parvo
- Rubella
- Syphilis
- Toxoplasmosis
- Varicella
- Zika
- Lithium
- Mercury
- Retinoic acid
- Tetracycline
- Tobacco
- Warfarin

early in pregnancy, often before the pregnancy is recognized. To avoid some agents such as alcohol and illicit drugs, some pregnant clients must be committed to making substantial lifestyle changes. The Organization of Teratology Information Specialists is a source of information about drug use (includes therapeutic, illicit, and herbal), infections and vaccines, and maternal medical conditions, as well as exposure to common substances such as caffeine, suntan beds, or fish (https://www.mothertobaby.org). As of 2021, this website also has fact sheets nurses can provide to expectant clients regarding various substance exposures that may be cause for concern.

Infections. For infections that cannot be prevented by immunization, the nurse may counsel the client to avoid situations in which acquiring the disease is more likely. Rubella infection during pregnancy may result in severe damage to the fetus. Rubella immunization 28 days before conception virtually eliminates the risk of infection. Pregnancy should be avoided for at least 4 weeks (28 days) after receiving a measles, mumps, and rubella (MMR) vaccine.

Drugs and Other Substances. In 2015, the U.S. Food and Drug Administration's Pregnancy and Lactation Labeling Rule (PLLR), changed the content and format of labeling information for prescription drugs and biologic products in the United States.. This rule eliminated the use of pregnancy categories A, B, C, D, and X from drug labels and replaced them with more meaningful information to assist the health care provider

evaluate benefit and risk of the drug and counsel pregnant and nursing clients to assist them in making informed and educated decisions regarding the medication. (USFDA, 2021).

Establishing whether an illicit drug can cause prenatal damage is difficult because clients who use these substances often have other problems that complicate analysis of fetal effects. For example, clients may use multiple drugs and have poor nutritional status, untreated sexually transmitted infections (STIs), inadequate prenatal care, and stressful lives. In addition, illicit drugs are unlikely to be pure, and substances used to dilute them may themselves be harmful. Legal drugs may be combined with illegal drugs, and users may abuse legal drugs.

Drugs are often metabolized and excreted in urine, including drugs in the fetal system. Fetal blood levels of drugs often remain high because the fetus swallows amniotic fluid containing excreted drug products, even after the drug has been eliminated by the mother's body.

The best action is for the client to eliminate use of nontherapeutic drugs and substances such as alcohol. If therapeutic drugs are required, the health care provider may be able to prescribe an alternative drug with a lower risk to the fetus or may eliminate nonessential therapeutic drugs such as acne medications.

Ionizing Radiation. Nonurgent radiologic procedures may be done during the first 2 weeks after the menstrual period begins, before ovulation occurs. For urgent procedures during pregnancy, the lower abdomen should be shielded with a lead apron, if possible. The radiation dose is kept as low as possible to reduce fetal exposure. Ultrasonography and magnetic resonance imaging are the imaging techniques of choice for pregnant women (ACOG, 2017).

Maternal Hyperthermia. An important teratogen is maternal hyperthermia. The mother's temperature may rise unavoidably during illness. Nurses should caution pregnant clients to avoid deliberate exposure to heat sources such as saunas and hot tubs. Temperatures vary widely among public hot tubs, and a specific guideline for duration of exposure is difficult. The important factor is how high the client's body temperature rises and for how long, not just the sauna or hot tub temperature. Pregnant clients should limit sauna or hot tub exposure to no more than 10 minutes and should keep the head and chest out of the water. It may take only 10 to 20 minutes in a sauna or hot tub to raise body temperature to 102 degrees F (38.9 degrees C). Exposure to temperatures of 37.8°C (100°F) or higher is not advised (MotherToBaby, 2019).

Manipulating the Fetal Environment

Appropriate medical therapy can help a pregnant client prevent fetal damage that could result from illness. For example, a client who has diabetes should try to keep blood glucose levels normal and stable before and during pregnancy for the best possible fetal outcomes. A client with PKU should return to a special phenylalanine-free diet before conception to prevent high levels of phenylalanine in the body that will damage the fetus.

Consuming folic acid before and during pregnancy can decrease the risk of neural tube defects in the fetus (CDC, 2021). Neural tube defects occur early in gestation, often before the pregnancy is realized. Because nearly half of the pregnancies in the United States are unplanned, all women of childbearing age should consume at least 0.4 mg (400 mcg) of folic acid daily. Higher dosages—4 mg (4000 mcg)—may be prescribed for clients who have delivered a child with a neural tube defect (CDC, 2021). Nurses should provide client education regarding the need for a supplement of folic acid before conception to help reduce this serious birth defect.

Mechanical Disruptions to Fetal Development

Mechanical forces that interfere with normal prenatal development include oligohydramnios and fibrous amniotic bands.

Oligohydramnios, an abnormally small volume of amniotic fluid, reduces the cushion surrounding the fetus and may result in deformations such as clubfoot. Prolonged oligohydramnios can interfere with fetal lung development by interfering with normal branching and development of the alveoli. Oligohydramnios may not be the primary fetal problem but related to other fetal anomalies. Oligohydramnios also may be a sign of reduced placental blood flow that may occur in certain complications of pregnancy.

Fibrous amniotic bands may result from tears in the inner sac (amnion) of the fetal membranes and can result in fetal deformations or intrauterine limb amputation. Congenital anomalies associated with Amniotic Band Syndrome (ABS) include disruption, deformation, and malformations of organs that were intended to develop normally (Singh & Gorla, 2020).

? KNOWLEDGE CHECK

13. What are the usual characteristics of multifactorial disorders?
14. What factors can vary the likelihood that a multifactorial disorder will occur or recur?
15. How can a client avoid exposing the fetus to teratogens?
16. Why should a client with phenylketonuria (PKU) adhere to a low-phenylalanine diet before and during pregnancy?
17. Why is adequate folic acid intake before conception important?

GENETIC COUNSELING

Genetic counseling provides information and support to help people understand the genetic disorder they are concerned about and the risk for its occurrence in their family and make informed decisions about testing and treatment.

Availability

Genetic counseling is often available through facilities that provide maternal-fetal medicine services. State departments of mental health, intellectual disability, and rehabilitation services also may provide counseling services. Local chapters of the March of Dimes are an important source of information about birth defects and counseling services. Fact sheets and other information about birth defects and their prevention are available at the March of Dimes

website: https://www.marchofdimes.com. Organizations that focus on specific birth defects provide valuable support and assistance in obtaining needed services for individuals and families affected by the disorder.

Focus on the Family

Genetic counseling focuses on the family, not merely on the affected individual. One family member may have a birth defect, but study of the entire family is often needed for accurate counseling. This may involve obtaining medical records and performing physical examinations and laboratory studies on numerous family members. Counseling is impaired if family members are unwilling to provide medical records and will not agree to examinations and laboratory studies. In addition, those who seek counseling may be unwilling to request cooperation from other family members or share newly acquired genetic information.

Process of Genetic Counseling

Genetic counseling may be a slow process and is not always straightforward. Several visits spread over months may be needed. Multiple family members may be part of the process. Tests for rare disorders may be performed at only one or a few laboratories in the world, and several weeks may be needed to complete them. Despite a comprehensive evaluation, a diagnosis may never be established. An accurate diagnosis is crucial to provide families with the best information about the risks for a specific birth defect, prognosis for the person affected, and options available to prevent or manage the disorder (Box 4.4). Even if the counseling does not provide clear information, expanding knowledge may allow a definitive diagnosis later, and families are encouraged to contact the center for updates.

Individuals or families may request genetic counseling before or during pregnancy or after a child has been born with a defect. A genetic evaluation may include many factors, such as:

- A complete medical history of the affected person, including prenatal and perinatal history
- The medical history of other family members
- Laboratory, imaging, and other studies
- Physical assessment of a child with the birth defect and other family members, as needed
- Examination of photographs, particularly for family members who are deceased or unavailable
- Construction of a genogram, or pedigree, to identify relationships among family members and their relevant medical history

If a diagnosis is established, genetic counseling educates the family about the following:

- What is known about the cause of the disorder
- The natural course of the disorder
- The likelihood the disorder will occur or recur in other family members
- Current availability of prenatal diagnosis for the disorder
- The ways a couple may be able to avoid having an affected child
- Availability of treatment and services for the person with the disorder

BOX 4.4 Diagnostic Methods That May be Used in Genetic Counseling

Preconception Screening
Family history to identify hereditary patterns of disease or birth defects
Examination of family photographs
Physical examination for obvious or subtle signs of birth defects
Carrier testing
Persons from ethnic groups with a higher incidence of some disorders
Persons with a family history suggesting they may carry a gene for a specific disorder
Chromosomal analysis
DNA analysis

Prenatal Diagnosis for Fetal Abnormalities
Maternal serum tests to screen for abnormalities
Maternal serum analytes (i.e., alpha-fetoprotein)
Noninvasive prenatal screening (NIPS or NIPT)
Analysis of cell-free fetal DNA
Chorionic villus sampling
Amniocentesis
Ultrasonography
Percutaneous umbilical blood sampling

Postnatal Diagnosis for an Infant with a Birth Defect
Physical examination and measurements
Imaging procedures (e.g., ultrasonography, radiography, echocardiography)
Chromosome analysis
DNA analysis
Tests for metabolic disorders (phenylketonuria, cystic fibrosis)
Hemoglobin analysis for disorders such as sickle cell disease
Immunologic testing for infections
Autopsy

Genetic counseling is nondirective. The counselor does not tell the individual or parents what decision to make but educates them about options for dealing with the disorder. Genetic counseling after testing can help the client better understand test results and treatment options, address emotional concerns, and provide referrals to other health care providers and advocacy and support groups (CDC, 2020).

When risks and probabilities are discussed, these numbers should be stated in terms the individual or parents can understand, and their understanding should be verified. A 1-in-100 risk may sound higher to many people than a 1-in-5 risk. However, when the same numbers are framed in terms of percentages, the 1% risk is obviously much lower than the 20% risk.

Supplemental Services

Comprehensive genetic counseling includes services of professionals from many disciplines, such as biology, medicine, nursing, social work, and education. These professionals provide family support and referrals to parent support groups, grief counseling personnel, and intervention for problems that accompany the birth of a child with a birth defect, for example, socioeconomic and family dysfunction.

CLIENT EDUCATION
Birth Defects

1. *How can this birth defect be genetic? No one else in our family has ever had anything like it.*
   Autosomal recessive disorders are carried by parents who themselves are unaffected. The abnormal gene may have been passed down through many generations, but the risk for an affected child is nonexistent until two carrier parents mate.

2. *Isn't the chance this birth defect will happen to another of our children only one in a million?*
   Autosomal recessive disorders have a 25% (1 in 4) chance for recurring in children of the same parents. Autosomal dominant disorders may pose a 50% risk for recurrence unless they resulted from a new mutation in the parental germ cells.

3. *Isn't this birth defect very likely to recur? We'd better not have any more children.*
   Some birth defects are associated with a relatively high risk for recurrence; others have a low risk. Prenatal diagnosis may offer parents a way to avoid having an affected child, or some disorders may be treated before birth. New genetic knowledge may provide therapies not available just a short time ago. Parents' values and perceptions of risks for recurrence affect the final decision.

4. *Because we've already had a child with this birth defect (an autosomal recessive defect), will the next three not have the defect?*
   If both parents are carriers for an autosomal recessive disorder, a 25% (1 in 4) risk exists for their child to be affected that is constant with each conception. The chance their child will neither be affected nor be a carrier is constant with each conception. Each child has a 25% (1 in 4) chance for receiving both copies of the normal gene (unaffected and not a carrier) and a 50% (2 in 4) chance of receiving a single abnormal gene from one parent (a carrier but not affected with the disorder).

5. *If I undergo amniocentesis or another prenatal diagnostic test, can the test detect all birth defects?*
   Although many disorders can be prenatally diagnosed, not all can be diagnosed in the same fetus. Testing is offered for one or more specific disorders after a careful family history is taken to determine appropriate tests.

6. *If the prenatal test results are normal, will my baby be normal?*
   Normal results from prenatal testing exclude those specifically tested disorders. Every healthy couple has approximately a 5% risk of having a child with a birth defect, some of which are not obvious at birth. This baseline risk remains, even if all prenatal test results are normal.

7. *Will I have to have an abortion if my prenatal tests show my baby is abnormal?*
   Abortion may be an option for parents whose fetus is affected with a birth defect, but most parents are reassured by normal test results. If results are abnormal, some parents appreciate the time to prepare for a child with special needs. Better medical management can be planned for a newborn who is expected to have problems. Prenatal diagnosis gives many parents the confidence to have children despite their increased risk for having a child with a birth defect.

Nursing Care of Families Concerned about Birth Defects

Nurses have an important role in helping families concerned about birth defects. Some nurses work directly with family members who are undergoing genetic counseling. Many more nurses are generalists who bring their knowledge about birth defects and their prevention to those they encounter in everyday practice.

Nurses as Part of a Genetic Counseling Team

Many genetic counseling teams include nurses. Genetic nursing may include the following:

- Providing counseling after additional education in this area
- Guiding a client or couple through prenatal diagnosis
- Supporting parents as they make decisions after receiving abnormal prenatal diagnostic results
- Helping the family deal with the emotional impact of a birth defect
- Assisting parents who have had a child with a birth defect to locate needed services and support
- Coordinating services of other professionals such as social workers, physical and occupational therapists, psychologists, and dietitians
- Helping families find appropriate support groups to help them cope with the daily stresses associated with a child who has a birth defect

Nurses in General Practice

Nurses who work in women's health care and those who work in antepartum, intrapartum, newborn, or pediatric settings often encounter families who are concerned about birth defects. These families may include a member with a birth defect. Other families may think they have an increased risk for having a child with a birth defect. Generalist nurses provide care and support that complements that given by nurses who work on a genetic counseling team.

Women's Health Nurses

The nurse who provides care in women's health may encounter families who should be referred for genetic counseling. The ideal time to provide counseling is before conception so the childbearing couple has more options if risks are identified. Personal and family histories are taken and updated during primary care visits, and the nurse may identify factors that could affect a future child before conception. For example, the nurse may identify a client who belongs to a group in which the sickle cell gene is more frequent and subsequently arrange for testing to determine carrier status. If testing reveals the client is a carrier for the gene, that client can be advised that a child could be conceived having sickle cell disease if the partner is also a carrier. If the partner has not been tested, the nurse can arrange for testing. The carrier may want to advise blood relatives of the need for testing.

Antepartum Nurses

Antepartum nurses often identify those who may benefit from genetic counseling. The antepartum nurse also may assist families with decision-making, education about tests, management of abnormal results, and needed emotional support.

THERAPEUTIC COMMUNICATIONS

Assisting a Client Who May Benefit from Genetic Counseling

Paula is a 41-year-old White biologic female who is 8 weeks pregnant with her first child after more than 10 years of infertility. Barbara is a nurse who works with Paula's obstetrician.

Paula: I know all about the risks at my age. I'm not so much worried about my own health as the baby's.

Barbara: You seem to be concerned that the baby might not be all right. (*Clarifying*)

Paula: Sure, who wouldn't be? I know I'm more likely to have a baby with Down's syndrome at my age.

Barbara: Yes, the risks for having an infant with a chromosomal abnormality increase after the mother is 35 years old. Do you plan to have prenatal diagnosis to see if the fetus has this kind of problem? (*Paraphrasing and giving information. Barbara also uses a closed-ended question that tends to block communication because it is usually answered with a simple "yes" or "no."*)

Paula: Oh, yes. I know what's available from surfing the internet, and my doctor has asked me if I want that blood test. When we waited so long to have children, I just assumed I'd have whatever tests were recommended. Now I just don't know.

Barbara: You're reconsidering prenatal testing now? (*Reflecting*)

Paula: Well, not exactly reconsidering. It's just that I've waited so long for a baby, and this may be our only one.

Barbara: [*Waiting quietly but attentively because Paula seems to be thinking.*] (*Using silence*)

Paula: I'm just worried about testing. I know blood tests aren't risky. I also know most prenatal tests have a low risk, but what if I lose a normal baby? It took me so long to finally get pregnant, and I'm running out of time. I might not get another chance.

Barbara: It must be a very difficult decision. (*Reflecting*)

Paula: It is. Even if I have testing and the baby has Down's syndrome, I'm not so sure I'd have an abortion. The outlook for people with Down's syndrome is much better than it used to be. Why have testing if I wouldn't do anything about an abnormal baby?

Barbara: You certainly have some valid concerns. How does your partner feel about testing? (*Questioning using an open-ended question*)

Paula: Oh, Bill is all for it. He keeps reminding me the baby is probably normal and I probably won't have a miscarriage if I have testing. His cousin had a child with Down's syndrome, and Bill doesn't think we should knowingly bring a child with a serious birth defect into the world. What would you do if you were in my place?

Barbara: I can't answer that question because I'm not in your place. Let's review some of the issues so you can make the

Continued

THERAPEUTIC COMMUNICATIONS—cont'd

Assisting a Client Who May Benefit from Genetic Counseling

best decision for yourself and your family. First, you know you have an increased risk for having a baby with a chromosomal defect such as Down's syndrome because of your age. Second, the odds the baby will be normal are higher than the risk the baby will be abnormal. Third, amniocentesis poses a small but real risk for causing a miscarriage. Fourth, you are undecided about whether you would end a pregnancy if the fetus were abnormal. Other issues to consider are time limitations and the option of screening with a sample of your blood. The blood test the doctor told you about is done on your blood 8 to 10 weeks from now. The results of that test may reassure you but they may result in the need to make decisions about more complex testing such as amniocentesis. (*Summarizing*)

Paula: I know. I'm running out of time in more ways than one.

Barbara: If you like, I can set up an appointment with a genetic counselor. The counselor can provide you with the most accurate assessment of your risk for having a child with a birth defect and also the risks of any indicated prenatal diagnosis procedure. Then you can decide whether to have testing.

Paula: I think I'd like that, as long as I don't have to be committed to a particular decision before I go.

BOX 4.5 Indications for Genetic Counseling Referral

Maternal age 35 years of age or older when the infant is born

Paternal age 40 years or older

Members of a group with an increased incidence of a specific disorder

Carriers of autosomal recessive disorders

Females who are carriers of X-linked disorders

Couples related by blood (consanguineous relationship)

Family history of birth defect or intellectual disability

Family history of unexplained stillbirth

Clients who experience multiple spontaneous abortions

Pregnant clients exposed to known or suspected teratogens or other harmful agents either before or during pregnancy

Pregnant clients with abnormal prenatal screening results such as multiple-marker screen or suspicious ultrasound findings

---

BOX 4.6 Examples of Problems in Genetic Counseling and Prenatal Diagnosis

Inadequate medical records

Uncertain gestational age or inadequate prenatal care

Family members' refusal to share information

Records that are incomplete, vague, or uninformative

Inconclusive testing

Too few family members available when family studies are needed

Inadequate number of live fetal cells obtained during amniocentesis

Failure of fetal cells to grow in culture if other testing techniques are not useful

Ambiguous prenatal test results that are neither clearly normal nor clearly abnormal

Unexpected results from prenatal diagnosis

Finding an abnormality other than the one for which the person was tested

Nonpaternity revealed with testing

Inability to determine the severity of a prenatally diagnosed disorder

Inability to rule out all birth defects

Client misunderstanding of the mathematical risk as it is presented

---

Identifying Families for Referral. Nurses in antepartum settings often identify a client or family for whom referral for genetic counseling is appropriate at the first prenatal visit (Box 4.5). The personal and family history of the client and partner may disclose factors that increase their risks for having a child with a birth defect. In addition to the usual medical history about disorders such as hypertension and diabetes, the client should be questioned about a family history of birth defects, diseases that seem to "run in the family," intellectual disability, and developmental delay.

Some people are reluctant to disclose that they have a family member with intellectual disability or a birth defect. The nurse can gently probe for sensitive information by asking questions about whether any family members have learning differences. The use of words that are lay-oriented and caring often elicits more information than clinical terms that may seem harsh, for example, "low IQ."

Helping the Family Decide about Genetic Counseling. If genetic counseling is appropriate, the physician or nurse–midwife discusses it with the client and refers the family to an appropriate center. However, the final decision rests with the person affected. The nurse can help the client and family weigh issues that are important to them as they decide.

Genetic counseling can raise uncomfortable issues such as whether to undergo prenatal diagnosis, what to do if a condition cannot be prenatally diagnosed, and what options are acceptable if prenatal diagnosis shows abnormal results. Counseling may open family conflicts if information from other family members is needed or if family values differ on issues such as abortion of an abnormal fetus. In addition, the tests can show unexpected results (Box 4.6).

Teaching about Lifestyle. Nurses can teach a pregnant client about harmful lifestyle factors that can be modified to reduce the risk for defects to offspring. The nurse can support the client in making difficult lifestyle changes such as stopping alcohol consumption, reducing or eliminating smoking, and improving the diet. Use of liberal praise can motivate a client to continue efforts to promote an optimal outcome. However, a negative attitude from nurses or other professionals may make the client feel like a failure, and the client may abandon efforts to create a healthier lifestyle.

Providing Emotional Support. Until they know prenatal test results are normal, possibly a period spanning several days or weeks, many clients delay telling friends or family about their pregnancy or investing in it emotionally. When results are abnormal, clients face more difficult decisions about whether to terminate or continue the pregnancy.

Helping the Family Deal with Abnormal Results. Because prenatal diagnostic tests are performed to detect disorders involving serious physical and often mental defects, the client whose test results are abnormal must confront painful decisions. For many of these disorders, no effective prenatal or postnatal treatment exists. Only two choices may be available: continuing or terminating the pregnancy. In addition, the decision to terminate a pregnancy must be made in a short time. Making no decision is effectively a decision to continue the pregnancy. Although the physician or genetic counselor discusses abnormal results and available options, the nurse reinforces the information given to these anxious families and supports them.

When test results are abnormal, nurses should expect the couple to grieve. Even if a pregnancy was unplanned, the client who undergoes prenatal diagnosis has already made the initial decision to continue the pregnancy. If results are abnormal, the client must decide again whether to continue or end the pregnancy. Both parents will experience similar feelings of grief and loss when an abnormal diagnosis is detected prenatally.

Intrapartum and Neonatal Nurses

Nurses working in intrapartum and neonatal settings encounter families who have given birth to an infant with a birth defect that may have been unexpected. Stillborn infants sometimes have birth defects that contributed to their intrauterine death. In addition to the loss of their baby, these parents face pain because of the associated abnormality. An autopsy may be performed to document all anomalies and establish the most accurate diagnosis of the birth defect for future counseling. Nursing care for families who experience a perinatal loss, whether a result of the infant's death or the loss of the expected normal infant, is addressed in Chapter 11.

Nurses who care for these families in the intrapartum and neonatal settings will find the parents anxious, depressed, and sometimes hostile because of the unexpected event. The family's usual coping mechanisms may be inadequate for the situation, or new coping mechanisms may not have been developed. Diagnostic studies are often recommended soon after the birth of an infant with an abnormality to establish a diagnosis and give parents accurate information about the abnormality and the options available to them. However, a high anxiety level reduces their ability to understand the often massive amount of information received. The nurse is in a position to evaluate the family's perception of the problem, help them understand the diagnostic tests, reinforce correct information, and correct misunderstandings. In addition, the nurse is often most therapeutic by simply being an available, active listener, helping ease the family's pain over the event.

Nurses should encourage families to contact lay support groups, which are significant sources of support because members fully understand the daily problems encountered in the care of a child with a birth defect. Such groups can help the parents manage the stress and chronic grief associated with prolonged care of these children. Support groups also can help the parents see the positive aspects and victories when caring for their child with special needs. Internet sites regarding specific birth defects are often available to offer parent education and support.

Pediatric Nurses

Children with birth defects typically have numerous recurrent medical problems. They usually are hospitalized more often and for longer periods than children without birth defects. Travel to specialized hospitals may be needed for their care, adding to the family's stress. These families often incur substantial expenses for medical care and equipment not covered by insurance or public assistance programs. Transportation costs to reach distant health care facilities may be difficult to pay. Household income may be lost because one parent stops working to care for the child.

Family dysfunction is common, and the strain of caring for a child with a serious birth defect may lead to divorce. Siblings often feel left out of their parents' attention because the needs of this child demand so much of their parents' time.

The nurse case manager can reduce the family's stress by helping them locate appropriate support services. The nurse can contact social services departments to help the family find financial and other resources needed to care for the child. If parents have not connected with a lay support group, a nurse can encourage them to do so.

▌ SUMMARY CONCEPTS

- The 46 human chromosomes are long strands of DNA, each containing up to several thousand individual genes.
- With the exception of those genes located on the X and Y chromosomes in males, genes are inherited in pairs that may be identical or different. Some genes are dominant and some are recessive.
- Many genes can be analyzed by the products they produce, their DNA, or their close association with another gene that is more easily analyzed.

- Cells for chromosome analysis must be living cells. Specimens should be handled carefully to preserve viability if analysis of dividing cells in the metaphase of cell division is necessary. Other techniques, such as FISH, permit study of cells without requiring active cell division, allowing rapid test results.
- Chromosome abnormalities are either numerical, with the addition or deletion of an entire chromosome or chromosomes, or structural, with deletion, addition, rearrangement, or fragility of the chromosome material.

- Single gene disorders are associated with a fixed risk for occurrence or recurrence. The type of single gene abnormality (autosomal dominant, autosomal recessive, or X-linked) determines the risk.
- Multifactorial disorders occur because of a genetic predisposition combined with environmental factors.
- The risk for occurrence or recurrence of multifactorial disorders is not fixed, but varies according to the number of close relatives affected, severity of the defect in affected persons, sex of the affected person, and geographic location.
- Relatively few agents that can enter the fetal environment are known to be definitely teratogenic or definitely safe.
- The risk for fetal damage from environmental agents can be decreased by reducing exposure to the agent or manipulating the fetal environment.
- The purpose of genetic counseling is to educate individuals or families with accurate information so they can make informed decisions about reproduction and appropriate care for affected members.
- The nurse cares for people with concerns about birth defects by identifying those needing referral, teaching, and coordinating services and offering emotional support.

REFERENCES & READINGS

American College of Obstetricians and Gynecologists (ACOG). (2017). *Guidelines for diagnostic imaging during pregnancy and lactation. (ACOG Committee Opinion No. 723).*

American College of Obstetricians and Gynecologists (ACOG). (2020). *Carrier screening in the age of genomic medicine. (ACOG Committee Opinion No. 690).* https://www.acog.org/clinical/clinical-guidance/committee-opinion/articles/2017/03/carrier-screening-in-the-age-of-genomic-medicine.

Centers for Disease Control and Prevention (CDC). (2020). *Genetic counseling.* https://www.cdc.gov/genomics/gtesting/genetic_counseling.htm.

Centers for Disease Control and Prevention (CDC). (2021). *Folic acid.* https://www.cdc.gov/ncbddd/folicacid/index.html.

Driscoll, D. A., & Simpson, J. L. (2021). Genetic screening and diagnosis. In M. B. Landon, H. L. Galan, E. R. M. Jauniaux, D. A. Driscoll, V. Berghella, W. A. Grobman, et al. (Eds.), *Gabbe's obstetrics* (8th ed., pp. 180–201). Elsevier.

Gravholt, C. H., Chang, S., Wallentin, J. F., Moore, P., & Skakkebaek, A. (2018). Klinefelter syndrome: Integrating genetics, neuropsychology, and endocrinology. *Endocrine Reviews, 39*(4), 389–423.

Mayo Clinic. (2017). *Turner syndrome.* https://www.mayoclinic.org/diseases-conditions/turner-syndrome/symptoms-causes/syc-20360782#:~:text=Turner%20syndrome%2C%20a%20condition%20that,to%20develop%20and%20heart%20defects.

MotherToBaby. (2019). *Hyperthermia.* https://mothertobaby.org/fact-sheets/hyperthermia-pregnancy/.

National Human Genome Research Institute (NHGRI). (2020). *Genetic discrimination.* https://www.genome.gov/about-genomics/policy-issues/Genetic-Discrimination#:~:text=Other%20Laws-,Genetic%20Information%20Nondiscrimination%20Act%20of%202008,and%20employment%20(Title%20II).

National Human Genome Research Institute (NHGRI). (2021a). *Educational resources: Gene regulation.* https://www.genome.gov/genetics-glossary/Gene-Regulation.

National Human Genome Research Institute (NHGRI). (2021b). *Educational resources; sex linked traits.* https://www.genome.gov/genetics-glossary/Sex-Linked.

National Human Genome Research Institute (NHGRI). (2021c). *Educational resources: Autosomal dominant.* https://www.genome.gov/genetics-glossary/Autosomal-Dominant.

National Human Genome Research Institute (NHGRI). (2021d). *Educational resources: fragile x syndrome.* https://www.genome.gov/genetics-glossary/Fragile-X-Syndrome.

National Tay-Sachs and Allied Diseases Association (NTSAD). (2021). *Tay-Sachs disease.* https://www.ntsad.org/index.php/the-diseases/tay-sachs.

Singh, A. P., & Gorla, S. R. (2020). Amniotic band syndrome. In *StatPearls.* StatPearls Publishing. https://pubmed.ncbi.nlm.nih.gov/31424867/.

U.S Food and Drug Administration. (2021). *Pregnancy and lactation labeling (Drugs) final rule.* https://www.fda.gov/drugs/labeling-information-drug-products/pregnancy-and-lactation-labeling-drugs-final-rule.

5

Conception and Prenatal Development

Jennifer Rodriguez

After studying this chapter, you should be able to:
1. Describe formation of the female and male gametes.
2. Explain the process of human conception.
3. Explain implantation and nourishment of the embryo before development of the placenta.
4. Describe normal prenatal development from conception through birth.
5. Explain structure and function of the placenta, the umbilical cord, and fetal membranes with amniotic fluid.
6. Describe prenatal circulation and the circulatory changes after birth.
7. Explain the mechanisms and trends in multifetal pregnancies.

THE FAMILY BEFORE BIRTH

A basic understanding of conception and prenatal development helps the nurse provide care to parents during normal childbearing and better understand problems such as infertility and birth defects. This chapter addresses formation of the gametes and the process of conception, prenatal development, and important auxiliary structures that support normal prenatal development. The reason for the occurrence of multifetal pregnancy (e.g., twinning) is also discussed.

GAMETOGENESIS

Gametogenesis is the development of ova in the female and sperm in the male (Table 5.1). Production of **gametes** (reproductive or germ cells) requires a process different from formation of **somatic cells** or other body cells. Somatic cells reproduce by a process called *mitosis*. Each somatic cell has 46 paired chromosomes: 22 pairs of **autosomes** (non-sex chromosomes) and 1 pair of **sex chromosomes** (X or Y chromosomes). During mitosis, the cell divides into two new cells, each having 46 chromosomes like the parent cell.

Gametogenesis requires a special reduction division called *meiosis*. Unlike **mitosis**, in which the **diploid** number (46) of chromosomes is retained in the new cells, **meiosis** halves the number of chromosomes to arrive at the **haploid** number of 23. Only 1 of each chromosome pair (22 autosomes and 1 sex chromosome) is directed to the gamete. In addition, with the exception of the X and Y chromosomes in males, each chromosome exchanges some material with its mate so the new

chromosome in the gamete contains some material from the female parent and some from the male parent. This process, which is called *crossing over,* allows variation in genetic material while keeping constant the total amount of chromosome material from generation to generation. When the sperm and ovum unite at conception, the "halves" form a new cell and restore the chromosome number to 46.

Oogenesis

Oogenesis is the formation of female gametes (Fig. 5.1A) within the ovary. Oogenesis begins during prenatal life when primitive ova (oogonia) multiply by mitosis. Each oogonium contains 46 chromosomes. Before birth, these oogonia enlarge to form primary oocytes, each surrounded by a layer of follicular cells. These are called *primary follicles.* The primary oogonium begins its first meiotic division during fetal life but does not complete the process until puberty. The primary follicle and its oogonium, which still contains 46 chromosomes, remain dormant throughout childhood.

By the 30th week of gestation, female fetuses have all the ova they will ever have. Many of these ova regress during childhood. When a female's reproductive cycles begin at puberty, some of the primary follicles present at birth begin maturing. The process of gamete maturation continues throughout the reproductive years until the climacteric. When the oocyte matures, two meiotic divisions reduce the chromosome number from 46 paired chromosomes to 23 unpaired chromosomes: 22 autosomes and 1 X chromosome. Shortly before **ovulation**, or release of the mature ovum from the ovary, the primary oocyte completes its first meiotic division, which began during fetal life. The result is

TABLE 5.1 Comparison of Female and Male Gametogenesis

	Oogenesis	Spermatogenesis
Time during which primary germ cells are produced	Fetal life; no others develop after ~ 30 wk of gestation	Continuously after puberty
Hormones that control process	• GnRH • FSH • LH • Estrogen	• GnRH • FSH • LH • Testosterone • Estrogen (small amounts converted from testosterone) • Growth hormone
Number of mature germ cells that develop from each primary cell	One	Four
Quantity	One during each reproductive cycle of about 28 days	~35–200 million released with each ejaculation
Size	Large; visible to naked eye; abundant cytoplasm to nourish embryo until implantation	Tiny compared with ovum; little cytoplasm; head is almost all nuclear material (chromosomes)
Motility	Relatively nonmotile; transported by action of cilia and currents within fallopian tubes	Independently motile by means of whip-like tail; mitochondria in middle piece provide energy for motility
Chromosome complement	23 total: 22 autosomes plus 1 X sex chromosome	23 total: 22 autosomes, plus either an X or a Y sex chromosome

FSH, Follicle-stimulating hormone; *GnRH,* gonadotropin-releasing hormone; *LH,* luteinizing hormone.

a secondary oocyte containing 23 chromosomes. The primary cell's cytoplasm is divided unequally with this division, and most of it is retained by the secondary oocyte. The remainder of cytoplasm plus the other half of the chromosomes go into a tiny, nonfunctional polar body that soon degenerates.

At ovulation, the secondary oocyte begins to form a mature ovum (second meiotic division). Each of the 23 chromosomes divides without replication of the deoxyribonucleic acid (DNA). The second meiotic division is prolonged, and the mature ovum remains suspended in metaphase, the middle part of cell division. If fertilization occurs, the second meiotic division is completed, resulting in a mature ovum with 23 chromosomes and a second tiny polar body containing the 23 discarded chromosomes that degenerate. If the ovum is not fertilized, it does not complete the second meiotic division and degenerates. In oogenesis, one primary oocyte results in a single mature ovum.

When the mature ovum is released from the ovary, it is surrounded by two layers: the zona pellucida and the cells of the corona radiata. These layers protect the ovum and prevent fertilization by more than one sperm. For fertilization to occur, the sperm must penetrate these two layers to reach the ovum's cell nucleus.

Spermatogenesis

Spermatogenesis (formation of sperm, or male gametes, in the testes; see Fig. 5.1B) begins during puberty in the male and requires approximately 70 days to be completed. Primitive sperm cells, or spermatogonia, develop during the prenatal period and begin multiplying by mitosis during puberty. Unlike the female, the male continues to produce new spermatogonia that can mature into sperm throughout his lifetime. Although male fertility gradually declines with age, they can father children in their fifties, sixties, and beyond.

Each spermatogonium contains 46 paired chromosomes. In the mature male, a spermatogonium enlarges to become a primary spermatocyte containing all 46 chromosomes. The first meiotic division forms two secondary spermatocytes and reduces the number to 23 unpaired chromosomes in each gamete: 22 autosomes and 1 X or Y sex chromosome in each spermatocyte. Each chromosome of the secondary spermatocyte divides to retain 23 chromosomes in the second meiotic division, forming two spermatids. Therefore 50% of the four spermatids resulting from the two meiotic divisions of the spermatogonium carry an X chromosome and 50% carry a Y chromosome. The spermatids gradually evolve into mature sperm.

The gamete from a male determines the genetic sex of the new baby because the ovum carries only an X chromosome. Each mature sperm contains 23 chromosomes: 22 autosomes and either an X or a Y chromosome. If an X-bearing spermatozoon fertilizes the ovum, the baby is genetically female. If a Y-bearing spermatozoon fertilizes the ovum, the baby is genetically male.

The mature sperm has three major sections: a head, middle portion, and tail (Fig. 5.2). The head is almost entirely a cell nucleus and contains the male chromosomes that join the chromosomes of the ovum. The middle portion supplies energy for the tail's whip-like action. The movement of the tail propels the sperm toward the ovum.

? KNOWLEDGE CHECK

1. What is the purpose of meiosis in the gametes?
2. How many mature ova can be produced by each oogonium? When does meiosis occur in the female?
3. How many mature spermatozoa can be produced by each spermatogonium? When does meiosis occur in the male?

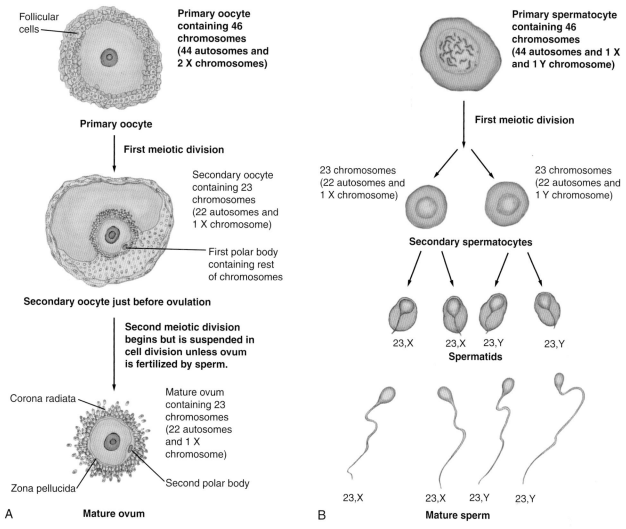

FIG. 5.1 Gametogenesis. A, Formation of the mature ovum. B, Formation of mature sperm.

CONCEPTION

Natural conception is the interaction of many factors, including correct timing between release of a mature ovum at ovulation and **ejaculation** (semen expulsion) of enough healthy, mature, motile sperm into the vagina. Although exact viability is unknown, the ovum may survive no longer than 24 hours after its release at ovulation. Most sperm survive no more than 24 hours in the female reproductive tract, although a few may remain fertile in the female's reproductive tract for up to 80 hours (Blackburn, 2018; Hall & Hall, 2021).

Preparation for Conception in the Female

Before ovulation, several oocytes begin to mature under the influence of follicle-stimulating hormone (FSH) and luteinizing hormone (LH) from the female's anterior pituitary gland. Each maturing oocyte is contained within a sac called the **graafian follicle**, which produces estrogen and progesterone to prepare the **endometrium** (uterine lining) for a possible pregnancy. Eventually, one follicle outgrows the others. The less mature oocytes permanently regress.

Release of the Ovum

Ovulation occurs approximately 14 days before the next menstrual period would begin. The follicle develops a weak spot on the surface of the ovary and ruptures, releasing the mature ovum with its surrounding cells onto the surface of the ovary. The collapsed follicle is transformed into the **corpus luteum**, which maintains high estrogen and progesterone secretion necessary to make final preparation of the uterine lining for a fertilized ovum.

Ovum Transport

The mature ovum is released on the surface of the ovary, where it is picked up by the fimbriated (fringed) ends of the fallopian tube. The ovum is transported through the tube by the muscular action of the tube and movement of cilia within the tube. Fertilization normally occurs in the distal third of the fallopian tube (ampulla) near the ovary. The ovum, fertilized or not, enters the uterus approximately 4 days after its release from the ovary.

Preparation for Conception in the Male

The male preparation for fertilizing the ovum consists of ejaculation, movement of the sperm in the female reproductive tract, and preparation of the sperm for actual fertilization.

Ejaculation

When a male ejaculates during sexual intercourse, 35 to 200 million sperm are deposited in the upper vagina and over the cervix (Blackburn, 2018; Hall & Hall, 2021). The sperm are suspended in 2 to 5 milliliters (mL) of seminal fluid, which nourishes and protects the sperm from the acidic environment of the vagina (Blackburn, 2018; Hall & Hall, 2021). Many sperm are lost as the ejaculate drips from the vaginal introitus. Other sperm are inactivated by acidic vaginal secretions or digested by vaginal enzymes and phagocytes. The seminal fluid coagulates slightly after ejaculation to hold the semen deeply in the vagina. Many sperm are relatively immobile for approximately 15 to 30 minutes until other seminal enzymes dissolve the coagulated fluid and allow the sperm to begin moving upward through the cervix.

Transport of Sperm in the Female Reproductive Tract

The whip-like movement of the tails of spermatozoa propels them through the cervix, uterus, and fallopian tubes. Uterine contractions induced by prostaglandins in the seminal fluid enhance movement of the sperm toward the ovum. Only sperm cells enter the cervix. The seminal fluid remains in the vagina.

Many sperm are lost along the way. Some are digested by enzymes and phagocytes in the female reproductive tract, whereas others simply lose their direction, moving into the wrong tube or past the ovum and out into the peritoneal cavity.

Preparation of Sperm for Fertilization

Sperm are not immediately ready to fertilize the ovum when they are ejaculated. During the trip to the ovum, the sperm undergo changes enabling one of them to penetrate the protective layers surrounding the ovum, a process called *capacitation*. During capacitation, a glycoprotein coat and seminal proteins are removed from the acrosome, which is the tip of the sperm head. After capacitation, the sperm look the same but are more active and can better penetrate the corona radiata and zona pellucida surrounding the ovum.

Sperm must also undergo an acrosome reaction to further prepare them to fertilize the ovum. The sperm that reach the ovum release hyaluronidase and acrosin to digest a pathway through the corona radiata and zona pellucida. Their tails beat harder to propel them toward the center of the ovum. Eventually, one spermatozoon penetrates the ovum.

Fertilization

Fertilization occurs when one spermatozoon enters the ovum and the two nuclei containing the parents' chromosomes merge (Fig. 5.3).

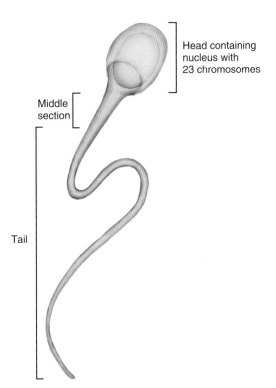

Head containing nucleus with 23 chromosomes

Middle section

Tail

FIG. 5.2 Mature sperm.

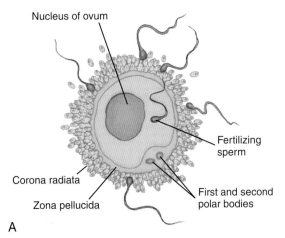

Nucleus of ovum

Corona radiata

Zona pellucida

Fertilizing sperm

First and second polar bodies

A

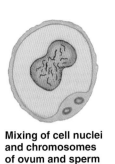

Mixing of cell nuclei and chromosomes of ovum and sperm

B

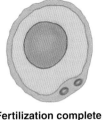

Fertilization complete

C

FIG. 5.3 Process of Fertilization. **A,** A sperm enters the ovum. **B,** The 23 chromosomes from the sperm mingle with the 23 chromosomes from the ovum, restoring the diploid number to 46. **C,** The fertilized ovum is now called a *zygote* and is ready for the first mitotic cell division.

Entry of One Spermatozoon into the Ovum

Entry of a spermatozoon into the ovum has three results. First is the zona reaction, in which changes in the zona pellucida surrounding the ovum prevent other sperm from entering. Second, the cell membranes of the ovum and sperm fuse and break down, allowing the contents of the sperm head to enter the cytoplasm of the ovum. Third, the ovum, which has been suspended in the middle of its second meiotic division since just before ovulation, completes meiosis. This results in a nucleus with 23 chromosomes and the expulsion of a second nonfunctional polar body. The mature ovum now contains 23 unpaired chromosomes (22 autosomes and 1 X chromosome) in its nucleus.

Fusion of the Nuclei of Sperm and Ovum

Once a spermatozoon has penetrated the ovum, fusion of their nuclei begins. The sperm head enlarges, and the tail degenerates. The nuclei of the gametes move toward the center of the ovum, where the membranes surrounding their nuclei touch and dissolve. The 23 chromosomes from the sperm mingle with the 23 from the ovum, restoring the diploid number to 46. Fertilization is complete, and cell division can begin when the nuclei of the sperm and ovum unite.

KNOWLEDGE CHECK

4. Where does fertilization usually occur?
5. What are the functions of the seminal fluid?
6. What occurs when a spermatozoon penetrates the ovum?
7. When is fertilization complete and a new human conceived?

PREEMBRYONIC PERIOD

The preembryonic period is the first 2 weeks after conception (Fig. 5.4). Around the fourth day after conception, the fertilized ovum, now called a **zygote**, enters the uterus.

Initiation of Cell Division

The zygote divides into 2, then 4, then 8 cells, and so on until the 16-cell stage. The cells become tightly compacted with each division, so they occupy about the same amount of space as the original zygote. When the **conceptus** (cells and membranes resulting from fertilization of the ovum) is a solid ball of 16 cells, it is called a **morula** because it resembles a mulberry.

The outer cells of the morula secrete fluid, forming a *blastocyst,* a sac of cells with an inner cell mass placed off center within the sac. The inner cell mass develops into the **fetus**. Part of the outer layer of cells develops the fetal membranes and the **placenta**, or the fetal structure that provides nourishment, removes wastes, and secretes necessary hormones for continuation of the pregnancy.

Entry of the Zygote into the Uterus

When the blastocyst contains approximately 100 cells, it enters the uterus. It lingers in the uterus another 2 to 4 days before beginning implantation. The endometrium, now called the *decidua,* is in the secretory phase of the reproductive cycle, 1½ weeks before the next menstrual period would otherwise begin. The endometrial glands are secreting at their maximum, providing rich fluids to nourish the conceptus before placental circulation is established. The endometrial spiral arteries are well developed in the secretory phase, providing easy access for the development of the placental blood supply.

Implantation in the Decidua

The conceptus carries a small supply of nutrients for early cell division. Nevertheless, implantation at the proper time and location in the uterus is critical for continued development. Implantation, or **nidation**, is a gradual process that occurs between days 6 and 10 after conception. During the relatively long process of implantation, embryonic structures continue to develop.

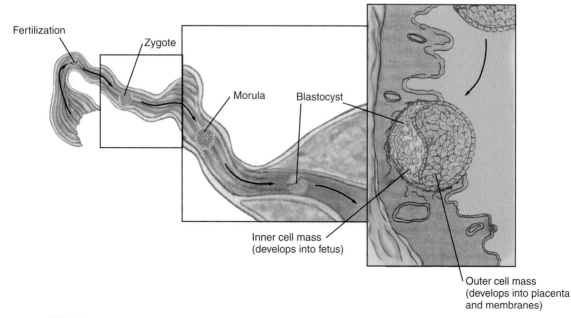

FIG. 5.4 Prenatal Development from Fertilization through Implantation of the Blastocyst. Implantation gradually occurs from day 6 through day 10. Implantation is complete on day 10.

Maintaining the Decidua

Implantation and survival of the conceptus require a continuing supply of estrogen and progesterone to maintain the decidua in the secretory phase. The zygote secretes human chorionic gonadotropin (hCG), which causes the corpus luteum to persist and continue secretion of estrogen and progesterone until the placenta takes over this function.

Location of Implantation

The conceptus must be in the right place at the right time for normal implantation to occur. The site of implantation is important because it is where the placenta develops. Normal implantation occurs in the upper uterus, slightly more often on the posterior wall than the anterior wall (Moore et al., 2021). The upper uterus is the best area for implantation and placental development for three reasons:

- The upper uterus is richly supplied with blood for optimal fetal gas exchange, nutrition, and waste elimination.
- The uterine lining is thick in the upper uterus, preventing the placenta from attaching too deeply into the uterine muscle and facilitating easy expulsion of the placenta after full-term birth.
- Implantation in the upper uterus limits blood loss after birth because strong interlacing muscle fibers in this area compress open endometrial vessels after the placenta detaches.

Mechanism of Implantation

Enzymes produced by the conceptus erode the decidua, tapping maternal sources of nutrition. Primary chorionic villi are tiny projections on the surface of the conceptus extending into the endometrium, now called the *decidua basalis,* which lies between the conceptus and the wall of the uterus. The chorionic villi eventually form the fetal side of the placenta. The decidua basalis forms the maternal side of the placenta (see Fig. 5.7A).

At this early stage, nutritive fluid passes to the embryo by *diffusion* (the passive movement across a cell membrane from an area of higher concentration to one of lower concentration) because the circulatory system is not yet established. The conceptus is fully embedded within the uterine decidua by 10 days, and the site of implantation is almost invisible.

As the conceptus implants, usually near the time of the next expected menstrual period, a small amount of bleeding ("spotting") may occur at the site. Implantation bleeding may be confused with a normal menstrual period, particularly if the menstrual periods are usually light.

KNOWLEDGE CHECK

8. When does implantation occur?
9. What are the advantages of implantation in the upper uterus?
10. How is the embryo nourished before the placenta develops?

EMBRYONIC PERIOD

The embryonic period of development extends from the beginning of the third week through the eighth week after conception (Fig. 5.5). Basic structures of all major body organs are completed during the embryonic period (Table 5.2).

Differentiation of Cells

The **embryo** (developing baby from the beginning of the third week through the eighth week after conception) progresses from undifferentiated cells with essentially identical functions to differentiated, or specialized, body cells. By the end of the eighth week, all major organ systems are in place, and many are functioning, although in a simple way.

Development of the specialized structures is controlled by three factors: (1) genetic information in the chromosomes received from the parents, (2) interaction between adjacent tissues, and (3) timing. Although basic instructions are carried within the chromosomes, one tissue may induce change toward greater specialization in another, but only if a signal between the two tissues occurs at a specific time during development. In this way, structures develop with appropriate sizes and relationships to each other.

During the embryonic period, structures are vulnerable to damage from **teratogens** because these structures are developing rapidly. Normal development of one structure often requires normal and properly timed development of another structure. Unfortunately, the client may not be aware of the pregnancy during this sensitive time. For this reason, the possibility of pregnancy should be explored before the prescription of drugs or administration of diagnostic procedures such as radiography. Some agents may be damaging at one time during pregnancy but not at another. Others may be damaging at any time during pregnancy.

Weekly Developments

Development occurs simultaneously in all embryonic organ systems. Prenatal development proceeds in patterns that continue after birth:

- Cephalocaudal (head to toe)
- Central to peripheral direction (from center outward)
- Simple to complex (early cells may become any cell of the body before they become specialized into specific structures with specific functions)
- General to specific (upper extremities begin as limb buds before detailed development of bones, joints, muscles, ligaments, and fingers)

Full-term ranges from 36 to 40 weeks of **fertilization age** calculated from date of conception or 38 to 42 weeks of **gestational age** (after last menstrual period). Because conception occurs approximately 2 weeks after the first day of the last menstrual period in a 28-day menstrual cycle, the fertilization age used in this chapter is approximately 2 weeks shorter than the gestational age. Nevertheless, gestational age is most commonly used in practice because the last menstrual period provides a known marker, whereas the date of conception

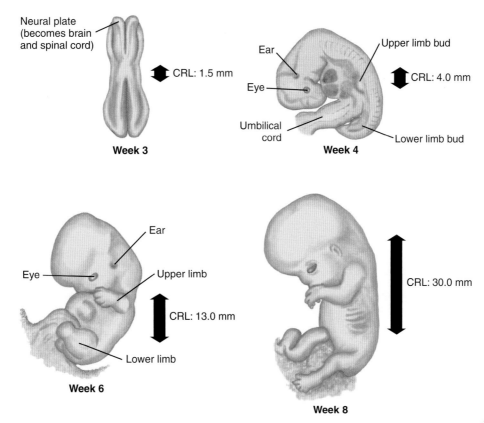

FIG. 5.5 Embryonic Development from Week 3 Through Week 8 After Fertilization. A, Week 3. B, Week 4. C, Week 6. D, Week 8. *CRL,* Crown–rump length.

may be unknown. Ultrasonography provides added information to identify the most accurate fetal age (see Chapter 9).

Week 2

Implantation is complete by the end of the second week after fertilization. The most growth occurs in the outer cells, or trophoblast, which eventually become the fetal part of the placenta. The inner cell mass becomes flattened into the embryonic disc and will later develop into the baby. Cells that eventually form part of the fetal membranes develop.

Week 3

For many, the first menstrual period is missed during the third week after conception. The embryonic disc develops three layers, called *germ layers,* which, in turn, give rise to major organ systems of the body (Table 5.3). The three germ layers are the ectoderm, the mesoderm, and the endoderm.

The central nervous system (CNS) begins developing during the third week. A thickened, flat neural plate appears, extending toward the cephalic end of the embryonic disc. The neural plate develops a longitudinal groove that folds to form the neural tube. At the end of the third week, the neural tube is fused in the middle but still open at each end.

Early heart development consists of a pair of parallel heart tubes that fuse longitudinally. The primitive, or tubular, heart begins beating at 22 to 23 days, resulting in a wave-like flow of blood. By the end of the fourth week, coordinated contractions result in the unidirectional flow of blood characteristic

of the mature heart. Vessels developing in the chorionic villi and membranes join the heart tube. Primitive blood cells arise from the endoderm lining the distal blood vessels.

Week 4

The shape of the embryo changes during the fourth week after conception. It folds at the head and tail end and laterally, resembling a C-shaped cylinder. A "tail" is apparent during the embryonic period because the brain and spinal cord develop more rapidly than other systems. The tail disappears as the rest of the body catches up with growth of the CNS. The neural tube closes during the fourth week. If the neural tube does not close, defects such as anencephaly and spina bifida result.

Formation of the face and upper respiratory tract begins. Beginnings of the internal ear and the eye are apparent. The upper extremities appear as buds on the lateral body walls. Because the embryo is sharply flexed anteriorly, the heart is near the embryo's mouth. Partitioning of the heart into four chambers begins during the fourth week and is completed by the end of the sixth week.

The lower respiratory tract begins growth as a branch of the upper digestive tract, which is a simple tube at this time. Gradually, the esophagus and trachea complete separation. The trachea branches to form the right and left bronchi. These bronchi, in turn, branch to form the three lobes of the right lung and two lobes of the left lung. Continued branching of the bronchi eventually forms the terminal air sacs, or alveoli.

TABLE 5.2   Timetable of Prenatal Development Based on Fertilization Age[a]

Nervous/Sensory System	Cardiorespiratory System	Digestive System	Genitourinary System	Musculoskeletal System	Integumentary System
3 Weeks: 1.5-mm CRL					
• Flat neural plate begins closing to form neural tube. • Neural tube still open at each end.	• Heart consists of two parallel tubes that fuse into a single tube. • Contractions of heart tube begin. • Chorionic villi of early placenta connect with heart.	• Endoderm (inner germ layer) will become digestive tract.		• Paired, cube-shaped swellings (somites) appear and will form most of head and trunk skeleton. • Muscle, bone, and cartilage develop from mesoderm.	• Epidermis (outer skin layer) will develop from ectoderm (outer germ layer). • Dermis (deep skin layer) and connective tissue will develop from mesoderm (middle germ layer).
4 Weeks: 4-mm CRL					
• Neural tube closed at each end. • Cranial end of neural tube will form brain; caudal end will form spinal cord. • Eye development begins as an outgrowth of forebrain. • Nose development begins as two pits. • Inner ear begins developing from hindbrain.	• Heart begins partitioning into four chambers and begins beating. • Blood circulating through embryonic vessels and chorionic villi. • Tracheal development begins as a bud on upper gut and branches into two bronchial buds.	• Development of primitive gut as embryo folds laterally. • Stomach begins as a widening of tube-shaped primitive gut. • Liver, gallbladder, and biliary ducts begin as a bud from primitive gut.	• Primordial germ (reproductive) cells are present on embryonic yolk sac.	• Upper limb buds are present and look like flippers. • Lower limb buds appear.	• Mammary ridges that will develop into mammary glands appear.
6 Weeks: 13-mm CRL					
• Development of pituitary gland and cranial nerves. • Head sharply flexed because of rapid brain growth. • Eyelid development beginning. • External ear development begins in neck region as six swellings.	• Blood formation primarily in liver. • Three right and two left lung lobes develop as outgrowths of right and left bronchi. • Partitioning of heart into four chambers completed.	• Most intestines are contained within the umbilical cord because liver and kidneys occupy most of abdominal cavity. • Stomach nearing final form. • Development of upper and lower jaws.	• Kidneys are near bladder in pelvis. • Kidneys occupy much of abdominal cavity. • Primordial germ cells incorporated into developing gonads. • Male and female gonads are identical in appearance.	• Arms are paddle-shaped, and fingers are webbed. • Feet and toes develop similarly, but a few days later than arms and hands. • Bones cartilaginous, but ossification of skull begins.	• Mammary glands begin development. • Tooth buds for primary (deciduous) teeth begin developing.
8 Weeks: 30-mm CRL					
• Spinal cord stops at end of vertebral column. • Taste buds begin developing. • Eyelids fuse. • Ears have final form but are low-set.	• Heart partitioned into four chambers. • Heartbeat detectable with ultrasound. • Additional branching of bronchi.	• Stomach has reached final form. • Lips are fused. • Intestines remain in umbilical cord.	• Testes begin developing under influence of Y chromosome. • Ovaries will develop if a Y chromosome is not present. • External genitalia begin to differentiate but still appear quite similar.	• Fingers and toes still webbed but distinct by end of week 8. • Bones begin to ossify. • Joints resemble those of adults.	• Auricles of ear low-set but beginning to assume final shape.

TABLE 5.2	Timetable of Prenatal Development Based on Fertilization Age[a]—cont'd				
Nervous/Sensory System	Cardiorespiratory System	Digestive System	Genitourinary System	Musculoskeletal System	Integumentary System
10 Weeks: 61-mm CRL; weight, 14 g					
• Head flexion still present, but straighter. • Eyelids closed and fused. • Top of external ear slightly below eye level.	• May be possible to detect heartbeat with Doppler transducer. • Blood produced in spleen and lymphatic tissue.	• Intestines contained within abdominal cavity as growth of this cavity catches up with digestive system development. • Digestive tract patent from mouth to anus.	• Kidneys in their adult position. • Male and female external genitalia have different appearance but are still easily confused.	• Toes distinct; soles face each other.	• Fingernails begin developing. • Tooth buds for permanent teeth begin developing below those for primary teeth.
12 Weeks: 87-mm CRL; weight, 45 g					
• Surface of brain is smooth, without sulci (grooves) or gyri (convolutions). • Nasal septum and palate complete development.	• Heartbeat should be detected with Doppler transducer.	• Sucking reflex present. • Bile formed by liver.	• Kidneys begin producing urine. • Male and female external genitalia can be distinguished by appearance.	• Limbs are long and thin. • Involuntary muscles of viscera develop.	• Downy lanugo begins developing at end of this week.
16 Weeks: 140-mm CRL; weight, 200 g					
• Face is human-looking because eyes face forward rather than to the side.	• Pulmonary vascular system developing rapidly.	• Fetus swallows amniotic fluid and produces meconium (bowel contents).	• Urine excreted into amniotic fluid.	• Lower limbs reach final relative length, longer than upper limbs. • Fetal movement may be perceived, especially if this is not the first pregnancy.	• External ears have enough cartilage to stand away from head somewhat. • Blood vessels easily visible through delicate skin. • Fingerprints developing.
20 Weeks: 160-mm CRL; weight, 460 g					
• Myelination of nerves begins and continues through first year of postnatal life.	• Heartbeat should be detectable with regular fetoscope.	• Peristalsis well developed.	• More than 40% of nephrons are mature and functioning. • Testes contained in abdomen but begin descent toward scrotum. • Primordial follicles of ovary reach peak of 5–7 million and then gradually decline.	• Fetal movements felt by client and may be palpable by an experienced examiner.	• Skin is thin and covered with vernix caseosa. • Brown fat production complete. • Nipples begin development.

Continued

TABLE 5.2   Timetable of Prenatal Development Based on Fertilization Age[a]—cont'd

Nervous/Sensory System	Cardiorespiratory System	Digestive System	Genitourinary System	Musculoskeletal System	Integumentary System
24 Weeks: 230-mm CRL; weight, 820 g					
• Spinal cord ends at level of first sacral vertebra because of more rapid growth of vertebral canal.	• Primitive thin-walled alveoli (air sacs) have developed and are surrounded by capillary network. • Surfactant production begins in lungs. • Respiration possible.		• Testes descending toward inguinal rings.	• Fetus is active. • Fetal movements become progressively more noticeable to both client and examiner.	• Body appearance lean. • Skin wrinkled and red. • Fingerprints and footprints developed. • Fingernails present. • Eyebrows and lashes present.
28 Weeks: 270-mm CRL; weight, 1300 g					
• Major sulci and gyri are present. • Eyelids no longer fused after 26 weeks. • Responds to bitter substances on tongue.	• Erythrocyte formation completely in bone marrow. • Sufficient alveoli, surfactant, and capillary network to allow respiratory function, although respiratory distress syndrome is common. • Many infants born at this time survive with intensive care.		• Testes descended through inguinal canal into scrotum by end of week 26.		• Skin slightly wrinkled but smoothing out as subcutaneous fat is deposited under it.
32 Weeks: 300-mm CRL; weight, 2100 g					
• Maturation of parasympathetic nears that of sympathetic nervous system, resulting in fetal heart rate variability on electronic fetal monitor tracing.	• Surfactant production nears mature levels. • Respiratory distress still possible if born at 32 weeks. • Fetal heart rate variability gradually increases toward full term.				• Skin smooth and pigmented. • Large vessels visible beneath skin. • Fingernails reach fingertips. • Lanugo disappearing.
38 Weeks: 360-mm CRL, weight, 3400 g					
• Sulci and gyri developed. • Visual acuity ~20/600 at birth.	• Newborn infant has ~1/8–1/6 number of alveoli of an adult. • Well-developed ability to exchange gas.		• Both testes usually palpable in scrotum at birth. • The newborn female's ovaries contain ~1 million follicles. No new ones are formed after birth; their numbers continue to decline after birth.		• Fetus plump and skin smooth. • Vernix caseosa present in major body creases. • Lanugo present on shoulders and upper back only. • Fingernails extend beyond fingertips. • Ear cartilage firm.

CRL, Crown–rump length; g, gram(s).
[a]Fertilization age is about 2 wks less than gestational age.

TABLE 5.3 Derivatives of the Three Germ Layers

Ectoderm	Mesoderm	Endoderm
• Brain and spinal cord	• Cartilage	• Lining of gastrointestinal and respiratory tracts
• Peripheral nervous system	• Bone	
	• Connective tissue	
	• Muscle tissue	
• Pituitary gland	• Heart	• Tonsils
• Sensory epithelium of eye, ear, and nose	• Blood vessels	• Thyroid
	• Blood cells	• Parathyroid
	• Lymphatic system	• Thymus
	• Spleen	• Liver
• Epidermis	• Kidneys	• Pancreas
• Hair	• Adrenal cortex	• Lining of urinary bladder and urethra
• Nails	• Ovaries	
	• Testes	
• Subcutaneous glands	• Reproductive system	• Lining of ear canal
• Mammary glands	• Lining membranes (pericardial, pleural, and peritoneal)	
• Tooth enamel		

The alveoli proliferate and become surrounded by a rich capillary network enabling oxygen and carbon dioxide exchange at birth.

Week 5

The head is very large because the brain grows rapidly during the fifth week after fertilization. The heart is beating and developing four chambers. Upper limb buds are paddle shaped with obvious notches between the fingers. Lower limbs form slightly later than upper limbs. Lower limbs are also paddle shaped, but the area between the toes is not as well defined as is the division between the fingers.

Week 6

The rapidly developing head is bent over the chest. The heart reaches its final four-chambered form. Upper and lower extremities continue to become more defined.

The eyes continue to develop, and the beginnings of the external ears appear as six small bumps on each side of the neck. Facial development begins with eyes, ears, and nasal pits widely separated and aligned with the body walls. Gradually the embryo grows such that the face comes together in the midline and the external ears assume their proper position on the sides of the head.

Week 7

General growth and refinement of all systems occur 7 weeks after conception. The face becomes more human looking. The eyelids begin to grow, and the extremities become longer and better defined. The trunk elongates and straightens, although a C-shaped spinal curve remains in the newborn at birth.

The intestines have been growing faster than the abdominal cavity during the embryonic period. The relatively large liver and kidneys also occupy much of the abdominal cavity. Therefore, most of the intestines are contained within the

umbilical cord while the abdominal cavity grows to accommodate them. The abdomen is large enough to contain all its normal contents by 10 weeks.

Week 8

The embryo has a definite human form, and refinements to all systems continue. The ears are low-set but approaching their final location. The eyes are pigmented but not yet fully covered by eyelids. Fingers and toes are stubby but well-defined. The external genitalia begin to differentiate, but male and female characteristics are not distinct until 10 weeks after conception, or 12 weeks after the last menstrual period.

KNOWLEDGE CHECK

11. Why is the embryo particularly susceptible to damage from teratogens?
12. What is the difference between *fertilization age* and *gestational age*? Which term is more commonly used, and why?
13. How does the lower respiratory tract develop?
14. Why are the intestines mostly contained within the umbilical cord until the 10th week?

FETAL PERIOD

The fetal period is the longest part of prenatal development. It begins 9 weeks after conception and ends with birth. All major systems are present in their basic form. Dramatic growth and refinement in the structure and function of all organ systems occur during the fetal period (Fig. 5.6). Teratogens may damage already formed structures but are less likely to cause major structural alterations. The CNS is vulnerable to damaging agents through the entire pregnancy.

Weeks 9 Through 12

The head is approximately half the total length of the fetus at the beginning of this period. The body begins growing faster than the head, changing the proportions. The extremities approach their final relative lengths, although the legs remain proportionately shorter than the arms. The first fetal movements begin but are too slight for the client to detect.

The face is broad with a wide nose and widely spaced eyes. The eyes close at 9 weeks and reopen at 26 weeks after conception. The ears appear low-set because the mandible is still small.

The intestinal contents partly contained within the umbilical cord enter the abdomen by 11 weeks as the capacity of the abdominal cavity catches up with them in size. Blood formation occurs primarily in the liver during week 9 but shifts to the spleen by the end of week 12. The fetus begins producing urine during this period and excretes it into the amniotic fluid.

Internal differences in males and females begin to be apparent in the seventh week. External genitalia look similar until the end of the 9th week. By the end of week 12, the sex can be determined by the appearance of the external genitalia.

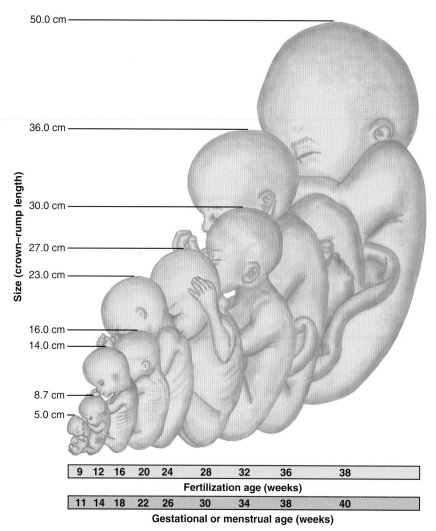

FIG. 5.6 Fetal Development from Week 9 Through Week 38 of Fertilization Age. The gestational age, measured from the first day of the last menstrual period, is approximately 2 weeks longer than the fertilization age.

Weeks 13 Through 16

The fetus grows rapidly in length, so the head becomes smaller in proportion to the total length. Movements strengthen, and those who have been pregnant before may be able to detect them. This phenomenon is referred to as *quickening.* The face looks human because the eyes face fully forward. The ears approach their final position at the sides of the head and in line with the eyes.

Weeks 17 Through 20

Fetal movements feel like fluttering or "butterflies." These subtle sensations may not be recognized. The fetus is unlikely to survive outside of the uterus at the age of 20 weeks.

Changes in the skin and hair are evident. *Vernix caseosa,* a fatty, cheese-like secretion of the fetal sebaceous glands, covers the skin to protect it from constant exposure to amniotic fluid. *Lanugo* is fine, downy hair covering the fetal body that helps the vernix adhere to the skin. Both vernix and lanugo diminish as the fetus reaches term. Eyebrows and head hair appear.

Brown fat is a special heat-producing fat deposited during this period. It is located on the back of the neck, behind the sternum, and around the kidneys (see Chapter 20, Fig. 20.4).

Weeks 21 Through 24

While continuing to grow and gain weight, the fetus still appears thin because of minimal subcutaneous fat. The skin is translucent and red because the capillaries are close to its fragile surface.

The lungs begin to produce surfactant, a surface-active lipid that makes it easier for the baby to breathe after birth. Surfactant reduces surface tension in the lung alveoli and prevents them from collapsing with each breath. Production of surfactant begins at approximately 20 weeks but does not reach levels that increase likelihood of survival outside the uterus until 26 to 28 weeks after conception. Surfactant production increases during late pregnancy, particularly during the last 2 weeks (Hall & Hall, 2021; Moore et al., 2020). The capillary network surrounding the alveoli is increasing but still very immature, although some gas exchange is possible. A fetus born at this gestational age is less likely to survive because of inadequate gas exchange. Other systems are extremely immature as well, such as blood vessels in the brain that may bleed.

Weeks 25 Through 28

The fetus is more likely to survive if born during this period because of maturation of the lungs, pulmonary capillaries, and CNS. The fetus becomes plumper with smoother skin as subcutaneous fat is deposited under the skin. The skin gradually becomes less red. The eyes, which closed during the 9th week, reopen. Head hair is abundant. Blood formation shifts from the spleen to the bone marrow.

During early pregnancy, the fetus floats freely within the amniotic sac, but the fetus usually assumes a head-down position during this time for two reasons:

- The uterus is shaped like an inverted egg. The overall shape of the fetus in flexion is similar, with the head being the small pole of the egg shape and the buttocks, flexed legs, and feet being the larger pole.
- The fetal head is heavier than the feet, and gravity causes the head to drift downward in the pool of amniotic fluid.

The head-down position is also most favorable for birth.

Weeks 29 Through 32

The skin is pigmented according to race and is smooth. Larger vessels are visible over the abdomen, but small capillaries cannot be seen. Toenails are present, and fingernails extend to the fingertips. The fetus has more subcutaneous fat, which rounds the body contours. If the fetus is born during this period, chances of survival are good with specialized neonatal care.

Weeks 33 Through 38

Growth of all body systems continues until birth, but the rate of growth slows as full-term approaches. The fetus is mainly gaining weight. The pulmonary system matures to enable efficient and unlabored breathing after birth.

The well-nourished term fetus at 38 or more weeks is rotund with abundant subcutaneous fat. At birth, males are slightly heavier than females. The skin is pink to brownish pink, depending on race. Lanugo may be present over the forehead, upper back, and upper arms. Vernix often remains in major creases such as the groin and axillae.

The testes are in the scrotum. Breasts of both male and female infants are enlarged, and breast tissue is palpable beneath the areola and nipple because of maternal hormone effects.

KNOWLEDGE CHECK

15. Why does the fetus usually assume a head-down position in the uterus?
16. What is the purpose of each of the following fetal structures or substances: Vernix caseosa? Lanugo? Brown fat? Surfactant?

AUXILIARY STRUCTURES

Three auxiliary structures sustain the pregnancy and permit prenatal development: the placenta, the umbilical cord, and fetal membranes. These structures develop simultaneously with the baby's development.

Placenta

The placenta is a thick, disc-shaped organ. The placenta has two components: maternal and fetal (Fig. 5.7). It is involved in metabolic, transfer, and endocrine functions. The fetal side is smooth, with branching vessels covering the membrane-covered surface. The maternal side is rough where it attaches to the uterus (see Chapter 12, Fig. 12.14A–B).

The umbilical cord is normally inserted on the fetal side of the placenta, near the center. It may, however, insert off-center or even on the fetal membranes (Fig. 5.8).

During early pregnancy, the placenta is larger than the embryo or fetus, but the fetus grows faster than the placenta, so the placenta is approximately one-sixth the weight of the fetus at the end of a full-term pregnancy.

Maternal Component

Development. When conception occurs, cells of the endometrium undergo changes to promote early nutrition of the embryo and enable most of the uterine lining to be shed after birth. These changes convert endometrial cells into the decidua. In addition to providing nourishment for the embryo, the decidua may prevent uncontrolled invasion of fetal placental tissue into the uterine wall.

The three decidual layers are (1) the decidua basalis, which underlies the developing embryo and forms the maternal side of the placenta; (2) the decidua capsularis, which overlies the embryo and bulges into the uterine cavity as the embryo and fetus grow; and (3) the decidua parietalis, which lines the rest of the uterine cavity. By approximately 22 weeks of gestation, the decidua capsularis fuses with the decidua parietalis, filling the uterine cavity.

Circulation on the maternal side. Maternal and fetal blood normally do not mix in the placenta, although they flow very close to each other. Exchange of substances occurs within the intervillous spaces of the placenta. When in the intervillous space, the mother's blood is briefly outside the circulatory system. Approximately 150 mL of maternal blood is contained within the intervillous space. Blood in the intervillous space is changed approximately three to four times per minute, requiring circulation of 450 to 750 mL per minute for placental perfusion.

Maternal blood spurts into the intervillous spaces through 80 to 100 spiral arteries in the decidua. After the oxygenated and nutrient-bearing maternal blood washes over the chorionic villi containing the fetal vessels, it returns to the maternal circulation through the endometrial veins for elimination of fetal waste products.

Fetal Component

Development. The fetal side of the placenta develops from the outer cell layer (trophoblast) of the blastocyst at the same

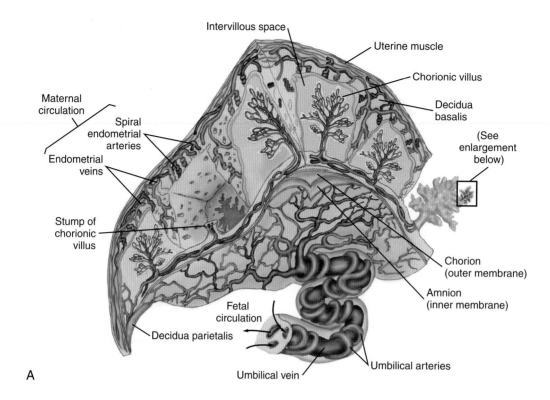

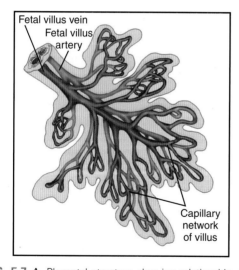

FIG. 5.7 A, Placental structure showing relationship of placenta. *Arrows* indicate the direction of blood flow between the fetus and placenta through the umbilical arteries and vein. Maternal blood bathes the fetal chorionic villi within the intervillous spaces to allow exchange of oxygen, nutrients, and waste products without gross mixing of maternal and fetal blood. **B,** Structure of a chorionic villus; its fetal capillary network is illustrated.

time the inner cell mass develops into the embryo and fetus. The primary chorionic villi are the initial structures that eventually form the fetal side of the placenta.

Circulation on the fetal side. The umbilical cord contains the umbilical arteries and vein to transport blood between the fetus and placenta. Chorionic villi are bathed by oxygen- and nutrient-rich maternal blood in the intervillous spaces. Each chorionic villus is supplied by a tiny fetal artery carrying deoxygenated blood and waste products from the fetus. The vein of the chorionic villus returns oxygenated blood and nutrients to the embryo and fetus.

Capillaries in the chorionic villi are separated from actual contact with the mother's blood by the membranes of each villus. This arrangement allows contact close enough for exchange and prevents mixing of maternal and fetal blood. The closed fetal circulation is important because the blood types of mother and fetus may not be compatible.

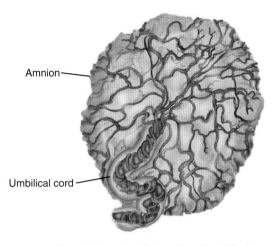

Amnion

Umbilical cord

Normal placenta with insertion of umbilical cord near center and branching of fetal umbilical vessels over the surface

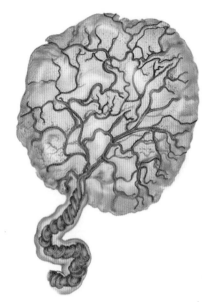

Placenta with cord inserted near margin of placenta

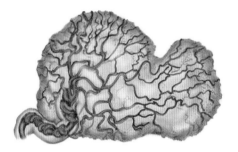

Placenta with a small accessory lobe

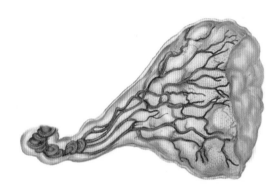

Velamentous insertion of umbilical cord. Cord vessels branch far out on membranes. When membranes rupture, fetal umbilical vessels may be torn and the fetus can hemorrhage.

FIG. 5.8 Placental variations.

The placental arteries and veins converge in the blood vessels of the umbilical cord. Two umbilical arteries and one umbilical vein transport blood between the fetus and the fetal side of the placenta. Blood is circulated to and from the fetal side of the placenta by the fetal heart.

Metabolic Functions

The placenta produces some nutrients needed by the embryo and for placental functions. Substances synthesized include glycogen, cholesterol, and fatty acids (Moore et al., 2020).

Transfer Functions

Exchange of oxygen, nutrients, and waste products across the chorionic villi occurs through several methods (Table 5.4). Placental transfer of harmful substances also may occur. Most substances that enter the mother's bloodstream can enter the fetal circulation, and many agents enter it almost immediately.

Gas exchange. Respiration is a key function of the placenta. Oxygen and carbon dioxide pass through the placental membrane by simple diffusion. The average oxygen partial pressure (Po_2) of maternal blood in the intervillous space is 50 mm Hg. The average blood Po_2 in the umbilical vein (after oxygenation) is approximately 30 mm Hg (Hall & Hall, 2021).

The following three reasons explain how the fetus can thrive in this low-oxygen environment:

- Fetal hemoglobin can carry 20% to 50% more oxygen than adult hemoglobin.
- The fetus has a higher oxygen-carrying capacity because of a higher average hemoglobin level (14.5 to 22.5 g/dL) and hematocrit value (approximately 48% to 69%).
- Hemoglobin can carry more oxygen at low carbon dioxide partial pressure (Pco_2) levels than it can at high levels (Bohr effect). Blood entering the placenta from the fetus has a high Pco_2, but carbon dioxide diffuses quickly to

TABLE 5.4   Mechanisms of Placental Transfer

Mechanism	Description	Examples of Substances Transferred
Simple diffusion	Passive movement of substances across a cell membrane from an area of higher concentration to one of lower concentration	• Oxygen and carbon dioxide • Carbon monoxide • Water • Urea and uric acid • Most drugs and their metabolites
Facilitated diffusion	Passage of substances across a cell membrane by binding with carrier proteins that assist transfer	• Glucose
Active transport	Transfer of substances across a cell membrane against a pressure or electrical gradient or from an area of lower concentration to one of higher concentration	• Amino acids • Water-soluble vitamins • Minerals: calcium, iron, iodine
Pinocytosis	Movement of large molecules by ingestion within cells	• Maternal IgG class antibodies • Some passage of maternal IgA antibodies

IgA, Immunoglobulin A; *IgG,* immunoglobulin G.

the mother's blood, where the P_{CO_2} is lower, reversing the levels of carbon dioxide in the maternal and the fetal blood. Therefore the fetal blood becomes more alkaline, and the maternal blood becomes more acidic. This allows the mother's blood to release oxygen and the fetal blood to combine with oxygen readily.

The fetal P_{CO_2} is only approximately 2 to 3 mm Hg higher than the P_{CO_2} of maternal blood, but carbon dioxide is very soluble, allowing it to pass across the placental membrane into maternal blood at this low-pressure gradient.

Nutrient transfer. The growing fetus requires a constant supply of nutrients. Glucose, fatty acids, vitamins, and electrolytes pass readily across the placenta. Glucose is the major energy source for fetal growth and metabolic activities.

Waste removal. In addition to carbon dioxide, urea, uric acid, and bilirubin are readily transferred from fetus to mother for disposal. Because the placenta removes wastes for the fetus, metabolic defects such as phenylketonuria (PKU) are usually not evident until after birth.

Antibody transfer. Many in the immunoglobulin G (IgG) class of antibodies are passed from mother to fetus through the placenta. This confers passive (temporary) immunity to the fetus against diseases to which the mother is immune (e.g., measles). Passage of antibodies against disease is beneficial because the newborn does not produce antibodies for several months after birth. The preterm or small-for-gestational age infant has little protection provided by maternal antibodies because antibodies are transferred during late pregnancy and are poorly transferred if placental function is inadequate.

Passage of antibodies to fetus is not always beneficial. If maternal and fetal blood types are not compatible, the mother may already have or may produce antibodies against fetal erythrocytes. The mother's antibodies may then destroy the fetal erythrocytes, causing fetal anemia or even death. This situation may occur if the mother is Rh-negative and the fetus is Rh-positive.

Transfer of maternal hormones. Most maternal protein hormones do not reach the fetus in significant amounts. The female fetus exposed to androgenic hormones may have masculinization of the genitalia, and the genetic sex may be difficult to visually determine at birth.

Endocrine Functions

The placenta produces several hormones necessary for pregnancy. Human chorionic gonadotropin (hCG) causes the corpus luteum to persist for the first 6 to 8 weeks of pregnancy and secrete estrogens and progesterone. As the placenta develops further, it takes over estrogen and progesterone production, and the corpus luteum regresses. When a Y chromosome is present in the male fetus, hCG also causes the fetal testes to secrete testosterone, necessary for normal development of male reproductive structures.

Human placental lactogen, also called *human chorionic somatomammotropin,* promotes normal nutrition and growth of the fetus as well as maternal breast development for lactation. This placental hormone decreases maternal insulin sensitivity and glucose use, making more glucose available for fetal nutrition.

Steroid hormones secreted by the placenta include estrogens and progesterone. Estrogens cause enlargement of the uterus, enlargement of the breasts, growth of the ductal system of the breasts, and enlargement of the external genitalia. Progesterone is essential for normal continuation of the pregnancy. It modifies and maintains the endometrium to receive and nourish the conceptus and forms the decidua. Progesterone also reduces muscle contractions of the uterus to prevent spontaneous abortions. (See Chapter 6 for a more detailed list of the functions of estrogen and progesterone during pregnancy.) Other hormones produced by the placenta include human chorionic thyrotropin and human chorionic adrenocorticotropin.

KNOWLEDGE CHECK

17. Which structure takes over the functions of the corpus luteum?
18. What is the purpose of the intervillous spaces of the placenta?
19. Why should fetal and maternal blood not actually mix?
20. What factors enable the fetus to thrive in a low-oxygen environment?
21. What are the purposes of the following placental hormones: hCG? Human placental lactogen? Estrogen? Progesterone?

Fetal Membranes and Amniotic Fluid

The two fetal membranes are the *amnion* (inner membrane) and the *chorion* (outer membrane). The two membranes are so close they seem to be one membrane (the "bag of waters"), but they can be separated. If the membranes rupture in labor, amnion and chorion usually rupture together, releasing the amniotic fluid within the sac.

The amnion is continuous with the surface of the umbilical cord, joining the epithelium of the abdominal skin of the fetus. Chorionic villi proliferate over the entire surface of the gestational sac for the first 8 weeks after conception. A conceptus observed at this time looks like a shaggy sphere with the embryo suspended inside. As the embryo grows, it bulges into the uterine cavity. The villi on the outer surface gradually atrophy and form the smooth-surfaced chorion. The remaining villi continue to branch and enlarge to form the fetal side of the placenta.

Amniotic fluid protects the growing fetus and promotes prenatal development. Amniotic fluid protects the fetus by the following actions:
- Cushioning against impacts to the maternal abdomen
- Maintaining a stable temperature
- Promoting prenatal development by the following actions:
  - Allowing symmetric development as the major body surfaces fold toward the midline
  - Preventing the membranes from adhering to developing fetal parts
  - Allowing room and buoyancy for fetal movement

Amniotic fluid is derived from fetal urine and fluid transported from the maternal blood across the amnion. Cast-off fetal epithelial cells and vernix are suspended in the amniotic fluid. The water of the amniotic fluid changes by absorption across the amnion, returning to the mother. The fetus also swallows amniotic fluid and absorbs it in the digestive tract. Waste products are returned to the placenta through the umbilical arteries.

The volume of amniotic fluid increases during pregnancy and is approximately 700 to 800 mL at term. An abnormally small quantity of fluid (less than 50% of the amount expected for gestation or under 400 mL at term) is called *oligohydramnios* and may be associated with the following (Blackburn, 2018; Carlson, 2019; Hall & Hall, 2021):
- Poor placental blood flow
- Preterm rupture of the membranes
- Failure of fetal kidney development
- Blocked urinary excretion
- Poor fetal lung development (pulmonary hypoplasia)
- Malformations such as skeletal abnormalities from compression of fetal parts

Hydramnios (also called *polyhydramnios*) is the opposite situation, in which the quantity may exceed 2000 mL. Hydramnios may be associated with the following (Blackburn, 2018):
- Imbalanced water exchange among mother, fetus, and amniotic fluid that has no known cause

- Poorly controlled maternal diabetes mellitus resulting in large quantities of fetal urine excretion having an elevated glucose level
- Malformations of the CNS, cardiovascular system, or gastrointestinal tract that interfere with normal fluid ingestion, metabolism, and excretion
- Chromosomal abnormalities
- Multifetal gestation

FETAL CIRCULATION

The course of fetal blood circulation is from the fetal heart to the placenta for exchange of oxygen, nutrients, and waste products and back to the fetus for delivery to fetal tissues (Fig. 5.9A).

Umbilical Cord

The fetal umbilical cord is the lifeline between the fetus and placenta. It has two arteries carrying deoxygenated blood and waste products away from the fetus to the placenta, where these substances are transferred to the mother's circulation. The umbilical vein carries freshly oxygenated and nutrient-laden blood from the placenta back to the fetus. The umbilical arteries and vein are coiled within the cord to allow them to stretch and prevent obstruction of blood flow through them. The entire cord is cushioned by a soft substance called *Wharton's jelly* to prevent obstruction resulting from pressure.

Fetal Circulatory Circuit

Because the fetus does not breathe air, several alterations of the postnatal circulatory route are needed (see Fig. 5.9A). Also, the fetal liver does not have the metabolic functions it will have after birth because the mother's body performs these functions. Three shunts in the fetal circulatory system allow blood with the highest oxygen content to be sent to the fetal heart and brain: the ductus venosus, foramen ovale, and ductus arteriosus.

Ductus Venosus

Oxygenated blood from the placenta enters the fetal circulation through the umbilical vein. About one-third of the blood is directed away from the liver into the ductus venosus, which connects to the inferior vena cava. The rest of the umbilical vein flow goes through the liver before entering the inferior vena cava. Near the end of pregnancy the liver needs more perfusion, and 70% to 80% of the oxygenated blood goes to the liver first and then to the ductus venosus (Blackburn, 2018).

Blood from the ductus venosus or the portal system of the liver enters the inferior vena cava and joins blood from the lower part of the body. Little mixing of blood from the ductus venosus and the lower body occurs because it travels to the heart in separate streams within the inferior vena cava. As blood flows into the right atrium, a flap of tissue directs the blood from the more highly oxygenated stream across the atrium to the foramen ovale.

Foramen Ovale

The foramen ovale is a flap valve in the septum between the right and left atria of the fetal heart. As blood flows into the right atrium, 50% to 60% crosses the foramen ovale to the left atrium (Blackburn, 2018). In the left atrium it mixes with the small amount of blood entering from the pulmonary veins, flows to the left ventricle, and leaves through the aorta. The majority of the blood in the ascending aorta flows to the coronary, left carotid, and subclavian arteries. Therefore, most of the better-oxygenated blood bypasses the nonfunctioning lungs before birth and travels to the heart, brain, head, and upper body.

Blood that does not cross the foramen ovale moves to the right ventricle, but flow to the lungs is restricted by the narrow pulmonary artery and pulmonary blood vessels, causing a high pressure in the right side of the heart. Pressure is low on the left side of the heart because little resistance occurs as blood leaves the left ventricle to travel to the rest of the body and into the widely dilated placental vessels. This difference in pressures between the right and left atria allows blood to flow through the foramen ovale.

Pulmonary Blood Vessels

Blood from the superior vena cava and the less oxygenated blood from the inferior vena cava flow into the right atrium, to the right ventricle, and into the pulmonary artery. Most of the blood passes through the ductus arteriosus to the descending aorta, and 10% to 12% of the blood goes to the lungs. After 30 weeks of gestation, the amount of blood to the lungs increases (Blackburn, 2018). Blood flow to the lungs is limited because the pulmonary artery and other blood vessels are constricted, causing high pulmonary vascular resistance. Blood perfusing the lungs returns to the left atrium by the pulmonary veins.

Ductus Arteriosus

The ductus arteriosus connects the pulmonary artery and the descending aorta during fetal life. Dilation of the ductus arteriosus is maintained by prostaglandins from the placenta and low oxygen content of the blood.

Changes in Blood Circulation after Birth

Fetal circulatory shunts are not needed after birth because the infant oxygenates blood in the lungs and is not circulating

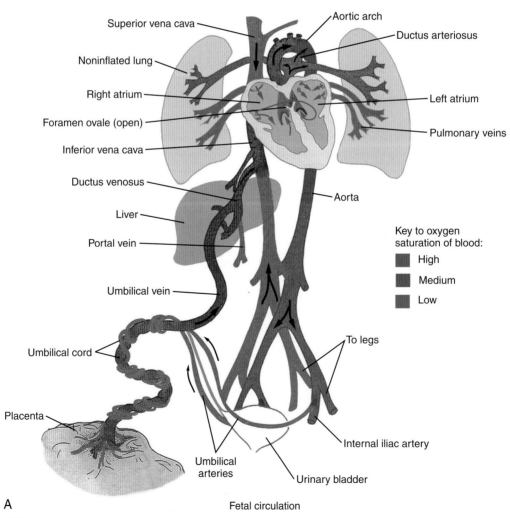

FIG. 5.9 A, Fetal circulation. Three shunts allow most blood from the placenta to bypass the fetal lungs and liver; they are the ductus venosus, ductus arteriosus, and foramen ovale.

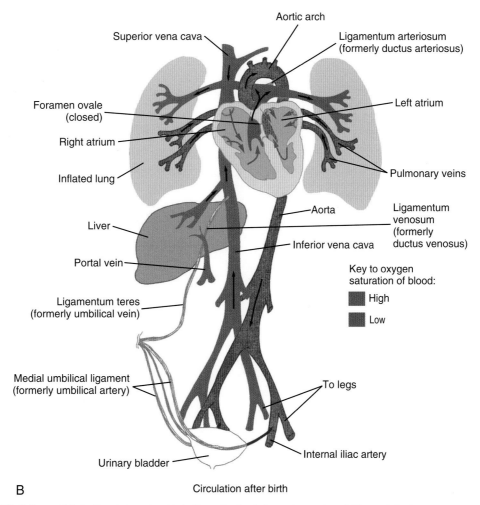

FIG. 5.9 cont'd B, Circulation after birth. Note the fetal shunts have closed. The umbilical vessels, ductus venosus, and ductus arteriosus will be converted to ligaments.

blood to the placenta (see Fig. 5.9B). As the infant breathes and the lungs expand, blood flow to the lungs increases, pressure in the right side of the heart falls, and the foramen ovale closes. The ductus arteriosus constricts as the arterial oxygen level rises. Persistent hypoxia may cause the ductus arteriosus to remain open for a prolonged period. The ductus venosus constricts when flow of blood from the umbilical cord stops.

Transition to the postnatal circulatory pattern is gradual. Functional closure begins when the infant breathes and the cord is cut, removing the placenta from the circulation. The foramen ovale and ductus venosus are permanently closed as tissue proliferates in these structures. The ductus venosus becomes a ligament, as do the umbilical vein and arteries.

❓ KNOWLEDGE CHECK

22. What are the purposes of the fetal membranes and amniotic fluid?
23. Trace the path of fetal circulation from the placenta through the fetal body and back to the placenta.

MULTIFETAL PREGNANCY

The incidence of multifetal pregnancy (multiple gestation) has increased in the United States. Much of the increase is a result of a rise in maternal age, which is associated with an increased incidence of twinning, and infertility treatments that induce multiple ovulations. The twin birth rate steadily increased from 1980 to reach an all-time high in 2014 of 33.9 twin births per 1000 births. After the 2014 high, the twin birth rate has decreased each year, landing at 32.7 in 2019 (Martin et al., 2021). Rates of high-order multiples (triplets or more) steadily increased between the mid-1990s and 2003, and a high of 193.5 per 100,000 births was recorded in 1998. These rates, however, have steadily declined, and in 2019, there were 94.1 per 100,000 live births (Martin et al., 2021).

Twinning is the most common form of multifetal pregnancy. The same processes that occur in twin pregnancies also may occur in higher-order multiple gestations. Twins are often called *identical* or *fraternal* by lay people but are more accurately described by their zygosity, or the number of ova and sperm involved. The two types of twins are *monozygotic* and *dizygotic* (Fig. 5.10).

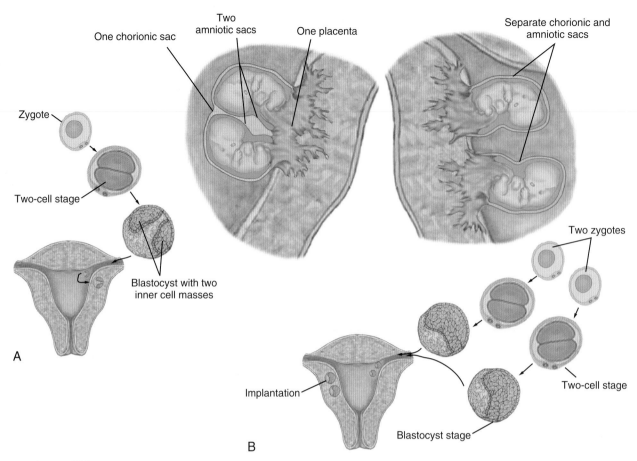

FIG. 5.10 **A,** Monozygotic twinning. The single inner cell mass divides into two inner cell masses during the blastocyst stage. These twins have a single placenta and chorion, but each twin develops in its own amnion. **B,** Dizygotic twinning. Two ova are released during ovulation, and each is fertilized by a separate spermatozoon. The ova may implant near each other in the uterus, or they may be far apart.

Monozygotic Twinning

Monozygotic twins are conceived by the union of a single ovum and spermatozoon, with later division of the conceptus into two. Monozygotic twins have identical genetic complements and are the same genetic sex. Nevertheless, they may not always look identical at birth because one twin may have grown much larger than the other or one may have a birth defect such as a cleft lip. Monozygotic twins have a higher rate of birth defects, preterm births, and low birth weight. Monozygotic twinning occurs essentially at random (about 1 in 250 natural [nonassisted] pregnancies), and a hereditary or racial component is not well established (Unal & Newman, 2021).

Monozygotic twinning occurs when a single conceptus divides early in gestation. The blastocyst in most monozygotic twins is formed with two inner cell masses instead of one. If this occurs, the fetuses usually have two amnions (inner membranes) but a single chorion (outer membrane) (Blackburn, 2018; Cunningham et al., 2022; Unal & Newman, 2021).

If the conceptus divides earlier, two separate but identical morulas (and then blastocysts) develop and implant separately. These monozygotic twins have two amnions and two chorions. Although the placentas develop separately, they may fuse and appear as one at birth. The chorions also may fuse during prenatal development. Examination of the placenta and membranes after birth may not identify whether twins are monozygotic or dizygotic. Tests such as DNA analysis or detailed blood typing may be needed to determine whether twins are monozygotic or dizygotic.

Late separation of the inner cell mass may result in twins having a single amnion and a single chorion. These twins are more likely to die because their umbilical cords become entangled during pregnancy. Incomplete separation of the inner cell mass may result in conjoined twins.

Dizygotic Twinning

Dizygotic twins arise from two ova fertilized by different sperm. Dizygotic twins may be the same or different genetic sex, and they may not have similar physical traits.

Dizygotic twinning may be hereditary in some families, presumably because of an inherited tendency of the females to release more than one ovum per cycle. Dizygotic twins are more common in some races. Infertility therapy increases the incidence of twins, usually dizygotic, because induction of ovulation often results in the release of multiple ova, with implantation of more than one zygote in the uterus. Conception after age 40 years is also associated with an increased incidence of spontaneous dizygotic twin births because multiple ova are more likely to be released near the climacteric.

Because dizygotic twins arise from two separate zygotes, their membranes and placentas are separate. The membranes, the placentas, or both may fuse during development if they implant closely. Dizygotic twins are not conjoined because they do not involve division of a single cell mass into two but arise from two separate conceptions.

High Multifetal Gestations

Pregnancies resulting in triplets or higher may arise from a single zygote or a combination of a single and multiple zygotes, or each may arise from a separate zygote. High multifetal pregnancies pose greater hazards to both the mother and fetuses. The incidence of long-term complications is higher as the number of fetuses increases.

SUMMARY CONCEPTS

- The purpose of gametogenesis is to produce ova and sperm with half the full number of chromosomes, or 23 unpaired chromosomes. When an ovum and sperm unite at conception, the number is restored to 46 paired chromosomes.
- Females have all the ova they will ever have at 30 weeks of prenatal life. No other ova are formed after this time.
- One primary oocyte can mature into one mature ovum with 23 unpaired chromosomes (22 autosomes and 1 X chromosome).
- Males can continuously produce new sperm from puberty through the rest of their life, although fertility gradually declines after age 40 years.
- One primary spermatocyte can result in production of four mature sperm. Two of the mature sperm have 22 autosomes and 1 X sex chromosome. Two have 22 autosomes and 1 Y sex chromosome.
- The male determines the baby's genetic sex because sperm carry either an X or a Y sex chromosome. The female contributes only an X chromosome to the baby.
- The basic structures of all organ systems are established during the first 8 weeks of pregnancy. During this period, teratogens may cause major structural and functional damage to the developing organs.
- The fetal period is one of growth and refinement of already established organ systems. Teratogens are less likely to cause major structural damage to the fetus but may cause major functional damage.
- The placenta is an embryonic or a fetal organ with metabolic, respiratory, and endocrine functions.

- Transfer of substances between mother and embryo or fetus occurs by four mechanisms: simple diffusion, facilitated diffusion, active transport, and pinocytosis.
- Most substances in the maternal blood can be transferred to the fetus.
- The fetal membranes contain the amniotic fluid, which cushions the fetus, allows normal prenatal development, and maintains a stable temperature.
- The umbilical cord is the lifeline between the fetus and the placenta. Two umbilical arteries carry deoxygenated blood and waste products to the placenta for transfer to the mother's blood. One umbilical vein carries oxygenated and nutrient-rich blood to the fetus. Coiling of the vessels and enclosure in Wharton's jelly reduce the risk for obstruction of the umbilical vessels.
- Three fetal circulatory shunts are needed to partially bypass the fetal liver and lungs: the ductus venosus, foramen ovale, and ductus arteriosus. These structures close functionally after birth but are not closed permanently until several weeks or months later.
- Multifetal pregnancy may be monozygotic or dizygotic. Twins are the most common form of multifetal pregnancy.
- Examination of the placenta and membranes alone cannot conclusively establish whether multiple fetuses are monozygotic or dizygotic.
- Dizygotic twins are more likely to occur in certain families and racial groups and especially in clients older than 40 years and those who take fertility treatments to induce ovulation.

Clinical Judgment and Next-Generation NCLEX® Examination-Style Questions

Complete the statements by selecting from the lists of options provided.

1. Oxygenated blood from the placenta enters the fetal circulation through the ___1___ umbilical ___2___. About one-third of the blood is directed away from the liver into the ___3___, which connects to the inferior vena cava. As blood flows into the right atrium, a flap valve in the septum between the right and left atria called the ___4___ directs the highly oxygenated blood into the left atria. Blood from the superior vena cava and the less oxygenated blood from the inferior vena cava flow into the right atrium, to the right ventricle, and into the pulmonary artery. Most of this blood bypasses the fetal lungs and is shunted into the descending aorta through the ___5___. The ___6___ umbilical ___7___ return the deoxygenated blood to the placenta for oxygenation.

Options for 1 and 6	Options for 2 and 7	Options for 3, 4 and 5
One	Artery(ies)	Ductus venosus
Two	Vein (s)	Liver shunt
Three		Ductus arteriosus
		Vena caval shunt
		Foramen ovale
		Septal shunt

REFERENCES

Blackburn, S. T. (2018). *Maternal, fetal, & neonatal physiology: A clinical perspective* (5th ed.). Elsevier.

Carlson, B. M. (2019). *Human embryology and developmental biology* (6th ed.). Mosby.

Cunningham, F. G., Leveno, K. J., Bloom, S. L., Dashe, J. S., Hoffman, B. L., Casey, B. M., & Spong, C. Y. (2022). *Williams obstetrics* (26th ed.). McGraw-Hill Companies.

Hall, J. C., & Hall, M. E. (2021). *Guyton and Hall textbook of medical physiology* (14th ed.). Elsevier.

Martin, J. A., Hamilton, B. E., Osterman, M. J. K., & Driscoll, A. K. (2021). Births: Final data for 2019. *National Vital Statistics Reports, 68*(13). https://www.cdc.gov/nchs/products/index.htm.

Moore, K. L., Persaud, T. V. N., & Torchia, M. G. (2020). *The developing human: Clinically oriented embryology* (11th ed.). Elsevier.

Moore, K. L., Persaud, T. V. N., & Torchia, M. G. (2021). *Before we are born: Essentials of embryology and birth defects* (10th ed.). Elsevier.

Unal, E. R., & Newman, R. (2021). Multiple gestations. In M. B. Landon, H. L. Galan, E. R. M. Jauniaux, et al. (Eds.), *Gabbe's Obstetrics: Normal and problem pregnancies* (8th ed., pp. 751–783). Elsevier.

Adaptations to Pregnancy

Dawn Piacenza

OBJECTIVES

After studying this chapter, you should be able to:

1. Describe the physiologic changes that occur during pregnancy.
2. Differentiate presumptive, probable, and positive signs of pregnancy.
3. Describe the psychological responses of the expectant individual to pregnancy.
4. Identify the process of parental role transition.
5. Explain the parental tasks of pregnancy.
6. Describe the transition processes by the partner to the role of parent.
7. Describe the responses of prospective grandparents and siblings to pregnancy.
8. Discuss factors that influence psychosocial adaptation to pregnancy, such as age, parity, social support, gender identification, absence of a partner, and abnormal situations.
9. Explain the ways in which different psychosocial adaptations affect nursing practice.

From the moment of conception, changes occur in the pregnant client's body. These changes are necessary to support and nourish the fetus, prepare for childbirth and lactation, and maintain the client's health. Pregnant clients are often puzzled by the physical changes and unprepared for associated discomforts. Many clients rely on nurses to provide accurate information and compassionate guidance throughout their pregnancy. To respond effectively, nurses must understand not only the physiologic changes but also how these changes affect the daily lives of expectant individuals.

CHANGES IN BODY SYSTEMS

Although pregnancy challenges each body system to adapt to increasing demands of the fetus, the most obvious changes are in the reproductive system.

Reproductive System
Uterus

Growth. The most dramatic change during pregnancy occurs in the uterus, which before conception is a small, pear-shaped organ entirely contained in the pelvic cavity. The nonpregnant uterus weighs up to 70 g (2.5 oz) and has a capacity of about 10 mL (one-third of an ounce). By **term** (37 to 40 weeks of gestation) the uterus weighs 1100 to 1200 g (2.4 to 2.6 lb.) and has a capacity of 5 L (Norwitz et al., 2019).

Uterine growth occurs as the result of hyperplasia and hypertrophy. Growth can be predicted for each **trimester** (one of three 13-week periods of pregnancy). Early in pregnancy, growth results from hyperplasia caused by estrogen and growth factors. In the latter half of pregnancy, uterine growth results mainly from hypertrophy as the muscle fibers stretch in all directions to accommodate the growing fetus. In addition to muscle growth, fibrous tissue accumulates in the outer muscle layer of the uterus and the amount of elastic tissue increases. These changes greatly increase the strength of the muscle wall (Cunningham et al., 2022).

Muscle fibers in the myometrium increase in both length and width. Although the uterine wall thickens during early pregnancy, the wall of the uterus thins to about 0.5 to 1 cm (0.2 to 0.4 inch), and the fetus can be palpated easily through the abdominal wall by term (Blackburn, 2018). As the uterus expands into the abdominal cavity, it displaces the intestines upward and laterally. The uterus gradually rotates to the right as a result of pressure from the rectosigmoid colon on the left side of the pelvis.

Pattern of Uterine Growth. The uterus grows in a predictable pattern that provides information about fetal growth (Fig. 6.1). This growth helps confirm the estimated due date (EDD), sometimes called the *estimated date of birth (EDB) or estimated date of confinement (EDC).* By 12 weeks of gestation, the fundus can be palpated above the symphysis pubis. At 16 weeks, the fundus reaches midway between the symphysis pubis and the umbilicus. It is located at the umbilicus at 20 weeks.

The fundus reaches its highest level at the xiphoid process at 36 weeks of gestation. It pushes against the diaphragm, and the expectant individual may experience shortness of breath, even during rest. By 40 weeks, the fetal head descends into the pelvic cavity, and the uterus sinks to a lower level. This descent of the fetal head is called **lightening** because it reduces pressure on the diaphragm and makes breathing easier. Lightening is more pronounced in first pregnancies.

Contractility. Throughout pregnancy, the uterus undergoes irregular contractions called **Braxton Hicks contractions**. During the contractions, the uterus temporarily tightens and then returns to its original relaxed state. During the first two trimesters, the contractions are infrequent and usually not felt by the client. Contractions occur more frequently during the third trimester and may cause some discomfort. They are called *false labor* when they are mistaken for the onset of early labor (see Chapter 15).

Uterine Blood Flow. As the uterus enlarges, an increase in the size and number of blood vessels expands blood flow dramatically. As pregnancy progresses, the delivery of nutrients needed for fetal growth and the removal of metabolic wastes depends on adequate perfusion of the placental intervillous spaces. During late pregnancy, blood flow to the uterus and placenta reaches 750 mL per minute and is 10% to 15% of maternal cardiac output (Burton et al., 2021). Almost 90% of the blood goes to the placenta (Ross et al., 2021). The total blood carried by the myometrial arteries enters the intervillous spaces, where oxygen and nutrients are transferred to the chorionic villi and hence to the fetus. Metabolic wastes from the fetus diffuse into venous structures of the client (see Chapter 5).

Cervix

The cervix also undergoes significant changes after conception. Water content and vascularity of the area increase. The most obvious changes occur in color and consistency. Increasing levels of estrogen cause **hyperemia** (congestion with blood) of the cervix, resulting in the characteristic bluish–purple color that extends to include the vagina and the labia. This discoloration, referred to as the **Chadwick sign**, is one of the earliest signs of pregnancy.

The cervix is largely composed of connective tissue that softens when the collagen fibers decrease in concentration. Before pregnancy, the cervix has a consistency similar to that of the tip of the nose. After conception the cervix softens, feeling more like the lips or earlobe. This cervical softening is referred to as **Goodell's sign**.

A less obvious change occurs as the cervical glands proliferate during pregnancy, and the glandular walls become thin and widely separated. As a result, the endocervical tissue resembles a honeycomb that fills with mucus secreted by the cervical glands. The mucus, which is rich in immunoglobulins, forms a plug in the cervical canal (Fig. 6.2). It blocks the ascent of bacteria from the vagina into the uterus during pregnancy to help protect the fetus and the uterine membranes from infection (Cunningham et al., 2022).

The mucous plug remains in place until term when the cervix begins to thin and dilate, allowing the mucous plug to be expelled. One of the earliest signs of labor may be "bloody show," which consists of the mucous plug and a small amount of blood. Bleeding is produced by disruption of the cervical capillaries as the mucous plug is dislodged when the cervix begins to thin and dilate.

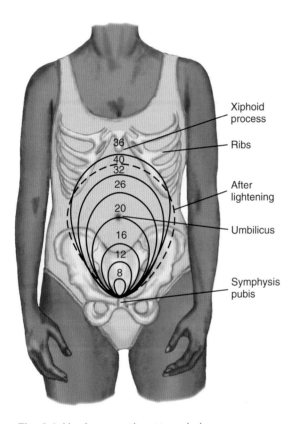

Xiphoid process

Ribs

After lightening

Umbilicus

Symphysis pubis

36
40
32
26
20
16
12
8

Fig. 6.1 Uterine growth pattern during pregnancy.

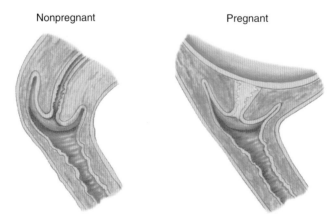

Nonpregnant

Pregnant

Fig. 6.2 Cervical changes that occur during pregnancy. Note the thick mucous plug filling the cervical canal.

Vagina and Vulva

Increased vascularity causes the vaginal walls to appear bluish purple. Softening of the abundant connective tissue allows the vagina to distend during childbirth. The vaginal mucosa thickens, and vaginal rugae (folds) become very prominent.

Vaginal cells contain increasing amounts of glycogen, which causes rapid sloughing and increased thick, white, vaginal discharge. The pH of the vaginal discharge is acidic (3.5 to 6) because of the increased production of lactic acid that results from the action of *Lactobacillus acidophilus* on glycogen in the vaginal epithelium (Cunningham et al., 2022). The acidic condition helps prevent growth of harmful bacteria in the vagina. However, the glycogen-rich environment favors the growth of *Candida albicans,* and persistent yeast infections (candidiasis) are common during pregnancy.

Increased vascularity, edema, and connective tissue changes make the tissues of the vulva and perineum more pliable. Pelvic congestion during pregnancy can lead to heightened sexual interest and increased orgasmic experiences.

Ovaries

Progesterone, called the "hormone of pregnancy," must be present in adequate amounts from the earliest stages to maintain pregnancy. Progesterone helps suppress contractions of the uterus and may also help prevent tissue rejection of the fetus (Cunningham et al., 2022; Norwitz et al., 2019). After conception, the corpus luteum of the ovaries secretes progesterone, mainly during the first 6 to 7 weeks of pregnancy (Cunningham et al., 2022). Between 6 and 10 weeks of gestation, the corpus luteum produces a smaller amount of progesterone as the placenta takes over production (Cunningham et al., 2022; Norwitz et al., 2019). The corpus luteum then regresses because it is no longer needed.

Ovulation ceases during pregnancy because the high circulating levels of estrogen and progesterone inhibit the release of follicle-stimulating hormone (FSH) and luteinizing hormone (LH), which are necessary for ovulation.

Breasts

During pregnancy the breasts change in both size and appearance (Fig. 6.3). Estrogen stimulates the growth of mammary ductal tissue, and progesterone promotes the growth of the lobes, lobules, and alveoli. The breasts become highly vascular, with a delicate network of veins often visible just beneath the surface of the skin. If the increase in breast size is extensive, striations ("stretch marks") similar to those that occur on the abdomen may develop.

Characteristic changes in the nipples and areolae occur during pregnancy. The nipples increase in size and become darker and more erect, and the areolae become larger and more pigmented. The degree of pigmentation varies with the complexion of the expectant individual. Clients with very light skin tones exhibit less change in pigmentation than those with darker skin.

Sebaceous glands called Montgomery tubercles become more prominent during pregnancy and secrete a substance that lubricates the nipples. In addition, a thick, yellowish fluid—**colostrum**—can be expressed within the first few months (Cunningham et al., 2022). Secretion of milk is suppressed during pregnancy by the high levels of estrogen and progesterone.

❓ KNOWLEDGE CHECK

1. What is the expected uterine growth at 16 weeks, 20 weeks, and 36 weeks of gestation?
2. How does uterine blood flow change during pregnancy?
3. What is the purpose of the cervical mucous plug?
4. What is the major purpose of progesterone in early pregnancy?
5. How do breasts change in size and appearance during pregnancy?

Cardiovascular System

During pregnancy, alterations occur in heart size and position, blood volume, blood flow, and blood components.

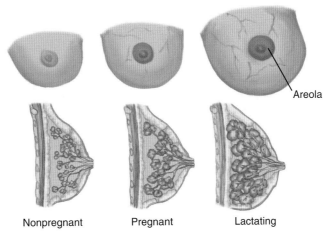

Nonpregnant   Pregnant   Lactating

Areola

Fig. 6.3 Breast changes that occur during pregnancy. The breasts increase in size and become more vascular, the areolae become darker, and the nipples become more erect.

Heart

Heart Size and Position. Cardiac changes are minor and reverse soon after childbirth. The muscles of the heart (myocardium) enlarge 10% to 15% during the first trimester (Blackburn, 2018). The heart is pushed upward to the left and rotated on its long axis as the uterus elevates the diaphragm during the third trimester. As a result of the change in position, the locations for auscultation of heart sounds may be shifted upward and laterally in late pregnancy.

Heart Sounds. Some heart sounds may be so altered during pregnancy that they would be considered abnormal in the nonpregnant state. The changes are first heard between 12 and 20 weeks and continue for 2 to 4 weeks after childbirth. The most common variations in heart sounds include splitting of the first heart sound and a systolic murmur that is found in more than 95% of pregnant clients (Mastrobattista & Monga, 2019). The murmur is best heard at the left sternal border. Up to 90% of pregnant individuals have a third heart sound (Blackburn, 2018).

Blood Volume

Total blood volume is a combination of plasma and components such as red blood cells (RBCs, erythrocytes), white blood cells (WBCs, leukocytes), and platelets (thrombocytes). Total blood volume increase begins by 6 weeks of gestation and reaches an average of 30% to 45% during pregnancy (Blackburn, 2018).

Plasma Volume

Plasma volume increases from 6 to 8 weeks until 32 weeks of gestation. The plasma volume is 40% to 60% (1200 to 1600 mL) greater than that in nonpregnant individuals (Blackburn, 2018). The increase is higher in multifetal pregnancies. The reason for the increase is unclear, but it may be related to vasodilation from nitric oxide, and estrogen, progesterone, and prostaglandin stimulation of the renin–angiotensin–aldosterone system, which causes sodium and water retention (Blackburn, 2018).

The increased volume is needed to (1) transport nutrients and oxygen to the placenta, where they become available for the growing fetus; (2) meet the demands of expanded tissue in the uterus and breasts; and (3) provide a reserve to protect the pregnant client from the adverse effects of blood loss that occurs during childbirth.

Red Blood Cell Volume. RBC volume increases by about 20% to 30% above prepregnancy values (Blackburn, 2018). Although both RBC volume and plasma volume expand, the increase in plasma volume is more pronounced and occurs earlier. The resulting dilution of RBC mass causes a decline in hemoglobin and hematocrit. This condition is frequently called **physiologic anemia of pregnancy** because it reflects dilution of RBCs in the expanded plasma volume, rather than an actual decline in the number of RBCs, and does not indicate true anemia.

Physiologic anemia should not be dismissed as unimportant, however. Frequent laboratory examinations may be needed to distinguish between physiologic and true anemia. Generally, iron deficiency anemia occurs when the hemoglobin is less than 11 grams per deciliter (g/dL) in the first and third trimesters or less than 10.5 g/dL in the second trimester (Cunningham et al., 2022). Iron supplementation is often prescribed for pregnant clients by the second trimester to prevent anemia.

Dilution of RBCs by plasma may have a protective function. By decreasing blood viscosity, dilution may counter the tendency to form clots (thrombi) that could obstruct blood vessels and cause serious complications. Hemodilution may also increase placental perfusion (Mastrobattista & Monga, 2019).

Cardiac Output

The expanded blood volume of pregnancy results in an increase in cardiac output, the amount of blood ejected from the heart each minute. It is based on *stroke volume* (the amount of blood pumped from the heart with each contraction) and *heart rate* (the number of times the heart beats each minute). Cardiac output increases 30% to 50%, with half of the rise occurring in the first 8 weeks of pregnancy, and it remains elevated throughout pregnancy (Casanova et al., 2019). The increase in cardiac output is the result of a gain in stroke volume and a heart rate acceleration that peaks at 15 to 20 beats per minute (bpm) by 32 weeks of gestation. Cardiac output is highest when the client is in a lateral position and is lower in the standing and supine positions (Antony et al., 2021).

Systemic Vascular Resistance

Systemic vascular resistance falls during pregnancy. This change is likely because of (1) vasodilation resulting from the effects of progesterone and prostaglandins; (2) the addition of the uteroplacental unit, which provides a greater area for circulation and low resistance; (3) increased heat production from fetal, placental, and maternal metabolism, which produces vasodilation; (4) decreased sensitivity to angiotensin II; and (5) endothelial prostacyclin and endothelial-derived relaxant factors such as nitric oxide (Blackburn, 2018).

Blood Pressure

The effect of decreased systemic vascular resistance is that blood pressure (BP) changes little during pregnancy despite the increase in blood volume.

Effect of Position. Because BP is affected by position during pregnancy, the client's position during measurements should be recorded so that the method of evaluation remains consistent. Systolic pressure remains largely unchanged or decreases slightly if it is measured when the client is sitting or standing. Diastolic pressure shows a decrease (about 10 to 15 mm Hg) that is greatest at 24 to 32 weeks of gestation. BP returns to usual levels by term (Blackburn, 2018). Arterial pressures are about 10 mm Hg lower when the pregnant client is in a side-lying or supine position than when sitting or standing (Antony et al., 2021).

Supine Hypotension. When the pregnant client is in the supine position, particularly in late pregnancy, the weight of the gravid (pregnant) uterus partially occludes the vena cava and the aorta (Fig. 6.4). The occlusion diminishes return of blood from the lower extremities and consequently reduces

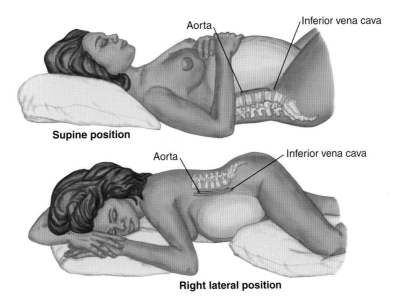

Fig. 6.4 Supine Hypotensive Syndrome. When the pregnant client is in the supine position, the weight of the uterus partially occludes the vena cava and the aorta. The side-lying position corrects supine hypotension.

cardiac return. Cardiac output may be reduced 25% to 30% when the client is in this position (Antony et al., 2021).

Collateral circulation developed in pregnancy generally allows blood flow from the legs and pelvis to return to the heart when the individual is in a supine position. As many as 5% to 10% of clients develop a drop in BP known as *supine hypotensive syndrome,* with symptoms of lightheadedness, dizziness, nausea, or *syncope* (a brief lapse in consciousness) (Antony et al., 2021). Blood flow through the placenta also decreases if the client remains in the supine position for a prolonged time, which could result in fetal hypoxia.

Turning to a lateral recumbent position alleviates the pressure on the blood vessels and quickly corrects supine hypotension. Pregnant clients should be advised to rest in the side-lying position to prevent or correct the occurrence of supine hypotension. If they must lie in the supine position for any reason, a wedge or pillow under one hip may be effective in decreasing supine hypotension.

Blood Flow

Five major changes in blood flow occur during pregnancy:
1. Blood flow is altered to include the uteroplacental unit.
2. Renal plasma flow increases markedly to remove the increased metabolic wastes generated by the client and fetus (Antony et al., 2021).
3. The individual's skin requires increased circulation to dissipate heat generated by increased metabolism during pregnancy.
4. Blood flow to the breasts increases, resulting in engorgement and dilated veins.
5. The weight of the expanding uterus on the inferior vena cava and iliac veins partially obstructs blood return from veins in the legs. Blood pools in the deep and superficial veins of the legs causing venous distention. Prolonged engorgement of the veins of the lower legs may lead to varicose veins of the legs, vulva, or rectum (hemorrhoids) and

increase the risk of developing deep-vein thrombosis or pulmonary embolism (Cunningham et al., 2022).

Blood Components

Although iron absorption is increased during pregnancy, sufficient iron is not always supplied by the diet. Iron supplementation is necessary to promote hemoglobin synthesis and ensure erythrocyte production adequate to prevent iron deficiency anemia.

Leukocytes increase during pregnancy ranging from 5000 cells/mm³ to 12,000 cells/mm³ or as high as 15,000 cells/mm³. Leukocytes increase further during labor and the early postpartum period, reaching levels of 25,000 cells/mm³ (Cunningham et al., 2022).

Pregnancy is a hypercoagulable state because of an increase in factors that favor clotting and a decrease in factors that inhibit clotting. Fibrinogen (factor I), fibrin split products, and factors VII, VIII, IX, and X rise by 50% (Casanova et al., 2019). These changes increase the ability to form clots. Fibrinolytic activity (to break down clots) decreases during pregnancy. The platelet count may decrease slightly but generally remains within the normal range (Blackburn, 2018). These changes offer some protection from hemorrhage during childbirth but also increase the risk of thrombus formation. The risk is a particular concern if the client must stand or sit for prolonged periods with stasis of blood in the veins of the legs.

? KNOWLEDGE CHECK

6. Why is expanded blood volume important during pregnancy?
7. How does physiologic anemia differ from iron deficiency anemia?
8. Why do some pregnant clients feel faint when they are in a supine position?
9. Why is circulation to the kidneys and skin increased during pregnancy?

Respiratory System

The major respiratory changes in pregnancy are the result of three factors: increased oxygen consumption, hormonal factors, and the physical effects of the enlarging uterus.

Oxygen Consumption

Oxygen consumption increases 20% in pregnancy. Half the increase is used by the uterus, the fetus, and the placenta, 30% by the heart and kidneys, and the rest by the respiratory muscles and breast tissues (Casanova et al., 2019). The tidal volume (the volume of gas moved into or out of the respiratory tract with each breath) increases by 30% to 40%. Although residual volume decreases by 20% to 25%, total lung capacity may remain unchanged or decreases by less than 5% (Cunningham et al., 2022). To compensate for the increased need, progesterone causes the client to take deeper breaths, although the respiratory rate remains unchanged. The partial pressure of carbon dioxide (P_{CO_2}) decreases. Increased excretion of hydrogen ions from the kidneys partially compensates for the resulting mild respiratory alkalosis. The hyperventilation and respiratory alkalosis facilitates transfer of carbon dioxide from the fetus to the client (Antony et al., 2021).

Hormonal Factors

Progesterone. Progesterone is considered a major factor in the respiratory changes of pregnancy. Progesterone, along with prostaglandins, helps decrease airway resistance by up to 50% by relaxing the smooth muscle in the respiratory tract. Progesterone is also believed to increase the sensitivity of the respiratory center in the medulla oblongata to carbon dioxide, thus stimulating the increase in minute ventilation. These two factors are responsible for the heightened awareness of the need to breathe experienced by many clients during pregnancy (Blackburn, 2018).

Estrogen. Estrogen causes increased vascularity of the mucous membranes of the upper respiratory tract. As the capillaries become engorged, edema and hyperemia develop within the nose, pharynx, larynx, and trachea. This congestion may cause nasal and sinus stuffiness, epistaxis (nosebleed), and deepening of the voice. Increased vascularity also causes edema of the eardrum and eustachian tubes and may result in a sense of fullness in the ears.

Physical Effects of the Enlarging Uterus

During pregnancy, the enlarging uterus lifts the diaphragm about 4 cm (1.6 inches). The elevation of the diaphragm does not impede its movement, however, which is increased by about 1 to 2 cm (0.4 to 0.8 inch) during respirations. The ribs flare, the substernal angle widens, and the transverse diameter of the chest expands by about 2 cm (0.8 inches) to compensate for the reduced space. These changes begin when the uterus is just beginning to enlarge. They result from the hormone relaxin, which causes relaxation of the ligaments around the ribs. Breathing becomes thoracic rather than abdominal, adding to the dyspnea that as many as 60% to 70% of clients experience beginning in the first or second trimester (Blackburn, 2018).

Gastrointestinal System

The gastrointestinal system undergoes changes that are clinically significant because they may cause discomfort for the expectant client.

Appetite

Unless the client is nauseated, appetite is often increased during pregnancy. This helps with consumption of the additional calories recommended. Food intake may increase by 15% to 20% beginning in early pregnancy (Blackburn, 2018).

Mouth

Elevated levels of estrogen cause hyperemia of the tissues of the mouth and gums and may lead to gingivitis and bleeding gums. Some clients develop a highly vascular hypertrophy of the gums, called *epulis.* The condition regresses spontaneously after childbirth.

Although the amount of saliva does not usually change, some clients experience *ptyalism,* or excessive salivation. The cause of ptyalism may be decreased swallowing associated with nausea or stimulation of the salivary glands by the ingestion of starch (Cunningham et al., 2022). Small, frequent meals and use of chewing gum and oral lozenges offer limited relief to some clients.

Many people think that pregnancy causes loss of minerals from teeth to meet fetal needs. However, this is not true, and the tooth enamel is stable during pregnancy. Tooth decay may occur because of changes in saliva and the nausea and vomiting of pregnancy. Periodontal disease may result in infections that precipitate preterm labor (Blackburn, 2018).

Esophagus

The lower esophageal sphincter tone decreases during pregnancy, primarily because of the relaxant activity of progesterone on the smooth muscles. These changes, along with upward displacement of the stomach, allow gastroesophageal reflux of acidic stomach contents into the esophagus and produce heartburn (**pyrosis**).

Stomach

Elevated levels of progesterone relax all smooth muscle, decreasing tone and motility of the gastrointestinal tract. The effect on emptying time of the stomach is unclear, with some studies showing a decrease and others showing no change during pregnancy. Gastric acidity is decreased during the first two trimesters and increased during the third trimester. The risk of gastric ulcers decreases during pregnancy.

Large and Small Intestines

Emptying time of the intestines increases, allowing more time for nutrient absorption. It may also cause bloating and abdominal distention. Calcium, iron, some amino acids, glucose, sodium, and chloride are better absorbed during pregnancy, but absorption of some of the B vitamins is reduced (Blackburn, 2018). Decreased motility in the large intestine allows time for more water to be absorbed, leading to constipation. Constipation may cause or exacerbate hemorrhoids if the expectant client must strain to have bowel movements. Flatulence may also be a problem.

Liver and Gallbladder

Although the size of the liver and gallbladder remains unchanged during pregnancy, estrogen and progesterone cause functional changes. The enlarging uterus pushes the liver upward and backward during the last trimester, and liver function is also altered. The serum alkaline phosphatase level rises to two to four times that in nonpregnant individuals. Serum albumin and total protein fall partly because of hemodilution (Williamson et al., 2019).

The gallbladder becomes hypotonic, and emptying time is prolonged. The bile becomes thicker predisposing to the development of gallstones. Reduced gallbladder tone also leads to a tendency to retain bile salts, which can cause itching (pruritus) (Cunningham et al., 2022).

Urinary System

Bladder

The client experiences frequency and urgency of urination throughout pregnancy. Although uterine expansion within the pelvis is one cause of these urinary changes, frequency begins before the uterus is big enough to exert pressure on the bladder. Hormonal influences, increased blood volume, and changes in renal blood flow and *glomerular filtration rate (GFR)*—the rate at which water and dissolved substances are filtered in the glomerulus—may play a significant role in urinary frequency. Stress and urge incontinence that begins at any time during pregnancy and continues until after delivery is experienced by 30% to 50% of pregnant clients (Blackburn, 2018). Although frequency and urgency are normal during pregnancy, they are also signs of infection and, if accompanied by burning sensation or pain, may indicate urinary tract infection.

Bladder capacity doubles by term, and the tone is decreased in response to progesterone (Blackburn, 2018). Nocturia is common because sodium and water are retained during the day and excreted during the night when the client is lying down. Pressure from the uterus pushes the base of the bladder forward and upward near the end of pregnancy. The bladder mucosa becomes congested with blood, and the bladder walls become hypertrophied as a result of stimulation from estrogen. Decreased drainage of blood from the base of the bladder results in edema of its tissues and renders the area susceptible to trauma and infection during childbirth.

Kidneys and Ureters

Changes in Size and Shape. During pregnancy, the kidneys change in both size and shape because of dilation of the renal pelves, calyces, and ureters above the pelvic brim. This dilation begins during the second month of pregnancy. The ureters become elongated and are compressed between the enlarging uterus and the bony pelvic brim.

The flow of urine through the ureters is partially obstructed, causing hydrostatic pressure against the renal pelvis. This occurs especially on the right side because the ureter turns toward the right during pregnancy and crosses the iliac and right ovarian veins. As much as 300 mL of urine may be present in the ureters (Blackburn, 2018). The resulting stasis of urine is important because it allows time for bacteria to multiply. The risk of bacteriuria, which may be asymptomatic, is increased, and pyelonephritis results in 30% of these clients (Antony et al., 2021).

Functional Changes of the Kidneys. Renal plasma flow increases by 50% to 80% during pregnancy. This change results from increases in plasma volume and cardiac output. The flow is highest when the client is in the left side-lying position. The GFR rises by as much as 50% because of the higher renal blood flow (Cunningham et al., 2022).

The increases in renal plasma flow and GFR are necessary for excretion of additional metabolic waste from the client and the fetus. Glucose excretion increases, and glycosuria is common during pregnancy. Small quantities of amino acids, water-soluble vitamins, and electrolytes are also excreted because the filtered load of these substances exceeds the ability of the renal tubules to reabsorb them. Bacteria thrive in urine that is rich in nutrients, increasing the risk of urinary tract infections during pregnancy.

Urine output increases throughout pregnancy. Mild proteinuria is common and does not necessarily indicate abnormal kidney function or preeclampsia (Blackburn, 2018). Protein level may be monitored throughout pregnancy to identify increases that would indicate a problem. Tests of renal function may be misleading during pregnancy. As a result of increased GFR, serum creatinine and blood urea nitrogen decrease and creatinine clearance levels increase (Antony et al., 2021).

🔲 KNOWLEDGE CHECK

10. Why do some clients experience dyspnea during pregnancy?
11. How does the respiratory system compensate for upward pressure exerted on the diaphragm by the enlarging uterus?
12. How does pregnancy affect the gastrointestinal system?
13. Why are pregnant clients at increased risk for urinary tract infection?

Integumentary System

Skin

Circulation to the skin increases to help dissipate excess heat produced by increased metabolism. Pregnant clients feel warmer and perspire more, particularly during the last trimester. Accelerated activity by the sebaceous glands fosters the development of acne. Additional changes include hyperpigmentation and vascular changes in the skin.

Hyperpigmentation. Increased pigmentation from elevated levels of estrogen, progesterone, and melanocyte-stimulating hormone occurs in 90% of pregnant clients (Cunningham et al., 2022; Rapini, 2019). Clients with dark hair or skin exhibit more hyperpigmentation compared with clients with very light coloring.

Areas of pigmentation include brownish patches called **melasma**, chloasma, or the "mask of pregnancy." Melasma involves the forehead, cheeks, and bridge of the nose and

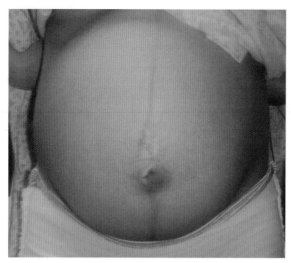

Fig. 6.5 Linea Nigra. A dark pigmented line from the fundus to the symphysis pubis.

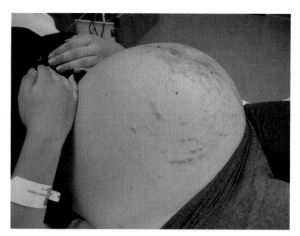

Fig. 6.6 Striae Gravidarum. Lineal tears that may occur in connective tissue.

occurs in about 70% of pregnant clients. It may also occur in nonpregnant individuals taking oral contraceptives. Melasma increases with exposure to sunlight, but use of sunscreen may reduce the severity. Although melasma usually resolves after delivery when estrogen and progesterone levels decline, it continues for months or years in about 30% of clients (Rapini, 2019).

The linea alba—the line that marks the longitudinal division of the midline of the abdomen—darkens to become the **linea nigra** (Fig. 6.5). This dark line of pigmentation may extend from the symphysis pubis to as high as the top of the fundus. Preexisting moles (nevi), freckles, and the areolae become darker as pregnancy progresses. Hyperpigmentation usually disappears after childbirth.

Cutaneous Vascular Changes. During pregnancy, blood vessels dilate and proliferate, which is an effect of estrogen. Changes in surface blood vessels are obvious during pregnancy, especially in clients with fair skin. These include angiomas (vascular spiders, telangiectasia) that appear as tiny red elevations branching in all directions and occur most often on areas exposed to the sun. Redness of the palms of the hands or soles of the feet, known as *palmar erythema,* is thought to occur due to excessive estrogen. Vascular changes may be emotionally distressing for the expectant client, but they are clinically insignificant and usually disappear shortly after childbirth.

Connective Tissue

Linear tears may occur in the connective tissue, most often on the abdomen, breasts, and buttocks, appearing as slightly depressed, discolored streaks called **striae gravidarum,** or "stretch marks" (Fig. 6.6). They occur in 50% to 80% of pregnant clients, and 10% have severe striae (Rapini, 2019). Some individuals may be concerned about striae because they do not disappear after childbirth, although the marks usually fade to lighter or silvery skin tones. Laser therapy is sometimes used after childbirth to reduce or eliminate severe striae. Many clients believe that striae can be prevented by massaging with

oil, vitamin E, or cocoa butter, but these substances have not been found to be effective. Antipruritic creams may be effective in controlling the itching that often occurs.

Hair and Nails

Because fewer follicles are in the resting phase, hair grows more rapidly and less hair falls out during pregnancy. After childbirth, hair follicles return to normal activity, and many clients become concerned at the rate of hair loss that occurs 3 to 4 months following childbirth. They need reassurance that more follicles have returned to the normal resting phase and excessive hair loss will not continue. Hair growth returns to normal within 6 to 12 months after childbirth (Casanova et al., 2019).

The nails may become brittle or softer or may develop transverse grooves. Some clients' nails grow faster or split or break more easily during pregnancy. These changes end after childbirth and no treatment is needed.

Musculoskeletal System

Calcium Storage

During pregnancy, fetal demands for calcium increase, especially in the third trimester. Absorption of calcium from the intestine doubles during pregnancy. Calcium is stored for use during the third trimester when fetal needs peak. Although 28 to 30 g of calcium from maternal bone stores is transferred to the fetus, this amount is small in comparison with total maternal stores and does not deplete the total bone density (Blackburn, 2018).

Postural Changes

Musculoskeletal changes are progressive. They begin early in pregnancy when relaxin and progesterone initiate relaxation of the ligaments. At 28 to 30 weeks, the pelvic symphysis separates (Casanova et al., 2019). The increased mobility of the pelvic joints causes the pregnant client to assume a wide stance with the "waddling" gait of pregnancy.

During the third trimester, as the uterus increases in size, the expectant client must lean backward to maintain balance (Fig. 6.7). This posture creates a progressive lordosis

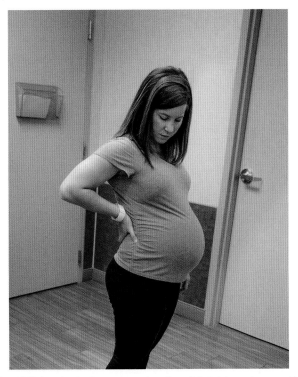

Fig. 6.7 Lordosis increases by the third trimester as the uterus grows larger, and the individual must lean backward to maintain balance.

or curvature of the lower spine and often leads to backache. Obesity or previous back problems increase the problem.

Abdominal Wall

The abdominal muscles may be stretched beyond their capacity during the third trimester, causing **diastasis recti**, separation of the rectus abdominis muscles (see Fig. 17.4). The extent of the separation varies from slight and clinically insignificant to severe, when a large portion of the uterine wall is covered only by the peritoneum, fascia, and skin.

Endocrine System

Numerous changes in hormones occur in pregnancy (Table 6.1).

Pituitary Gland

The anterior pituitary gland increases in size during pregnancy. Serum prolactin levels increase 10-fold by term to prepare the breasts for lactation (Blackburn, 2018). The hormones FSH and LH are not needed to stimulate ovulation during pregnancy and are suppressed by high levels of estrogen and progesterone.

The posterior pituitary releases oxytocin, which stimulates contractions of the uterus. This action is inhibited by progesterone, produced mainly by the placenta during pregnancy. In the second half of pregnancy, estrogen causes a gradual rise of oxytocin receptors in the uterus increasing contractions

TABLE 6.1	Hormones Related To Pregnancy	
Hormone	**Source**	**Major Effects**
Prolactin	Anterior pituitary	Primary hormone of milk production, insulin antagonist
Follicle-stimulating hormone (FSH)	Anterior pituitary	Initiates maturation of ovum, suppressed during pregnancy
Luteinizing hormone (LH)	Anterior pituitary	Stimulates ovulation of mature ovum in nonpregnant state, suppressed in pregnancy
Oxytocin	Posterior pituitary	Stimulates uterine contractions, stimulates milk-ejection reflex after birth, inhibited during pregnancy
Thyroxine (T4)	Thyroid	Increased during pregnancy to stimulate basal metabolic rate, used by fetus in early pregnancy
Cortisol	Adrenals	Increased during pregnancy, insulin antagonist, active in metabolism of glucose, protein, and fats
Aldosterone	Adrenals	Increased during pregnancy to conserve sodium and maintain fluid balance
Human chorionic gonadotropin (hCG)	Trophoblast	Prevents involution of corpus luteum to maintain production of estrogen and progesterone until placenta is formed
Estrogen	Corpus luteum of ovary, placenta	Suppresses FSH and LH; stimulates development of uterus and breasts; causes vascular changes in skin, uterus, respiratory tract, and bladder; causes hyperpigmentation; insulin antagonist; increases fat stores
Progesterone	Corpus luteum of ovary, placenta	Maintains uterine lining for implantation, relaxes smooth muscles, decreases uterine contractions, develops breasts for lactation, increases carbon dioxide sensitivity, increases resistance to insulin, inhibits FSH and LH, prevents fetal tissue rejection, retains sodium
Human chorionic somatomammotropin (human placental lactogen)	Placenta	Stimulates metabolism of fat to provide energy, antagonistic to insulin, promotes sodium retention, prepares breasts for lactation, acts as growth hormone
Relaxin	Corpus luteum, decidua, placenta	Inhibits uterine activity, softens connective tissue of cervix, relaxes cartilage and connective tissue

near term (Boron & Boulpaep, 2021). After childbirth, oxytocin plays an important role in keeping the uterus contracted to prevent excessive bleeding. Oxytocin also stimulates the milk-ejection reflex after childbirth. The pituitary gland returns to prepregnancy size by 6 months postpartum (Cunningham et al., 2022).

Thyroid Gland

Hyperplasia and increased vascularity cause the thyroid gland to enlarge during pregnancy. The availability of thyroid hormones increases by 40% to 100% (Cunningham et al., 2022).

Early in the first trimester, a rise in total thyroxine (T4) and thyroxine-binding globulin occurs. Levels of serum-unbound or free T4 rise early in pregnancy but return to normal nonpregnant levels by the end of the first trimester (Cunningham et al., 2022). Both T4 and triiodothyronine (T3) cross the placenta. Thyroid hormones are important for fetal neurologic function because the fetus does not begin to concentrate iodine until 10 to 12 weeks of gestation and synthesis and secretion of thyroid hormones does not begin until approximately 20 weeks of gestation (Cunningham et al., 2022).

Parathyroid Glands

Parathyroid hormone, which is important in calcium homeostasis, is decreased by 10% to 30% in the first trimester and increases by term. However, it remains in the normal range throughout pregnancy (Blackburn, 2018). Calcium supplies for transfer to the fetus are adequate.

Pancreas

Significant changes in the pancreas during pregnancy are the result of alterations in blood glucose levels and fluctuations in insulin production. Blood glucose levels are 10% to 20% lower than before pregnancy, and hypoglycemia may develop between meals and at night as the fetus continuously draws glucose from the client (Blackburn, 2018).

During the second half of pregnancy, tissue sensitivity to insulin begins to decline because of the effects of human chorionic somatomammotropin (hCS), prolactin, estrogen, progesterone, and cortisol. Fatty acids are used to meet energy needs. Fasting blood glucose level is decreased as glucose passes to the fetus. Postprandial (after a meal) blood glucose level is higher than before pregnancy because of insulin resistance, making more glucose available for fetal energy needs. In healthy clients, the pancreas produces additional insulin. In some clients, however, insulin production cannot be increased, and they experience periodic hyperglycemia or gestational diabetes (see Chapter 10).

Adrenal Glands

Although the adrenal glands enlarge only slightly during pregnancy, significant changes occur in two adrenal hormones: cortisol and aldosterone. The concentrations of both serum cortisol and free (unbound) cortisol, the metabolically active form, are higher. The increase is the result of the elevated estrogen level and a decrease in metabolic clearance rate doubling the half-life of cortisol (Blackburn, 2018). Cortisol regulates carbohydrate and protein metabolism. It stimulates gluconeogenesis (formation of glycogen from noncarbohydrate sources such as amino and fatty acids) whenever the supply of glucose is inadequate to meet the body's needs for energy.

Aldosterone regulates the absorption of sodium from the distal tubules of the kidneys. It increases very early in pregnancy to overcome the salt-wasting effects of progesterone. This helps maintain the necessary level of sodium in the greatly expanded blood volume to meet the needs of the fetus. Aldosterone level is closely related to water metabolism.

Changes Caused by Placental Hormones

Human Chorionic Gonadotropin. In early pregnancy, human chorionic gonadotropin (hCG) is produced by the trophoblastic cells surrounding the developing embryo. The primary function of hCG in early pregnancy is to prevent deterioration of the corpus luteum so that it can continue producing estrogen and progesterone until the placenta is sufficiently developed to assume this function. The presence of this hormone produces a positive pregnancy test result.

Estrogen. Early in pregnancy, estrogen is produced by the corpus luteum. The placenta produces estrogen for the remainder of pregnancy. The effects of estrogen during pregnancy include the following:

- Suppression of FSH and LH
- Stimulation of uterine growth
- Increased blood supply to uterine vessels
- Added deposit of fat stores to provide a reserve of energy
- Increased uterine contractions near term
- Development of the glands and ductal system in the breasts in preparation for lactation
- Hyperpigmentation
- Stimulation of vascular changes in the skin, breasts, upper respiratory tract, and bladder
- Antagonist to insulin

Progesterone. Progesterone is produced first by the corpus luteum and then by the fully developed placenta. Progesterone is the most important hormone of pregnancy. Its major effects include the following:

- Suppression of FSH and LH
- Maintenance of the endometrial layer for implantation of the fertilized ovum and prevention of menstruation
- Decreased uterine contractility to prevent spontaneous abortion
- Increased fat deposits
- Stimulation of development of the lobes, lobules, and ducts in the breast for lactation
- Relaxation of smooth muscles of the uterus, gastric sphincter, bowel, ureters, and bladder
- Increased respiratory sensitivity to carbon dioxide, stimulating ventilation
- Suppression of the immunologic response, preventing rejection of the fetus
- Antagonist to insulin
- Retention of sodium

Human Chorionic Somatomammotropin. Also called *human placental lactogen (hPL),* hCS is present early in pregnancy and increases steadily throughout pregnancy. Its primary function is to increase the availability of glucose for the fetus. A potent insulin antagonist, hCS reduces the sensitivity of cells to insulin and decreases maternal metabolism of glucose. This frees glucose for transport to the fetus, who needs a constant supply. In addition, hCS encourages the quick metabolism of free fatty acids to provide energy for the pregnant client. hCS also helps prepare the breasts for lactation and may act as a growth hormone.

Relaxin. Relaxin is produced by the corpus luteum, the decidua, and the placenta and is present by the first missed menstrual period. Relaxin inhibits uterine activity, softens connective tissue in the cervix, and relaxes cartilage and connective tissue to increase mobility of the pelvic joints (Blackburn, 2018).

Changes in Metabolism

During pregnancy, approximately 3.5 kg of fat and 30,000 kilocalories (kcal) are accumulated. In addition, the client, fetus, and placenta synthesize 900 g of new protein (Blackburn, 2018). The basal metabolic rate increases 10% to 20% by the third trimester (Cunningham et al., 2022).

Weight Gain. A correlation exists between inadequate weight gain in pregnancy and small-for-gestational age infants, as well as between excessive weight gain and increased risk for large-for-gestational age infants. Therefore clients of normal prepregnancy weight are encouraged to gain an average of 11.3 to 16 kg (25 to 35 lb.) during pregnancy (American College of Obstetricians and Gynecologists [ACOG], 2020). The fetus, placenta, and amniotic fluid make up less than half the recommended weight gain. The remainder is found in the increased size of the uterus and breasts, increased blood volume, increased interstitial fluid, and subcutaneous fat stores.

Water Metabolism. The amount of water needed during pregnancy increases to meet the needs of the fetus, placenta, amniotic fluid, and increased blood volume. Total body water increases by 6.5 to 8.5 L by term (Antony et al., 2021). The kidneys must compensate for the many factors that influence fluid balance. Increased GFR, prostaglandins, decreased concentrations of plasma proteins, and increased progesterone level all result in an increase in sodium excretion. However, increased concentrations of estrogen, deoxycorticosterone, hCS, and aldosterone all tend to promote the reabsorption of sodium. The net effect of the combined hormonal action is the maintenance of the sodium and water balance (Blackburn, 2018).

Edema. Because of hemodilution, colloid osmotic pressure decreases slightly, which favors the development of edema during pregnancy. Edema further increases toward term when the weight of the uterus compresses the veins of the pelvis. This process delays venous return, causing the veins of the legs to become distended, and increases venous pressure, resulting in additional fluid shifts from the vascular compartment to interstitial spaces.

Up to 70% of clients have dependent edema during pregnancy. The edema is obvious at the end of the day (particularly if a pregnant client stands for prolonged periods), and the force of gravity contributes to the pooling of blood in the veins of the legs. Generalized edema occurs if the client retains 4 to 5 L of water (Blackburn, 2018). Dependent edema is clinically insignificant if no other abnormal signs are present.

Carbohydrate Metabolism. Carbohydrate metabolism changes markedly during pregnancy when more insulin is needed as pregnancy progresses as a result of increased insulin resistance (Cunningham et al., 2022). See the section titled Pancreas for more information.

Sensory Organs
Eye

Corneal edema may cause clients who wear contact lenses to have some discomfort. The problem resolves after childbirth, and clients should not get new prescriptions for lenses for several weeks after delivery. Intraocular pressure decreases, which may cause improvement and a need for less medication in clients with glaucoma (Blackburn, 2018).

Ear

Changes in the mucous membranes of the eustachian tube from increased levels of estrogen may cause clients to have blocked ears and a mild, temporary hearing loss.

Immune System

Immune function is altered during pregnancy to allow the fetus, which is foreign tissue for the pregnant individual, to grow undisturbed without being rejected by the client's body. This may cause some autoimmune conditions such as rheumatoid arthritis and multiple sclerosis to improve during pregnancy (Cunningham et al., 2022). Resistance to some infections is decreased, however, and some viral and fungal infections occur more often during pregnancy (Blackburn, 2018).

> **? KNOWLEDGE CHECK**
>
> 14. What causes the progressive changes in posture and gait during pregnancy?
> 15. What are the reasons that clients do not ovulate and have menstrual periods during pregnancy?
> 16. Why does the pregnant client's need for insulin change during pregnancy?

CONFIRMATION OF PREGNANCY

Although many clients undergo early ultrasonography to confirm pregnancy, the diagnosis of pregnancy has traditionally been based on symptoms experienced by the client as well as signs observed by a health care provider. Fig. 6.8 summarizes physiologic changes that occur throughout pregnancy. (See Chapter 5 for a discussion on fetal growth and development.)

Gestational age 5-8 weeks

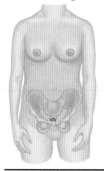

Client misses menstrual period. Nausea; fatigue. Tingling of breasts. Uterus is the size of a lemon; positive Chadwick, Goodell, and Hegar signs. Urinary frequency; increased vaginal discharge.

Gestational age 9-12 weeks

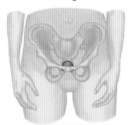

Nausea usually ends by 10–16 weeks. Uterus is size of an orange; palpable above symphysis pubis. Vulvar varicosities may appear. Fetal heartbeat may be heard with a Doppler.

Gestational age 13-16 weeks

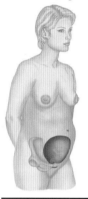

Fetal movements may be felt at about 16 weeks. Uterus has risen into the abdomen; fundus midway between symphysis pubis and umbilicus. Colostrum present; blood volume increases.

Gestational age 17-20 weeks

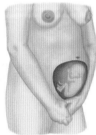

Fetal movements felt. Heartbeat can be heard with fetoscope. Skin pigmentation increases: areolae darken; melasma and linea nigra may be obvious. Braxton Hicks contractions palpable. Fundus at level of umbilicus at about 20 weeks.

Gestational age 21-24 weeks

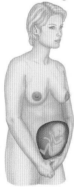

Relaxation of smooth muscles of veins and bladder increases the chance of varicose veins and urinary tract infections. Client is more aware of fetal movements.

Gestational age 25-28 weeks

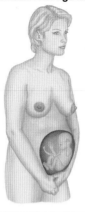

Period of greatest weight gain and lowest hemoglobin level begins. Lordosis may cause backache.

Gestational age 29-32 weeks

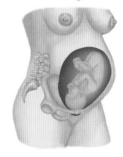

Heartburn common as uterus presses on diaphragm and displaces stomach. Braxton Hicks contractions more noticeable. Lordosis increases; waddling gait develops due to increased mobility of pelvic joints.

Gestational age 33-36 weeks

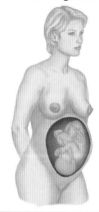

Shortness of breath caused by upward pressure on diaphragm; client may have difficulty finding a comfortable position for sleep. Umbilicus protrudes, pedal or ankle edema may be present. Urinary frequency noted following lightening when presenting part settles into pelvic cavity.

Gestational age 37-40 weeks

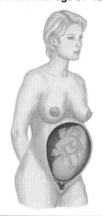

Client is uncomfortable; looking forward to birth of baby. Cervix softens, begins to efface; mucous plug is often lost.

Fig. 6.8 Maternal responses based on the date of the last menstrual period.

The signs and symptoms of pregnancy are grouped into three classifications: presumptive, probable, and positive indications. A diagnosis of pregnancy cannot be made solely on the presumptive or probable signs because they may have other causes, listed in Table 6.2. A definitive diagnosis of pregnancy can be based only on positive signs.

Presumptive Indications of Pregnancy

Most, but not all, presumptive indications are subjective changes that are experienced and reported by the client. These changes are the least reliable indicators of pregnancy because they can be caused by conditions other than pregnancy.

TABLE 6.2 Indications of Pregnancy and Other Possible Causes

Sign	Other Possible Causes
Presumptive Indications	
Amenorrhea	Emotional stress, strenuous physical exercise, endocrine problems, chronic disease, early menopause, anovulation, low body weight
Nausea and vomiting	Gastrointestinal virus, food poisoning, emotional stress
Fatigue	Illness, stress, sudden changes in lifestyle
Urinary frequency	Urinary tract infection
Breast and skin changes	Premenstrual changes, use of oral contraceptives
Chadwick sign	Infection or hormonal imbalance causing pelvic congestion
Quickening	Intestinal gas, peristalsis, or pseudocyesis (false pregnancy)
Probable Indications	
Abdominal enlargement	Abdominal or uterine tumors
Goodell's sign	Hormonal contraceptives or imbalance
Hegar's sign	Hormonal imbalance
Ballottement	Uterine or cervical polyps
Braxton Hicks contractions	Intestinal gas
Palpation of fetal outline	Large leiomyoma that feels like the fetal head, small soft leiomyoma that simulates fetal body parts
Uterine souffle	Confusion with the client's pulse
Positive pregnancy test	Hematuria, proteinuria, some medications, tumors that produce human chorionic gonadotropin (hCG), some drugs
Positive Indications	
Auscultation of fetal heart sounds	
Fetal movements detected by an examiner	
Visualization of embryo or fetus	

Amenorrhea

Absence of menstruation (**amenorrhea**) in a sexually active client who menstruates regularly is one of the first changes noted and strongly suggests that conception has occurred. Menses cease after conception because progesterone and estrogen, secreted by the corpus luteum, maintain the endometrial lining in preparation for implantation of the fertilized ovum. A small amount of bleeding from implantation of the blastocyst may cause the client to think they are having a period (Cunningham et al., 2022).

Nausea and Vomiting

Approximately 60% to 80% of pregnant clients experience nausea and vomiting that begins at 4 to 8 weeks of pregnancy and resolves at 10 to 16 weeks, but some clients experience it earlier and longer (Blackburn, 2018; Cunningham et al., 2022). Nausea and vomiting are believed to be caused by the increased hormones (such as hCG and estrogen) and decreased gastric motility (an effect of progesterone).

Fatigue

Many pregnant clients experience fatigue and drowsiness during the first trimester. The direct cause is unknown, but it may be from changes in hormones such as progesterone.

Urinary Frequency

Urinary frequency begins in the first few weeks of pregnancy and results from hormonal and fluid volume changes. It continues later as the expanding uterus exerts pressure on the bladder. Late in the third trimester, the fetus settles into the pelvic cavity and causes more frequency and urgency of urination as the uterus presses against the bladder.

Breast and Skin Changes

Breast changes begin by the sixth week of pregnancy. The expectant client experiences breast tenderness, tingling, feelings of fullness, and increased size and pigmentation of the areolae.

Many clients observe increased pigmentation of the skin (such as melasma, linea nigra, darkening of the areolae of the breasts) during pregnancy. These skin changes are the result of estrogen and progesterone on melanocytes (Blackburn, 2018).

Vaginal and Cervical Color Change

The cervix, vagina, and labia change from pink to a dark bluish purple. This color change, called the *Chadwick sign*, is another presumptive sign of pregnancy (Blackburn, 2018; Cunningham et al., 2022). It results from increased vascularity of the pelvic organs and is present by 8 weeks of pregnancy.

Fetal Movement

Unlike other presumptive indications of pregnancy, fetal movement (quickening) is not perceived until the second trimester. Although some clients become aware of fetal movement sooner, most expectant clients notice subtle fetal movements, which gradually increase in intensity between 16 and 20 weeks of gestation.

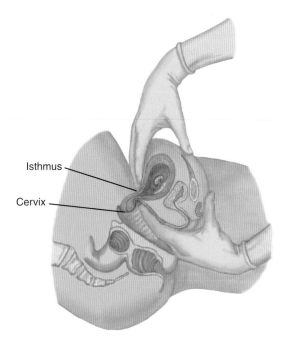

Isthmus

Cervix

Fig. 6.9 Hegar's sign demonstrates softening of the isthmus of the cervix.

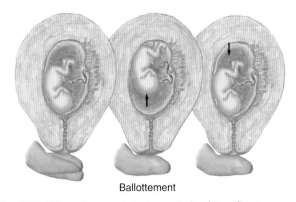

Ballottement

Fig. 6.10 When the cervix is tapped, the fetus floats upward in the amniotic fluid. A rebound is felt by the examiner when the fetus falls back.

Probable Indications of Pregnancy

Probable indications of pregnancy are objective findings that can be documented by an examiner. They are primarily related to physical changes in the reproductive organs. Although these signs are stronger indicators of pregnancy, a positive diagnosis cannot be made because they may have other causes.

Abdominal Enlargement

Enlargement of the abdomen during the childbearing years is a fairly reliable indication of pregnancy, particularly if it corresponds with a slow, gradual increase in uterine growth. Pregnancy is even more likely when abdominal enlargement is accompanied by amenorrhea.

Cervical Softening

In the early weeks of pregnancy, the cervix softens as a result of pelvic vasocongestion (**Goodell's sign**). Cervical softening is

noted during pelvic examination (Cunningham et al., 2022).

Changes in Uterine Consistency

About 6 to 8 weeks after the last menses, the lower uterine segment is so soft that it can be compressed to the thinness of paper. This is called **Hegar's sign** (Fig. 6.9). The body of the uterus can be easily flexed against the cervix.

Ballottement

Near midpregnancy, a sudden tap on the cervix during vaginal examination may cause the fetus to rise in the amniotic fluid and then rebound to its original position (Fig. 6.10). This movement, called *ballottement,* is a strong indication of pregnancy, but it may also be caused by other factors such as uterine or cervical polyps.

Braxton Hicks Contractions

Irregular, painless contractions occur throughout pregnancy, although many expectant clients do not notice them until the third trimester. They increase in strength and frequency as the pregnancy nears term, occurring as often as every 10 minutes (Cunningham et al., 2022). It is important to differentiate Braxton Hicks contractions from the contractions of preterm labor. This is often difficult, and the client should check with a health care provider if unsure, has more than five or six contractions in an hour, or has any other signs of early labor.

Palpation of the Fetal Outline

Unless the client is very obese, an experienced practitioner is able to palpate the outlines of the fetal body by the middle of pregnancy. Outlining the fetus becomes easier as the pregnancy progresses and the uterine walls thin to accommodate the growing fetus.

Uterine Souffle

Late in pregnancy, the *uterine souffle*—a soft, blowing sound—may be auscultated over the uterus. This is the sound of blood circulating through the dilated uterine vessels and it corresponds to the client's pulse. Therefore, to identify the uterine souffle, the client's pulse rate must be checked simultaneously. Uterine souffle differs from *funic souffle*—the soft, whistling sound heard over the umbilical cord and corresponding to the fetal heart rate.

Pregnancy Tests

Pregnancy tests detect hCG or the beta subunit of hCG, which is secreted by the placenta and present in maternal blood and urine shortly after conception. Immunoassay tests are available to test blood or urine for pregnancy in a laboratory or home. They can detect hCG at very low concentrations and are positive as early as 3 to 7 days after conception (Pagana et al., 2021). For home testing, the client obtains a urine sample and dips a strip or wick into the specimen and observes for a color or digital change. The first morning void is preferred because it is most concentrated. Instructions vary with different tests and directions should be read carefully when testing at home.

Inaccurate Pregnancy Test Results. When pregnancy test results are reported as negative and the client is in fact pregnant, the results are called *false-negative*. False-negative results may occur when the instructions are not followed properly, it is too early in the pregnancy, the urine is too dilute, or the client is taking medications such as diuretics. Hematuria, proteinuria, or some tumors may cause *false-positive* results, where the test indicates a pregnancy when the client is not pregnant. Some anticonvulsants, antiparkinsonian drugs, tranquilizers, and hypnotics may also cause a false-positive result (Pagana et al., 2021).

Positive Indications of Pregnancy

Only three signs are accepted as positive confirmation of pregnancy: auscultation of fetal heart sounds, fetal movement detected by an examiner, and visualization of the embryo or fetus.

Auscultation of Fetal Heart Sounds

Fetal heart sounds can be heard with a fetoscope by 18 to 20 weeks of gestation (Casanova et al., 2019). The electronic Doppler, which is used more often, detects heart motion and makes an audible sound by 10 weeks of gestation (Cunningham et al., 2022).

To distinguish the fetal heartbeat from the client's pulse, the examiner palpates the client's pulse while auscultating the fetal heartbeat. The normal fetal heart rate is 110 to 160 bpm. The fetal heart rate is muffled by the amniotic fluid, and the location changes because the fetus moves freely in the amniotic fluid.

Fetal Movements Detected by an Examiner

Fetal movements are considered a positive sign of pregnancy when felt or visualized by an experienced examiner who is not likely to be deceived by peristalsis in the large intestine.

Visualization of the Embryo or Fetus

Confirmation of pregnancy has become much simpler since the development of ultrasonography, which makes it possible to view the embryo or fetus and observe the fetal heartbeat very early in pregnancy. Positive confirmation of pregnancy is possible by transvaginal ultrasonography as early as 3 to 4 weeks of gestation (Casanova et al., 2019). Ultrasonographic testing is discussed further in Chapter 9.

❓ KNOWLEDGE CHECK

17. How do presumptive and probable indications of pregnancy differ?
18. Why is "fetal" movement felt by the pregnant client not a positive sign of pregnancy?
19. What are the most common causes of inaccurate pregnancy test results?

PSYCHOSOCIAL ADAPTATIONS TO PREGNANCY

Becoming a parent who is capable of loving and caring for a totally dependent infant is more than a biologic event. The process begins before conception and involves major changes in the client, the client's partner, and the entire family. Although each couple adapts to pregnancy in a unique way, the psychological responses of prospective parents change as the pregnancy progresses. Although the initial reaction may be uncertainty, by the time the infant is born, the client and partner have completed **developmental tasks**, maturation steps that allow further development. These help them become parents in the true sense of the word. Both social and cultural factors influence their adjustment to the pregnancy.

PSYCHOLOGICAL RESPONSES

A client's psychological response to pregnancy changes over time. Initially, there may be uncertainty or ambivalence about the pregnancy, and the client's primary focus is on themselves. Gradually, the focus shifts, and the client becomes increasingly concerned about protecting and providing for the fetus.

First Trimester
Uncertainty

During the early weeks, the client is unsure and seeks to confirm the pregnancy. The body is carefully observed for changes indicating pregnancy. Family and friends may be consulted about the probability, and over-the-counter pregnancy test kits may be used for validation.

Reaction to the uncertainty of pregnancy depends on the individual. An individual may be eager to find confirming signs, or may dread the possibility and hope for signs indicating there is no pregnancy. Usually, confirmation from a health care provider is sought during the first trimester of pregnancy.

Ambivalence

Pregnancy is often unexpected as almost half of pregnancies are unintended. Once the pregnancy is confirmed, many clients have conflicting feelings, or **ambivalence**, about being pregnant (Link, 2018). Some may feel that this is not the right time, even if the pregnancy is wanted and planned. Clients who had intended to become pregnant often say they thought it would take longer to occur and that they feel unprepared. Many pregnancies are desired but unplanned, and these clients may wish they had completed some goal before becoming pregnant.

Pregnancy causes permanent life changes for clients, and they often begin to examine expected changes and decide how they will cope with them. If it is the first pregnancy, clients may worry about the added responsibility and feel unsure of their ability to be a good parent. Multiparas may be apprehensive about how this pregnancy will affect their relationships with their other children and partners. Ambivalence has usually changed to acceptance by the second trimester.

The Self as Primary Focus

Throughout the first trimester, clients' primary thoughts are about themselves, not the fetus. Early physical responses to pregnancy, such as nausea and fatigue, confirm something is happening, but the fetus seems vague and unreal. Because no weight has been gained to confirm a growing, developing fetus, thoughts may be more about being pregnant than about the coming baby.

Physical changes and increased hormone levels may cause emotional lability (unstable moods). Mood can change quickly from contentment to irritation or from optimistic planning to an overwhelming sleepiness. These changes may be confusing to the partner and family, who are accustomed to more stability.

Nurses should concentrate on the client's physical and psychological needs during this period of self-focus. Teaching should be aimed at the common early changes of pregnancy and their normality. Ways of coping with morning sickness, sexuality, and mood swings are important subjects to explore. The nurse should assess how the client and family are managing these changes and explain that such changes are normal and generally do not indicate problems.

Second Trimester

Physical Evidence of Pregnancy

During the second trimester, physical changes occur that make the fetus "real". The uterus grows rapidly and can be palpated in the abdomen, weight increases, and breast changes are obvious. Ultrasound examination allows the client to see the fetus, and ultrasound pictures or videos can be shared with family and friends. During this time, fetal movement (**quickening**) is experienced. This is important because it confirms the presence of the fetus with each movement. As a result, the client no longer thinks of the fetus as simply a part of the body but now perceives it as separate from themselves.

The Fetus as Primary Focus

The fetus becomes the primary focus during the second trimester. The discomforts of the first trimester have usually decreased, and uterine and fetal size does not affect physical activity. Concern shifts to producing a healthy infant. Information about diet and fetal development may be of interest. A feeling of creative energy and satisfaction is common.

Narcissism and Introversion

At this time, many clients become increasingly concerned about their ability to protect and provide for the fetus. This concern is often manifested as **narcissism** (undue preoccupation with oneself) and **introversion** (concentration on the self and body). Selecting exactly the right foods to eat or the right clothes to wear may assume more importance than earlier in the pregnancy. Some individuals lose interest in their jobs, which may seem alien compared with the events taking place inside them. They may become less interested in current events as they focus on the pregnancy or may become fearful that world events threaten them and their fetus.

Particularly during the first pregnancy, the expectant client wonders about the infant, looking at their own baby pictures and those of the other parent, or hearing stories about what they were like as infants may be of interest. Although multiparas know more about infants in general, they are interested in this infant and concerned with this child's acceptance by siblings and grandparents. Expectant parents may also examine their relationships with others and how these ties will change after the birth.

The client often spends much time thinking about the fetus and daydreaming or fantasizing about what life will be like when it is born. They may call the baby by name and talk about the baby's personality. Some enjoy reading about fetal development to see what changes are happening each week. This intense introspection may be confusing to the partner and family because it is so different from the client's usual behavior.

Body Image

Rapid and profound changes take place in the body during the second trimester. Changes in body size and contour are obvious with thickening of the waist, bulging of the abdomen, and enlargement of the breasts. Increasing breast size in an individual with previously small breasts may be a happy side effect of pregnancy. Others with large breasts may be concerned about pregnancy changes causing their breasts to be too heavy or pendulous.

Changes may be welcomed because they signify growth of the fetus and give the client and partner a feeling of pride. They increase the client's **body image** (subjective view of oneself). For some, however, the change in body size and shape, coupled with hyperpigmentation of the skin and striae gravidarum, may contribute to a negative body image. Changes in body function such as altered balance, reduced physical endurance, and discomfort in the pelvis and lower back areas may also affect body image (see Nursing Care Plan).

◎ NURSING CARE PLAN

Body Image during Pregnancy

Assessment	**Nursing Diagnosis**
Shannon is a 34-year-old primiparous client in the 26th week of pregnancy. Both she and her husband have been runners for several years. With her physician's permission, she continued running until 6 weeks ago when she began to find it uncomfortable. Shannon says she now walks "like other old ladies." She expresses concern about the discoloration on her face and her increasing size and says she feels "fat, awkward, and ugly." She states, "I hate the way I look! I can't wait to get back into shape." She also has questions about what sexual activity is allowed during pregnancy.	Disturbed body image related to changes in body size, contour, and function secondary to pregnancy **Expected Outcomes** By the end of her next prenatal visit Shannon will: 1. Make statements that indicate acceptance of expected body changes during her pregnancy. 2. Express her feelings about body changes to her husband and the health care team.

◎ NURSING CARE PLAN—cont'd

Body Image during Pregnancy

3. Set realistic goals for weight loss and the resumption of a running program after childbirth.
4. Report continued mutually satisfactory sexual activity during pregnancy.

Interventions and Rationales

1. Acknowledge Shannon's feelings. "I can see you're disappointed about not being able to run and concerned about how pregnancy has changed your body." *Feelings must be acknowledged, reflected, and dealt with before the underlying cause can be addressed.*
2. Clarify her concerns. "You've always been an athlete. Pregnant clients often wonder if changes in pregnancy will affect them permanently." *An underlying unvoiced concern may be that pregnancy will change the client and make continuing athletics impossible. This altered perception of self may cause fear, grief, or both.*
3. Suggest that she share her feelings with her husband and seek his support. Model this interaction, if necessary: "I feel awkward and left out of a big part of our lives. I need some reassurance from you." *Although the client may assume the partner recognizes and understands the negative feelings, this may not be true.*
4. Discuss types of low-impact, moderate exercise, such as walking or swimming, that would be beneficial for Shannon. *Moderate daily exercise is encouraged during uncomplicated pregnancy.*
5. Describe the expected pattern of weight gain for the rest of the pregnancy and correlate this with the growth and development of the fetus. Explain that adipose tissue provides needed energy for birth and lactation. *Knowledge of the expected weight gain and understanding that weight gain shows the fetus is growing may allay unexpressed fears of excessive weight gain.*
6. Help Shannon make realistic plans to lose weight and recover her strength and endurance after childbirth.
   a. Explain the expected pattern of weight loss after childbirth.
   b. Demonstrate graduated exercises that increase muscle tone and strength.
   c. Discuss a diet that meets her needs for breastfeeding.
   Many clients are relieved to know that the added weight will be lost gradually. Breastfeeding requires additional calories and nutrients.
1. Explain that the discoloration on her face (melasma) is normal and usually disappears after pregnancy. Suggest she limit exposure to the sun and use sunscreen. *Knowledge of what is normal is comforting. Limiting exposure to the sun and using sunscreen may help decrease the severity.*
2. Determine Shannon's specific concerns about sexuality and respond to those in particular. *Concerns vary among couples. Some couples worry about harming the fetus or causing discomfort for the client.*
3. Reassure her that sexual activity poses no harm to either herself or the fetus in a normal pregnancy. Explain the anatomy of the vagina, cervix, and uterus. Suggest she bring her partner to the next visit if he has concerns. *Knowledge of the separation between the vagina and the fetus may relieve concern about the safety of vaginal intercourse during pregnancy.*
4. Suggest that alternative positions such as side-lying, client-superior, and vaginal entry from the back be used for intercourse during the third trimester. *When the client lays flat on their back, it can be uncomfortable and because the uterus is large and heavy, it increases the risk of supine hypotension.*

Evaluation

At the next prenatal visit, Shannon speaks with pride about how big the baby is growing and makes other statements showing more acceptance of body changes. She reports that her husband has shown increased concern about her feelings and has been very supportive since she shared her feelings with him. Shannon has explored other types of exercises and has found several she will use during the rest of her pregnancy. She begins to plan a realistic schedule of diet and exercise that she will follow after the birth. She relates mutually satisfying sexual experiences.

Changes in Sexuality

The sexual interest and activity of pregnant clients and their partners are unpredictable and may increase, decline, or remain unchanged. Physical comfort and sense of well-being are closely linked to interest in sexual activity. The culture of the couple is also important. Intercourse during pregnancy is allowed and encouraged in some cultures but strictly forbidden in others.

During the first trimester, freedom from worry about becoming pregnant or the need for contraception may provide a sense of freedom and enhance sexual interest in both partners. However, nausea, fatigue, and breast tenderness may interfere with erotic feelings. Fear of miscarriage may cause couples to avoid intercourse, particularly if the client has previously lost a pregnancy or has had infertility therapy. Nurses can reassure the couple that intercourse has not been associated with early pregnancy loss when no complications are present.

In the second trimester, clients experience increased sensitivity of the labia and clitoris and increased vaginal lubrication from pelvic vasocongestion. Nausea is no longer a concern by this time for most clients. Many have a general feeling of well-being and energy that may increase sexual responsiveness. Orgasm may occur more frequently and with greater intensity during pregnancy because of these changes. Although orgasm causes temporary uterine contractions, they are not harmful if the pregnancy has been normal.

During the third trimester, the "missionary position" (partner on top) may cause discomfort because of abdominal pressure. Heartburn, indigestion, and supine hypotensive syndrome also increase in this position. The pressure of the fetus low in the pelvis may add to the discomfort. Moreover, fatigue, ligament pain, urinary frequency, and shortness of breath may be problems.

The nurse can suggest alternative positions such as female-superior, side-to-side, or vaginal rear-entry for intercourse. The side-lying position may be the most comfortable and require the least amount of energy during the third trimester. Hugging, cuddling, kissing, and mutual massage or masturbation are other ways to express affection without vaginal intercourse.

As the uterus becomes larger, some clients believe their bodies are ugly and worry about their partner's reaction to their increased size. Sexual response varies widely among partners. Some partners report heightened feelings of sexual interest, but others perceive the client's body in late pregnancy as unattractive, and erotic feelings decrease. In addition, fear of harming the fetus or causing discomfort to the client may interfere with sexual activity.

Despite the need for information, many clients are reluctant to initiate a discussion about sexual activity. Unfortunately, most health care professionals do not introduce the topic. They may fear offending the client or may be uncomfortable with their own sexuality and embarrassed to begin a discussion. Providers often lack time for any but the most pressing assessments. The result may be that an important aspect of care is ignored.

A broad opening statement may help initiate discussion about sexual activity—for example, "Sometimes couples are concerned about having sex during pregnancy." Such statements introduce the subject in a way that lets the client feel comfortable either pursuing it or ignoring it.

The couple should be made aware of the normal changes in sexual desire that occur during pregnancy and the importance of communicating their feelings openly with each other to find solutions to problems. The nurse can reassure the couple that their feelings are normal.

Intercourse is safe throughout pregnancy if there are no complications. Bleeding, an incompetent cervix, placenta previa, rupture of membranes, and history of preterm labor in the present pregnancy are contraindications for intercourse. In addition, blowing into the vagina should be avoided at any time as it may cause an air embolus (Cunningham et al., 2022).

Third Trimester

Vulnerability

The sense of well-being and contentment that dominates the second trimester gives way to increasing feelings of vulnerability that peak in the third trimester during the seventh month (Cunningham et al., 2022). The expectant client may worry that the precious baby may be lost or harmed if not protected at all times. They may have fantasies or nightmares about having a deformed baby or harm coming to the infant and may become very cautious as a result. They may avoid crowds due to feeling unable to protect the infant from infectious diseases or potential physical dangers. They may need reassurance that such dreams and fears are not unusual in pregnancy.

Increasing Dependence

The expectant client often becomes increasingly dependent on the partner in the last weeks of pregnancy. The client may insist that the partner be easy to reach at all times and may call several times during the day. Reliance on others may increase at this time, which may result in seeking their help with decision- making. This may be frustrating if it is a marked change.

Individuals often have fears about the safety of the partner and that something will happen to him or her. The need for love and attention from the partner is even more pronounced in late pregnancy. When the partner assures the client of their concern and willingness to provide assistance, the client feels more secure and able to cope.

Although the client may not be able to explain the increasing dependence, anger and frustration may result if the partner does not understand and sympathize. Irritability may increase because of fatigue at this time as well. The nurse can encourage couples to discuss fears and feelings openly so that misunderstandings can be avoided.

Some pregnant clients have difficulty with tasks that require direct, sustained attention, particularly in the third trimester. They may feel that they have trouble concentrating or focusing on learning new material or skills at this time. Teaching should be clear and concise to help them learn most easily.

Preparation for Birth

Gradually, the feelings of vulnerability decrease as the client comes to terms with the situation. The fetus continues to grow, and fetal movements are no longer gentle. Pokes, jabs, and kicks are intrusive expressions of the baby's crowded condition and increasing activity. The relationship with the fetus changes during this time and clients start to see the baby as an individual and not a part of their own body. Although the client may not consciously acknowledge the increasing feelings of separateness, there is a longing to see and become acquainted with the baby.

Most pregnant clients are concerned about their ability to determine when they are in labor. They review the signs of labor and question friends and family members who are parents. Many couples are anxious about getting to the birth facility in time for the birth, and they may be worried about coping with labor.

During the last few weeks, the client becomes increasingly concerned about the due date and the experience of labor and delivery. Some fear labor and dread the due date, whereas others are so uncomfortable that they look forward to that day, expecting it to be the exact day the birth will occur. They often say they are tired of being pregnant and want the pregnancy to be over.

Clients pregnant for the first time are more likely to fear childbirth than multiparas. Common concerns include fear of childbirth pain or adverse outcomes for labor or the baby. Multiparas who had a previous negative pregnancy or birth experience have increased concerns during the current pregnancy. Worry may also increase if friends or relatives have had difficult pregnancies.

Clients may seek help for their fears by talking to members of their support system or by seeking information from health care professionals, books, television, or the internet.

Clients may watch TV or listen to podcasts that describe pregnancy and childbirth to learn more about what their own experience might be like. However, the information shared may not always be scientifically based, show practices that are evidence-based, or depict experiences that are most common.

During the third trimester some expectant clients prepare for the infant. "Nesting" behavior includes obtaining clothing and furniture and arranging a place for the infant to sleep. Negotiation of how the couple will share household tasks is among the plans made at this time. In addition, many couples complete childbirth education classes (see Chapter 7). Table 6.3 summarizes changes in client responses during pregnancy.

❓ KNOWLEDGE CHECK

20. Why might an expectant client say, "I am pregnant" during the first trimester and "I am going to be a parent" late in pregnancy?
21. How might pregnancy affect the sexual responses of a couple?

PARENTAL ROLE TRANSITION

Becoming a parent involves intense feelings of love, tenderness, and devotion that endure over a lifetime. How does an individual learn to be a parent? While concepts of what a "family" looks like have changed over time, many of the tasks and roles can be generalized to adoption, surrogacy, or transgender individuals.

TABLE 6.3 Progressive Changes in Responses to Pregnancy

First Trimester	Second Trimester	Third Trimester
Emotional Responses		
Uncertainty, ambivalence, focus on self, emotional lability	Wonder, increased narcissism, introversion, concern about changes in their body and sexuality	Vulnerability, increased dependence, acceptance that fetus is separate but totally dependent
Physical Validation		
No obvious signs of fetal growth	Quickening, enlarging abdomen	Obvious fetal growth, discomfort, decreased physical activity
Role		
May begin to seek safe passage for self and fetus	Seeks acceptance of fetus and their role as parent	Prepares for birth, sets up expectations of oneself as a parent
"Self-Statement"		
"I am pregnant."	"I am going to have a baby."	"I am going to be a parent."

Role transition is changing from one pattern of behavior and self-image into another. The transition into the parental role begins during pregnancy and increases with gestational age. The client must accept the pregnancy and the changes that will result. They develop a relationship with the unborn child, first as part of oneself and then as a separate individual. Near the end of pregnancy, they must prepare for the birth and for parenting the new baby.

Transitions Experienced throughout Pregnancy

The client undergoes transitions in relationships that continue throughout the pregnancy and becomes more aware of self and the changes occurring in life. The relationship with the client's partner changes as they both prepare for parenthood. The client needs mentors to provide reassurance that feelings and experiences that occur during pregnancy are normal, in addition to support from other new parents.

Steps in Parental Role Taking

Rubin (1984), in this classic work, observed specific steps that provide a framework for understanding the process of maternal role taking: mimicry, role play, fantasy, the search for a role fit, and grief work.

Mimicry

Mimicry involves observing and copying the behaviors of other pregnant individuals or new parents in an attempt to discover what the role is like. Mimicry often begins in the first trimester, when the client may wear maternity clothes before they are needed to understand the feelings of others in more advanced pregnancy and to see how others react. Clients may also mimic the waddling gait or posture of a person who is close to delivery long before these changes occur in their bodies.

Role Play

Role play consists of acting out some aspects of what parents actually do. The pregnant client searches for opportunities to hold or care for infants in the presence of another person. Role playing provides an opportunity to "practice" the expected role and receive validation of success from an observer. The client may be particularly sensitive to the responses of the partner and the client's parents.

Fantasy

Fantasies (mental images formed to prepare for the birth of a child) allow the client to consider a variety of possibilities and daydream or "try on" a variety of behaviors. Fantasies often revolve around how the infant will look and what characteristics the baby will have. The client may daydream about taking the child to the park or reading or singing songs to the child. There may also be vivid dreams at night.

At times, fantasies are fearful. What if something is wrong with the infant? What if the baby cries and will not stop? Some people dream about a stranger entering their life. The stranger may represent the fetus (James & Suplee, 2021). Fearful fantasies often provoke pregnant clients to respond by seeking information or reassurance. For instance, they may ask their partner if they will love the baby even if the baby is not perfect, or they may strive to learn all they can about caring for a baby who is difficult to console.

Fantasies may change during each trimester and may be different for primigravidas and multigravidas. Fantasies are most frequent during the third trimester. The nurse shows acceptance and understanding by listening to the client's fantasies. In addition, listening helps the nurse identify concerns that may need further discussion.

The Search for a Role Fit

The search for a role fit occurs once the client has established a set of role expectations and internalized a view of a "good" parent's behavior. They compare their self-expectations with behaviors seen in other parents. They imagine themselves acting in the same way and either reject or accept the behaviors, depending on how well they fit their idea of what is right. This process implies that clients have explored the role of parent long enough to have developed a sense of themselves in the role and to be able to select behaviors that reaffirm their view of how they will fulfill the role.

Grief Work

Although grief work seems incongruous with parental role taking, people often experience a sense of sadness when they realize that they must give up certain aspects of their previous selves and can never go back. A primigravida will never again be a carefree person who has not had a child and must relinquish some of the old patterns of behavior to take on a new identity as a parent. Even simple things such as going shopping or to the movies will require planning to include the infant or find alternative care. The multipara will have one more child claiming their attention. Changes may be particularly difficult for the adolescent parent, who is not used to planning ahead and may have to give up or change school plans as well.

Parental Tasks of Pregnancy

To become parents, pregnant clients spend a great deal of time and energy learning new behaviors. As clients work to establish a relationship with the infant, they must also reorder relationships with their partner and family. This psychological work of pregnancy has been grouped into four maternal tasks of pregnancy (Rubin, 1984):

1. Seeking safe passage for oneself and baby through pregnancy, labor, and childbirth
2. Gaining acceptance of the baby and oneself from the partner and family
3. Learning to give of oneself
4. Developing attachment and interconnection with the unknown child

Seeking Safe Passage

Seeking safe passage for oneself and the baby is the client's priority task. If clients cannot be assured of that safety, they cannot move on to the other tasks. Behaviors that ensure safe passage include seeking the care of a health care provider

and following recommendations about diet, vitamins, rest, and subsequent visits for care. In addition to following the advice of health care professionals, the pregnant client must also adhere to cultural practices that ensure safety for self and the baby.

Securing Acceptance

Securing acceptance is a process that continues throughout pregnancy. It involves reworking relationships so that the important persons in the family accept the client in the role of parent and welcome the baby into the family constellation.

In their first pregnancy, the parents of the baby must give up an exclusive relationship and make a place in their lives for a child. When the partner expresses pride and joy in each pregnancy, the client feels valued and comforted. This feeling is so important that many clients retain a memory of the partner's reaction to the announcement of pregnancy for many years.

Feeling support and acceptance from their parents is especially important. The pregnant client gains energy and contentment when their parents freely offer acceptance and support. Many expectant clients gain a sense of increased closeness with their parents during pregnancy.

Problems may occur if the family strongly desires a child with particular characteristics and the client believes that the family may reject an infant who does not meet the criteria. For example, if family members wish for a boy, will they accept a girl?

Learning to Give of Self

Giving is one of the most idealized components of parenthood but one that is essential. Learning to give to the new baby begins in pregnancy when clients allow their body to give space and nurturing to the fetus. This tests their ability to derive pleasure from giving by providing food, care, and acts of thoughtfulness for the family.

Pregnant clients also learn to give by receiving. Gifts received at "baby showers" are more than needed items. They also confirm continued interest and commitment from friends and family. Intangible gifts from others, such as companionship, attention, and support, help increase energy and affirm the importance of giving.

Committing Self to the Unknown Child

The process of **attachment** (development of strong affectional ties) begins in early pregnancy when the client accepts or "binds in" to the idea of pregnancy, even though the baby is not yet real to them. During the second trimester, the baby becomes real and feelings of love and attachment surge. This is especially true when quickening occurs or after an ultrasound shows recognizable parts of the baby.

Clients report feedback from their unborn infants during the third trimester and describe unique characteristics of the fetus with regard to sleep–wake cycles, temperament, and communication. Love of the infant becomes possessive and leads to feelings of vulnerability. Clients integrate the role of parent into their self-image. They become comfortable with the idea of themselves as parents and find pleasure in contemplating the new role.

Some clients delay attachment to the fetus until they feel sure the pregnancy is normal and will continue. This is especially true for those who have lost a pregnancy previously. They may begin to have feelings of attachment after they have passed a critical time that correlates to the time they lost a previous pregnancy (James & Suplee, 2021).

> **❓ KNOWLEDGE CHECK**
>
> 22. What does "looking for a fit" mean in role transition?
> 23. Why is grief work part of parental role transition?
> 24. How does the pregnant client seek safe passage for self and baby?

PARTNER ADAPTATION TO PREGNANCY

Expectant partners do not experience the biologic processes of pregnancy, but they also must make major psychosocial changes to adapt to a new role. These changes may be more difficult because the partner is often neglected by the health care team and peer groups, as attention is focused on the pregnant client. Concerns and anxieties may remain unknown because of the lack of focus on the partner.

Variations in Partner Adaptation

Wide variations exist in parental responses of the partner related to pregnancy. Some individuals are emotionally invested and comfortable as full partners exploring every aspect of pregnancy, childbirth, and parenting. Others are more task-oriented and view themselves as managers. They may direct the client's diet and rest periods and act as coaches during childbirth, but they remain detached from the emotional aspects of the experience. Some individuals are more comfortable as observers and prefer not to participate. In some cultures, men are conditioned to see pregnancy and childbirth as "women's work" and may not be able to express their true feelings about pregnancy and parenthood.

Readiness for parenthood is more likely if a stable relationship between the partners, financial security, and a desire for parenthood are present. Additional factors include partners' relationship with their parents, previous experience with children, and confidence in their ability to care for the infant.

Partners have many concerns during a pregnancy. Unplanned pregnancy is more likely to cause distress for parents-to-be, as might be expected. In addition, coping with the expectant client's emotional lability can be confusing and difficult. Common concerns include anxiety about the health of the client and baby, financial concerns, and apprehension about the role during the birth and about changes that will result when the baby arrives.

Financial concerns may be especially acute in a two-income family if the client develops complications that result in loss of expected income. A reduction in income coupled with an increase in expenses can result in added stress for both parents. Partners may seek a second job or work overtime to prepare for the increased financial needs. Other concerns include the responsibility parenthood will bring and whether the couple will be good parents.

Developmental Processes

The responses of the expectant partner are dynamic, progressing through phases that are subject to individual variation. Jordan (1990) describes three developmental processes that an expectant partner must address:

- Grappling with the reality of pregnancy and the new child
- Struggling for recognition as a parent from the family and social network
- Making an effort to be seen as relevant to childbearing

The Reality of Pregnancy and the Child

The pregnancy and the child must become real before a partner can assume the identity of parent. The process requires time and may be incomplete until the birth. Initially, the pregnancy is a diagnosis only, and changes in the expectant client's behavior, such as nausea and fatigue, are perceived as symptoms of illness that have little to do with having a baby.

A partner's initial reaction to the announcement of pregnancy may be pride and joy but may include ambivalence, particularly if the partner is unprepared for the added responsibility or commitment. Various experiences act as catalysts or "reality boosters" that make the child more real. The most frequently mentioned experiences are seeing the fetus on an ultrasound, hearing the baby's heartbeat, and feeling the baby move.

Preparing room for the baby and accumulating supplies also reinforce the reality of the coming child. These tasks often represent the first time that the partner has the opportunity to do something directly for the baby. The birth itself is the most powerful reality booster, and the infant becomes real with the opportunity to see and hold the baby.

The Struggle for Recognition as a Parent

Partners may be perceived by others as helpmates but not parents in their own right. Some individuals may be upset that their feelings are not validated and that they may not be recognized as parents as well as helpers. Many individuals accept that the focus should be on the birthing parent, but others are frustrated by the lack of understanding of their own experiences.

Support groups or classes for expectant parents are sometimes available. These groups allow them to talk with other people about changes resulting from the pregnancy and how these changes have affected them. Knowing experiences and feelings are shared by other individuals in the same situation is very helpful.

Expectant clients play an important role in helping their partners gain recognition as parents. Clients who openly share their physical sensations and emotions help their partner feel that they are part of the process. These clients often say "we" are pregnant and include their partners in all discussions and decisions.

Nurses must learn to view the client, partner, and baby together and not focus exclusively on the birthing parent and the fetus. Partners may be concerned about the physical symptoms experienced by the client. The nurse should encourage partners to ask questions about the pregnancy. Partners are entitled to as much advice and reassurance as the birthing parent. Partners who have sufficient information about pregnancy, birth, and newborn care are less likely to experience psychological stress as those who do not feel they have enough information. Internet resources such as that of the American College of Obstetricians & Gynecologists (2019) also provide valuable information for partners at https://www.acog.org.

The nurse can guide the couple in discussion of the role the partner will play during and after the birth. How actively will the partner participate during labor? Will the partner be involved in infant care from the start or wait until the baby is older? Will the partner change diapers and help with nighttime care? The expectant parents may be surprised to learn each other's views and may need to negotiate, taking the beliefs of each partner into consideration, to determine the roles each will play.

Creating the Role of the Involved Partner

Partners should be encouraged and guided to use various means to create a parenting role that is comfortable for them. They may seek closer ties with their parents to reminisce about their own childhoods. They may fantasize about their relationships with their children as they progress through the stages of childhood.

Expectant partners also observe others who are already parents and "try on" parenting behaviors to determine whether they are comfortable and fit their own concepts of the parental role. Some partners change their self-images and even their appearances to fit their new images (Link, 2018). In addition, many partners assertively seek information about infant care and growth and development so that they will be prepared.

Parenting Information. Expectant partners need information about infant care and parenting. Although adequate information may be given to them, partners may not be ready to learn at the time it is provided. As a result, they may have unrealistic expectations and be unprepared to care for the newborn. Nurses must review information about infant care and growth and development after the infant is born when the knowledge is immediately relevant.

Couvade. The term **couvade** refers to pregnancy-related symptoms and behavior in expectant partners. In primitive cultures, couvade took the form of rituals involving special dress, confinement, limitations of physical work, avoidance of certain foods, sexual restraint, and, in some instances, performance of "mock labor."

In modern practice, partners sometimes experience physical symptoms similar to those of pregnant client, such as loss of appetite, nausea, headache, fatigue, and weight gain. Symptoms are more likely to occur in early pregnancy and lessen as the pregnancy progresses. They may be caused by stress, anxiety, or empathy for the birthing partner. They are usually harmless but may persist and result in nervousness, insomnia, restlessness, and irritability. Although the symptoms are almost always unobserved by the health care team, anticipatory guidance is beneficial for both partners.

KNOWLEDGE CHECK

25. What are reality boosters? Why are they important for the partner's adjustment?
26. How can nurses help partners in their struggle for recognition as parents?
27. Why should information relating to newborn care presented in prenatal classes be repeated after the infant is born?

ADAPTATION OF GRANDPARENTS

The initial reaction of grandparents depends on factors such as their ages, the number and spacing of other grandchildren, and their perceptions of the role of grandparents.

Age

Age is a major determining factor in the emotional responses of prospective grandparents. Older grandparents have often already dealt with their feelings about aging and react with joy when they find they are to become grandparents. They look forward to being able to love grandchildren, who signify the continuity of life and family.

Younger grandparents may not be happy with the stereotype of grandparents as old persons. They may experience conflict when they must resolve their self-image with the stereotype. They often have career responsibilities and may not be accessible because of the continuing demands of their own lives.

Number and Spacing of Other Grandchildren

The number and spacing of other grandchildren also determine grandparents' reactions. A first grandchild may be an exciting event that creates great joy. If the grandparents have other grandchildren, another may be welcomed, but with less excitement. The subdued reaction may be disappointing to the couple, who may desire the same reaction as that expressed for the first grandchild.

Perceptions of the Role of Grandparents

Grandparents' beliefs about their importance to grandchildren vary widely. Many grandparents see their relationships with grandchildren as second in importance only to the parent–child relationship. They want to be involved in the pregnancy and often engage in rituals such as shopping and gift-giving showers that confirm their role as important participants. Many grandparents are intimately involved in child care and offer unconditional love to the child. They offer to care for older children while the client gives birth, and they assist during the first weeks after childbirth.

In the past, grandparents were often asked for advice about childbearing and child-rearing. Health care personnel have now become the "experts," and many grandparents have difficulty adjusting to this change. Some grandparents may withdraw, sensing that their participation is no longer valued. Other grandparents worry about their lack of familiarity with modern ways of childbearing and parenting. Special classes are often available to teach them about current childbearing practices.

On the other hand, some contemporary grandparents plan little participation in pregnancy or child care. They may say, "I've raised my children, and I don't plan to do it again." This attitude often results in conflict with the parents, who may feel hurt and wish for the grandparents' help during the third trimester and after the birth.

Nurses can assist families to verbalize their feelings about the grandparents' responses to the pregnancy by statements such as, "It may seem that the grandparents aren't interested in the baby, but perhaps they are uneasy about what their role should be." Parents and grandparents may need to negotiate how the grandparents can be involved without feeling that they must assume more care of the child than they desire. For instance, the couple may need suggestions to help the grandparents participate in family gatherings that do not involve babysitting or child care. Letting grandparents know that the parents want them to share in the joy the child brings without other expectations may ease the situation.

ADAPTATION OF SIBLINGS

Sibling adaptation to the birth of an infant depends largely on age and developmental level.

Toddlers

Children 2 years old or younger are unaware of the physiologic changes occurring during pregnancy and are unable to understand that a new brother or sister is going to be born. Toddlers have little perception of time; therefore many parents delay telling toddlers that a baby is expected until shortly before the birth.

Although preparing very young children for the birth of a baby is difficult, the nurse can make suggestions that may prove helpful. Any changes in sleeping arrangements should be made several weeks before the birth so the child does not feel displaced by the new baby. Family members should be prepared that toddlers may show feelings of jealousy or resentment. Toddlers need frequent reassurance that they are loved.

Older Children

Children from 3 to 12 years are more aware of changes in the expectant parent's body and may realize a baby is to be born. They may enjoy observing the growing abdomen, feeling the fetus move, and listening to the heartbeat. They may have questions about how the fetus will develop, how it was created, and how it will get out of the abdomen. Although they look forward to the baby's arrival, preschool children may expect the infant to be a full-fledged playmate and may be shocked and disappointed when the infant is small and helpless. They also need preparation for the fact that the client will go away for several days when the baby is born.

School-age children are often told about the pregnancy during the second trimester and benefit from being included in preparations for the new baby. They are interested in following the development of the fetus, preparing space for the infant to sleep, and helping to accumulate supplies the infant will need. They should be encouraged to feel the fetus move, and many come close to the abdomen and talk to the fetus.

School-age children may wonder how the birth will affect their role in the family. Parents should address these concerns and reassure the children about their continued importance. Providing time alone with the parents may help them gain a sense of security. Reading books about other children's experiences after the birth of a sibling may be helpful (Fig. 6.11).

Children as young as 3 years can benefit from sibling classes. The classes provide an opportunity for them to discuss what newborns are like and what changes the new baby will bring to the family. They are encouraged to bring a doll to these classes to simulate caring for the infant.

In some settings, siblings are permitted to be with the client during childbirth. They should attend a class that prepares them for the event. During the birth, a familiar person who has no other role but to support and care for younger siblings should be available to explain what is taking place and to comfort or remove them if events become overwhelming.

Adolescents

The response of adolescents also depends on their developmental level. Some are embarrassed because the pregnancy confirms the continued sexuality of their parents. Many adolescents are immersed in their own developmental tasks involving loosening ties to their parents and coming to terms with their own sexuality. They may be indifferent to the pregnancy unless it directly affects them or their activities. Other adolescents become very involved and want to help with preparations for the baby.

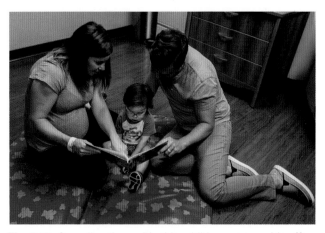

Fig. 6.11 Spending time with older children can provide affection, a sense of security, and preparation for the new baby.

? KNOWLEDGE CHECK

28. What determines the response of grandparents to the pregnancy?
29. How does the response to pregnancy differ for a toddler, a preschool child, and an adolescent?
30. How can parents prepare siblings for the addition of a newborn to the family?

FACTORS INFLUENCING PSYCHOSOCIAL ADAPTATIONS

Age

Pregnancy presents a challenge for teenagers, who must cope with the conflicting developmental tasks of pregnancy and adolescence at the same time. The major developmental task of adolescence is to form and become comfortable with a sense of self. On the other hand, one of the major tasks of pregnancy involves learning to "give of self," a process that includes sacrificing personal desires for the benefit of the fetus.

Nurses who work with pregnant teenagers should help them adjust to their changing bodies and the increasing presence of the developing fetus. Adolescents also need prompting to follow a lifestyle that promotes the best outcomes for them and their infants.

The pregnant client over age 35 years may also have some concerns. Pregnancy may mean a major change in lifestyle. Additionally, there may be medical conditions that impact the pregnancy as well. Concerns relating to the pregnant adolescent and the older client are discussed further in Chapter 11.

Multiparity

The assumption that a multipara needs less help than a primigravida is inaccurate, as pregnancy tasks are often more complex. The multipara does not have as much time to take special care of oneself as during the first pregnancy. Fatigue is more common, and the client may have serious concerns about the other children accepting the infant. The multipara may worry about finding time and energy for additional responsibilities. When seeking acceptance of the new baby, the multipara may find the family less excited than they were for the first child. The couple's celebration is also more subdued.

The client spends a great deal of time developing a new relationship with the first child, who may become demanding. This behavior may foster feelings of guilt as the client tries to expand love to include the second child. Developing attachment for the coming baby is hampered by feelings of loss between oneself and the first child. The client may sense that the child is growing up and away from them and may grieve for the loss of this special relationship.

Nurses cannot assume that the process is "old hat" and that information about labor, breastfeeding, and infant care is not needed. The parents may also need special assistance in integrating an additional infant into the family structure.

Social Support

Social support has been found to be a significant predictor of health-related quality of life during the perinatal period. Social support comes from the client's partner, family, friends, and coworkers. Generally, support from the client's partner and parents is particularly important.

Depression may occur in clients who have little support during pregnancy, and they are more likely to begin prenatal care late. The nurse should assess for signs of depression in all clients and refer them for help when necessary. (See Chapter 11 for a discussion of postpartum depression.) When social support is inadequate, the nurse can help the client explore potential sources such as support groups, childbearing education classes, church, work, or school. Some community programs employ nurses or paraprofessionals to visit expectant clients to provide teaching and social support.

Sexual and/or Gender Minority

The growing number of families that include members of sexual and/or gender minority (SGM) groups require that perinatal nurses know how to provide respectful and affirming care to all people. As a group, these individuals tend to suffer poorer health outcomes, partially due to stigma and discrimination (Griggs et al., 2021). Recent studies found that these individuals are more likely to experience lack of comprehensive prenatal care and an increased number of adverse pregnancy outcomes, including depression, miscarriage, and preterm birth (Gonzales et al., 2019).

Nurses can decrease barriers to care by creating an inclusive environment. This includes educating themselves, avoiding assumptions, and asking only questions that are relevant to care. One question that should be asked as soon as possible is which pronouns clients use for themselves. If the provider uses an incorrect pronoun, it is appropriate to acknowledge the error and apologize (ACOG, 2021).

Absence of a Partner

Pregnant single clients may have special concerns. Although some unmarried individuals have the financial and emotional support of a partner, others do not. They may experience more stress about telling their family and friends about the pregnancy. They may have to enlist more social support to substitute for that of a partner. Legal issues such as whom to list as the father on birth records and what arrangements must be made to allow paternal contact with the infant may be added concerns.

Single clients without partners may live below the poverty level. The lack of financial resources is more likely to delay prenatal care until the second or third trimester, and these clients are at increased risk for pregnancy complications and delivery of a low-birth-weight infant.

Nurses must recognize the single client's needs for accessible and affordable prenatal care. In addition, nurses must be prepared to offer specialized supportive care for single clients. Necessary social services may include Medicaid; the

Special Supplemental Nutrition Program for Women, Infants, and Children (WIC) for food vouchers; and transportation to prenatal appointments.

Some individuals are single by choice. They may have been inseminated to achieve pregnancy or choose not to continue the relationship with their partner. If the pregnancy was planned, these people may have fewer financial concerns.

Abnormal Situations

Other factors that influence psychosocial adaptation during pregnancy include abnormal situations such as intimate partner violence (see Chapter 2) and substance abuse (see Chapter 11). The nurse should assess all individuals for both of these risk factors during pregnancy so that appropriate referrals for help can be given.

SUMMARY CONCEPTS

- Pregnancy causes a predictable pattern of uterine growth. In general, the uterus can be palpated halfway between the symphysis pubis and the umbilicus at 16 weeks of gestation, at the level of the umbilicus at 20 weeks, and at the xiphoid process by 36 weeks.
- Thick mucus fills the cervical canal and protects the fetus from infection caused by bacteria ascending from the vagina.
- Plasma volume expands faster and to a greater extent than red blood cells, resulting in a dilution of hemoglobin concentration. This physiologic anemia does not reflect an inadequate number of red blood cells.
- Although blood volume increases, blood pressure is not elevated during normal pregnancy.
- The gravid uterus partially occludes the vena cava and aorta when the client is supine, causing supine hypotensive syndrome. This can be prevented or corrected if positioned laterally or if a wedge or pillow is placed under the client's hip tilting the uterus toward one side.
- During the last trimester the uterus pushes the diaphragm upward. To compensate, the ribs flare, the substernal angle widens, and the circumference of the chest increases.
- Increased progesterone level is associated with relaxation of smooth muscles, resulting in stasis of urine and increasing the risk of urinary tract infections and constipation.
- Increased renal plasma flow causes increased GFR and effectively removes additional metabolic wastes produced by the pregnant client and the fetus but often results in "spilling" of glucose and other nutrients into urine.
- Increased blood flow to the skin reduces heat generated by the increased metabolic rate.
- Forms of hyperpigmentation during pregnancy include melasma and linea nigra.
- Striae gravidarum occur from separation of connective tissue fibers.
- Increased estrogen and hCG and decreased gastric motility are associated with nausea in early pregnancy. Morning sickness will not harm the fetus and usually ends by 10 to 16 weeks.
- The expanding uterus causes progressive changes that can lead to muscle strain and backache during the last trimester.
- Progesterone maintains the uterine lining for implantation, prevents uterine contractions during pregnancy, and helps prepare the breasts for lactation.
- Presumptive and probable signs of pregnancy may be caused by conditions other than pregnancy and cannot be considered positive or diagnostic signs. Positive signs can have no other cause.
- Following conception, psychological responses progress during pregnancy from uncertainty and ambivalence to feelings of vulnerability and preparation for the birth of the infant.
- As the fetus becomes real, usually in the second trimester, individual focus shifts from self to the fetus and turns inward to concentrate on the processes taking place in the client's body.
- Sexual activity varies among couples and may be culturally influenced. It is safe throughout pregnancy if no complications are present.
- Changes in the body during pregnancy may result in a negative body image that affects sexual responses. This change may be especially troubling if the couple does not discuss emotions and concerns related to the changes in sexuality.
- Making the transition to the role of parent involves mimicking the behavior of other parents, role play, fantasizing about the baby, developing a sense of self as parent, and grieving the loss of previous roles.
- To complete the parental tasks of pregnancy the individual must seek safe passage for oneself and the fetus, gain acceptance from significant persons, and learn to be giving while forming an attachment to the unknown child.
- The partner's parenting responses change throughout pregnancy and depend on the ability to perceive the fetus as real, gain recognition for the role of parent, and create a role as involved parent.
- The most powerful reality boosters for the partner during pregnancy are hearing the fetal heartbeat, feeling the fetus move, and viewing the fetus on an ultrasound.
- In primitive cultures, *couvade* refers to pregnancy-related rituals performed by the partner. Today, it refers to a cluster of pregnancy-related symptoms experienced by the partner.
- The response of grandparents to pregnancy depends on their ages and beliefs about the role of grandparents as well as the number and ages of other grandchildren.
- The response of siblings to pregnancy depends on their ages and developmental levels.
- Completing the developmental tasks of pregnancy is more difficult for multiparas because they have less time, experience more fatigue, and must negotiate a new relationship with the older child or children.

Clinical Judgment And Next-Generation NCLEX® Examination-Style Questions

1. **Choose the most likely options for the information missing from the statements below by selecting from the lists of options provided.**

During pregnancy, the uterine fundus reaches the umbilicus at approximately ___1___ weeks' gestation. After that time, the fundal height is measured from the ___2___ to the top of the fundus in ___3___. That measurement is approximately equal to the weeks' gestation until ___4___ weeks, at which time the fetus drops into the pelvis, an occurrence know as ___5___.

Options for 1	Options for 2	Options for 3	Options for 4	Options for 5
12	Bottom rib	Centimeters	24	Ballottement
14	Symphysis pubis	Inches	36	Hegar's sign
20	Umbilicus	Finger width	40	Lightening
24	Xiphoid	Millimeters	42	Quickening

2. A client presents to the family medicine clinic with symptoms of pregnancy. **For each symptom, use an "X" to identify presumptive, probable, and positive signs of pregnancy.**

Symptom	Presumptive	Probable	Positive
Amenorrhea			
Fetal heart rate detected by Doppler or ultrasound			
Goodell's sign			
Positive pregnancy test			
Quickening			
Fetal movements palpated by examiner			

3. The nurse is assessing a client who is 30 weeks pregnant and presents at the clinic because she doesn't feel well. **For each assessment finding below, use an "X" to indicate whether the finding requires nursing follow-up (could be harmful to the client) or is expected (no follow-up required).**

	Expected	Requires Follow-Up
Darkening of a mole		
Decreased frequency of urination		
Spotting of bright red blood after intercourse		
Diarrhea		
Dizziness when supine		
Temperature of 100.8°F		
Severe backache with flank pain		

REFERENCES & READINGS

American College of Obstetricians and Gynecologists (ACOG). (2019). *A partner's guide to pregnancy.* https://www.acog.org/womens-health/faqs/a-partners-guide-to-pregnancy.

American College of Obstetricians and Gynecologists (ACOG). (2020). *Weight gain during pregnancy.* ACOG Committee Opinion (548). Published 2013, reaffirmed 2020.

American College of Obstetricians and Gynecologists (ACOG). (2021). *Health care for transgender and gender diverse individuals.* ACOG Committee Opinion (832).

Antony, K. M., Racusin, D. A., Aagaard, K., & Dildy, G. A. (2021). Maternal physiology. In M. Landon, H. Galan, E. Jauniaux, D. Driscoll, V. Berghella, W. Grobman, S. Kilpatrick, & A. Cahill (Eds.), *Gabbe's obstetrics: Normal and problem pregnancies* (8th ed., pp. 43–67). Elsevier.

Blackburn, S. T. (2018). *Maternal, fetal, and neonatal physiology: A clinical perspective* (5th ed.). Elsevier.

Boron, W. F., & Boulpaep, E. L. (2021). *Concise medical physiology.* Elsevier.

Burton, G. J., Sibley, C. P., & Jauniaux, E. R. M. (2021). Placental anatomy and physiology. In M. Landon, H. Galan, E. Jauniaux, D. Driscoll, V. Berghella, W. Grobman, S. Kilpatrick, & A. Cahill (Eds.), *Gabbe's obstetrics: Normal and problem pregnancies* (8th ed., pp. 2–25). Elsevier.

Casanova, R., Chuang, A., Goepfert, A. R., et al. (2019). *Beckmann and Ling's obstetrics and gynecology* (8th ed.). Lippincott Williams & Wilkins.

Cunningham, F. G., Leveno, K. J., Bloom, S. L., et al. (2022). *Williams' obstetrics* (26th ed.). McGraw-Hill Companies.

Gonzales, G., Quinones, L., & Attanasio, L. (2019). Health and access to care among reproductive-age women by sexual orientation and pregnancy status. *Women's Health Issues, 29*(1), 8–16. https://doi.org/10.1016/j.whi.2018.10.006.

Griggs, K. M., Waddill, C. B., Bice, A., & Ward, N. (2021). Care during pregnancy, childbirth, postpartum, and human milk feeding for individuals who identify as LGBTQ+. *The American Journal of Maternal Child Nursing, 46*(1), 43–53. https://doi.org/10.1097/NMC.0000000000000675.

James, D. C., & Suplee, P. D. (2021). Postpartum care. In K. Simpson, P. Creehan, N. O'Brien-Abel, C. Roth, & A. Rohan (Eds.), *AWHONN's perinatal nursing* (5th ed., pp. 509–563). Wolters Kluwer.

Jordan, P. L. (1990). Laboring for relevance: Expectant and new fatherhood. *Nursing Research, 39*(1), 11–16.

Link, D. G. (2018). Nursing care of the family during pregnancy. In S. Perry, M. Hockenberry, D. Lowdermilk, & D. Wilson (Eds.), *Maternal child nursing care* (6th ed., pp. 264–298). Mosby.

Mastrobattista, J. M., & Monga, M. (2019). Maternal cardiovascular, respiratory, and renal adaptation to pregnancy. In R. Resnik, C.

Lockwood, T. Moore, M. Greene, J. Copel, & R. Silver (Eds.), *Creasy & Resnik's maternal-fetal medicine: Principles and practice* (8th ed., pp. 141–147). Elsevier.

Norwitz, E. R., Mahendroo, M., & Lye, S. J. (2019). Physiology of parturition. In R. Resnik, C. Lockwood, T. Moore, M. Greene, J. Copel, & R. Silver (Eds.), *Creasy & Resnik's maternal-fetal medicine: Principles and practice* (8th ed., pp. 81–95). Elsevier.

Pagana, K. D., Pagana, T. J., & Pagana, T. N. (2021). *Mosby's diagnostic and laboratory test reference* (15th ed.). Elsevier.

Rapini, R. P. (2019). The skin and pregnancy. In R. Resnik, C. Lockwood, T. Moore, M. Greene, J. A. Copel, & R. M. Silver (Eds.), *Creasy & Resnik's maternal-fetal medicine: Principles and practice* (8th ed., pp. 1258–1268). Elsevier.

Ross, M. G., Desai, M., & Ervin, M. G. (2021). Fetal development, physiology, and effects on long-term health. In M. Landon, H. Galan, E. Jauniaux, D. Driscoll, V. Berghella, W. Grobman, S. Kilpatrick, & A. Cahill (Eds.), *Gabbe's Obstetrics: Normal and problem pregnancies* (8th ed., pp. 26–42). Elsevier.

Rubin, R. (1984). *Maternal identity and the maternal experience.* Springer.

Williamson, C., Mackillop, L., & Heneghan, M. A. (2019). Diseases of the liver, biliary system, and pancreas. In R. Resnik, C. Lockwood, T. Moore, M. Greene, J. Copel, & R. Silver (Eds.), *Creasy & Resnik's maternal-fetal medicine: Principles and practice* (8th ed., pp. 1173–1191). Elsevier.

7

Antepartum Assessment, Care, and Education

Dawn Piacenza

OBJECTIVES

After studying this chapter, you should be able to:

1. Compute gravida, para, and estimated due date.
2. Describe preconception, initial, and subsequent antepartum assessments in terms of history, physical examination, and risk assessment.
3. Describe multifetal pregnancy adaptations and complications associated with these pregnancies.
4. Describe the common discomforts of pregnancy in terms of causes and measures to prevent or relieve them.
5. Apply the nursing process to care of the antepartum patient.
6. List the goals of perinatal education.
7. Describe various types of education for childbearing families.
8. Explain the purposes of a birth plan.
9. Describe techniques for pain relief taught in childbirth classes.

The objective of antepartum care is to promote optimum health of the client and infant. Prenatal care involves early and continuing risk assessments, health education, counseling, and social support. The care provided during this period requires the clinician to be knowledgeable of normal and abnormal pregnancy events and outcomes. Careful coordination of medical, obstetric, and psychosocial care begins before conception and continues throughout pregnancy.

ANTEPARTUM ASSESSMENT AND CARE

Ideally, antepartum care begins before conception and continues on a regular basis until birth. Although no prospective controlled trials have demonstrated the efficacy of prenatal care overall, inadequate antepartum care is associated with low birth weight and an increased incidence of prematurity. Prenatal visits provide clinicians with the opportunity to address primary health care concerns, as well as assess pregnancy risks and potential or existing complications (Gregory et al., 2021).

In 2019, birth certificate data show 77.6% of individuals giving birth received early prenatal care in the first trimester, while 6.4% of individuals began prenatal care in the third trimester or did not receive any prenatal care (Martin et al., 2021). The *Healthy People 2030* goal is for at least 80.5% of individuals to begin prenatal care in the first trimester (U.S. Department of Health and Human Services, 2020).

Preconception and Interconception Care

Ideally, the first visit takes place before conception. Preconception care (the period of time prior to conception) and interconception care (the period of time between pregnancies) are important to identify problems or risk factors that might harm the client or the infant once pregnancy occurs and to provide education to help promote a healthy pregnancy. The early weeks of pregnancy are particularly important because the fetal organs are forming and are especially sensitive to harm. Many individuals do not begin prenatal care until after this sensitive period, and injury may already have transpired. Interconception care is especially important for clients who have had previous pregnancy or birth complications. It also identifies and treats risk factors which have occurred since the last pregnancy.

Any visit to a health care provider by a client of childbearing age should be seen as an opportunity for preconception or interconception care due to the incidence of unintended pregnancies. This care can be part of developing a reproductive life plan which includes deciding the desired number and spacing of pregnancies. Such a plan helps individuals make changes to improve birth outcomes (Gregory et al., 2021). Chronic conditions such as asthma, obesity, diabetes, or hypothyroidism should be addressed before pregnancy occurs. Previous reproductive problems and family history (of both parents) for possible genetic conditions are explored. Genetic testing may be indicated by the family history (see Chapter 4).

During a preconception visit, the health care provider obtains a complete history and performs a physical examination. The client is assessed for health problems (e.g., diabetes, hypertension, sexually transmitted infections [STIs], or psychological problems), harmful habits (such as use of alcohol or drugs), or social problems (such as intimate partner violence) that might adversely affect pregnancy. If problems are discovered, intervention may be started immediately to avoid complications or worsening of the client's condition or situation because of pregnancy. Screening for rubella, varicella, and hepatitis B is performed, and the vaccines are given, if indicated. The client should be instructed to wait at least 1 month after receiving rubella and varicella vaccines before conceiving to minimize risk to the fetus (Centers for Disease Control [CDC], 2019).

If the client is taking prescription and over-the-counter (OTC) medications, vitamins, or other supplements, their effect on pregnancy is evaluated and changes made, if necessary. Approximately 75% of individuals report taking at least one medication during pregnancy (CDC, 2020). Potentially teratogenic medications should be evaluated and changed to less harmful medications, if possible, before attempting pregnancy.

Use of complementary or alternative therapies is addressed because some therapies may be generally considered safe but are harmful during pregnancy. Avoidance of common teratogens or other harmful substances is discussed. Clients who are obese can obtain help to lose weight before conceiving. Referral to smoking cessation programs may be indicated.

The client is advised to consume 400 to 800 mcg (0.4 to 0.8 mg) of folic acid daily for at least 1 month before conception and 2 to 3 months after conception to decrease the risk for neural tube defects (Adams, 2021; CDC, 2020; U.S. Preventive Services Task Force, 2017). A daily intake of 600 mcg (0.6 mg) is recommended for the rest of pregnancy. Clients who have previously given birth to an infant with a neural tube defect should consult with their provider about increasing the dosage to 4000 mcg (4 mg) of folic acid daily during the 4 weeks before pregnancy and throughout the first trimester. Individuals on antiepileptic medications are advised to take 1000 mcg of folic acid during this time frame as well (Berger & West, 2021).

Initial Prenatal Visit

If a preconception visit has occurred recently, many initial prenatal assessments will have been completed. If not, the provider will complete a thorough history and physical examination. The obstetric nurse may play an essential role in this intake visit as well, verifying history, uncovering potential risk factors, and providing early pregnancy education. The following are the primary objectives of the first antepartum visit:

- Establish trust and rapport with the childbearing family.
- Verify or rule out pregnancy.
- Evaluate the pregnant client's physical and psychological health relevant to childbearing.
- Assess the growth and health of the fetus.
- Establish baseline data for comparison with future observations.
- Evaluate the psychosocial needs of the client and family.
- Assess the need for counseling or teaching.
- Negotiate a plan of care to promote optimal health of the client and baby.

History

Obstetric History. The obstetric history provides essential information about previous pregnancies and may alert the health care provider to possible problems in the present pregnancy. Components of this history include the following:

- Gravida, para (term and preterm deliveries), abortions (spontaneous or elective termination of pregnancies before the 20th week of gestation; spontaneous abortion is frequently called *miscarriage*), and living children
- Length of previous gestations
- Weight of infants at birth
- Labor experiences, type of deliveries, locations of births, and names of providers
- Types of anesthesia and any difficulties with anesthesia during childbirths or previous surgeries
- Medical complications such as hypertension, diabetes, infection, bleeding, or psychologic complications
- Infant complications
- Methods of infant feeding used in the past and currently planned
- Special concerns

Gravida refers to a client who is or has been pregnant, regardless of the length of the pregnancy. A **primigravida** is a client pregnant for the first time. A **multigravida** has been pregnant more than once. **Para** refers to the number of pregnancies which have ended at 20 or more weeks, regardless of whether the infant was born alive or stillborn. A multiple gestation pregnancy, such as twins or triplets, is still one pregnancy and therefore one para. A **nullipara** is a client who has never completed a pregnancy to 20 weeks or more. A **primipara** has delivered one pregnancy of at least 20 weeks. A **multipara** has delivered two or more pregnancies of at least 20 weeks.

There are two methods of summarizing a client's obstetric history (gravida and para). The first uses two digits, gravida (the number of times they have been pregnant) and para (the number of completed pregnancies of 20 weeks or more). The second method, described by the acronym GTPAL, is more informative because it uses five digits: G = pregnancies or gravida, T = term pregnancies delivered, P = preterm pregnancies delivered, A = abortions (spontaneous and induced), and L = living children (Box 7.1).

Nurses should use caution when discussing gravida and para with the expectant client in the presence of a significant other or family members. Although the antepartum record may indicate a previous pregnancy or childbirth, this information may not have been shared with family, and the right to privacy could be jeopardized by asking probing questions in their presence. The pregnancy may have terminated in elective or spontaneous abortion or in the birth of an infant who

BOX 7.1 Calculation of Gravida and Para

A method for calculating gravida and para is to separate pregnancies and their outcome using the acronym GTPAL: G = gravida, T = term, P = preterm, A = abortions, and L = living children.

The following examples illustrate the use of this method:

- Jennie is 6 months pregnant. Past pregnancy history includes one spontaneous and one elective abortion in the first trimester, as well as a son who was born at 40 weeks of gestation and a daughter who was born at 34 weeks of gestation. Using the two-digit method, Jennie is gravida 5, para 2. The two abortions are counted in the gravida but not included in the para because they occurred before 20 weeks of gestation. Using the five-digit method, GTPAL is 5-1-1-2-2. (G = all pregnancies, including the current one; T = 1, the son born at 40 weeks; P = 1, the daughter born at 34 weeks; A = 2, the spontaneous and elective abortions in the first trimester; and L = 2, the number of current living children).

- Lani gave birth to twins at 32 weeks of gestation and to a stillborn infant at 24 weeks of gestation. Approximately 2 years later, this client experienced a spontaneous abortion at 12 weeks of gestation. If pregnant now, the gravida is 4, para 2 (the twins count as 1 parous experience, and the stillborn infant counts as 1 parous experience because the pregnancy extended past 20 weeks gestation, the spontaneous abortion does not count as a parous experience because the pregnancy ended before 20 weeks gestation). If the GTPAL acronym is used, G = 4, T = 0 (no pregnancies went to term), P = 2 (the twins count as 1 and the stillborn infant counts as 1 pregnancy ending in preterm birth), A = 1 (the 12 weeks spontaneous abortion), L = 2 (the two living children).

was placed for adoption. The confidentiality of the pregnant individual should always be protected. The nurse should wait until the client is alone if it is necessary to clarify information about past obstetric history.

Menstrual History and Estimated Due Date. A complete menstrual history is necessary to establish the estimated due date (EDD) and therefore the gestational age of the fetus at any given time. The EDD is important in deciding when to schedule certain tests or procedures commonly performed during pregnancy. Common practice is to estimate the EDD on the basis of the first day of the last menstrual period (LMP), although ovulation and conception occur approximately 2 weeks after the beginning of menstruation in a regular 28-day cycle. The average duration of pregnancy from the first day of the LMP is 40 weeks, or 280 days.

Nägele's rule is often used to establish the EDD. This method involves subtracting 3 months from the date the LMP began, adding 7 days, and then correcting the year, if appropriate. For example:

- LMP: August 30, 2022
- Subtract 3 months: May 30, 2022
- Add 7 days and change the year: June 6, 2023

Calculations of EDD may be inaccurate in some situations. For example, the Nägele's rule is less accurate when the client's menstrual cycle is very irregular. To determine EDD quickly, many health care providers also use a gestational wheel or an EDD calculator tool application designed for electronic medical records or smart phones (Cunningham et al., 2022). Ultrasound measurements taken early in pregnancy (before 20 weeks of gestation) can more accurately determine the gestational age.

Gynecologic and Contraceptive History. Any previous gynecologic problems should be identified. STIs should be treated. Infertility problems with past or the current pregnancy should be discussed.

A detailed history of contraceptive methods is important. Studies have shown no increased risk for congenital malformations when clients conceive while using hormonal contraceptives (Cunningham et al., 2022). Any client who becomes pregnant should stop taking hormonal contraceptives and consult with a health care provider.

Pregnancy with an intrauterine device (IUD) in place is unusual, but it can cause complications such as spontaneous abortion, infection, and preterm delivery. The client should be evaluated for ectopic pregnancy. As soon as the pregnancy is confirmed, the IUD should be removed promptly by a provider. An individual who shows signs of infection with an IUD in place should receive intensive antibiotic treatment and have the uterus evacuated (Cunningham et al., 2022).

Medical and Surgical History. Chronic conditions can affect the outcome of the pregnancy and should be investigated. Infections, surgical procedures, and trauma may complicate the pregnancy or childbirth and should be documented. The history includes the following:

- Age and ethnic background (risk for specific genetic problems such as sickle cell disease, thalassemia, cystic fibrosis, and Tay-Sachs disease)
- Childhood diseases and immunizations
- Chronic illnesses (onset and treatment) such as asthma, heart disease, hypertension, diabetes, renal disease, and lupus
- Previous illnesses, surgical procedures, and injuries (particularly of the pelvis and back)
- Previous infections such as hepatitis, STIs, tuberculosis, and presence of group B *Streptococcus*
- History of and treatment for anemia, including any previous blood transfusions
- Bladder and bowel function (problems or changes)
- Amount of caffeine and alcohol consumed each day
- Tobacco use in any form (number of years and daily amount)
- Prescription, OTC, and illicit drugs (name, dose, frequency)
- Complementary or alternative therapies used
- Appetite, general nutrition, history of eating disorders
- Contact with pets, particularly cats (increased risk for infections such as toxoplasmosis)
- Allergies and drug sensitivities
- Occupation and related risk factors

Family History. A family history provides valuable information about the general health of the family, including chronic diseases such as diabetes and heart disease and infections such as tuberculosis and hepatitis. In addition, it may reveal information about patterns of genetic or congenital anomalies.

Partner's Health History. The partner's history may include significant health problems such as genetic abnormalities, chronic diseases, and infections. Use of drugs such as cocaine and alcohol may affect the family's ability to cope with pregnancy and childbirth. Tobacco use by the partner increases the risk for upper respiratory tract infections for both the client and the infant from exposure to passive smoke.

In addition, the blood type and Rh factor of the biological father are important if the client is Rh-negative or type O because blood incompatibility between the client and fetus is possible.

Psychosocial History. The psychosocial history, including mental health, substance abuse, risk for violence or abuse, and coping abilities, should be elicited during the initial visit.

Physical Examination

Many clients have not had a recent physical examination before becoming pregnant. Therefore, a thorough evaluation of all body systems is necessary to detect previously undiagnosed physical problems which may affect the pregnancy outcome. It also establishes baseline levels to guide the treatment of the expectant client and fetus throughout pregnancy.

Vital Signs

Blood Pressure. Position, anxiety, pain, and the use of alcohol or tobacco products can affect blood pressure (BP). BP should be obtained using an appropriate size cuff with the individual seated and the arm supported in a horizontal position at heart level. The same arm should be used for each assessment. There may be differences between BP values obtained manually and BP values obtained with automatic cuffs. Documentation should include the position, arm used, pressures obtained, and type of sphygmomanometer used. The nurse may notice a normal decrease in BP during first and second trimesters, which normalizes by the third trimester (see Chapter 6). A BP of 140/90 mm Hg or higher early in pregnancy may indicate chronic hypertension or other hypertensive disorders and requires additional evaluation (see Chapter 10).

Pulse. The normal adult heart rate (HR) is 60 to 100 beats per minute (bpm). Tachycardia (HR > 100 bpm) is associated with anxiety, hyperthyroidism, and infection and should be investigated. Apical pulse should be assessed for at least 1 minute to determine the amplitude and regularity of the heartbeat and presence of murmurs. Pedal pulses are assessed to determine the presence of circulatory problems in the legs. Pedal pulses should be strong, equal, and regular.

Respirations. Respiratory rate during pregnancy is in the range of 12 to 24 breaths per minute. Tachypnea may indicate respiratory tract infection or cardiac disease. Breath sounds should be equal bilaterally, chest expansion should be symmetric, and lung fields should be free of abnormal breath sounds.

Temperature. Normal temperature during pregnancy is 36.6°C to 37.6°C (97.8°F to 99.6°F). Fever suggests infection and may require medical management.

Cardiovascular System. Additional assessment of the cardiovascular system includes observation for venous congestion, which can develop into varicosities and edema. Venous congestion is most commonly noted in the legs, the vulva (as varicosities), or the rectum (as hemorrhoids). Edema of the legs may be a benign condition that reflects pooling of blood in the extremities caused by occlusion of the pelvic veins and inferior vena cava by the large uterus. This results in a shift of intravascular fluid into interstitial spaces. When pressure exerted by a finger leaves a persistent depression, pitting edema is present (see Fig. 17.5).

Musculoskeletal System. Body mechanics and changes in posture and gait should be addressed. Poor body mechanics during pregnancy may place strain on the muscles of the lower back and legs. Many joints have increased mobility during pregnancy, which contributes to posture changes, potentially leading to lower back pain.

Height and Weight. An initial weight is recorded to establish a baseline for evaluation of weight gain throughout pregnancy. The body mass index should be calculated. Individuals who are underweight before pregnancy are at risk for having low-birth-weight infants (Adams, 2021).

Obesity is a special concern during pregnancy (see Chapter 10). Obesity increases the incidence of hypertensive disorders, gestational diabetes, postpartum hemorrhage, poor labor progression, cesarean delivery, anesthesia complications, wound infection, and birth of large-for-gestational age infants (Cunningham et al., 2022). Obese clients often need closer observation and careful management of complications during pregnancy. Tests for fetal well-being may be important during the third trimester.

Abdomen. The contour, size, and muscle tone of the abdomen should be assessed. The fundal height should be measured if the fundus is palpable above the symphysis pubis (Fig. 7.1). The fetal heart rate should be auscultated, counted, and recorded if the pregnancy is advanced enough (10 to 12 weeks by Doppler; 18 to 20 weeks by fetoscope).

Neurologic System. A complete neurologic assessment is not necessary for clients who have a negative history and are free of signs or symptoms indicating a problem. However, deep tendon reflexes should be evaluated because hyperreflexia is associated with complications of pregnancy (see Chapter 10).

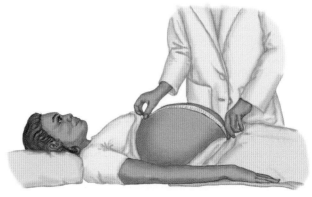

Fig. 7.1 Uterine measurements include the distance between the upper border of the symphysis pubis and the top of the fundus.

Carpal Tunnel Syndrome. Carpal tunnel syndrome is believed to result when edema compresses the median nerve at the point where it passes through the carpal tunnel of the wrist. Symptoms include pain, burning, numbness, or tingling of the hand and wrist. Splinting of the wrist at night may provide improvement. It resolves by 3 months after childbirth for most clients (Blackburn, 2018).

Integumentary System. Skin color should be consistent with ethnicity. Pallor may result from anemia, and jaundice may indicate hepatic disease. Lesions, bruising, rashes, areas of hyperpigmentation related to pregnancy (melasma, linea nigra), and stretch marks (striae) should be noted. Nail beds should be pink with instant capillary return.

Endocrine System. The thyroid enlarges moderately during the second trimester. However, gross enlargement, nodules, or tenderness may indicate thyroid disease and requires further medical evaluation.

Gastrointestinal System

Mouth. Mucous membranes should be pink, smooth, glistening, and uniform. Lips should be free of ulcerations. Gums may be red, tender, and edematous and may bleed more easily. Teeth should be in good repair. Dental plaque may increase, and a temporary increase in tooth mobility may occur (Blackburn, 2018).

The client should be referred for regular dental care. The second trimester may be the most comfortable time for dental care. However, if necessary, dental care can be performed during the third trimester if the client is positioned to avoid supine hypotension syndrome.

Intestine. A warm stethoscope for assessing bowel sounds is most comfortable for the pregnant client. Bowel sounds may be diminished because of the effects of progesterone on smooth muscle. Bowel sounds are often increased if a meal is overdue or diarrhea is present. Problems with constipation can be discussed during abdominal examination.

Urinary System. A clean-catch midstream urine sample is tested for urinary tract infection (UTI) and indicators of other complications. Although a trace amount of protein may be present in the urine, the amount should not increase. Its presence may indicate kidney disease, preeclampsia, or contamination by vaginal secretions. Small amounts of glucose may indicate physiologic "spilling," which occurs during normal pregnancy. Ketones may be found in the urine after heavy exercise or as a result of inadequate intake of food and fluid. Increased bacteria in urine is associated with UTI, which is common during pregnancy. A baseline urinalysis or culture may detect any underlying bacterial infections that warrant treatment to prevent more serious infections, such as pyelonephritis, from occurring (Antony et al., 2021; Cunningham et al., 2022).

Reproductive System

Breasts. Breast size and symmetry, condition of the nipples (erect, flat, inverted), and presence of colostrum should be noted. Any lumps, dimpling of the skin, or asymmetry of the nipples requires further evaluation. Breast tissue changes during pregnancy frequently cause increased tenderness and sensitivity during breast examination.

External Reproductive Organs. The skin and mucous membranes of the perineum, vulva, and anus are inspected for excoriations, growths, ulcerations, lesions, varicosities, warts, chancres, and perineal scars. Enlargement, tenderness, redness, or discharge from the Bartholin or Skene glands may indicate gonorrheal or chlamydial infection. The examiner should obtain a specimen for culture of any discharge from lesions or inflamed glands to determine the causative organisms and to provide effective care.

Internal Reproductive Organs. A speculum inserted into the vagina permits the examiner to see the walls of the vagina and the cervix. The cervix should be pink in a nonpregnant individual and bluish purple in a pregnant individual (**Chadwick's sign**). The external cervical os is closed in nulliparous clients, but one fingertip may be inserted into the cervix of multiparous individuals. The cervix feels relatively firm except during pregnancy, when marked softening is noted (**Goodell's sign**). Routine cervical cultures for gonorrhea and chlamydial infection are generally obtained during the initial pregnancy examination. The examiner also collects a specimen for a Papanicolaou (Pap) test to screen for cervical cancer if indicated.

A bimanual examination involves the use of both hands, one on the abdomen and the other in the vagina, to palpate the internal genitalia. The examiner palpates the uterus for size, contour, tenderness, and position. The uterus should be movable between the two examining hands and should feel smooth and enlarged according to gestational age. The ovaries, if palpable, should be about the size and shape of almonds and nontender.

Pelvic Measurements. Pelvic measurements may be assessed at this time to determine whether the shape and size of the bony pelvis are adequate for a normal vaginal birth (see Fig. 16.5).

Laboratory Data

Table 7.1 lists laboratory tests commonly performed during pregnancy and describes the purpose and significance of each test. Table 7.2 shows laboratory values for pregnant and nonpregnant clients.

Risk Assessment

Risk assessment begins at the initial visit when the health care provider identifies which factors might put the expectant client or fetus at risk for complications and determines the need for specialized care. Individuals with identified risk factors may require closer surveillance to monitor client and fetal well-being. Furthermore, risk factors change as pregnancy progresses, and risk assessment should be updated throughout pregnancy. Table 7.3 lists major risk factors and their implications.

> **❓ KNOWLEDGE CHECK**
>
> 1. Why is a preconception visit important?
> 2. Why are medical, surgical, psychological and obstetric histories necessary?
> 3. Why is it important for all caregivers to be consistent when measuring BP?
> 4. What are major risk factors during pregnancy?

Subsequent Visits

Ongoing antepartum care is important to the successful outcome of pregnancy. Although the recommended number

TABLE 7.1 **Common Laboratory Tests**		
Test	**Purpose**	**Significance**
Complete blood count	To detect infection, anemia, or cell abnormalities	More than 15,000/mm³ white blood cells or decreased platelets require follow-up.
Hemoglobin (Hgb) or hematocrit (Hct)	To detect anemia; often checked several times during pregnancy	Low Hgb or Hct may indicate need for added iron supplementation.
Blood grouping, Rh factor, and antibody screen	To determine blood type to screen for maternal-fetal blood incompatibility	Identifies possible causes of incompatibility which may result in jaundice in neonate. If the father is Rh-positive and the client is Rh-negative and unsensitized, Rho (D) immune globulin will be given to the client at 28 wk.
Venereal Disease Research Laboratory (VDRL) test or rapid plasma reagin	To screen for syphilis	Treat, if results are positive. Retest, as indicated.
Rubella titer	To determine immunity	If the client is not immune, then immunize postpartum.
Tuberculin skin test	To screen for tuberculosis	If positive, refer for additional testing or therapy.
Genetic testing (for sickle cell anemia, cystic fibrosis, Tay-Sachs disease, and other genetic conditions)	Offered if an increased risk for certain genetic conditions exists	If the client is positive, check the partner. Counsel as appropriate for test results.
Hepatitis B screen	To detect presence of antigens	If antigens are present, infants should be given hepatitis immune globulin and vaccine soon after birth.
HIV screen	Encouraged at first visit to detect HIV antibodies	Positive results require retesting, counseling, and treatment to lower risk for infant infection.
Urinalysis	To detect renal disease or infection	Requires further assessment if positive for more than trace protein (renal damage, preeclampsia, or normal), ketones (fasting or dehydration), or bacteria (infection).
Papanicolaou (Pap) test	To screen for cervical neoplasia	Refer for treatment if abnormal cells are present.
Vaginal–rectal culture	To detect chlamydia and gonorrhea (in early pregnancy) and group B streptococci (in late pregnancy)	Treat and retest as necessary; treat chlamydia and gonorrhea when discovered and group B streptococci during labor.
Multiple marker screen: Maternal serum alpha-fetoprotein, human chorionic gonadotropin, and estriol. Inhibin A and nuchal translucency may also be measured	To screen for fetal anomalies	Abnormal results may indicate increased risk for chromosomal abnormality (e.g., trisomy 13, 18, or 21) or structural defects (e.g., neural tube defects or gastroschisis).
Glucose challenge test	To screen for gestational diabetes	If the initial testing is elevated, a 3-hr glucose tolerance test is recommended.

Data from Cunningham, F. G., Leveno, K. J., Bloom, S. L., Dashe, J. S., Hoffman, B. L., Casey, B. M., & Spong, C. Y. (2022). *Williams obstetrics* (26th ed.). McGraw-Hill.

of visits can be reduced for clients without complications, the usual schedule for prenatal assessment in normal pregnancy is as follows (American Academy of Pediatrics [AAP] & American College of Obstetricians and Gynecologists [ACOG], 2017; Cunningham et al., 2022):

- Conception to 28 weeks—every 4 weeks
- 29 to 36 weeks—every 2 weeks
- 37 weeks to birth—weekly

Although the preceding schedule is the traditional model of prenatal care, other options do exist. "Centering Pregnancy" is an example of an evidence-based alternative method of care. The method involves 10 sessions of 1.5 to 2 hours with groups of 8 to 12 clients meeting with a facilitator, who may be a nurse or other health care provider, beginning at 12 to 16 weeks of pregnancy and ending soon after childbirth. Individuals assess their own BP and weight during the first 30 minutes of the session, promoting personal ownership and responsibility. Each visit includes a separate, individualized assessment with the health care provider. Then they participate in a group educational discussion with peers who are of similar gestational ages (ACOG, 2019). The social support provided by the group is an important benefit. Clients participating in this form of care have been satisfied with their care, reported a greater positive influence on stress, and had favorable pregnancy outcomes. More information is available at www.centeringhealthcare.org.

Vital Signs

Significant deviations from baseline values for vital signs indicate the need for further assessment. BP should be measured in the same arm, with the client in the same position each time.

Weight

Weight should be recorded and evaluated for expected progress. Inadequate weight gain may indicate the pregnancy is

TABLE 7.2 Laboratory Values in Nonpregnant and Pregnant Individuals

Value	Nonpregnant	Pregnant
Red blood cell count (million/mm³)	4.0–5.2	2.71–4.55 Decreases slightly because of hemodilution
Hemoglobin (g/dL)	12–15.8	9.5–15 (consider anemia if <11.0 in 1st or 3rd trimester; <10.5 in 2nd trimester)
Hematocrit, packed cell volume (%)	35.4–44.4	28–41
White blood cell (mm³)	3500–9100	5600–16,900
Platelets (mm³)	165,000–415,000	146,000–429,000
Prothrombin time (s)	12.7–15.4	9.5–13.5
Activated partial thromboplastin time (seconds)	26.3–39.4	22.6–38.9
D-dimer (µg/mL)	0.22–0.74	0.05–1.7
Blood glucose, fasting (mg/dL)	70–100	≤95
Creatinine (mg/dL)	0.5–0.9	0.4–0.9
Creatinine clearance, 24-hr urine (mL/min)	91–130	50–166
Fibrinogen (mg/dL)	233–496	244–696

Cunningham, F.G., Leveno, K.J., Bloom, S.L., Dashe, J.S., Hoffman, B.L., Casey, B.M., & Spong, C.Y. (2022). *Williams obstetrics* (26th ed.). McGraw-Hill.

not as advanced as was thought or the fetus is not growing as expected. A sudden, rapid weight gain may indicate excessive fluid retention.

Urine

Urine may be tested at each visit for protein, glucose, and ketones. Urine is also checked for nitrates to identify UTI and the need for a urine culture.

Fundal Height

Measuring fundal height is an inexpensive and noninvasive method of evaluating fetal growth and confirming gestational age. It is performed at each visit once the fundus is high enough to be palpated in the abdomen. The bladder should be empty to avoid elevation of the uterus. The client lies down with their knees slightly flexed. The top of the fundus is palpated, and a tape measure is stretched from the top of the symphysis pubis, over the abdominal curve, to the top of the fundus (see Fig. 7.1).

From 20 weeks until 32 weeks of gestation, the fundal height, measured in centimeters, is approximately equal to the gestational age of the fetus in weeks. If a discrepancy between fundal height and weeks of gestation is present, additional assessment is necessary. The EDD may be incorrect and the pregnancy more or less advanced than thought. The number of fetuses present, fetal growth, the amount of amniotic fluid, presence of leiomyomata (fibroids), or gestational trophoblastic disease (hydatidiform mole) will affect the fundal height. Ultrasonography may be performed to obtain further information.

Leopold Maneuvers

Leopold maneuvers provide a systematic method for palpating the fetus through the abdominal wall during the latter part of pregnancy. These maneuvers provide valuable information about the location and presentation of the fetus (see Procedure 15.1).

Fetal Heart Rate

The fetal heart rate should be between 110 and 160 bpm. The location of the fetal heart sounds helps determine the position in which the fetus is entering the pelvis. For example, fetal heart sounds heard in an upper quadrant of the abdomen suggest the fetus is in breech presentation.

Fetal Activity

Fetal movements (**quickening**) are usually first noticed by the expectant client at 16 to 20 weeks of gestation and gradually increase in frequency and strength. In the last trimester, the client may be asked to count fetal movements, commonly called *kick counts*. In general, fetal activity is a reassuring sign of a physically healthy fetus. Obese individuals may have decreased perception of fetal movements.

Signs of Labor

The client should be asked about signs of labor at each visit. A discussion of contractions, bleeding, and rupture of membranes will help them learn to identify preterm labor. The client should be cautioned to call the health care provider or go to the hospital if labor is suspected. During the third trimester, a discussion of the normal course of labor is important to prepare the client.

Ultrasonographic Screening

Ultrasonography is a commonly used prenatal diagnostic procedure (see Chapter 9). During early pregnancy, ultrasonography helps determine gestational age, fetal number, and cardiac activity. Ultrasound during the second and third trimesters can be useful when there is a discrepancy between the client's last menstrual period and uterine size to detect fetal anatomic defects, to observe for abnormal fetal growth, to check placental location and amniotic fluid volume estimates, and to determine fetal sex. Ultrasound also may be used to measure cervical length in clients at risk for preterm delivery (Adams, 2021).

Glucose Screening

Initial screening for diabetes in pregnant clients may be through medical history, clinical risk factors, and/or laboratory tests (ACOG, 2018b). For clients with significant history or risk factors, the blood glucose level is assessed at 24 to 28 weeks of gestation with a 1-hour oral glucose challenge test. If the result is 130 to 140 mg/dL or higher, the client receives a 3-hour oral glucose tolerance test to determine whether they

TABLE 7.3   Summary of Major Risk Factors in Pregnancy

Factors	Associated Problems
Demographic Factors	
<19 yr of age	Preterm birth, low birth weight, intrauterine growth restriction, perinatal mortality, congenital anomalies, anemia, HIV, sexually transmitted infections, insufficient prenatal care, preeclampsia, and substance abuse
>35 yr of age	Gestational diabetes, hypertension, prolonged labor, cesarean birth, congenital anomalies, infant mortality, placenta previa
Low socioeconomic status or dependence on public assistance	Preterm labor, maternal and neonatal mortality, low birth weight, chromosomal disorders, fetal growth disorders, insufficient prenatal care
Multiparity	Abnormal fetal presentation, antepartum or postpartum hemorrhage, cesarean birth
Social and personal factors	
Low prepregnancy weight	Low birth weight
Obesity	Preterm birth, hypertension, gestational diabetes, stillbirth, failure to progress in labor, macrosomia, cesarean birth, wound infections, anesthesia complications, postpartum hemorrhage, thromboembolism
Height <152 cm (5 ft)	Cesarean birth due to cephalopelvic disproportion
Smoking	Spontaneous abortion, low birth weight, placental abruption, placenta previa, preterm birth, perinatal mortality, sudden infant death syndrome
Use of alcohol or illicit drugs	Congenital anomalies, neonatal withdrawal syndrome, fetal alcohol spectrum disorder, risky lifestyle behaviors
Domestic violence	Poor pregnancy weight gain, infection, anemia, tobacco use, stillbirth, pelvic fracture, placental abruption, fetal injury, preterm delivery and low birth weight. Violence may escalate, causing severe maternal injury or death
Obstetric Factors	
Birth of previous infant >4000 g (8.8 lb)	Maternal gestational diabetes, cesarean birth; birth injury, neonatal hypoglycemia
Previous fetal or neonatal death	Maternal psychological distress
Rh sensitization	Jaundice, fetal anemia, erythroblastosis fetalis, kernicterus
Previous preterm birth	Repeated preterm birth
Existing Medical Conditions	
Diabetes mellitus	Preeclampsia, cesarean birth, preterm birth, infant either small or large for gestational age, neonatal hypoglycemia, congenital anomalies
Hypothyroidism	Gestational hypertension, low birth weight, mental and motor developmental delay, placental abruption, postpartum hemorrhage
Hyperthyroidism	Spontaneous abortion, heart failure, thyroid storm, preeclampsia, growth restriction, fetal or neonatal thyrotoxicosis, stillbirth
Cardiac disease	Congestive heart failure, arrhythmias, stroke, maternal mortality, growth restriction, preterm birth
Renal disease	Maternal renal failure, preeclampsia, preterm delivery, perinatal mortality, growth restriction
Concurrent infections	Severe fetal implications (heart disease, blindness, deafness, bone lesions) if maternal disease occurred in first trimester, increased incidence of spontaneous abortion or congenital anomalies associated with some infections. If occurring after 20 wks, preterm delivery and increased fetal and maternal morbidity and mortality
Psychological conditions	Perinatal mood disorders (anxiety, depression)

Cunningham, F. G., Leveno, K. J., Bloom, S. L., Dashe, J. S., Hoffman, B. L., Casey, B. M., & Spong, C. Y. (2022). *Williams obstetrics* (26th ed.). McGraw-Hill; Simpson, K. R., Creehan, P. A., O'Brien-Abel, N., Roth, C. K., & Rohan, A. J. (2021). *Perinatal nursing* (5th ed.). Wolters Kluwer.

have gestational diabetes. In high-risk individuals or high-risk populations, laboratory screening at the initial visit is also indicated and includes a fasting glucose test and a hemoglobin A1C (ACOG, 2018b; Adams, 2021) (see Chapter 10).

Isoimmunization

Antibody tests may be repeated in the third trimester in clients who are Rh-negative if the father of the baby is Rh-positive. If unsensitized, the client should receive Rho (D) immune globulin (RhoGAM) prophylactically at 28 weeks of gestation; after any invasive procedure, such as amniocentesis, or abdominal trauma; and again within 3 days after birth. The client should

be counseled to notify their provider of any episodes of vaginal bleeding or abdominal trauma during the pregnancy.

Pelvic Examination

During the last month of pregnancy, the obstetric provider may perform a pelvic examination to determine cervical changes. The descent of the fetus and the presenting part are also assessed at this time.

Psychosocial Assessments

The client's psychosocial adaptation should be assessed at each visit (Table 7.4). The nurse should ask about mood

TABLE 7.4   Psychosocial Assessment

Normal Findings (Findings of Concern)	Sample Questions	Nursing Implications
Psychological Response		
First trimester: Uncertainty, ambivalence, mood changes, self as primary focus Second trimester: Wonder, joy, focus on fetus Third trimester: Vulnerability, preparing for birth (fear, anger, apathy, ambivalence, lack of preparation)	"How do you and your partner feel about being pregnant?" "How will pregnancy change your lives?" "How do you feel about the changes in your body?" "How are you getting ready for the baby?"	Use active listening and reflection to establish a sense of trust. Reevaluate negative responses (fear, apathy, anger) in subsequent assessments.
Availability of Resources		
Financial concerns (lack of funds or insurance) Availability of grandparents, friends, family (family geographically or emotionally unavailable)	"What are your plans for prenatal care and birth?" "How do your parents feel about being grandparents?" "Who else can you depend on besides your family?" "Who helps you when there is a problem?"	Determine adequacy of financial means. Refer to resources such as a public clinic for care, Program for Women, Infants, and Children (WIC) for food. Help the couple discover alternative resources if family is unavailable. Identify family conflicts early to allow time for resolution.
Changes in Sexual Practices		
Mutual satisfaction with changes (excessive concern with comfort or safety, excessive conflict)	"How has your sexual relationship changed during this pregnancy?" "How do you cope with the changes?" "What concerns you most?"	Offer reassurance that intercourse is safe if pregnancy is normal. Suggest alternative positions and open communication.
Educational Needs		
Many questions about pregnancy, childbirth, and infant care (no questions, absence of interest in educational programs)	"How do you feel about caring for an infant?" "What are your major concerns?" "Where do you get information about pregnancy?"	Respond to needs which are expressed. Refer couple to appropriate child and parenting classes or reliable websites for accurate information.
Cultural Influences		
Ability of either the client or family to speak English or availability of fluent interpreters Cultural influences that support a healthy pregnancy and infant (harmful cultural beliefs or health practices)	"What foods and practices are recommended during pregnancy?" "What is forbidden?" "What is most important to you in your care?" "How do your religious beliefs affect pregnancy?"	Locate fluent interpreters, if needed. Avoid labeling beliefs as "superstition." Reinforce beliefs which promote a good pregnancy outcome. Elicit help from accepted sources of information to overcome harmful practices.

swings, body image, dreams, and concerns. In addition to assessment for normal psychosocial changes in pregnancy, ACOG (2018d) recommends all clients be screened at least once during the perinatal period for depression and anxiety.

Multifetal Pregnancy

A multifetal pregnancy is a pregnancy in which two or more embryos or fetuses are present simultaneously.

Diagnosis

Multifetal pregnancies are more likely in individuals who are over 35 years of age or in those who have a personal or family history of multifetal pregnancies. Advances in reproductive technology have contributed to an increased incidence of multifetal gestation (Cunningham et al., 2022).

Clients with multifetal pregnancies are larger than expected for the weeks of gestation, report increased fetal movements, and gain more weight. The fundal height is often 4 cm larger than expected on the basis of gestational age computed from the last menstrual period (Casanova et al., 2019). When more

than one fetus is suspected, diagnosis should be confirmed with ultrasonography. Separate fetuses and heart activities may be seen as early as 6 weeks of gestation (Cunningham et al., 2022).

Physiologic Adaptation to Multifetal Pregnancy

The degree of physiologic change is greater with multiple fetuses than with a single fetus. For example, with twins, blood volume increases 500 mL more than the amount needed for a single fetus. This increases the workload of the heart and may contribute to fatigue and activity intolerance. The additional size of the uterus intensifies the mechanical effects of pregnancy. The uterus may achieve a volume of ≥10 L and weigh >9 kg (20 lb) (Cunningham et al., 2022). Respiratory difficulty increases because the overdistended uterus causes greater elevation of the diaphragm.

The uterus may also cause more compression of the large vessels, resulting in more pronounced and earlier supine hypotension. Greater compression of the ureters can occur, edema, and slight proteinuria are common. Compression of the bowel makes constipation and hemorrhoids persistent problems. Nausea and vomiting occur three times as often as in single-fetus pregnancies because of the increased hormones (Cunningham et al., 2022). Fatigue and backache are also increased.

Antepartum Care in Multifetal Pregnancy

Early diagnosis of multifetal pregnancy allows time for the family to be educated about the many ways in which the pregnancy will differ from those involving a single fetus. Special antepartum classes can explain the need for increased nutrition, rest, and fetal monitoring. Instruction about signs of preterm labor, a common complication, should begin early. Discussions of the possible need to reduce activity and take frequent rest periods as well as the potential family stress caused by a high-risk pregnancy should be included.

Individuals with multifetal pregnancies have more frequent antepartum visits to allow early detection of common complications. These include preeclampsia, preterm labor, placental abruption, congenital anomalies, low birth weight, and postpartum hemorrhage (Casanova et al., 2019; Cunningham et al., 2022). Ultrasound scanning may be performed every 4 to 6 weeks beginning at 24 weeks of gestation to assess the growth of each fetus. Assessment of cervical lengths using ultrasound may help determine increased risk for preterm delivery (Cunningham et al., 2022).

Nutritional education is essential. Adequate calories, iron, calcium, folic acid, and vitamins are important. Clients with a normal prepregnancy weight are advised to gain 37 to 54 pounds during a twin pregnancy (ACOG, 2020c; Bowers, 2021).

The client may have many concerns and may need more support than others with only one fetus. Discomforts of pregnancy, which are merely annoying to others, are increased during multifetal pregnancies. Preterm birth is the most frequent complication in multifetal pregnancies; therefore, teaching about signs of labor and how to respond should begin early in pregnancy.

In addition, the financial burden of medical and hospital care during and after pregnancy is increased. Concerns about the effect of more than one newborn on the family should be discussed. The client may need referral for assistance in these areas.

? KNOWLEDGE CHECK

5. What is the recommended schedule for antepartum visits?
6. How does fundal height relate to gestational age?
7. How does adaptation differ in multifetal pregnancies?

Common Discomforts of Pregnancy

Many individuals experience discomforts of pregnancy that are not serious but detract from their feeling of comfort and well-being (see Patient Teaching: Discomforts of Pregnancy).

PATIENT TEACHING

Discomforts of Pregnancy

Nausea and Vomiting
- Eat crackers, dry toast, or dry cereal before arising in the morning; then get out of bed slowly.
- Eat small amounts of high-carbohydrate, low-fat foods every 2 hours and a total of five to six small meals per day to prevent an empty stomach.
- Eat a protein snack before bedtime.
- Suck on hard candy.
- Drink fluids frequently but separately from meals. Try small amounts of ice chips, water, and clear liquids like gelatin or frozen juice bars. Avoid coffee.
- Avoid fried, high-fat, greasy, or spicy foods and those with strong odors such as onion and cabbage. Instead, try bland foods, which may be more easily tolerated.
- If cooking odors are bothersome, open a window to help disperse them.
- Experimenting with different foods may be helpful, such as ginger (tea, cookies, soda), peppermint (tea or candy), tart and salty combinations such as potato chips and lemonade or green apples, or sweet and salty combinations.
- Take prenatal vitamins at bedtime because they may increase nausea if taken in the morning.
- Use an acupressure band over a point approximately three finger widths above the wrist crease on the inner arm.
- Nap and rest more frequently, if possible, because fatigue may increase nausea.

- Check with your health care provider before taking any herbal remedies.
- Notify your health care provider for severe nausea and vomiting or signs of dehydration (dry, cracked lips, elevated pulse, fever, concentrated urine).

Heartburn
- Eat small meals every 2 to 3 hours and avoid fatty, acidic, or spicy foods.
- Eliminate or curtail smoking and drinking coffee and carbonated beverages, which stimulate acid formation in the stomach.
- Avoid citrus fruits and juices, tomato-based products, chocolate, and peppermint if they increase symptoms.
- Try chewing gum.
- Avoid bending over or lying flat.
- Wear loose-fitting clothes.
- Take deep breaths and sip water to help relieve the burning sensation.
- Use antacids, but avoid those that are high in sodium and cause fluid retention (such as Alka-Seltzer, baking soda). Antacids high in calcium (such as Tums) are effective but may cause rebound hyperacidity. Take calcium–magnesium-based antacids after meals and at bedtime. Avoid antacids containing phosphorus, sodium, or aluminum. Liquid antacids may be more effective, as they coat the esophagus.

Continued

PATIENT TEACHING—cont'd

- Remain upright for 1 to 2 hours after eating to reduce reflux and relieve symptoms.
- Avoid eating or drinking for 2 to 3 hours before bedtime and sleep with an extra pillow to elevate your head.

Backache

- Maintain correct posture with the head up and the shoulders back.
- Avoid high-heeled shoes because they increase lordosis and back strain.
- Do not gain excess weight.
- Do not lift heavy objects.
- To pick up objects, squat rather than bend from the waist.
- When sitting, use foot supports, arm rests, and pillows behind the back.
- Exercise: Tailor sitting, shoulder circling, and pelvic rocking strengthen the back and help prepare for labor.
- Application of heat or acupuncture may help.
- Standing with one foot in front of the other and rocking back and forth may help.

Round Ligament Pain

- Use good body mechanics and avoid very strenuous exercise.
- Do not make sudden movements or position changes.
- Do not stretch and twist at the same time. When getting out of bed, turn to the side first without twisting and then get up slowly.
- Bend toward the pain, squat, or bring the knees up to the chest to relieve pain by relaxing the ligament.
- Apply heat and lie on the right side if discomfort persists.

Urinary Frequency and Loss of Urine

- Restrict fluids in the evening but take adequate amounts during the day.
- Limit intake of natural diuretics such as coffee, tea, and other sources of caffeine.
- Perform Kegel exercises to help maintain bladder control:
  - Identify the muscles to be exercised by stopping the flow of urine midstream. Do not routinely perform the exercise while urinating, however, because it might cause urinary retention and increase the risk of urinary tract infection.
  - Slowly contract the muscles around the vagina and hold for 10 seconds. Relax for at least 10 seconds.
  - Repeat the contraction–relaxation cycle 30 or more times each day.

Varicosities

- Avoid constricting clothing and crossing the legs at the knees, which impede blood return from the legs.
- Rest frequently with the legs elevated above the level of the hips and supported with pillows.
- Apply support hose or elastic stockings that reach above the varicosities before getting out of bed each morning. Putting them on later makes them less effective because pooling begins on rising.
- If working in one position for prolonged periods, walk around for a few minutes at least every 2 hours to stimulate blood flow and relieve discomfort.
- Walk frequently to stimulate circulation in the legs.

- Do foot circles and flex your feet toward your head frequently if sitting for long periods.

Constipation

- Self-care measures generally are as effective as laxatives but do not interfere with absorption of nutrients or lead to laxative dependency.
- Drink at least eight glasses of liquids including water, juice, or milk each day. These should not include coffee, tea, or carbonated drinks because of their diuretic effect. After drinking diuretic beverages, drink a glass of water to counteract its effect.
- Add foods high in fiber to help maintain bowel elimination. Include unpeeled fresh fruits and vegetables, whole-grain breads and cereals, bran muffins, oatmeal, potatoes with skins, dried beans, and fruit juices. Four pieces of fruit and a large salad provide enough fiber requirements for 1 day.
- Restrict consumption of cheese, which causes constipation.
- Curtail the intake of sweets, which increases bacterial growth in the intestine and can lead to flatulence.
- Do not discontinue taking iron supplements if they have been prescribed. If constipation persists, consult your health care provider about use of stool softeners.
- Exercise stimulates peristalsis and improves muscle tone. Walking briskly for at least 20 to 30 minutes per day, swimming, or riding a stationary bicycle may be helpful.
- Establish a regular pattern by allowing a consistent time each day for elimination. One hour after meals is ideal to take advantage of the gastrocolic reflex (the peristaltic wave in the colon that is induced by taking food into the fasting stomach).
- Use a footrest during elimination to provide comfort and decrease straining.

Hemorrhoids

- Avoid constipation to prevent straining, which causes or worsens hemorrhoids. Drink plenty of water, eat foods rich in fiber, and exercise regularly.
- To relieve existing hemorrhoids, take frequent tepid baths. Apply cool witch hazel compresses or anesthetic ointments.
- Lie on your side with the hips elevated on a pillow.
- If pain or bleeding persists, call your health care provider.

Leg Cramps

- To prevent cramps, elevate the legs frequently to improve circulation.
- To relieve cramps, extend the affected leg, keeping the knee straight. Bend the foot toward the body, or ask someone to assist. If alone, stand and apply pressure on the affected leg with the knee straight. These measures lengthen the affected muscles and relieve cramping.
- Avoid excessive foods high in phosphorus, such as soft drinks.
- Check with your health care provider regarding the need for supplemental calcium, magnesium, or sodium chloride.

Dependent Edema

- Apply support stockings before getting out of bed.
- Sit or lie with the legs elevated often.

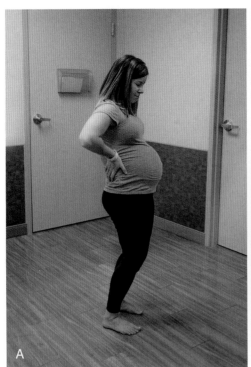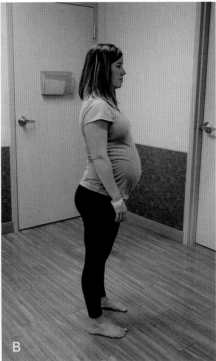

Fig. 7.2 Posture during pregnancy may cause or alleviate backache. **A,** Incorrect posture. The neck is jutting forward, the shoulders are slumping, and the back is sharply curved, creating back pain and discomfort. **B,** Correct posture. The neck and shoulders are straight, the back is flattened, and the pelvis is tucked under and slightly upward.

Nausea and Vomiting

Nausea and vomiting of pregnancy are frequently called *morning sickness* because these symptoms are more acute on arising. However, they may occur at any time and may continue throughout the day. Symptoms may be aggravated by odors (such as from cooking), fatigue, and emotional stress. Clients need reassurance that although morning sickness is distressing, it is common, temporary, and will not harm the fetus. Approximately 50% to 80% of clients experience nausea and vomiting beginning at 4 to 10 weeks gestation and resolving by 20 weeks in most clients (ACOG, 2018c; Kelly & Savides, 2019). Morning sickness should be distinguished from *hyperemesis gravidarum*—severe vomiting accompanied by weight loss, dehydration, electrolyte imbalance, and ketosis (see Chapter 10).

Nausea and vomiting that significantly interfere with the client's intake of nutrients may decrease the nutrients available to the fetus. Eating small, frequent meals and high-protein snacks may help alleviate symptoms. Vitamin B$_6$ (pyridoxine), doxylamine, and phenothiazines may be prescribed by the health care provider, if necessary (Cunningham et al., 2022). Many nonpharmacologic alternative therapies may be helpful, including ginger, peppermint tea, and acupressure. Although these therapies may be helpful in some clients, the efficacy of many of these alternative remedies is not significant. The health care provider should be consulted before complementary and alternative methods are used.

Heartburn

Heartburn, an acute burning sensation in the epigastric and sternal regions, occurs in up to 80% of pregnant clients (Blackburn, 2018). It is caused by reverse peristaltic waves, which produce regurgitation of stomach contents into the esophagus. The underlying causes are diminished gastric motility, displacement of the stomach by the enlarging uterus, relaxation of the lower esophageal and gastric sphincters, and increased intraabdominal and intragastric pressure as pregnancy progresses. If common remedies and dietary changes are not effective, the provider may prescribe histamine-2 receptor inhibitors (Blackburn, 2018).

Backache

Backache occurs in more than two-thirds of pregnant clients (Blackburn, 2018). Increased joint mobility, lumbar lordosis, and relaxed ligaments contribute to the problem. Teaching correct posture and body mechanics can help prevent back pain (Fig. 7.2). Stooping or bending puts a great deal of strain on the muscles of the lower back. Instruction should include correct and incorrect methods of lifting and exercises to relax the shoulders and help prevent backache (Fig. 7.3).

Round Ligament Pain

Round ligament pain is a sharp pain in the inguinal area or on the side, usually on the right. It results from softening and stretching of the ligament from hormones and uterine growth. In some instances, it may be difficult for the client to distinguish from uterine contractions. Careful assessment to rule out contractions followed by reassurance are appropriate measures.

Urinary Frequency

Although urinary frequency is a common complaint during pregnancy, the condition is temporary and is managed by

Shoulder circling

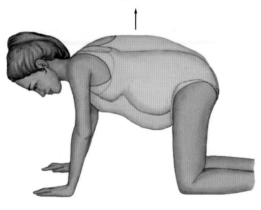

The fingertips are placed on the shoulders, then the elbows are brought forward and up during inhalation, back and down during exhalation. Repeat five times.

Tailor sitting

The woman uses her thigh muscles to press her knees to the floor. Keeping her back straight, she should remain in the position for 5 to 15 minutes.

Pelvic tilt or pelvic rocking

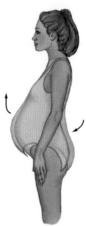

This exercise can be performed on hands and knees, with the hands directly under the shoulders and the knees under the hips. The back should be in a neutral position, not hollowed. The head and neck should be aligned with the straight back. The woman then presses up with the lower back and holds this position for a few seconds, then relaxes to a neutral position. Repeat 5 times. The exercise may also be performed in a standing position when the pelvis is rotated forward to flatten the lower back.

Fig. 7.3 Exercises to prevent backache.

most clients without undue distress. Urinary incontinence, especially in the third trimester, may occur. Kegel exercises may be helpful in maintaining bladder control.

Varicosities

Varicosities occur in 40% of pregnancies (Blackburn, 2018). They are seen more often in clients who are obese, are multiparas, or have a family history of varicose veins. During pregnancy, the weight of the uterus partially compresses the veins returning blood from the legs, and estrogen causes elastic tissue to become more fragile. As blood pools, the vessels dilate and become engorged, inflamed, and painful. Varicose veins are exacerbated by prolonged standing, during which the force of gravity makes blood return more difficult.

Varicosities are usually confined to the legs but may involve the veins of the vulva or rectum (hemorrhoids). Varicosities may range from barely noticeable blemishes with minimal discomfort at the end of the day to large, tortuous veins

producing severe discomfort with any activity. They usually improve after childbirth but do not go away completely.

Hemorrhoids

Hemorrhoids are varicosities of the rectum and may be external (outside the anus) or internal (above the sphincter). Some common causes are vascular engorgement of the pelvis, constipation, straining with bowel movements, and prolonged sitting or standing. Pushing during the second stage of labor aggravates the problem, which may continue into the postpartum period. Hemorrhoids often shrink and become less troublesome postpartum.

Constipation

Occasional constipation is not harmful, although it can cause feelings of abdominal fullness and flatulence and aggravate painful hemorrhoids. Intestinal motility is reduced during pregnancy as a result of progesterone, pressure from the enlarged uterus, and decreased activity. The result may be hard, dry stools and decreased frequency of bowel movements. Iron supplementation often increases constipation. Increasing fluid and fiber intake may help to decrease this condition.

Leg Cramps

Painful contractions of the muscles of the legs occur in 25% to 50% of pregnant clients (Blackburn, 2018). Cramps often occur during sleep when the muscles are relaxed or when the client stretches and extends their feet with the toes pointed. Venous congestion in the legs during the third trimester also contributes to leg cramps. Nonpharmacologic treatments including dorsiflexion of the foot, heat or cold application, and increased hydration.

❓ KNOWLEDGE CHECK

8. What are some relief methods for morning sickness?
9. How can backache be decreased during pregnancy?

APPLICATION OF THE NURSING PROCESS: FAMILY RESPONSES TO PHYSICAL CHANGES OF PREGNANCY

The nursing process focuses on identifying each family's unique responses to the physiologic changes of pregnancy, determining factors that might interfere with their ability to adapt to changes, and finding solutions to identified problems.

Assessment

Assess the client's responses to the physiologic processes of pregnancy and explore the family's preparation for the birth. Use structured interviews and planned teaching sessions, as well as more informal spontaneous discussions during assessments. Review the history and physical examination to obtain important data. Gather information from the expectant client, as well as from their partner and significant family members, if appropriate.

Identification of Client Problems

When analyzing data, nurses should use all their critical thinking skills before reaching a conclusion about the most significant client problems or opportunities.

Much of the time, the nurse will work with the family to enhance their opportunity for health improvement during the antepartum period. Most families express an intense desire to protect the health of the unborn child and the well-being of the client.

Planning: Expected Outcomes

If the expected outcomes have been achieved, the client will:
- Explain self-care practices which promote safety and well-being for the client and the fetus.
- Describe relief measures for common discomforts of pregnancy.
- Identify personal habits or behaviors that could adversely affect their health or the health of the fetus and develop a plan to modify these behaviors.

Interventions
Teaching Health Behaviors

Teaching should be addressed at each visit and should focus on the client's immediate questions and concerns. Common concerns are discussed here.

Bathing. Bathing protects pregnant individuals from infections and promotes comfort by dissipating heat produced by the increased metabolism. During the last trimester, when balance is altered by a changing center of gravity, the client is prone to falls. Advise them to use nonskid pads in the tub or shower.

Tubs and Saunas. Although warm baths and showers help relax tense and tired muscles, pregnant individuals should avoid activities that may cause hyperthermia. Hyperthermia, particularly during the first trimester, may be associated with fetal anomalies. Caution the client not to be in a sauna for more than 15 minutes or a hot tub for more than 10 minutes and to keep the head, chest, shoulders, and arms out of the water (Casanova et al., 2019).

Douching. Some individuals douche because they believe it increases cleanliness and prevents infection. However, despite increased vaginal discharge during pregnancy, douching is unnecessary at any time. Douching increases the risk for ectopic pregnancy, cervical cancer, STIs, pelvic inflammatory disease, and endometritis. Bacterial vaginosis occurs more often in those who douche. In pregnancy, bacterial vaginosis has been associated with spontaneous abortion, preterm birth, premature rupture of membranes, and chorioamnionitis (Cunningham et al., 2022). Discuss the client's reasons for douching and explain it is unnecessary.

Breast Care. Instruct the expectant client to avoid using soap on the nipples because it removes the natural lubricant secreted by Montgomery glands in the areola. Advise wearing of a well-fitting supportive bra to help prevent loss of tone as the breasts become heavier during pregnancy. Wide bra straps distribute the weight evenly across the shoulders and provide greater comfort.

Inform the client that breast stimulation increases oxytocin secretion and may cause uterine contractions. Therefore, breast stimulation is unsafe if the client has a history of preterm labor or existing signs of preterm labor such as rhythmic pelvic pressure or regular uterine contractions. No breast or nipple preparation is necessary during pregnancy for breastfeeding (Smith et al., 2019). Nurses and providers should promote and discuss the benefits of breastfeeding early in pregnancy and throughout prenatal care.

Clothing. Recommend practical, comfortable, and non-constricting clothing. Tight jeans or pantyhose, which may impede venous circulation, should be avoided or worn only for short periods. Suggest the client wear low heels because they do not interfere with balance. High heels increase the curvature of the lower spine (lordosis) increasing backache and making the client more likely to fall.

Exercise. Exercise during pregnancy is generally beneficial and can strengthen muscles, reduce backache and stress, and provide a feeling of well-being. The amount and type of exercise recommended depend on the physical condition of the individual and the stage of pregnancy. Exercise tolerance is often decreased, but mild to moderate exercise is generally not a problem.

Teach clients who have no medical or obstetric complications to exercise in moderation for at least 20 to 30 minutes or more on most if not all days of the week (ACOG, 2020a; Casanova et al., 2019). Recreational sports can be continued if no risk for falling or abdominal trauma is present. Joint and ligament laxity and lumbar lordosis increase the risk for injury, especially in the third trimester. Contact sports and exercise with a high risk for falling such as rock climbing or skiing should be avoided. Exercise in the supine position should be discontinued after the first trimester to avoid supine hypotensive syndrome.

Walking is an ideal exercise because it stimulates muscular activity, gently increases respiratory and cardiovascular effort, and does not result in fatigue or strain. Swimming and water exercises are excellent during pregnancy because the buoyancy of the water helps prevent injuries. Riding a stationary bike and yoga are also helpful. Exercise classes especially for pregnant individuals are often available and offer companionship with others having similar experiences.

Instruct the client not to begin strenuous exercise programs or intensify training during pregnancy. Those who have been exercising strenuously before pregnancy should consult the health care provider but may be able to continue some of their usual routine. As pregnancy progresses, the exercise program may need modification because the change in the client's center of gravity makes them more prone to falls. Therefore, an activity may be safe in the first trimester but not in the third trimester.

Pregnant individuals should avoid becoming overheated during exercise because heat is transmitted to the fetus, causing an increase in fetal oxygen needs. Clients should allow a cool-down period after exercising. To prevent dehydration, it is important to take liquids frequently while exercising.

Exercise should be tailored to the way the client feels to avoid becoming overly fatigued. Generally, if a person cannot carry on a conversation while exercising, they are doing too much. The individual should stop exercising and seek medical advice if they have chest pain, dizziness, headache, vaginal bleeding, decreased fetal movement, or signs of labor while exercising.

Sleep and Rest. Problems sleeping may begin as early as the first trimester and continue throughout pregnancy (Cunningham et al., 2022). Finding a comfortable position for rest may be difficult by the third trimester. Backache, abdominal discomfort and contractions, leg cramps, fetal movement, and urinary frequency may interfere with sleep.

Suggest the client use pillows to support the abdomen and back to enhance sleep (Fig. 7.4). Emphasize frequent rest periods are beneficial, even if the client does not fall asleep. Suggest relaxation exercises to use during the day and before bed. In addition, avoiding caffeine and limiting fluids at night may be helpful.

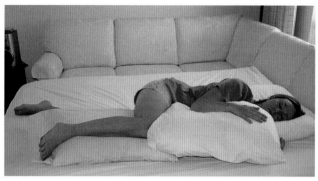

Fig. 7.4 During the third trimester, pillows supporting the abdomen and back provide a comfortable position for rest.

Sexual Activity. Sexual intercourse is generally safe for the healthy pregnant individual.

Nutrition. A discussion of nutrition should be part of each visit. The nurse should assess the client's diet and use of prenatal vitamins and answer any questions they may have (see Chapter 8).

Employment. Most individuals of childbearing age in the United States are employed outside the home, and most continue to work during pregnancy. Clients with uncomplicated pregnancies can usually continue working until they begin labor, if they wish (AAP & ACOG, 2017). However, the level of physical activity involved and the risk for exposure to environmental toxins and industrial hazards should be considered.

Safety. Work should not lead to undue fatigue. Frequent rest periods with the feet elevated are essential. Clients with jobs that require constant standing or sitting should change positions often or walk briefly to stimulate circulation and reduce fatigue. Tasks that require balance may be hazardous as the center of gravity shifts. Heavy lifting should be avoided.

Working clients have many home responsibilities. The fatigue and stress of both the home and employment workloads may be difficult during pregnancy. If possible, the expectant client should adapt their home and employment workloads during pregnancy to reduce fatigue and stress (Gregory et al., 2021).

Exposure to Teratogens. Intrauterine exposure to toxic substances is of particular concern during the first trimester, the period of organogenesis. Advise clients to investigate their own occupational hazards. For example, nurses and hospital personnel may be exposed to chemotherapy drugs, radiation, anesthetic gases, and infectious diseases such as cytomegalovirus infection; hair and nail salon workers may be exposed to hair spray and nail products; laundry and dry-cleaning workers may be exposed to fetotoxic compounds; and farm workers may be exposed to pesticides. In addition, some individuals are exposed to passive smoking in the workplace, which is harmful to both client and fetus.

Travel. Car travel is safe during normal pregnancies. Generally, no more than 6 hours in a 24-hour period of car travel is recommended during pregnancy (Gregory et al., 2021). Suggest the client stop to walk every 2 hours to increase venous return from the legs and consider compression stockings. Hydration is also important.

Instruct the client to fasten the seat belt snugly with the lap belt under their abdomen and across their thighs and the shoulder belt in a diagonal position across their chest and above the bulge of the uterus. This position is uncomfortable for some individuals, and it causes concern about internal injuries if a collision occurs. However, it is safer to wear the belt than to leave it off and risk ejection from the vehicle during an accident.

Travel by plane is generally safe for up to 36 weeks in the absence of complications of pregnancy. Support stockings, periodic movement of the legs and ambulation, avoidance of restrictive clothing, and adequate hydration may help avoid venous thrombosis. The seat belt should be worn at all times because air turbulence is unpredictable (ACOG, 2018a). The belt should be buckled below the abdomen (AAP & ACOG, 2017). Advise the client to walk at least every hour to maintain adequate peripheral circulation and avoid thromboembolism. The client should not travel to remote locations where medical care is unavailable. Suggest they take a copy of their medical records if traveling a long distance.

Immunizations. In general, immunizations with live virus vaccines (such as measles, mumps, rubella, and varicella) are contraindicated during pregnancy because they may have teratogenic effects on the fetus. Inactivated vaccines are safe and can be used in those who have a risk for developing diseases such as tetanus and influenza. Inactivated influenza vaccine is especially important for individuals who are pregnant during flu season because they can have serious complications from the disease. It can be given at any point in pregnancy (ACOG, 2021; CDC, 2019). Recent recommendations include administration of the COVID-19 vaccine to pregnant clients to decrease complications for both the client and the fetus. Evidence suggests that COVID-19 vaccination is safe before, during, and after pregnancy (ACOG & Society for Maternal-Fetal Medicine, 2021). The CDC (2019) recommends administration of the Tdap vaccination between 27 and 36 weeks of pregnancy. (See the CDC website at www.cdc.gov/vaccines for current information.)

Teaching Necessary Lifestyle Changes

Many expectant parents are willing to make changes in lifestyle to avoid adversely affecting the fetus.

Prescription and Over-the-Counter Drugs. Advise pregnant clients to consult with their health care providers before taking any medications or herbal supplements. This applies to OTC medications as well as prescription drugs. Some nonsteroidal antiinflammatory drugs such as aspirin should be avoided because they may increase bleeding. When prescription medications are necessary, the health care provider weighs the risks against the benefits to decide if a drug can be used safely or if changes are necessary. Medications taken during the first trimester are of particular concern because of the risk to developing fetal organs.

Complementary and Alternative Therapies. Some complementary and alternative therapies are very safe and helpful during pregnancy. Estimations predict over one-third of pregnant individuals in the United States use some type of alternative therapies during pregnancy. Many have not been studied adequately. Ask about any complementary or alternative therapies used and advise the client to discuss them with their health care provider.

Tobacco. An important aspect of prenatal care is assessment of and intervention for smoking. Approximately 7.2% of clients in the United States smoke at some time during their pregnancy (Drake et al., 2018). A *Healthy People 2030* objective is to increase the number of clients who stop smoking during the first trimester and do not restart for the entire pregnancy from 20.2% to 22.4% (DHHS, 2020).

Identify clients who smoke and explain the effects of smoking during pregnancy. Every nurse should screen for tobacco use and refer clients to smoking cessation programs as needed. Make every effort to motivate expectant individuals to stop smoking and to avoid contact with others who smoke. Secondhand smoke during pregnancy increases the risk for miscarriage, preterm birth, low birth weight, sudden infant death syndrome, and other complications (AAP, 2017; ACOG, 2020b; Samet & Sockrider, 2021). The following approach to smoking cessation is often effective:

1. *Ask* the client at each visit if they smoke, if the amount of smoking has changed, and if they would like to quit. Pregnancy is a time when individuals are motivated to make changes to benefit their health and the health of the fetus.
2. *Advise* the client about the importance of not smoking.
3. *Assess* the client's willingness to try to stop smoking. Discuss motivational information if the individual is not willing to quit at this time. Refer the client to a smoking cessation program if they are willing to try to stop smoking.
4. *Assist* the client in making a plan to stop smoking, and provide practical counseling on how to solve the problems they may encounter—for example, avoiding others who smoke and being aware of activities they associate with smoking may be helpful. Advise them total abstinence is essential to success.
5. *Arrange* follow-up visits or phone calls to discuss the client's progress and any problems they may have experienced and to offer encouragement. Telephone support may be beneficial in preventing smoking relapse in individuals who have stopped smoking (AAP, 2017; ACOG, 2020b).

Include the client's partner in discussions of smoking cessation and the effects of smoking on the fetus. The partner's support is especially important in helping the pregnant client quit smoking. The partner who smokes may be interested in joining a cessation program too.

Approximately 50% to 60% of clients who stop smoking during pregnancy begin smoking again within 1 year after they give birth (ACOG, 2020b). Explain the effects of smoking on infants and provide continued support for smoking cessation during the postpartum period.

Although nonpharmacologic methods of smoking cessation are best, nicotine replacement therapy may be used if other methods are unsuccessful (Cunningham et al., 2022).

Use of nicotine replacement therapy during pregnancy should occur only under the close supervision of the health care provider (AAP & ACOG, 2017; ACOG, 2020b).

Alcohol. Alcohol is a known teratogen, and alcohol use during pregnancy is a leading cause of intellectual disability in the United States. Alcohol may produce a characteristic cluster of developmental anomalies known as fetal alcohol spectrum disorders. Conclusive data about fetal effects of social or moderate drinking are not available, but no amount of alcohol consumed during pregnancy is known to be safe. Therefore, the best advice for pregnant clients or those who plan to become pregnant is to abstain from all alcohol.

Illicit Drugs. Use of street or recreational drugs such as cocaine, heroin, and methamphetamines are harmful to the fetus. Advise the pregnant client to seek help to discontinue all illicit drug use.

Teaching about Signs of Possible Complications

Instruct the pregnant client and their family about signs and symptoms which should be reported immediately because they indicate a serious danger (see "Critical to Remember: Signs of Possible Pregnancy Complications"). The client should be instructed to call their health care provider or go to the hospital immediately if complications are suspected.

Although making the expectant client aware of signs of complications during pregnancy is crucial, the nurse should take care not to overly worry them. Avoid the term *danger signs* when talking to the client and their family, because it may be frightening. It is less alarming to say, "The signs I am about to explain to you are unusual, but if you notice them, notify your health care provider at once because they require immediate attention."

Providing Resources

Provide the client with sources for more information. These may include internet websites such as the March of Dimes at www.marchofdimes.org for information about pregnancy and infants. The Association of Women's Health, Obstetric, and Neonatal Nurses, American College of Nurse-Midwives, and ACOG provide online information for all obstetric and gynecologic health topics, including pregnancy, at www.health4mom.org, www.our-momentoftruth.com, and www.acog.org/patients, respectively.

A free service providing information about pregnancy and infants through 1 year is available by text to mobile phones. The service can be accessed by going to the website at www.text4baby.org. The service is supported by both private and governmental agencies and provides three text messages weekly with health tips appropriate to the week of pregnancy or age of the infant.

Evaluation

Interventions can be considered to effectively meet the established outcomes if the client and family (1) discuss and practice self-care measures to promote safety and health of the client and fetus, (2) explain methods to help relieve common discomforts of pregnancy, and (3) identify a plan early in pregnancy to modify habits or behaviors that could adversely affect health. If interventions are ineffective, the nurse collaborates with the family to define new plans and work out additional interventions.

APPLICATION OF THE NURSING PROCESS: PSYCHOSOCIAL CONCERNS

Assessment

The purpose of a psychosocial assessment is to monitor the adaptation of the family to pregnancy, which may require a major

---

CRITICAL TO REMEMBER

Signs of Possible Pregnancy Complications

Signs	Possible Causes
Vaginal bleeding with or without discomfort	Spontaneous abortion, placenta previa, placental abruption, lesions of the cervix or vagina, "bloody show"
Escape of fluid from the vagina	Rupture of membranes
Swelling of the fingers (rings become tight) or puffiness of the face or around the eyes	Excessive edema, preeclampsia
Continuous pounding headache	Chronic hypertension or preeclampsia
Visual disturbances (such as blurred vision, dimness, flashing lights, spots before the eyes)	Worsening preeclampsia
Seizures	Eclampsia
Persistent or severe abdominal or epigastric pain	Ectopic pregnancy (if early), worsening preeclampsia, placental abruption
Chills or fever	Infection
Painful urination	Urinary tract infection, pyelonephritis
Persistent vomiting	Hyperemesis gravidarum
Change in frequency or strength of fetal movements	Fetal compromise or death
Signs or symptoms of preterm labor: Uterine contractions, cramps, constant or irregular low backache, pelvic pressure, watery vaginal discharge	Labor onset

transition in role function and relationships. For some families, pregnancy offers the potential for growth. For others, an alteration in family processes requires guidance and information. Specific needs can be discovered during a thorough psychosocial assessment. Table 7.4 identifies areas for assessment, provides sample questions, and indicates nursing implications.

Identification of Client Problems

Most families strive to maintain the health of the expectant individual and fetus and to complete developmental tasks that help the couple to take on the parent role. Perhaps the most encompassing client issue is the opportunity for improved family coping, because of the desire to meet added family needs and assume parenting roles.

Planning: Expected Outcomes

Expected outcomes include:
- The expectant parents will verbalize emotional responses appropriate to each trimester.
- The family will describe methods to help the expectant parents complete the developmental processes of pregnancy.
- The family will identify cultural factors which may produce conflicts and collaborate to reduce those conflicts.

Interventions

Providing Information

Provide the prospective parents with information and anticipatory guidance to prepare them for the progressive changes which occur during pregnancy, and reassure them that their feelings and behaviors are normal. Guidance also gives them an opportunity to ask questions and explore their feelings. Common subjects include the following:
- The emotional changes that occur during pregnancy
- The developmental tasks of the client
- Role transition
- The developmental processes of the prospective coparent

Adapting Nursing Care to Pregnancy Progress

Adapt nursing care to the changes that occur in each trimester of pregnancy. During the first trimester, focus on the client's acceptance of the pregnancy. Tailor teaching to their feelings (physical and psychological), as this is a period of self-focus. The second trimester is a time to concentrate more on the fetus and how the client and family will adapt to the changes resulting from the birth. Ask about any fantasies about the baby and relationships with significant others. The focus is on the client's discomforts and readiness to give birth during the third trimester. Observe for signs the client is having difficulty with any of the tasks or steps throughout pregnancy.

Discussing Resources

Initiate a discussion of the adequacy of the financial situation and support systems, and help couples without financial resources or insurance coverage find a convenient location to obtain prenatal care. This is particularly important for clients who have little knowledge about how to gain access to government-sponsored care. Emotional resources include those that help the new family adjust to the demands of pregnancy and parenting.

Discuss the responses and participation of the grandparents. Although emotional responses vary, the family unit is strengthened and the attachment of the grandparents to the child is enhanced when grandparents actively participate in the pregnancy.

If family members who traditionally offer help in times of stress are unavailable, refer the prospective parents to community resources such as support groups and childbirth education, sibling, breastfeeding, and new parenting classes.

Helping the Family Prepare for Birth

During the last trimester, discuss lifestyle changes that will occur when the infant is born. Unanticipated changes that accompany this dramatic life event may add stress and disrupt family processes. Help the prospective parents make practical plans for the infant, such as obtaining clothing and needed equipment and choosing the method of feeding.

Assist the parents in planning sibling preparation. Older siblings should be prepared several weeks or even months before the birth. They often benefit from participating in planning for the baby. Younger children have a poor concept of time and can be prepared shortly before birth.

Suggest the expectant parents consider how they will divide household chores, parenting tasks, and child care, especially if the client will return to work after childbirth. If these issues are not resolved, the couple can experience frustration and anger when one parent, usually the client, assumes total care of the infant and attempts to complete all household tasks. Exhaustion and frustration can overwhelm the joys of parenting when one parent must provide all care.

Modeling Communication Technique

When disagreements are evident, discuss and model therapeutic communication techniques that include all significant family members. Techniques to clarify, summarize, and reflect feelings can defuse negative feelings that might result in family disruption.

Identifying Conflicting Cultural Factors

Explore possible areas of conflict related to cultural beliefs and health practices that affect pregnancy.

Expectant clients are reassured when nurses support beneficial health beliefs before confronting them with concerns about health care practices. For example, "The foods you are choosing are very good for you and the baby. I am worried, though, because you missed your last appointment."

If a conflict occurs because of differences in time orientation, acknowledge the problem, convey understanding of the differences, and emphasize the importance of calling when appointments cannot be kept. Many families do not realize when they miss an appointment, another family misses the opportunity for health care.

Evaluation

When the family verbalizes concerns and emotions at each visit, the initial goal is met. Continued interest and involvement of the partner and significant family members are evidence that the family has completed the developmental tasks of pregnancy. Participation with health care workers to find a compromise if differing cultural beliefs cause conflict confirms the family will identify and initiate measures to reduce conflicts.

PERINATAL EDUCATION CLASSES

The goals of perinatal education are to help parents become knowledgeable consumers, take an active role in maintaining health during pregnancy and birth, and learn coping techniques for pregnancy, childbirth, and parenting. Meeting these goals helps reduce their fear of the unknown and increases their abilities to make informed decisions regarding childbirth and parenting with confidence and satisfaction. Although much perinatal education is accomplished during the prenatal visits, many classes are available and valuable. Perinatal education classes are strongly recommended by the AAP and ACOG (2017) because they can have a beneficial effect on patients' experience.

Expectant families have many choices for prenatal education classes. Their decisions are based on the classes available in the area, costs, and types of information they need. Small classes with few clients and their partners are ideal but may be too expensive or unavailable. The teacher is usually a nurse who has experience in maternity nursing and is certified by a nationally known organization such as Lamaze International or the International Childbirth Education Association.

Although most people think of perinatal education primarily as preparation for the birth experience, classes are available for all areas of pregnancy, childbirth, and parenting.

Nurses help the client and their partner find classes suited to their educational needs by providing a list and description of classes in the community and suggesting they talk with others who have taken various classes. The couple may wish to interview teachers to learn about their preparation and philosophies. Some couples want classes that focus on avoidance of medication as the primary goal of childbirth. Many prefer those that consider a variety of tools, including medication, for coping with pain.

Preconception Classes

Classes for individuals or couples who are thinking about having a baby are designed to help them have a healthy pregnancy from the beginning. Information about nutrition before conception, healthy lifestyle, signs of pregnancy, and choosing a caregiver is presented. The effects of pregnancy and childbirth on a client's relationships and career are discussed. Preconception classes emphasize early and regular prenatal care beginning before pregnancy and ways to reduce risk factors for poor pregnancy outcomes.

Education in First Trimester

First-trimester classes cover information on adapting to pregnancy and understanding what to expect in the months ahead (Box 7.2). Emphasis is placed on how to have a healthy pregnancy by obtaining prenatal care and avoiding hazards to the fetus.

One important task for expecting individuals during early pregnancy is to choose the provider and setting that is most appropriate. Some clients may wish to prepare a birth plan (Box 7.3).

BOX 7.2 Topics Covered in Early Pregnancy Classes

Pregnancy changes
   Anatomy and physiology
   Physiologic and psychological changes
   Fetal development
   Hazards to the client and fetus (e.g., drugs, alcohol, smoking, environmental hazards)
   Prenatal care (e.g., what to expect at each visit)
   Communication with the provider
   Prenatal screening tests
Self-care
   Hygiene
   Nutrition
   Exercise and body mechanics
   Discomforts of pregnancy
   Warning signs and actions to take
   Sexuality
   Work and pregnancy
Infant care
   Selection of a pediatric provider
   Infant development
   Infant feeding
Birth
   Birth options (such as birth plan, costs)
   Preterm labor

BOX 7.3 Birth Plan

Help couples prepare a plan for their birth experience if they wish. The birth plan, sometimes called a *family preference plan*, describes the couple's desires as they consider their choices in childbirth. The plan may be unwritten and very simple or a list of very specific items to be included in the childbirth experience. Cultural wishes can be incorporated into the birth plan.

The birth plan is a tool for expanding communication with health care professionals. It helps couples learn about their options and make informed choices and ensures their wishes are known before labor begins. It may help the couple choose the provider, setting, and classes most conducive to meeting specific needs. The couple should discuss the plan with the health care provider during pregnancy and with the nurse in the labor and delivery unit when they are admitted. This may result in a more satisfying birth experience even if not everything goes according to the expectations.

Help the couple learn about locally available choices and explain any restrictions. For example, insurance coverage may dictate which facility they must use. Those without insurance are concerned about the cost of various options. In addition, the health care provider or birth agency may have set policies on certain issues. Complications during labor and birth may necessitate changes in the plan.

If the couple has not chosen a health care provider, suggest they interview several physicians or nurse–midwives to learn about the provider's usual practices and possible exceptions. If they have a provider, emphasize the importance of discussing their plan with that provider. With discussion, the couple and provider can create a plan that is satisfactory to all.

Education in Second Trimester

Second-trimester classes focus on changes occurring during middle pregnancy and what to expect during the third trimester. Teachers discuss childbirth choices and information to help students become more knowledgeable consumers. With a Centering Pregnancy model of care, much of the perinatal education is incorporated into the regular prenatal visit. Exercise classes help clients keep fit and healthy during pregnancy. Written consent from the primary caregiver may be required to ensure the client can participate safely. The instructor should understand the special needs of pregnancy and teach low-impact exercises preceded by warm-up routines. Clients should avoid excessive heart rate elevation to prevent diversion of blood away from the uterus.

The client with a high-risk pregnancy may have activity restrictions and may be unable to attend regular perinatal classes. If possible, help them arrange for individual instruction. Online courses or podcasts, DVDs, written materials, and phone or e-mail contact with an instructor are ways they can learn and practice techniques without attending classes.

Education in Third Trimester

During the third trimester, clients may enroll in prenatal classes to cope with vulnerabilities and fears regarding the upcoming birth.

In childbirth preparation classes during the third trimester, clients and their support persons learn self-help measures, what to expect during labor and birth, and how to prepare for the big day (Boxes 7.4 and 7.5). Although once referred to as "natural childbirth classes," they are now called *prepared childbirth classes* to denote the client's preparation for all aspects of childbirth.

Clients and their support persons learn coping methods to help them approach childbirth in a positive manner. Teachers do not promise prevention of all pain in labor. However, the increased confidence and the techniques learned in prepared childbirth classes may help increase tolerance of pain during labor and increase satisfaction with their birth experience. Class series range from a 1-day class to 3 to 12 meetings, depending on the content included. Supervised practice of relaxation, breathing techniques, and coping strategies in "labor rehearsals" may be part of every class.

Most classes cover information about both pharmacologic and nonpharmacologic methods of coping with labor pain. While some clients plan to have epidural anesthesia during childbirth, they may also rely on nonpharmacologic pain relief measures until pharmacologic pain relief is available.

By learning what to expect during labor and birth, clients and their support persons are able to rehearse the experience in their minds in preparation for the actual event. They practice coping techniques during simulated contractions. Realistic, valid class information and discussion of possible variations are essential so couples are adequately prepared.

Prepared childbirth classes based in birth facilities include detailed information on what to expect in that particular setting but may not cover unavailable options. A tour of birthing units may be offered as part of the class or as a separate class.

BOX 7.4   Topics Included in Prepared Childbirth Classes

Some topics may be presented in separate classes.
Physical and psychological changes of the last trimester
    Common discomforts and concerns
    Nutrition
    Exercise and body mechanics
    Sexuality
    Danger signs and actions to take
Labor and birth
    Anatomy and physiology of labor
    Plans for the birth (e.g., options, birth plan)
    Signs of labor and when to go to the hospital
    Hospital admission, procedures, and policies
    Physical and emotional aspects of labor
    Labor variations (e.g., back labor)
    Medical procedures (e.g., induction, augmentation, amniotomy, episiotomy, vacuum extraction)
    Birthing process
    Recovery
    Tour of birthing unit
    Role of the labor partner
    Techniques for support
Coping techniques for labor
    Relaxation and breathing techniques
    Comfort measures
    Labor rehearsals
    Pain relief (pharmacologic and nonpharmacologic)
Complications
    Fetal testing
    Preterm labor
    Hypertension
    Cesarean birth
High-risk pregnancy

Coping Techniques

Relaxation. Tension and anxiety during labor cause tightening of abdominal muscles, impeding contractions and increasing pain by stimulation of nerve endings which heightens awareness of pain. Prolonged muscle tension causes fatigue and increased pain perception. When anxiety and tension are high, uterine contractions are less effective and the length of labor increases. The ability to relax during labor is an important component of coping effectively with childbirth. Relaxation conserves energy, decreases oxygen use, and enhances other pain relief techniques. Most childbirth preparation classes teach clients exercises to help them recognize and release tension. The labor partner assists by identifying symptoms of tension and providing feedback to help the client relax. For example, tightening of shoulders, frowning, or jiggling a foot may be observed when stressed. The partner helps focus on areas the client finds difficult to release. Positive feedback from the partner and teacher encourages increased relaxation.

Relaxation exercises should be practiced frequently to be useful during labor. Couples begin practice sessions in a quiet, comfortable setting. Later, they practice in other places to simulate the noise and unfamiliar setting of the hospital.

BOX 7.5 What to Take to the Hospital

Items to Be Included in the Labor Bag

Focal point
Lotion, oil, or powder to make massage more comfortable
Warm socks for cold feet
Colored washcloths for washing face (white ones might be lost)
Hand-held fan
Elastic bands and clips for hair
Tennis balls in a sock for sacral pressure
Sugar-free sour lollipop for dry mouth
Mouthwash
Lip balm, unflavored
Instruction sheets or reminder checklists
Paper and pencil
Playing cards or simple games for early labor
Camera
Snack for labor partner
Cell phone/charger and telephone numbers for calls after birth
Earbuds for phone (to listen to music)
Pillows (use colored pillowcases to prevent loss)

Items for After Birth

Robe and nightgown or pajamas which open in the front (for breastfeeding)
Nursing bras
Slippers
Shampoo, conditioner, comb, toothbrush, toothpaste
Loose-fitting clothes to wear home
Clothes for the baby to wear home
Baby blankets
Car seat

Relaxation exercises may be combined with other techniques such as imagery and massage.

Breathing. Historically, specific breathing techniques were taught in childbirth preparations classes. Today, breathing is taught in conjunction with relaxation techniques. Many classes teach a variety of techniques to allow participants to pick and choose those which work best for them. The cleansing breath, a deep inhalation followed by complete exhalation is used at the beginning and end of each contraction. This oxygenates the client and fetus. With slow abdominal breathing, the patient is told to release tension, breathe in through the nose until they cannot comfortably take in any more air and then breathe out through the mouth. Breathing techniques maintain oxygenation and provide a distraction for the client (see Chapter 13).

Conditioning. Many techniques for prepared childbirth are based partially on theories of conditioned response, in which certain responses to stimuli become automatic through frequent association. Clients learn to associate uterine contractions with relaxation by practicing those techniques with mental images of contractions. Because effective conditioning requires a great deal of practice, individuals are encouraged to practice their techniques daily. For some, the intensity of real uterine contractions is surprisingly different from what they visualized during practice sessions. They may have difficulty with relaxation as a result and may need to use other methods along with conditioning.

Labor Partner. Almost all types of childbirth preparation encourage the participation of someone who remains with the client throughout labor. This person may be called a *labor partner, support person, coach,* or *labor companion.* The presence of a labor partner may help the client cope more effectively, decrease distress during labor, and result in greater satisfaction with the childbirth experience. This support person shares the experience and helps the client remain focused and calm during labor.

The person who takes on this role may be the baby's father, partner, relative, friend, or doula. The labor partner generally attends classes with the client to learn about labor, birth, and techniques to assist during labor. By practicing together, the client and partner learn to work smoothly as a team during labor. Classes may increase confidence for support persons, who learn specific techniques to use during labor. Many clients hire a doula to assist with labor support. The doula may attend or teach the childbirth class. Encourage couples to think about the support person's labor role before labor begins and then encourage the partner in whatever role is chosen. Labor partners should not feel responsible for more than is included in the role. Teachers should discuss the duties of the labor nurse and encourage labor partners to seek assistance when they are uncertain. The labor nurse may have helpful suggestions and adaptations of techniques.

Class discussion of complications should include the role of the support person in these situations.

Methods of Childbirth Education

Although all methods of prepared childbirth education use some combination of pain management techniques, each method has unique aspects. Many classes have a holistic approach, providing a variety of techniques from which couples can choose what works best for them. The nurse should give the family a list and description of classes in their community and the philosophies of each class.

Lamaze Childbirth Education. The Lamaze method is often called **psychoprophylaxis** because it uses the mind to block pain. It involves concentration and conditioning to help the client respond to contractions with relaxation and various techniques to decrease pain. The Lamaze method is the most popular method used today. A variety of techniques are taught, and clients should feel free to choose among them (see Chapter 13). Clients should not be taught that there is only one right way of responding to labor.

KNOWLEDGE CHECK

10. What are the goals of perinatal education?
11. What information is typically covered in preconception classes? Early pregnancy classes? Second-trimester classes?
12. What techniques are commonly taught in childbirth preparation classes during the third trimester?
13. How is the client in labor helped by having a labor partner?

BOX 7.6   Topics Included in Breastfeeding Classes
Anatomy and physiology Preparation for breastfeeding First feedings Positioning and latch-on Establishment of milk supply Prevention and solutions for problems: Engorgement, sore   nipples, nipple confusion, insufficient milk supply, mastitis Nutrition Use of bottles and storage of breast milk Breast pumps Role of support person(s) Work and breastfeeding Weaning

Breastfeeding Classes

Prenatal breastfeeding education is important because of the short time available after birth to help breastfeeding clients in the birth facility. Classes help increase a client's confidence in their ability to breastfeed successfully. Teachers are often certified lactation consultants who have special education and advanced knowledge about breastfeeding.

Breastfeeding classes include information about the various aspects of lactation and help support persons attending learn methods of providing assistance during breastfeeding (Box 7.6). Resources for additional help are provided in case the client encounters difficulties. Some teachers hold additional sessions after the birth to provide ongoing counseling at a time when clients may experience unexpected problems. These sessions allow discussion of problems as they occur.

Additionally, lactation consultants may offer individual sessions to address learning on a one-to-one basis. They are available to address less common situations, such as induced lactation in the absence of pregnancy or chest feeding when a transgender man carries and births his own baby.

Classes for Partners

Classes for partners often focus on the supportive role in pregnancy, birth, and parenting. They provide an opportunity for partners to meet other people and ask questions they might not ask in classes which include expectant clients. Some involve practicing infant care techniques with dolls. Classes are often taught by nurses who are experienced partners, or new partners are invited to come and share their experiences.

Classes for Siblings

Sibling classes are usually for children aged 3 to 12 years. The classes teach them about newborn characteristics and help decrease anxiety about the approaching birth (Fig. 7.5).

Many young children have never seen a newborn and are expecting a child near their own age who can be a playmate. A visit with a newborn infant allows them to see newborns at close range and learn to be safe helpers. Videos and stories promote discussion about normal feelings of jealousy and

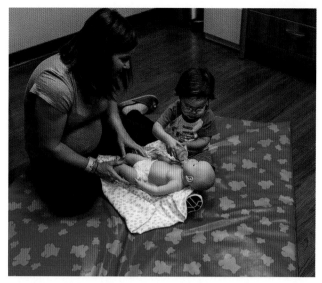

Fig. 7.5 During sibling classes, children learn about the new babies coming into their lives.

BOX 7.7   Topics Included in Parenting and Infant Care Classes

Normal newborn appearance: marks, rashes, normal behavior
General care: diapering, cord care, circumcision care, bathing
Behavior cues
Feeding methods and problems, schedules, colic
Other concerns: crying, comforting techniques, sleeping
    through the night
Safety: car seats, positioning for sleep, "baby-proofing" the
    home
Baby equipment
Early growth and development: expectations, infant stimula-
    tion, immunization
Illness: signs of common conditions, taking a temperature,
    calling the physician
Infant cardiopulmonary resuscitation
Family and relationship changes

anger. Emphasis is placed on the important role of being the older sibling and explaining the new baby could not replace them in their parents' affection.

A separate parent discussion may provide suggestions for further preparation and ways to cope with the transition after birth. Concerns about sibling rivalry and meeting the needs of more than one child are common topics.

Special sibling classes may be held for children who will be present at the birth. These classes help prepare the child for the sights and sounds of birth. The child's support person also attends the class.

Parenting and Infant Care Classes

Content for parenting classes typically includes information parents need during the early weeks after the birth (Box 7.7). Baby equipment such as infant car seats is often displayed. Practice with dolls may be included. Classes may continue after the birth of the infant.

Postpartum Classes

Although the postpartum period is discussed briefly in prepared childbirth classes, in some areas the client also can attend classes after birth. Content frequently focuses on exercise and nutrition but may also include the physiologic and psychological changes of the postpartum period, role transition, and sexuality. Signs of postpartum depression may be discussed, with emphasis on when the individual should seek help. Some classes are informal support groups led by a knowledgeable professional.

SUMMARY CONCEPTS

- The preconception, interconception, or initial prenatal visit includes a complete history and physical examination to determine potential risks to the client and fetus and obtain baseline data for a plan of care.
- Assessment of risk for problems is performed at each prenatal visit because pregnancies considered low risk in early pregnancy may later become high risk.
- Multifetal pregnancies impose greater physiologic changes than a single-fetus pregnancy and require extra vigilance to detect possible complications.
- Families need information related to self-care, health promotion, and coping with the common discomforts of pregnancy.
- Nurses use the nursing process and critical-thinking skills to assist the parents to make necessary changes in lifestyle.

- Education for childbearing helps couples become knowledgeable consumers and active participants in pregnancy and childbirth.
- Many classes are available for pregnant clients and their support persons. Preconception and early pregnancy classes emphasize ways to have a healthy pregnancy. Classes conducted in later pregnancy focus on preparation for childbirth, breastfeeding, and early parenting.
- Classes for partners and siblings help all family members prepare for the birth.
- Education, relaxation, breathing, and conditioning are used to increase coping ability for childbirth.
- Having a labor partner or support person increases a client's satisfaction with childbirth.

Clinical Judgment and Next-Generation NCLEX® Examination-Style Questions

A 33-year-old pregnant client presents to the New OB clinic for an initial prenatal visit. The nurse completes the assessments and the electronic medical record with the following data:

Past medical history:
- No known drug allergies
- + Chronic hypertension diagnosed 2 years ago; managed with losartan
- No other chronic medical conditions

Family history:
- + for hypertension, type II diabetes, heart disease

Obstetrical history:
- LMP: 8/12/2022; menstrual cycle regular, 28–32 days long
- Past pregnancies:

Date of birth	Gestational Age at Birth (wk)	Sex	Type of Birth	Singleton/ Multiple Birth	Complications	Currently Living?
9/6/2013	41	M	Spont Vag	Single	None	Yes
6/24/2015	40	F	Spont Vag	Single	None	Yes
7/14/2017	8	?	Vag	?	Spont Abortion	No
5/25/2018	29	M	C/S	Monozygotic twin	Preterm birth	Yes
5/25/2018	29	M	C/S	Monozygotic twin	Preterm birth	No; died at 2 wks age

Laboratory Results

Blood type: O
D(Rh) type: Neg
Antibody screen: Neg
Hct/Hgb: 34/12
Rubella: Nonimmune
VDRL: Nonreactive
Chlamydia: Neg

Current Complaints

Client complains of nausea and morning sickness.

1. **Choose the best option for the information missing from the statement below by selecting from the options provided.**
   The client is a gravida __**1**__, para __**2**__. The number of term births is __**3**__, the number of preterm births is __**4**__, the number of abortions is __**5**__, and the number of living children is __**6**__. The estimated due date for this pregnancy is __**7**__.

Options for 1 and 2	Options for 3 and 4	Options for 5 and 6	Options for 7
2	1	1	Dec. 12, 2022
3	2	2	May 5, 2023
4	3	3	May 19, 2023
5	4	4	Oct. 12, 2023
6	5	5	Nov. 5, 2023
7	6	6	Nov. 19, 2023

2. **Which of the lab values require further action by the nurse? Choose all that apply.**
   A. Blood type: O
   B. D(Rh) type: Neg
   C. Antibody screen: Neg
   D. Hct/Hgb: 34/12
   E. Rubella: nonimmune
   F. VDRL: Nonreactive
   G. Chlamydia: Neg

3. **Which of the following relief measures should the nurse suggest for the client's complaint of nausea and morning sickness? Choose all that apply.**
   A. Eat a dry carbohydrate such as crackers before getting out of bed in the morning, then arise slowly.
   B. Take prenatal vitamins first thing in the morning.
   C. Avoid an empty or overdistended stomach by eating several small meals during the day.
   D. Eat a high-fat diet and limit carbohydrates.
   E. Use an acupressure band on the wrist.
   F. Drink peppermint or ginger tea.
   G. Drink at least 8 oz of water with every meal.

REFERENCES & READINGS

Adams, E. D. (2021). Antenatal care. In K. Simpson, P. Creehan, N. O'Brien-Abel, C. Roth, & A. Rohan (Eds.), *AWHONN's perinatal nursing* (5th ed., pp. 18–47). Wolters Kluwer.

American Academy of Pediatrics. (2017). *The dangers of secondhand smoke.* http://www.healthychildren.org/english/health-issues/conditions/tobacco/pages/dangers-of-secondhand-smoke.aspx.

American Academy of Pediatrics & American College of Obstetricians and Gynecologists. (2017). In *Guidelines for perinatal care* (8th ed.).

American College of Obstetricians and Gynecologists (ACOG) & Society for Maternal-Fetal Medicine. (2021). *ACOG and SMFM recommend COVID-19 vaccination for pregnant individuals.* https://www.acog.org/news/news-releases/2021/07/acog-smfm-recommend-covid-19-vaccination-for-pregnant-individuals.

American College of Obstetricians and Gynecologists. (2021). *Influenza vaccination during pregnancy.* Committee Opinion, 732. published 2018; reaffirmed 2021.

American College of Obstetricians and Gynecologists (ACOG). (2018a). *Air travel during pregnancy.* ACOG Committee Opinion, 746.

American College of Obstetricians and Gynecologists (ACOG). (2018b). *Gestational diabetes mellitus.* Practice Bulletin, 190.

American College of Obstetricians and Gynecologists (ACOG). (2018c). *Nausea and vomiting of pregnancy.* ACOG Practice Bulletin, 189.

American College of Obstetricians and Gynecologists (ACOG). (2018d). *Screening for perinatal depression.* ACOG Committee Opinion, 757.

American College of Obstetricians and Gynecologists (ACOG). (2019). *Group prenatal care.* ACOG Committee Opinion, 731.

American College of Obstetricians and Gynecologists (ACOG). (2020a). *Physical activity and exercise during pregnancy and the postpartum period.* ACOG Committee Opinion, 804. published 2015, reaffirmed 2020.

American College of Obstetricians and Gynecologists (ACOG). (2020b). *Tobacco and nicotine cessation during pregnancy.* ACOG Committee Opinion, 807.

American College of Obstetricians and Gynecologists (ACOG). (2020c). *Weight gain during pregnancy.* ACOG Committee Opinion, 548. published 2013, reaffirmed 2020.

Antony, K. M., Racusin, D. A., Aagaard, K., & Dildy, G. A. (2021). Maternal physiology. In S. Gabbe, J. Niebyl, J. Simpson, M. Landon, H. Galan, R. Jauniaux, et al. (Eds.), *Obstetrics: Normal and problem pregnancies* (8th ed., pp. 43–67). Elsevier.

Berger, D. S., & West, E. H. (2021). Nutrition during pregnancy. In S. Gabbe, J. Niebyl, J. Simpson, M. Landon, H. Galan, R. Jauniaux, et al. (Eds.), *Obstetrics: Normal and problem pregnancies* (8th ed., pp. 108–121). Elsevier.

Blackburn, S. T. (2018). In *Maternal, fetal, and neonatal physiology: A clinical perspective* (5th ed.). Elsevier.

Bowers, N. A. (2021). Multiple gestation. In K. Simpson, P. Creehan, N. O'Brien-Abel, C. Roth, & A. Rohan (Eds.), *AWHONN's perinatal nursing* (5th ed., pp. 249–295). Wolters Kluwer.

Casanova, R., Chuang, A., Goepfert, A. R., et al. (2019). In *Beckmann and Ling's obstetrics and gynecology* (8th ed.). Lippincott Williams & Wilkins.

Centers for Disease Control and Prevention. (2019). *Guidelines for vaccinating pregnant women.* http://www.cdc.gov.

Centers for Disease Control and Prevention. (2020). *Research on medicines and pregnancy.* http://www.cdc.gov/pregnancy/meds/treatingfortwo/research.html.

Cunningham, F. G., Leveno, K. J., Bloom, S. L., et al. (2022). In *Williams obstetrics* (26th ed.). McGraw-Hill.

Drake, P., Driscoll, A. K., & Mathews, T. J. (2018). Cigarette smoking prevalence during pregnancy: Data from the birth certificate, 2016. *National Vital Statistics Reports*, 65(1).

Gregory, K. D., Ramos, D. E., & Jauniaux, E. R. M. (2021). Preconception and prenatal care. In S. Gabbe, J. Niebyl, J. Simpson, M. Landon, H. Galan, R. Jauniaux, et al. (Eds.), *Obstetrics: Normal and problem pregnancies* (8th ed., pp. 88–107). Elsevier.

Kelly, T. F., & Savides, T. J. (2019). Gastrointestinal disease in pregnancy. In R. Resnik, C. Lockwood, T. Moore, M. Greene, J. Copel, & R. Silver (Eds.), *Creasy & Resnik's maternal-fetal medicine: Principles and practice* (8th ed., pp. 1158–1172.e4). Elsevier.

Martin, J. A., Hamilton, B. E., Osterman, M. J. K., & Driscoll, A. K. (2021). Births: Final data for 2019. *National Vital Statistics Reports*, 68(13). http://www.cdc.gov/nchs/products/index.htm.

Samet, J. M., & Sockrider, M. (2021). *Secondhand smoke exposure: Effects in children.* http://www.uptodate.com.

Smith, L. J., King, T. L., & Jevitt, C. M. (2019). Breastfeeding and the mother-newborn dyad. In T. King, M. Brucker, J. Kriebs, J. Fahey, C. Gegor, & H. Varney (Eds.), *Varney's midwifery* (6th ed., pp. 1233–1268). Jones & Bartlett Learning.

U.S. Department of Health and Human Services. (2020). *Healthy people 2030.* https://health.gov/healthypeople/objectives-and-data/browse-objectives/pregnancy-and-childbirth.

U.S. Preventive Services Task Force. (2017). *Folic acid for the prevention of neural tube defects: U.S. Preventive services task force final recommendation statement.* https://www.uspreventiveservicestaskforce.org/.

Nutrition for Childbearing

Nan Ketcham, Heather S. Hendrikson

At no other point in a client's life is nutrition as important as it is during pregnancy and lactation. At this time, clients must nourish not only themselves but also the baby. Nutrition may affect the size of the fetus and determine whether it has adequate stores of some nutrients after birth. If clients fail to consume sufficient nutrients during pregnancy, their own stores of some nutrients may be depleted to meet the needs of the fetus, who also may be deprived of essential nutrients.

Nurses interact with pregnant clients and can provide education about nutrition on a continuing basis. This is especially important because many clients do not understand the nutritional needs of pregnancy. Nurses may provide nutrition counseling before conception to clients who are considering becoming pregnant. Such counseling increases the chances a client will be nutritionally healthy at the time of conception and will continue to practice good nutrition throughout pregnancy. It also may increase the level of nutrition the parent provides for the entire family. Therefore, nutritional education is an essential part of nursing care.

WEIGHT GAIN DURING PREGNANCY

Weight gain during pregnancy can affect the health of both the client and the child. Insufficient weight gain during pregnancy has been associated with preterm birth and decreased birth weight leading to small-for-gestational-age (SGA) infants (Bodner & Himes, 2019; Goldstein et al., 2017). Low weight gain in the second trimester is especially associated with poor infant birth weight, even if overall gain is within the recommended range (Grodner et al., 2020). Approximately 21% of clients gain less than the recommended amount during pregnancy (Centers for Disease Control and Prevention [CDC], 2021b). Lower caloric intake and decreased intake of important nutrients are more likely present when poor maternal weight gain occurs.

Excessive weight gain is also an issue. It is associated with increased birth weight leading to large-for-gestational-age (LGA) infants, macrosomia, and later obesity for the infant while increasing maternal preeclampsia, gestational diabetes, cesarean delivery, and postpartum weight retention risks (Goldstein et al., 2017). Approximately 48% of clients gain more than the recommended amount during pregnancy (CDC, 2021b). The nutrient intake is even more important than the weight gain itself. Weight gain from a diet lacking in essential nutrients is not as beneficial as weight gain from a balanced diet. It could be inadequate in nutrients such as protein, iron, or folic acid, which could cause anemia, neural tube defects, or inadequate fetal nutrient stores.

Recommendations for Total Weight Gain

Recommendations for weight gain during pregnancy have changed and continue to evolve in an effort to improve maternal and infant outcomes. There are multiple factors to take into consideration when determining weight gain adequacy for individual clients.

Weight gain recommendations are based on the client's prepregnancy body mass index (BMI). BMI is calculated by dividing the weight in kilograms by the height in meters squared. Another method is to divide the weight in pounds by the height in inches squared and multiply the result by 703 (CDC, 2021a). For example, if a client weighs 56 kg (124 lb) before pregnancy and is 163 cm (64 inches) tall, the BMI is 21, which shows normal weight for height. A calculator to measure BMI is available at https://www.nhlbi.nih.gov/health/educational/lose_wt/BMI/bmicalc.htm.

Recommendations vary according to the client's BMI before pregnancy (Table 8.1). The recommended weight gain

TABLE 8.1 Recommended Weight Gain during Pregnancy

Weight before Pregnancy	Total Gain	Range and Mean of Weekly Gain (Second and Third Trimesters)
Underweight (BMI <18.5)	12.5–18 kg (28–40 lb)	Range: 0.44–0.58 kg (1–1.3 lb) Mean: 0.51 kg (1 lb)
Normal weight (BMI 18.5–24.9)	11.5–16 kg (25–35 lb)	Range: 0.35–0.5 kg (0.8–1 lb) Mean: 0.42 kg (1 lb)
Overweight (BMI 25–29.9)	7–11.5 kg (15–25 lb)	Range: 0.23–0.33 kg (0.5–0.7 lb) Mean: 0.28 kg (0.6 lb)
Obese (BMI ≥30)	5–9 kg (11–20 lb)	Range: 0.17–0.27 kg (0.4–0.6 lb) Mean: 0.22 kg (0.5 lb)

BMI, Body mass index.
Note: Weight gain during the first trimester should be 0.5 to 2 kg (1.1 to 4.4 lb).
From American College of Obstetricians and Gynecologists (ACOG). (2020b). Weight gain during pregnancy. *ACOG Committee Opinion 548.* Published 2013, reaffirmed 2020. American College of Obstetricians and Gynecologists (ACOG). (2021). Obesity in pregnancy. *ACOG Practice Bulletin 230.* Published 2015, reaffirmed 2021.

during pregnancy is 11.5 to 16 kg (25 to 35 lb) for clients who begin pregnancy at normal BMI (American College of Obstetricians and Gynecologists [ACOG], 2020b; Institute of Medicine [IOM], 2009). The range allows for individual differences because no precise weight gain is appropriate for everyone. It provides a target and allows for variations in individual needs. Of note, approximately one-third (32%) gain adequate weight during pregnancy with the rest exceeding or not meeting weight gain goals (CDC, 2021b).

Low prepregnancy weight is associated with preterm labor, SGA, and increased perinatal mortality (Cunningham et al., 2022). Clients who are underweight should gain more to meet the needs of pregnancy as well as their own need to gain weight. They should gain 12.5 to 18 kg (28 to 40 lb).

Obesity is an increasing problem with over half of pregnant clients in the United States being overweight or obese (Agency for Healthcare Research and Quality [AHRQ], 2018; Martin et al., 2021). Obese clients have more challenges getting pregnant and are at higher risk for early and recurrent pregnancy loss, still birth, preterm delivery, birth defects, macrosomia, gestational diabetes, hypertension, preeclampsia, induction of labor, failed induction of labor, cesarean birth, maternal death, postpartum hemorrhage, wound complications, thromboembolic disorders, and other postpartum complications (Cunningham et al., 2022). Their children have an increased risk for childhood obesity. Overweight and obese clients should be advised to lose weight before conception to achieve the best pregnancy outcomes. Weight loss is not generally recommended during pregnancy.

The current recommended total weight gain for overweight clients is 6.8 to 11.3 kg (15 to 25 lb). Although, studies show overweight clients who gained 2.7 to 6.4 kg (6 to 14 lb) had similar fetal growth, perinatal and neonatal outcomes, and less postpartum weight retention as overweight clients

who gained weight within the current recommended range. For an overweight client who is not gaining weight within the recommended range but has adequate fetal growth, the evidence does not support encouraging weight gain just to meet the recommended goal (ACOG, 2020b).

The weight gain for obese clients is 5 to 9.1 kg (11 to 20 lb). Obesity is defined as a BMI of 30 or greater, but there are three classes of obesity. Class I obesity (BMI of 30 to 34.9), class II obesity (BMI of 35 to 39.9) and class III obesity (BMI of 30 to 34.9) are not individually addressed with different weight gain targets. Due to limited data, current guidelines for obese clients do not suggest lower weight gains for more severe degrees of obesity. Clients with an obese BMI are noted to be similar to those with an overweight BMI. If weight gain is below the target and fetal growth is appropriate, it is not suggested to encourage weight gain just to meet the goal (ACOG, 2020b).

Adolescents (less than 20 years of age) should gain weight according to their prepregnancy BMI using adult rather than pediatric BMI categories. Using adult BMI classifications may place adolescents in a lighter group who have historically been advised to gain more weight to improve birth outcomes (IOM, 2009). Studies are ongoing to determine the best criteria for prepregnancy BMI classification in adolescents. Inappropriate weight gain in teens, like adults, is directly correlated to negative maternal and neonatal outcomes such as preterm delivery, SGA, or LGA (Sámano et al., 2018).

Another consideration is the client who is pregnant with more than one fetus. Infants of a multifetal pregnancy are often born before term and tend to weigh less than those born of single pregnancies. Clients with greater weight gain may help prevent low birth weight (CDC, 2021b). The recommended gain for clients of normal prepregnancy weight who are carrying twins is 16.8 to 24.5 kg (37 to 54 lb); overweight, 14.1 to 22.7 kg (31 to 50 lb); and obese, 11.3 to 19.1 kg (25 to 42 lb) at term. There is insufficient data to determine the weight gain range for underweight clients or multifetal pregnancies with triplets or higher (ACOG, 2020b; IOM, 2009).

Pattern of Weight Gain

The pattern of weight gain is as important as the total increase in weight. Early and adequate prenatal care allows assessment of weight gain on a regular basis throughout pregnancy. The general recommendation is approximately 0.5 to 2 kg (1.1 to 4.4 lb) during the first trimester, when the client may be nauseated and the fetus needs few nutrients for growth. During the rest of the pregnancy, the weekly expected weight gain for various prepregnancy weights is shown in Table 8.1. Pregnancy weight gain trackers, similar to growth charts, can help clients and providers visually follow the weight gain week to week.

Maternal and Fetal Weight Distribution

Clients often wonder why they should gain so much weight when the fetus weighs only 3.2 to 3.6 kg (7 to 8 lb). The nurse should explain the distribution of weight to help them understand this need. The bulk of maternal weight gain is attributed to amniotic fluid, placenta, increased breast tissue, uterine tissue, body fluids, blood volume, and stores of fat, protein, and other nutrients.

Factors Influencing Weight Gain

The nurse can positively influence the expectant client's weight gain by teaching how the diet affects fetal growth. A discussion of the effects of maternal intake on fetal growth and storage of nutrients often motivates clients to improve their nutrition. Knowledge of factors that may negatively influence nutrient intake and weight gain helps the nurse devise plans for improving nutrition.

> ### KNOWLEDGE CHECK
> 1. How does weight gain during pregnancy relate to the birth weight of the infant?
> 2. How much weight should the average client gain during pregnancy? What factors might change this?
> 3. What pattern of weight gain is recommended for the average client?

NUTRITIONAL REQUIREMENTS

Nutrient needs increase during pregnancy to meet the demands of the client and fetus. The amount of increase for each nutrient varies. In most cases, the increases are not large and are relatively easy to obtain through the diet.

Dietary Reference Intakes

In the United States **dietary reference intakes** (DRIs) are used to estimate nutrient needs. DRIs include the following four categories:

- Recommended dietary allowance (RDA)—The amount of a nutrient sufficient to meet the needs of almost all (97% to 98%) healthy people in a life stage group. The actual needs of individuals (particularly for calories and protein) may vary according to body size, previous nutritional status, and usual activity level.
- Adequate intake (AI)—The nutrient intake assumed to be adequate when an RDA cannot be determined.
- Tolerable upper intake level (UL)—The highest amount of a nutrient taken by most people without probable adverse health effects.
- Estimated average requirement (EAR)—The amount of a nutrient estimated to meet the needs of half the healthy people in life stage group.

Tables of recommendations are based on a reference individual, a hypothetical person of medium size. These tables are used to calculate nutrient needs based on age, gender, and life stage. Recommendations for energy, carbohydrate, and protein intakes are shown in Table 8.2. Recommendations for vitamin and mineral intake and food sources are shown in Table 8.3.

Energy

The energy provided by foods for body processes is calculated in kilocalories. **Kilocalories** (commonly called *calories* [the

term used in this book]) refers to a unit of heat and is used to show the energy value in foods. Calories are obtained from carbohydrates and proteins, which provide four calories in each gram, and fats, which provide nine calories in each gram.

Carbohydrates

Carbohydrates may be simple or complex. The most common simple carbohydrate is sucrose (table sugar), which is a source of energy but provides no other nutrients. Fruits and vegetables contain simple sugars along with other nutrients. Complex carbohydrates are present in starches such as cereal, pasta, and potatoes. They supply vitamins, minerals, and fiber. They should be the major source of carbohydrates in the diet because of their value in providing other nutrients.

Another type of carbohydrate is fiber, the nondigestible product of plant foods and an important source of bulk in the diet. Fiber absorbs water and stimulates peristalsis, causing food to pass more quickly through the intestines. Fiber helps prevent constipation and also slows gastric emptying, causing a sensation of fullness.

Fats

Fats provide energy and fat-soluble vitamins. When decreasing calories is necessary, a reduction, but not elimination, of carbohydrates and fats is important. If carbohydrate and fat intake provides insufficient calories, the body uses protein to meet energy needs. This use decreases the amount of protein available for building and repairing tissue.

Clients often restrict fat to prevent weight gain. However, essential fatty acids such as alpha-linolenic acid and linoleic acid help in fetal neurologic and visual development. Docosahexaenoic acid (DHA) is also important for fetal visual and cognitive development. These fatty acids are found in canola oil, soybean oil, and walnuts, as well as some seafood such as sea bass or salmon.

Calories

Approximately 80,000 additional calories are needed during pregnancy. These extra calories furnish energy for production and maintenance of the fetus, placenta, added maternal tissues, and increased basal metabolic rate. Most pregnant clients need a daily caloric intake of 2200 to 2900 calories, depending on their age, activity level, and prepregnancy BMI (American Academy of Pediatrics [AAP] & ACOG, 2017; CDC, 2021a; Cunningham et al., 2022).

During the first trimester of pregnancy, no added calories are needed. However, the daily caloric intake for pregnancy should increase by 340 calories during the second trimester and 452 calories during the third trimester (ACOG, 2020b; Cunningham et al., 2022; IOM, 2006). This increase can be achieved relatively easily with a variety of foods to assist in meeting specific nutrient needs and only a small increase in total food intake. As noted in Table 8.4, to meet the increased calorie needs of the second and third trimesters, a pregnant client could add one healthy snack per day to their current diet.

TABLE 8.2   Recommendations for Daily Energy, Carbohydrate, and Protein Intakes for Clients Aged 14 to 50 Years

Nonpregnant Adult Female	Pregnancy	Lactation
Energy Varies greatly according to body size, age, and physical activity level *Example:* Client, 30 years, active, height 1.65 m (65 inches), weight 50.4 kg (111 lb), body mass index (BMI) 18.5 needs 2267 kcal Same client, weight 68 kg (150 lb), BMI 24.99 needs 2477 kcal	First trimester: No change from nonpregnant needs Second trimester: 340 kcal above nonpregnant needs Third trimester: 452 kcal above nonpregnant needs	First 6 months: 330 kcal above nonpregnant needs (with an additional 170 kcal drawn from maternal stores) Second 6 months: 400 kcal above nonpregnant needs
Carbohydrate 130 g	175 g	210 g
Protein 46 g	71 g	71 g

Data from Institute of Medicine (IOM), Food and Nutrition Board (FNB). (2005). Dietary reference intakes for energy, carbohydrate, fiber, fat, fatty acids, cholesterol, protein, and amino acids (macronutrients). *The National Academies Press.*

TABLE 8.3   Recommendations for Vitamins and Minerals

Adult Females: Nonpregnant	Pregnancy and Lactation	Sources	Importance in Pregnancy
Vitamins **Vitamin A** Ages 14–50: 700 mcg (RDA)*	*Pregnancy:* Ages 14–18: 750 mcg Ages 19–50: 770 mcg *Lactation:* Ages 14–18: 1200 mcg Ages 19–50: 1300 mcg	Dark green, yellow, or orange vegetables; whole or fortified low-fat or nonfat milk; egg yolk; butter and fortified margarine	Fetal growth and cell differentiation. Excessive intake causes spontaneous abortions or serious fetal defects. Isotretinoin (Accutane), a vitamin A derivative for acne, should not be taken during pregnancy because it causes fetal defects.
Vitamin D Ages 14–50: 600 IU (15 mcg) (RDA)	*Pregnancy and lactation:* Ages 14–50: 600 IU (15 mcg) (RDA)	Fortified milk, margarine, and soy products; butter; egg yolks Synthesized in skin exposed to sunlight Vegans and those who are not exposed to sun and who do not eat fortified foods need supplements.	Necessary for metabolism of calcium. Inadequate amounts may cause neonatal hypocalcemia and hypoplasia of tooth enamel. Excessive intake causes hypercalcemia and possible fetal deformities. Supplements should be taken with caution.
Vitamin E Ages 14–50: 15 mg (RDA)	*Pregnancy:* Ages 14–50: 15 mg *Lactation:* Ages 14–50: 19 mg (RDA)	Vegetable oils, whole grains, nuts, dark green leafy vegetables	Rarely deficient in pregnant clients, but deficiency can cause anemia in mother and fetus.
Vitamin K Ages 14–18: 75 mcg Ages 19–50: 90 mcg (AI)	*Pregnancy and lactation:* Ages 14–18: 75 mcg Ages 19–50: 90 mcg (AI)	Dark green leafy vegetables Also produced by normal bacterial flora in small intestine	Newborns are temporarily deficient and receive one dose by injection at birth to prevent hemorrhage.

Continued

TABLE 8.3 Recommendations for Vitamins and Minerals—cont'd

Adult Females: Nonpregnant	Pregnancy and Lactation	Sources	Importance in Pregnancy
Vitamin B₆ (Pyridoxine) Ages 14–18: 1.2 mg Ages 19–50: 1.3 mg (RDA)	*Pregnancy:* Ages 14–50: 1.9 mg *Lactation:* Ages 14–50: 2 mg (RDA)	Chicken, fish, pork, eggs, peanuts, whole grains, cereals	Increased metabolism of amino acids during pregnancy.
Vitamin B₁₂ Ages 14–50: 2.4 mcg (RDA)	*Pregnancy:* Ages 14–50: 2.6 mcg *Lactation:* Ages 14–50: 2.8 mcg (RDA)	Meat, fish, eggs, milk, fortified soy and cereal products	Cell division, increased formation of red blood cells (RBCs), and protein synthesis.
Folic Acid Ages 14–50: 400 mcg (RDA)	*Pregnancy:* Ages 14–50: 600 mcg *Lactation:* Ages 14–50: 500 mcg (RDA)	Dark green leafy vegetables, legumes (beans, peanuts), orange juice, asparagus, spinach, and fortified cereal and pasta May be lost in cooking	Increased maternal RBC formation, tissue growth. Deficiency in first weeks of pregnancy may cause spontaneous abortion and neural tube defects.
Thiamin Ages 14–18: 1 mg Ages 19–50: 1.1 mg (RDA)	*Pregnancy and lactation:* Ages 14–50: 1.4 mg (RDA)	Lean pork, whole or enriched grain products, legumes, organ meats, seeds, nuts	Forms coenzymes necessary to release energy, aids in nerve and muscle functioning. Increased need because of greater intake of calories.
Riboflavin Ages 14–18: 1 mg Ages 19–50: 1.1 mg (RDA)	*Pregnancy:* Ages 14–50: 1.4 mg *Lactation:* Ages 14–50: 1.6 mg (RDA)	Milk, meat, fish, poultry, eggs, enriched grain products, dark green vegetables	Forms coenzymes necessary to release energy, aids in nerve and muscle functioning. Increased need because of greater intake of calories.
Niacin Ages 14–50: 14 mg (RDA)	*Pregnancy:* Ages 14–50: 18 mg *Lactation:* Ages 14–50: 17 mg (RDA)	Meats, fish, poultry, legumes, enriched grains, milk	Forms coenzymes necessary to release energy, aids in nerve and muscle functioning. Increased need because of greater intake of calories.
Vitamin C Ages 14–18: 65 mg Ages 19–50: 75 mg (RDA)	*Pregnancy:* Ages 14–18: 80 mg Ages 19–50: 85 mg *Lactation:* Ages 14–18: 115 mg Ages 19–50: 120 mg (RDA)	Citrus fruit, peppers, strawberries, cantaloupe, green leafy vegetables, tomatoes, potatoes Destroyed by heat and oxidation	Formation of fetal tissue, collagen formation, tissue integrity, healing, immune response, and metabolism.
Choline Ages 14–18: 400 mg Ages 19–50: 425 mg	*Pregnancy:* Ages 14–50: 450 mg *Lactation:* Ages 14–50: 550 mg	Eggs, meats, seafood, nuts, beans, lentils, peas	Membrane biosynthesis, tissue expansion, neurotransmission and brain development, gene expression

TABLE 8.3   Recommendations for Vitamins and Minerals—cont'd

Adult Females: Nonpregnant	Pregnancy and Lactation	Sources	Importance in Pregnancy
Minerals			
Iron Ages 14–18: 15 mg Ages 19–50: 18 mg (RDA)	*Pregnancy:* Ages 14–50: 27 mg *Lactation:* Ages 14–18: 10 mg Ages 19–50: 9 mg (RDA)	Meats, dark green leafy vegetables, enriched bread and cereal, dried fruits, tofu, legumes, nuts, blackstrap molasses	Expanded maternal blood volume, formation of fetal RBCs, and storage in fetal liver for use after birth.
Calcium Ages 14–18: 1300 mg Ages 19–50: 1000 mg (AI)	*Pregnancy and lactation:* Ages 14–18: 1300 mg Ages 19–50: 1000 mg (AI)	Dairy products, salmon, sardines with bones, legumes, fortified juice, tofu, broccoli	Mineralization of fetal bones and teeth.
Phosphorus Ages 14–18: 1250 mg Ages 19–50: 700 mg (RDA)	*Pregnancy and lactation:* Ages 14–18: 1250 mg Ages 19–50: 700 mg	Dairy products, lean meat, fish, poultry, cereals; high in processed foods, snacks, carbonated drinks	Mineralization of fetal bones and teeth; excessive intake causes binding of calcium in intestines and prevents calcium absorption.
Zinc Ages 14–18: 9 mg Ages 19–50: 8 mg (RDA)	*Pregnancy:* Ages 14–18: 12 mg Ages 19–50: 11 mg *Lactation:* Ages 14–18: 13 mg Ages 19–50: 12 mg (RDA)	Meat, poultry, seafood, eggs, nuts, seeds, legumes, wheat germ, whole grains, yogurt	Fetal and maternal tissue growth, cell differentiation and reproduction, DNA and RNA synthesis, metabolism, acid-base balance.
Magnesium Ages 14–18: 360 mg Ages 19–30: 310 mg Ages 31–50: 320 mg (RDA)	*Pregnancy:* Ages 14–18: 400 mg Ages 19–30: 350 mg Ages 31–50: 360 mg *Lactation:* Ages 14–18: 360 mg Ages 19–30: 310 mg Ages 31–50: 320 mg (RDA)	Whole grains, nuts, legumes, dark green vegetables, small amounts in many foods	Cell growth and neuromuscular function; activates enzymes for metabolism of protein and energy.
Iodine Ages 14–50: 150 mcg (RDA)	*Pregnancy:* Ages 14–50: 220 mcg *Lactation:* Ages 14–50: 290 mcg (RDA)	Seafood, iodized salt	Important in thyroid function. Deficiency may cause abortion, stillbirth, congenital hypothyroidism, neurologic conditions.

DNA, Deoxyribonucleic acid; *RNA*, ribonucleic acid.

*Dietary reference intakes are listed as recommended dietary allowance (RDA) or adequate intake (AI).

Data from Institute of Medicine (IOM), Food and Nutrition Board (FNB). (1997). Dietary reference intakes for calcium, phosphorus, magnesium, vitamin D, and fluoride. *The National Academies Press*; IOM, FNB. (1998). Dietary reference intakes for thiamin, riboflavin, niacin, vitamin B$_6$, folate, vitamin B$_{12}$, pantothenic acid, biotin, and choline. *The National Academies Press*; IOM, FNB. (2000). Dietary reference intakes for vitamin C, vitamin E, selenium, and carotenoids. *The National Academies Press*; IOM, FNB. (2001). Dietary reference intakes for vitamin A, vitamin K, arsenic, boron, chromium, copper, iodine, iron, manganese, molybdenum, nickel, silicon, vanadium, and zinc. The National Academies Press; IOM (2011). Dietary reference intakes for calcium and vitamin D. *The National Academies Press*.

Nutrient Density. The quantity and quality of the various nutrients in each 100 calories of food is the **nutrient density**. Foods of high nutrient density have large amounts of quality nutrients per serving. During pregnancy, the increased need for most nutrients may not be met unless calories are selected carefully. The term *empty calories* refers to foods high in calories but low in other nutrients. Many snack foods contain excessive calories and low nutrient density and are high in fat, sodium, and added sugar. Increased calories should be "spent" on foods that provide the nutrients needed in increased amounts during pregnancy.

TABLE 8.4	Extra Foods Needed to Meet Pregnancy Requirements*
Energy (kcal)	1 slice whole wheat bread, 1 T peanut butter, ½ banana, *and* ½ c low-fat milk in second trimester; add 1 oz cheddar cheese and 1–2 carrots in third trimester
Protein	3 oz meat or poultry *or* 3 c milk *or* 3½ oz cheddar cheese *or* 1 c cottage cheese *or* 3¾ oz peanuts *or* 1⅔ c pinto or kidney beans
Iron	1 c raisin bran, *or* 1 c beef chuck + 1 c pinto beans, + 3 eggs
Thiamin	1½ oz pork *or* 2½ oz peanuts *or* 1⅔ c brown rice *or* 1½ c orange juice
Riboflavin	¾ c low-fat milk *or* ¾ c low-fat cottage cheese *or* ¾ c cooked spinach *or* 2 chicken drumsticks *or* 4 oz lean beef
Niacin	2 T peanut butter *or* 3 oz ground beef *or* 1½ oz salmon; also made by body from tryptophan
Vitamin C	2 T orange juice *or* 1½ peaches *or* 1 banana *or* 1½ pear *or* 1 c watermelon *or* ¼ c tomato juice

c, Cup; *kcal*, calories; *oz*, ounce; *T*, tablespoon.
*Examples of foods that would meet the additional requirements of pregnancy for clients between the ages of 19 and 50 years.
Data from U.S. Department of Agriculture, Agricultural Research Service. (2016). U.S. Department of Agriculture, Agricultural Research Service, Nutrient Data Laboratory. *USDA National Nutrient Database for Standard Reference, Release 28*. Version Current: September 2015, slightly revised May 2016. https://data.nal.usda.gov/system/files/sr_28_doc.pdf

Clients often use sugar substitutes to reduce their caloric intake. Saccharin (Sweet'N Low), sucralose (Splenda), aspartame (Equal or NutraSweet), acesulfame potassium (Sweet One), neotame (Newtame), Advantame, luo han guo fruit extracts (monk fruit), and steviol glycosides (Stevia) are considered and approved as safe for use in moderation. Of note, people with phenylketonuria (PKU), a rare disease, have difficulty metabolizing phenylalanine, which is a component of aspartame, and should avoid intake. While these nonnutritive sweeteners are approved by the U.S. Food and Drug Administration (FDA), there is limited research that addresses the safety on healthy pregnancies (Procter & Campbell, 2014).

Protein

Protein is necessary for metabolism, tissue synthesis, and tissue repair. The daily protein from RDA is 46 g for females, depending on age and size. A protein intake of approximately 71 g each day is recommended during the second half of pregnancy because of expansion of blood volume and growth of maternal and fetal tissues (Grodner et al., 2020). This is an increase of 25 g of protein daily. Emerging data show there may be even higher protein needs in pregnancy and those needs increase over the course of pregnancy (National Academies of Sciences, Engineering, and Medicine [NASEM], 2020).

Protein is generally abundant in diets in most industrialized nations. Diets low in calories may also be low in protein.

If calories are low and protein is used to provide energy, fetal growth may be impaired.

The nurse should teach clients at risk for low-protein diets how to determine intake and increase food sources of protein. When clients need to increase intake, they should eat more protein-rich foods rather than use high-protein powders or drinks. Protein substitutes increase protein intake but do not have the other nutrients provided by foods.

Vitamins

Although most people do not eat as much of every vitamin and mineral each day as recommended, true deficiency for most nutrients are uncommon in North America.

Fat-Soluble Vitamins

Fat-soluble vitamins (A, D, E, and K) are stored in the liver, fat (adipose) tissue, and skeletal muscle. Deficiency is not as likely to occur, but excessive intake of these vitamins can be toxic. For example, too much vitamin A can cause fetal defects. The nurse should ask about vitamins and medications taken by pregnant clients and counsel them about the dangers of excess vitamins (see Table 8.3).

Water-Soluble Vitamins

Water-soluble vitamins (B_6, B_{12}, and C; folic acid; thiamin; riboflavin; and niacin) are not stored in the body as easily as fat-soluble vitamins. Therefore, they should be included in the daily diet. Because excess amounts are excreted in urine, the chances of toxicity from excessive intake are lower, but toxicity can occur with megadoses.

Water-soluble vitamins are easily transferred from food to water during cooking. Foods should be steamed, microwaved, or prepared in only small amounts of water. The remaining water can be used in other dishes such as soups.

Folic Acid

Folic acid (also called *folate*) can decrease the occurrence of neural tube defects such as spina bifida and anencephaly in infants. It also may help prevent cleft lip, cleft palate, and some heart defects (Cunningham et al., 2022). Adequate intake of folic acid is especially important before conception and during the first trimester because the neural tube closes before many clients realize they are pregnant. Because approximately half of pregnancies are unplanned, all clients of childbearing age should consume at least 400 micrograms (mcg) (0.4 milligram [mg]) of folic acid every day. Once pregnancy occurs, daily intake of 600 mcg (0.6 mg) of folic acid is recommended.

Although the CDC recommends a daily folic acid intake of 400 mcg (0.4 mg) for clients capable of childbearing (CDC, 2018), the U.S. Preventive Services Task Force (USPSTF) recommends 400 to 800 mcg (0.4 to 0.8 mg) each day. The dose should be taken for at least 1 month before conception and for 2 to 3 months after conception, then 600 mcg (0.6 mg) of folic acid daily for the rest of the pregnancy (USPSTF, 2017). For clients who have previously had a child with a neural tube defect, the recommended dose is 4 mg (4000 mcg) daily during the months before conception (CDC, 2018; Cunningham et al., 2022).

Clients often do not realize the importance of folic acid in their diet before pregnancy begins, and many do not meet the recommended level in spite of a national campaign to make the public aware of this problem. Inadequate intake of folic acid is the most prevalent vitamin deficiency during pregnancy. One-third of births occur in clients ages 18 to 24 years. This same age group has lower intake of supplements containing folic acid than older clients (CDC, 2018). More education is necessary to increase folic acid use in clients of childbearing age. Fortunately, since food fortification with folic acid was begun, folic acid deficiency has decreased.

A *Healthy People 2030* goal is to increase the proportion of clients of childbearing age who have optimal red blood cell folate concentrations by getting enough folic acid through food or supplements. The concentration of folate in a client's red blood cells shows whether there is an adequate amount of folic acid (U.S. Department of Health and Human Services [DHHS], 2020). To help achieve adequate intake in the United States and Canada, folic acid is added to breads, cereals, and other products containing enriched flour and, more recently, corn mesa products.

Choline

Choline is an organic, water-soluble compound, not a vitamin nor a mineral. It is often grouped with the water-soluble B vitamins because of its similarities. Choline requirements increase in pregnancy and lactation and is critical for placental function, epigenetic programming, and neurodevelopment, with the most notable attribute being on fetal brain and spinal cord development. Studies indicate supplementing the maternal diet with additional choline improves several pregnancy outcomes and protects against certain neural and metabolic insults.

Choline is found in both animal and plant food sources. Eggs, meats, and seafood are concentrated sources while nuts, legumes, and cruciferous vegetables (broccoli) are a fairly good source. Choline is found throughout many food groups and subgroups, but it is absent from most prenatal vitamins. Less than 10% of pregnant clients achieve target intake levels of choline. Encourage pregnant clients to obtain choline from food sources and, if supplementation is desired, to speak with their health care provider (Korsmo et al., 2019; U.S. Department of Agriculture [USDA] & DHHS, 2020; NASEM, 2020).

KNOWLEDGE CHECK

4. How many additional calories should a client consume each day during pregnancy?
5. How much protein is recommended during pregnancy?
6. Which vitamins are in the fat-soluble and water-soluble groups? What is the difference in the way the body stores them?
7. Why should all clients of childbearing age consume 400 mcg of folic acid daily?

Minerals

Although most minerals are supplied in sufficient amounts in normal diets, there is an increased need for several key minerals during pregnancy. The intake of these minerals may be inhibited by food choices, absorption, or intolerance.

Iron

Iron helps form some enzymes necessary for metabolism and is important in the formation of hemoglobin (Hgb). Hgb is an iron-rich protein inside of red blood cells (RBCs) giving them their red color. Hgb carries oxygen to the body and helps remove carbon dioxide. With a growing fetus and increased maternal blood supply, there is an increased demand for Hgb during pregnancy. The pregnant client needs 27 mg of iron daily (an increase from 18 mg for nonpregnant clients). The additional iron is needed to cover the increased production of RBCs and for transfer to the fetus. Fetal stores of iron, which double during the last weeks of pregnancy, are critical because the infant's intake of iron is low for the first 4 to 6 months after birth. Iron will be transferred to the fetus even if the client is anemic, but infants will have less stored iron and an increased risk for anemia during the first year (Blackburn, 2018).

Even though iron is better absorbed during pregnancy, it is probably the only nutrient that cannot be supplied completely and easily by the diet. Iron is present in many foods but in small amounts (Table 8.5). The average person's daily diet contains approximately 6 mg of iron for each 1000 calories. In addition, some clients restrict their intake of meats and grains in an effort to cut down on fat, carbohydrates, and calories. Menstrual bleeding causes loss of iron. Therefore, clients frequently enter pregnancy with low iron stores (Cunningham et al., 2022). A *Healthy People 2030* goal is to reduce iron deficiency among childbearing individuals age 12 to 49 years to 7.2% from a baseline of 11% (DHHS, 2020).

Iron from animal sources (called **heme iron**) is more easily absorbed than iron from plant and fortified food sources (called **nonheme iron**). Absorption of iron is affected by intake of other substances. Calcium in milk and dairy products and tannins in tea and red wine decrease iron absorption if they are consumed during the same meal. Coffee binds iron, preventing it from being fully utilized. Antacids, phytates (in grains and vegetables), oxalic acid (in spinach), and ethylenediaminetetraacetic acid (EDTA; a food additive) also decrease absorption. Foods cooked in iron pans have more iron. Foods containing ascorbic acid (vitamin C) consumed with iron containing foods increase the absorption. Ingesting meat, fish, or poultry (heme iron) with nonheme iron foods increases absorption (Grodner et al., 2020).

Because of the difficulty in obtaining enough iron in the diet, health care providers recommend iron supplements in conjunction with a healthy diet containing iron sources. Clients who are anemic, have more than one fetus, or begin supplementation late may need 60 to 120 mg daily (AAP & ACOG, 2017; Cunningham et al., 2022). Supplementation may begin during the second trimester when the need increases and morning sickness has usually ended.

TABLE 8.5 Foods High in Iron Content*

Food and Amount	Average Amounts of Iron Supplied (mg)
Meats and Poultry (3-oz serving)	
Beef (average)	2
Chicken	1
Turkey	2
Legumes	
Kidney beans (1 c)	3
Lentils (1 c)	6.6
Chickpeas (garbanzo beans) (1 c)	4.7
Lima beans (1 c)	4.5
Peas, green (1 c)	2.4
Peanuts, dry roasted (4 oz)	1.8
Sunflower seeds (¼ c)	1.2
Grains	
Rice, white enriched cooked (1 c)	2.8
Bread, wheat (slice)	1
Bagel, plain enriched, medium	3.8
Enriched cereals	7–18
Fruits	
Raisins (1 c)	2.7
Apricots, dried (10 halves)	0.9
Prune juice (1 c)	3
Vegetables (1 c)	
Broccoli	1
Collards	2.2
Tomatoes, stewed	3.4
Other	
Tofu, hard, 3.5 oz.	2.75

c, Cup; *oz*, ounce.

*The recommended daily allowance for iron during pregnancy is 27 mg. Although many clients take supplements because they do not eat enough iron-containing foods in their daily diet to meet this need, iron in foods is often better absorbed. Therefore, the nurse should suggest ways a client can increase their dietary iron.

Data from U.S. Department of Agriculture, Agricultural Research Service. (2016). *USDA National Nutrient Database for Standard Reference, Release 28.* Retrieved from www.ars.usda.gov/northeast-area/beltsville-md/beltsville-human-nutrition-research-center/nutrient-data-laboratory/docs/usda-national-nutrient-database-for-standard-reference/.

Iron taken between meals is absorbed more completely, but many clients find it difficult to tolerate iron without some food. Iron taken at bedtime may be easier to tolerate. For best results, it should be taken with water or a source of vitamin C such as orange juice, but not with coffee, tea, or milk. Side effects occur more often with higher doses and include nausea, vomiting, heartburn, epigastric pain, constipation, diarrhea, and black stools.

Clients should be reminded to keep iron and all other medicines out of the reach of children. Accidental iron overdose is a significant cause of childhood poisoning.

Calcium

Calcium is necessary for bone formation, maintenance of cell membrane permeability, coagulation, and neuromuscular function. It is transferred to the fetus, especially in the last trimester, and is important for mineralization of fetal bones and teeth. Calcium absorption and retention increase during pregnancy, and it is stored for use in the third trimester when fetal needs are highest.

Although a small amount of calcium is removed from the client's bones, it is insignificant, and overall mineralization of the client's bones is usually not affected. A common myth is calcium is removed from teeth during pregnancy. In reality, the calcium in teeth is stable and not affected by pregnancy.

Dairy products are the best source of calcium. Whole, low-fat, and nonfat milk all contain the same amount of calcium and may be used interchangeably to increase or reduce calorie intake. Clients with **lactose intolerance** (lactase deficiency resulting in gastrointestinal problems when dairy products are consumed) need other sources of calcium such as reduced-lactose dairy products or nondairy alternatives (Box 8.1). Non-cow milk dairy alternatives could include products made from soy, rice, almond, or coconut. These products are typically lower in calcium but can be calcium-fortified. Clients should be instructed to check the nutrition label to verify the calcium content.

Calcium is also present in legumes, nuts, dried fruits, broccoli, and dark green leafy vegetables. Although spinach and chard contain calcium, they also contain oxalates, which decrease calcium availability, making them poor sources. Caffeine increases excretion of calcium. Large amounts of fiber interfere with calcium absorption. More calcium is needed by clients younger than 18 years because their bone density is incomplete. The recommendations for calcium intake during pregnancy and lactation are the same as those for nonpregnant people.

Clients who do not eat dairy products because of lactose intolerance or to avoid eating animal products or for other reasons should take supplements unless they can meet their needs with other calcium-rich foods or dairy alternatives. Calcium should be taken with vitamin D, which increases its absorption. It is better absorbed when taken with meals, separately from iron supplements. It is also suggested to take prenatal vitamins at a different time from individual calcium supplements. The body can absorb approximately 500 mg of calcium at one time. Taking the prenatal vitamin and calcium supplement at the same time would exceed that amount.

Sodium

Sodium needs are increased during pregnancy to provide for an expanded blood volume and the needs of the fetus. Although sodium is not restricted during pregnancy, excessive amounts should be avoided. Clients are advised a moderate intake of salt or the salting of foods to taste is acceptable, but intake of high-sodium foods should be limited (Box 8.2).

Iodine

Iodine requirements increase in pregnancy and is important in the neurocognitive development and growth of the fetus.

BOX 8.1 Calcium Sources Approximately Equivalent to 1 Cup of Milk* (~300 mg of Calcium)

¾ cup (c) yogurt
1½ ounces (oz) hard cheese
1½ c low-fat cottage cheese
1 c calcium-fortified orange juice
1¾ c ice cream
3 c sherbet
3½ c pinto beans
½ block tofu
4½ c broccoli
1 c cooked collard greens (frozen)
6 oz canned salmon with bones
3 oz canned sardines with bones

* This list can be used to counsel clients who are vegans or lactose intolerant. Lactose-intolerant clients often can manage small amounts of yogurt and cheese without distress. Although the amounts of some foods listed are more than would be likely to be eaten within 1 day, they serve for comparison.
Data from U.S. Department of Agriculture, Agricultural Research Service. (2016). U.S. Department of Agriculture, Agricultural Research Service, Nutrient Data Laboratory. *USDA National Nutrient Database for Standard Reference, Release 28.* Version Current: September 2015, slightly revised May 2016. https://data.nal.usda.gov/system/files/sr_28_doc.pdf

BOX 8.2 High-Sodium Foods*

Products containing the words *salt*, *soda*, or *sodium*, such as table salt, garlic salt, monosodium glutamate, bicarbonate of soda (baking soda)
Salty tasting foods, including sauerkraut and snack foods such as popcorn, potato chips, pretzels, crackers
Condiments and relishes such as catsup, chili sauce, horse-radish, mustard, soy sauce, bouillon, pickles, green and black olives
Smoked, dried, and processed foods such as ham, bacon, lunch meats, corned beef
Canned soups, meats, and vegetables unless the label states the contents are low in sodium
Canned tomato and vegetable juices
Packaged mixes for sauces, gravies, cakes, and other baked foods

* During pregnancy, foods high in sodium should be consumed in moderation. Expectant mothers should be taught to read labels and avoid or limit products in which sodium is listed among the first ingredients.

While it is present in adequate amounts in the diets of most clients of childbearing age, national surveys show there may be a subset of pregnant and lactating clients who have mild to moderate inadequate iodine intake. Clients who do not regularly consume dairy products, eggs, seafood, or use iodized table salt would be at highest risk. Inadequate iodine can lead to damage of the developing brain of the fetus and neonatal hypothyroidism with cretinism (a condition characterized by physical deformity and learning disabilities that is caused by congenital thyroid deficiency) in its severest form (Procter & Campbell, 2014; USDA & DHHS, 2020).

Pregnant clients should make effort to consume dairy products, eggs, seafood, and iodized table salt to meet the increased needs of pregnancy. It is not recommended to start using table salt but to ensure the table salt used in cooking or added to foods is iodized. If clients do not regularly consume dairy products, eggs, or seafood due to vegan diet, cultural or religious purposes, or intolerance or allergy, they may need a separate supplement containing iodine, as many prenatal vitamins do not contain iodine (Procter & Campbell, 2014; USDA & DHHS, 2020; NASEM, 2020).

Nutritional Supplementation
Purpose

Food is the best source of nutrients. Health care providers usually prescribe prenatal vitamin–mineral supplements, and they are seen as an important part of pregnancy by many clients. However, with adequate diets, supplements may not be needed except for iron and folic acid, which are often not obtained in adequate amounts through normal food intake. Expectant clients who are vegetarians, are lactose intolerant, or have special problems in obtaining nutrients through diet alone may need supplements. Assessment of each client's individualized needs determines whether supplementation is appropriate.

Disadvantages and Dangers

Because they believe supplements are a harmless way to improve their diets, some clients take large amounts without consulting a health care provider. No standardization or regulation of the amounts of ingredients contained in supplements is available at this time. Label information for some supplements may not be accurate, and the supplement may not fulfill the health claims made for it.

The use of supplements may increase the intake of some nutrients to doses much higher than recommended. Excessive amounts of some vitamins and minerals may be toxic to the fetus. For example, excessive levels of vitamin A can cause fetal anomalies of the bones, urinary tract, and central nervous system. High doses of some vitamins or minerals may interfere with the ability to use others. If clients understand this, they are less likely to exceed recommended doses.

Some clients believe their nutrient needs can be met by vitamin–mineral supplements and are less concerned about their food intake. The word supplement literally means something that completes or enhances something else when added to it. Supplements do not generally contain protein and calories and may lack many necessary nutrients. Nurses should emphasize supplements are not food substitutes and do not contain all the nutrients needed during pregnancy. In fact, some nutrients important to pregnancy and provided by foods may be unknown at this time.

Water

Water is important during pregnancy for the expanded blood volume and as part of the increased maternal and fetal tissues. Clients should drink approximately 10 cups (2400 mL) of fluids that are mostly water each day (Procter & Campbell,

TABLE 8.6 Food Plan for Pregnancy and Lactation

Food and Amounts per Serving	Recommended Intake for Pregnancy*	Recommended Intake for Lactation[†]
Whole grains (1 oz = 1 slice bread, ½ c rice or pasta)	6–8 oz	7 oz
Vegetables	2½–3 c	3 c
Fruits	1½–2 c	2 c
Dairy group (1 c milk or yogurt, 1 ½ oz hard cheese, 2 c cottage cheese)	3 c	3 c
Protein group (1 oz meat/poultry/fish, 1 egg, ¼ c cooked beans, ¼ c tofu, 1 T peanut butter)	5–6½ oz	6 oz

c, Cup; *oz*, ounce; *T*, tablespoon.

*Example for a client 5 feet, 4 inches tall weighing 125 lb before pregnancy. Specific individualized food plans can be found at https://www.choosemyplate.gov.

[†]Amounts are for exclusive breastfeeding.

Data from https://www.choosemyplate.gov.

2014). Fluids low in nutrients (e.g., carbonated beverages, coffee, tea, or juice drinks with high amounts of sugar and little real juice) should be limited because they are filling and replace other more nutritional foods and drinks.

MyPlate

The USDA MyPlate provides a guide for healthy eating for adults and children. Guidelines for pregnancy and lactation are discussed later and are summarized in Table 8.6. Pregnant clients can go to the website https://www.choosemyplate.gov to get an individualized diet plan specifically adapted for them and their needs during pregnancy.

Whole Grains

Breads, cereals, rice, and pastas provide complex carbohydrates, fiber, vitamins, and minerals. At least half of the daily servings should be whole grains because they provide more nutrients than processed grain products. Although foods can be enriched to replace some nutrients lost during processing, not all nutrients are restored by enrichment. MyPlate recommendations are for 6 oz each day for adult women. Pregnant females should have 6 to 8 oz, and lactating females should have 8 oz daily.

Vegetables and Fruits

Vegetables and fruits are important sources of vitamins, minerals, and fiber. The daily recommendation for vegetables for nonpregnant adult females is 2.5 cups, 2.5 to 3 cups for pregnancy, and 3 cups for lactation. Adult females should have 1.5 to 2 cups of fruit daily. Pregnant and lactating females should also have 2 cups of fruit daily. A wide range of vegetables and fruits provides the best nutrition. Dark green, orange, or dark yellow vegetables are especially nutritious.

Dairy Group

The dairy group includes foods such as milk, yogurt, and cheese. They contain approximately the same nutrient values whether they are whole (4% fat), low fat (2% fat), or nonfat/skim (0% fat), but calories and fat are reduced in the latter two. The dairy group has especially good sources of calcium with a boost of protein. Adult females and those who are pregnant or lactating need 3 cups or the equivalent from this group.

Protein Group

Many adults think of meat, poultry, fish, and eggs as the only sources of protein. However, legumes (e.g., beans, peas, lentils), nuts, and soybean products, such as tofu, are also good sources. Adult females should consume 5 to 5.5 oz or the equivalent each day. Pregnant females need 5.5 to 6.5 oz, and with lactation 6 oz of protein foods are needed daily. A typical portion of meat, fish, and poultry varies in size. A 3-oz portion is about the size of a deck of playing cards.

Other Elements

Concentrated sugars, fats, and oils should be eaten sparingly. They provide calories for energy but few other nutrients. An adequate allowance for oils for adult females is 5 to 6 tsp of unsaturated oils (24 to 28 grams fat/day). Pregnant females need 6 to 8 tsp (28 to 37 grams fat/day), and lactating females need 6 tsp (28 grams fat/day) of unsaturated fats daily. Foods containing saturated fats and trans–fatty acids should be avoided.

Food Precautions
Fish and Seafood

Although fish are an excellent source of nutrients supporting fetal growth and development, certain precautions should be taken. Some species of fish have high levels of mercury, which can damage the fetal central nervous system. Pregnant and lactating clients should avoid those fish, which include shark, swordfish, king mackerel, marlin, orange roughy, tile fish (Gulf of Mexico), and bigeye tuna. Other types of fish have smaller amounts of mercury and can be eaten at 6 to 12 oz weekly (AAP & ACOG, 2020; USDA & DHHS, 2020).

Foodborne Illness

Pregnant clients and their fetuses are more susceptible to foodborne illnesses due to hormones and decreased cell-mediated immune function. Examples of foodborne illness are listeriosis (caused by the bacteria *Listeria monocytogenes*) and toxoplasmosis (caused by the bacteria *Toxoplasma gondii*). Pregnant clients are ten times more likely than the general population to get listeriosis. Listeriosis can cause miscarriage, stillbirth, and preterm labor. Babies born with listeriosis may have serious infections of the blood or brain causing lifelong health problems or even death in newborns (ACOG 2018a; USDA & DHHS, 2020).

Clients can become infected with *Listeria* by eating contaminated food, by handling contaminated food, or by touching contaminated surfaces and utensils and then accidentally transferring the bacteria from their hands to their mouths. Infants can become infected in utero or at birth. The bacteria can contaminate a variety of food, such as raw meat, poultry, or eggs; ready-to-eat processed meat such as hot dogs and deli meat (both factory-sealed packages and products sold at deli counters); raw sprouts; refrigerated pâtés; ready-to-eat smoked seafood and raw seafood; prepared or stored salads (including coleslaw and fresh fruit salad); melons; soft cheeses made with unpasteurized milk; unpasteurized juice; and unpasteurized milk and milk products. Pasteurization, cooking, and most disinfecting agents kill *Listeria* (ACOG 2018a; FDA, 2020; USDA & DHHS, 2020).

While listeriosis is one of the most common foodborne illnesses, there are multiple other bacteria that can make clients ill. Eating raw or undercooked meat or unwashed fruits or vegetables may cause toxoplasmosis with severe consequences to the fetus. Toxoplasmosis also can be contracted by contact with cat feces. Food safety and cleanliness decrease the incidence of foodborne illness in this higher risk population, and it is important for nurses to assist families in their awareness.

⚡ SAFETY CHECK

Food Safety during Pregnancy and Lactation

Do not eat shark, swordfish, king mackerel, orange roughy, tilefish, and bigeye tuna.

Eat up to 12 oz of shrimp, salmon, pollock, catfish, and canned light tuna (but only 6 oz of white albacore tuna) each week.

Do not eat raw or undercooked fish, meat, poultry, or eggs.

Avoid luncheon meats and hot dogs unless reheated until steaming hot.

Avoid soft cheeses unless made with pasteurized milk.

Do not consume refrigerated pâté, meat spreads, or smoked seafood.

Do not consume raw (unpasteurized) milk or milk products.

❓ KNOWLEDGE CHECK

8. Which minerals are often below the recommended amounts in the diets of pregnant clients?
9. Why is excessive use of vitamin–mineral supplements unnecessary and possibly dangerous?
10. How much fluid should a client drink each day during pregnancy?
11. How much of each food group is recommended during pregnancy?

FACTORS INFLUENCING NUTRITION

Age, knowledge about nutrition, exercise, and cultural background all influence the food choices clients make and their nutritional status. The nurse should consider these factors when counseling clients about their diets.

Age

Age is an important consideration. Adolescents, who are not fully mature, need nutritional support for their own growth. Older clients in good health have the same nutritional requirements as younger pregnant clients. They may have more knowledge about nutrition through life experiences or may need as much teaching as younger clients. Older clients are more likely to be financially secure than very young clients.

Nutritional Knowledge

Once pregnancy is confirmed, even clients who have not previously been attentive to their diets often want to learn about the relationship between what they eat and the effect on the fetus. Although clients know they should "eat well" during pregnancy, they may have little idea of what "eating well" means. Some lack basic understanding of nutrition and have misconceptions based on common food myths that interfere with good nutritional choices. They may seek information about nutrition from a multitude of media sources such as books, magazine articles, television, and the internet. Clients benefit by receiving nutritional education from nurses.

Exercise

Moderate exercise during pregnancy is encouraged. Physical activity during pregnancy maintains fitness and can reduce excessive weight gain and gestational diabetes. Clients who exercise more strenuously or are athletes may need modifications of their diet to meet additional nutritional needs after the first trimester. Extra calories may be needed to restore the energy used during exercise. For those that exercise more strenuously, greater than 30 minutes per day, a carbohydrate serving such as fruit, yogurt, or pasta before and after exercise may be sufficient. It is important to include protein in the post exercise snack or meal along with the carbohydrate. Clients younger than 18, athletes, or those who strenuously exercise regularly may require higher calories due their own potential growth. Additional fluids should be taken during and after exercise as well.

Culture

Culture defines how people in a society behave in relation to others and physical objects. It can be termed as the way of life for a group. Many factors can influence culture including customs, beliefs, faith or religion, attitudes, language, rituals, behaviors, art, music, ethnicity, and food. Many people in the United States are not culture-pure but are a combination of cultures that have evolved over time. A client's culture can also be influenced by the partner's culture, thus making culturally unique individuals.

Food is important in all cultures and often has special meaning during pregnancy and childbirth when certain foods may be favored or discouraged. Nurses need to be aware of the diverse habits of different cultures so they can provide culturally appropriate nutritional counseling. Before making assumptions about the influence of a client's culture on their diet, the nurse should assess each client individually. Not all clients follow food practices considered typical for their cultures.

For first- and even second-generation immigrants, the nurse should assess clients' age, how long they have lived in North America, and whether they have adopted any common American eating habits. Greater exposure to the North American diet may cause younger members of a group to make more dietary changes compared with their older relatives. Some clients who usually follow an American diet may return to some aspects of their traditional cultural diet during pregnancy.

Nurses often give clients pamphlets during nutritional teaching, but before giving a client printed material, the nurse should determine whether they prefer to read English or their native language. People who cannot read may not readily admit it to others. In addition, the reading level may be too complicated for a client with little education. Having an interpreter discuss the material with the client helps determine how well they can read and aids in other teaching. Cultural food preferences during pregnancy can be affected by beliefs and practices based on cold–hot body balance, taboo foods that are to be restricted or avoided, specific foods customary to ingest during pregnancy and lactation, and ethnicity, geographic region, and religion. These cultural aspects are discussed further below with examples. It is critical for nursing to focus on the effects of cultural diversity on food practices, especially during pregnancy, to better assess intake to ensure the client receives adequate nutrition.

People of many cultures believe certain foods, conditions, and medicines are "hot" or "cold" and should be balanced to preserve health. Foods considered hot in one culture may not fit in that category in another culture, and the designation does not necessarily match the temperature or spiciness of the food. In the Chinese culture, this belief is expressed with terms such as *yin* for cold and *yang* for hot and may influence what the client eats during pregnancy and the postpartum period. In the Hispanic culture, pregnancy is considered hot, and to balance this, the client would ingest more cold foods. Hot foods include many protein-containing foods, so the clinician could suggest rich protein foods that are not regarded as hot. Some clients who practice cold–hot body balance view prenatal vitamins or iron supplements as hot. The nurse educator could encourage the client to take the supplements with a cold liquid like juice.

Food taboos may determine what clients eat during the childbearing period. For example, Samoan clients avoid eating octopus or raw fish during pregnancy. Haitians believe they should eat for two and eat a hearty diet with lots of red fruits and vegetables. They also believe eating white foods such as milk, white beans, and lobster after birth will increase the lochia. Some Asians believe vitamin preparations containing iron harden the bones, making birth more difficult. Chinese clients may avoid spicy foods such as chili peppers but eat bird's nests, considered a delicacy (Callister, 2021).

Special foods may be customary during pregnancy or after birth. Punjabi clients may drink milk to prevent melasma. A Korean family may bring the postpartum client a hot beef and seaweed soup to cleanse the body and increase breast milk production (Callister, 2021).

Cultural preferences for foods are extremely varied. For example, some African Americans follow a diet historically specific to the southeastern United States. This diet is also known as soul food. Common foods include okra, collard greens, mustard greens, ham hocks, black-eyed peas, and hominy or grits. The diet of other Black Americans may vary according to the geographic area in which they live. Lactose intolerance is common and results in a lack of calcium if other sources are not present in the diet. Intake of high-sodium and fried foods may present health problems.

Some Jewish clients follow a strictly kosher diet. They avoid meat from animals without cloven hooves or do not chew their cud, which excludes pork and pork products. The meat must be processed to remove all blood and cannot be eaten in the same meal as milk. Muslim clients also do not eat pork and may fast on certain days. Although the religion exempts pregnant and nursing clients from obligatory fasting, the client must make up the fasting days at another time. Some choose to fast, regardless, for spiritual reasons or so they do not have to make up the days later.

NUTRITIONAL RISK FACTORS

The nurse should identify factors that may interfere with a client's ability to meet the nutritional needs of pregnancy.

Socioeconomic Status
Poverty
Low-income clients may have deficient diets because of lack of financial resources and nutritional education. Carbohydrate foods are often less expensive than meats, dairy products, fresh fruits, and vegetables. Therefore, the diet may be high in calories but low in vitamins and minerals. A referral to Temporary Assistance for Needy Families (TANF), Supplemental Nutrition Assistance Program (SNAP), or Special Supplemental Nutrition Program for Women, Infants, and Children (WIC) may be helpful if a client's food intake is inadequate due to financial constraints. The SNAP-Ed program and the USDA's Eating Healthy on A Budget help families plan and prepare healthy, inexpensive meals. Vitamin–mineral supplementation may be important, especially if the diet is likely to be inconsistent. Low-income families may experience food shortages at the end of the month when resources are depleted or when food is shared with a large number of people. Providing clients with information for food banks or pantries, community meal programs, or other resources or assistance programs can help better ensure food security for this at-risk population.

Food Supplement Programs
The WIC program is administered by the USDA to provide nutritional assessment, counseling, and education to low-income clients and children up to age 5 years who are at nutritional risk. This supplemental nutrition program also provides vouchers for foods such as milk, cheese, tofu, eggs, whole wheat bread, brown rice, tortillas, fruits and vegetables, iron-fortified cereal, juice, legumes, peanut butter, and

formula to qualified clients and their children. Eligibility is based on an income at or below 185% of the federal poverty level. Clients are eligible throughout pregnancy and for 6 months after birth if formula feeding or 1 year if breastfeeding. Children at risk for poor nutrition may be eligible until 5 years of age. Further information is available at https://www.fns.usda.gov/wic.

？ KNOWLEDGE CHECK

12. When the nurse assesses cultural influences on nutrition during pregnancy, what factors should be considered?
13. For what nutritional problems should the nurse assess when caring for low-income clients?

Vegetarianism

A **vegetarian** diet is composed of only or mostly plant foods. It occurs in a variety of forms. **Vegan** dietary patterns avoid all animal products, including honey. The **lactovegetarian** diet avoids animal products except for milk products, the **ovovegetarian** dietary pattern avoids animal products except for eggs, and the **lacto-ovovegetarian** diet avoids animal products except for milk products and eggs. There are several other more limited plant-based diets. The raw food diet consists exclusively of vegetables, including sprouted cereals and pulses, fresh and dried fruits, and seeds, as well as milk and eggs. All foods are typically eaten raw. The fruit diet consists exclusively of fresh and dried fruits, seeds, and some vegetables. The macrobiotic diet consists of cereals, pulses, vegetables, seaweed, and soy products. Fish is consumed by some who adhere to the macrobiotic diet (Melina et al., 2016; Sebastiani et al., 2019).

Vegetarian dietary patterns have increased over the last few decades to help lower the risk of chronic disease, such as coronary heart disease, cancer, and diabetes; to therapeutically manage those diseases; out of animal compassion; out of environment protection; and for cultural reasons. While a well-planned vegetarian or vegan diet is considered safe in pregnancy and lactation, the client needs awareness of a balanced intake of key nutrients. Nutrients at highest risk include protein, calcium, vitamin D, iron, zinc, iodine, omega-3 fatty acids, and vitamin B_{12}. Those practicing vegetarian dietary patterns should pay particular attention to obtaining these nutrients in food or supplement form (Melina et al., 2016; Sebastiani et al., 2019). Additional vegetarian and vegan resources for clients and clinicians can be found at https://www.dietaryguidelines.gov and https://www.USDA.gov.

Meeting the Nutritional Requirements of the Pregnant Vegetarian

Energy. Vegetarian diets may be low in calories and fat, and some do not meet the energy needs of pregnancy. The diets are high in fiber and may cause a feeling of fullness before enough calories are eaten. A pregnant client can increase caloric intake by eating snacks and higher calorie foods. If carbohydrate and fat intake is too low, the body may use protein for energy, making it unavailable for other purposes.

Protein. Although most vegetarians get enough protein, this area needs consideration, especially in vegan diets. **Complete proteins** contain all the **essential amino acids** (amino acids the body cannot synthesize from other sources). Animal proteins are complete, but plant proteins (with the exception of soybeans) are **incomplete proteins**, lacking one or more of the essential amino acids.

However, even a diet with only plant proteins can meet the needs of pregnancy. Combining incomplete plant proteins with other plant foods with complementary amino acids allows intake of all essential amino acids. Dishes with grains (e.g., wheat, rice, corn) and legumes (e.g., garbanzo, navy, kidney, or pinto beans; peas; peanuts) are combinations that provide complete proteins. Complementary proteins do not have to be eaten at the same meal if they are consumed in a single day.

Incomplete proteins also can be combined with small amounts of complete protein foods, such as cheese or milk, to provide all amino acids. Therefore, clients who include even small amounts of animal products meet their protein needs more easily.

Many vegetarians use tofu, made from soybeans, which provides protein, calcium, and iron. Meat analogs with a texture similar to meat but made from vegetable protein are available. Some look and taste like hamburgers, bacon, lunch meats, chicken patties, and other commonly eaten foods. Meat analogs may be fortified with nutrients that are often low in vegan diets.

With the increase in overall protein needs in pregnancy, vegetarian clients should increase their protein intake by 10%. This can be achieved by adding 1.5 cups of lentils per day or 2.5 cups of soy milk per day. Excessive or high protein supplementation is not recommended (Sebastiani et al., 2019).

Calcium. Vegetarians who include milk products in their diet may meet the pregnancy needs for calcium. Vegans obtain calcium from dark green vegetables and legumes, but their high-fiber diet may interfere with calcium absorption. Calcium-fortified juices or soy products such as soy milk or tofu may help meet the requirements. Low-dose calcium supplements may be necessary.

Vitamin D. Vitamin D deficiencies exist among the general population, especially those with dark skin and vegetarians. Levels of this vitamin depend on sunlight exposure and intake of foods high in vitamin D. Foods fortified with vitamin D include cow's milk, some fruit juices, breakfast cereals, soy or other plant-based milks, and margarines. Eggs have some vitamin D, and mushrooms treated with ultraviolet light can be a significant source. Vitamin D supplementation may be needed based on foods consumed and type of vegetarian diet (Melina et al., 2016; Sebastiani et al., 2019).

Iron. Although the ability to absorb iron increases in pregnancy and continues to improve in the second and third trimester, iron from plants in the vegetarian diet is not as readily absorbed. Absorption is enhanced by eating a source of vitamin C in the same meal in which nonheme iron is consumed or by preparing food in iron pans. Plant-based foods that can increase iron intake include soy, beans, seeds, nuts, and green leafy vegetables. Iron supplements can be particularly important for vegetarian clients during pregnancy.

Zinc. Because the best sources of zinc are meat and fish, vegetarians may have lower levels of this mineral. Fortified cereals, nuts, soy, grains, and legumes increase zinc intake. To help increase absorption, adopting food preparation methods such as soaking, germination, fermentation, and sourdough leavening of bread reduce phytate levels in zinc rich foods. Zinc supplementation is available as needed (Sebastiani et al., 2019).

Iodine. Plant-based diets are often lower in iodine, and during pregnancy, iodine needs increase. The key vegan sources of iodine are iodized salt and sea vegetables. Sea salt, kosher salt, and salty seasonings are not generally iodized. Vegan clients of childbearing age are recommended to supplement with 150 mcg/day of iodine (Melina et al., 2016).

Fatty Acids. Dietary intakes of omega-3 fatty acids, eicosapentaenoic acid (EPA), and docosahexaenoic acid (DHA) are lower in vegetarians and absent in vegans. A balanced amount of omega-3 and omega-6 fatty acids are important to produce sufficient amounts of DHA and EPA. A vegetarian diet may be at a disadvantage in optimizing this ratio because there are limited omega-3 fatty acids in plant-based foods. Food sources include seeds (flax, chia, camelina, canola, and hemp), walnuts, and their oils. Low-dose microalgae-based DHA supplements of 100 to 200 mg/day are suggested for pregnant and lactating vegetarians (Melina et al., 2016; Sebastiani et al., 2019).

Vitamin B_{12}. Vitamin B_{12} is obtained only from animal products. Because vegetarian diets contain large amounts of folic acid, anemia from inadequate intake of vitamin B_{12} may not be apparent at first. Vegans may eat fortified foods such as cereal and soy products or take B_{12} supplements at 4 mcg/day dissolved under the tongue or chewed slowly for increased absorption.

Bariatric Surgery

As obesity and morbid obesity rates have increased over the years, so has the incidence of bariatric surgery to help offset the associated chronic disease morbidity and mortality. There are several procedures included under the bariatric surgery umbrella, which are in two groups. There are gastric volume restrictive surgeries that decrease the size of the stomach, often by using a gastric banding or sleeve procedure. The band or ring diameter is controlled by a saline reservoir, which can be increased or decreased after the initial procedure. It is not uncommon to deflate the band by decreasing or removing the saline during pregnancy and lactation. The second group is restrictive malabsorption. One example of this procedure is where the stomach and duodenum are bypassed and the jejunum brought up and connect to a small, separated pouch of the stomach. Due to the significant and rapid weight loss, clients are encouraged to avoid pregnancy for at least 12 to 24 months after bariatric surgery (ACOG, 2017).

Bariatric surgery clients are at increased risk of malnutrition and nutrient deficiencies in protein, iron, folate, calcium, vitamin B_{12}, and vitamin D. A broad evaluation for deficiencies in micronutrients should be considered at the beginning of pregnancy in clients who have had bariatric surgery, which would include serum testing of complete blood count and metabolic panel and measurement of iron, ferritin, calcium, vitamin B_{12}, folate, vitamin K, vitamin A, and vitamin D levels. Treatment for any deficiencies should be initiated. If there are no deficits, a complete blood count and metabolic panel and measurement of iron, ferritin, calcium, and vitamin D levels every trimester are recommended. Intake strategies of small frequent meals, nutrient-dense foods, and powder or liquid supplements are encouraged, but due to the decreased food intake and tolerance, pregnant post-bariatric surgery clients often require supplementation. Individual supplementation as indicated of vitamin B_{12}, vitamin D, vitamin K, vitamin A, folic acid, iron, calcium, and protein are most typical. Supplements can be administered orally, intramuscularly, or intravenously as needed (ACOG, 2017; Cunningham et al., 2022; Kominiarek & Rajan, 2016).

Clients who become pregnant after bariatric surgery may have lower risk for gestational diabetes, gestational hypertension, and preeclampsia but could have an increased risk for preterm delivery and SGA infants. The long-term effects of the surgery on pregnancy outcomes are unknown, and more data is needed to determine specific care guidelines for this nutritionally at-risk population (Al-Nimr et al., 2019; Stand & Huffman, 2016).

Nausea and Vomiting of Pregnancy

Morning sickness usually disappears soon after the first trimester, although some clients experience nausea at other times of the day and for a longer time. Most clients can consume enough food to maintain nutrition sufficiently. They are often able to manage frequent small meals better than three large meals. Protein and complex carbohydrates are often tolerated best, but fatty foods increase nausea. Drinking liquids between meals instead of with meals can minimize the nausea experienced after eating. Eating a bedtime protein snack helps maintain glucose levels through the night. A carbohydrate food such as dry toast or crackers eaten before getting out of bed in the morning helps prevent nausea. Peppermint or ginger tea may relieve nausea in some clients.

Anemia

Anemia is a common concern during pregnancy. Hgb values decrease during the second trimester of pregnancy as a result of plasma increases diluting the blood. This physiologic anemia is normal (see Chapter 6). During the third trimester, Hgb levels generally rise to near prepregnant levels because of increased absorption of iron from the gastrointestinal tract, even though iron is transferred to the fetus primarily during this time.

A client may begin pregnancy with anemia or develop it during pregnancy. They are considered anemic if their Hgb is less than 11 grams per deciliter (g/dL) during the first and third trimesters or if their Hgb is less than 10.5 g/dL during the second trimester (Cunningham et al., 2022).

If fetal iron stores during the third trimester are sufficient, anemia will not develop in the newborn for the first 4 to 6 months after birth. However, if the client's intake of iron is insufficient, Hgb levels may not rise during the third trimester, iron deficiency anemia may develop, and transfer of iron to the fetus may be decreased. Anemic clients need iron supplements and help choosing foods high in iron (see Table 8.5).

Abnormal Prepregnancy Weight

In addition to teaching about dietary changes, the nurse should be alert for problems associated with abnormal prepregnancy weight. The client who is below normal weight may not have enough money for food or may have an eating disorder. Obese clients may have other health problems such as hypertension, which may affect the nurse's nutritional counseling plan.

Eating Disorders

Eating disorders include **anorexia nervosa** (refusal to eat because of a distorted body image and feelings of obesity) and **bulimia** (overeating followed by induced vomiting, fasting, or use of laxatives or diuretics). Ideally these disordered behaviors should be addressed before the client is pregnant with a goal of eating well and maintaining a healthy weight for several months. Eating disorders can be a threat to pregnancy and fetal development and require close supervision during pregnancy. They are associated with miscarriage, low birth weight, preterm birth, congenital anomalies, and postpartum depression. Clients with anorexia often have amenorrhea and have difficulty conceiving. Clients with bulimia or subclinical anorexia are more likely to become pregnant. All pregnant clients should be asked about eating disorders, and nurses should assess for behaviors of disordered eating as both maternal and neonatal adverse outcomes are significant (Mantel et al., 2020).

Some clients with these disorders eat normally during pregnancy for the sake of the fetus. For others, the normal weight gain of pregnancy may be very stressful as old fears about obesity are reactivated. They may return to their previous eating patterns during pregnancy or in the early postpartum period when they do not lose weight immediately. Explaining that clients often lose weight during breastfeeding may encourage them to breastfeed and eat a good diet during lactation. Clients with eating disorders need a great deal of individual counseling to ensure they meet the increased nutrient needs of pregnancy and understand normal postpartum weight loss. Assessment of weight gain at each prenatal visit is especially important (Cunningham et al., 2022).

Food Cravings and Aversions

Clients may have a strong preference or a strong dislike for certain foods only during pregnancy. Cravings for pickles, ice cream (not necessarily together), pizza, chocolate, cake, candy, spicy foods, and dairy products are common. Food aversions often include those to coffee, alcoholic beverages, highly seasoned or fried foods, and meat. The cause of cravings and aversions is not known, but they may be a result of changes in the sense of taste and smell. They are generally not harmful, and some, like aversion to alcohol, may be beneficial.

Satisfying food cravings during pregnancy is thought important in many cultures. For example, clients from India may believe cravings during pregnancy should be satisfied because they come from the fetus (Callister, 2021). Ethiopian clients may believe unfulfilled food cravings during pregnancy may cause miscarriage.

Pica

Some people have cravings for nonnutritive substances. The practice of eating substances not usually considered part of a normal diet is called **pica**. Ice, clay or dirt, and laundry starch or cornstarch are the most common materials, but other items such as chalk, baking soda, antacid tablets, coffee grounds, freezer frost, toothpaste, burnt matches, or ashes may be included (Cunningham et al., 2022).

Pica is practiced by approximately 30% of pregnant clients globally. In the United States it is more common in clients from inner cities, rural areas, and the southeastern regions; African Americans; clients who live in poverty and have poor nutrition; and those with a childhood or family history of the practice. However, pica is not limited to any one socioeconomic group or geographic area. While pica may be present before pregnancy, pica during pregnancy has been related to iron deficiency and food insecurity (Roy et al., 2018).

While the cause of pica is unknown, cultural values may influence pica practices. Pica may be related to beliefs regarding the effects of the substance on labor or the baby. Clay and dirt are not sources of iron and may decrease the absorption of iron and other minerals. Iron deficiency is often associated with pica, and the client should be tested to see if additional iron supplementation will be needed (Roy et al., 2018; Sadeghi et al., 2020).

Substances eaten may be contaminated with parasites, other organisms, or toxins such as lead. Clay and dirt may cause constipation or intestinal blockage. Eating large amounts of ice may cause dental problems. Pica also may decrease the intake of foods and essential nutrients. Some clients fear their eating habits are harmful but are unable to ignore the cravings. They often hide their eating practices from caregivers who might disapprove.

Multiparity and Multifetal Pregnancy

The number and spacing of pregnancies and the presence of more than one fetus influence nutritional requirements. The client who has had previous pregnancies may begin a pregnancy with a nutritional deficit. In addition, they may be too busy meeting the needs of the family to be attentive to their own nutritional needs.

Pregnancies spaced at least 18 months apart are healthier for the client and the fetus. An interval of less than 6 months between pregnancies increases the risk for preterm and low-birth-weight infants, as well as maternal morbidity and mortality (ACOG, 2018b).

Closely spaced pregnancies may not allow a client to remedy any nutritional deficits originating during a previous pregnancy. If they have inadequate nutrient stores, nutritional needs must be met from daily diet intake and supplementation alone. Morning sickness from a new pregnancy soon after delivery may further interfere with an expectant client's ability to eat an adequate diet.

A client with a multifetal pregnancy must provide enough nutrients to meet the needs of each fetus without depleting the maternal stores. More calories will be needed to meet necessary weight gain and energy needs. In 1990 the IOM updated recommendations for pregnancy weight gain. According to the guidelines, a client with a normal prepregnancy weight should gain 17 to 25 kg (37 to 54 lb) with a twin pregnancy, a gain of 5.5 to 9 kg (12 to 19 lb) more than expected for a single-fetus pregnancy. When clients meet the recommended weight gain, they are less likely to deliver their twins before 32 weeks of gestation and the infants are more likely to weigh more than 2500 g (5.5 lb) and have less maternal complications such as preeclampsia (Lipworth et al., 2021; Pécheux et al., 2019).

Clients carrying triplets should gain a total of 23 to 27 kg (50 to 60 lb). Those pregnant with more than one fetus should consume an additional 300 calories per day for each fetus (CDC, 2021b). Additional vitamin–mineral supplementation may also be necessary.

Substance Abuse

Substance abuse often accompanies a lifestyle that is unlikely to promote healthy eating habits. The expense of supporting a substance abuse habit decreases money available to purchase food. Therefore, nutrition in pregnant clients who abuse substances should be explored fully. Usually, more than one substance is involved, and the effects of various combinations of substances on nutrition are not fully understood. The damaging effects of smoking, alcohol, and illicit drug use on the fetus are discussed further in Chapter 11.

Smoking

Cigarette smoking increases maternal metabolic rate and decreases appetite, which may result in a lower weight gain. As the amount of smoking increases, infant birth weight decreases despite an adequate diet. Smoking decreases the availability of some vitamins and minerals, and vitamin–mineral supplements are important during pregnancy. Counseling to help clients stop smoking or at least decrease the number of cigarettes smoked during pregnancy is essential.

Caffeine

The evidence regarding the effect of caffeine on nutrition during pregnancy is conflicting, and more research is needed. Currently, it appears caffeine intake of 200 to 300 mg/day is not a major contributing cause of miscarriage or preterm birth. Until more is known about its effects on nutrition and the fetus, caffeine intake should be limited during pregnancy to 200 to 300 mg/day (ACOG, 2020a; March of Dimes, 2020; USDA & DHHS, 2020). An 8-oz cup of brewed coffee contains approximately 137 mg, brewed tea contains 48 mg/8 oz, cola beverages contain 37 mg/12 oz, and cocoa mix contains 8 to 12 mg/packet or 3 tsp (March of Dimes, 2020). The nurse should discuss other sources of caffeine, including some over-the-counter medications.

Alcohol

Because of the association between drinking and fetal alcohol spectrum disorders, clients should avoid alcohol completely during pregnancy. Alcohol affects the absorption of vitamin B_{12}, folic acid, and magnesium and often takes the place of food in the diet. Vitamin–mineral supplementation may be necessary for clients who had large intakes of alcohol before pregnancy, even if they stop drinking after conception, because their nutrient stores may be depleted. According to the USDA and the DHHS (2020), alcohol consumption should be stopped during pregnancy, and alcohol abstinence should continue while breastfeeding.

Drugs

The use of drugs other than those prescribed during pregnancy increases danger to the fetus and may interfere with nutrition. Even some prescribed medications have risks during pregnancy that should be weighed against their benefits. The interaction of various drugs with nutrients is not fully understood.

Marijuana increases appetite, but clients may not satisfy their hunger with foods of good nutrient quality. Heroin alters metabolism and may cause a client to become malnourished. Cocaine acts as an appetite suppressant, interfering with nutrient intake. Vasoconstriction from cocaine use decreases nutrient flow to the fetus. Cocaine users also tend to drink more caffeine and alcoholic beverages. Amphetamines and methamphetamines depress appetite. Clients who use amphetamines for dieting should be warned these drugs should be discontinued during pregnancy.

Adolescence

Adolescent pregnancies are associated with higher risk for complications for both the expectant client and the fetus. Pregnant adolescents who are younger than 4 years **gynecologic age** (number of years since menarche) and those who are undernourished at the time of conception have the greatest nutritional needs (Larson et al., 2020). Maternal growth may interfere with placental blood flow and transfer of nutrients to the fetus. As a result, adolescents may add weight and fat to their own body rather than use it for support of the fetus. This leads to a tendency to have smaller infants even with good weight gain in the client.

Weight Gain

As noted earlier in this chapter in the section titled Weight Gain during Pregnancy, weight gain goals for adolescents are based on prepregnancy BMI, using adult BMI and not pediatric BMI. According to the IOM, adolescent expected weight gain is the same as adult pregnancies. Further research is needed to determine whether these weight gain goals are appropriate in teens to optimize pregnancy outcomes. Several studies have concluded that more than 70% of teenage pregnancy participants showed inappropriate gestational weight gain, which could have a significant impact on pregnancy outcomes (Sámano et al., 2018). Inappropriate weight gain includes gaining too much and too little weight during pregnancy, which is similar to current adult pregnancies. Adequate nutrition and appropriate weight gain in teen pregnancies will aid in improving maternal and fetal outcomes.

Nutrient Needs

The nutrient DRIs needed by pregnant adolescents are the same as those for older clients for most nutrients. Adolescents need more calcium, phosphorus, magnesium, and zinc to meet their own growth needs. Individualized assessment of gynecologic age, nutritional status, and daily diet may indicate the need for increases in other areas as well.

Common Problems

The diets of teenagers before pregnancy are often low in vitamin A, folic acid, calcium, iron, and zinc. Although they may get three or four servings of vegetables daily, one or two may be potatoes and often are French fries. Teens average only 1.5 servings of fruits and dairy a day. Foods high in sugar and fat are common (Larson et al., 2020). These habits often lead to inadequate stores of nutrients for pregnancy. Supplements may be prescribed, but the adolescent may not take them regularly. This combination of poor intake and unreliable supplementation may further deplete nutrient stores and general nutritional status.

Adolescents are often concerned about body image. If weight is a major focus for teenagers and their peers, they are more likely to restrict calories to prevent weight gain during pregnancy. Teens tend to skip meals, especially breakfast. The fetus requires a steady supply of nutrients, and the expectant client's stores may be used if intake is not sufficient to meet fetal needs.

Teenagers are often in a hurry and want fast and convenient foods. Meals may be irregular and often eaten away from home. A significant part of the adolescent diet may consist of fast foods from restaurants or snack machines. These foods are often high in fat, sweeteners, and sodium and low in vitamins, minerals, and fiber. Peer pressure is an important influence on nutritional status. Choosing fast foods that do not make them appear different from their peers yet meet their added nutrient needs is important for the pregnant adolescent.

Teaching the Adolescent

Teaching the adolescent about nutrition can be a challenge for nurses. It is essential to establish an accepting, relaxed atmosphere and show willingness to listen to the teenager's concerns. The teenager's lifestyle, pattern of eating, and food likes and dislikes should be explored to determine whether changes are needed in the diet.

The adolescent's home life may affect nutritional status. Clients may live at home where the whole family may eat together or may eat with the family only occasionally because they are often away at mealtimes. Some pregnant adolescents are homeless or in unstable situations. The number of other people in the home and the sufficiency of the food available also affect the dietary intake.

The nurse should keep suggestions to a minimum and focus on only the most important changes. If adolescents believe they must eliminate all their favorite foods, they are likely to rebel. Asking for the adolescent's input increases the likelihood of following suggestions. When changes are necessary the nurse should explain why they are important for both the fetus and the expectant client. Teenagers, like other pregnant clients, often makes changes for the sake of their unborn baby that they would not consider for themselves alone.

The teenager's likes and dislikes should be considered, and snacks should be included in the meal plan. The need to be like their peers is of major importance to the adolescent, especially when they are going through the changes of pregnancy. With education about appropriate choices, teens can eat fast foods with their friends and still maintain a nourishing diet. Giving them plenty of examples of alternatives from which they can choose should be very helpful (Table 8.7 and "Client Education: Fast Foods and Nutrition").

Other Risk Factors

Clients who follow food fads may not meet the nutritional requirements for pregnancy. Those who have followed a severely restricted diet for a long time may have depleted nutrient stores. Nurses can help them understand the necessary changes to help ensure successful pregnancies.

Clients with complications of pregnancy such as diabetes, heart disease, and preeclampsia may need dietary alterations. Those with other medical conditions such as extreme obesity, history of bariatric surgery, cystic fibrosis, and celiac disease may need nutritional counseling from a dietitian. Clients with phenylketonuria should follow a low-phenylalanine diet before conception and during pregnancy to prevent cognitive impairment and other defects in the infant. This is true even if they have not routinely followed the diet during adulthood (March of Dimes, 2020).

TABLE 8.7 Nutritious Choices from Snack Machines*	
Food	Nutrients Provided
Yogurt, white or chocolate milk	Protein, calcium
Fruit juices, fresh fruits (usually apples or oranges), dried fruit	Vitamins, fiber
Vegetables such as baby carrots	Vitamins, fiber
Popcorn (best without butter or salt)	Fiber
Peanuts, almonds (roasted)	Protein, vitamins, calcium, iron
Granola or granola bars, trail mix, sunflower seeds	Fiber, protein
Crackers and cheese	Protein, calcium
Crackers and peanut butter	Protein

*Snack machines generally dispense foods high in calories, fats, and sodium and low in nutrients. Some of the foods listed here are somewhat high in calories, but all provide other worthwhile nutrients.

CLIENT EDUCATION
Fast Foods and Nutrition

Add cheese to hamburgers to increase calcium and protein. Include lettuce and tomato for vitamins A and C.

Avoid dressings on hamburgers because they tend to be high in calories and fat.

To reduce fat and calories, choose broiled, roasted, and barbecued foods (e.g., chicken breast, roast beef). Avoid fried foods (e.g., French fries, fried zucchini, onion rings, fried cheese) because they are high in fat and the high heat may destroy some vitamins. Breaded foods such as chicken nuggets and breaded clams are high in calories and absorb more oil if they are fried.

Try wraps instead of sandwiches to decrease calories.

Baked potatoes with broccoli, cheese, and meat fillings provide better nutrition than French fries or baked potatoes with sour cream and butter.

Pizza is high in calories, but the cheese provides protein and calcium. Ask for vegetable toppings or add a salad to increase vitamins.

Salad bars are often available at fast food restaurants and provide vitamins and minerals without adding too many calories. Use only a small amount of salad dressing, which is high in fat.

Milk, milkshakes, and orange juice provide more nutrients than carbonated beverages, which are high in sodium and calories.

Avoid pickles, olives, and other salty foods. Too much sodium may increase swelling of the ankles. Add only small amounts of salt to foods to prevent or decrease swelling.

KNOWLEDGE CHECK

14. What suggestions can the nurse give the vegan about diet during pregnancy?
15. How can lactose-intolerant clients increase their intake of calcium?
16. What other conditions present nutritional risk factors during pregnancy?
17. What nutritional problems may the adolescent have during pregnancy?

NUTRITION AFTER BIRTH

Nutritional requirements after birth depend on whether the client breastfeeds or formula-feeds the infant. The nurse should review the client's nutritional knowledge when returning to the prepregnancy diet and teach the breastfeeding client how to adapt a diet to meet the needs of lactation.

Nutrition for the Lactating Client

There are less evidenced-based nutrient recommendations for lactation than there are for pregnancy. Breastfeeding is often considered successful if the infant grows appropriately. Nonetheless, the lactating client must nourish both themselves and the baby as they did during pregnancy for optimal outcomes. Therefore, the need for highly nutritious diet continues during this time. Most DRIs for lactation are higher than those for pregnant adults, which are higher than for nonpregnant clients. Lactating mothers with poor diets may have reduced milk levels of fatty acids, selenium, iodine, vitamin A, and some B vitamins (NASEM, 2020).

The client's weight, BMI, body fat percentage, and weight gain during pregnancy do not influence milk production. The quantity and caloric value of breast milk does not change with mild to moderate dieting and exercise, although it is recommended to allow breast milk supply to be well established before starting dieting or exercise (Kominiarek & Rajan, 2016).

Energy

During the first 6 months the total calories needed is 500 calories per day to meet the needs of lactation. The estimated energy requirement (EER) is 330 calories each day in addition to normal needs for client according to age, weight, and height. In addition to the calories consumed, approximately 170 calories per day are drawn from the client's fat stores. This provides a total of 500 calories each day above prepregnancy requirements to meet the needs of lactation. The use of calories from fat stores aids in postpartum weight loss.

The EER for the second 6 months of lactation is 400 calories more than prepregnancy needs. After 6 months, it is assumed maternal pregnancy energy stores have been used, and the calories should come from the client's daily intake (IOM, 2006). The caloric value of the breast milk produced does not change based on the caloric intake of the mother. Milk volume is usually adequate even when a client's diet is less than optimal, but volume may be reduced, and maternal nutrient stores will be depleted with very low caloric intake.

Protein

The DRI for protein during lactation is 71 g each day. Although there is no change from the pregnancy DRI of 25 additional grams of protein per day, it is important for the client to maintain protein intake throughout the breastfeeding period.

Fats

There is no evidence stating changes in maternal fat intake influence the quantity of fat in breast milk, but it has been shown repeatedly the type of the fat consumed by the client will influence the fatty acid composition of milk. The long-chain polyunsaturated omega-3 and omega-6 fatty acids are healthful and present in human milk. Therefore, they should be included in the client's diet and supplemented as needed for some, such as vegans, during lactation (DHHS, 2020; NASEM, 2020).

Vitamins and Minerals

The DRIs for 20 vitamins and minerals increase in pregnancy and lactation with only calcium, phosphorus, vitamin D, vitamin K, biotin, fluoride, magnesium, sodium, and chloride recommended intakes remaining the same as nonpregnant clients. During lactation, 17 of the vitamin and mineral recommended intakes increase even higher than during pregnancy. Lactating clients who eat a well-balanced diet generally consume adequate amounts of essential nutrients to meet the infant's and their own needs. Although the quality of the milk is not affected by the mother's intake of most minerals, the vitamin content may be decreased if the diet is consistently low in vitamins. While vitamin deficiencies are not common, fortunately, breast milk content does respond to maternal supplementation (Kominiarek & Rajan, 2016).

Vitamin D is low in breast milk, and supplements are recommended for exclusively breastfed infants (AAP & ACOG, 2017). Iron is also low in breast milk, but term infants are typically born with iron stores lasting for the first 6 months of life, making iron supplementation of most infants unnecessary, although infants born preterm or to iron-deficient mothers will need supplementation before 6 months of age. Milk levels of other nutrients such as calcium remain constant because some nutrients are drawn from the mother's stores if the intake is poor. Many health care providers recommend that clients continue to take their prenatal vitamin–mineral supplements during lactation.

Fluid

Total water intake DRIs increase in pregnancy and during lactation. It is recommended the client be aware of this higher need, which often increases in the early breastfeeding period, and drink volumes to relieve thirst. Eight to ten cups of non-caffeinated fluid is adequate. Drinking large quantities of fluids, as was once recommended, is not necessary.

Alcohol

Not drinking alcohol during lactation is the safest option. If alcohol is consumed, it is recommended to wait until the infant is at least 3 months of age. No more than 1 standard drink per day is not harmful to the infant, especially if the client waits at least 2 hours after a single drink. Removing milk from the breasts does not speed the elimination of alcohol from the milk. It is the alcohol level in the client's blood that determines the level in the breast milk. If additional alcohol is consumed, the infant could take previously expressed milk (Academy of Nutrition and Dietetics [AND], 2020; USDA & DHHS, 2020).

Caffeine

Caffeine should be limited during lactation to about 300 mg per day, which is equivalent to approximately 2 to 3 cups of coffee. Caffeine content of coffee, tea, soda, and a variety of energy drinks vary. Other sources of caffeine include some medication and weight-loss aids. Newborns typically are more sensitive to caffeine. Infants affected by caffeine intakes may be irritable or have trouble sleeping (AND, 2020; USDA & DHHS, 2020).

Other Items for Consideration

Lactating mothers should continue to avoid fish with high mercury levels just as in pregnancy. Herbal teas, remedies, and supplements should be avoided unless approved by a lactation consultant or medical provider. Illicit drugs and tobacco should be avoided as well (AND, 2020; USDA & DHHS, 2020).

Specific Nutritional Concerns

Some clients have difficulty consuming all required nutrients and need special counseling or considerations. This group includes clients who are dieting, adolescents, vegans, those who avoid dairy products, those with a history of bariatric surgery, and those whose diet is inadequate for other reasons.

Dieting. Clients who are concerned about losing weight after pregnancy need special consideration. After the initial losses in the first month, weight gradually decreases as maternal fat is used to meet a portion of the energy needs of lactation. However, breastfeeding does not necessarily result in weight loss, and some clients maintain or even gain weight during lactation. This is more likely when weight gain during pregnancy was excessive.

Dieting should be postponed for at least 3 weeks after birth to allow for recovery after childbirth and to establish a milk supply if they are breastfeeding. Gradual weight loss is preferable and should be accomplished by a combination of moderate exercise and a diet high in nutrients not below 1500 to 1800 calories per day. Weight loss of approximately 0.45 to 0.68 kg (1 to 1.5 lb) a week, not exceeding 5 lb per month, is generally considered safe and will not compromise milk supply (AND, 2020; USDA & DHHS, 2020). Nursing mothers should avoid appetite suppressants, which may pass into the milk. They should not use liquid diet drinks or diets, which severely restrict any nutrient, because they will not meet the infant's needs.

Adolescence. The problems of the adolescent diet continue to be of concern during lactation. Adolescents may be deficient in the same nutrients as other clients during lactation and may have a low iron intake. If they dislike or cannot afford fruits and vegetables, their intake of vitamins A and C may be inadequate. While adherence and consistency may be an issue with teens, they may benefit from a multivitamin supplement during lactation.

Vegan Diet. The milk of vegan clients may contain inadequate amounts of vitamin B_{12}, and they may need supplements. Calcium adequacy may also be a challenge because of the possible decreased intake and absorption from a plant-based diet. It is recommended to consider consuming an addition 200 mg of calcium per day in the diet to offset potential absorption limitations. Vegans can meet their need for other nutrients during lactation by diet alone with careful planning. Those who are not knowledgeable about nutrition should take supplements.

Avoidance of Dairy Products. The recommendation for calcium is the same for pregnancy and lactation, which is the same as nonpregnant clients. The calcium content of breast milk is not affected by maternal intake. During lactation, calcium is removed from the mother's bones. Research found that mothers who breastfed for 4 months or longer had bone density changes; however, with calcium supplementation, bone density increased higher than those mothers who did not take calcium supplements during lactation, and it is replaced, to some extent, when they are no longer breast-feeding (Cullers et al., 2019). Clients who do not eat dairy products should obtain calcium from other sources or take a calcium supplement. Unless they consume foods fortified with vitamin D or are exposed to sunlight, they may require vitamin D supplementation, which is necessary for calcium absorption.

Bariatric Surgery. Clients who have a history of bariatric surgery are encouraged to breastfeed if they desire, the same as the general population. Continued laboratory evaluation of micronutrients, as during pregnancy, is recommended and completed up to every 3 months while lactating; however breast milk nutrients and composition has been found to be similar in clients with a history of bariatric surgery compared with clients of differing BMI categories who had not experienced weight reduction surgery (Jans et al., 2018). For clients with a gastric banding procedure, it is suggested to keep the band deflated at least until successful establishment of breast-feeding.

Inadequate Diet. Clients with cultural or other food prohibitions may need help choosing a diet adequate for lactation. Low-income clients may need referral to agencies such as WIC. If the client must take medications that interfere with absorption of certain nutrients, their diet should be high in foods containing those nutrients.

Nutrition for the Nonlactating Client

Postpartum clients who are not breastfeeding can return to their prepregnancy diet, provided it meets recommendations for their age group. Their diet should contain enough protein and vitamin C to promote healing. Many health care providers suggest clients continue to take their prenatal vitamin–mineral supplements until their supply is finished. This ensures adequate intake during the time of involution and helps renew nutrient stores.

The nurse should assess the client's understanding of the amount of food needed from each food group. A review of important nutrient sources for calcium and iron may be relevant. If the client was anemic during pregnancy, the client should continue to take an iron supplement until the Hgb level returns to normal.

Weight Loss

When the baby is born, the client can expect to lose about 4.5 to 5.8 kg (10 to 13 lb) immediately followed by approximately 3.2 to 5 kg (7 to 11 lb) weight loss during the first week. The greatest weight loss can be expected during the first 3 months after birth. If weight gain during pregnancy has not been excessive, the client will probably lose all but about 1 kg (2.2 lb) within a year with a well-balanced diet (Blackburn, 2018). The client should decrease caloric intake to normal nonpregnant levels to avoid retaining weight. Suggestions for sensible calorie reduction combined with exercise are appropriate.

Clients who gain excess weight during pregnancy may have difficulty losing it after birth and may need help from a dietitian to plan a weight loss program. Those who do not

lose the weight gained during pregnancy may begin the next pregnancy overweight, and this may lead to further retention of weight after birth.

Clients are sometimes so involved with the needs of the infant that they fail to eat properly. They may snack instead of planning meals for themselves, especially if they are home alone with the baby during the early weeks. The nurse should remind them snacking often involves high caloric intake without meeting nutritional needs. During the postpartum period, clients need to ensure their own good health so they are able to care for their baby. Therefore, meals and snacks should be high in nutrient content.

> ### ? KNOWLEDGE CHECK
>
> 18. How do the nutritional needs of the lactating client compare with those who are not lactating?
> 19. What changes should the client who is not breastfeeding make after the birth of the baby?

APPLICATION OF THE NURSING PROCESS: NUTRITION FOR CHILDBEARING

The nursing process focuses on determining any factors that might interfere with the client's ability to meet the nutrient needs of pregnancy, postpartum, and lactation and finding solutions to any problems identified. This process primarily involves client and family education.

Assessment
Interview

The interview provides an opportunity to develop rapport and identify any specific problems affecting dietary intake.

Appetite. Begin the interview by discussing the client's appetite. Has it changed during the pregnancy? How does it compare with their appetite before pregnancy? Morning sickness may decrease food intake during the first trimester. Determine the severity and duration of nausea and vomiting. Hyperemesis gravidarum is the most serious form of this problem and may require intravenous correction of fluid and electrolyte imbalance and parenteral nutrition (see Chapter 10).

Eating Habits. Assess the usual pattern of meals to discover poor food habits such as skipping breakfast, eating only snack foods for lunch, or eating fast foods for most meals. Determine who cooks for the family. If someone else does the cooking, discuss nutritional needs during pregnancy with that person. If the client does the cooking, the likes and dislikes of other family members may influence what is served, especially if there is little understanding of nutritional needs during pregnancy.

Food Preferences. Ask the client about food preferences and dislikes. Some people experience aversions to certain foods, such as meats, only during pregnancy. Careful counseling helps work around dislikes and aversions to find ways of obtaining the nutrients needed. For example, if the client dislikes most vegetables, fruits may often be substituted.

Discussing likes and dislikes provides an opening to ask about food cravings and pica. Cravings may be for nutritional foods or foods low in nutrient density or eaten in amounts that interfere with intake of other foods. Ask about pica in a matter-of-fact manner to avoid giving an impression of disapproval. Food items such as ice are included in pica, and the nurse should ask about it as well. Also determine whether the client eats large amounts of a particular food or group of foods.

When assessing for pica the nurse might say, "Have you had any cravings for special things to eat during your pregnancy?" This can be followed with, "People sometimes eat things like ice, clay, dirt, and laundry starch during pregnancy. Have you tried these?"

Potential Problems. Identify any obvious areas of potential deficiency. For example, the client might eat little meat, avoid vegetables, be lactose intolerant, or follow a fad diet. Assess the client's knowledge about nutritional needs during pregnancy. Inquire how long the vegetarian has followed that diet, determine which foods are included, and determine the awareness of changes necessary during pregnancy.

Psychosocial Influences

Psychosocial factors should be assessed because they can affect dietary intake. People who are fatigued, stressed, and anxious during pregnancy may consume more high-calorie foods but have lower intake of some important nutrients. The diets of postpartum clients are also affected by psychosocial factors. Those with stress, weight-related concerns, negative body image, and depressive symptoms are less likely to eat healthful diets.

Identify cultural or religious considerations that affect the diet. Do these apply only during pregnancy or at all times? Assess whether the client follows all or only certain restrictions, and determine the effect on their nutrient intake.

Identify other factors that affect nutrition. Those with low incomes may not know about sources of assistance. Smoking habits, alcohol intake, and other substance abuse may become obvious during the interview. Determine whether any medications are taken that interfere with nutrient absorption. Other questions include the amount of time the client has for food preparation and the frequency of fast food intake.

Provide an opportunity for the client to ask about special dietary concerns. This may bring out fears about weight gain, worry about specific foods could hurt the fetus, or other issues that have not yet been addressed.

Diet History

Diet histories provide information about a client's usual intake of nutrients. Food intake records, 24-hour diet histories, and food frequency questionnaires can form a basis for counseling about any changes required to meet pregnancy needs. They also help clients become more aware of their eating habits.

Food Intake Records. Food intake records are used to report foods eaten over one or more days. Instruct the client to list everything they eat throughout the day. The list is more accurate if it is written immediately after eating. Some clients eat more nutritious foods during the recording period when they are concentrating on good diet and then return to a less wholesome diet later.

24-Hour Diet History. Ask the client to recall what they ate at each meal and snack during the previous 24 hours. Use specific questions about the size of portions, ingredients, and food preparation for each meal. Models of food items and measuring utensils may be helpful to determine portion sizes. Inquire about beverages and snacks between meals and at bedtime. Ask if this sample is typical of their usual daily food intake. If it is not, ask what foods are more representative of the usual intake. Analyze the diet to determine whether the client has met the recommendations for specific food groups, calories, and protein. Detailed analysis for individual nutrients is unnecessary because it is time-consuming and because daily variation in intake occurs.

The food history may be inaccurate if clients cannot remember what they ate or are mistaken about amounts of food. Expectant clients may alter their reported intake to make it appear they are eating better. They may be embarrassed about their inability to follow the diet prescribed because of lack of money or cooking facilities. The atmosphere created by the nurse is important in helping clients feel free to be honest.

Food Frequency Questionnaires. Food frequency questionnaires, which contain lists of common foods, may provide information about diet over a longer period. Review the questionnaire with the client and ask how often they eat each food. Foods consumed daily and weekly are the most common source of nutrients. Analyze the list to determine whether foods from each food group are eaten in adequate amounts to meet pregnancy needs and determine whether any major groups are omitted.

Physical Assessment

Information about nutritional status can be obtained during the physical assessment. This assessment includes measurement of weight and examination for signs of nutritional deficiency.

Weight and Height at Initial Visit. Weigh the client at the first prenatal visit to provide a baseline value for future comparison. Ask if the client has gained or lost weight. Measure height without shoes because the client may not have had a recent accurate measurement. Determine the BMI from the prepregnancy weight and height to draw conclusions about the nutritional condition. If the client's weight is low for height, nutritional reserves are marginal.

Weight at Subsequent Visits. Assessment of weight gain at each prenatal visit provides an easy method of estimating whether nutrition is adequate and serves as a basis for counseling. Weigh the client at each visit on the same scale with approximately the same amount of clothing.

Record the weight on a weight grid at each visit throughout the pregnancy (Fig. 8.1). This grid allows examination of the pattern of weight gain. It helps keep track of the amount of gain between individual visits and provides the total gain to date.

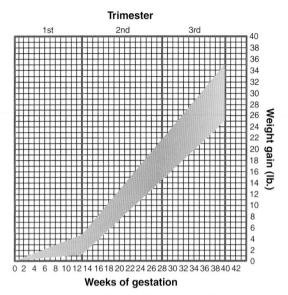

Fig. 8.1 Weight Gain Grid for Pregnancy. The normal range for weight gain is 11.5 to 16 kg (25 to 35 lb).

Be careful not to overemphasize weight gain. In some instances, a client may be afraid caregivers will be disapproving if they gain weight and consequently may diet or fast a day or two before the prenatal visit.

Signs of Nutrient Deficiency. Observe for indications of nutritional status or any signs of deficiency. For example, bleeding gums may indicate inadequate intake of vitamin C. Actual deficiency states, however, are not likely to occur in clients in most industrialized countries. The exception is iron deficiency anemia, which is common in a mild form. Signs and symptoms include pallor, low Hgb level, fatigue, and increased susceptibility to infection.

Laboratory Tests

Laboratory tests for in-depth analysis of nutrient intake are generally impractical. Analysis of specific nutrients is expensive, and normal laboratory values during pregnancy have not been determined for all laboratory tests. Hemoglobin (Hgb), hematocrit (Hct), and, in some cases, serum ferritin tests are most often used to determine anemia.

Ongoing Nutritional Status

At each prenatal visit (1) reassess the client's dietary status; (2) ask if there are any questions about diet or if the client is having any difficulty; (3) check the weight gain to see whether it is within the expected pattern; (4) evaluate Hgb and Hct levels to detect anemia, if appropriate; and (5) explain what assessments are being made and why.

Identification of Client Problems

Although some clients consume more calories than necessary during pregnancy and risk obesity as a result, others are likely to eat fewer nutrients than recommended. The problem may be related to many factors, the most common of which is general lack of knowledge of nutrition. Analysis of the data collected enables the nurse to identify actual and potential client problems and develop an individualized plan of care.

Planning: Expected Outcomes

The expected outcomes for an actual or potential nutritional problem in pregnancy include the following:
- The client's daily diet will include the recommended amount of food from each food group for pregnancy.
- The client with a normal BMI before pregnancy will gain approximately 0.5 to 2 kg (1.1 to 4.4 lb) during the first trimester and 0.35 to 0.5 kg (0.8 to 1 lb) per week during the second and third trimesters for a total gain of 11.5 to 16 kg (25 to 35 lb).

Interventions
Identifying Problems

After analyzing food likes and dislikes and taking a 24-hour diet history, identify any obvious deficient areas and determine the client's knowledge about the nutrient needs of pregnancy. If the client is experiencing pica, try to find foods to replace the substances being eaten. Crunchy foods may replace some ice ingestion. Other clients are willing to make substitutions such as nonfat dry milk powder for laundry starch or baby powder.

Explaining Nutrient Needs

Use the client's diet history as a basis to introduce information about nutrition during pregnancy. Explain the recommended servings from each food group, help the client analyze their own diet so they understand the process, and determine whether the number of servings recommended for each food group are being met. Explain which important nutrients are provided in each food group and why they are necessary for mother and fetus.

Calculate a rough estimate of calories, protein, iron, folic acid, and calcium in the diet to help identify whether the client eats enough of these foods on a regular basis. Compare the usual sources of these nutrients with the diet history and list of favorite foods. Suggest ways the client can increase deficient nutrients by increasing foods that are good sources. Advise the client that adequate nutrition, especially intake of iron and folic acid, may help reduce fatigue during pregnancy and after birth.

Providing Reinforcement

Give frequent positive reinforcement when the client is eating appropriately. Assist in evaluating weaknesses in the diet and planning ways to remedy them (Fig. 8.2). Ask what problems the client foresees in obtaining the nutrients needed. Explore a variety of options to overcome expected problems and ask about how these changes will affect the rest of the family. Perhaps the changes needed to meet the needs of the pregnancy would be beneficial to the entire family.

If the client can read, give printed materials in the preferred language on nutrition during pregnancy and review them with client. If the information can be taken home, it can be reviewed to ensure everyone is eating properly. A small

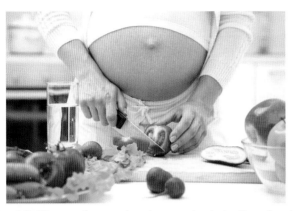

Fig. 8.2 Clients often make changes in their diets for the sake of their unborn children that they would not consider for themselves alone. (Courtesy YanLev, Photographer. © 2012 Photos.com, a division of Getty Images. All rights reserved.)

pamphlet with pictures might be placed on the refrigerator to help everyone remember what foods are needed each day.

Demonstrate portion sizes by utilizing plastic models of frequently eaten foods. These are available for various common and ethnic foods and help people understand how to incorporate cultural foods into the pregnancy food plan.

Evaluating Weight Gain

Compare the client's weight with a weight gain chart to ascertain whether the client has gained the appropriate amount of weight for this point in the pregnancy. Discuss the importance and expected pattern of weight gain and explain the need to eat foods high in nutrient density when increasing calories. If the client's weight is greatly outside of normal ranges, discuss necessary diet modifications with the primary health care provider. For example, an obese client is expected to gain some weight, but the amount should be individualized according to the needs of the client.

Although slight variations from the recommended weight gain have little significance, possible reasons for larger differences should be examined carefully. For clients of normal weight, a monthly gain of less than 1 kg (2.2 lb) should lead to a discussion of diet and possible problems in food intake. A gain of more than 2.9 kg (6.5 lb) per month may signify edema or problems with increased calorie consumption. However, errors in calculation of gestation may reflect a pattern of weight gain different from what was expected.

Encouraging Supplement Intake

If vitamin–mineral supplements have been prescribed, determine whether the client takes them regularly and, if

not, explore reasons and possible solutions. Iron supplements often cause constipation, but dietary changes such as increased intake of fluids and fiber can help prevent this problem (Box 8.3). If the client is forgetting to take the supplement, suggest taking vitamin–mineral supplements with meals or iron tablets with orange juice at bedtime just before nightly dental hygiene. If the client is avoiding iron supplements because of side effects such as nausea, a reminder to take them with meals or snacks may help. Even though taking iron supplements with food decreases the absorption of the iron, it is preferred to not using the supplements at all. Let the client know black stools are a harmless side effect of iron supplements.

Making Referrals

The nurse can provide adequate nutritional counseling for most clients, but some situations warrant referral to other sources. Refer clients with health problems affecting nutrition (such as diabetes, celiac disease, extreme weight problems) to a dietitian with follow-up by the nurse. Clients with inadequate financial resources to buy food can be referred to public assistance programs such as WIC. At the next visit, determine whether the client/family obtained the help needed and whether other assistance is necessary.

Evaluation

Ongoing evaluation of diet and pattern of weight gain throughout the pregnancy determines whether the goals have been met. The client should eat the recommended amounts of foods from each food group daily. The client should gain approximately 0.5 to 2 kg (1.1 to 4.4 lb) during the first trimester and 0.35 to 0.5 kg (0.8 to 1 lb) per week during the rest of the pregnancy. Total weight gain should be about 11.5 to 16 kg (25 to 35 lb).

SUMMARY CONCEPTS

- Nutritional education during the childbearing period may have long-term positive effects on the client, the infant, and the entire family.
- Weight gain during pregnancy is an important determinant of fetal growth. Poor weight gain in pregnancy is associated with low-birth-weight and SGA infants.

- Excessive weight gain may lead to increased birthweight, gestational diabetes, labor complications, and postpartum weight retention.
- The recommended weight gain during pregnancy for clients of normal prepregnancy weight is 11.5 to 16 kg (25 to 35 lb). The amount is greater for clients who are

underweight or who carry more than one fetus, and it is less for those who are overweight or obese.

- The pattern of weight gain is also important. The client should gain 0.5 to 2 kg (1.1 to 4.4 lb) during the first trimester and 0.35 to 0.5 kg (0.8 to 1 lb) per week thereafter.
- The recommended increase in daily energy intake during pregnancy is 340 calories in the second trimester and 452 calories in the third trimester. Calorie increases should be attained by choosing foods high in nutrient density to meet the other needs of pregnancy.
- Protein should be increased to 71 g daily during pregnancy and lactation, which is 25 g more than nonpregnancy needs.
- Some clients may not eat enough foods high in vitamins and minerals to meet recommendations.
- Fat-soluble vitamins (A, D, E, K) are stored in the liver, fat (adipose) tissue, and skeletal muscle. Excess consumption may result in toxic effects.
- Daily intake of water-soluble vitamins and folic acid is necessary because excesses are not stored but excreted.
- Minerals that may not be consumed at recommended amounts during pregnancy are iron and calcium. Iron is often added as a supplement, and calcium is added for clients with low intake.
- Vitamin–mineral supplements should be used carefully to prevent excessive intake and toxicity. Increased intake of some nutrients interferes with use of others.
- Pregnant and lactating clients should drink approximately 8 to 10 cups of fluids each day. They should eat 6 to 8 oz of whole grains, 2.5 to 3 cups of vegetables, 2 cups of fruits, 3 cups of the dairy group, and 6 to 6.5 oz of protein foods daily.
- Culture can influence diet during pregnancy. The nurse should learn whether a client follows specific dietary practices and whether the food practices are consistent with good nutrition.

- Low-income clients may not have enough money or knowledge to meet the nutrient needs of pregnancy. Nurses should refer them for financial assistance and nutritional counseling.
- Pregnant vegetarians may need help choosing a diet with adequate nonanimal sources of nutrients.
- Bariatric surgery clients are encouraged to avoid pregnancy for the first 12 to 24 months post procedure and require additional micronutrient evaluation with potential supplementation during pregnancy and lactation.
- Lactose-intolerant clients should increase calcium intake from foods other than cow or other animal milk, such as calcium-rich vegetables and fortified plant-based milks and other products.
- Abnormal prepregnancy weight, anemia, eating disorders, pica, multiparity, substance abuse, closely spaced pregnancies, and multifetal pregnancies are all nutritional risk factors that warrant adaptations of diet during pregnancy and lactation.
- Adolescents may skip meals and eat snacks and fast foods of low nutrient density. They are subject to peer pressure which may decrease their nutritional intake.
- Lactating clients need an additional daily intake of 330 calories during the first 6 months, with the remaining 170 calories drawn from maternal stores for a total of 500 calories per day. During the second 6 months of breastfeeding, an added daily intake of 400 calories is needed.
- Lactating clients should avoid alcohol and excess caffeine.
- The postpartum client who does not breastfeed should resume prepregnant caloric intake and eat a well-balanced diet to enhance recovery from childbirth. Weight loss should be accomplished slowly and sensibly.

▌ Clinical Judgment And Next-Generation NCLEX® Examination-Style Questions

Nutrition in Pregnancy

The school nurse evaluates a 17-year-old high school senior, who identifies as female, using pronouns she/her/hers. During a visit to the clinic, she complaints of nausea and "just being so tired." The client reports that she wakes up most mornings the past 2 weeks so sick she can barely get out of bed. The client states she does not want to eat because she hates to throw up. Student states she is sleeping 10 to 12 hours a night and wants to nap during the day. When questioned by the nurse, the client denies having a period for about 2 months and upon further questioning, the nurse determines that it is possible the client is about 11 weeks pregnant. The pregnancy is confirmed with a urine pregnancy test. The school nurse refers the client to the high school pregnancy clinic where they complete an assessment and begin prenatal care with the resident nurse midwife.

Physical assessment reveals the client weighs 48.5 kgs (106.7 lb) and is 65 inches tall. Her apical pulse is 106, respiratory rate (RR) 18, blood pressure (BP) 106/66, temperature (temp) 98.4, and oxygen saturation (SpO$_2$) is 98% at initial assessment. Fetal heart rate (FHR) by ultrasound is 144 bpm. The client denies taking any medications, supplements, alcohol, or tobacco use. The client states no allergies to food or medications. The client states this is the first pregnancy (G1P0) and has only been sexually active with one partner and only for a few months. Denies use of any contraception.

The client is single, lives with her parents, is a cheerleader, has a GPA 3.6, and plans to attend community college after graduation in a few months. The client denies being in a long-term relationship and begs the midwife to "not tell anyone about this pregnancy, not my parents, not anybody!" Prenatal laboratories are drawn, and a second appointment at the pregnancy clinic is made for 2 weeks to assess nausea and review laboratory work. Daily prenatal vitamins have been given to the client to begin taking each morning.

1. **Highlight or place a check mark next to the assessment findings that require follow-up by the nurse.**
   Single 17-year-old female
   High school student
   Lives with parents
   HR 106
   RR 18
   BP 106/66
   Urine pregnancy test
   FHR 144 bpm
   Medication use
   Supplement use
   Alcohol/tobacco use
   Height
   Weight
   Contraception
   Nausea
   Sleep pattern

2. **Use an X to indicate whether the nursing actions listed below are <u>indicated</u> (appropriate or necessary), <u>contraindicated</u> (could be harmful), or <u>nonessential</u> (make no difference or are not necessary) for the client's care at this time.**

Nursing Action	Indicated	Contraindicated	Non-Essential
Educate client about the relation of nutrition and fetal growth.			
Provide education regarding foods that contain iron, calcium, folic acid, and protein.			
Ask client to complete a food diary for 7 days.			
Suggest vitamin supplementations such as vitamin D, iron, folate, and calcium.			
Refer client to a registered dietitian to answer questions and provide further education.			
Discuss the need for fluid intake during pregnancy including water, diet sodas, electrolyte-enhanced sports drinks, iced tea, and coffee.			

Nursing Action	Indicated	Contraindicated	Non-Essential
Encourage food intake including age-appropriate foods such as hamburgers, fries, chicken nuggets, fried vegetables, and cheese sticks.			
Encourage client to eat three healthy meals a day to increase nutrition and avoid snacking.			
Provide a scale for home weight-monitoring and encourage daily weights for the pregnant client.			

3. **Indicate which nursing response listed in the far-left column is appropriate for the client's question. Note that not all actions will be used.**

Nurse's Responses	Client Questions	Appropriate Nurse's Response for Each Client Question
1. "Normal weight gain during pregnancy is 25–35 lb. You are currently underweight so you should plan on gaining around 30–35 lb. to help you have a healthy baby."	"I don't like taking any medicines, why do I need to take these prenatal vitamins?"	
2. "Protein is important to help your baby grow. You should be eating foods high in protein since you need about 25 g of protein in your diet every day more than you did before you were pregnant."	"How am I supposed to eat a healthy diet when I feel sick all the time?"	
3. "Fried foods like chicken nuggets, fries, and fried cheese sticks are high in fat and calories. Candy, sugary soda, and cookies are high in sugar and calories. Foods high in fat can make your nausea worse."	"What foods do I need to avoid?"	

Nurse's Responses	Client Questions	Appropriate Nurse's Response for Each Client Question
4. "Morning sickness is a temporary condition that usually goes away after the first trimester of pregnancy. It may be relieved with ginger or peppermint tea. Eating small frequent meals help maintain your blood sugar level and may make eating more tolerable. A nighttime high-protein snack may help maintain your glucose level during the night. Try eating crackers or other carbohydrate before you get out of bed in the morning, and that may help with nausea in the morning."	"I don't want to gain weight. How can I keep from gaining weight while I am pregnant?"	
5. "Folic acid is needed to help your baby develop. Folic acid is available in your diet, but many people do not eat enough foods high in folate."		
6. "Reading food labels will be helpful to identify foods high in protein, carbohydrates, sugars, or fats. Selecting foods low in fat and sugar content provide nutrients you need to help your baby grow and helps you avoid high-calorie foods that are not as nutritious."		
7. "Oats, whole grains, fruits, and vegetables are high in fiber to help prevent constipation."		

The client misses the 2-week follow-up clinic appointment and states she just did not feel like coming to the clinic. The client returns to the clinic 6 weeks after the first appointment and is now at 17 weeks' gestational age. Current weight was 48.8 kg, and the client states nausea is no longer a problem.

Vital Signs (VS): Heart rate 88, RR 18, temp 97.6, BP 102/66, FHR 152 bpm by ultrasound. Client's parent is present at this visit and expresses concern that the client is not eating "healthy meals" but only little snacks all day long. Client's laboratory from first visit showed Hgb 9.8 g/dL. The midwife asks the client to provide a 24-hour diet history from the previous day. The client provides the following information:

Breakfast: a banana and a diet soda; morning snack: a banana, a cheese stick, and a diet soda; lunch: fries and a hot dog and diet soda; afternoon snack: peanut butter and apple slices; dinner: a hamburger and fries from a local fast-food restaurant after cheer practice with lemonade; bedtime snack: cookies and a glass of milk. Client states these are their favorite foods and eats the same things almost every day.

Client states the prenatal vitamins are causing nausea, so she only takes them a "couple times a week." The client's parent stated that the client is also constipated and complains of a stomach ache 2 or 3 days a week. Client admits bowel pattern has changed and now only has a bowel movement a couple of times a week. A stool softener has been added to the client's medication list and client has been encouraged to add more fruits, vegetables, and fluids to her diet.

4. **Highlight or place a check mark next to the assessment findings that require follow-up by the nurse.**
   Maternal vital signs
   Lab results
   Fetal heart rate
   Parent present at visit
   24-hour food history
   Medication use
   Supplement use
   Weight
   Nausea
   Constipation

5. **For each client response, use an X to indicate whether the nurse's teaching was <u>effective</u> (helped the client understand nutritional needs in pregnancy), <u>ineffective</u> (did not help the client understand nutritional needs in pregnancy), or <u>unrelated</u> (not related to the health teaching about nutritional needs in pregnancy).**

Client Response	Effective	Ineffective	Unrelated
"I need to add calcium to my diet. Dairy products, salmon, and calcium fortified juice will help me add calcium to my diet."			
"I should take my iron in the morning with milk to help prevent me from being nauseated when I take it."			
"Because the prenatal vitamins make me feel sick, I should not take vitamin supplementation."			

Client Response	Effective	Ineffective	Unrelated
"I can consume plain milk, yogurt, cheese, beef, nuts, tofu, and green leafy vegetables to increase my protein, iron, and calcium."			
"Oats, whole grains, watermelon, prunes, vegetables are high in fiber that can help with constipation."			
"Fruit juice, coffee, iced tea, and soda will help me increase my fluids during my pregnancy."			

Client Response	Effective	Ineffective	Unrelated
"Since I like sandwiches, ham and turkey lunch meat should be a staple in my refrigerator."			
"If I develop nausea, I need to write down what I ate so I can make a list of foods to avoid."			
"I need to ensure I take my prenatal vitamin with orange juice because it enhances the amount of iron I get from the medication."			

REFERENCES & READINGS

Academy of Nutrition and Dietetics (AND). (2020). *Adult nutrition care manual.* http://www.nutritioncaremanual.org.

Agency for Healthcare Research and Quality (AHRQ). (2018). *Screening for and management of obesity.* www.ahrq.gov/ncepcr/tools/healthier-pregnancy/fact-sheets/obesity.html.

Al-Nimr, R. I., Hakeem, R., Moreschi, J. M., Gallo, S., McDermid, J. M., Pari-Keener, M., et al. (2019). Effects of bariatric surgery on maternal and infant outcomes of pregnancy - An evidence analysis center systematic review. *Journal of the Academy of Nutrition and Dietetics, 119*(11), 1921–1943. https://doi.org/10.1016/j.jand.2019.02.008.

American Academy of Pediatrics & American College of Obstetricians and Gynecologists (AAP & ACOG). (2017). *Guidelines for perinatal care* (8th ed.).

American Academy of Pediatrics & American College of Obstetricians and Gynecologists (AAP & ACOG). (2020). *Practice advisory: Seafood consumption during pregnancy.* Published 2014, reaffirmed 2020.

American College of Obstetricians and Gynecologists (ACOG). (2017). *Bariatric surgery and pregnancy.* ACOG Practice Bulletin, 105. Published June 2009, reaffirmed 2017.

American College of Obstetricians and Gynecologists (ACOG). (2018a). *Listeria and pregnancy: FAQ501.* www.acog.org/womens-health/faqs/listeria-and-pregnancy.

American College of Obstetricians and Gynecologists (ACOG). (2018b). *Optimizing postpartum care.* ACOG Committee Opinion, 736. Published 2016, reaffirmed 2018.

American College of Obstetricians and Gynecologists (ACOG). (2020a). *Moderate caffeine consumption during pregnancy.* ACOG Committee opinion, 462. Published 2010, reaffirmed 2020.

American College of Obstetricians and Gynecologists (ACOG). (2020b). *Weight gain during pregnancy.* ACOG Committee Opinion, 548. Published 2013, reaffirmed 2020.

American College of Obstetricians and Gynecologists (ACOG). (2021). *Obesity in pregnancy.* ACOG Practice Bulletin, 230. Published 2015, reaffirmed 2021.

Blackburn, S. T. (2018). *Maternal, fetal, and neonatal physiology: A clinical perspective* (5th ed.). Elsevier.

Bodner, L. M., & Himes, K. P. (2019). Maternal nutrition. In R. Resnik, C. Lockwood, T. Moore, M. Greene, J. Copel, & R. Silver (Eds.), *Creasy & Resnik's maternal-fetal medicine: Principles and practice* (8th ed., pp. 181–189.e3). Elsevier.

Callister, L. C. (2021). Integrating cultural beliefs and practices when caring for childbearing women and families. In K. Simpson, P. Creehan, N. O'Brien-Abel, C. Roth, & A. Rohan (Eds.), *AWHONN's perinatal nursing* (5th ed., pp. 18–47). Wolters Kluwer.

Centers for Disease Control and Prevention (CDC). (2018). *Frequently asked questions about folic acid.* www.cdc.gov/ncbddd/folicacid/faqs/.

Centers for Disease Control and Prevention (CDC). (2021a). *About adult BMI.* www.cdc.gov/healthyweight/assessing/bmi/adult_bmi/.

Centers for Disease Control and Prevention (CDC). (2021b). *Weight gain during pregnancy.* www.cdc.gov/reproductivehealth/maternalinfanthealth/pregnancy-weight-gain.htm.

Cullers, A., King, J. C., Van Loan, M., Gildengorin, G., & Fung, E. B. (2019). Effect of prenatal calcium supplementation on bone during pregnancy and 1 y postpartum. *The American Journal of Clinical Nutrition, 109*(1), 197–206. https://doi.org/10.1093/ajcn/nqy233.

Cunningham, F. G., Leveno, K. J., Bloom, S. L., Dashe, J. S., Hoffman, B. L., Casey, B. M., & Spong, C. Y. (2022). *Williams' obstetrics* (26th ed.). McGraw-Hill Companies.

Goldstein, R. F., Abell, S. K., Ranasinha, S., Misso, M., Boyle, J. A., Black, M. H., et al. (2017). Association of gestational weight gain with maternal and infant outcomes: A systematic review and meta-analysis. *Journal of the American Medical Association, 317*(21), 2207–2225. https://doi.org/10.1001/jama.2017.3635.

Grodner, M., Escott-Stump, S., & Dorner, S. (2020). *Nutritional foundations & clinical applications: A nursing approach* (8th ed., pp.142, 180–183). Elsevier.

Institute of Medicine (IOM). (2006). *Dietary reference intakes: The essential guide to nutrient requirements.* The National Academies Press.

Institute of Medicine (IOM). (2009). *Weight gain during pregnancy: Reexamining the guidelines.* http://iom.edu/Reports/2009/Weight-Gain-During-Pregnancy-Reexamining-the-Guidelines.aspx.

Institute of Medicine (IOM). (2011). *Dietary reference intakes for calcium and vitamin D.* The National Academies Press.

Institute of Medicine (IOM), Food and Nutrition Board (FNB). (1997). *Dietary reference intakes for calcium, phosphorus, magnesium, vitamin D, and fluoride.* The National Academies Press.

Institute of Medicine (IOM), Food and Nutrition Board (FNB). (1998). *Dietary reference intakes for thiamin, riboflavin, niacin, vitamin B$_6$, folate, vitamin B$_{12}$, pantothenic acid, biotin, and choline.* The National Academies Press.

Institute of Medicine (IOM), Food and Nutrition Board (FNB). (2000). *Dietary reference intakes for vitamin C, vitamin E, selenium, and carotenoids.* The National Academies Press.

Institute of Medicine (IOM), Food and Nutrition Board (FNB). (2001). *Dietary reference intakes for vitamin A, vitamin K, arsenic, boron, chromium, copper, iodine, iron, manganese, molybdenum, nickel, silicon, vanadium, and zinc.* The National Academies Press.

Institute of Medicine (IOM), Food and Nutrition Board (FNB). (2005). *Dietary reference intakes for energy, carbohydrates, fiber, protein and amino acids (macronutrients).* The National Academies Press.

Jans, G., Devlieger, R., De Preter, V., Ameye, L., Roelens, K., Lannoo, M., et al. (2018). Bariatric surgery does not appear to affect women's breast-milk composition. *The Journal of Nutrition, 148*(7), 1096–1102. https://doi.org/10.1093/jn/nxy085.

Kominiarek, M. A., & Rajan, P. (2016). Nutrition recommendations in pregnancy and lactation. *Medical Clinic of North America, 100*(6), 1199–1215. https://doi.org/10.1016/j.mcna.2016.06.004.

Korsmo, H. W., Jiang, X., & Caudill, M. A. (2019). Choline: Exploring the growing science on its benefits for moms and babies. *Nutrients, 11*(8), 1823. https://doi.org/10.3390/nu11081823.

Larson, N., Leak, T., & Stang, J. (2020). Nutrition in adolescence. In J. Raymond, & K. Morrow (Eds.), *Krause and Mahan's food & the nutrition care process* (15th ed., pp. 341–361). Elsevier.

Lipworth, H., Melamed, N., Berger, H., Geary, M., McDonald, S. D., et al. (2021). Maternal weight gain and pregnancy outcomes in twin gestations. *American Journal of Obstetrics and Gynecology*, 1.e1–1.e12. https://doi.org/10.1016/j.ajog.2021.04.260.

Mantel, A., Hirschberg, A. L., & Stephansson, O. (2020). Association of maternal eating disorders with pregnancy and neonatal outcomes. *JAMA Psychiatry, 77*(3), 285. https://doi.org/10.1001/jamapsychiatry.2019.3664.

March of Dimes. (2020). *Caffeine in pregnancy.* Retrieved from https://www.marchofdimes.org/pregnancy/caffeine-in-pregnancy.aspx.

Martin, J. A., Hamilton, B. E., Osterman, M. J. K., & Driscoll, A. K. (2021). Births: Final data for 2019. *National Vital Statistics Reports, 68*(13). www.cdc.gov/nchs/products/index.htm.

Melina, V., Craig, W., & Levin, S. (2016). Position of the academy of nutrition and dietetics: Vegetarian diet. *Journal of the Academy of Nutrition and Dietetics, 116*(12), 1970–1980. https://doi.org/10.1016/j.jand.2016.09.025.

National Academies of Sciences, Engineering, and Medicine (NASEM). (2020). *Nutrition during pregnancy and lactation: Exploring new evidence: Proceedings of a workshop.* The National Academies Press. https://doi.org/10.17226/25841.

Pécheux, O., Garabedian, C., Drumez, E., Mizrahi, S., Cordiez, S., Deltombe, S., et al. (2019). Maternal and neonatal outcomes according to gestational weight gain in twin pregnancies: Are the institute of medicine guidelines associated with better outcomes? *European Journal of Obstetrics & Gynecology and Reproductive Biology, 234*, 190–194. https://doi.org/10.1016/j.ejogrb.2019.01.010.

Procter, S. B., & Campbell, C. G. (2014). Position of the academy of nutrition and dietetics: Nutrition and lifestyle for a healthy pregnancy outcome. *Journal of the Academy of Nutrition and Dietetics, 114*(7), 1099–1103. https://doi.org/10.1016/j.jand.2014.05.005.

Roy, A., Fuentes-Afflick, E., Fernald, L. C. H., & Young, S. L. (2018). Pica is prevalent and strongly associated with iron deficiency among Hispanic pregnant women living in the United States. *Appetite, 120*, 163–170. https://doi.org/10.1016/j.appet.2017.08.033.

Sadeghi, E., Yas, A., Rabiepoor, S., & Sayyadi, H. (2020). Are anemia, gastrointestinal disorders, and pregnancy outcome associated with pica behavior? *Journal of Neonatal-Perinatal Medicine, 13*(4), 521–527. https://doi.org/10.3233/NPM-190257.

Sámano, R., Chico-Barba, G., Martínez-Rojano, H., Godínez, E., Rodríguez-Ventura, A. L., Ávila-Koury, G., et al. (2018). Pre-pregnancy body mass index classification and gestational weight gain on neonatal outcomes in adolescent mothers: A follow-up study. *PLoS ONE, 13*(7), e0200361. https://doi.org/10.1371/journal.pone.0200361.

Sebastiani, G., Barbero, A. H., Borrás-Novell, C., Casanova, M. A., Aldecoa-Bilbao, V., Andreu-Fernandez, V., et al. (2019). The effects of vegetarian and vegan diet during pregnancy on the health of mothers and offspring. *Nutrients, 11*(3), 557. https://doi.org/10.3390/nu11030557.

Stand, J., & Huffman, L. G. (2016). Position of the academy of nutrition and dietetics: Obesity, reproduction, and pregnancy outcomes. *Journal of the Academy of Nutrition and Dietetics, 116*(4), 677–691. https://doi.org/10.1016/j.jand.2016.01.008.

U.S. Department of Agriculture, Agricultural Research Service. (2016). *U.S. Department of Agriculture, Agricultural Research Service, Nutrient Data Laboratory.* USDA National Nutrient Database for Standard Reference, Release, 28.

U.S. Department of Agriculture and U.S. Department of Health and Human Services (USDA & DHHS). (2020). *Dietary Guidelines for Americans* (9th ed.). 2020–2025. https://www.dietaryguidelines.gov/sites/default/files/2020-12/Dietary_Guidelines_for_Americans_2020-2025.pdf.

U.S. Department of Health and Human Services (DHHS). (2020). *Healthy People 2030.* Author.

U.S. Food and Drug Administration (FDA). (2020). *Get the facts about Listeria.* www.fda.gov/animal-veterinary/animal-health-literacy/get-facts-about-listeria.

U.S. Preventive Services Task Force. (2017). Folic Acid Supplementation for the Prevention of Neural Tube Defects US Preventive Services Task Force Recommendation Statement. *Journal of the American Medical Association, 317*(2), 183–189.

Prenatal Diagnosis and Fetal Assessment During the Antepartum Period

Rebecca L. Cypher, Courtney M. Kujansuu

After studying this chapter, you should be able to:

1. Explain the difference between prenatal screening and diagnostic tests.
2. Discuss types of ultrasounds performed during pregnancy.
3. Compare and contrast the purpose of screening and diagnostic procedures discussed in this chapter.
4. Formulate specific indications for fetal diagnostic procedures.
5. Differentiate six methods of antepartum fetal testing (APFT).
6. Describe the role of the nurse in prenatal testing and APFT.

Prenatal testing and antepartum fetal surveillance (antepartum fetal testing - APFT) are the basis of contemporary obstetric care. In the early development of prenatal testing, fundamental approaches were used to verify fetal life; assess fetal size, growth, and position; and quantify amniotic fluid volume. Over several decades, expansion in fetal development research, innovative technologic advances in obstetric imaging and fetal therapy, and the sustained evolution of novel prenatal testing methods is bridging the gap in care between a fetus and an obstetric client. Clinicians are better equipped to establish fetal well-being; screen for genetic, structural, and chromosomal anomalies; and make diagnoses with greater accuracy related to the fetal condition. Nurses play an important role in this aspect of prenatal care by fostering an environment where communication, coordination, and expertise are vital to shared decision-making, continuity of care, and optimizing health care delivery.

GENERAL CONCEPTS IN PRENATAL SCREENING AND DIAGNOSIS

Advanced technologies have resulted in the discovery of more genetic conditions, which in turn has opened the door to more complex prenatal testing options (Hoskovec & Stevens, 2018). Today's perinatal clients are concerned about fetal health and well-being. Fortunately, 21st-century pregnancy care provides clients with previously unavailable information as well as updated testing options. The primary objective of prenatal screening and diagnosis is to detect genetic disorders or abnormalities that could affect an obstetric client, fetus, and newborn (American College of Obstetrics and Gynecology [ACOG], 2020b).

Screening Versus Diagnostic Testing

There are two categories of health care testing: screening and diagnostic. Nurses should know the differences between these categories to provide effective communication between and among clinicians and clients. Screening is primarily used to identify individuals who have a higher likelihood of having an abnormality or disease. Screening tests are not 100% accurate due to a risk for false-negative and false-positive results. A false-negative is when a result is normal but a disease or condition is present. For example, a screening test for chromosomal abnormalities is negative but trisomy 21 is diagnosed after birth. A false-positive occurs when there is a positive screening result but a chromosomally normal fetus is found with further testing. Therefore follow-up testing in the form of diagnostic testing may be necessary to confirm the presence or absence of the specific disease or condition. Most of the screening tests done during pregnancy are serum analyte screens, which are laboratory analysis of the pregnant client's blood for specific substances. To decrease the false negative and false positive results, these tests should be timed to the appropriate gestational age based on the specific condition for which the fetus is at risk.

Diagnostic testing is more precise for a given condition and usually provides "yes or no" answers about a condition or chromosomal abnormality. With shared decision-making, these tests are reasonable when a screening test is positive and diagnostic testing results will change management of the client or provide meaningful information about future prognosis. Think in terms of breast cancer; on a self-breast examination (screening) a new lump is discovered. After a thorough client and family history, as well a physical examination, a mammogram is obtained. Results of this mammogram prompt a diagnostic surgical breast biopsy. A pathology report confirms stage I invasive breast cancer, and this client is offered treatment options.

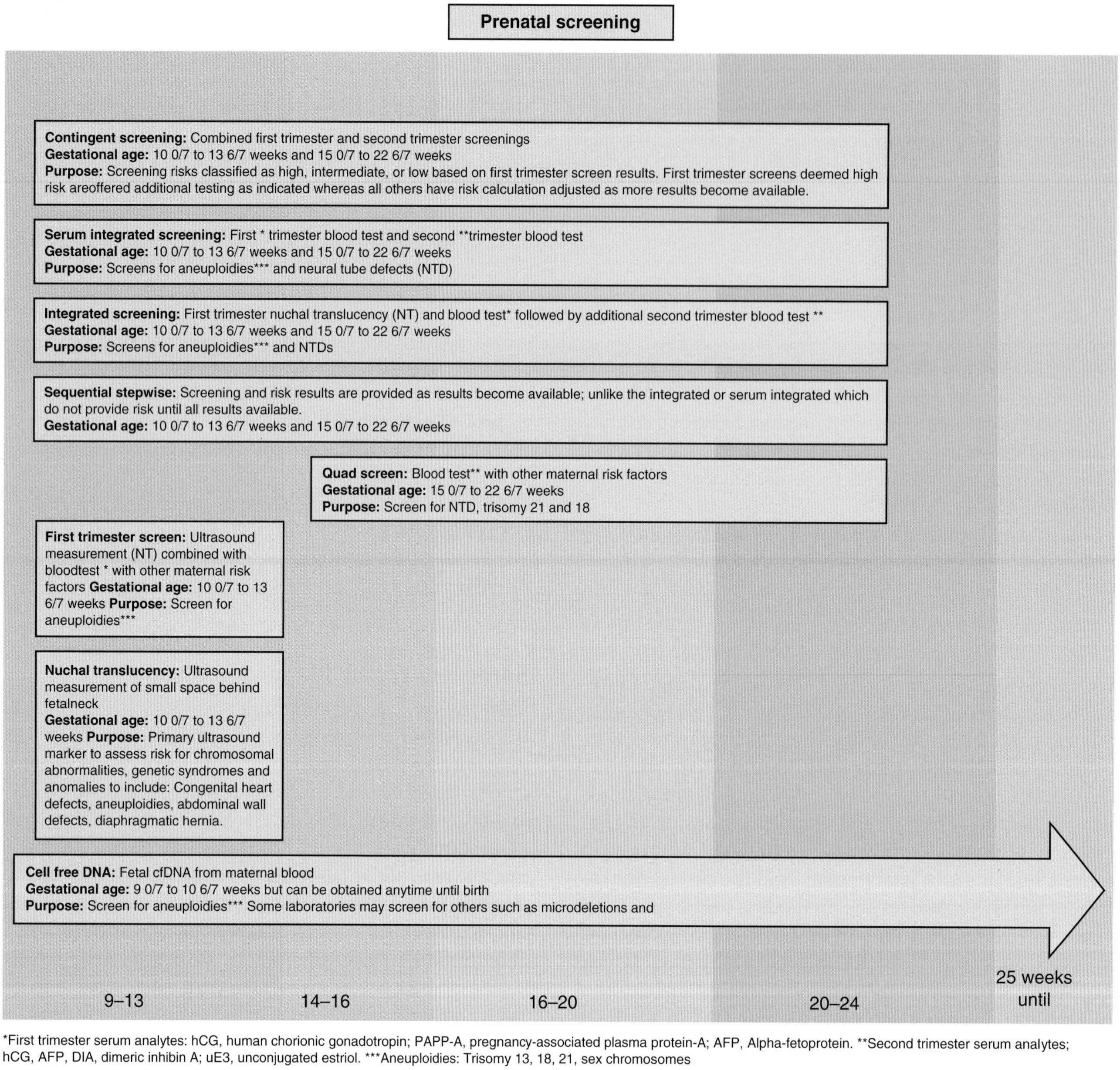

Prenatal screening

Contingent screening: Combined first trimester and second trimester screenings
Gestational age: 10 0/7 to 13 6/7 weeks and 15 0/7 to 22 6/7 weeks
Purpose: Screening risks classified as high, intermediate, or low based on first trimester screen results. First trimester screens deemed high risk areoffered additional testing as indicated whereas all others have risk calculation adjusted as more results become available.

Serum integrated screening: First * trimester blood test and second **trimester blood test
Gestational age: 10 0/7 to 13 6/7 weeks and 15 0/7 to 22 6/7 weeks
Purpose: Screens for aneuploidies*** and neural tube defects (NTD)

Integrated screening: First trimester nuchal translucency (NT) and blood test* followed by additional second trimester blood test **
Gestational age: 10 0/7 to 13 6/7 weeks and 15 0/7 to 22 6/7 weeks
Purpose: Screens for aneuploidies*** and NTDs

Sequential stepwise: Screening and risk results are provided as results become available; unlike the integrated or serum integrated which do not provide risk until all results available.
Gestational age: 10 0/7 to 13 6/7 weeks and 15 0/7 to 22 6/7 weeks

Quad screen: Blood test** with other maternal risk factors
Gestational age: 15 0/7 to 22 6/7 weeks
Purpose: Screen for NTD, trisomy 21 and 18

First trimester screen: Ultrasound measurement (NT) combined with bloodtest * with other maternal risk factors **Gestational age:** 10 0/7 to 13 6/7 weeks **Purpose:** Screen for aneuploidies***

Nuchal translucency: Ultrasound measurement of small space behind fetalneck
Gestational age: 10 0/7 to 13 6/7 weeks **Purpose:** Primary ultrasound marker to assess risk for chromosomal abnormalities, genetic syndromes and anomalies to include: Congenital heart defects, aneuploidies, abdominal wall defects, diaphragmatic hernia.

Cell free DNA: Fetal cfDNA from maternal blood
Gestational age: 9 0/7 to 10 6/7 weeks but can be obtained anytime until birth
Purpose: Screen for aneuploidies*** Some laboratories may screen for others such as microdeletions and

| 9–13 | 14–16 | 16–20 | 20–24 | 25 weeks until |

*First trimester serum analytes: hCG, human chorionic gonadotropin; PAPP-A, pregnancy-associated plasma protein-A; AFP, Alpha-fetoprotein. **Second trimester serum analytes; hCG, AFP, DIA, dimeric inhibin A; uE3, unconjugated estriol. ***Aneuploidies: Trisomy 13, 18, 21, sex chromosomes

Fig. 9.1 *First-trimester serum analytes: *AFP,* Alpha-fetoprotein; *hCG,* human chorionic gonadotropin; *PAPP-A,* pregnancy-associated plasma protein-A.

**Second-trimester serum analytes; hCG, AFP, DIA, dimeric inhibin A; uE3, unconjugated estriol.

***Aneuploidies: Trisomy 13, 18, 21, sex chromosomes.

Modified from Alldred, S. K., Takwoingi, Y., Guo, B., Pennant, M., Deeks, J. J., Neilson, J. P., & Alfirevic, Z. (2017). First and second trimester serum tests with and without first trimester ultrasound tests for Down's syndrome screening. *Cochrane Database of Systematic Reviews.* https://doi.org/10.1002/14651858. cd012599; American College of Obstetrics and Gynecology. (2019). Prenatal genetic testing chart. https://www.acog.org/womens-health/infographics/prenatal-genetic-testing-chart; American College of Obstetrics and Gynecology (ACOG). (2020b). *Screening for fetal chromosomal abnormalities.* ACOG Practice Bulletin 226.; Gil, M. M., Accurti, V., Santacruz, B., Plana, M. N., & Nicolaides, K.H. (2017). Analysis of cell-free DNA in maternal blood in screening for aneuploidies: Updated meta-analysis. *Ultrasound in Obstetrics & Gynecology, 50*(3), 302–314. https://doi.org/10.1002/uog.17484.

Single time point screening approaches include preimplantation genetic diagnosis (PGD); first-trimester screening (FTS); second-trimester triple, quadruple ("quad"), or penta screens; and cell-free DNA (cfDNA) (Fig. 9.1). Currently, penta screening is only offered in selected laboratories and is not a mainstream screening test. Some screening tests combine samples from the first and second trimesters and include *integrated, sequential,* and *contingent screening* (ACOG, 2020b). Diagnostic testing options include chorionic villus sampling (CVS), amniocentesis, and percutaneous umbilical blood sampling (PUBS).

Who Is Offered Prenatal Testing?

In the United States, prenatal testing for fetal chromosomal and genetic disorders, as well as fetal anomalies, is offered routinely to all pregnant clients regardless of age, family history, or obstetric history (ACOG, 2020b; Hoskovec & Stevens, 2018). Initial counseling is performed by obstetric providers. Genetic counseling by specially trained professionals is another communication process found in prenatal testing. These individuals can assist clients in understanding and adapting to the medical, psychosocial, and familial implications of genetic diseases (Hoskovec & Stevens, 2018). Screening and diagnostic tests are voluntary from a client perspective. Each client has a choice to decline or pursue available testing based on personal values, goals, and preferences (Cypher, 2019). Decisions may be based on family or ethnic traditions, and culture. Additionally, a client may ask for assistance from a trusted person, such as a spouse or significant other, family members, religious affiliations, or other health care providers. In a shared decision-making environment, unbiased, nondirective counseling about benefits and limitations of each test, as well as informed client consent, is provided before testing (ACOG, 2020a; ACOG, 2020b; Cypher, 2019; Knutzen & Stoll, 2019). These basic concepts are important because obstetric clients who receive well-informed counseling are more likely to decline prenatal testing. This is a reflection of clients being enabled to make informed prenatal decisions (Knutzen et al., 2013). Obstetric clients are advised there are no right or wrong answers when deciding to pursue prenatal screening and diagnosis.

Clinicians often have questions about the education and counseling process.

1. *Why do obstetric clients pursue screening and diagnostic testing?* Through a shared decision-making process prenatal screening and diagnostic testing can offer vital information to both clients and health care team members. For some clients, a normal result can provide reassurance. For others, waiting for results can impart fear, anxiety, and concern.

2. *What will a client do with the results?* If a screening test is positive the client has choices to pursue further testing during the pregnancy or decline testing until after birth. If diagnostic testing shows an abnormal result, this knowledge may give clients time to learn about the disorder, allow for referrals to specialists of the identified disorder, and seek information about an infant's future health care. Alternatively, obstetric clients can choose to electively end a pregnancy.

3. *Will test results influence prenatal management?* Some tests detect structural anomalies such as spina bifida (e.g., myelomeningocele). These conditions can sometimes be surgically repaired in utero. Screening and diagnosis may identify a condition, such as a congenital heart defect, which may necessitate a planned transfer to a specialized facility which can provide immediate evaluation and treatment at the time of birth.

Nursing Role in Prenatal Screening and Diagnosis

In addition to client and family education, nurses play an important role in prenatal testing including scheduling and assisting with invasive procedures. Nurses serve as one of the clients' primary resources of electronic and written information, often helping clients to understand available options and answering questions (Chard & Norton, 2016; Driscoll & Simpson, 2021). Finally, nurses are a crucial source of emotional support to perinatal clients and their support system.

ULTRASOUND

Ultrasound is one of the most valuable diagnostic tools in the obstetric field and is used consistently with prenatal testing (Richards, 2021). Prior to a discussion on individual prenatal screening and diagnostic tests, baseline knowledge related to obstetric sonography is needed. This procedure is often seen in the antepartum and intrapartum setting where nurses play an important role in client education and assisting other clinicians. Using high-frequency sound waves, real-time images of maternal structures, placenta, amniotic fluid, and fetus are visualized. More precisely, sound waves from an ultrasound transducer penetrate to the level of the structure being evaluated. Sound waves bounce back to a computer screen with images displayed as a type of video. Ultrasound may be paused at different points for obtaining measurements, or if closer imaging of specific structure needs to be acquired. Examinations are performed only when there is a valid medical reason and with the lowest possible settings to obtain adequate diagnostic information (Pellerito et al., 2018). Perinatal clients often have at least two ultrasound examinations during pregnancy; a dating ultrasound, typically performed during a first-trimester obstetric appointment to confirm pregnancy and estimated due date (EDD) and a second ultrasound between 18 and 22 weeks of gestation to assess fetal anatomy, growth and potential structural abnormalities. When an ultrasound examination is performed, clients are counseled about ultrasonography limitations regardless of ultrasound location, examiner's skill, or sophistication of equipment (ACOG, 2020c). Clients are informed that ultrasound carries unknown theoretical risks and is only performed for specific indications. There is a possibility, though small, that effects from these sound waves may have a biologic impact on the fetus (Richards, 2021).

Types of Ultrasound Images

Ultrasound images may appear as two- (2D), three- (3D), or four-dimensional (4D). Two dimensional provides a flat picture of an image because sound waves are sent straight down and reflected back to the transducer. Three-dimensional ultrasound provides a more advanced imaging technology so clinicians can visualize a structure's width, height, and depth. This type of ultrasound also provides greater detail of typical features and assists in identifying abnormalities. Although 3D ultrasound is not considered a requirement in routine obstetrics at this time, some facilities use 3D as an adjunct to 2D ultrasound, particularly when identifying fetal facial anomalies such as cleft lips (ACOG, 2020b; Richards, 2021) (Fig. 9.2).

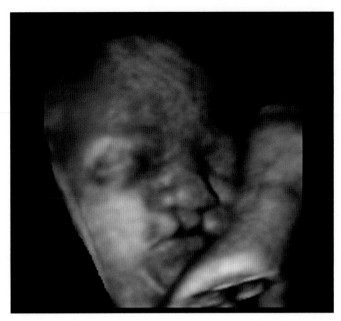

Fig. 9.2 Three-dimensional ultrasound image of a bilateral cleft lip. (From Goetzinger, K. R., & Odibo, A. O. (2017). Ultrasound evaluation of fetal aneuploidy in the first and second trimesters. In M. Norton, L. Scoutt, V. Feldstein (Eds.). *Callen's ultrasonography in obstetrics and gynecology.* (6th ed., pp. 57–81). Elsevier.)

Four-dimensional allows for live streaming video of images, such as fetal heart wall motion.

Transvaginal and Transabdominal Ultrasound

Obstetric ultrasounds are performed transvaginally or transabdominally. A client's bladder may need to be full when either approach is used in the first trimester to allow for better visualization. Transvaginal ultrasound requires a specially shaped transducer with a disposable probe cover containing ultrasound gel. The transducer is inserted into the vagina to create sharper images. Transvaginal ultrasound is commonly used in the first trimester for determining gestational age but is sometimes used in later gestations for cervical length measurements and definitive images of placental location. In contrast, a transabdominal approach uses one of several types of transducers depending on the gestational age, indication for ultrasound, and structure. A water-soluble transmission gel or lotion is applied to a client's abdomen as a lubricant to increase transmission of sound waves. After gel is applied, a transducer is maneuvered back and forth to visualize multiple structures or to view a single structure from different angles (Fig. 9.3). Ultrasound imaging results are documented for each examination and placed in a client's medical record. Ultrasound still images and those obtained with other media types, such as video, are uploaded into a secure clinic or hospital system connection for storage and review for future evaluations.

Ultrasound Categories

Three categories of obstetric ultrasound include standard (or basic), limited, and specialized (detailed or target). Basic obstetric ultrasound provides information about (ACOG, 2020c):

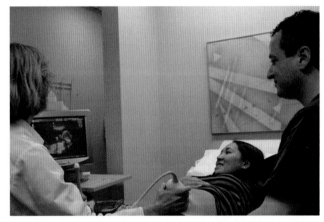

Fig. 9.3 An obstetric client and birthing partner watching the screen during a fetal anatomy ultrasound. (From Leifer, G. (2019). Prenatal care and adaptations to pregnancy. In G. Leifer (Ed.). *Introduction to maternity and pediatric nursing.* (8th ed., pp. 47–83). Elsevier.)

- Anatomy (cervix, uterus, adnexa)
- Number of fetuses
- Biometry (measurements of specific fetal structures) which estimates gestational age and fetal weight or determines whether a structure is a normal or abnormal size
- Fetal anatomy survey
- Fetal presentation
- Presence or absence of fetal cardiac activity
- Placental location
- Amniotic fluid volume

Limited obstetric ultrasound offers data about a specific problem or concern that requires further evaluation (ACOG, 2020c). These are usually reserved for clients who have already completed a basic obstetric ultrasound. An example is confirming the presence of a four-chamber fetal heart when a client is morbidly obese. In this scenario, a basic examination may have had inadequate views of fetal heart structures because excess adipose tissue decreases the ability for sound waves to penetrate to the structure's level. In this case clients are generally asked to come back in 2 to 4 weeks for a limited ultrasound to ensure four chambers are visualized (Reddy et al., 2014; Richards, 2021).

Specialized obstetric ultrasounds are accomplished when a specific fetal structure or organ system requires a more comprehensive assessment than what a basic examination affords (ACOG, 2020c; Wax et al., 2014). Examples of indications for detailed obstetric ultrasound include the following:

- Suspected or known fetal structural anomaly (e.g., gastroschisis)
- Suspected or known fetal genetic or chromosomal abnormality (e.g., trisomy 13)
- History of previous pregnancy with anatomic, genetic, or chromosomal abnormality (e.g., congenital heart defect such as a hypoplastic left heart)
- Fetal growth abnormalities (e.g., growth restriction or macrosomia)
- Maternal-fetal complications affecting the fetus (e.g., Rh sensitization)

This type of targeted ultrasound is performed by specially trained staff, such as maternal-fetal medicine physicians and sonographers.

Nonmedical Obstetric Ultrasound

In recent years, 3D and 4D ultrasounds have been used in nonmedical locations for client entertainment pictures and videos (i.e., "keepsake images"). This type of prenatal ultrasound is especially popular for identification of fetal sex. Ultrasound for research and diagnostic purposes have been used for several decades and there is a lack of current reliable evidence demonstrating a causal relationship between sonography and fetal harm (ACOG, 2020c; American Institute of Ultrasound Medicine [AIUM], 2020). However, ultrasound technology involves delivery of sound waves, which cannot be assumed to be harmless. Therefore there are theoretical concerns related to adverse bioeffects. Another concern is nonclinically indicated ultrasounds can provide false reassurance to clients because major, as well as subtle, abnormalities may be missed, especially if performed by noncredentialed entities. In these same circumstances, if an abnormality is identified, the person performing the ultrasound usually does not have adequate knowledge or resources to discuss the abnormality, provide follow-up appointments, or have the infrastructure to refer a client to a higher level of obstetric care (ACOG, 2020c; Richards, 2021).

Professional and government organizations have criticized ultrasound for nondiagnostic purposes by noncredentialed providers because this is an unapproved use of a medical device (AIUM, 2020; U.S. Food and Drug Administration [FDA], 2014; Pellerito et al., 2018). Therefore nonmedical use of obstetric ultrasound is discouraged, limiting the use to medical and obstetric reasons. Managing client expectations may also be encountered at appointments. Clients may frequently ask for early identification of fetal sex during an

---

BOX 9.1 Indications for First-Trimester Ultrasound

Evaluate pelvic structures (uterus, adnexa, and cul-de-sac)
Confirm intrauterine pregnancy
Assess for ectopic pregnancy
Estimate gestational age
Verify cardiac activity
Diagnose multiple gestations, including number of fetuses, chorionicity, and amnionicity
Assess pelvic pain or source of vaginal bleeding
Evaluate suspected gestational trophoblastic disease
Identify ultrasound markers (e.g., nuchal translucency) or severe fetal anomalies (e.g., anencephaly)
Adjunct to chorionic villus sampling

Adapted from Mei, J. Y., Afshar, Y., & Platt, L. D. (2019). First-trimester ultrasound. *Obstetrics and Gynecology Clinics, 46*(4), 829–852. https://doi.org/10.1016/j.ogc.2019.07.011; Pellerito, J., Bromley, B., Allison, S., Chauhan, A., Destounis, S., Dickman, E., Kline-Fath, B., Mastrobattista, J., Neumyer, M., Rundek, T., Sakhel, K., Shwayder, J., Toi, A., Wax, J., & Wilkins, I. (2018). AIUM-ACR-ACOG-SMFM-SRU practice parameter for the performance of standard diagnostic obstetric ultrasound examinations. *Journal of Ultrasound in Medicine, 37*(11), E13–E24. https://doi.org/10.1002/jum.14831; Reddy, U. M., Abuhamad, A. Z., Levine, D., Saade, G. R., & Fetal Imaging Workshop Invited Participants. (2014). Fetal imaging: Executive summary of a joint Eunice Kennedy Shriver National Institute of Child Health and Human Development, Society for Maternal-Fetal Medicine, American Institute of Ultrasound in Medicine, American College of Obstetricians and Gynecologists, American College of Radiology, Society for Pediatric Radiology, and Society of Radiologists in Ultrasound fetal imaging workshop. *American Journal of Obstetrics and Gynecology, 210*(5), 387–397.

---

anatomy scan. Clinicians are encouraged to have an open conversation with clients that although fetal genitalia are observed during this examination, this is not the purpose of the examination, nor are printed images a requirement though oftentimes expected.

First-Trimester Ultrasonography

Major advancements in high-resolution ultrasonography have shifted from first-trimester imaging visualization of pelvic and embryonic structures and establishing an EDD to a higher level of care. With transvaginal sonography, a gestational sac may be seen at approximately 4½ weeks based on menstrual age. The first structure to be seen in a gestational sac is a yolk sac. Early in the sixth week, an embryo is identified in a normal pregnancy with measurement of the crown rump length. Cardiac activity can also be identified when the crown rump length is 3 to 5 mm. Either a transabdominal or transvaginal approach may be used for this measurement.

Transvaginal ultrasonography allows clearer visualization of the uterus, gestational sac, embryo, and pelvic structures such as the ovaries and fallopian tubes.

Purpose

A variety of clinical indications for performing first-trimester ultrasound is presented in Box 9.1 (Mei et al., 2019; Pellerito et al., 2018; Reddy et al., 2014).

BOX 9.2   Indications for Second- and Third-Trimester Ultrasound

Confirm fetal viability
Evaluate fetal anatomy, including umbilical cord, vessels, insertion site, and placenta location
Determine gestational age
Assess serial fetal growth over several scans
Quantify amniotic fluid amount
Compare fetal growth and amniotic fluid volumes in multifetal gestations
Evaluate four or five markers in a biophysical profile (BPP)
Locate precise placental location when placenta previa is suspected
Determine fetal presentation

Adapted from Pellerito, J., Bromley, B., Allison, S., Chauhan, A., Destounis, S., Dickman, E., Kline-Fath, B., Mastrobattista, J., Neumyer, M., Rundek, T., Sakhel, K., Shwayder, J., Toi, A., Wax, J., & Wilkins, I. (2018). AIUM-ACR-ACOG-SMFM-SRU practice parameter for the performance of standard diagnostic obstetric ultrasound examinations. *Journal Of Ultrasound in Medicine*, *37*(11), E13–E24. https://doi.org/10.1002/jum.14831; Reddy, U. M., Abuhamad, A. Z., Levine, D., Saade, G. R., & Fetal Imaging Workshop Invited Participants. (2014). Fetal imaging: Executive summary of a joint Eunice Kennedy Shriver National Institute of Child Health and Human Development, Society for Maternal-Fetal Medicine, American Institute of Ultrasound in Medicine, American College of Obstetricians and Gynecologists, American College of Radiology, Society for Pediatric Radiology, and Society of Radiologists in Ultrasound fetal imaging workshop. *American Journal of Obstetrics and Gynecology, 210*(5), 387–397.

Procedure

A perinatal client is placed in lithotomy position for transvaginal ultrasound. A transvaginal probe encased in a disposable cover and coated with a gel that provides lubrication and promotes conductivity is inserted into a vagina. This procedure generally takes less than 15 to 30 minutes depending on the information being gathered by the clinician.

Second-Trimester and Third-Trimester Ultrasonography

Transabdominal ultrasonography is most often used during the second and third trimesters. This is related to the uterus extending out of a pelvis, allowing for sharper and clearer images of the fetus and placenta.

Purposes

Most commonly, ultrasonography is used throughout the second and third trimesters to assess fetal anatomy and biometry. Other indications are listed in Box 9.2 (AIUM, 2020; Pellerito et al., 2018):

Establishing Gestational Age

Gestational age determination with ultrasonography is increasingly less accurate after the first trimester because a combination of individual growth potential and intrauterine environment can cause greater variations among fetuses. Two methods improve gestational age determination accuracy in later pregnancy:

- Multiple calculations are obtained from fetal head biparietal diameter, head circumference, abdominal circumference, and femur length measurements.
- If the perinatal client is between 28 weeks of gestation or beyond, two or three ultrasound measurements taken 2 weeks apart will allow for a comparison against standard fetal growth curves. If measurements are done after 32 weeks of gestation, fetal age is subject to greater error (ACOG, 2020c).

Procedure

For transabdominal ultrasound, a client is assisted into a supine position, with the head and knees supported. The client is tilted with a pillow or rolled towel placed under the left or right hip to prevent aortocaval syndrome (hypotension) from a gravid uterus. Transmission gel is applied to the abdomen, and images or video are obtained. An ultrasound can take minutes to hours depending on the type of ultrasound being performed.

Nursing Role in Ultrasound

While nurses can assist with basic tasks like client positioning, they can also be an essential part of a clinic setting where obstetric ultrasounds are performed depending on the clinical environment. One example is a perinatal nurse coordinator in a high-risk obstetric clinic. This individual may be responsible for obtaining medical records, assisting with scheduling and follow-up appointments, acting as a primary point of contact for clients, coordinating referrals to other specialties, and case managing for more complex obstetric complications (e.g., congenital heart disorders) (Braley et al., 2020). Another expanded role for experienced nurses is limited obstetric ultrasound in a predefined clinical situation, such as biophysical profiles in a prenatal clinic or triage. Performance of this task must be within the scope of practice as defined by a state board of nursing and as allowed by institutional policies. Adherence to current guidelines from professional organizations such as those put forth by the Association of Women's Health, Obstetric and Neonatal Nurses (AWHONN) and unit-specific policies is recommended. Specialized education, including didactic and hands-on training, is required (AWHONN, 2016).

KNOWLEDGE CHECK

1. What are three categories of obstetric ultrasound? What are the two routes for obstetric ultrasound?
2. Describe indications for first-, second-, and third-trimester ultrasound.
3. Why are clients placed in a supine position with a lateral tilt during ultrasounds?
4. Explain a nurse's role when an obstetric client is having an ultrasound.

PRENATAL SCREENING TESTS

Preimplantation Genetic Testing

Preimplantation genetic testing is an option available to clients who have undergone successful in vitro fertilization. This type

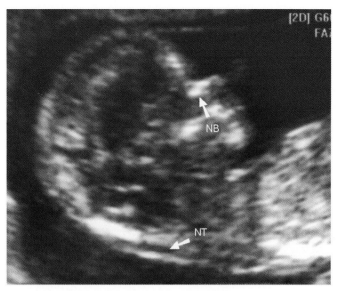

Fig. 9.4 Normal nuchal translucency (NT) and nasal bone (NB) in a 12-week fetus. (From Richards, D. S. (2021). Obstetric ultrasound. In M. Landon, V. Berghella, A. Cahill, D. Driscoll, H. Galan, W. Grobman, E. Jauniax, & S. Kilpatrick (Eds.). *Gabbe's obstetrics: Normal & problem pregnancies* (8th ed., pp. 156–179). Elsevier.)

of testing analyzes cells from an embryo after fertilization and prior to subsequent transfer of selected embryos to the uterus based on testing results and client preference. Preimplantation genetic testing looks for chromosomal abnormalities, such as trisomy 21, and specific genetic conditions that may be inherited from one or both parents. Examples include, but are not limited to, sickle cell anemia, cystic fibrosis, Duchenne muscular dystrophy, fragile X syndrome, and Tay-Sachs disease. Results are usually received within 1 to 2 days. This type of testing will not provide a definitive diagnosis because cells are obtained from an early embryo. Confirmatory testing such as CVS or amniocentesis is recommended to validate a diagnosis (ACOG, 2020a; Sullivan-Pyke & Dokras, 2018; Wapner & Dugoff, 2019).

First-Trimester Screening

FTS includes a nuchal translucency (NT) measurement via ultrasound with serum analyte quantification of pregnancy-associated plasma protein-A (PAPP-A) and human chorionic gonadotropin (hCG) (ACOG, 2020b). This gestational age specific test screens for trisomy 21 and trisomy 18. hCG is a hormone produced by an embryo. This serum analyte level usually doubles every 2 days for the first 4 weeks of pregnancy, peaking at 8 to 10 weeks of gestation, and then declines for the remainder of the pregnancy. Increased levels of serum hCG have been associated with trisomy 21 in the fetus, whereas fetal trisomy 13 and 18 demonstrate decreased levels (ACOG, 2020b; Blackburn, 2018). PAPP-A is a glycoprotein made by the placenta and is released directly into the pregnant client's bloodstream. This protein is detectable in blood serum at approximately 6 weeks of gestation and peaks at 14 weeks. Low first-trimester PAPP-A serum levels are linked to trisomy 21 (ACOG, 2020b; Blackburn, 2018).

NT is an ultrasound measurement of the fluid-filled space at the back of a fetal neck (Fig. 9.4). An enlarged NT, often defined as 3.0 mm or greater, or above the 99th percentile for gestational age, is associated with trisomy 21 as well as structural abnormalities such as congenital heart defects (ACOG, 2020b; Driscoll & Simpson, 2021) (Fig. 9.5). This measurement can only be obtained between approximately 10 to 14 weeks of gestation and is sometimes performed when a fetal crown rump length is obtained for gestational age dating (ACOG, 2020b). A crown rump length is measured from the top of the head to an embryo's rump (Fig. 9.6). This is the most precise gestational age dating method during the first trimester.

In addition to FTS, an independent ultrasound marker sometimes used to detect structural anomalies associated with trisomy 21 is nasal bone assessment. Midface hypoplasia and a flattened nose is one characteristic feature often found in individuals with trisomy 21. At 11 to 14 weeks of gestation, the presence or absence of a nasal bone can be an important ultrasound finding. Unfortunately, nasal bone imaging is technically difficult and has not been shown to improve trisomy 21 prediction when combined with FTS or NT (ACOG, 2020b; Driscoll & Simpson, 2021; Richards, 2021; Wapner & Dugoff, 2019).

Cell-Free Fetal DNA

Advances in human genomics have resulted in the development of cfDNA screening, which is used in a variety of clinical fields to include, but not limited to, obstetrics and oncology. In pregnancy, small fragments of cfDNA that originate from maternal and fetal cell breakdown at the placental level mix freely in circulation (ACOG, 2020b; Driscoll & Simpson, 2021). cfDNA is found in a client's bloodstream as early as 5 to 7 weeks of gestation but is a more suitable source of fetal genetic material after 9 to 10 weeks of gestation. Shortly after birth, the cells dissipate (ACOG, 2020b; Norton & Rink, 2016). Hence, this test can be performed at approximately 10 weeks of gestation and has no gestational age cutoff. Results

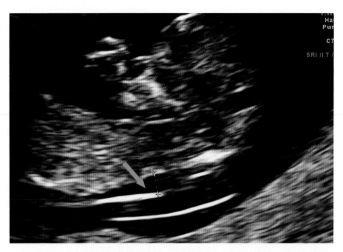

Fig. 9.5 Abnormal nuchal translucency with measurement of >3 mm in a 12-week fetus (*green arrow*). (From Richards, D. S. (2021). Obstetric ultrasound. In M. Landon, V. Berghella., A. Cahill, D. Driscoll, H. Galan, W. Grobman, E. Jauniax, & S. Kilpatrick (Eds.). *Gabbe's obstetrics: Normal & problem pregnancies* (8th ed., pp. 156–179). Elsevier.)

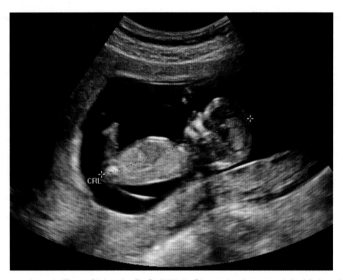

Fig. 9.6 Crown rump length (From Richards, D. S. (2021). Obstetric ultrasound. In M. Landon, V. Berghella., A. Cahill, D. Driscoll, H. Galan, W. Grobman, E. Jauniax, & S. Kilpatrick (Eds.). *Gabbe's obstetrics: Normal & problem pregnancies* (8th ed., pp. 156–179). Elsevier.)

are usually returned within 1 week. This type of screening, sometimes referred to as *noninvasive prenatal screening*, is a serum analyte test which targets trisomy 21, trisomy 18, trisomy 13, sex chromosome composition, and selected microdeletions and microduplications (ACOG, 2020b; Dar et al., 2016; Gregg et al., 2016). However, approximately 3% to 13% of cfDNA disseminated in a client's circulation is of fetal origin (ACOG, 2020b; Gregg et al., 2016; Norton & Rink, 2016). This makes analysis of cfDNA challenging because the test cannot distinguish between fetal and maternal DNA, leading to false results (ACOG, 2020b; Wapner & Dugoff, 2019). Identification of structural anomalies like neural tube defects (NTDs) cannot be done with cfDNA (ACOG, 2020b; Driscoll & Simpson, 2021).

Initially, cfDNA screening in the obstetric population was designed for high-risk clients, including those 35 years or older at birth or ultrasound findings indicating an increased risk for aneuploidy. Cell-free fetal DNA screening has a high sensitivity and specificity for trisomy 21 in this population. Sensitivity means if the test result is negative, trisomy 21 is unlikely in the pregnancy. If cfDNA screening is positive and the test is highly specific, trisomy 21 is probably present. Subsequently, cfDNA screening is now offered to clients regardless of risk status though there appears to be a larger proportion of false-positive tests among low-risk perinatal clients (ACOG, 2020b; Wapner & Dugoff, 2019).

Before cfDNA screening is ordered, a baseline ultrasound is performed which may aid in timing and appropriateness of the test. Findings such as gestational age, vanishing twin syndrome, and multiple gestations can affect the results of cfDNA or negate this form of screening in the pregnant client (ACOG, 2020b). Anyone with a positive screening result is offered follow-up diagnostic testing such as CVS or

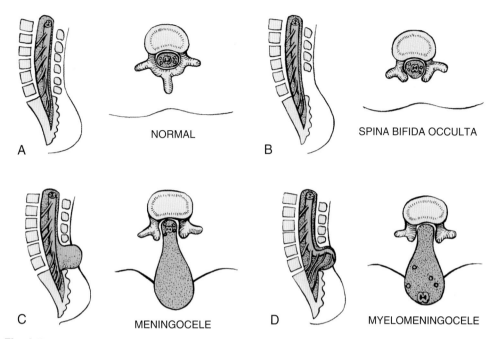

Fig. 9.7 In normal fetal development the spinal cord is enclosed in a protective sheath of bone and meninges. In some cases, a neural tube fails to close resulting in neural tube defects (occulta, meningocele, and myelomeningocele). (From Hockenberry, M. J. (2017). The child with neuromuscular or muscular dysfunction. In S. Perry, D. Lowdermilk, K. Cashion, K. Alden, E. Olshansky, M. Hockenberry, D. Wilson, & C. Rodgers. (Eds.). *Maternal child nursing care* (6th ed., pp. 1455–1483). Elsevier.)

amniocentesis to confirm a disease or condition (ACOG, 2020b; Gregg et al., 2016).

Second-Trimester Multiple-Marker Screening

Second-trimester multiple-marker screening reports a client's risk for trisomy 21, trisomy 18, and open NTDs. NTDs are congenital anomalies affecting the brain and spinal cord. Different types of NTDs can occur, and each has a different level of severity. Two of the more common types of open NTDs are anencephaly and spina bifida. Anencephaly is abnormal development of the brain and skull affecting brain function and is severe enough to result in fetal or neonatal death. In spina bifida, an occulta, meningocele, or myelomeningocele, may be found (Fig. 9.7). A spina bifida occulta simply means a defect is not visible externally and is most frequently found in the lumbosacral area. With a meningocele, the meninges protrude from the spinal canal while a myelomeningocele has both the spinal cord and meninges extending through the defect (Fig. 9.8). Complications of spina bifida include a range of minor physical disabilities with little functional impairment to severe physical and intellectual disabilities requiring specialized care and equipment (National Institute of Neurological Disorders and Stroke, 2021). However, since the introduction of folic acid to food products and additional supplementation in prenatal vitamins, the rate of NTDs has dramatically decreased in the past several decades.

Second-trimester screening requires blood to be drawn from the pregnant client so specific serum analytes can be measured. Screening is performed between 15 0/7 and 22 6/7 weeks of gestation. Optimal timing is between 16 and 18 weeks of gestation to improve screening for open NTDs.

Serum analytes include (1) hCG, (2) alpha-fetoprotein (AFP), (3) inhibin-A, and (4) unconjugated estriol (uE3). These hormones and proteins are produced by the fetus and the placenta and eventually cross over into the client's circulation. Quad screens determine the level of all four analytes. The penta screen adds hyperglycosylated hCG. Results are based on computer risk calculations of the serum analyte level, gestational age, a client's current weight, ethnicity, presence of diabetes, and number of fetuses. All results are reported as negative or positive. Incorrect information, such as gestational age, will decrease result accuracy, delaying future testing options if applicable (ACOG, 2020b; Driscoll & Simpson, 2021; Wapner & Dugoff, 2019).

The fetal liver and placenta produce uE3. Levels of this protein rise throughout the pregnancy. Trisomy 18 and 21 are associated with lower levels of uE3. Inhibin-A is a glycoprotein that originates in the placenta. Levels of this protein gradually rise through pregnancy. Levels of inhibin-A that are two times higher than normal are associated with trisomy 21 (Wapner & Dugoff, 2019). Alpha-fetoprotein (AFP) is also a glycoprotein produced early in the first-trimester yolk sac and later from the fetal gastrointestinal system. This protein is transported from fetal plasma into fetal urine, which is then excreted into amniotic fluid. Although a portion of AFP is swallowed and digested by the fetus, the remainder crosses fetal membranes through diffusion into the pregnant client's circulation. Normally, AFP levels increase until 10 to 14 weeks of gestation and then decline (Blackburn, 2018). Elevated AFP measurements are most associated with NTDs. Other circumstances associated with elevated and low AFP are found in Table 9.1.

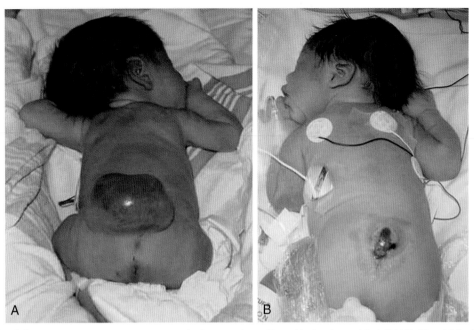

Fig. 9.8 Myelomeningocele. A, Intact sac. B, Ruptured sac. (From Hockenberry, M. J. (2017). The child with neuromuscular or muscular dysfunction. In S. Perry, D. Lowdermilk, K. Cashion, K. Alden, E. Olshansky, M. Hockenberry, D. Wilson, & C. Rodgers. (Eds.). (6th ed., pp. 1455–1483). Elsevier.)

TABLE 9.1	Abnormal Alpha-Fetoprotein Levels
Elevated AFP Levels	Neural Tube Defects
	Underestimation of gestational age
	Undiagnosed multiple gestation
	Fetal demise
	Conditions associated with fetal edema (e.g., cystic hygroma)
	Abdominal wall defects (e.g., gastroschisis)
	Low client BMI: inaccurate elevation
	Unexplained elevation after comprehensive assessment
Decreased AFP Levels	Chromosomal trisomy (e.g., trisomy 21)
	Gestational trophoblastic diseases
	Inaccurate gestational age or client weight
	Client obesity: inaccurately low

Adapted from Driscoll, D. A., & Simpson, J. L. (2021). Genetic screening and diagnosis. In M. Landon, V. Berghella., A. Cahill, D. Driscoll, H. Galan, W. Grobman, E. Jauniax, & S. Kilpatrick (Eds.). *Gabbe's obstetrics: Normal & problem pregnancies* (8th ed., pp. 180–203). Elsevier.

Combined First-Trimester and Second-Trimester Screening Tests

Combined first- and second-trimester screening tests allow for a higher detection rate than FTS alone. This means second-trimester screening tests can be joined with components of FTS. Combined testing can be either integrated, sequential, or contingent and include measurements of serum analytes,

NT, or both elements. *Integrated screening* combines NT measurement and PAPP-A with a quad screen. The first portion of this test is done between 11 and 13 6/7 weeks of gestation, followed by the second step being performed between 15 and 22 weeks of gestation. The *sequential stepwise screening* combines NT measurement, hCG, and PAPP-A with results from the quad screen. *Serum integrated screening* combines PAPP-A results with the quad screen, but NT measurement is omitted. Results for integrated, sequential stepwise, and serum integrated screening are not available to the client until the second trimester (ACOG, 2020b). With contingent screening, a pregnancy is categorized as low, intermediate, or high risk based on first-trimester screening. Depending on the risk status, clients are offered further diagnostic testing, continued screening the in the second trimester, or no testing.

> **❓ KNOWLEDGE CHECK**
>
> 5. What is an NT measurement? What chromosomal abnormality is associated with an increased NT measurement?
> 6. List specific conditions that can be identified with cell-free DNA.
> 7. Name four serum analytes measured with a second-trimester screening test.
> 8. What conditions are associated with elevated AFP levels?
> 9. What is multiple-marker screening? Why is it performed?

PRENATAL DIAGNOSTIC TESTS

The prenatal diagnostic (as opposed to screening) tests are chorionic villi sampling (CVS), amniocentesis and percutaneous umbilical cord blood sampling (PUBS). Only CVS can be performed during the first trimester; amniocentesis and PUBS cannot be performed until the second or third trimester. A disadvantage of second-trimester screening and

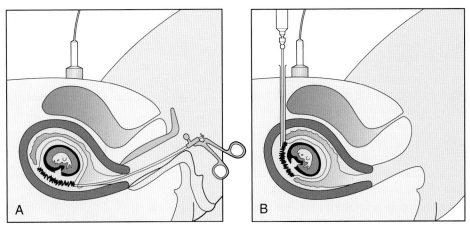

Fig. 9.9 Chorionic villus sampling. A, Transcervical approach. B, Transabdominal approach. (From Odibo, A. O., & Acharya, G. (2019). Invasive diagnostic procedures. In P. Pandya, D. Oepkes, N. Sebire, & R. Wapner. (Eds.). *Fetal medicine: Basic science and clinical practice* (3rd ed., pp. 225–252). Elsevier.)

diagnostic testing is the delay in obtaining results. This can lead to a prolonged interval between screening and diagnosis, which may impact the pregnancy decision-making process (ACOG, 2020a; Wapner & Dugoff, 2019). Additionally, delaying diagnostic procedures until the second trimester, when client perception of fetal movement is more pronounced, may cause increased emotional stress (ACOG, 2020a; Wapner & Dugoff, 2019).

Chorionic Villus Sampling

Chorionic villi are microscopic projections which develop from the chorion and burrow into endometrial tissue during placental formation. These villi are located in the placenta's intervillous spaces. The finger-like projections maximize the surface area for nutrient and gas exchange between the pregnant client and fetus. Additionally, chorionic villi typically contain fetal chromosomal, metabolic, and genetic material (Blackburn, 2018). Therefore first-trimester CVS allows for diagnostic results to be obtained earlier in pregnancy compared with amniocentesis. CVS is performed between 10 and 13 weeks of gestation in an ambulatory setting to diagnose fetal chromosomal, metabolic, or deoxyribonucleic acid (DNA) abnormalities. Two acceptable routes for aspiration of placental tissue can be used: transcervical or transabdominal (Fig. 9.9). Both methods require ultrasound guidance to confirm FHR, gestational age, and location of the uterus, cervix, and placenta. However, client choice and technical difficulty are often considered when deciding between a transcervical or transabdominal technique (ACOG, 2020a; Driscoll & Simpson, 2021; Wapner & Dugoff, 2019). For example, a transabdominal approach may be used in clients with active herpes to avoid transmission to a fetus. Final CVS results can be reported in 5 to 7 days (ACOG, 2020a; Wapner & Dugoff, 2019). Clients can be provided reassurance when results are normal. If abnormal results are detected, pregnancy management options are discussed with the client and include continuing the pregnancy or elective termination. When time is a factor, a technique called fluorescence in-situ hybridization

(FISH) may be used for chromosome analysis. This offers an opportunity for rapid screening of aneuploidies resulting in a turnaround time of 24 to 48 hours. Unfortunately, FISH is not diagnostic because the test cannot detect other chromosomal abnormalities such as structural rearrangements. Clients are counseled to wait for final CVS results before making decisions about pregnancy management (ACOG, 2020a).

Procedure

As with all diagnostic procedures, a client will receive counseling about the general procedure and genetic counseling about the specific abnormality for which CVS sampling is being performed. The risks and benefits of the procedure are carefully explained, and a signed informed consent is obtained. Transcervical CVS is performed by inserting a flexible catheter through the cervix. The transabdominal approach is performed using an 18- or 20-gauge spinal needle with a stylet attached. Both procedures require the insertion site to be aseptically prepared.

Ultrasound is used to guide the catheter or needle placement. A sample of chorionic villi, usually between 10 and 30 mL, is aspirated into a syringe containing culture medium. A second aspiration may be needed if an insufficient sample is obtained (Wapner & Dugoff, 2019). RhoGAM is administered to Rh-negative clients after CVS to prevent alloimmunization (i.e., isoimmunization). (Moise, 2021; Chapter 10).

Clients are often concerned about CVS procedure safety and pregnancy loss risk. There are varying opinions and research studies about pregnancy loss rates with CVS. In general, if CVS is performed by experienced, specially trained physicians, the pregnancy loss rate is approximately 1% (Beta et al., 2019). Limb reduction defects were once associated with CVS when the procedure was performed at less than 9 to 10 weeks of gestation. Improvements in technique and timing of procedure shows no increased risk for this type of defect when CVS is performed at 10 weeks of gestation or later (ACOG, 2020a). Other CVS complications include culture failure in growing chromosomes, subchorionic hematomas, infection, and spontaneous rupture of membranes (ACOG, 2020a; Wapner & Dugoff, 2019).

Chorionic Villus Sampling: Nursing Responsibilities

Nurses are responsible for educating clients about postprocedure complaints. Postprocedure spotting usually appears red in the first 2 days and transitions to brown. Spotting generally resolves without any intervention. A small amount of bleeding occurs more commonly in clients who had a transcervical CVS procedure and less frequently with a transabdominal approach (ACOG, 2020a). Uterine cramping is an expected complaint during and immediately after the procedure. Postprocedure recommendation includes resting for 24 hours and avoiding exercise, heavy lifting, and sexual intercourse for several days. Clients receive written and/or verbal instructions to report signs of spotting or heavy bleeding similar to a menstrual period, clot or tissue passage, uterine cramping increasing in intensity, leaking of amniotic fluid, or temperature greater than 100.4°F.

> **? KNOWLEDGE CHECK**
>
> 10. What is the major advantage of CVS compared with amniocentesis?
> 11. What is the difference between the transcervical and transabdominal technique?
> 12. What are common client complaints after a CVS procedure?

Amniocentesis

Amniocentesis is an invasive procedure that has been the foundation of prenatal diagnosis for several decades. The procedure involves aspiration of amniotic fluid from the uterus and is performed for a variety of indications in the second and third trimesters (Fig. 9.10). These include identification of chromosomal, metabolic, or genetic abnormalities. Less commonly, amniocentesis can be performed to diagnose fetal infection or as a therapeutic procedure for amniotic fluid volume disorders such as polyhydramnios. Occasionally, amniocentesis for fetal chromosomal analysis may be utilized for investigative purposes in the case of fetal demise (ACOG & Society of Maternal-Fetal Medicine [SMFM], 2020).

Amniocentesis for prenatal diagnosis is usually performed midtrimester, around 15 to 20 weeks of gestation, when an adequate amount of amniotic fluid and viable fetal cells are available (ACOG, 2020a). Amniocentesis can also be performed in later gestations depending on the clinical scenario. Amniocentesis prior to 15 weeks of gestation has mostly been abandoned in clinical practice for the following reasons (Chard & Norton, 2016; Wapner & Dugoff, 2019):

1. Increased degree of difficulty and failed procedure rate because of incomplete fusion of the amnion and chorion membrane early in pregnancy. This results in "tenting," where the needle is unable to penetrate the amniotic membrane.
2. Inadequate samples because the amount of amniotic fluid is less at early gestational ages.

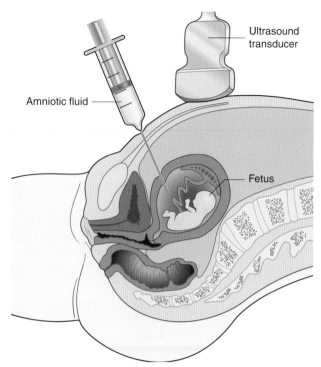

Fig. 9.10 Amniocentesis (From Odibo, A. O., & Acharya, G. (2019). Invasive diagnostic procedures. In P. Pandya, D. Oepkes, N. Sebire, & R. Wapner. (Eds.). *Fetal medicine: Basic science and clinical practice* (3rd ed., pp. 225–252). Elsevier.)

3. Higher cell culture failure rates.
4. Increased rates of pregnancy loss and amniotic fluid leakage.

Compared with CVS, the most significant disadvantage of performing amniocentesis for prenatal diagnosis is that final test results are not available for a minimum of 10 to 14 days. This is due to the amount of time required for fluid analysis and cell growth (ACOG, 2020a; Driscoll & Simpson, 2021; Wapner & Dugoff, 2019). Much like CVS, FISH testing may also be used, but results are interpreted only as preliminary findings. Another disadvantage of amniocentesis is the procedure takes place in the second trimester, when the pregnancy is more apparent and fetal movement has been perceived. The client bonding process has started, making decisions about pregnancy continuation versus termination more emotionally and physically difficult.

Procedure

Ultrasound is used to locate the fetus, placenta, and pockets of amniotic fluid, which are free of fetal body parts and the umbilical cord. The abdomen is prepared aseptically. A small amount of local anesthetic may be injected subcutaneously into the skin for client comfort, but clients will still feel pressure and cramping as the needle enters the myometrium. A 20- to 22-gauge spinal needle with stylet is inserted into the fluid pocket, under continuous ultrasound guidance. A syringe is then attached to the needle to allow for aspiration of 1 to 2 mL of amniotic fluid; the syringe is immediately discarded to prevent contamination of the sample with cells from the pregnant client which may enter the needle as it penetrates client tissues. Another syringe is then connected, and approximately 20 mL or more of fluid is removed. The amount aspirated is determined by the number of diagnostic tests being performed on the amniotic fluid.

Fetal cardiac activity and fetal movement are documented postprocedure. If amniocentesis is performed at a gestational age which is considered viable, electronic fetal monitoring may be implemented to assess fetal heart rate and uterine activity. Like CVS, RhoGAM is administered to Rh-negative clients to prevent hemolytic disease in a fetus or newborn (ACOG, 2020a; Moise, 2021).

Pregnancy loss after amniocentesis is also a concern for clients. Like CVS, accurate data reflecting pregnancy loss rates vary. Most agree that miscarriage rates have decreased due to ultrasound equipment enhancements and optimization of the procedure technique. Pregnancy loss is generally quoted as less than 1% in facilities where experienced physicians perform frequent amniocentesis procedures (ACOG, 2020a; Driscoll & Simpson, 2021). Approximately, 1% to 2% of clients may experience vaginal spotting or continuous leakage of amniotic fluid post procedure. Unlike spontaneous preterm premature rupture of membranes caused by infection, vaginal bleeding, or uterine distention, rupture of membranes after amniocentesis is associated with a needle puncture site between the uterus and amniotic membranes. This is often short-lived as the membranes usually reseal quickly and is not typically associated with adverse perinatal and neonatal outcomes (ACOG, 2020a). Incidences of infection and needle injuries to the fetus are extremely rare.

Amniocentesis: Nursing Responsibilities

Nurses may be included as part of a health care team during amniocentesis. Client positioning, and labeling and sending specimens for laboratory analysis may be a part of the nurse's responsibility. Postprocedure education mirrors that provided to CVS clients as common complaints and warning signs are similar. Clients may verbalize uterine cramping, which may last several hours after the amniocentesis is performed. Some clients experience low abdominal discomfort lasting 24 to 48 hours. A small amount of amniotic fluid leakage may be noted the first day. Postprocedure instructions include resting the day of the amniocentesis and resumption of normal activities the next day.

Fetal Lung Maturity

Previously, amniocentesis was a common practice to assess for FLM, especially in those with suboptimal dating for establishing an EDD. In modern obstetric practice, there is a lack of reliable data to predict newborn pulmonary and nonrespiratory outcomes, even in the event of mature fetal lung laboratory testing (ACOG, 2021d). Routine use of amniocentesis for FLM is no longer practiced today due to an increased administration of antenatal steroids, enhanced ultrasound technology, and improved neonatal capabilities in an intensive care setting. Additionally, contemporary research has demonstrated that documentation of FLM does not equate to other physiologic processes being adequately developed (ACOG, 2021b; Bates et al., 2010; Tita et al., 2018). In today's

obstetric environment where there is more focus on morbidity and mortality of the pregnant client and neonate, delaying birth due to immature fetal lungs may not be in the best interest of the client.

However, a foundational understanding of FLM and laboratory testing is an important aspect of obstetric nursing education. One of the last systems to mature structurally and physiologically in a fetus is the pulmonary system. A complex substance, surfactant, plays a critical role in fetal lung maturation. Primarily composed of phospholipids, surfactant has many functions but primarily reduces surface tension on the alveoli's inner walls allowing them to stay slightly open during exhalation. Additionally, surfactant stabilizes lung volume, alters lung mechanics, and maintains gas exchange in the lung. Without adequate surfactant, lung walls adhere to one another, making alveoli inflation during inhalation difficult, increasing the amount of pressure required to keep alveoli open (Blackburn, 2018). If this situation is not corrected, impaired oxygenation eventually leads to respiratory distress syndrome and other complications, which increase neonatal morbidity and mortality rates.

Nurses can conduct a visual inspection of amniotic fluid for color and particles as this can offer preliminary information about surfactant levels before laboratory analysis. Amniotic fluid is yellow and clear in the first and second trimesters and becomes colorless in the third trimester. By 35 weeks of gestation, amniotic fluid is cloudy, with particles of vernix appearing at around 36 to 37 weeks of gestation (Verpoest et al., 1976). Generally, amniotic fluid with obvious vernix or cloudy fluid that does not permit reading of newsprint through the specimen tube is considered a mature lecithin-to-sphingomyelin (L/S ratio) (Clements et al., 1972).

Primary laboratory methods historically used to evaluate FLM include L/S ratio, presence or absence of phosphatidylglycerol (PG), and lamellar body counting. Lecithin is a phospholipid component of fetal lung fluid and surfactant; concentrations gradually increase throughout pregnancy, peaking 34 to 35 weeks of gestation. Sphingomyelin is an amniotic membrane lipid with a relatively stable concentration in amniotic fluid during the entire pregnancy (Blackburn, 2018). By 35 weeks of gestation, lecithin concentration markedly increases over sphingomyelin. An L/S ratio of 2:1 or greater generally indicates adequate surfactant and mature fetal lungs. In clients with diabetes, an L/S ratio 2:1 may not be indicative of lung maturity, and further testing may be required. Another component of surfactant which can be evaluated for in FLM is establishing the presence of PG. The presence of PG supports the likelihood of fetal lungs maturity (Blackburn, 2018; Greenberg & Druzin, 2021). Counting lamellar bodies is sometimes used for evaluating FLM. Lamellar bodies are the storage form of surfactant produced by type II pneumocytes. This test utilizes a hematology analyzer, which is used for platelet counting, to evaluate amniotic fluid. Values less than 15,000 per microliter reflect immature fetal lungs while 50,000 or more are associated with maturity (Abdou et al., 2020).

Percutaneous Umbilical Blood Sampling

PUBS, also referred to as *cordocentesis,* is a procedure that is performed in the second and third trimesters for diagnostic and therapeutic purposes. The most common indications for this procedure are diagnosis and management of allo-immunization and hydrops, though this procedure can also be used to obtain blood for other laboratory testing such as chromosomal analysis, genetic disorders, and infectious diseases (e.g., cytomegalovirus). Furthermore, this procedure is intended for intrauterine blood transfusions for fetal anemia and direct medication administration for fetal arrhythmias (Too & Berkowitz, 2018). A PUBS procedure is comparable to amniocentesis in that a spinal needle, usually 21 or 22 gauge, is inserted via ultrasound guidance into the umbilical vein or intrahepatic vein (Fig. 9.11). An umbilical vein is preferable over other locations because the vessel is larger and less likely to cause complications such as fetal bradycardia or bleeding. Other problems include umbilical cord lacerations, umbilical cord hematomas, thrombosis, infection, preterm labor resulting in an emergent birth of a compromised fetus, preterm premature rupture of membranes, and pregnancy loss. Although PUBS is used in some high-risk centers on a case-by-case basis, there may be alternatives, such as CVS, amniocentesis, or Doppler flow studies, that are safer, easier, and faster (Driscoll & Simpson, 2021; Too & Berkowitz, 2018; Wapner & Dugoff, 2019).

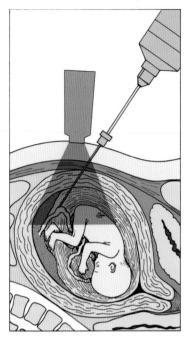

Fig. 9.11 Percutaneous blood sampling. (From Cashion, K. (2017). Assessment of high-risk pregnancy. In S. Perry, D. Lowdermilk, K. Cashion, K. Alden, E. Olshansky, M. Hockenberry, D. Wilson, & C. Rodgers. (Eds.). *Maternal child nursing care* (6th ed., pp. 226–243). Elsevier.)

KNOWLEDGE CHECK

13. What are second- and third-trimester indications for amniocentesis?
14. Name potential complications associated with amniocentesis.
15. Describe surfactant's role in fetal lung maturity.
16. What are the most common indications for PUBS and potential risks associated with this procedure?

ANTEPARTUM FETAL TESTING

Today, an assortment of antepartum fetal testing (APFT) methods has been refined as a means of assuring fetal well-being and identifying fetuses at risk for adverse outcomes. In some pregnancies, fetal well-being may need to be assessed more frequently during the antepartum period, especially with a viable gestational age in a high-risk pregnancy. The primary goal of antepartum surveillance is identification of fetuses at risk for permanent neurologic injury or stillbirth so timely interventions can be performed in an effort to decrease perinatal morbidity and mortality rates (ACOG, 2021a; Signore et al., 2009). This is related to data that abnormal fetal surveillance results may be associated with changes in fetal acid–base status leading to adverse outcomes. Though testing results reflect neither the severity nor duration of the interruption in oxygenation and are weakly correlated with adverse short-term and long-term neonatal outcomes (ACOG, 2021a). More importantly no test can predict stillbirths related to acute unpreventable circumstances such as

an umbilical cord prolapse (ACOG, 2021a). Nevertheless, despite widespread use of APFT, there continues to be inadequate evidence to demonstrate an improvement in perinatal outcome except for fetal Doppler flow ultrasound (ACOG, 2021a; O'Neil & Thorp, 2012).

Common methods of fetal surveillance include the following:

1. Fetal movement counting (FMC)
2. Nonstress test (NST)
3. Contraction stress test (CST)/oxytocin challenge test (OCT)
4. Biophysical profile (BPP)
5. Modified biophysical profile (MBPP)
6. Doppler flow studies

The type of antepartum surveillance method selected is based on risk factors, gestational age, and available technology. Shared decision-making in the clinical context guide timing and frequency of antepartum fetal surveillance (ACOG, 2021a). All methods are considered screening tests, and none are considered better than another. Each one offers a different endpoint considered in the decision-making process. Nevertheless, like all screening tests, a false-negative rate or false-positive rate is possible. Normal APFT results are encouraging in most situations, as reflected in the low false-negative rate for surveillance tests as a whole. False-negative results in APFT are defined as a stillbirth occurring within 1 week of a *normal* antepartum fetal test result (Kaimal, 2019). In some cases, when an abnormal result is obtained, a test is more likely to indicate a false-positive, which means an antepartum test is abnormal, but an unaffected fetus is

TABLE 9.2	Indications for Antepartum Fetal Assessment		
Client	**Fetal**	**Obstetric**	**Placental**
Hypertensive disorders (chronic, gestational, preeclampsia)	Decreased fetal movement	Abnormal serum markers on prenatal testing	Chronic placental abruption
Diabetes (type 1, type 2, gestational)	Growth restriction	Previous intrauterine fetal demise	Vasa previa
Renal disease (creatinine >1.4 mg/dL)	Fetal anomalies	≥41 0/7 weeks gestation	Velamentous cord insertion
Systemic lupus erythematosus	Multiple gestation	Cholestasis	Single umbilical artery
Antiphospholipid Syndrome			Polyhydramnios (single deepest pocket [SDP] ≥12 cm or AFI ≥30 cm)
>35 years of age			Isolated oligohydramnios (SDP <2 cm)
Substance abuse			
Alcohol ≥5 drinks/week			
Polysubstance			
Prepregnancy BMI ≥35 kg/m²			
Sickle cell disease			
Inadequately controlled thyroid disease			
In vitro fertilization			

Adapted from American College of Obstetrics and Gynecology. (2021a). ACOG Practice Bulletin. No. 229. Antepartum fetal surveillance. *Obstetrics & Gynecology, 137*(6) 1134–1136. https://doi.org/10.1097/aog.0000000000004411; American College of Obstetrics and Gynecology. (2021c). ACOG Committee Opinion. No 828. Indications for outpatient antenatal fetal surveillance. *Obstetrics & Gynecology, 137*(6), 1148–1151. https://doi.org/10.1097/aog.0000000000004408; Signore, C., Freeman, R. K., & Spong, C. Y. (2009). Antenatal testing–A reevaluation. *Obstetrics & Gynecology, 113*(3), 687–701. https://doi.org/10.1097/aog.0b013e318197bd8a.

delivered (Miller et al., 2022). True positives occur when an abnormal result corresponds with a compromised fetus at the time of birth (ACOG, 2021a; O'Neil & Thorp, 2012).

Risk Identification

Several risk factors can have a connection to fetal compromise or stillbirth because there is a presumed alteration in the maternal-fetal oxygenation pathway. Indications for APFT are found in Table 9.2, though this is not an exhaustive list. Briefly, oxygen is carried from the environment to a fetus along a pathway that includes a client's lungs, heart, vasculature, uterus, placenta, and umbilical cord (Fig. 9.12). Interruptions can occur anywhere along this pathway (Miller et al., 2022). For example, severe hypertension in pregnancy can cause an oxygenation interruption at the level of the pregnant client's vascular system, uterus, and placenta. Elevated blood pressures reduce intravascular volume and cause vasoconstriction in systemic and placental vasculature. Insufficient exchange of oxygen, carbon dioxide, nutrients, and waste products between client and fetal circulation may consequently lead to a fetal physiologic response such as a minimal variability or late decelerations (see Chapter 14). In some clinical situations, APFT may identify fetal hypoxia early enough for treatment to begin before fetal oxygenation reaches a critical level. Using an example of critically elevated blood pressures such as 180/102 and 176/110, administration of an antihypertensive agent lowers a client's blood pressure, which in turn allows for improved blood flow to the fetus and adequate oxygen exchange. Otherwise, if recurrent interruptions in the

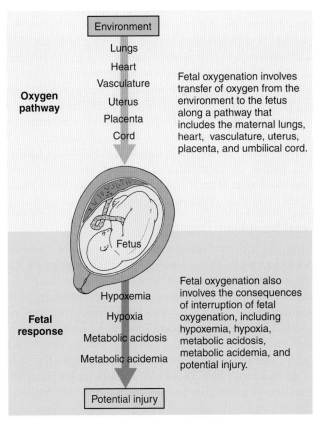

Fig. 9.12 Maternal-fetal oxygenation pathway. (From Miller, L.A., Miller, D.A., & Cypher, R.L. (2022). *Mosby's pocket guide to fetal monitoring: A multidisciplinary approach* (9th ed.). Elsevier.)

oxygenation pathway continue, decreased oxygen content in the blood (hypoxemia) progresses to hypoxia or decreased oxygen in fetal tissues. Anaerobic metabolism is triggered, and lactic acid is produced, resulting in metabolic acidosis, metabolic acidemia, and finally, potential neurologic injury or death (Miller et al., 2022).

Gestational Age and Frequency of Assessment

The gestational age to initiate APFT has not been defined and is generally individualized to the earliest threshold for neonatal survival based on risk status (ACOG, 2021a; ACOG, 2021c; Devoe & Jones, 2002; Greenberg & Druzin, 2021). Several factors go into decisions as to when to begin testing. Antepartum fetal surveillance is traditionally initiated at around 32 weeks of gestation for high-risk pregnancies. Though earlier testing may be recommended for several reasons, including other risk factors such as pre-existing client comorbidities and previous testing results in a current pregnancy. Antepartum testing, especially methods using electronic fetal heart monitoring (EFM), is not initiated until the gestational age is sufficient to expect infant survival if intervention and birth becomes necessary (ACOG, 2021a; Devoe et al., 2002; Miller et al., 2022; Raju et al., 2014). Frequency of testing is individualized to a client and fetus, the current clinical situation, and a health care team's judgment. Typically, antepartum testing is conducted weekly or biweekly. More frequent intervals of APFT may be warranted if the clinical status of the pregnant client or fetus deteriorates (ACOG, 2021a; Signore et al., 2009). For example, a perinatal client may be receiving biweekly NSTs and measurement of amniotic fluid due to gestational hypertension. This client is subsequently admitted to an inpatient antepartum unit to evaluate worsening blood pressures and to perform a 24-hour urine collection. NST frequency may be increased to twice daily while the client is hospitalized. Sometimes, an isolated situation warrants outpatient APFT, but continued surveillance is not necessary. For example, an NST may be performed due to a client report of decreased fetal movement. If an NST is reactive and the client is reassured, no further testing is indicated.

Fetal Movement Counting

For obstetric clients, perception of fetal movement is an indicator of fetal life, and absence of movement potentially signals an adverse perinatal outcome. As a fetus becomes more hypoxic related to interruptions in the oxygenation pathway, activity is reduced to conserve oxygen consumption and maintain energy supplies. Over time, fetal movement may no longer be felt, and a stillbirth may occur (ACOG, 2021a; Mangesi et al., 2015; Signore et al., 2009). Ingestion of medications, such as narcotics, barbiturates, benzodiazepines, or methadone, as well as alcohol, beta-blockers, tobacco, and corticosteroids for FLM, have also been associated with altered fetal movement (ACOG, 2021a; Treanor, 2021; Devoe & Jones, 2002; Greenberg & Druzin, 2021). See Table 9.3 for more information regarding substance use and fetal effects.

TABLE 9.3 **Substance Use and Fetal Effects**	
Substance	**Impact on Fetus**
Alcohol	Cardiac anomalies
Anticholinergics	Fetal heart rate increases, tachycardia
Beta blockers	Fetal heart rate increases, bradycardia
Beta sympathomimetics	Fetal heart rate increases, tachycardia
Caffeine	Increased fetal activity, fetal heart rate increases, tachycardia
Cocaine	No effect on fetal heart rate baseline, decreased accelerations, increased decelerations
Decongestants	Fetal heart rate increases, tachycardia
Opioids and methadone	Decreased fetal heart rate accelerations, fetal movement, and fetal breathing
Sedatives	Decreased fetal movement
Tobacco and nicotine	Decreased fetal reactivity, movements, and heart rate variability

Adapted from Abernathy, A. (2017). Transient fetal tachycardia after intravenous diphenhydramine administration. *Obstetrics & Gynecology, 130*(2), 374–376. https://doi.org/10.1097/AOG.0000000000002147; Anastasio, G. D., & Harston, P. R. (1992). Fetal tachycardia associated with maternal use of pseudoephedrine, an over-the-counter oral decongestant. *The Journal of the American Board of Family Practice, 5*(5), 527–528; Baxi, L. V., Gindoff, P. R., Pregenzer, G. J., & Parras, M. K. (1985). Fetal heart rate changes following maternal administration of a nasal decongestant. *American Journal of Obstetrics & Gynecology, 153*(7), 799–800. https://doi.org/10.1016/0002-9378(85)90351-5; Collazos, J. C., Acherman, R. J., Law, I. H., Wilkes, P., Restrepo, H., & Evans, W. N. (2007). Sustained fetal bradycardia with 1:1 atrioventricular conduction and long QT syndrome. *Prenatal Diagnosis, 27*(9), 879–881. https://doi.org/10.1002/pd.1784; Neilson, J. P., West, H. M., Dowswell, T. (2014). Betamimetics for inhibiting preterm labour. *Cochrane Database of Systematic Reviews, 2*, CD004352. https://doi.org/10.1002/14651858.CD004352.pub3; Signore, C., Freeman, R. K., & Spong, C. Y. (2009). Antenatal testing–A reevaluation. *Obstetrics & Gynecology, 113*(3), 687–701. https://doi.org/10.1097/aog.0b013e318197bd8a.

Quantifying fetal movement is considered a method to evaluate well-being because movement generally reflects an intact and functioning central nervous system and adequate oxygenation (Turner et al., 2021). Various FMC methods have been suggested. Unfortunately, an optimal number of fetal movements or duration for counting has not been proposed (American Academy of Pediatrics [AAP] & ACOG, 2017; ACOG, 2021a; Mangesi et al., 2015).

One approach to FMC is a "count to 10" method. Clients are instructed to rest in a quiet location and count distinct fetal movements, such as kicks or rolls. Client perception of 10 distinct movements in a 1- to 2-hour period is reflective of a nonhypoxic fetus at that point in time. The count

Fetal Movement Chart

This chart will help to keep track of your baby's well-being. Carefully count the number of movements your baby makes during the same hour every evening, when babies are typically most active. For example, between 9 and 10 p.m.

If your baby has not moved for 12 hours, please contact 602.406.3521. Be sure to bring this chart with you when visiting your doctor.

Daily Chart of Baby Kicks

DAYS OF WEEK	MONDAY	TUESDAY	WEDNESDAY	THURSDAY	FRIDAY	SATURDAY	SUNDAY
DATE							
KICKS							
DATE							
KICKS							
DATE							
KICKS							
DATE							
KICKS							
DATE							
KICKS							
DATE							
KICKS							
DATE							
KICKS							
DATE							
KICKS							
DATE							
KICKS							

Fetal movement (kick count) chart. Courtesy of St. Joseph's Hospital and Medical Center, Phoenix, AZ.

Fig. 9.13 Fetal movement count sheet example (From Cashion, K. (2017). Assessment of high-risk pregnancy. In S. Perry, D. Lowdermilk, K. Cashion, K. Alden, E. Olshansky, M. Hockenberry, D. Wilson, & C. Rodgers. (Eds.). *Maternal child nursing care* (6th ed., pp. 226–243). Elsevier.)

is discontinued once 10 movements are perceived (ACOG, 2021a; Moore & Piacquadrio, 1989). Fetal movement is then recorded on paper or a mobile phone application. (Fig. 9.13). In situations where a preidentified number of kicks is not met, a client will be advised to seek further evaluation.

Some clients have difficulty recognizing fetal movement related to fetal position, obesity, amniotic fluid volume abnormalities, and placental location (Carroll et al., 2019; O'Neil & Thorp, 2012; Sheikh et al., 2014). For example, an anterior placenta or a breech position may alter the client's perception of movement. In these situations, a nurse can assist the client in uterine palpation for fetal movement. Ultrasound may be used to assist a client in distinguishing fetal movement. Time of the day can potentially influence FMC results. Fetal movement generally peaks between 9:00 PM and 1:00 AM, which is attributed to a fall in the pregnant client's glucose level (Patrick et al., 1982). In this scenario, clients may need to select a different time of day to perform counting.

? KNOWLEDGE CHECK

17. What is the primary goal of APFT?
18. Name the six methods used for antepartum surveillance.
19. List primary indications for initiating APFT.
20. Describe one method of FMC as if you are explaining this procedure to a client.

Nonstress Test

NSTs are one of the primary means of fetal surveillance and are used widely in obstetric practice. NSTs involve placement of an EFM to continuously record FHR and uterine activity; refer to Nursing Procedure 9.1. Early observations of NST results demonstrated when normal oscillations and fluctuations in baseline FHR (variability) and accelerations were present, fetal well-being could be established (Lee et al., 1975; Rochard et al., 1976). An NST identifies FHR accelerations, which indicate an intact central nervous system and normal autonomic regulation of the FHR, as well as being predictive of the absence of fetal metabolic acidemia at the time of observation (Macones et al., 2008; Miller et al., 2022; Powell et al., 1979). If the fetal heart does not accelerate spontaneously with movement or with stimuli, further assessment by a clinician is warranted.

Accelerations are defined as visually apparent FHR increases that reach a peak of 15 beats per minute (bpm) above baseline, with an entire acceleration lasting a minimum of 15 seconds but less than 2 minutes ("15 × 15"). Before 32 weeks of gestation, accelerations are defined as visually apparent FHR increases that reach a peak of 10 bpm above baseline with an entire acceleration lasting at least 10 seconds ("10 × 10") (Macones et al., 2008). This is because preterm fetuses may not have the physiologic maturity to generate accelerations that meet the 15 x 15 criteria. In the antepartum period, accelerations can either be spontaneous or elicited with abdominal manipulation of the fetus during Leopold's maneuver or an acoustic stimulation device. Sometimes monitoring may show uterine activity not perceived by a client. These contractions, which are often mild on palpation and irregular, reflect normal structural and functional changes in the myometrium (Blackburn, 2018). However, if contraction frequency increases, appears to be more coordinated, or changes intensity, further assessment is recommended especially in preterm gestations.

Procedure

NSTs are noninvasive and can be performed in a hospital or clinic setting. Clients are placed in a comfortable position, such as side-lying or semi-Fowler's with a lateral tilt. This type of positioning reduces aortocaval compression risk which, in turn, can manifest into hypotension in a client and abnormal FHR changes. Fetal position is assessed with Leopold's maneuvers to allow correct EFM placement and maximize the ability to obtain a continuous tracing. An ultrasound transducer and Toco transducer are applied and secured to a client's abdomen to detect FHR and uterine activity (Fig. 9.14). Although NST contains the word *stress*, a fetus is not physically challenged by factors such as increased client activity or contractions to obtain necessary data. Clients remain on continuous fetal monitoring for a minimum of 20 minutes. If there is an absence of an acceleratory response or accelerations do not meet criteria, an NST can be extended another 20 minutes for a total of 40 minutes. This additional time accounts for normal fetal sleep–wake cycles when fetal movement and normal FHR characteristics are decreased (ACOG, 2021a; Liston et al. 2018).

After 10 to 20 minutes, fetal stimulation may be required to elicit a fetal response. One simple method uses an artificial larynx to provide vibroacoustic stimulation. An artificial larynx is placed on a client's abdomen near the fetal head.

NURSING PROCEDURE 9.1
External Fetal Monitor

1. Review institutional policy for EFM and how a device interfaces with computer documentation if necessary. Verify date and time for the equipment are consistent with computer documentation. Become familiar with proper operation of the monitoring equipment by reviewing the manufacturer's guidelines.
2. Perform a function test following manufacturer's instructions. Press the "TEST" button and observe the result. A correct function test ensures a bedside monitor is calibrated properly so accurate data can be interpreted. Each manufacturer sets standards for indicators of proper function.
3. Explain the basic EFM procedure to the client.
4. Transducer belts are placed around the client's abdomen before transducer placement. After Leopold's maneuver, apply ultrasound gel, which improves sound transmission between a Doppler ultrasound transducer and monitoring device. Place the transducer on the abdomen along the fetal back. Move the transducer until a clear signal is heard. Most bedside units have a green light or flashing light to indicate an adequate signal.
5. Place the tocodynamometer on the uterine fundus or an area where contractions are palpated the strongest.
6. Apply transducer belts or adhesive ring to secure transducers in place. Be sure to keep the belts smooth under the client's back because this will improve comfort and improve transmission contact of external transducers. Adequate contact improves tracing quality and may reduce the number of adjustments needed.
7. Assess FHR and UA in accordance with institutional policies and professional guidelines.

EFM, Electronic fetal monitoring; *FHR,* fetal heart rate; *UA,* uterine activity.

Acoustic stimulation is applied for one to two seconds and can be repeated up to three times for progressively longer durations, up to three seconds long if no response is obtained (ACOG, 2021a; Treanor, 2021). Fetuses will respond to externally applied sound and vibration by displaying more FHR accelerations with increased amplitude and duration (Walker et al., 1971; Read & Miller, 1977). Cellular phones placed on a client's abdomen and loud noises or vibration near a client (e.g., vacuum cleaner) may also elicit a similar response. Occasionally, a client may be asked to press an event marker, recording a symbol on an EFM tracing each time fetal movement is perceived. This is not a requirement for interpretation of an NST. Fetal heart rate and uterine activity is recorded either on a paper tracing from the EFM, electronically, or both.

Interpretation

NSTs are interpreted as reactive or nonreactive. A reactive NST contains two or more FHR accelerations which meet the criteria previously described within a 20-minute period (Fig. 9.15). Documentation of accelerations in relationship to fetal movement is not required for a reactive NST. Nonreactive NSTs are defined as less than two accelerations during a 40-minute period (Fig. 9.16). Variable decelerations

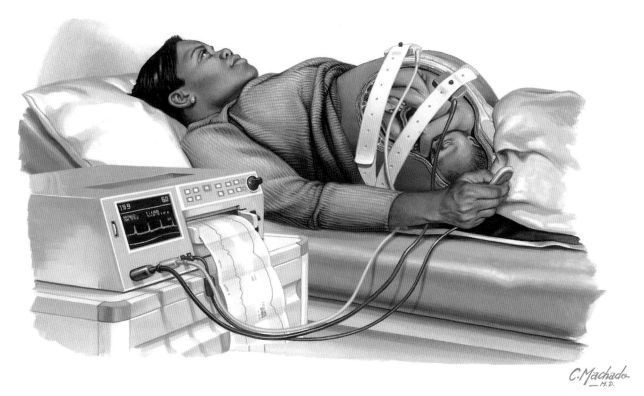

Fig. 9.14 Electronic fetal monitoring being used for a nonstress test. Note that the top tocodynamometer is placed on the fundus to measure uterine contractions. The bottom Doppler ultrasound transducer is placed over the fetal back to measure heart rate. The client is holding a device to mark fetal movement on the tracing. This is not a requirement for nonstress test interpretation. (From Smith, R. (2018). Nonstress Testing. In R. Smith (Ed.) *Netter's obstetrics & gynecology* (3rd ed., pp. 427–429). Elsevier.)

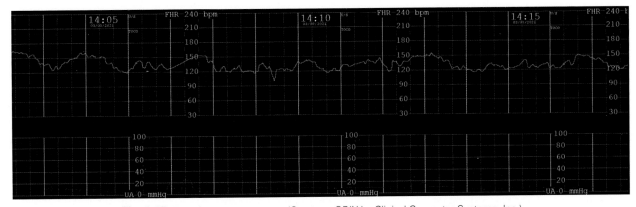

Fig. 9.15 Reactive nonstress test. (Courtesy OBIX by Clinical Computer Systems, Inc.)

are sometimes observed in NSTs and are associated with umbilical cord compression. Variable decelerations that are not recurrent and last less than 30 seconds require no further intervention or monitoring, though a physician, midwife, or nurse practitioner is notified prior to discontinuing this test (AAP & ACOG, 2017, ACOG, 2021a; Liston et al., 2018). However, if variable decelerations become recurrent, defined as three or more in 20 minutes, a client is generally monitored for an extended period to allow for further evaluation of the entire clinical picture and current fetal status. Recurrent variable decelerations and decelerations that persist for 1 minute or longer during an NST have been associated with

an increased cesarean birth risk for indeterminate and abnormal FHR patterns, as well as stillbirth (ACOG, 2021a; Liston et al., 2018; Treanor, 2021). Nurses may interpret and document NST results if hospital or clinic directed educational and competency requirements have been met.

Contraction Stress Test and Oxytocin Challenge Test

CSTs determine fetal well-being by monitoring FHR responses to contractions when uteroplacental sufficiency is in question. CSTs may be referred to as an oxytocin challenge test (OCT), in which intravenous oxytocin is used

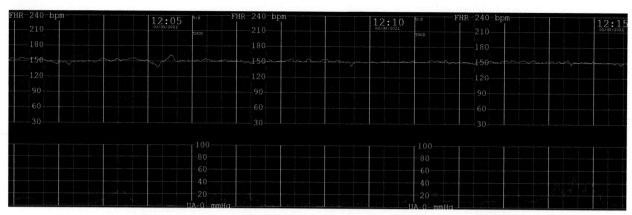

Fig. 9.16 Nonreactive nonstress test. (Courtesy OBIX by Clinical Computer Systems, Inc.)

to elicit contractions or nipple stimulation test, in which client manipulation of the nipple produces contractions. While BPPs and Doppler flow studies have mostly replaced this test in clinical practice, a CST may be appropriate if there is concern about fetal status (Esplin, 2020; Liston et al., 2018). Examples include a pregnancy complicated by both hypertensive disease and type 1 diabetes or fetal conditions such as growth restriction and postdates pregnancy. The physiologic premise of this test is based on the knowledge that normal uterine contractions transiently restrict blood flow to the intervillous spaces of the placenta. In turn, this alters oxygen delivery to the chorionic villli and fetus. Simply stated, uteroplacental blood flow is temporarily interrupted as a result of blood vessel compression during contractions. A healthy oxygenated fetus can tolerate uterine activity and maintain a FHR with normal characteristics, such as a stable baseline rate and accelerations. In a compromised fetus, this exchange may result in the appearance of late decelerations, which are reflective of transient fetal hypoxemia.

Late decelerations are defined as a gradual FHR decrease (≥30 seconds) from the FHR baseline with a nadir (lowest part of a deceleration) occurring after a contraction peaks. This is followed by a gradual recovery to baseline after a contraction subsides (Macones et al., 2008, Chapter 14). If contractions continue, a fetus could progressively deteriorate from hypoxemia down a pathway of leading to potential neurologic injury or death (Miller et al., 2022).

Procedure

CSTs are typically performed in a hospital environment where interventions, such as administration of intravenous medication or an expedited birth, can occur in the event of an emergency. Relative contraindications for performing this test include clients in whom vaginal birth is not recommended at the time of the test. Examples include placenta previa, preterm premature rupture of membranes, preterm labor, history of preterm birth, previous classic cesarean birth, or multiple gestations (AAP & ACOG 2017; ACOG, 2021a). Procedure steps are much like those of NSTs. Initial monitoring will determine whether an adequate contraction pattern is spontaneously present. An adequate contraction pattern is defined as three contractions within a 10-minute

timeframe. Each contraction must be 40 seconds or longer in duration and palpable to the nurse. Contractions do not need to be perceived as painful by the client. An adequate contraction pattern with continuous FHR and uterine activity is required to interpret CST results. If spontaneous contractions are sufficient, additional uterine stimulation is not necessary. When adequate contractions are not present, oxytocin or nipple stimulation is required. Regardless of which method is used, success rates for achieving an adequate contraction pattern to interpret test results are similar (Greenberg & Druzin, 2021).

For an OCT, an intravenous infusion of dilute exogenous oxytocin is required to stimulate uterine activity. Oxytocin is administered by a continuous infusion pump per hospital policy. One sample protocol starts oxytocin at 0.5 mU/min to 1 mU/min, with increases every 15 to 20 minutes until sufficient contractions are recorded (AAP & ACOG, 2017; Miller et al., 2022; Treanor, 2021). Oxytocin is discontinued once an adequate contraction pattern with interpretable data is visualized. If there is evidence of tachysystole (more than five contractions in a 10-minute segment averaged over a 30-minute period) and/or FHR decelerations, oxytocin is decreased or discontinued (Simpson, 2020).

An alternative to oxytocin infusion is nipple stimulation. When breasts are stimulated, endogenous oxytocin is released from the posterior pituitary gland and uterine contractions will occur (Blackburn, 2018). Before starting this procedure, a nurse can apply warm packs to a client's breasts for approximately 10 minutes to improve relaxation and circulation. The client is instructed to brush the palm of a hand across one nipple or roll a nipple using the palmar surface of the index finger and thumb. Nipple stimulation can be performed through clothing or skin to skin. One example protocol involves a client rubbing the nipple for 2 minutes or until a contraction begins. Uterine activity is evaluated and if there are no contractions or inadequate contractions to meet predefined criteria, a client is instructed to rest for 2 to 5 minutes. This is followed by a second cycle of 2 minutes of stimulation on the opposite nipple. If after four cycles an adequate contraction pattern is not recorded, the process is continued for another 10 minutes. If this is unsuccessful, an additional 10 minutes of bilateral nipple stimulation is advised. If nipple stimulation does not produce the required uterine contraction pattern, an

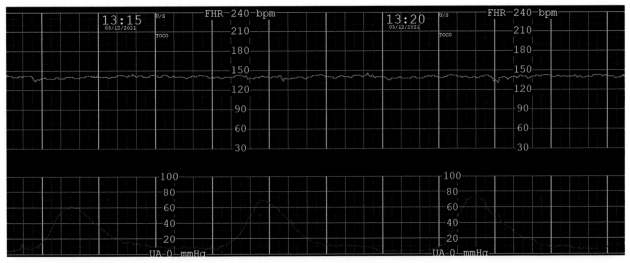

Fig. 9.17 Negative contraction stress test via nipple stimulation. (Courtesy OBIX by Clinical Computer Systems, Inc.)

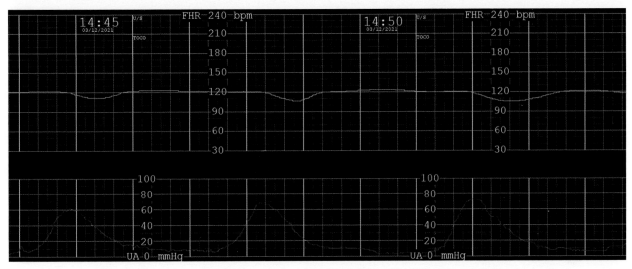

Fig. 9.18 Positive contraction stress test. (Courtesy OBIX by Clinical Computer Systems, Inc.)

OCT may become necessary. Nipple stimulation is stopped when three or more contractions lasting longer than 40 seconds occur in a 10-minute time frame or in cases of tachysystole or decelerations (Liston et al., 2018; Miller et al., 2022; Treanor, 2021).

The interpretation criteria for CST are as follows (AAP & ACOG, 2017; ACOG, 2021a):

- *Negative*—No late or significant variable decelerations (Fig. 9.17)
- *Positive*—Late decelerations present with a minimum of 50% of contractions, even when fewer than three contractions occur in 10 minutes (Fig. 9.18)
- *Equivocal-suspicious*—Intermittent late decelerations or significant variable decelerations (Fig. 9.19)
- *Equivocal*—FHR decelerations in the presence of contractions that are more frequent than every 2 minutes or last longer than 90 seconds (Fig. 9.20)
- *Unsatisfactory*—Fewer than three contractions in 10 minutes or an uninterpretable tracing (Fig. 9.21)

A negative CST has been consistently associated with positive fetal outcomes as long as an acute event (e.g., placental abruption) does not occur (Lagrew, 1995; Freeman et al., 1982; Signore et al., 2009). Negative CSTs can be repeated in 1 week, although more frequent monitoring with NSTs or BPPs may be necessary in certain conditions such as postterm pregnancy, diabetes, growth abnormalities, or hypertension (ACOG, 2021a). Positive CSTs are linked to an increased incidence of growth restriction, late decelerations in labor, meconium-stained fluid, low 5-minute Apgar scores, and stillbirth (Lagrew, 1995). In the event of a positive CST result, the health care team will discuss management options with a client including, but not limited to, further testing or an expedited birth after an evaluation of the entire clinical situation. An equivocal, equivocal suspicious, or unsatisfactory CST result prompts further assessment, including repeat testing within 24 hours, prolonged continuous monitoring, or using adjunct methods of testing unless other clinical factors indicate a need for an expedited birth (ACOG, 2021a; Greenberg & Druzin, 2021).

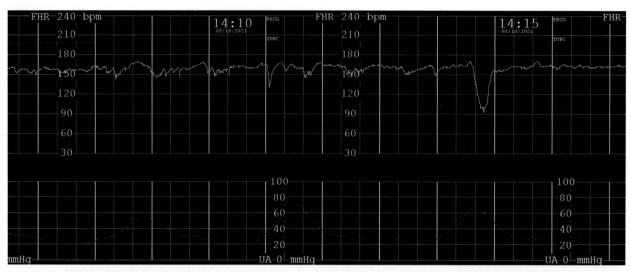

Fig. 9.19 Equivocal-suspicious contraction stress test. (Courtesy OBIX by Clinical Computer Systems, Inc.)

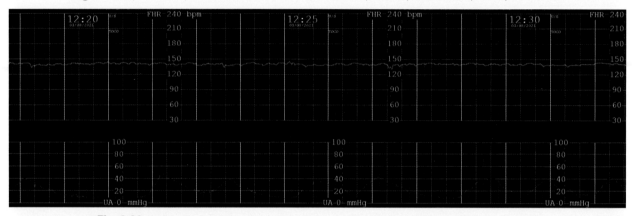

Fig. 9.20 Equivocal contraction stress test. (Courtesy OBIX by Clinical Computer Systems, Inc.)

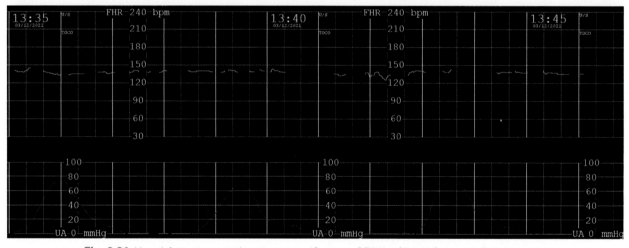

Fig. 9.21 Unsatisfactory contraction stress test. (Courtesy OBIX by Clinical Computer Systems, Inc.)

KNOWLEDGE CHECK

21. Define a reactive and nonreactive NST.
22. Why are contractions necessary for CST interpretation?
23. Identify the five results of a CST interpretation and explain the management plan for each finding.

Biophysical Profile

BPPs combine EFM with an ultrasound assessment of specific fetal behavioral and physiologic characteristics. These include fetal movement, fetal tone, fetal breathing movement, and amniotic fluid amount. These biophysical characteristics reflect both the central and autonomic nervous systems and, if

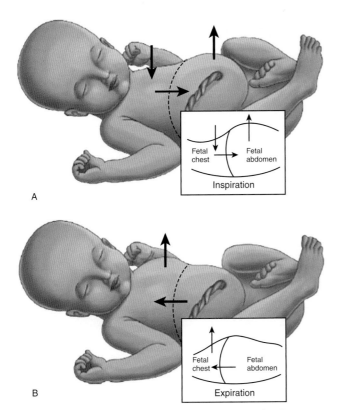

A

B

Fig. 9.22 Fetal breathing. (From Antepartum fetal assessment (2022). In F. Cunningham, K. Leveno, S. Bloom, J. Dashe, B. Hoffman, B. Casey, & C. Spong (Eds). *William's obstetrics* (26th ed.). McGraw-Hill Companies.)

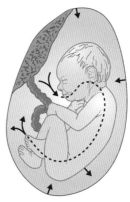

Fig. 9.23 Amniotic fluid is swallowed by the fetus, absorbed through gastrointestinal tract, and excreted through fetal urine. (From Ioannides, A. S. (2020). Placental and fetal growth and development. In I. Symonds, & S. Arulkumaran (Eds.). *Essentials and gynaecology* (6th ed., pp. 41–55). Elsevier.)

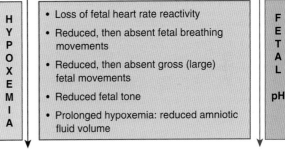

Fig. 9.24 Effects of gradual hypoxemia and worsening of fetal acidosis.

present, represent normal neurologic function and adequate oxygenation (Vintzileos et al., 1987). Individual BPP components combine short-term (acute) and long-term (chronic) indicators of fetal well-being and sufficient oxygenation. Short-term indicators of adequate oxygenation include FHR reactivity and fetal breathing movement, while the long-term indicators include amniotic fluid volume, gross body movements, and tone (Manning et al., 1980). Each component is susceptible to oxygenation pathway interruptions, which may lead down a pathway to hypoxia and eventually neurologic injury if not corrected (ACOG, 2021a; Blackburn, 2018; Manning et al., 1980). Unlike NSTs and CSTs, which assess FHR characteristics, a BPP allows for a complete assessment of oxygenation in the intrauterine environment.

Biophysical characteristics emerge at different stages of fetal development. Fetal tone is established at approximately 7 to 8 weeks of gestation. Spontaneous fetal movement can be observed on ultrasound at around 9 weeks of gestation, starting with flexion–extension of the vertebral column. Fetal breathing can be detected at 10 weeks of gestation and becomes more apparent by 19 to 20 weeks of gestation. Sometimes referred to as "practice breathing," this biophysical characteristic is often rhythmic and reflects diaphragmatic, laryngeal, and intercostal muscle contractions (Fig. 9.22). Amniotic fluid production by the fetal renal system is present at approximately 10 weeks of gestation. Physiologically, a fetus swallows amniotic fluid, and in turn fluid is absorbed

in the fetal gastrointestinal tract. Fetal urine is subsequently excreted by a fetus, and the process is repeated (Fig. 9.23). Finally, FHR reactivity is established by the conclusion of the second trimester (Blackburn, 2018; Manning, 1995; Vintzileos & Knuppel, 1994).

Interruptions of the oxygen pathway at one or more points can lead to acute or chronic periods of hypoxia which in turn prompts the fetus to decrease biophysical activities in reverse order of pregnancy development (Fig. 9.24). Physiologically, this phenomenon preserves energy and oxygen consumption. Fetal heart rate reactivity disappears first, followed by fetal breathing movement. If hypoxia continues, decreased fetal movement and loss of fetal tone will occur. During this process, oligohydramnios or decreased amniotic fluid levels develop, because uteroplacental circulation is not adequate to oxygenate fetal kidneys. Shunting occurs, and blood is redirected from areas not critical to fetal life (e.g., kidneys, gastrointestinal tract, and extremities) to vital organs (e.g., heart, brain, and adrenal glands). If oxygen pathway interruptions continue, blood flow to the fetal kidneys ceases. Therefore oligohydramnios in fetuses with normal renal structures and intact amniotic membranes suggests prolonged fetal hypoxia and is a strong indication of fetal compromise (Manning, 1995; Vintzileos & Knuppel, 1994).

TABLE 9.4   Biophysical Profile Scoring Criteria

Fetal Biophysical Variables	2 Points	0 Points
Movement	At least three episodes of trunk or limb movement	Less than three episodes of trunk or limb movement
Tone	At least one episode of active extension with return to flexion of the fetal limb or trunk; opening and closing of the hand is deemed normal tone	Absent movement or slow extension/flexion
Breathing movement	At least one breathing episode lasting a minimum of 30 seconds	Absent breathing movement or less than 30 seconds of sustained breathing movement
Amniotic fluid	At least one pocket of amniotic fluid that measures at least 2 cm in two perpendicular planes	Absent amniotic fluid pockets or a pocket measure less than 2 cm in two perpendicular planes
Nonstress test (NST)	Reactive	Nonreactive

Adapted from Manning, F. A. (1995). Dynamic ultrasound-based fetal assessment: The fetal biophysical profile score. *Clinical Obstetrics and Gynecology, 38*(1), 26–44. https://doi.org/10.1097/00003081-199503000-00006; Manning, F., Platt, L., & Sipos, L. (1980). Antepartum fetal evaluation: Development of a fetal biophysical profile. *American Journal of Obstetrics and Gynecology, 136*(6), 787–795. https://doi.org/10.1016/0002-9378(80)90457-3.

TABLE 9.5   Interpretation and Management for Biophysical Profiles

Score	Interpretation	Management
10 of 10 8 of 10 (normal AFV) 8 of 8 (NST not done)	Risk of fetal asphyxia extremely rare	No indication for intervention Individualize based on client, obstetric, or fetal factors only (i.e., worsening preeclampsia)
8 of 10 (Abnormal AFV)	No acute asphyxia; probable chronic fetal compromise	Establish intact membranes and functioning renal tissue Consider birth for oligohydramnios or further testing depending on gestational age and client or obstetric factors
6 of 10 (Normal fluid)	Equivocal test, possible fetal asphyxia	Mature fetus: consider birth Immature fetus: repeat testing within 24 hours
6 of 10 (Abnormal fluid)	Probable asphyxia	Consider birth for oligohydramnios or further testing Individualize to client, obstetric, or fetal factors
4 of 10	Probable fetal asphyxia	Consider birth Shared decision-making for neonatal consult and future management prior to birth
2 of 10	Fetal asphyxia almost certain	Consider birth Shared decision-making for neonatal consult and future management prior to birth
0 of 10	Fetal asphyxia certain	Consider birth Shared decision-making for neonatal consult and future management prior to birth

Adapted from Cypher, R. L., & Foglia, L. M. (2020). Periviability: A review of key concepts and management for perinatal nursing. *The Journal of Perinatal & Neonatal Nursing, 34*(2), 146–154. https://doi.org/10.1097/JPN.0000000000000473; Manning, F. A. (1995). Dynamic ultrasound-based fetal assessment: The fetal biophysical profile score. *Clinical Obstetrics and Gynecology, 38*(1), 26–44. https://doi.org/10.1097/00003081-199503000-00006; Treanor, C. M. (2021). Antenatal fetal assessment and testing. In A. Lyndon, & K. Wisner (Eds.). *Fetal heart rate monitoring: Principles and practices.* (6th ed., pp. 277–308). Kendall-Hunt.

Procedure and Interpretation

NSTs are the EFM portion of BPPs and are generally performed prior to the ultrasound to determine whether an FHR tracing is reactive or nonreactive. Sometimes, NSTs are performed after an ultrasound, especially if any of the biophysical characteristics criteria are not met. Observation of the four biophysical characteristics is conducted over a 30-minute period and no longer. This type of ultrasound is typically performed by sonographers, advanced practice nurses, or physicians. As mentioned previously, nurses may perform BPPs according to state and local level guidance.

A scoring technique is used to interpret data, with each parameter receiving a score of 2 (normal) or 0 (abnormal) (Table 9.4). Scores for all five BPP components are totaled together for interpretation and management (Table 9.5). Biophysical scores of 8 or 10 correlate with normal fetal oxygenation. A BPP score of 6 is considered equivocal. With equivocal scores, extending the testing period, retesting within 24 hours, or adding adjunct testing, such as a CST, may be done before making pregnancy management decisions (ACOG, 2021a; Greenberg & Druzin, 2021; Kaimal, 2019). Scores of 0 to 4 in situations where previous APFT results were normal may justify birth depending on the clinical scenario and gestational age. Abnormal scores of 0 to 4 are usually associated with hypoxemia or acidemia, which leads to poor perinatal and neonatal outcomes. Regardless of a score, if oligohydramnios is observed, further evaluation is warranted (ACOG, 2021a).

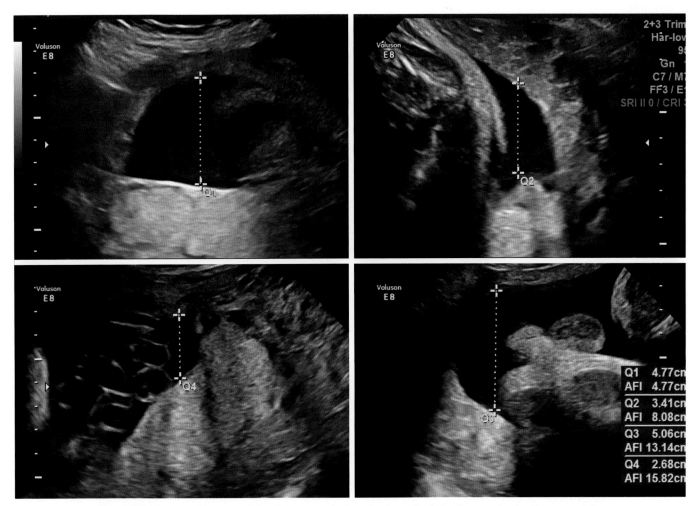

Fig. 9.25 Ultrasound images of the deepest vertical pocket in each of the four quadrants. The sum of the measurements is referred to as an amniotic fluid index. In this image the first quadrant measures 4.77 cm, the second quadrant is 3.41 cm, the third quadrant is 5.06 cm, and the fourth quadrant is 2.68 cm. The total amniotic fluid index is 15.82 cm. (From Richards, D. S. (2021). Obstetric ultrasound. In M. Landon, V. Berghella, A. Cahill, D. Driscoll, H. Galan, W. Grobman, E. Jauniax, & S. Kilpatrick (Eds.). *Gabbe's obstetrics: Normal & problem pregnancies* (8th ed., pp. 156–179). Elsevier.)

Modified Biophysical Profile

MBPP is a variation of a BPP. Modified BPPs combine an NST with ultrasound measurement of amniotic fluid. Remember, NSTs are a short-term indicator of how well a fetus is oxygenated, and amniotic fluid level is a long-term reflection of adequate oxygenation in which shunting has not taken place. This method is generally performed weekly or biweekly, depending on the indication for testing. Unlike a BPP, this test is not as time consuming and does not require the same level of ultrasound skills (AAP & ACOG, 2017; O'Neill & Thorp, 2012), although it may be beyond the scope of nursing practice for the RN in many states.

Procedure and Management

An NST is performed with this test. Amniotic fluid amount is assessed by one of two methods. The first includes measurement of the largest pocket of amniotic fluid in four quadrants (Fig. 9.25). These measurements are totaled together to report an amniotic fluid index (AFI). Oligohydramnios is an AFI of less than 5 cm for this procedure.

Single deepest pocket measurement is an alternative to a complete AFI. The pocket measured must be free of umbilical cord and fetal parts. If a single deepest pocket is 2 cm or less, oligohydramnios is identified (AAP & ACOG, 2017; ACOG, 2021a). Results are interpreted as normal if an NST is reactive and oligohydramnios is not observed. Abnormal MBPPs have either a nonreactive NST or oligohydramnios, or both conditions are present (AAP & ACOG, 2017; ACOG, 2021a). Further evaluation is indicated if test results are abnormal.

Fetal Doppler Flow Ultrasound

Fetal Doppler flow ultrasound is an assessment of placental condition. This noninvasive procedure assesses hemodynamic components of vascular resistance in high-risk pregnancies with fetal growth restriction (ACOG, 2021a). Doppler flow is also used to detect fetal anemia when Rh alloimmunization is suspected (Moise, 2021). With Doppler flow studies, a skilled clinician or sonographer measures cardiac cycle differences between peak-systolic

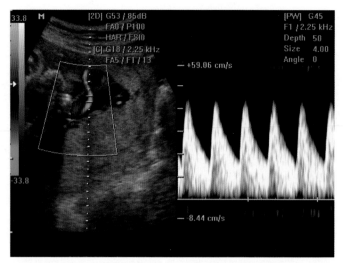

Fig. 9.26 Doppler flow evaluation of umbilical cord. The red and blue colors represent the coiling of the umbilical cord arteries and vein. Red represents blood flow toward the ultrasound transducer, and the blue color is blood flow that is going away from the transducer. (From Richards, D. S. (2021). Obstetric ultrasound. In M. Landon, V. Berghella, A. Cahill, D. Driscoll, H. Galan, W. Grobman, E. Jauniax, & S. Kilpatrick (Eds.). *Gabbe's obstetrics: Normal & problem pregnancies* (8th ed., pp. 156–179). Elsevier.)

and end-diastolic blood flow velocity, referred to as the *S/D ratio*. Also, the amount of blood flow resistance and pulsatility index in various fetal vessels can be calculated (ACOG, 2021a; O'Neil & Thorp, 2012). Color may be added to assist in assessing blood flow velocity (Fig. 9.26). One of the most common vessels observed with Doppler flow are umbilical arteries, which allows for assessment of blood flow from the fetus to the placenta. Measurements also can be taken of the middle cerebral artery, umbilical veins, ductus venosus, and other structures (Kaimal, 2019; O'Neil & Thorp, 2012). In fetal growth restriction, more attention is paid to middle cerebral artery measurements because of this shunting phenomenon. Hypoxic fetuses shunt blood flow to the brain by reducing the amount of resistance in fetal cerebrovascular vessels. This allows for an increase in blood flow to a fetal brain (Bahtiyar & Copel, 2019).

Fetal Doppler flow ultrasound results are reported as normal, elevated, absent, or reversed (Fig. 9.27). A growth-restricted fetus may have elevated, absent, or reversed end-diastolic flow when deterioration occurs from an interruption in the oxygenation pathway. The sequence of events for abnormal Doppler flow starts with increased resistance in placental vasculature and indicates poor placental function. This leads to decreased diastolic velocities that eventually become absent. Once absent diastolic flow occurs, blood flow resistance continues to increase, and an elastic component to fetal vasculature is added to this sequence of events. This causes reversed end-diastolic flow, and placental circulation starts to recoil or "reverse" after being distended (Kaimal, 2019). Increased resistance occurs when approximately 30%

of fetal vasculature is abnormal (Morrow et al., 1989). Absent and reversed end-diastolic Doppler images are abnormal and have been linked to altered fetal acid–base status and poor perinatal outcomes, including stillbirth (Kaimal, 2019; Miller et al., 2022; O'Neil & Thorp, 2012). Clients with normal Doppler flow results are typically evaluated weekly. In the same week, an NST or MBPP may be performed. Increased frequency of Doppler examinations and other adjuncts of fetal assessment occur when abnormal results are identified. As with other methods of APFT, Doppler flow study results are interpreted in the context of an entire clinical scenario, including results of other surveillance methods to make pregnancy management decisions.

Nursing Responsibilities

Similar to prenatal screening and diagnostic tests, a nurse provides an appropriate level of individualized client and family education and support based on the clinical situation (Chard & Norton, 2016). Tools such as educational pamphlets covering APFT can reinforce key points such as indications for testing and surveillance methods.

❓ KNOWLEDGE CHECK

24. What are four biophysical characteristics observed with ultrasound during a BPP, and what do they reflect?
25. Why is amniotic fluid volume an important parameter in BPPs and MBPPs?
26. Describe the process of shunting in relationship to fetal oxygenation.

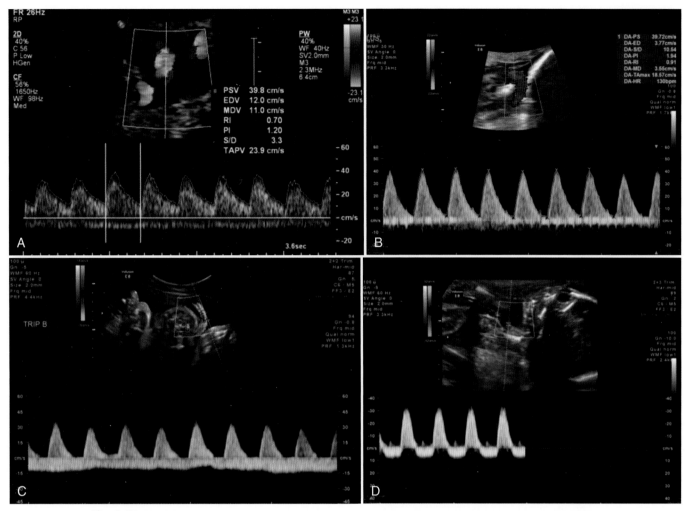

Fig. 9.27 Doppler ultrasound of the umbilical artery demonstrating progressive worsening of blood flow velocity. A, Normal blood flow pattern. B, Increased systolic to diastolic blood flow velocity. C, Absent systolic to diastolic blood flow velocity. D, Reverse end-diastolic blood flow. (From Bahtiyar, M. O., & Copel, J. A. (2019). Assessment of fetal health. In R. Resnik, C. Lockwood, T. Moore, M. Greene, J. Copel, & R. Silver (Eds). *Creasy and Resnik's maternal-fetal medicine: Principles and practice.* (8th ed., pp. 266–273). Elsevier.)

SUMMARY CONCEPTS

- There are two categories of prenatal testing. Screening detects or identifies individuals who are at risk for an abnormality or disease. Diagnostic testing identifies or confirms a diagnosis and is the most accurate test.
- Ultrasound is widely used during pregnancy for a variety of indications to include, but not limited to, determine gestational age and fetal size, evaluate for various fetal and placental conditions, and use as an adjunct to other fetal surveillance tests and procedures, such as amniocentesis.
- First-trimester screenings incorporate the levels of human chorionic gonadotropin and pregnancy-associated plasma protein-A in the pregnant client's blood with ultrasound nuchal translucency measurement to identify fetal chromosomal anomalies such as trisomy 21.
- Second-trimester multiple-marker screening is performed between 15 and 22 6/7 weeks of gestation and is used to report a client's risk for trisomy 21, trisomy 18, and open NTDs.

- Measurement of human chorionic gonadotropin, alpha-fetoprotein, inhibin-A, and unconjugated estriol 3 levels in the client's serum are calculated with gestational age, weight, ethnicity, presence of diabetes, and number of fetuses to determine test results.
- Chorionic villus sampling is an invasive procedure performed in the first trimester to obtain chromosomal, metabolic, and genetic disorder information.
- Amniocentesis is another invasive procedure performed in the second and third trimesters. Amniotic fluid is removed for prenatal testing, and as a therapeutic measure for excess amniotic fluid volume.
- The primary goal of antepartum fetal testing is to decrease risk for permanent neurologic injury or stillbirth in high-risk pregnancies.
- Methods of APFT include fetal movement counting, non-stress test, contraction stress test, biophysical profile, modified biophysical profile, and fetal Doppler flow ultrasound.

- A simple evaluation tool for fetal well-being is the pregnant client's perception of fetal movement.
- Fetal activity becomes reduced when a fetus becomes hypoxic, to conserve energy and oxygen. Pregnant clients are advised to seek further evaluation for complaints of decreased fetal movement.
- Fetal heart rate accelerations reflect normal autonomic regulation and an intact central nervous system, as well as being predictive of the absence of fetal metabolic acidemia.
- Nonstress tests are a form of antepartum surveillance in which a presence or absence of fetal heart rate accelerations is assessed.
- Contraction stress tests evaluate fetal heart rate response to uterine contractions. Healthy oxygenated fetuses can tolerate temporary disruptions in oxygenation, whereas compromised fetuses will demonstrate fetal heart rate decelerations.
- Biophysical profiles assess fetal heart rate reactivity and four fetal biophysical characteristics observed on ultrasound: breathing motion, gross movements, muscle tone, and amniotic fluid amount.
- A modified biophysical profile consists of a nonstress test and measurement of amniotic fluid volume.
- Fetal Doppler flow ultrasound is a method of measuring blood flow patterns in fetal circulation. Flow that is normal is associated with adequate fetal oxygenation. Absent or reversed flow is abnormal and is associated with a poor fetal prognosis.

Clinical Judgment And Next-Generation NCLEX® Examination-Style Questions

Two days ago, a client, 37 years old $G_3 P_0$ at 35 weeks gestation, presented to the clinic. Medical history includes type 2 diabetes that has been well controlled this pregnancy. Obstetric history includes two spontaneous abortions at 8 and 12 weeks of gestation. Current pregnancy has been uncomplicated until current visit. The client reported a weight gain of 8 lb over 2 days and a constant headache. Initial blood pressure assessed was 145/96, and 10 minutes later the blood pressure was reassessed at 138/88. The head-to-toe assessment revealed 3+ deep tendon reflexes. Client admits to smoking half a pack of cigarettes a day and denies alcohol or recreational drug use.

Laboratory work was drawn to rule out preeclampsia (multiorgan disease process involving vasoconstriction that results in elevated blood pressure, end organ damage, decreased placental perfusion, and decreased fetal oxygenation when left uncontrolled). The client was sent home from the prenatal clinic with orders to decrease activity level and rest frequently over the next few days.

Today (2 days after prenatal clinic visit), the client arrives in Labor and Delivery complaining of decreased fetal movement and headache. The OB provider orders a nonstress test (NST).

1. **Choose the most likely options for the information missing from the statement below by selecting from the lists of options provided.**

   The nurse performing the NST knows there must be ___1___ in a ___2___-minute period in order for the nonstress test to be reactive.

Option 1	Option 2
Two 15 x 15 accelerations (peak at least 15 bpm above baseline and last for at least 15 seconds)	10
Minimal baseline variability	20
Two 10 x 10 accelerations (peak at least 10 bpm above baseline and last for at least 10 seconds)	30
Moderate baseline variability	40

The NST was reactive. The client's blood pressure was 142/90 initially, with repeat assessment 10 minutes later at 140/87. The provider ordered Tylenol 650 mg po and to discharge the client home with fetal movement counts to be performed daily.

2. **Choose the most likely options for the information missing from the statement below by selecting from the lists of options provided.**

   Fetal movement counts serve as an indicator of fetal ___1___ based on the premise that the fetus will ___2___ when oxygenating appropriately. Fetal movement ___3___ at night; therefore fetal movement counts should occur at the same time every day to give an accurate assessment.

Option 1	Option 2	Option 3
Growth	Curl into the fetal position	Increases
Distress	Move	Decreases
Well-being	Lie still	Remains unchanged

3. **For each client response, use an X to indicate whether the nurse's teaching was effective (helped the client understand how to perform fetal movement counts), ineffective (did not help the client understand how to perform fetal movement counts), or unrelated (not related to the health teaching about fetal movement counts).**

Client Response	Effective	Ineffective	Unrelated
"It does not matter what time of day I do my fetal movement counts, just as long as I complete them every day."			
"If I smoke right before I complete my fetal movement counts, my baby may not move as much."			
"I need to complete fetal movement counts at the same time every night."			
"If my baby does not move at least 10 times in 1 hour, then I need to call my doctor."			
"It does not matter how many times my baby moves, just as long as I feel movement occur daily."			
"If I take my prenatal vitamin regularly, it will help my baby move more."			

REFERENCES & READINGS

Abdou, A. M., Badr, M. S., Helal, K. F., Rafeek, M. E., Abdelrhman, A. A., & Kotb, M. (2020). Diagnostic accuracy of lamellar body count as a predictor of fetal lung maturity: A systematic review and meta-analysis. *European Journal of Obstetrics & Gynecology and Reproductive Biology, 5*, 100059. https://doi.org/10.1016/j.eurox.2019.100059.

Abernathy, A. (2017). Transient fetal tachycardia after intravenous diphenhydramine administration. *Obstetrics & Gynecology, 130*(2), 374–376. https://doi.org/10.1097/AOG.0000000000002147.

Alldred, S. K., Takwoingi, Y., Guo, B., Pennant, M., Deeks, J. J., Neilson, J. P., et al. (2017). First and second trimester serum tests with and without first trimester ultrasound tests for Down's syndrome screening. *Cochrane Database of Systematic Reviews, 11*, CD011975. https://doi.org/10.1002/14651858.cd012599.

American Academy of Pediatrics & American College of Obstetricians and Gynecologists. (2017). *Guidelines for perinatal care* (8th ed.).

American College of Obstetrics and Gynecology (ACOG). (2019). *Prenatal genetic testing chart.* https://www.acog.org/womens-health/infographics/prenatal-genetic-testing-chart.

American College of Obstetrics and Gynecology (ACOG). (2020a). *Prenatal diagnostic testing for genetic disorders.* ACOG Practice Bulletin 162. Published 2016, reaffirmed 2020.

American College of Obstetrics and Gynecology (ACOG). (2020b). *Screening for fetal chromosomal abnormalities.* ACOG Practice Bulletin 226.

American College of Obstetrics and Gynecology (ACOG). (2020c). *Ultrasound in pregnancy.* ACOG Practice Bulletin 175. Published 2016, reaffirmed 2020.

American College of Obstetrics and Gynecology (ACOG). (2021a). *Antepartum fetal surveillance.* ACOG Practice Bulletin 229.

American College of Obstetrics and Gynecology (ACOG). (2021b). *Avoidance of nonmedically indicated early-term deliveries and associated neonatal morbidities.* ACOG Committee Opinion 765. Published 2019, reaffirmed 2021.

American College of Obstetrics and Gynecology (ACOG). (2021c). *Indications for outpatient antenatal fetal surveillance.* ACOG Committee Opinion 828.

American College of Obstetrics and Gynecology (ACOG). (2021d). *Management of suboptimally dated pregnancies.* ACOG Committee Opinion 688. Published 2017, reaffirmed 2021.

American College of Obstetrics and Gynecology and Society of Maternal-Fetal Medicine. (2020). *Management of stillbirth.* ACOG Obstetric Care Consensus 10.

American Institute of Ultrasound in Medicine (AIUM). (2020). *Prudent use and safety of diagnostic ultrasound in pregnancy.* https://www.aium.org/resources/statements.aspx.

Anastasio, G. D., & Harston, P. R. (1992). Fetal tachycardia associated with maternal use of pseudoephedrine, an over-the-counter oral decongestant. *Journal of the American Board of Family Practice, 5*(5), 527–528.

Association of Women's Health, Obstetric and Neonatal Nurses. (2016). *Ultrasound examinations performed by registered nurses in obstetric, gynecologic, and reproductive medicine settings: Clinical competencies and education guide* (4th ed.).

Bahtiyar, M. O., & Copel, J. A. (2019). Doppler ultrasound: Select fetal and maternal applications. In R. Resnik, C. Lockwood, T. Moore, M. Greene, J. Copel, & R. Silver (Eds.), *Creasy and Resnik's maternal-fetal medicine: Principles and practice* (8th ed., pp. 266–273). Elsevier.

Bates, E., Rouse, D. J., Mann, M. L., Chapman, V., Carlo, W. A., & Tita, A. T. (2010). Neonatal outcomes after demonstrated fetal lung maturity prior to 39 weeks of gestation. *Obstetrics & Gynecology, 116*(6), 1288. https://doi.org/10.1097/AOG.0b013e3181fb7ece.

Baxi, L. V., Gindoff, P. R., Pregenzer, G. J., & Parras, M. K. (1985). Fetal heart rate changes following maternal administration of a nasal decongestant. *American Journal of Obstetrics and Gynecology, 153*(7), 799–800. https://doi.org/10.1016/0002-9378(85)90351-5.

Beta, J., Zhang, W., Geris, S., Kostiv, V., & Akolekar, R. (2019). Procedure–related risk of miscarriage following chorionic villus sampling and amniocentesis. *Ultrasound in Obstetrics and Gynecology, 54*(4), 452–457. https://doi.org/10.1002/uog.20293.

Blackburn, S. T. (2018). *Maternal, fetal, & neonatal physiology: A clinical perspective* (5th ed.). Elsevier.

Braley, K., Dadlani, G., Geiger, J., Douglas, K., & Mehta, M. (2020). Introduction to fetal echocardiography. *Progress in Pediatric Cardiology, 58*(2020), 101278. https://doi.org/10.1016/j.ppedcard.2020.101278.

Carroll, L., Gallagher, L., & Smith, V. (2019). Risk factors for reduced fetal movements in pregnancy: A systematic review and meta-analysis. *European Journal of Obstetrics & Gynecology and Reproductive Biology, 243,* 72–82.

Cashion, K. (2017). Assessment of high-risk pregnancy. In S. Perry, D. Lowdermilk, K. Cashion, K. Alden, E. Olshansky, M. Hockenberry, et al. (Eds.), *Maternal child nursing care* (6th ed., pp. 226–243). Elsevier.

Chard, R. L., & Norton, M. E. (2016). Genetic counseling for patients considering screening and diagnosis for chromosomal abnormalities. *Clinics in Laboratory Medicine, 36*(2), 227–236. https://doi.org/10.1016/j.cll.2016.01.005.

Clements, J. A., Platzker, A. C., Tierney, D. F., Hobel, C. J., Creasy, R. K., Margolis, A. J., et al. (1972). Assessment of the risk of the respiratory-distress syndrome by a rapid test for surfactant in amniotic fluid. *New England Journal of Medicine, 286*(20), 1077–1081. https://doi.org/10.1056/nejm197205182862004.

Collazos, J. C., Acherman, R. J., Law, I. H., Wilkes, P., Restrepo, H., & Evans, W. N. (2007). Sustained fetal bradycardia with 1:1 atrioventricular conduction and long QT syndrome. *Prenatal Diagnosis, 27*(9), 879–881. https://doi.org/10.1002/pd.1784.

Cypher, R. L. (2019). Shared decision-making: A model for effective communication and patient satisfaction. *Journal of Perinatal and Neonatal Nursing, 33*(4), 285–287. https://doi.org/10.1097/JON.0000000000000441.

Cypher, R. L., & Foglia, L. M. (2020). Periviability: A review of key concepts and management for perinatal nursing. *Journal of Perinatal and Neonatal Nursing, 34*(2), 146–154. https://doi.org/10.1097/JPN.0000000000000473.

Dar, P., Shani, H., & Evans, M. I. (2016). Cell-free DNA: Comparison of technologies. *Clinics in Laboratory Medicine, 36*(2), 199–211. https://doi.org/10.1016/j.cll.2016.01.015.

Devoe, L. D., & Jones, C. R. (2002). Nonstress test: Evidence-based use in high-risk pregnancy. *Clinical Obstetrics and Gynecology, 45*(4), 986–992. https://doi.org/10.1097/00003081-200212000-00005.

Driscoll, D. A., & Simpson, J. L. (2021). Genetic screening and diagnosis. In M. Landon, V. Berghella, A. Cahill, D. Driscoll, H. Galan, W. Grobman, et al. (Eds.), *Gabbe's obstetrics: Normal & problem pregnancies* (8th ed., pp. 180–203). Elsevier.

Esplin, M. (2020). The golden hours of fetal heart rate monitoring: Systematic approach to the critical times of labor and delivery. *Clinical Obstetrics and Gynecology, 63*(3), 668–677. https://doi.org/10.1097/grf.0000000000000545.

Food and Drug Administration. (2014). *Avoid fetal "keepsake" images, heartbeat monitors.* https://www.fda.gov/consumers/consumer-updates/avoid-fetal-keepsake-images-heartbeat-monitors.

Freeman, R. K., Anderson, G., & Dorchester, W. (1982). A prospective multi-institutional study of antepartum fetal heart rate monitoring: II. Contraction stress test versus nonstress test for primary surveillance. *American Journal of Obstetrics and Gynecology, 143*(7), 778–781. https://doi.org/10.1016/0002-9378(82)90009-6.

Gil, M. M., Accurti, V., Santacruz, B., Plana, M. N., & Nicolaides, K. H. (2017). Analysis of cell-free DNA in maternal blood in screening for aneuploidies: Updated meta-analysis. *Ultrasound in Obstetrics and Gynecology, 50*(3), 302–314. https://doi.org/10.1002/uog.17484.

Goetzinger, K. R., & Odibo, A. O. (2017). Ultrasound evaluation of fetal aneuploidy in the first and second trimesters. In M. Norton, L. Scoutt, & V. Feldstein (Eds.), *Callen's ultrasonography in obstetrics and gynecology* (6th ed., pp. 57–81). Elsevier.

Greenberg, M. B., & Druzin, M. L. (2021). Antepartum fetal evaluation. In M. Landon, V. Berghella, A. Cahill, D. Driscoll, H. Galan, W. Grobman, et al. (Eds.), *Gabbe's obstetrics: Normal & problem pregnancies* (8th ed., pp. 514–538). Elsevier.

Gregg, A. R., Skotko, B. G., Benkendorf, J. L., Monaghan, K. G., Bajaj, K., Best, R. G., et al. (2016). Noninvasive prenatal screening for fetal aneuploidy, 2016 update: A position statement of the American College of Medical Genetics and Genomics. *Genetics in Medicine, 18*(10), 1056–1065. https://doi.org/10.1038/gim.2016.97.

Hockenberry, M. J. (2017). The child with neuromuscular or muscular dysfunction. In S. Perry, D. Lowdermilk, K. Cashion, K. Alden, E. Olshansky, M. Hockenberry, et al. (Eds.), *Maternal child nursing care* (6th ed., pp. 1455–1483). Elsevier.

Hoskovec, J. M., & Stevens, B. K. (2018). Genetic counseling overview for the obstetrician-gynecologist. *Obstetrics and Gynecology Clinics of North America, 45*(1), 1–12. https://doi.org/10.1016/j.ogc.2017.10.008.

Ioannides, A. S. (2020). Placental and fetal growth and development. In I. Symonds, & S. Arulkumaran (Eds.), *Essentials and Gynaecology* (6th ed., pp. 41–55). Elsevier.

Kaimal, A. J. (2019). Assessment of fetal health. In R. Resnik, C. Lockwood, T. Moore, M. Greene, J. Copel, & R. Silver (Eds.), *Creasy and Resnik's maternal-fetal medicine: Principles and practice* (8th ed., pp. 549–563). Elsevier.

Knutzen, D., & Stoll, K. (2019). Beyond the brochure: Innovations in clinical counseling practices for prenatal genetic testing options. *Journal of Perinatal and Neonatal Nursing, 33*(1), 12–25. https://doi.org/10.1097/JON.0000000000000374.

Knutzen, D. M., Stoll, K. A., McClellan, M. W., Deering, S. H., & Foglia, L. M. (2013). Improving knowledge about prenatal screening options: Can group education make a difference? *Journal of Maternal-Fetal and Neonatal Medicine, 26*(18), 1799–1803. https://doi.org/10.3109/14767058.2013.804504.

Lagrew, D. C. (1995). The contraction stress test. *Clinical Obstetrics and Gynecology, 38*(1), 11–25. https://doi.org/10.1097/00003081-199503000-00005.

Lee, C. Y., Di Lereto, P. C., & O'Lane, J. M. (1975). A study of fetal heart rate acceleration patterns. *Obstetrics & Gynecology, 45*(2), 142–146.

Liston, R., Sawchuck, D., & Young, D. (2018). No. 197a-fetal health surveillance: Antepartum consensus guideline. *Journal of Obstetrics and Gynaecology Canada, 40*(4), e251–e271. https://doi.org/10.1016/j.jogc.2018.02.007.

Macones, G. A., Hankins, G. D., Spong, C. Y., Hauth, J., & Moore, T. (2008). The 2008 National Institute of Child Health and Human Development workshop report on electronic fetal monitoring: Update on definitions, interpretation, and research guidelines. *Obstetrics & Gynecology, 112*(3), 661–666. https://doi.org/10.1097/aog.0b013e3181841395; *Journal of Obstetric, Gynecologic, & Neonatal Nursing, 37*(5), 510–515. https://doi.org/10.1111/j.1552-6909.2008.00284.x.

Mangesi, L., Hofmeyr, G. J., Smith, V., & Smyth, R. M. D. (2015). Fetal movement counting for assessment of fetal wellbeing. *Cochrane Database of Systematic Reviews* (10). https://doi.org/10.1002/14651858.CD004909.pub3. Art. No: CD004909.

Manning, F. A. (1995). Dynamic ultrasound-based fetal assessment: The fetal biophysical profile score. *Clinical Obstetrics and Gynecology, 38*(1), 26–44. https://doi.org/10.1097/00003081-199503000-00006.

Manning, F. A., Platt, L. D., & Sipos, L. (1980). Antepartum fetal evaluation: Development of a fetal biophysical profile. *American Journal of Obstetrics and Gynecology, 136*(6), 787–795. https://doi.org/10.1016/0002-9378(80)90457-3.

Mei, J. Y., Afshar, Y., & Platt, L. D. (2019). First-trimester ultrasound. *Obstetrics and Gynecology Clinics of North America, 46*(4), 829–852. https://doi.org/10.1016/j.ogc.2019.07.011.

Miller, L. A., Miller, D. A., & Cypher, R. L. (2022). *Mosby's pocket guide to fetal monitoring: A multidisciplinary approach* (9th ed.). Elsevier.

Moise, K. J. (2021). Red cell alloimmunization. In M. Landon, V. Berghella, A. Cahill, D. Driscoll, H. Galan, W. Grobman, et al. (Eds.), *Gabbe's obstetrics: Normal & problem pregnancies* (8th ed., pp. 784–799). Elsevier.

Moore, T. R., & Piacquadio, K. (1989). A prospective evaluation of fetal movement screening to reduce the incidence of antepartum fetal death. *American Journal of Obstetrics and Gynecology, 160*(5), 1075–1080. https://doi.org/10.1016/0002-9378(89)90164-6.

Morrow, R. J., Adamson, S. L., Bull, S. B., & Ritchie, J. K. (1989). Effect of placental embolization on the umbilical arterial velocity waveform in fetal sheep. *American Journal of Obstetrics and Gynecology, 161*(4), 1055–1060. https://doi.org/10.1016/0002-9378(89)90783-7.

National Institute of Neurological Disorders and Stroke. (2021). *Spina bifida fact sheet.* https://www.ninds.nih.gov/disorders/patient-caregiver-education/fact-sheets/spina-bifida-fact-sheet.

Neilson, J. P., West, H. M., & Dowswell, T. (2014). Betamimetics for inhibiting preterm labour. *Cochrane Database of Systematic Reviews, 2*, CD004352. https://doi.org/10.1002/14651858.CD004352.pub3.

Norton, M. E., & Rink, B. D. (2016). Changing indications for invasive testing in an era of improved screening. *Seminars in Perinatology, 40*(1), 56–66. https://doi.org/10.1053/j.semperi.2015.11.008.

Norton, M. E., & Rink, B. D. (2017). Genetics and prenatal genetic testing. In M. Norton, L. Scoutt, & V. Feldstein (Eds.), *Callen's ultrasonography in obstetrics and gynecology* (6th ed., pp. 24–56). Elsevier.

Odibo, A. O., & Acharya, G. (2019). Invasive diagnostic procedures. In P. Pandya, D. Oepkes, N. Sebire, & R. Wapner (Eds.), *Fetal medicine: Basic science and clinical practice* (3th ed., pp. 225–252). Elsevier.

O'Neill, E. R., & Thorp, J. (2012). Antepartum evaluation of the fetus and fetal well-being. *Clinical Obstetrics and Gynecology, 55*(3), 722–730. https://doi.org/10.1097/grf.0b013e318253b318.

Patrick, J., Campbell, K., Carmichael, L., Natale, R., & Richardson, B. (1982). Patterns of gross fetal body movements over 24-hour observation intervals during the last 10 weeks of pregnancy. *American Journal of Obstetrics and Gynecology, 142*(4), 363–371. https://doi.org/10.1016/S0002-9378(16)32375-4.

Pellerito, J., Bromley, B., Allison, S., Chauhan, A., Destounis, S., Dickman, E., et al. (2018). AIUM-ACR-ACOG-SMFM-SRU practice parameter for the performance of standard diagnostic obstetric ultrasound examinations. *Journal of Ultrasound in Medicine, 37*(11), E13–E24. https://doi.org/10.1002/jum.14831.

Powell, O. H., Melville, A., & MacKenna, J. (1979). Fetal heart rate acceleration in labor: Excellent prognostic indicator. *American Journal of Obstetrics prend Gynecology, 134*(1), 36–38. https://doi.org/10.1016/0002-9378(79)90792-0.

Raju, T. N., Mercer, B. M., Burchfield, D. J., & Joseph, G. F. (2014). Periviable birth: Executive summary of a joint workshop by the Eunice Kennedy Shriver National Institute of Child Health and Human Development, Society for Maternal-Fetal Medicine, American Academy of Pediatrics, and American College of Obstetricians and Gynecologists. *American Journal of Obstetrics and Gynecology, 210*(5), 406–417. https://doi.org/10.1016/j.ajog.2014.02.027.

Read, J. A., & Miller, F. C. (1977). Fetal heart rate acceleration in response to acoustic stimulation as a measure of fetal well-being. *American Journal of Obstetrics and Gynecology, 129*(5), 512–517. https://doi.org/10.1016/0002-9378(77)90088-6.

Reddy, U. M., Abuhamad, A. Z., Levine, D., Saade, G. R., & Fetal Imaging Workshop Invited Participants. (2014). Fetal imaging: Executive summary of a joint Eunice Kennedy Shriver National Institute of Child Health and Human Development, Society for Maternal-Fetal Medicine, American Institute of Ultrasound in Medicine, American College of Obstetricians and Gynecologists, American College of Radiology, Society for Pediatric Radiology, and Society of Radiologists in ultrasound fetal imaging workshop. *American Journal of Obstetrics and Gynecology, 210*(5), 387–397. https://doi.org/10.1016/j.ajog.2014.02.028.

Richards, D. S. (2021). Obstetric ultrasound. In M. Landon, V. Berghella, A. Cahill, D. Driscoll, H. Galan, W. Grobman, et al. (Eds.), *Gabbe's obstetrics: Normal & problem pregnancies* (8th ed., pp. 156–179). Elsevier.

Rochard, F., Schifrin, B. S., Goupil, F., Legrand, H., Blottiere, J., & Sureau, C. (1976). Nonstressed fetal heart rate monitoring in the antepartum period. *American Journal of Obstetrics and Gynecology, 126*(6), 699–706. https://doi.org/10.1016/0002-9378(76)90523-8.

Sheikh, M., Hantoushzadeh, S., & Shariat, M. (2014). Maternal perception of decreased fetal movements from maternal and fetal perspectives, a cohort study. *BMC Pregnancy and Childbirth, 14*(1), 1–7. https://doi.org/10.1186/1471-2393-14-286.

Signore, C., Freeman, R. K., & Spong, C. Y. (2009). Antenatal testing–A reevaluation. *Obstetrics & Gynecology, 113*(3), 687–701. https://doi.org/10.1097/aog.0b013e318197bd8a.

Simpson, K. R. (2020). Cervical ripening and labor induction and augmentation, 5th ed. *Nursing for Womens Health, 24*(4), s1–s41. https://doi.org/10.1016/j.nwh.2020.04.005.

Sullivan-Pyke, C., & Dokras, A. (2018). Preimplantation genetic screening and preimplantation genetic diagnosis. *Obstetrics and Gynecology Clinics of North America, 45*(1), 113–125. https://doi.org/10.1016/j.ogc.2017.10.009.

Tita, A. T., Jablonski, K. A., Bailit, J. L., Grobman, W. A., Wapner, R. J., Reddy, U. M., et al. (2018). Neonatal outcomes of elective early-term births after demonstrated fetal lung maturity. *American Journal of Obstetrics and Gynecology, 219*(3), 296.e1-e8. https://doi.org/10.1016/j.ajog.2018.05.011.

Too, G., & Berkowitz, R. L. (2018). Cordocentesis and fetal transfusion. In J. Copel, M. D'Alton, H. Feltovich, E. Gratacos, D. Krakow, A. Odibo, et al. (Eds.), *Obstetric imaging: Fetal diagnosis and care* (2nd ed., pp. 475–478). Elsevier.

Treanor, C. M. (2021). Antenatal fetal assessment and testing. In A. Lyndon, & K. Wisner (Eds.), *Fetal heart rate monitoring: Principles and practices* (6th ed., pp. 277–308). Kendall-Hunt.

Turner, J. M., Flenady, V., Ellwood, D., Coory, M., & Kumar, S. (2021). Evaluation of pregnancy outcomes among women with decreased fetal movements. *JAMA Network Open, 4*(4), e215071. https://doi.org/10.1001/jamanetworkopen.2021.5071.e215071.

Verpoest, M. J., Seelen, J. C., & Westerman, C. F. (1976). Changes in appearance of amniotic fluid during pregnancy: The macroscore. *Journal of Perinatal Medicine, 4*(1), 12–25. https://doi.org/10.1515/jpme.1976.4.1.12.

Vintzileos, A. M., Gaffney, S. E., Salinger, L. M., Kontopoulos, V. G., Campbell, W. A., & Nochimson, D. J. (1987). The relationships among the fetal biophysical profile, umbilical cord pH, and Apgar scores. *American Journal of Obstetrics and Gynecology, 157*(3), 627–631. https://doi.org/10.1016/S0002-9378(87)80018-2.

Vintzileos, A. M., & Knuppel, R. A. (1994). Multiple parameter biophysical testing in the prediction of fetal acid-base status. *Clinics in Perinatology, 21*(4), 823–848. https://doi.org/10.1016/s0095-5108(18)30321-x.

Walker, D., Grimwade, J., & Wood, C. (1971). Intrauterine noise: A component of the fetal environment. *American Journal of Obstetrics and Gynecology, 109*(1), 92–95. https://doi.org/10.1016/0002-9378(71)90840-4.

Wapner, R. J., & Dugoff, L. (2019). Prenatal diagnosis of congenital disorders. In R. Resnik, C. J. Lockwood, T. Moore, M. Greene, J. Copel, & R. Silver (Eds.), *Creasy and Resnik's maternal-fetal medicine: Principles and practice* (8th ed., pp. 549–563). Elsevier.

Wax, J., Minkoff, H., Johnson, A., Coleman, B., Levine, D., Helfgott, A., et al. (2014). Consensus report on the detailed fetal anatomic ultrasound examination indications, components, and qualifications. *Journal of Ultrasound in Medicine, 33*(2), 189–195.

Complications of Pregnancy

Nan Ketcham, Kristin L. Scheffer, Reneé Jones, Karen S. Holub,
Jessica L. McNeil-Santiel

OBJECTIVES

After studying this chapter, you should be able to:

1. Describe the development and management of hemorrhagic conditions of early pregnancy, including spontaneous abortion, ectopic pregnancy, and gestational trophoblastic disease.
2. Explain physiology and management of placenta previa and placental abruption.
3. Discuss the effects and management of hyperemesis gravidarum.
4. Describe the pathophysiology, effects, and management of hypertensive disorders of pregnancy.
5. Compare Rh and ABO blood incompatibilities in terms of etiology, fetal and neonatal complications, and management.
6. Describe the effects of pregnancy on glucose metabolism.
7. Discuss the effects and management of preexisting diabetes mellitus during pregnancy.
8. Explain the physiology and management of gestational diabetes mellitus during pregnancy.
9. Describe the effects of obesity during pregnancy.
10. Explain the effects of specific anemias and the required management during pregnancy.
11. Identify the effects, management, and nursing considerations of specific preexisting autoimmune and neurologic conditions.
12. Discuss the effects of selected prenatal infections.
13. Explain nursing considerations for each complication of pregnancy.

Although childbearing is usually a normal process, complications may arise, threatening the well-being of the client, the fetus, or both. Conditions complicating pregnancy are divided into two broad categories: (1) those related to pregnancy and (2) those that can occur at any time and complicate a pregnancy when they occur concurrently.

Common pregnancy-related complications are hemorrhagic conditions that occur in early pregnancy, hemorrhagic complications of the placenta in late pregnancy, hyperemesis gravidarum (HG), hypertensive disorders of pregnancy, and blood incompatibilities. Concurrent conditions include diabetes mellitus, cardiac disease, obesity, anemias, autoimmune disorders, neurologic disorders, and infections. Cardiovascular complications of pregnancy are discussed in Chapter 19.

PREGNANCY COMPLICATIONS

HEMORRHAGIC CONDITIONS OF EARLY PREGNANCY

The three most common causes of hemorrhage during the first half of pregnancy are abortion, ectopic pregnancy, and gestational trophoblastic disease.

Abortion

Abortion is the loss of pregnancy before the fetus is viable, or capable of living outside the uterus. According to the World Health Organization and the National Center for Health Statistics, a fetus of less than 20 weeks of gestation or one weighing less than 500 grams (g) is not viable (Cunningham et al., 2022). Ending of pregnancy before this time is considered an abortion. Abortion may be either spontaneous or induced. *Abortion* is an accepted medical term for either a spontaneous or an induced ending of pregnancy, although the lay term *miscarriage* is sometimes used to denote spontaneous abortion. Elective termination of pregnancy, or induced abortion, is described in Chapter 28.

Spontaneous Abortion

Spontaneous abortion (miscarriage) is the termination of pregnancy without action taken by the client or another person.

Incidence and Etiology. Determining the exact incidence of spontaneous abortion is difficult because many unrecognized losses occur in early pregnancy, but it averages approximately 8% to 15% with any pregnancy (Linnakaari et al., 2019). The incidence of spontaneous abortion increases with the age of the pregnant client. The incidence is 12% for clients

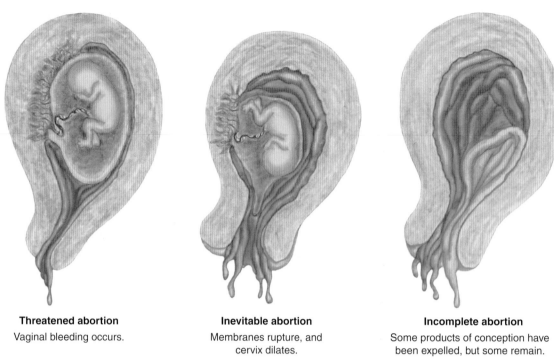

Threatened abortion	**Inevitable abortion**	**Incomplete abortion**
Vaginal bleeding occurs.	Membranes rupture, and cervix dilates.	Some products of conception have been expelled, but some remain.

Fig. 10.1 Three types of spontaneous abortion, also called miscarriage.

younger than 20 years, rising to 50% for clients older than 42 years. About 80% of miscarriages occur in the first 12 weeks of pregnancy, with the rate declining rapidly thereafter (Cunningham et al., 2022; Jauniaux & Simpson 2021).

The most common cause of miscarriage is karyotype abnormalities that are often incompatible with life. Chromosomal abnormalities account for approximately 50% to 60% of spontaneous abortions within the first 12 weeks (Jacobson & Connolly, 2019). Embryonic causes such as monosomy X (45,X) or autosomal trisomy contribute to chromosomal abnormalities. Another chromosomal abnormality is anembryonic (no embryo) or a "blighted ovum" causing a miscarriage (Jacobson & Connolly, 2019).

Additional causes include genitourinary tract infections, viruses, and parasites; however, incidence is uncommon (Cunningham et al., 2022). Endocrine disorders such as hypothyroidism, diabetes, and obesity increase the risk of spontaneous abortion (Jauniaux & Simpson, 2021). There is a greater miscarriage risk with intake of caffeine equal to 500 mg (Cunningham et al., 2022). Finally, heavy alcohol consumption and heavy smoking may play a role in miscarriage (Cunningham et al., 2022; Jauniaux & Simpson, 2021).

Spontaneous abortion is divided into six subgroups: threatened, inevitable, incomplete, complete, missed, and recurrent. Fig. 10.1 illustrates threatened, inevitable, and incomplete abortions.

Threatened Abortion. Vaginal bleeding before 20 weeks of gestation without dilation of the cervix or passage of fetal or placental tissue is a threatened abortion.

Clinical Manifestations. The first sign of threatened miscarriage is vaginal bleeding, which is rather common during early pregnancy. Approximately 25% of pregnant clients experience "spotting" or bleeding in early pregnancy,

and up to 50% of these pregnancies end in spontaneous abortion (Cunningham et al., 2022). Vaginal bleeding, which may be brief or last for weeks, may be accompanied by uterine cramping, persistent backache, or feelings of pelvic pressure. These added symptoms are more likely to be associated with loss of pregnancy. If a miscarriage does not occur, later problems such as prematurity, low-birth-weight infant or fetal-growth restriction, fetal death, and abnormal placentation may occur in pregnancies with early bleeding (Cunningham et al., 2022).

Therapeutic Management. Bleeding during the first half of pregnancy should be considered a threatened abortion, and clients should be advised to notify their provider if brownish or red vaginal bleeding is noted. When a client reports bleeding in early pregnancy, the nurse obtains a detailed history with the length of gestation (or first day of the last menstrual period) and the onset, duration, amount, and color of vaginal bleeding. Any accompanying discomfort such as cramping, backache, or abdominal pain also is noted.

Transvaginal ultrasound examination is performed to determine whether an embryo or fetus is present with a heartbeat (viability) and the approximate gestational age. Serum beta-human chorionic gonadotropin (b-hCG) and progesterone levels provide added information about the viability of the pregnancy (i.e., whether the levels are appropriate for gestation period).

The client may be advised to limit sexual activity until bleeding has ceased and should be instructed to count the number of perineal pads used and note the quantity and color of blood on the pads. Evidence of tissue passage, which indicates progression beyond a threatened abortion, and drainage with a foul odor, which suggests infection, should be reported.

Inevitable Abortion. Miscarriage is usually inevitable (i.e., it cannot be stopped) when membranes rupture and the cervix dilates.

Clinical Manifestations. Rupture of membranes generally is experienced as a loss of fluid from the vagina and subsequent uterine contractions and active bleeding. Incomplete evacuation of the products of conception can result in excessive bleeding or infection.

Therapeutic Management. Natural expulsion of uterine contents is common in inevitable abortion. **Vacuum curettage** (removal of uterine contents with a vacuum curette) is used to clear the uterus if the natural process is ineffective or incomplete. If the pregnancy is more advanced or if bleeding is excessive, a **dilation and curettage (D&C)** (stretching the cervical os to permit scraping the uterine walls) may be needed. Intravenous (IV) sedation or other anesthesia provides pain management for the procedure.

Incomplete Abortion. Incomplete abortion occurs when some but not all of the products of conception are expelled from the uterus.

Clinical Manifestations. The major manifestations of an incomplete miscarriage are active uterine bleeding and severe abdominal cramping. The cervix is open, and some fetal and/or placental tissues are passed.

Therapeutic Management. Retained tissue prevents the uterus from contracting firmly, thereby allowing excessive bleeding from uterine blood vessels. Initial treatment should focus on stabilizing the client's cardiovascular state. A blood specimen is drawn for blood type and screen or crossmatch, and an IV line is inserted for fluid replacement and drug administration. When the client's condition is stable, a D&C usually is performed to remove the remaining tissue. If the bleeding is later in pregnancy when the fetal tissue is larger, a greater cervical **dilation and evacuation (D&E)**, followed by vacuum or surgical curettage, is required. This procedure may be followed by IV administration of oxytocin (Pitocin) or intramuscular (IM) administration of methylergonovine (Methergine) to contract the uterus and control bleeding. Other less invasive treatments include the administration of misoprostol either vaginally or orally. This treatment can have unpredictable bleeding and the client may elect to have a D&C.

A D&C may not be performed if the pregnancy has advanced beyond 14 weeks because of the danger of excessive bleeding. In this case oxytocin or prostaglandin is administered to stimulate uterine contractions until all products of conception (fetus, membranes, placenta, and amniotic fluid) are expelled.

Complete Abortion. Complete abortion occurs when all products of conception are expelled from the uterus.

Clinical Manifestations. After passage of all products of conception, uterine contractions and bleeding subside, and the cervix closes. The uterus feels smaller than the length of gestation would suggest. The symptoms of pregnancy are no longer present, and the pregnancy test becomes negative as hormone levels fall. The client may be encouraged to bring in the products of conception in order to determine blood clot versus tissue. A transvaginal ultrasound may be obtained to confirm absence of a gestational sac.

Therapeutic Management. Once complete abortion is confirmed, no additional intervention is required unless excessive bleeding or infection develops. The client should be advised to rest and watch for further bleeding, pain, or fever. Sexual intercourse should be delayed until after a follow-up visit with the health care provider.

Missed Abortion. Missed abortion occurs when the fetus dies during the first half of pregnancy but is retained in the uterus.

Clinical Manifestations. When the fetus dies, the early symptoms of pregnancy (nausea, breast tenderness, urinary frequency) disappear. The uterus stops growing and decreases in size, reflecting the absorption of amniotic fluid and **maceration** (discoloration, softening, and eventual tissue degeneration) of the fetus. Vaginal bleeding of a red or brownish color may or may not occur.

Therapeutic Management. An ultrasound examination confirms fetal death by identifying a gestational sac or fetus that is too small for the presumed gestational age. No fetal heart activity can be found. Pregnancy tests for hCG show a decline in placental hormone production.

In most cases, the contents of the uterus would eventually be expelled spontaneously, but this is emotionally difficult once the client knows the fetus is not alive. Therefore the uterus usually is emptied by the most appropriate method for the size when the diagnosis of missed abortion is made. For a first-trimester missed abortion, a D&C usually can be done. If the missed abortion occurs during the second trimester, when the fetus is larger, a D&E may be done, or vaginal prostaglandin E_2 (PGE_2) or misoprostol (Cytotec) may be needed to induce uterine contractions that expel the fetus. A D&C may be needed to remove the placenta.

Two major complications of missed abortion are infection and disseminated intravascular coagulation (DIC). Signs such as elevation in temperature, vaginal discharge with a foul odor, and abdominal pain indicate uterine infection. Cultures are obtained, antimicrobial therapy is initiated, and the uterus is evacuated. See Chapter 19 for information on DIC.

Recurrent Pregnancy Loss. Recurrent pregnancy loss is defined as three or more consecutive pregnancy losses less than 20 weeks of gestation or less than 500 g (Cunningham et al., 2022).

Clinical Manifestations. The primary causes of repeated pregnancy loss are believed to be genetic or chromosomal abnormalities (Jauniaux & Simpson, 2021; Williams & Scott, 2019). Anomalies of the reproductive tract, such as a septate uterus (the uterus is divided by a wall of tissue), Asherman syndrome (adhesions or scarring form in the uterus), chronic endometritis, and polycystic ovarian syndrome as well as systemic diseases such as systemic lupus erythematosus antiphospholipid syndrome, and diabetes mellitus have been implicated in recurrent pregnancy loss.

Therapeutic Management. The first step in management of recurrent pregnancy loss is examination of the reproductive system to determine whether anatomic defects are the cause. If the cervix and uterus are normal, the client and partner are usually referred for genetic screening to identify chromosomal factors that would increase the possibility of recurrent miscarriages.

Additional therapeutic management of recurrent pregnancy loss depends on the cause. For instance, treatment may involve assisting the client to develop a regimen to maintain normal blood glucose level if diabetes mellitus is a factor. Antimicrobials are prescribed for the client with infection.

Recurrent pregnancy loss may be caused by **cervical incompetence**, also called **cervical insufficiency**, an anatomic defect that results in painless dilation of the cervix in the second trimester. In this situation, a **cerclage** procedure—suturing of the cervix to prevent early dilation—may be performed. The cerclage is most likely to be successful if done before much cervical dilation or bulging of the membranes through the cervix has occurred. Sutures may be removed near term in preparation for vaginal delivery, or they may be left in place if a cesarean birth is planned. Prophylactic antibiotics are ordered if the client is at increased risk for infection. Preterm labor may still occur after the fetus is viable.

Nursing Considerations for Spontaneous Abortions

Rho(D) immune globulin (RhoGAM) is given to the unsensitized Rho(D)-negative client to prevent development of anti-Rh antibodies. A microdose (50 mcg) is given to the client whose fetus is less than 13 weeks of gestational age at the time of the miscarriage.

Nurses should consider the psychological needs of the client experiencing any type of spontaneous abortion. Vaginal bleeding is frightening, and waiting and watching are often difficult (although possibly the only treatment recommended). Many clients and their families feel an acute sense of loss and grief with threatened or actual pregnancy loss. Grief often includes feelings of guilt and speculation about whether the client could have done something to prevent the situation.

The nurse should offer accurate information and avoid false reassurance. Nurses may help by emphasizing threatened and actual pregnancy loss usually occurs as the result of factors or abnormalities that cannot be avoided. Anger, disappointment, and sadness are common emotions, although the intensity of these feelings may vary. For many parents, the fetus has not yet taken on specific physical characteristics, but they grieve for their fantasies of the unseen, unborn child. Recognizing the meaning of the loss to each client and their significant other is important. Nurses should listen carefully to what the client says. The couple may want to express their sadness but may think family, friends, and often health care personnel are uncomfortable or diminish their loss. Nurses should convey their acceptance of the feelings expressed or demonstrated by the couple. Providing information and simple brief explanations of what has occurred and what will be done facilitates the family's ability to grieve.

Many hospitals have grief support programs families may attend for 12 weeks or as needed to assist with the grief process. Family support, knowledge of the grief process, spiritual counselors, and support from other bereaved couples may provide needed assistance during this time. See Chapter 11 for more on perinatal loss.

> **❓ KNOWLEDGE CHECK**
>
> 1. What are the signs of threatened abortion, and how do they differ from those of inevitable abortion?
> 2. What are the major causes of recurrent spontaneous abortion?
> 3. What interventions can nurses provide for families experiencing grief as a result of early pregnancy loss?

Ectopic Pregnancy

Ectopic pregnancy is an implantation of a fertilized ovum in an area outside the uterine cavity. Although implantation can occur in the abdomen or cervix, 97% of ectopic pregnancies occur in the fallopian tube (Cunningham et al., 2022). Fig. 10.2 shows the common sites of ectopic implantation.

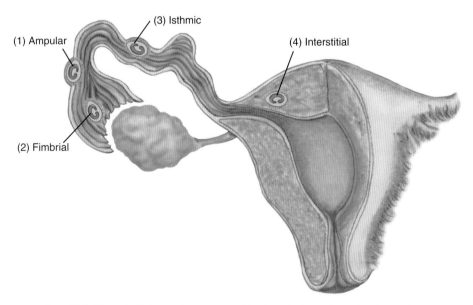

(1) Ampular
(3) Isthmic
(4) Interstitial
(2) Fimbrial

Fig. 10.2 Sites of tubal ectopic pregnancy. Numbers indicate the order of prevalence.

BOX 10.1 Risk Factors for Ectopic Pregnancy

History of previous ectopic pregnancies
History of sexually transmitted infections (gonorrhea, chlamydia)
Failed tubal ligation and tubal reconstruction after ligation
Assisted reproductive techniques
Intrauterine device contraceptives
Multiple induced abortions

Ectopic pregnancy remains a significant cause of maternal death from hemorrhage. In addition, tubal damage caused by an ectopic pregnancy reduces the client's chances of subsequent pregnancies. With improved diagnostic tests such as laboratory b-hCG assays and transvaginal sonography (TVS), earlier diagnosis can improve the client's chances of survival.

Incidence and Etiology

A common factor for the development of ectopic pregnancy in the fallopian tube is scarring of the fallopian tubes because of pelvic infection, inflammation, or surgery. Tubal adhesions from a previous tubal infection, appendicitis, or endometriosis increases the risk of an ectopic pregnancy (Cunningham et al., 2022). A failed tubal ligation, even if performed many years ago, and a history of previous ectopic pregnancy also increase the risk for an ectopic pregnancy in the fallopian tube. Greater incidences of ectopic pregnancies occur in clients who conceived with assisted reproduction, most likely related to the tubal factors that contributed to infertility. Contraception such as intrauterine contraceptive devices or low-dose progesterone agents are associated with increased risk for ectopic pregnancy (Cunningham et al., 2022).

Additional causes of ectopic pregnancy are delayed or premature ovulation, with the tendency of the fertilized ovum to implant before arrival in the uterus and altered tubal motility in response to changes in estrogen and progesterone levels that occur with conception. Multiple induced abortions increase the risk for tubal pregnancy, possibly because of salpingitis (infection of the fallopian tube) that occurred after induced abortion (Box 10.1). Regardless of the cause of tubal pregnancy, the effect is transport of the fertilized ovum through the fallopian tube is interrupted.

Clinical Manifestations

The classic triad of symptoms indicating an ectopic pregnancy includes the following:
- Missed menstrual period
- Abdominal pain
- Vaginal bleeding

More subtle signs and symptoms depend on the site of implantation. If implantation occurs in the distal end of the fallopian tube, which can contain the growing embryo longer, the client may at first exhibit the usual early signs of pregnancy and consider oneself to be normally pregnant. Several weeks into the pregnancy, intermittent abdominal pain and small amounts of vaginal bleeding occur, and initially this could be mistaken for threatened abortion. Because routine ultrasound examination in early pregnancy is common, however, it is not unusual to diagnose an ectopic pregnancy before onset of symptoms.

If implantation has occurred in the proximal end of the fallopian tube, rupture of the tube may occur within 2 to 3 weeks of the missed period because the tube is narrow in this area. Symptoms include sudden severe pain in one of the lower quadrants of the abdomen as the tube tears open and the embryo is expelled into the pelvic cavity, often with profuse abdominal hemorrhage. Radiating pain under the scapula may indicate bleeding into the abdomen caused by phrenic nerve irritation. **Hypovolemic shock** (acute peripheral circulatory failure from loss of circulating blood) is a major concern because systemic signs of shock may be rapid and extensive without external bleeding.

Diagnosis

The combined use of transvaginal ultrasound examination and determination of beta-hCG usually results in early detection of ectopic pregnancy. An abnormal pregnancy is suspected if beta-hCG is present but at lower levels than expected. Institutions set their threshold at greater than 1500 mIU/mL. If a gestational sac cannot be visualized when beta-hCG is present or greater than 1500 mIU/mL, a diagnosis of ectopic pregnancy may be made with great accuracy (Cunningham et al., 2022). Visualization of an intrauterine pregnancy, however, does not absolutely rule out an ectopic pregnancy. The client may have an intrauterine pregnancy and concurrently have an ectopic pregnancy. **Laparoscopy** (examination of the peritoneal cavity by means of a laparoscope) occasionally may be necessary to diagnose rupture of an ectopic pregnancy. A characteristic bluish swelling within the tube is the most common finding.

Therapeutic Management

Management of tubal pregnancy depends on whether the tube is intact or ruptured.

Medical management with methotrexate may be an option for the client with an early ectopic pregnancy if the tube is unruptured (Cunningham et al., 2022). The goal of medical management is to preserve the tube and improve the chance of future fertility. Methotrexate, a chemotherapeutic agent, is a folic acid antagonist inhibiting cell replication and targets rapidly dividing cells, such as the trophoblastic cells in early pregnancy. Successful medical management is associated with small ectopic size, low initial serum beta-hCG levels, and absent fetal cardiac activity (Cunningham et al., 2022). It may be given in a single dose or multiple dose protocol (Cunningham et al., 2022).

Surgical management of a tubal pregnancy that is unruptured may involve a **linear salpingostomy**, removal of the ectopic pregnancy from the tube in an effort to salvage the tube or a **salpingectomy**—removal of the tube. Salvaging the tube is particularly important when the client is concerned about future fertility, although the same cause may affect both tubes.

When ectopic pregnancy results in rupture of the fallopian tube, the goal of therapeutic management is to control the bleeding and prevent hypovolemic shock. Ruptured ectopic pregnancy is a major emergency. When the client's cardiovascular status is stable, salpingectomy with ligation of bleeding vessels may be required.

Nursing Considerations

Nursing care focuses on prevention or early identification of hypovolemic shock, pain control, and psychological support for the client who experiences ectopic pregnancy. Nurses monitor for signs and symptoms suggesting tubal rupture or bleeding (e.g., pelvic, shoulder, or neck pain; dizziness or faintness; increased vaginal bleeding). Nurses administer ordered analgesics and evaluate their effectiveness so pain can be adequately controlled. The nurse administers Rho(D) immune globulin to Rho-negative clients.

If the plan of care includes methotrexate, the nurse should be aware methotrexate is a chemotherapeutic agent. Facility protocols for chemotherapy should be followed, including appropriate personal protective equipment (double glove) and verification of client name, medication, and dosage by another nurse. Air should not be expelled from the syringe because it could aerosolize the medication. Urine is considered toxic for 72 hours. The client should be taught to be careful to avoid getting urine on the toilet seat and to flush the toilet twice with the lid closed when voiding. Additional client teaching includes adverse side effects such as nausea and vomiting and the importance of informing the health care team of any physical changes. Transient abdominal pain occurs during methotrexate therapy, probably because of expulsion of the products of conception from the tube. The client should be instructed to refrain from drinking alcohol (which decreases the effectiveness of methotrexate), taking vitamins containing folic acid, using nonsteroidal antiinflammatory drugs, and having sexual intercourse until beta-hCG is not detectable in the blood. If the treatment is successful, this hormone disappears from plasma within 2 to 3 weeks. Maintaining follow-up appointments is essential to identify whether the hCG titer becomes negative and remains negative (Cunningham et al., 2022). Continued presence of hCG in the serum requires follow-up to identify whether the ectopic pregnancy is still present (Cunningham et al., 2022).

The client and family will need psychological support to process the intense emotions which may include anger, grief, guilt, and self-blame. Anxiety about the ability to become pregnant in the future is common. Because ectopic pregnancy may occur when a client has undergone an assisted reproductive procedure, the anxiety about becoming pregnant again and if similar risks exist for another pregnancy may be heightened. The nurse should clarify the provider's explanation and use therapeutic communication techniques to assist the client to cope with anxiety.

Gestational Trophoblastic Disease (Hydatidiform Mole)

Hydatidiform mole is one form of **gestational trophoblastic disease**, which occurs when trophoblasts (outer cells of the fertilized ovum which attach it to the uterine wall) develop abnormally (Cohn et al., 2019; Cunningham, 2022). The placenta does not develop normally, and, if a fetus is present, there will be a fatal chromosome defect. Gestational trophoblastic disease is characterized by proliferation and edema of the chorionic villi. The fluid-filled villi form grapelike clusters of tissue and rapidly grow large enough to fill the uterus to the size of an advanced pregnancy. The molar pregnancy may be complete, with no fetus present, or partial, in which fetal tissue or membranes are present.

Incidence and Etiology

In the United States and Europe, the incidence of hydatidiform mole is 1 in every 1000 to 1200 pregnancies (Cohn et al., 2019; Soper, 2021). Age is a factor, with the frequency of molar pregnancies highest at both ends of reproductive life. Clients who have had one molar pregnancy have a greater risk to have another in a subsequent pregnancy (Cunningham et al., 2022; Soper, 2021). The incidence is higher among Asian, Hispanic, and Native Americans (Cunningham et al., 2022). Persistent gestational trophoblastic disease may undergo malignant change (choriocarcinoma) and may metastasize to sites such as the lung, vagina, liver, and brain.

A complete mole is thought to occur when the ovum is fertilized by a sperm that duplicates its own chromosomes and the chromosomes in the ovum are inactivated. In a partial mole, the maternal contribution is usually present, but the paternal contribution is doubled, and therefore the karyotype is triploid (69,XXY or 69,XYY) (Soper, 2021). If a fetus is identified with the partial mole, it is grossly abnormal because of the abnormal chromosomal composition.

Clinical Manifestations

Routine use of ultrasound allows earlier diagnosis of hydatidiform mole, usually before the more severe manifestations of the disorder develop. Possible signs and symptoms of molar pregnancy include the following:

- Higher levels of beta-hCG than expected for gestation
- Characteristic "snowstorm" ultrasound pattern that shows the vesicles and the absence of a fetal sac or fetal heart activity in a complete molar pregnancy
- A uterus that is larger than expected for gestational age
- Vaginal bleeding, which varies from dark-brown spotting to profuse hemorrhage
- Excessive nausea and vomiting or hyperemesis gravidarum (HG) may be related to high levels of beta-hCG from the proliferating trophoblasts
- Early development of preeclampsia before 24 weeks of gestation in an otherwise normal pregnancy

Diagnosis

Measurement of beta-hCG levels detects the abnormally high levels of the hormone before treatment. After treatment, beta-hCG levels are measured to determine whether they fall and then disappear. Increased hCG levels greater than expected for the gestational age and abnormal ultrasound findings support the diagnosis of molar pregnancy (Soper, 2021).

In addition to the characteristic pattern showing the vesicles, ultrasound examination allows a differential diagnosis to be made between two types of molar pregnancies: (1) a partial mole to include some fetal tissue and membranes and (2) a complete mole composed only of enlarged villi but contains no fetal tissue or membranes.

Therapeutic Management

Medical management includes two phases: (1) evacuation of the trophoblastic tissue of the mole and (2) continuous follow-up of the client to detect malignant changes of any remaining trophoblastic tissue. At the same time, the client is treated for any other problems such as preeclampsia or HG.

Before evacuation, chest radiography is performed to detect metastatic disease. Along with a quantitative hCG level, a complete blood count, laboratory assessment of coagulation status, and blood type screening or crossmatching are also necessary. Blood chemistry examinations are done to evaluate renal, hepatic, and thyroid function (Cunningham et al., 2022; Ngan et al., 2018; Soper, 2021).

The mole usually is removed by vacuum aspiration. IV oxytocin is given during and following the procedure to contract the uterus (Ngan et al., 2018; Soper, 2021). The tissue obtained is sent for laboratory evaluation. Although a hydatidiform mole is usually a benign process, choriocarcinoma may occur (Cohn et al., 2019).

Follow-up is critical to detect changes suggestive of trophoblastic malignancy (Cohn et al., 2019). A baseline hCG is obtained within 48 hours after evacuation and repeated every 1 to 2 weeks until it is no longer detectable (Cunningham et al., 2022; Soper, 2021). The client is then followed with monthly hCG levels for 6 to 12 additional months (Cunningham et al., 2022; Ngan et al., 2018; Soper, 2021). A persistent or rising beta-hCG level suggests continued gestational trophoblastic disease. Pregnancy must be avoided during the follow-up because the normal rise of beta-hCG level in pregnancy would obscure evidence of choriocarcinoma (Cohn et al., 2019).

Nursing Considerations

Bleeding is a possible complication with a molar pregnancy, but emotional care of the client is also essential. The clients who have had a hydatidiform mole experience emotions similar to those experiencing any other type of pregnancy loss. In addition, they may be anxious about follow-up evaluations, the possibility of malignant change, and the need to delay pregnancy for at least 1 year (Soper, 2021).

APPLICATION OF THE NURSING PROCESS: HEMORRHAGIC CONDITIONS OF EARLY PREGNANCY

Regardless of the cause of early antepartum bleeding, nurses play a vital role in its management. Nurses are responsible for monitoring the condition of the pregnant client and for collaborating with the other members of the health care team to provide treatment.

Assessment

Confirmation of pregnancy and length of gestation are important initial data to obtain. Physical assessment focuses on determining the amount of bleeding and the description, location, and severity of pain. Estimate the amount of vaginal bleeding by examining the linen and peripads. When necessary, accurately assess the bleeding by weighing the linen and peripads (1 g weight equals 1 mL volume).

When assessing how much blood was lost before arriving at the birth facility, ask the client to compare the amount lost with a common liquid measure such as a tablespoon or a cup. Ask also how long the bleeding episode lasted and what was done to control the bleeding.

Bleeding may be accompanied by pain. Uterine cramping usually accompanies spontaneous abortion; deep, severe pelvic pain is associated with ruptured ectopic pregnancy. In ruptured ectopic pregnancy, bleeding may be concealed, and pain could be the only symptom.

Vital signs and urine output will assist the nurse in assessment of the client's cardiovascular status. Rising pulse and respiratory rates and falling urine output are associated with hypovolemia. The blood pressure usually falls late in hypovolemic shock. Check laboratory values for hemoglobin (Hgb) and hematocrit (Hct) and report abnormal values to the health care provider. Check laboratory values for coagulation factors to identify added risks for hemorrhage.

Because vaginal bleeding and necessary medical interventions may be associated with infections, assess for fever, elevated pulse rate, malaise, and prolonged or malodorous vaginal discharge. Determine the family's knowledge of needed follow-up care and how to prevent complications such as infection.

Identification of Client Problems

A variety of collaborative problems should be considered in the client who has a bleeding disorder of early pregnancy. Current diagnostic techniques often permit early diagnosis before hemorrhage occurs. An applicable problem for the client with these early pregnancy disorders is a need for client teaching about diagnostic and therapeutic procedures, signs and symptoms of additional complications, measures to prevent infection, and importance of follow-up care.

Planning: Expected Outcomes

Goals and expected outcomes for this collaborative problem are the client will do the following:

- Verbalize understanding of diagnostic and therapeutic procedures
- Verbalize measures to prevent infection
- Verbalize signs of infection to report to the health care provider
- Maintain follow-up care

Interventions

Provide Information about Tests and Procedures

The client and their families experience less anxiety if they understand what is happening. Explain planned diagnostic procedures such as transvaginal or transabdominal ultrasonography. Include the purpose of the tests, how long they will take, and whether the procedures cause discomfort. Briefly describe the reasons for blood tests, such as evaluation of hCG, Hgb, Hct, or coagulation factors. Explain diagnostic and therapeutic measures should be performed quickly to prevent excessive blood loss. If surgical intervention is necessary, reinforce the explanations from the anesthesia professional about planned anesthesia. Obtain needed consents before procedures. Administer Rho(D) immune globulin to appropriate Rh-negative clients.

Teach Measures to Prevent Infection

The risk for infection is greatest during the first 72 hours after spontaneous abortion or operative procedures. Personal hygiene should include daily showers and careful handwashing before and after changing perineal pads. Perineal pads, applied in a front-to-back direction, should be used instead of tampons until bleeding has subsided. In most cases, intercourse may be resumed in 4 to 6 weeks along with contraception. For some conditions, pregnancy may need to be avoided for 6 to 12 months.

Provide Dietary Information

Nutrition and adequate fluid intake help maintain the body's defense against infection, and the nurse should promote an adequate and culturally sensitive diet. The client who has a hemorrhagic complication is at risk for infection. Intake of foods should be high in iron to increase Hgb and Hct values. These foods include liver, red meat, dried fruits, dried peas and beans, and dark green leafy vegetables (Raymond & Morrow, 2021). Foods high in vitamin C include citrus fruits, broccoli, strawberries, cantaloupe, cabbage, and green peppers. Adequate fluid intake (2500 mL/day) promotes hydration after bleeding episodes and maintains digestive processes.

Iron supplementation is often prescribed. Less gastric upset is experienced when iron is taken with meals. Iron supplements having a slow release may be better tolerated. A diet high in fiber and fluid helps reduce the commonly associated constipation.

Teach Signs of Infection to Report

Ensure that the client has a thermometer at home and knows how to use it. Temperature should be checked every 8 hours for the first 3 days at home. Teach the client to seek medical help if the temperature rises above 100.4°F (38°C). Instruct the client to report other signs of infection, such as vaginal discharge with foul odor, pelvic tenderness, or persistent general malaise.

Reinforce Follow-Up Care

The client with gestational trophoblastic disease, such as hydatiform mole, requires follow up every 1 to 2 weeks for evaluation of serum beta-hCG levels (Cunningham et al., 2022). Immunologic or genetic testing and counseling may be advised for couples having recurrent abortions. All couples who have had a pregnancy loss should be seen by health care professionals and counseled.

At this time, acknowledge the family's grief, which often manifests as anger. They often need repeated reassurance the loss was not a result of anything they did or anything they neglected to do since feelings of guilt are common.

Couples who do not desire pregnancy right away will need contraception. Reliable contraception for at least 1 year will be essential for clients who have had a molar pregnancy. Teach the couple how to use the prescribed contraceptive method correctly to enhance effectiveness.

Evaluation

Interventions are deemed successful and the goals and expected outcomes are met if the client does the following:

- Verbalizes understanding of diagnostic and therapeutic procedures
- Verbalizes measures to prevent infection
- Verbalizes signs of infection that should be reported to a health care professional
- Helps develop and participate in a plan of longer-term follow-up care

HEMORRHAGIC CONDITIONS OF LATE PREGNANCY

After 20 weeks of pregnancy, the two major causes of hemorrhage are the disorders of the placenta called placenta previa and placental abruption.

Placenta Previa

Placenta previa is an abnormal implantation of the placenta in the lower uterus covering or lying close to the cervical os. High-resolution ultrasound allows more accurate measurement of the distance between the internal cervical os and the lower border of the placenta. In years past there were three classifications of placenta previa (total, partial, and marginal) depending on how much of the internal cervical os is covered by the placenta. The current classification system is

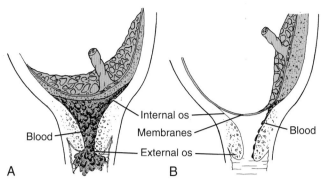

Fig. 10.3 (A) Placenta Previa. (B) Low-lying placenta. From Olshansky, E. F. (2020). *Maternity & women's health care* (12th ed.). Elsevier.

placenta previa and low-lying placenta (Cunningham et al., 2022). Placenta previa is the covering of the cervical os in the third trimester of pregnancy. Low-lying placenta previa is implanted in the lower uterus, but its lower border is within 2 cm from the internal cervical os. (Fig. 10.3A and B)

Placenta previa often appears to move upward and away from the internal cervical os (placental migration) as the fetus grows and the upper uterus develops more than the lower uterus (Cunningham et al., 2022). However, the placenta does not move as the chorionic villi remain anchored into the decidua. As the uterus and the placenta grows, it expands toward the fundus away from the cervical os (Cunningham et al., 2022).

Incidence and Etiology

The average incidence of placenta previa is 1 in 200 to 300 births (Francois & Foley, 2021; Hull et al., 2019). It is more common in older clients, multiparas, clients with previous placenta previa, previous cesarean births, or other uterine surgery. Other risk factors include cigarette smoking, non-White race, elevated serum alpha-fetoprotein (MSAFP) levels, and assisted reproductive technology (ART) (Cunningham et al., 2022; Gyamfi-Bannerman, 2018).

Clinical Manifestations

The classic sign of placenta previa is the sudden onset of *painless* uterine bleeding in the last half of pregnancy (Francois & Foley, 2021; Hull et al., 2019). Many cases of placenta previa are diagnosed by ultrasound examination before any bleeding occurs. Bleeding results from tearing of the placental villi from the uterine wall as the lower uterine segment thins and the internal os begins to dilate near term. Bleeding is painless because it does not occur in a closed cavity and does not cause pressure on adjacent tissue. It may be scant or spotting versus perfuse. The bleeding can begin as a dark brown blood on a peripad or bright red, and the bleeding can be intermittent or continuous. Bleeding may not occur until labor starts, when cervical changes disrupt placental attachment. The admitting nurse may be unsure whether the bleeding is just heavy "bloody show" or a sign of a placenta previa.

Digital examination of the cervical os or stimulation of contractions when a placenta previa is present can cause additional placental separation or tear the placenta itself, causing severe hemorrhage and impairment of oxygenation for the client and fetus. *When a pregnant client presents with vaginal bleeding, no manual vaginal examinations should be performed, and administration of oxytocin should be postponed until the location and position of the placenta are verified by ultrasonography.*

Therapeutic Management

When the diagnosis of placenta previa is confirmed, the client is evaluated to determine the amount of hemorrhage, and electronic fetal monitoring (EFM) is initiated to evaluate the fetus. Fetal gestational age is a third consideration.

Options for management include conservative management if the client's cardiovascular status is stable and the fetus is immature and stable based on ultrasound examination and heart rate monitoring. Delaying birth until 36 to 36 6/7 weeks may increase birth weight and maturity, and administration of corticosteroids to the client speeds maturation of the fetal lungs, if needed (Gyamfi-Bannerman, 2018). Conservative management may take place in the home or the hospital.

Home Care. The medical decision on home care versus inpatient care is difficult. General criteria for home care include the following (Cunningham et al., 2022; Hull et al., 2019):

- Absence of bleeding and abdominal pain for at least 48 hours.
- The client is able to limit activity at home.
- Home is located within a short distance from the hospital.
- Emergency systems are available for immediate transport to the hospital 24 hours a day.
- The client can verbalize understanding of the risks associated with placenta previa and how to manage care.

Nursing Considerations

Home Care. Nurses are often responsible for helping the client and family understand the provider's plan of care. Nurses help the client and family develop a workable plan for home care that may include limited activity or bed rest except for toileting and showering, the presence of another adult to manage the home and be present if an emergency arises, and a procedure to follow if heavy bleeding begins. Teaching includes emphasizing the importance of (1) assessing color and amount of vaginal discharge or bleeding, especially after each urination or bowel movement; (2) assessing fetal activity (kick counts) daily; (3) assessing uterine activity at prescribed intervals; and (4) refraining from sexual intercourse to prevent disruption of the placenta. Home care nurses may be responsible for making daily phone contact to assess the client's perception of uterine activity (cramping, regular or sporadic contractions), bleeding, fetal activity, and adherence to the prescribed treatment plan. In addition, they may make home visits for comprehensive assessments with portable equipment, such as nonstress tests (NSTs). The client and family are instructed to report a decrease in fetal movement or an increase in uterine contractions or vaginal bleeding.

Nurses should provide specific, accurate information about the condition of the fetus. For example, parents are reassured when they hear the fetal heart rate (FHR) is within the expected range and daily kick counts are normal. Nurses may need to help the family understand the provider's plan of care. For instance, the nurse may explain why a cesarean birth is necessary and why blood transfusion may be required.

Inpatient Care. Stable clients may be admitted to the antepartum unit if they do not meet the criteria for home care or if they require additional care to meet the goal of greater fetal maturity. When the expectant client is confined to the hospital, nursing assessments focus on determining whether there are bleeding episodes or signs of preterm labor. Periodic EFM is necessary to determine whether there are fetal heart activity changes associated with fetal compromise. A significant change in fetal heart activity, an episode of vaginal bleeding, or signs of preterm labor should be reported immediately to the provider.

At times, conservative management is not an option. For instance, delivery may be scheduled if the fetus is older than 36 weeks of gestation and the lungs are mature. Immediate delivery may be necessary regardless of fetal immaturity if bleeding is excessive, or if signs of hypovolemia or fetal compromise are present. If cesarean birth is necessary, nurses should prepare the expectant client for surgery. The preoperative procedures are often performed quickly if the client is hemorrhaging, and the family may be anxious. Nurses should use whatever time is available to keep the family informed. Additional personnel will be needed to prepare the client for cesarean birth. Preparations include one or more IV lines, type and crossmatch of blood, administration of preoperative antibiotics, anesthesia, Foley catheter insertion, and fetal monitoring. Neonatology or a team from the neonatal intensive care is usually notified and is present in the operating room for neonatal resuscitation.

Abruptio Placentae

Separation of a normally implanted placenta before the fetus is born is called *abruptio placentae, placental abruption,* or *premature separation of the placenta.* When this occurs, there is bleeding between the placenta and the wall of the uterus with possible formation of a hematoma (clot). As the clot expands, further separation occurs. Hemorrhage may be apparent (vaginal bleeding) or concealed (Cunningham et al., 2022; Francois & Foley, 2021; Hull et al., 2019). The severity of the complication depends on the amount of bleeding and the size of the hematoma. If bleeding continues, the hematoma expands and obliterates intervillous spaces. Fetal vessels are disrupted as placental separation occurs, resulting in fetal and maternal bleeding.

Placental abruption is a dangerous condition for both the pregnant client and the fetus, affecting oxygenation. The major dangers for the client are hemorrhage with consequent hypovolemic shock and clotting abnormalities. The major dangers for the fetus are blood loss affecting oxygenation and prematurity.

Incidence and Etiology

Placental abruption occurs in about 1 in 100 to 200 births. (Cunningham et al., 2022; Francois & Foley, 2021).The risk of reoccurrence in additional pregnancies is 5% to 10% after one previous abruption and 20% to 25% after two (Francois & Foley, 2021).

The cause is not always known, but several factors that increase the risk have been identified. In addition to a history of a previous abruption, hypertension (chronic or preeclampsia), preterm rupture of the amniotic membranes, the use of cocaine or cigarette smoking by the pregnant client, increased client age and parity and abdominal trauma increase the risk for an abruption. (Cunningham et al., 2022, Francois & Foley, 2021; Hull et al., 2019).

Clinical Manifestations

Although verification of placental abruption may be quickly evident, it is not always a dramatic or acute event. Classic signs and symptoms of placental abruption include the following:

- Bleeding, which may be evident vaginally or concealed behind the placenta
- Uterine pain or tenderness that may be localized at the site of the abruption
- Uterine irritability with frequent low-intensity contractions and poor relaxation between contractions
- Abdominal or low back pain that may be described as aching or dull
- High uterine resting tone identified with use of an intrauterine pressure catheter
- "Board-like" abdomen—the abdomen feels firm to touch because of the blood that can be concealed
- "Port wine"–colored amniotic fluid
- FHR patterns (fetal tachycardia, bradycardia, loss of variability, late decelerations, change in FHR baseline from tachycardia to normal baseline with minimal to absent variability, sinusoidal pattern) or fetal death
- Signs of hypovolemic shock

Cases of placental abruption are divided into two main types: (1) those in which hemorrhage is concealed and (2) those in which hemorrhage is apparent. In either type, the placental abruption may be complete or partial. In cases of concealed hemorrhage, the bleeding occurs behind the placenta but the margins remain intact, causing formation of a hematoma. The hemorrhage is apparent when bleeding separates or dissects the membranes from the endometrium and blood flows out through the vagina. Amniotic fluid often has a classic "port wine" color. Fig. 10.4 illustrates placental abruption with external and concealed bleeding. Apparent bleeding does not always correspond to the actual amount of blood lost, and signs of shock (tachycardia, hypotension, pale color, and cold, clammy skin) may be present when little or no external bleeding occurs. Also, the client may have an undiagnosed hypertensive disorder that masks hypovolemia until late hypotension occurs.

Abdominal pain is also related to the type of separation. It may be sudden and severe when bleeding occurs into the myometrium (uterine muscle) or intermittent and difficult to distinguish from labor contractions. The uterus may become exceedingly firm (board-like) and tender, making palpation of the fetus difficult. Ultrasound examination is helpful to

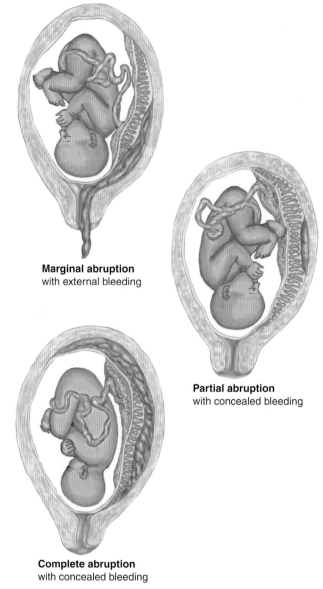

Marginal abruption
with external bleeding

Partial abruption
with concealed bleeding

Complete abruption
with concealed bleeding

Fig. 10.4 Types of placental abruption.

rule out placenta previa as the cause of bleeding, but it cannot be used to diagnose placental abruption reliably because the separation and bleeding may not be obvious on ultrasonography (Gyamfi-Bannerman, 2018).

Therapeutic Management

Any client who exhibits signs of placental abruption should be hospitalized and evaluated at once. Evaluation focuses on the cardiovascular status of the expectant client and the condition of the fetus.

If the condition is mild (the client is stable) and the fetus is under 34 weeks with no signs of compromise, conservative management may be initiated. This includes admission to an antepartum unit, administration of steroids to accelerate fetal lung maturity, initiation of a saline lock, fetal monitoring, and client observation for deterioration.

Immediate delivery of the fetus is necessary if signs of fetal compromise exist or if the client exhibits signs of excessive

bleeding, either obvious or concealed. Intensive monitoring of both the client and the fetus is essential because rapid deterioration of either can occur. Blood products for replacement should be available, and two large-bore IV lines should be started for replacement of fluid (lactated ringers) and blood at a rate to ensure urine output of 30 to 60 mL/hour and a hematocrit of 21% to 24% (Salera-Vieira, 2021). Blood loss should be quantified via a scale. All soiled pads or linens should be weighed and the dry weight subtracted. One gram of weight equals 1 mL of blood loss.

Pregnant clients who have experienced abdominal trauma are at increased risk for placental abruption. They may be observed for up to 24 hours after significant trauma such as a motor vehicle accident, even if they are not having any signs of bleeding, because it may take this long for a placental abruption to develop. For the Rh-negative client, Rho(D) immune globulin is administered to prevent possible client Rh sensitization. Although the Kleihauer-Betke (K-B) test is not useful for the diagnosis of abruption, it may be useful to determine the required dosage of Rho(D) immune globulin (Hull et al., 2019).

Nursing Considerations

Placental abruption is frightening for a client as they may experience severe pain and be aware of the danger to oneself and to the fetus. The client should be carefully assessed for signs of concealed hemorrhage (frequent contractions with short duration, board-like abdomen, abdominal pain, and/or cardiovascular instability).

If immediate cesarean delivery is necessary, the client may feel powerless as the health care team quickly prepares for surgery. Although time may be limited, nurses should explain the anticipated procedures to the client and family as much as possible to reduce their fear and anxiety. Excessive bleeding and fetal hypoxia are always major concerns with placental abruption; nurses should continuously monitor both the client and the fetus.

Complications of Late Pregnancy Hemorrhage

Placental abruption may be further complicated by DIC; hypovolemic shock is a potential complication with placenta previa and placental abruption. Both of these conditions are covered in Chapter 19.

> ⚡ **SAFETY CHECK**
>
> Signs of concealed hemorrhage in placental abruption include the following:
> - Increase in fundal height
> - Hard, board-like abdomen
> - High uterine baseline tone on electronic monitoring strip, especially when an intrauterine pressure catheter is used
> - Abdominal pain
> - Systemic signs of early hemorrhage (tachycardia in the pregnant client and fetus, tachypnea, falling blood pressure, falling urine output, restlessness)
> - Recurrent late decelerations in fetal heart rate or decreasing baseline variability; absence of accelerations
> - Slight or absent vaginal bleeding

HYPEREMESIS GRAVIDARUM

HG is believed to be an extreme form of nausea and vomiting of pregnancy ("morning sickness") diagnosed after other causes have been ruled out. Although there is not a set of defined criteria for diagnosis, the most common symptoms include persistent vomiting that is not due to any other condition, a loss of 5% or more of prepregnancy weight, dehydration, elevated levels of blood and urine ketones, alkalosis from loss of hydrochloric acid in the gastric fluids, and hypokalemia (American College of Obstetricians and Gynecologists [ACOG], 2022b; Cunningham et al., 2022). The client may also have liver and thyroid abnormalities, as well as electrolyte imbalances (ACOG, 2022b).

Etiology, Risk Factors, and Complications

The cause of HG is not known, but increased levels of human chorionic gonadotropin (hCG) and estrogen are associated with this condition (ACOG, 2022b; Gregory et al., 2021). There is ongoing debate on the role of psychological conditions in HG (ACOG, 2022b; Cunningham et al., 2022). Risk factors include hyperthyroidism, HG with a previous pregnancy, female fetus, and multiple gestation (ACOG, 2022b; Cunningham et al., 2022; Gregory et al., 2021). Association with *Helicobacter pylori* is not conclusive (Cunningham et al., 2022).

Complications from HG are rare, but they do occur. Potential client complications associated with severe cases include renal failure, esophageal rupture, and Wernicke encephalopathy (caused by a deficiency of thiamine) (ACOG, 2022b; Gregory et al., 2021). Fetal effects of HG are determined by the severity of the nausea and vomiting. Mild to moderate vomiting is not associated with increased risk for the fetus (ACOG, 2022b). However, if the pregnant client does not have adequate weight gain, the newborn may be underweight as well (Kelly & Savides, 2019).

Therapeutic Management

According to ACOG (2022b), some cases of HG may be prevented or minimized by enhancement of preconception nutritional status with a prenatal vitamin for 1 month prior to conception and with early recognition and treatment of nausea and vomiting in pregnancy. Although there is little published evidence to support dietary changes such as small low-fat meals, dry carbohydrate such as crackers before getting out of bed, and avoiding spicy foods, many clients find these modifications helpful. If taking the prenatal vitamin with iron before bed does not alleviate symptoms associated with this medication, the provider may substitute folic acid supplements (ACOG, 2022b; Gregory et al., 2021). Ginger and acupressure have demonstrated improvement of symptoms and may be helpful in mild to moderate cases (Hu et al., 2022; Khorasani et al., 2020; Mobarakabadi et al., 2020; Sharifzadeh et al., 2018).

If these measures are not effective, first-line pharmacologic treatment is usually vitamin B_6 (pyridoxine) with or without doxylamine. Additional medications that may be used include dopamine antagonists (metoclopramide and phenothiazines), antihistamines (dimenhydrinate and diphenhydramine), serotonin 5-HT3 inhibitors (ondansetron), and steroids, although steroids should be avoided before 10 weeks of gestation due to a weak association with cleft lip and cleft palate and used with caution after that time (ACOG, 2022b).

Inpatient management is most often required when vomiting persists despite outpatient management and the client is not able to tolerate oral liquids. Dehydration, ketonemia, electrolyte deficits, and acid–base imbalances are treated with IV hydration (Cunningham et al., 2022). Thiamine is added to the IV fluid to prevent Wernicke encephalopathy and is continued for 2 to 3 days followed by IV multivitamins for the client who has vomited for 3 weeks or more (ACOG, 2022b; Cunningham et al., 2022). In the rare situation where symptoms are prolonged and the client is unable to maintain a stable weight, enteral feedings may be initiated. Total parenteral nutrition and peripherally inserted central lines are associated with increased morbidity for the client and should only be used in extreme cases (ACOG, 2022b).

Nursing Considerations

Nurses may be responsible for assessing and intervening for the client with HG in the hospital or the home. Nursing assessment of the client with HG includes careful determination of intake and output and signs of dehydration. Intake includes IV fluids and enteral (or parenteral) nutrition, as well as oral nutrition, which is resumed with control of vomiting. Output includes the amount and character of emesis and urinary output. As a rule of thumb, the normal urinary output is about 1 mL/kg/hour (1 mL/2.2 lb/hour). Signs of dehydration should be assessed each shift while hospitalized or as prescribed by the provider for the client on homecare. These include decreased fluid intake (less than 2000 mL/day), decreased urinary output, increased urine specific gravity (more than 1.025), dry skin or dry mucous membranes, and nonelastic skin turgor.

Laboratory data may be evaluated to determine fluid, electrolyte, and metabolic status. Elevated levels of Hgb and Hct may occur as a result of dehydration, which results in hemoconcentration. Concentrations of phosphate, magnesium, sodium, and potassium are monitored. The urine should be assessed for ketones every shift in the hospitalized client or as prescribed for the client on homecare. The provider is informed of abnormal values.

Whether at home or at the hospital, the client weighs daily, first thing in the morning, and in similar clothing each day. Weight loss and the presence of ketones in the urine suggest that fat stores and protein are being metabolized to meet energy needs.

Nursing interventions focus on reducing nausea and vomiting, maintaining nutrition and fluid balance, and providing emotional support.

Reducing Nausea and Vomiting

The client will often have a diet order for NPO, advance as tolerated. Prescribed medications may include antiemetics, as well as medications to control heartburn and reflux. These should be administered in a timely manner. Environmental factors may be a significant stimulus for nausea and vomiting and should be controlled. The client's room should be quiet and away from any areas with strong odors. Staff caring for the client should be free from perfumes and other fragrances, as well as cigarette smoke. Care should be provided in a quiet, calm manor. Any containers or linen with emesis, urine, or stool should be removed from the room as soon as possible. Clean receptacles such as emesis basins should be easily accessible to the client. The room and bathroom should be kept clean, but cleaning products and air fresheners with strong odors should be avoided.

Maintaining Nutrition and Fluid Balance

IV fluids are administered as prescribed by the provider. Small oral feedings of clear liquids are started when nausea and vomiting subside. When oral fluids and adequate food intake are tolerated, IV fluids are gradually discontinued.

Once the nausea and vomiting subside, food and drink preferences should be assessed; the client should be encouraged to consume any food or beverage they can tolerate provided it is safe in pregnancy. Ice pops, broth, and gelatin are often offered first, and many clients find one or more of these acceptable. Bland foods such as baked, broiled, or boiled chicken; crackers; and dry toast are good options when the client progresses to solid foods. Clients with nausea and vomiting should eat small amounts every 1 to 2 hours, if possible, to avoid an empty stomach, as well as one which is overdistended. When food is offered, small portions do not appear overwhelming. Food should be attractively presented, and those with strong odors should be eliminated from the diet because food smells often incite nausea. High-protein, low-fat foods and easily digested carbohydrates provide important nutrients and help prevent low blood glucose levels, which can cause nausea. Soups and other liquids should be taken between meals to avoid distending the stomach and triggering vomiting. Sitting upright after meals reduces gastric reflux.

Continued inability to tolerate oral feedings or continued episodes of vomiting should be reported to the provider.

Providing Emotional Support

The relationship of emotional and psychological conditions to HG is debated. Belief that nausea and vomiting is a normal discomfort of pregnancy and that the extreme, HG, has a psychiatric etiology or origin has contributed to stigma of the disease and possibly to the underappreciation, underdiagnosis, and inadequate treatment of the condition (ACOG, 2022b; Dean et al., 2018; Fiaschi et al., 2019; Hsiao et al., 2021).

Although the role is unclear, there is evidence of an association, especially with depression and anxiety (Dekkers et al., 2020), but the evidence and expert opinions regarding whether psychological conditions are etiologic factors, risk factors, or the result of HG is inconsistent (ACOG, 2022b; Kelly & Savides, 2019; Cunningham et al., 2022; Dean et al., 2018; Dekkers et al., 2020). Regardless of the cause–effect relationship and timing of psychological conditions, clients with HG and their families need emotional support, active listening, teaching, and sometimes referrals.

Specifically, nurses should offer an opportunity for the client to express feelings in an atmosphere of compassion and empathy; listen, as loneliness and isolation are common for these clients. Reassure the client that you believe the symptoms are real and uncontrollable; try to alleviate feelings of guilt. Ask the client what, if anything, helps and specifically what can nurses do to help. Take complaints seriously and try to address them. Encourage the client to balance rest and activity as much as possible. Monitor for depression and posttraumatic stress disorder. Ask the provider for a mental health referral if needed. Teach the family about hyperemesis and how they can help. HER Foundation is an international organization that provides support, research, advocacy, and education on hyperemesis. Information is available for clients, family and friends, and health care providers at https://www.hyperemesis.org.

> **? KNOWLEDGE CHECK**
>
> 9. How do "morning sickness" and HG compare?
> 10. What are the nursing goals in therapeutic management of HG?

HYPERTENSIVE DISORDERS OF PREGNANCY

Hypertension is one of the most common medical complications of pregnancy and a leading cause of morbidity and mortality. Literature states 7% to 18% of pregnancy deaths are related to hypertension (American Academy of Pediatrics (AAP) & ACOG, 2017; ACOG, 2019c; Cunningham et al., 2022; World Health Organization [WHO], 2018). Hypertension is defined as a systolic blood pressure (BP) of 140 mm Hg or greater or a diastolic BP of 90 mm Hg or greater. The following are categories of hypertensive disorders in pregnancy (Table 10.1; AAP & ACOG, 2017; ACOG, 2019c; ACOG, 2020e; Burgess, 2021; Cunningham et al., 2022; Druzin et al., 2013; Harper et al., 2019):

- Gestational hypertension: Onset of hypertension after 20 weeks of pregnancy without proteinuria or other symptoms of preeclampsia. Gestational hypertension should be considered a working diagnosis because it may progress to preeclampsia. If gestational hypertension persists after 12 weeks postpartum, chronic hypertension is diagnosed.
- Preeclampsia: Onset of hypertension after 20 weeks of pregnancy that may be accompanied by proteinuria. Preeclampsia has been defined both with and

TABLE 10.1 Classification of Hypertension in Pregnancy

Classification	Characteristics
Chronic hypertension	1. BP ≥140 mm Hg systolic or ≥90 mm Hg diastolic predating conception 2. Identified before 20 weeks' gestation 3. Persists beyond the 12th week postpartum 4. Use of antihypertensive medications before pregnancy
Superimposed preeclampsia or eclampsia on chronic hypertension	1. New-onset proteinuria in a client with hypertension before 20 weeks' gestation 2. Sudden increase in proteinuria if already present in early gestation 3. Sudden increase in previously well controlled BP 4. Development of HELLP syndrome 5. Development of headache, vision changes, or epigastric pain 6. Change in laboratory values indicating multiorgan involvement (platelets less than 100,000, elevated liver enzymes, decreased kidney function, etc.).
Gestational hypertension	1. Systolic pressure of ≥140 mm Hg or a diastolic pressure ≥90 mm Hg without proteinuria occurring after 20th week gestation 2. Transient diagnosis with normalization of BP by 12th week postpartum 3. May represent preproteinuric phase of preeclampsia or recurrence of chronic hypertension abated in midpregnancy 4. May evolve to preeclampsia 5. Retrospective diagnosis
Preeclampsia	Occurring after 20th week of pregnancy 1. BP ≥140 mm Hg systolic or ≥90 mm Hg diastolic or higher 2. Proteinuria 300 mg protein or higher in a 24-hour urine specimen *or* ≥ +2 urine dipstick *or* protein/creatinine ratio ≥0.3 mg/dL
Preeclampsia with severe features	One or more of the following criteria are present: 1. Blood pressure of ≥160 mm Hg systolic or ≥110 mm Hg diastolic or higher on two occasions at least 15 minutes apart. Shortened time interval allows for more timely antihypertensive medication administration. 2. Cerebral or visual disturbances 3. Pulmonary edema 4. Impaired liver function—elevated liver enzymes to twice normal concentration, severe persistent right upper quadrant, or epigastric pain unresponsive to medication and not accounted for by alternative diagnoses, or both 5. Thrombocytopenia—platelets less than 100,000 6. Renal insufficiency—serum creatinine greater than 1.1mg/dL or doubling of serum creatinine in the absence of other renal disease
Eclampsia	1. Presence of new-onset focal/multifocal or tonic–clonic seizures in a pregnant client with preeclampsia (rule out idiopathic seizure disorder, drug use, or other central nervous system pathologic processes such as intracranial hemorrhage, bleeding arteriovenous malformation, ruptured aneurysm) 2. New-onset seizures 48–72 hours postpartum (other central nervous system pathologic process is the likely reason for the seizure after 7 days)
HELLP Syndrome (subset of severe preeclampsia)	1. Hemolysis; elevated liver enzymes; low platelets

Data from American College of Obstetricians and Gynecologists. (2020e, June). Practice Bulletin, Number 222: Gestational Hypertension and Preeclampsia: *Obstetrics and gynecology, 135*(6), e237–e260. https://doi.org/10.1097/AOG.0000000000003891.

without proteinuria. If no proteinuria is present, then diagnosis is associated with other signs and symptoms including thrombocytopenia, impaired hepatic or renal function, pulmonary edema, or cerebral or visual disturbances.

- Eclampsia: Progression of preeclampsia to generalized seizures that cannot be attributed to other causes. Seizures may occur during antepartum, intrapartum, or postpartum periods.
- Chronic hypertension: Hypertension that is present before pregnancy, diagnosed before 20 weeks of gestation, or continuing beyond 12 weeks postpartum.

- Chronic hypertension with superimposed preeclampsia: Chronic hypertension as defined previously with sudden changes in BP or protein, signs of multiorgan involvement, or development of further complications.

Preeclampsia

Preeclampsia is a pregnancy-specific, multiorgan disease process that is characterized by hypertension that develops after 20 weeks of gestation in a client with previously normal BP. In addition to hypertension, renal involvement may cause proteinuria (≥300 mg in a 24-hour urine collection, which correlates with a random urine dipstick evaluation of ≥2+)

(ACOG, 2020e). Many clients also experience generalized edema as a result of endothelial disruption. Edema, although common in preeclampsia, is considered nonspecific because it occurs in many pregnancies not complicated by hypertension. Two categories of preeclampsia were defined in past literature: mild and severe. The characterization of "mild" can be misleading because morbidity and mortality are significantly increased even in the absence of severe disease. Therefore the term *mild preeclampsia* has been replaced with *preeclampsia without severe features* (Cunningham et al., 2022; Harper et al., 2019). The only known cure for preeclampsia is birth of the fetus and delivery of the placenta. Morbidity can be minimized for the pregnant client and the fetus if preeclampsia is detected early and managed carefully (Cunningham et al., 2022; Harper et al., 2019).

Incidence and Risk Factors

Preeclampsia affects 5% to 8% of all pregnancies, and no known medications prevent its occurrence (Burgess, 2021; Cunningham et al., 2022). The implications of a preeclampsia diagnosis are significant for the pregnant client and the fetus. Adverse outcomes associated with preeclampsia, seen in Table 10.2, are thought to occur as a consequence of endothelial dysfunction, vasospasm, and ultimately ischemia (Burgess, 2021; Cunningham et al., 2022; Harper et al., 2019). Pregnant clients experiencing hypertensive disorders of pregnancy are at an increased risk of developing gestational hypertension, preeclampsia, or HELLP (hemolysis, elevated liver enzymes, and low platelets) in future pregnancies. There is also evidence of increased incidence of cardiovascular, neurovascular, renal, metabolic, and central nervous system disease and associated morbidity and mortality in later life (Cunningham et al., 2022).

Although the cause of preeclampsia is not understood, several factors are known to increase a client's risk (Box 10.2). While some factors such as obesity and prepregnancy diabetes may be interrelated, the individual predictive value of identified risk factors for screening and risk stratification has not been verified (ACOG, 2020e; Burgess, 2021; Cunningham et al., 2022; Harper et al., 2019).

Pathophysiology

Preeclampsia presents with generalized vasoconstriction and vasospasm resulting in poor tissue perfusion and ultimately multiorgan failure during pregnancy as summarized in Table 10.3. Several hypotheses regarding the etiology of this multisystem disease exist. Evidence suggests that the pathologic process begins with an abnormal cardiovascular and uteroplacental response to pregnancy (Witcher & Shah, 2019). Placenta pathology reveals abnormal trophoblast invasion, leading to narrowing of the spiral arteries, which decreases uteroplacental perfusion and fetal oxygenation (Fig. 10.5A and B). This diminished perfusion leads to a release of placental microparticles that generates a systemic inflammatory response and results in widespread endothelial damage. Other hypotheses include (1) a dysregulation of the immune

response to fetal and placental antigens leading to inflammatory changes and decreased adaptation to pregnancy changes or (2) a genetic predisposition for disease development (Burgess, 2021; Cunningham et al., 2022; Harper et al., 2019; Witcher & Shah, 2019).

In normal pregnancy, vascular volume and cardiac output increase significantly, along with a decrease in systemic and peripheral vascular resistance. Despite the increased volume and changes in cardiac output, BP does not rise in normal pregnancy. Pregnant clients develop resistance to the effects of vasoconstrictors, such as angiotensin II, and demonstrate decreased peripheral vascular resistance as a result of increased hormonal influences.

In preeclampsia, however, peripheral and systemic vascular resistance increase due to a sensitivity to angiotensin II and a decrease in availability of prostacyclin and

TABLE 10.2 Complications Associated with Preeclampsia

Complications in the Pregnant Client

Cardiovascular	1. Decreased intravascular volume
	2. Severe hypertension including hypertensive crisis
	3. Pulmonary edema
	4. Congestive heart failure
	5. Cardiomyopathy
	6. Future cardiac disease and dysfunction
Pulmonary	1. Pulmonary edema
	2. Hypoxemia/academia
Renal	1. Oliguria
	2. Acute kidney injury/renal failure
	3. Impaired drug metabolism and excretion
Hematologic	1. Hemolysis of red blood cells
	2. Decreased oxygen-carrying capacity
	3. Thrombocytopenia
	4. Coagulation defects (disseminated intravascular coagulation)
	5. Anemia
Neurologic	1. Seizures
	2. Cerebral edema
	3. Intracerebral hemorrhage
	4. Stroke
	5. Visual disturbances, blindness
Hepatic	1. Hepatocellular dysfunction/failure
	2. Hepatic rupture
	3. Hypoglycemia
	4. Coagulation defects
	5. Impaired drug metabolism and excretion
Uteroplacental	1. Abruption
	2. Decreased uteroplacental perfusion

Fetal Complications
1. Intrauterine growth restriction
2. Intrauterine fetal death
3. Fetal intolerance to labor
4. Preterm birth
5. Low birth weight
6. Decreased oxygenation

BOX 10.2 Risk Factors for Pregnancy-Related Hypertension

First pregnancy
New genetic material—males who fathered preeclamptic
   pregnancies are more likely to father further preeclamptic
   pregnancies
Age greater than or equal to 35 years old
African American race
History of thrombophilia such as hyperhomocysteinemia
   (elevated levels of homocysteine that increase the risk for
   developing clots, heart attack, and stroke); factor V Leiden;
   or protein C and protein S deficiencies
In vitro fertilization
History of preeclampsia
Chronic hypertension
Renal disease
Obesity—body mass index greater than 30
Diabetes mellitus
Metabolic syndrome
HIV-positive
Antiphospholipid syndrome
Systemic lupus erythematosus
Multifetal pregnancy
Obstructive sleep apnea
Hydatidiform mole or fetal hydrops

Information from ACOGe, 2020; Burgess, 2021; Cunningham et al.,
2018; Harper et al., 2019; Witcher et al., 2019.

endothelial-derived nitric oxide, which promote vasodilation. The increase in vascular resistance may be the body's attempt to maintain homeostasis and provide end organ perfusion particularly when the client is experiencing a hypovolemic intravascular state, which results from the multisystem pathology of preeclampsia. Widespread endothelial damage increases capillary permeability and allows colloid proteins, such as albumin, to leak into interstitial spaces further compounding the hypovolemic state of preeclampsia. Arterial vasospasm decreases the diameter of blood vessels, creating additional endothelial cell damage, and ultimately increasing capillary permeability. Vasoconstriction also results in impeded blood flow and elevated BP. As a result, circulation to all body organs, including the kidneys, liver, brain, and placenta, is decreased. The following changes are most significant (Burgess, 2021; Cunningham et al., 2022; Harper et al., 2019; Witcher et al., 2019):

- Decreased renal perfusion reduces the glomerular filtration rate. Blood urea nitrogen, creatinine, and uric acid levels rise.
- Decreased renal perfusion results in glomerular damage, allowing protein to leak across the glomerular membrane, which is normally impermeable to protein molecules. As the damage progressively worsens, the size of the protein molecule crossing the membrane incrementally increases.
- Loss of protein from the kidneys reduces colloid osmotic pressure and allows fluid to shift to interstitial spaces. This may result in edema and a reduction in intravascular volume, which causes increased viscosity of the blood and a rise in hematocrit level. Generalized edema often occurs.

- In preeclampsia, the normal response to reduced intravascular volume (releasing additional angiotensin II and aldosterone which trigger the retention of both sodium and water) does not occur. Preeclamptic clients are more susceptible to the effects of the renin-angiotensin-aldosterone system, creating a pathologic systemic vasoconstriction process: the release of angiotensin II results in further vasospasm and hypertension while aldosterone increases fluid retention, and edema worsens.
- Reduced liver circulation impairs function and leads to hepatic edema and subcapsular hemorrhage, which can result in hemorrhagic necrosis or rupture. This is manifested by elevation of liver enzymes. Epigastric pain is a common symptom.
- Vasoconstriction of cerebral vessels leads to pressure-induced rupture of thin-walled capillaries, resulting in small cerebral hemorrhages. Symptoms of arterial vasospasm include headache and visual disturbances such as blurred vision, "spots" before the eyes, and hyperactive deep tendon reflexes (DTRs).
- Dysfunction of the endothelial cells leads to decreased cerebral blood flow causing ischemia, edema, and eventually tissue infarction. Cerebral edema may present as posterior reversible encephalopathy syndrome (PRES). PRES presents with neurologic symptoms such as seizures, decreased level of consciousness, headache, and vision changes. Diagnosis is made by radiologic confirmation showing edema in the posterior portion of the brain. Treatment includes managing the hypertension to prevent ischemia, which may lead to subsequent irreversible damage (Witcher & Shah, 2019).
- Decreased colloid oncotic pressure can lead to pulmonary capillary leakage that results in pulmonary edema. Dyspnea is the primary symptom.
- Decreased placental circulation results in infarctions that increase the risk for placental abruption and HELLP syndrome. In addition, the fetus is likely to experience intrauterine growth restriction, persistent hypoxemia, and acidosis when blood flow through the placenta is reduced.

Preventive Measures

Prenatal Care. Early and regular prenatal care with attention to weight gain patterns and close monitoring of BP and urinary protein level may minimize morbidity and mortality by allowing early detection of preeclampsia.

Attempts at prevention in clients at high risk for recurrence have included low-dose aspirin, vitamin C and E, calcium supplements, exercise, salt-restricted diet, and fish oil supplements. Calcium supplementation appears to reduce the risk for preeclampsia in high-risk clients with low calcium intake. Exercise studies provided inconclusive results. Vitamin C and E, salt restriction, and fish oil supplements have failed to show an impact on the incidence or severity of preeclampsia. Low-dose aspirin, 81 mg/day, has proven most efficacious in decreasing inflammation, promoting normal blood vessel development, and inhibiting clot formation (ACOG, 2018c;

TABLE 10.3 Preeclampsia Pathophysiology as a Multiorgan System Disease

System	Effect of Preeclampsia	Clinical Implications
Vascular Bed 1. Endothelial dysfunction 2. Altered coagulation 3. Altered response to vasoactive substances	• Increased release of cellular fibronectin, growth factors, VCAM-1, factor VIII antigen, and peptides • Endothelial cell injury initiates coagulation either by intrinsic pathway (contact adhesion) or extrinsic pathway (tissue factor) • Decreased production of prostacyclin and alteration in prostacyclin/thromboxane ratio	• Endothelial dysfunction presents before clinical signs of the disease • Increased thrombus formation, including pulmonary and cerebral emboli • Vasoconstriction and vasospasm • Increased sensitivity to vasoactive substance • Capillary permeability, which contributes to edema formation
Cardiovascular and Pulmonary 1. ↑ Vascular resistance 2. ↑ Cardiac output and stroke volume 3. ↓ Colloid osmotic pressure	• Arteriolar narrowing • ↑ Sympathetic activity • ↑ Levels of endothelin-1, a vasoconstrictor • ↑ Sensitivity to endogenous pressors, including vasopressin, epinephrine, and norepinephrine • ↑ Capillary permeability • Further depletion of intravascular colloids through capillary permeability and renal excretion of proteins	• Increased blood pressure • Hyperdynamic cardiac activity • Epidurals can be used safely, however ephedrine to correct hypotension should be used with caution. • Subendocardial hemorrhages are present in >50% of clients who die of eclampsia • At risk for pulmonary edema, myocardial ischemia, left ventricular dysfunction
Renal 1. Proteinuria 2. Altered function	• Slight decrease in glomerular size • Diameter of glomerular capillary lumen decreased • Glomerular endothelial cells are greatly enlarged and may occlude the capillary lumen • Glomerular capillary endotheliosis • Thickening of renal arterioles	• Proteinuria plus hypertension is the most reliable indicator of fetal jeopardy, indicative of glomerular dysfunction • ↑ Serum uric acid secondary to a ↓ urate clearance (uric acid better predictor of outcome than blood pressure) • ↓ Creatinine clearance with an elevation of serum creatinine levels • ↑ BUN mirrors changes in creatine clearance and also a function of protein intake and liver function • Urine sediment analysis may not be beneficial • At risk for oliguria, ATN, renal failure
Hepatic 1. Hepatic dysfunction 2. Hepatic rupture	• Changes consistent with hemorrhage into hepatic tissue • Later changes consistent with hepatic infarction • ↑ Hepatic artery resistance • Fibrin deposition • Hepatocellular necrosis	• Elevations of liver function tests; association of microangiopathic anemia and elevations of AST/ALT carries ominous prognosis for the pregnant client and fetus • HELLP syndrome • Possible elevations in bilirubin • Signs of liver failure; malaise, nausea, epigastric pain, hypoglycemia, hemolysis, anemia
Hematologic 1. Thrombocytopenia 2. Altered platelet function 3. Hemolysis	• ↑ Platelet destruction • ↑ Platelet aggregation • ↓ Platelet life span • Hemolytic anemia • Destruction of RBCs in microvasculature	• Platelets <100,000 increased risk for coagulopathy • Platelets <50,000 increased risk for hemorrhage • Platelets <20,000 increased risk for spontaneous bleeding • Decreased oxygen-carrying capacity and organ oxygenation
Central Nervous System (CNS) 1. Hyperreflexia	• May indicate increasing CNS involvement, but not diagnostic of disease • Alteration of cerebral autoregulation with seizures • ↑ Intracranial pressures	• Cerebral edema with severe disease • Signs of CNS alterations: headache, dizziness, changes in vital signs, diplopia, scotomata, blurred vision, amaurosis, tachycardia, alteration in level of consciousness

Continued

TABLE 10.3	Preeclampsia Pathophysiology as a Multiorgan System Disease—cont'd	
System	**Effect of Preeclampsia**	**Clinical Implications**
Fetal/Neonatal 1. Fetal intolerance to labor 2. Preterm birth 3. Oligohydramnios 4. IUGR 5. IUFD 6. Abruptio placentae	• Alteration in placental function • At risk for indicated preterm birth secondary to disease process	• Must monitor signs for fetal compromise • Monitoring for IUGR and IUFD • At risk for abruptio placentae, oligohydramnios, indeterminate or abnormal fetal heart rate patterns
Uteroplacental 1. Spiral arteries 2. Changes consistent with hypoxia	• Abnormal invasion • Retain nonpregnant characteristics • Limited vasodilatation • Vessel necrosis	• Decreases in uteroplacental perfusion • Increased risk for fetal compromise and IUGR

AST/ALT, Aspartate aminotransferase/alanine aminotransferase; *ATN,* acute tubular necrosis; *BUN,* blood urea nitrogen; *HELLP,* hemolysis, elevated levels of liver enzymes, and low platelet levels; *IUFD,* intrauterine fetal death; *IUGR,* intrauterine growth restriction; *VCAM-1,* vascular cell adhesion protein 1.
From Simpson, K. R., Creehan, P. A., O'Brien-Abel, N., Roth, C. K., & Rohan, A. J. (2021). *AWHONN's perinatal nursing* (5th ed.). Lippincott Williams & Wilkins. Copyright © 2014, 2008, 2001, 1996 by the Association of Women's Health, Obstetrics and Neonatal Nurses (AWHONN). p. 107.

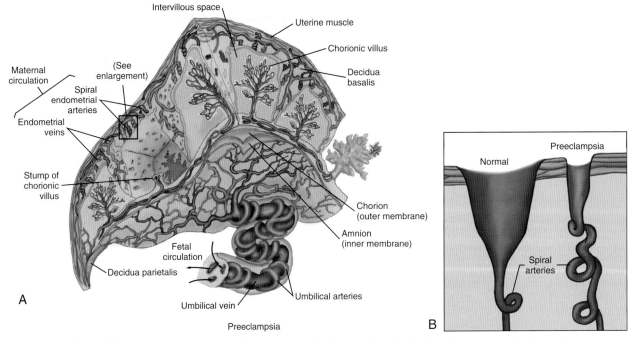

Fig. 10.5 Abnormal development of the spiral arteries in preeclampsia leads to decreased perfusion and oxygenation.

Burges, 2021; Cunningham et al., 2022; Harper et al., 2018; U.S. Preventive Services, 2021).

Clinical Manifestations of Preeclampsia

Diagnostic Criteria. Preeclampsia is hypertension (systolic BP ≥140 mm Hg or diastolic ≥90 mm Hg) occurring after 20 weeks of pregnancy in clients with previously normal BP usually accompanied by proteinuria. BP measurements should be measured uniformly at each office visit. BP should be measured with the client seated, feet flat on the floor and arm supported, with the appropriate-size cuff placed at heart level. After a 10-minute rest period, BP should be assessed with a sphygmomanometer and a stethoscope to provide best audible identification of Korotkoff sounds. The diastolic pressure should be recorded at Korotkoff phase V, disappearance of sound. Hospitalizing the client for serial observations of BP may identify true elevations from those induced by anxiety.

Proteinuria can be identified using a clean-catch specimen or a 24-hour urine collection. Clean-catch urine specimens are used to prevent contamination of the specimen by vaginal secretions or blood. Clients with urinary tract infections (UTIs) often have erythrocytes and leukocytes in their urine, which would elevate urine protein level in the absence of preeclampsia. Diagnostic values of 2+ or greater dipstick reading or 300 mg or greater in a 24-hour urine sample indicate developing preeclampsia. A protein-to-creatinine ratio of 0.3 mg or greater is also diagnostic (ACOG, 2020e).

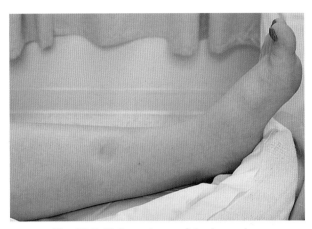

Fig. 10.6 Pitting edema of the lower leg.

In the absence of proteinuria, the following criteria are used to diagnose preeclampsia in a hypertensive client (AAP & ACOG, 2017; ACOG, 2020e; Burges, 2021; Cunningham et al., 2022):

- Thrombocytopenia—platelets less than 100,000/μL
- Renal insufficiency—serum creatinine greater than 1.1 mg/dL or a doubling of the serum creatinine concentration in the absence of other renal disease
- Impaired liver function—elevated blood concentrations of liver transaminases to twice normal concentration
- Pulmonary edema
- Cerebral or visual symptoms

When the retina is examined, vascular constriction and narrowing of the small arteries are obvious in most clients with preeclampsia. The vasoconstriction that can be seen in the retina is occurring throughout the body. DTRs may be very brisk (hyperreflexia), suggesting cerebral irritability secondary to decreased brain perfusion and edema.

Laboratory studies may identify liver and renal dysfunction if preeclampsia is severe. Coagulation may be impaired, as evidenced by a decrease in the number of platelets, which are often in the high–normal range in a client without preeclampsia.

Although it is a nonspecific sign that may have many causes, generalized edema often occurs with preeclampsia and may be severe. Edema may first manifest as a rapid weight gain caused by fluid retention. It may present in the lower legs, which is common in pregnancy, and in the hands and face (Fig. 10.6). Substantial edema may alter the client's appearance. Edema may not be present in all clients who develop preeclampsia, and it may be severe in clients who do not have the disorder.

Symptoms. Preeclampsia is dangerous for the client and the fetus for two reasons: (1) it can develop and worsen rapidly, and (2) the earliest symptoms are often not noticed by the client. By the time symptoms are noticeable, the disease may have progressed to an advanced state and valuable treatment time lost.

Certain symptoms such as continuous headache, drowsiness, or mental confusion indicate poor cerebral perfusion and may be precursors of seizures. Visual disturbances such as blurred or double vision or spots before the eyes indicate arterial spasms and edema in the retina. In rare instances, blindness can occur. Pathologic lesions present on the retina are caused by ischemia, infarction, or detachment. Numbness or tingling of the hands or feet occurs when nerves are

compressed by retained fluid. Some symptoms such as epigastric pain or "upset stomach" are particularly ominous because they indicate distention of the hepatic capsule and increase the risk for liver rupture. Decreased urinary output indicates poor perfusion of the kidneys and may precede acute renal failure (Cunningham et al., 2022).

Therapeutic Management of Preeclampsia

The only cure for preeclampsia is delivery of the baby and placenta. However, the decision about delivery will be based on the severity of the hypertensive disorder and the degree of fetal maturity. Delivery is indicated in the client with preeclampsia without severe features at 37 weeks of gestation. If the fetus is less than 34 weeks of gestation, steroids to accelerate fetal lung maturity may be given and an attempt made to delay birth for 48 hours. However, if the condition of the pregnant client or fetus deteriorates, the infant should be delivered, regardless of gestational age or administration of steroids. Vaginal birth is the preferred delivery method, reserving cesarean section for the usual obstetric implications (Cunningham et al., 2022; Harper et al., 2019).

Home Care. Management in the home may be possible for select clients. The client should be willing to adhere to a prescribed treatment plan that includes reduced activity (sedentary activity most of the day), home BP monitoring, and follow-up visits to the provider every 3 to 4 days. The client who is prescribed home care should be taught how to perform BP checks and to report symptoms suggesting worsening preeclampsia, such as visual disturbance, severe headache, or epigastric pain. Symptoms suggesting fetal compromise, such as reduced fetal movement, should also be reported. If the client is hospitalized with preeclampsia, the home care in the following section is adapted for inpatient care (Burges, 2021; Cunningham et al., 2022).

Activity Restrictions. The client should rest frequently, although full bed rest is not required for preeclampsia. The lateral position decreases pressure on the vena cava, thereby increasing cardiac return and circulatory volume and improving perfusion of the vital organs and the placenta. Although the efficacy of bed rest is not clearly established, it remains a usual and reasonable recommendation for preeclampsia management (Burges, 2021; Cunningham et al., 2022).

Blood Pressure. If BP monitoring is prescribed, the family should be taught to use electronic BP equipment, readily available in retail stores. BP should be checked in the same arm and in the same position at least twice weekly. An appropriate-size cuff should be used.

Weight. Daily weight should be obtained each morning, preferably on the same scale and in clothing of similar weight. Increasing weight is an indicator of the degree of fluid retention occurring.

Urinalysis. A provider may order urine analysis for protein. Typically, the first voided midstream specimen of the day is used. A 24-hour urine specimen collected at home or in the hospital may be ordered for the most accurate urine protein levels.

Fetal Assessment. Because vasoconstriction can reduce placental flow, the client will have increased fetal assessments to observe for evidence of fetal compromise. Fetal compromise can be evidenced by reduced fetal movement noted by the client ("kick counts"). Additional surveillance may include ultrasonography for fetal growth and quantity of amniotic fluid or as part of a biophysical profile (BPP), as well as assessment of umbilical artery blood flow and resistance (Doppler velocimetry). A diminishing amount of amniotic fluid suggests placental impairment (Cunningham et al., 2022; Harper et al., 2019). See Chapter 9 for discussion of fetal surveillance methods.

Diet. The diet should have ample protein and calories. A regular diet without salt or fluid restriction is usually prescribed. Clients who also have chronic hypertension or diabetes should have diet management appropriate for these disorders.

A nurse should reevaluate the client's compliance with prescribed care and the understanding of signs or symptoms to promptly report at each contact, whether by phone or home care visit. The client should go to the hospital for evaluation promptly if unable to contact the provider about signs or symptoms of concern.

Preeclampsia with Severe Features

Diagnostic Criteria. Some clinical findings suggest an increased risk for morbidity and mortality resulting in a diagnosis of preeclampsia with severe features. These features include one or more of the following (AAP & ACOG, 2017; ACOG, 2020e; Cunningham et al., 2022; Druzin et al., 2013):

- Systolic blood pressure of 160 mm Hg or greater or a diastolic blood pressure of 110 mm Hg or greater on at least two occasions at least 15 minutes apart. Shortened time interval allows for more timely antihypertensive medication administration.
- Thrombocytopenia (platelet count less than 100,000/μL)
- Impaired liver function as indicated by abnormally elevated liver enzymes (to twice normal concentration), severe persistent right upper quadrant, or epigastric pain unresponsive to medication and not accounted for by alternative diagnoses, or both
- Progressive renal insufficiency (serum creatinine concentration greater than 1.1 mg/dL or a doubling of the serum creatinine concentration in the absence of other renal disease)
- Pulmonary edema
- Cerebral or visual disturbances

Nursing assessments focus on identification of disease progression and timely notification of the provider of such findings.

Management of Preeclampsia with Severe Features. Preeclampsia with severe features requires inpatient hospitalization. Current recommendations for management depend on disease severity and include progression toward delivery, even if the gestation is less than 34 weeks.

Antepartum Management. Goals of management are to improve placental blood flow and fetal oxygenation as well as prevent seizures and other complications, such as stroke, as the client's condition is stabilized before birth. A decreased volume of amniotic fluid is considered significant because it suggests reduced placental blood flow, even if BPs are not high. Ultrasound may be done to evaluate fetal blood flow through the umbilical cord and placenta.

Activity and Fetal Monitoring. Clients are encouraged to reduce daily physical activity by having frequent rest periods while elevating their legs or resting in bed in a lateral position.

Ensuring the environment is kept quiet helps to decrease external stimuli (e.g., lights, noise) that might precipitate a seizure. EFM is indicated during hospitalization. The frequency of monitoring is individualized based on the client's status (e.g., twice a day, three times per day, or continuously).

Medications. Clients who have preeclampsia with severe features may require antihypertensive or anticonvulsant medications. Some will require both. These medications may be initiated during the antepartum, intrapartum, or postpartum period.

Antihypertensive Medications. Antihypertensive therapies are reserved for clients with systolic BP 160 mm Hg or greater or diastolic BP 110 mm Hg or greater to decrease the risk for stroke. Antihypertensive medications are recommended to slowly reduce the client's BP. The following medications are considered first line because of their efficacy and preservation of uteroplacental blood flow:

- Labetalol—Has less tachycardia and fewer adverse effects; contraindicated in clients with asthma, heart disease, heart block, bradycardia, or congestive heart failure; associated with hypoglycemia and small for gestational age infants.
- Hydralazine (Apresoline)—Higher doses are associated with hypotension, headaches, and fetal distress.
- Nifedipine—May be associated with reflex tachycardia and headaches; because of mechanism of action, a synergistic effect with magnesium sulfate may result in hypotension and neuromuscular blockade.

Caution is essential when antihypertensive medications are given to the client receiving magnesium sulfate because hypotension may result, reducing placental perfusion (Burges, 2021; Cunningham et al., 2022).

Anticonvulsant Medications. Magnesium sulfate is the drug most often used to prevent seizures. Phenytoin (Dilantin), lorazepam (Ativan), levetiracetam (Keppra), and midazolam (Versed) are not recommended as first-line agents because of their decreased efficacy compared with magnesium. However, in cases in which magnesium sulfate is inappropriate, such as in cases of myasthenia gravis, compromised renal function, or significant cardiac or pulmonary concerns, or when seizures recur after a second magnesium sulfate loading dose, these agents may be indicated (Burges, 2021; Cunningham et al., 2022). Current recommendations are to administer magnesium sulfate for seizure prophylaxis in the client who has preeclampsia with severe features. Use of magnesium in the client who has preeclampsia without severe features remains controversial (ACOG, 2020e; Druzin et al., 2013). Magnesium acts by blocking neuromuscular transmission of acetylcholine, which decreases the amount liberated and reduces central nervous system (CNS) irritability, blocks cardiac conduction, and relaxes smooth muscle. Magnesium is not an antihypertensive medication, but it relaxes smooth muscle, including the uterus, and thus reduces vasoconstriction, possibly resulting in modest BP reduction. Decreased vasoconstriction promotes circulation to the vital organs of the pregnant client and increases placental circulation. Increased circulation to the kidneys leads to diuresis as interstitial fluid is shifted into the vascular compartment and excreted.

DRUG GUIDE

Magnesium Sulfate

Classification

Anticonvulsant

Action

Decreases acetylcholine released by motor nerve impulses, thereby blocking neuromuscular transmission. Depresses central nervous system irritability and relaxes smooth muscle, decreasing frequency and intensity of uterine contractions. Slows cardiac conduction. Produces flushing, hypotension, and vasodilation.

Indications

Prevention and control of seizures in preeclampsia with severe features, prevention of uterine contractions in preterm labor, and neuroprotection of preterm fetus.

Dosage and Route

A common IV administration protocol for preeclampsia includes a loading dose and a continuous infusion using a controlled infusion pump. The IV loading dose is 4 to 6 g of magnesium sulfate administered over 15 to 30 minutes. The continuing maintenance infusion is 1 to 2 g/hour. Doses are individualized as needed. A mainline IV infusion with no medication is maintained, and the magnesium sulfate is piggybacked into the port closest to the IV site. Deep IM injection is acceptable but is painful, and the rate of absorption cannot be controlled. It is recommended to reconstitute magnesium with Xylocaine 2% when administering IM. Dosing for IM injection is 10 g (5 g in each buttock), followed by 5 g every 4 hours.

Onset of Action

IV: Immediate. IM: 1 hour.

Excretion

Renal clearance. In clients with normal kidney function, magnesium is excreted in approximately 4 hours.

Contraindications and Precautions

Contraindicated in persons with myocardial damage, greater than first-degree heart block without a pacemaker, myasthenia gravis, or impaired renal function.

Reactions

Side effects include flushing, sweating, and feeling tired or weak. Toxic effects may include hypotension, lethargy, mental confusion, slurred speech, visual disturbances, depressed DTRs, respiratory depression or arrest, adventitious lung sounds, and electrocardiogram changes leading up to cardiac arrest.

Nursing Implications

Monitor BP closely during administration. Assess the client for respiratory rate above 12 breaths per minute, clear bilateral lung sounds, presence of DTRs, and urinary output greater than 30 mL/hour before administering magnesium. Maintain strict intake and output. Notify provider if insufficient urine output or signs of toxicity occur. Place resuscitation equipment (suction and oxygen) in the room. Ensure calcium gluconate, which acts as an antidote to magnesium, is readily available (ACOG, 2020e; Burges, 2021; Cunningham et al., 2022; Harper et al., 2019; Magnesium Sulfate: Drug Information, 2021; Shepherd et al., 2017).

Magnesium is administered by IV infusion, which allows for immediate onset of action and does not cause the discomfort associated with IM administration. Magnesium is administered via a secondary line so the medication can be discontinued at any time while the primary line remains functional. The Institute for Safe Medication Practices (ISMP, 2018) lists magnesium sulfate as a high-risk medication. Therefore two nurses perform independent double checks verifying the orders and checking pump settings prior to initiation, with dosing changes, and client handoff.

Although magnesium sulfate is not risk-free, it is the drug of choice in preventing seizures during pregnancy (AAP & ACOG, 2017; ACOG, 2020e; Burges, 2021). Fetal magnesium levels are nearly identical with those of the pregnant client. As a result, the fetal monitor tracing may show decreased FHR variability and reactivity. No cumulative effect occurs, however, because the fetal kidneys excrete magnesium effectively.

The therapeutic serum level for magnesium is 4.8 to 8.4 mg/dL, although it is elevated in terms of normal laboratory values. Adverse reactions to magnesium sulfate usually occur if the serum level becomes too high. The most significant adverse reaction is CNS depression, including depression of the respiratory center. Magnesium is excreted solely by the kidneys, and the reduced urine output that often occurs in preeclampsia allows magnesium to accumulate to toxic levels

in the client. Frequent assessment of serum magnesium levels, DTRs, respiratory rate, and oxygen saturation can identify CNS depression before it progresses to respiratory depression or cardiac dysfunction. Monitoring urine output identifies oliguria that could allow magnesium to accumulate and reach excessive levels.

Intrapartum Management. Half of eclamptic seizures occur during labor or in the first 48 hours after birth. The other half occur antenatally (Burges, 2021). The fetus and the client should be monitored continuously to detect signs of decreased oxygenation and imminent seizures. The client should be kept in a lateral position to promote circulation through the placenta, and efforts should focus on decreasing stimuli that may cause agitation and precipitate seizures.

Oxytocin to stimulate uterine contractions and magnesium sulfate to prevent seizures are often administered simultaneously during labor when a client has preeclampsia. The client will have two secondary infusions in addition to the primary infusion line, one for oxytocin and one for magnesium. Antibiotics or other drugs may require additional lines. Multiple infusion pumps ensure that different medications and fluids are administered at the prescribed volume and dose. Equipment, IV lines, and IV sites should be checked carefully for correct placement and function.

Opiate analgesics or epidural analgesia may be administered to provide comfort and reduce painful stimuli that could precipitate a seizure. However, some clients who have preeclampsia with severe features also have coagulation abnormalities that may contraindicate use of epidural analgesia.

Continuous fetal monitoring identifies changes in FHR patterns that suggest compromise (see Chapter 14). Late decelerations and decreased variability are associated with reduced placental perfusion. The nurse continuously assesses the FHR pattern for any indeterminate or abnormal pattern. Interventions implemented are tailored to the fetal heart pattern identified, such as repositioning the client, stopping the oxytocin infusion, altering other IV infusion rates, or administering oxygen to the client. A neonatal resuscitation team is often called to the birth.

Postpartum Management. After birth, careful assessment of the client's blood loss and signs of shock are essential because the hypovolemia caused by preeclampsia may be aggravated by blood loss during the delivery. The nurse should also be alert for signs of postpartum hemorrhage due to uterine atony caused by the smooth muscle relaxant effect of magnesium sulfate. Assessments for signs and symptoms of preeclampsia should be continued for at least 48 hours, and administration of magnesium along with its associated care usually is continued to prevent seizures for 24 hours.

Signs that the client is recovering from preeclampsia include the following:

- Diuresis—increased urinary output, which causes a rapid reduction in edema and rapid weight loss
- Decreased protein in the urine
- Return of blood pressure to normal
- Resolution of abnormal laboratory values

Therapeutic Management of Eclampsia. Eclampsia is a potentially preventable extension of preeclampsia with severe features marked by one or more generalized seizures, occurring more frequently in the last trimester (Burges, 2021; Cunningham et al., 2022). Early identification of preeclampsia allows intervention before the condition reaches the seizure stage in most cases. Generalized seizures are characterized by muscles alternately contracting and relaxing. These tonic–clonic movements last for an unspecified timeframe. Breathing stops during a generalized seizure. Gradually the muscle movements decrease until they finally stop and the client lies still. The client enters in an unresponsive state (**postictal state**) and is unlikely to remember the seizure when consciousness resumes. This unresponsive state may be transient, or may result in a coma for an unspecified time depending on the severity of the insult (Cunningham et al., 2022). Transient FHR patterns such as bradycardia, loss of variability, or late and/or prolonged decelerations are anticipated. Fetal tachycardia may occur as the fetus compensates for the period of apnea during the seizures.

The client's blood volume is often severely reduced in eclampsia, increasing the risk for poor placental perfusion. Fluid shifts from the intravascular space to the interstitial space, including the lungs, causing pulmonary edema and possibly heart failure as forward blood flow from the heart is impeded. Renal blood flow is severely reduced, resulting in oliguria (less than 30 mL/hour urine output) and possibly renal failure. Cerebral hemorrhage may accompany eclampsia because of the high BP and coagulation deficits. The client's lungs should be auscultated at regular intervals assessing for adventitious breath sounds. A pulse oximeter provides continuous readings of oxygen saturation. Furosemide (Lasix) may be administered if pulmonary edema develops. Administration of oxygen via a nonrebreather face mask at 10 L/min improves oxygenation of the pregnant client and the fetus. Digitalis may be needed to strengthen contraction of the heart if circulatory failure results. Frequent assessments, usually at least hourly, of the previously mentioned parameters are indicated in the preeclamptic/eclamptic client.

Because eclampsia stimulates uterine irritability, the client should be monitored carefully for ruptured membranes, signs of labor, or placental abruption. While the client is postictal, position laterally to prevent aspiration and improve placental circulation. Aspiration of gastric contents increases the risk of pulmonary edema and morbidity after an eclamptic seizure (Burges, 2021; Cunningham et al., 2022). Equipment to suction the client's airway should be immediately available. The side rails should be raised and padded to prevent a fall and possible injury. After initial stabilization, the nurse should anticipate orders for chest radiography and arterial blood gas determination to identify aspiration and possibly an order for head computed tomography (CT) to identify any cerebral hemorrhage (Burges, 2021). HELLP syndrome is associated with preeclampsia with severe features. DIC is an added complication of unexpected bleeding that may occur with coagulation abnormalities of preeclampsia with severe features or eclampsia. Laboratory studies are performed at frequent intervals to identify both falling and recovering coagulation values, as well as to identify hemolysis and elevated levels of liver enzymes. After the client and fetus have been stabilized, the fetus usually is delivered, either by induction of labor if the client's cervix is favorable or by cesarean if remote from term.

KNOWLEDGE CHECK

11. What are the fetal complications associated with preeclampsia?
12. What are the signs and symptoms of preeclampsia? Why is reduced activity a part of management?
13. What is the effect of vasoconstriction on the brain?
14. What are the effects of magnesium sulfate, including the primary adverse effect?
15. What are the major complications of eclampsia?

APPLICATION OF THE NURSING PROCESS: PREECLAMPSIA

Assessment

Nursing assessment is one of the most important components of successful management of preeclampsia. Careful assessment helps determine whether the condition is responding to

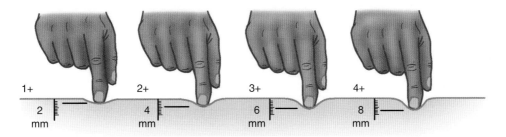

Fig. 10.7 Assessment of pitting edema of lower extremities. (A) +1. (B) +2. (C) +3. (D) +4. From Ball, J. W. et al. (2015). *Seidel's guide to physical examination* (8th ed.). Mosby.

medical management or whether the disease is worsening. A 1:1 nurse-to-client ratio is needed for the unstable client who has preeclampsia with severe features.

Weigh the client on admission and daily. Check vital signs and auscultate lung fields at least every 4 hours for crackles, adventitious breath sounds that indicate pulmonary edema. Assess the location and severity of edema at least every 4 hours. Although it is somewhat subjective, the relative degree of edema can be described using the method demonstrated in Fig. 10.7. Maintain strict intake and output monitoring. If the client is unable to ambulate to the restroom or void on a bedpan, insertion of an indwelling catheter to measure hourly urine output is initiated. Check the urine for protein as ordered. Apply an external electronic fetal monitor to identify changes in FHR resulting in indeterminate or abnormal patterns. Consider medications given to the pregnant client and their relationship to the FHR pattern.

Check reflexes such as bicep, triceps, and patellar reflexes for hyperreflexia, which indicates cerebral irritability. Determine whether clonus is present with hyperactive reflexes by dorsiflexing the client's foot sharply and then releasing it while holding the knee in a flexed position. **Clonus** (rapidly alternating muscle contraction and relaxation) may occur when reflexes are hyperactive. If clonus or hyperreflexia are present, notify the provider. Procedure 10.1 illustrates how to assess and rate DTRs and clonus.

Question the client carefully about symptoms, such as headache, visual disturbances, epigastric pain, nausea or vomiting, or a sudden increase in edema. Detailed questions are needed to identify important symptoms. Ask targeted questions such as the following:

- "Do you have a headache? Describe it for me."
- "Do you have any pain in the abdomen? Show me where it hurts, and describe it."
- "Do you see spots before your eyes? Flashes of light?"
- "Do you have double vision? Is your vision blurred? Does the light bother you?"
- "Are you still able to wear your rings? Did you remove them because your hands were swollen? When did that happen?"

Assessments for Magnesium Toxicity

Obstetric units have protocols that address routine assessments and their frequency when magnesium is being administered. Reflexes may be slightly hypotonic but should not be absent at

therapeutic levels of magnesium. Absent reflexes suggest CNS depression that precedes respiratory depression if magnesium levels are too high. Determining the respiratory rate and oxygen saturations by pulse oximetry identifies the adequacy of respirations. Checking urine output identifies oliguria (below 30 mL/hour), which may result in magnesium toxicity as the drug accumulates. Assess the client's level of consciousness (alert, drowsy [expected], confused, oriented, disoriented). Table 10.4 summarizes nursing assessments and their implications.

Psychosocial Assessment

The development of preeclampsia places added stress on the childbearing family. If the condition is not severe and the gestation period is early, the client may be instructed to reduce activity at home. Hospitalization or activity restriction may complicate caring for other children. This creates anxiety about the condition of the fetus and that of the client. Many families do not understand the seriousness of the disease. The possibility that a preterm birth may be necessary to reduce harm to the client and infant increases the family's concerns about the outcome.

Explore how the family will function while the client is hospitalized or has restricted activity. Determine how the client is adapting to the "sick role" and being dependent on others instead of functioning independently. Ask how much support is available and who is willing to participate. Determine whether referrals to manage loss of income are needed. Finally, determine the priority concerns of the family.

Identification of Client Problems

Analysis of the data collected can lead to both nursing diagnoses and collaborative problems for potential complications. Both provider-prescribed and nurse-prescribed interventions are used to minimize the complications. Potential complications for the client with preeclampsia are listed in Table 10.2.

Planning: Expected Outcomes

Client-centered goals should be collaborative due the interdisciplinary needs of the client with the potential complications of eclamptic seizures and magnesium toxicity. The nurse should confer with providers and use established protocols for treatment. Planning should reflect the nurse's responsibility to do the following:

- Perform actions that minimize the risk for seizures and prevent injury if seizures do occur.

10.1 NURSING PROCEDURE

Assessing Deep Tendon Reflexes

Explain the procedure to the client and support person, and wash your hands with warm water.

1. You will need a reflex hammer to best assess reflexes. The patellar reflex is less reliable if the client has epidural analgesia. Upper extremity reflexes should be assessed.

2. Support the client's arm and provide instruction to completely relax it while it is being held so that the arm is fully supported by the nurse and slightly flexed when assessing the bicep reflex. If you have difficulty identifying the correct tendon to tap, have the client flex and extend the arm until you can feel it moving beneath your thumb. Have the client fully relax again after you identify the tendon.

3. Place your thumb over the client's tendon, as illustrated, to allow you to feel as well as see the tendon response when it is tapped. Strike your thumb with the small end of the reflex hammer. The normal response is slight flexion of the forearm or brief twitch of the bicep muscle.

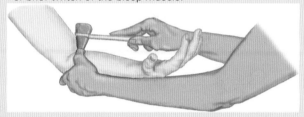

4. The patellar, or "knee-jerk," reflex can be assessed with the client in two positions, sitting or lying. When the client is sitting, allow the lower legs to dangle freely to flex the knee and stretch the tendons. If the patellar tendon is difficult to identify, have the client flex and extend the lower legs slightly until you palpate the tendon. Strike the tendon directly with the broad end of the reflex hammer just below the patella.

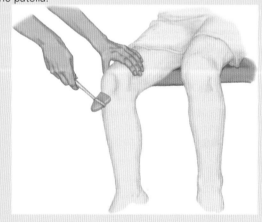

5. When the client is supine, the weight of the leg should be supported to flex the knee and stretch the tendons. An accurate response requires that the limb be relaxed and the tendon partially stretched. Strike the partially stretched tendons just below the patella. Slight extension of the leg or a brief twitch of the quadriceps muscle of the thigh is the expected response.

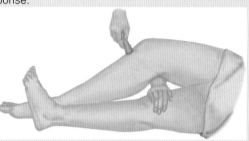

6. To assess for clonus, the client's lower leg should be supported, as illustrated, and the foot well dorsiflexed to stretch the tendon. Hold the flexion. If clonus is absent, no movement will be felt. When clonus (indicating hyperreflexia) is present, rapid rhythmic tapping motions of the foot are present.

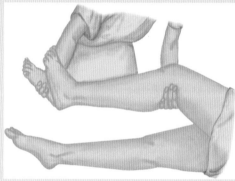

Deep Tendon Reflex Rating Scale

0	Reflex absent
+ 1	Reflex present, hypoactive
+ 2	Normal reflex
+ 3	Brisker than average reflex
+ 4	Hyperactive reflex; clonus may also be present

- Monitor for signs of impending seizures.
- Consult with the provider if signs of impending seizures are observed.
- Support the family of the client with eclampsia.
- Monitor for signs of magnesium toxicity.
- Consult with the provider if signs of magnesium toxicity are observed.
- Perform actions that reduce the possibility of magnesium toxicity.

Interventions

Interventions for Seizures

Monitor for Signs of Impending Seizures. Assess for changes in the following:

- Hyperreflexia, possibly accompanied by clonus
- Increasing signs of cerebral irritability (headache, visual disturbances)
- Epigastric or right upper quadrant pain, nausea, or vomiting

TABLE 10.4 Nursing Assessments for Preeclampsia and Magnesium Toxicity

Assessment	Implications
Daily weight	Provides estimate of fluid retention.
Blood pressure	Determines worsening condition, response to treatment, or both.
Respiratory rate, pulse oximeter readings	Drug therapy (magnesium sulfate) causes respiratory depression, and drug should be decreased or withheld and provider notified if respiratory rate is <12 breaths per minute or as specified by hospital policy. Pulse oximeter readings should be ≥95% in the pregnant client and ≥92% in the nonpregnant client.
Breath sounds	Identifies sounds of excess moisture in lungs associated with pulmonary edema.
Deep tendon reflexes and clonus	Hyperreflexia and clonus indicate increased cerebral irritability and edema; hyporeflexia is associated with magnesium excess.
Edema	Provides estimation of interstitial fluid.
Urinary output	Output of at least 30 mL/hour indicates adequate perfusion of the kidneys. Magnesium levels may become toxic if urinary output is inadequate.
Urine protein	Normal protein in random dipstick urine sample is negative or trace. Higher protein levels suggest greater leaking of protein secondary to glomerular damage with worsening preeclampsia. A 24-hour urine sample is most accurate for quantitative urine protein level.
Level of consciousness	Drowsiness or dulled sensorium indicates therapeutic effects of magnesium; no responsive behavior or muscle weakness is associated with magnesium excess.
Headache, epigastric pain, visual problems	These symptoms indicate increasing severity of condition caused by cerebral edema, vasospasm of cerebral vessels, and liver edema. Eclampsia may develop quickly.
Fetal heart rate and baseline variability	Rate should be between 110 and 160 bpm. Decreasing baseline variability may be caused by therapeutic magnesium level or by inadequate placental perfusion.
Laboratory data	Significant signs of increasing severity of disease are elevated serum creatinine level, elevated uric acid, elevated levels of liver enzymes, or decreased number of platelets (thrombocytopenia). Serum magnesium levels should be in therapeutic range designated by the provider.

Although none of these signs are a predictor of imminent seizure, nurses should be alert for subtle changes and be prepared for seizures in all clients with preeclampsia.

Initiate Preventive Measures. In the presence of cerebral irritability, generalized seizures may be precipitated by excessive visual or auditory stimuli. Nurses should reduce external stimuli by doing the following:

- Keep the door to the room closed. Heightened surveillance of client status is needed regardless of the specific room location that is available.
- Keep lights low and noise to a minimum. This may include blocking incoming telephone calls, instructing visitors to silence cell phones and electronic devices, and turning the noises of the electronic monitors (fetal monitor, pulse oximeter, IV pump) as low as possible.
- Group nursing assessments and care to allow the client periods of undisturbed quiet.
- Collaborate with the client and family to restrict visitors.

Prevent Seizure-Related Injury. Hard side rails should be padded and the bed kept in the lowest position with the wheels locked to prevent trauma during a seizure.

Oxygen and suction equipment should be assembled and ready to use to suction secretions and to provide oxygen if it is not already being administered. Check equipment and connections at the beginning of each shift because sufficient time for setup will not exist if seizures occur.

The following equipment should be readily available: an Ambu bag with mask, reflex hammer, pulse oximeter, stethoscope, and syringes and needles. Medications that should be readily available include magnesium sulfate and calcium gluconate.

Protect the Client and the Fetus during a Seizure. Nurses should protect the client and the fetus during a seizure. The nurse's primary responsibilities are the following:

- Remain with the client and press the emergency bell for assistance.
- If not lateral already, attempt to turn the client when the tonic phase begins. A side-lying position permits greater circulation through the placenta and may prevent aspiration.
- Note the time and sequence of the seizure. Eclampsia is marked by a tonic–clonic seizure that may be preceded by facial twitching that lasts for a few seconds. A tonic contraction of the entire body is followed by the clonic phase.
- Maintain a patent airway after the seizure and suction the client's mouth and nose to prevent aspiration. Administer oxygen by nonrebreather facemask at 10 L/min to increase oxygenation of the placenta and all organs.
- Notify the provider that a seizure has occurred. This is an obstetric emergency that is associated with cerebral hemorrhage, placental abruption, severe fetal hypoxia, and death.
- Administer medications and prepare for additional medical interventions as directed by the provider.

These interventions are also relevant if the client has a generalized seizure disorder that is unrelated to hypertension.

Provide Information and Support for the Family. Explain to the family what has happened without minimizing the seriousness of the situation. A generalized seizure is frightening for anyone who witnesses it. Explain that the client will be unconscious and then may be drowsy for some time afterward. Acknowledge that the seizure indicates worsening of the condition and that it will be necessary for the provider to determine future management, which may include delivery of the infant.

Interventions for Magnesium Toxicity

Monitor for Signs of Magnesium Toxicity. Magnesium excess depresses the entire CNS, including the brainstem, which controls respirations and cardiac function, and the cerebrum, which controls memory, mental processes, and speech. Carbon dioxide accumulates if the respiratory rate is reduced, leading to respiratory acidosis and further CNS depression, which could culminate in respiratory arrest.

Signs of magnesium toxicity include the following (Burges, 2021):
- Respiratory depression, with a rate of fewer than 12 breaths per minute
- Chest pain or shortness of breath
- Decreasing pulse oximeter values:
  - Less than 95% during pregnancy
  - Less than 92% during postpartum phase
- Absence of DTRs
- Visual disturbances (blurred vision, seeing double, etc.)
- Altered sensorium (confused, lethargic, slurred speech, drowsy, disoriented)
- Oliguria
- Hypotension
- Serum magnesium value greater than 8.4 mg/dL
- Respiratory/cardiac arrest

Respond to Signs of Magnesium Toxicity. Magnesium may need to be discontinued if signs of toxicity are present. Additional magnesium may worsen the condition. Notify the provider of the client's condition for additional orders. If the urinary output falls below 30 mL/hour, the provider may alter the drug dosage to maintain a therapeutic range.

Calcium opposes the effects of magnesium at the neuromuscular junction, and it should be readily available whenever magnesium is administered. Magnesium toxicity can be reversed by IV administration of 1 g (10 mL of 10% solution) of calcium gluconate over 3 minutes (Druzin, 2013).

Evaluation

Collect and compare data with established norms and then determine whether the data are within normal limits. For seizures, interventions are deemed successful if the following occur:
- Reflexes remain within normal limits (+1 to +3).
- The client is free of visual disturbances, headache, and epigastric or right upper quadrant pain.
- The client remains free of seizures or free of preventable injury if a seizure occurs.

For magnesium toxicity, determine whether respiratory rates remain at least 12 breaths per minute, DTRs are present

and not hyperactive, and plasma levels of magnesium do not exceed the therapeutic range of 4.8 to 8.4 mg/dL.

HEMOLYSIS, ELEVATED LIVER ENZYMES, AND LOW PLATELETS SYNDROME

The syndrome of hemolysis, elevated liver enzymes, and low platelets (HELLP syndrome) is a life-threatening occurrence that complicates approximately 10% of clients who have preeclampsia with severe features. While the majority of the clients affected by HELLP also have preeclampsia with severe features, hypertension and proteinuria may be absent. HELLP syndrome typically occurs during the last trimester or postpartum period (Lee et al., 2019).

Hemolysis is believed to occur as a result of the fragmentation and distortion of erythrocytes during passage through small, damaged blood vessels. Liver enzyme levels increase when hepatic blood flow is obstructed by fibrin deposits. Hyperbilirubinemia and jaundice may occur as a result of liver impairment. Vasospasm causes vascular damage. Platelets aggregate at sites of damage resulting in low platelet levels (thrombocytopenia), which increases the risk for bleeding, frequently in the liver.

The prominent symptom of HELLP syndrome is pain in the right upper quadrant, the lower right chest, or the midepigastric area. This tenderness may result from liver distention or rupture, ischemia, or hematoma development. Additional signs and symptoms include nausea, vomiting, malaise, headaches, and visual changes. A sudden increase in intraabdominal pressure, including that caused by a seizure, or by palpation of the liver could lead to rupture of a subcapsular hematoma, resulting in internal bleeding and hypovolemic shock. Hepatic rupture can lead to fetal and maternal mortality (Sibai, 2021; Lee et al., 2019).

Clients with HELLP syndrome should be managed in a setting with intensive care facilities. Treatment includes magnesium sulfate to control seizures and hydralazine or labetalol to control BP. Fluid replacement is managed to avoid worsening the client's reduced intravascular volume without causing fluid overload, which could result in pulmonary edema or ascites. Other treatments include antithrombotic agents (low-dose aspirin or heparin), immunosuppressive agents (steroids), and blood component replacement as indicated (AAP & ACOG, 2017; Cunningham et al., 2022; Sibai, 2021).

Cervical ripening with labor induction may be performed if the gestation is at least 34 weeks. Delivery may be delayed if the gestation is less than 34 weeks and the client's condition is stable, to allow for steroid administration to stimulate fetal lung maturation. If the client is near term and has a favorable cervix, induction of labor is preferred to avoid the bleeding and clotting complications that are more likely to occur with cesarean birth. Anesthesia choices are likely to be complicated by laryngeal edema (intubation difficulties), low platelet counts that may reduce safety of epidural block, and coagulation abnormalities that can have an impact on safety of pudendal blocks. Cesarean birth may be necessary if the client is remote from term or has an unfavorable cervix. Adverse outcomes associated with HELLP include increased rate of preterm delivery, wound hematomas, increased need for transfusion, and higher rates of morbidity and mortality (AAP & ACOG, 2017; Sibai, 2021).

CHRONIC HYPERTENSION

A diagnosis of chronic hypertension is made if hypertension precedes pregnancy or is identified before 20 weeks of gestation. The diagnosis also can be based on BP that remains elevated beyond the 12th week postpartum. Chronic hypertension is most often associated with advanced age, obesity, and comorbidities such as diabetes. Heredity plays a role in the development of chronic hypertension. However, hypertension may be secondary to another problem, such as renal disease or an autoimmune disorder (Centers for Disease Control and Prevention [CDC], 2020a; Cunningham et al., 2022).

Elevated circulating hormones, prostaglandins, and progesterone cause a decrease in BP during early pregnancy; therefore the client's BP may appear normal when prenatal care begins. Antihypertensive therapy is reserved for clients with consistently elevated systolic pressures greater than or equal 160 mm Hg or diastolic pressures greater than or equal to 110 mm Hg (ACOG, 2020e). Antihypertensive therapy continues during pregnancy unless hypotension develops due to vasodilation of pregnancy. Antihypertensive medications should be chosen carefully because they may reduce placental blood flow. Labetalol and Nifedipine have proven effective and safe to use in pregnancy. Methyldopa (Aldomet) is less effective and has a higher incidence of adverse effects. Angiotensin-converting enzyme (ACE) inhibitors are not recommended in pregnancy but may be used in the postpartum period. Hydralazine is a vasodilator reserved for hypertensive crisis. Diuretics are considered second-line agents, because they may decrease blood volume, which may lead to oligohydramnios or fetal growth restriction. In cases of pulmonary edema, diuretics may be necessary (ACOG, 2019c).

The most common complication is the development of preeclampsia, which occurs in approximately 25% of pregnant clients with chronic hypertension (Harper et al., 2019). New-onset proteinuria or a significant rise in preexisting proteinuria identifies the development of superimposed preeclampsia. The rise in BP with preeclampsia is likely to be greater in these clients. Development of signs and symptoms indicating multiorgan development (headache, epigastric pain, or visual changes) are correlated to abnormal renal, hepatic, or hematologic laboratory values (Cunningham et al., 2022; Harper et al., 2019).

A dietitian should be consulted about the appropriate diet and weight gain because many of these clients are obese and frequently have diabetes. A reduced salt intake may be advised, unlike recommendations for the client with preeclampsia alone. More frequent prenatal visits will be needed. Regular fetal surveillance by BPP and kick counts (see Chapter 9) is recommended to identify fetal compromise, such as poor growth patterns or decreasing amount of amniotic fluid.

> ## KNOWLEDGE CHECK
> 20. What does the acronym HELLP stand for? What are the prominent signs and symptoms of HELLP syndrome? Why should the liver not be palpated in a client with HELLP syndrome?
> 21. Compare preeclampsia with chronic hypertension in terms of onset and treatment.

MATERNAL-FETAL BLOOD INCOMPATIBILITY

When a person is exposed to a red blood cell (RBC) antigen that is not on their RBCs, they develop antibodies against it. The process of the development of RBC antibodies is known as *red cell alloimmunization* and may also be called sensitization. The antibodies attack and destroy any RBC with the foreign antigen. To destroy the antigen, the entire RBC is destroyed. The antibodies do not affect the RBC without the foreign antigen. Although 360 RBC antigens have been identified by the International Society of Blood Transfusion (Storry et al., 2019) many of these are rare and clinically insignificant (Cunningham et al., 2022). The most significant antigens during pregnancy are the D antigen (Rh) and ABO antigens. Exposure to the Rh antigen most often occurs from transfusion with incompatible blood or during pregnancy and childbirth. A client with blood type O may be sensitized to A and B antigens before pregnancy from exposure to bacteria with similar antigens (Cunningham et al., 2022).

Rh Incompatibility

Rh-negative blood is an autosomal recessive trait, and a person must inherit the same gene from both parents to be Rh-negative. The Rh factor incompatibility during pregnancy is possible only when two specific circumstances coexist: (1) the mother is Rh-negative, and (2) the fetus is Rh-positive. For such a circumstance to occur, the father of the fetus must be Rh-positive. Rh incompatibility is a problem that affects the fetus; it causes no harm to the pregnant client.

Pathophysiology

People who are Rh-positive have the D antigen on their RBCs, whereas people who are Rh-negative do not have the antigen. When exposed to the antigen, the Rh-negative client's body develops antibodies to destroy the invading antigen. Destruction of Rh-positive cells occurs in the Rh-negative person after they have become sensitized (developed antibodies) to the Rh-positive antigens.

Generally, the Rh antigen does not cross an intact placenta; sensitization of the pregnant client occurs when the Rh-positive blood of the fetus enters the client's circulation. Theoretically, the blood of the fetus does not mix with the blood of the client during pregnancy. In reality, the placenta is not a perfect barrier; it is possible to have some antenatal mixing of blood, which can initiate the production of antibodies in the pregnant client. Unlike antigens, antibodies readily cross the placenta and attack the fetus's Rh-positive blood (ACOG, 2021b). Sensitization also can occur during a spontaneous or elective abortion or during antepartum procedures such as amniocentesis and chorionic villus sampling. A rapid immune response against Rh-positive blood occurs with an uncomplicated birth or with an extensive fetal-maternal hemorrhage in complications such as placenta previa or placental abruption.

Most exposure of the pregnant client to fetal blood occurs during the third stage of labor, when active exchange of blood may occur from damaged placental vessels. In this case the client's first child is not usually affected because antibodies are formed after the birth of the infant. However, since the antibodies remain in the client's body and cross an intact placenta, subsequent Rh-positive fetuses may be affected, unless the Rho(D) immune globulin is administered to prevent antibody formation after the birth of each Rh-positive infant.

Fetal and Neonatal Implications

If antibodies to the Rh factor are present in the pregnant client's blood, they cross the placenta and destroy Rh-positive fetal erythrocytes (RBCs). The fetus becomes deficient in RBCs, which are needed to transport oxygen to fetal tissue. As fetal RBCs are destroyed, fetal bilirubin levels increase (icterus gravis), which can lead to neurologic disease (**kernicterus** [staining of brain tissue], leading to bilirubin encephalopathy). This hemolytic process results in rapid production of erythroblasts (immature RBCs), which cannot carry oxygen. The entire syndrome is known as **hemolytic disease of the fetus and newborn (HDFN)**, formerly termed erythroblastosis fetalis. The fetus may become so anemic that generalized fetal edema (hydrops fetalis) results and can end in fetal heart failure.

Prenatal Assessment and Management

Pregnant clients should have a blood test to determine blood type and Rh factor at the initial prenatal visit. Rh-negative clients should have an indirect Coombs' test to determine whether they are sensitized (have developed antibodies) as a result of previous exposure to Rh-positive blood. If the indirect Coombs' test is negative, it is repeated at 28 weeks of gestation to identify whether they have developed subsequent sensitization.

Rho(D) immune globulin is administered to the unsensitized Rh-negative client at 28 weeks of gestation to prevent sensitization, which may occur from small leaks of fetal blood across the placenta. Rho(D) immune globulin is a commercial preparation that effectively prevents the formation of active antibodies against Rh-positive erythrocytes. Administration of Rho(D) immune globulin is repeated after birth if the client delivers a Rh-positive infant.

> ### ⚡ SAFETY CHECK
>
> All unsensitized Rh-negative clients should receive Rho(D) immune globulin after abortion, ectopic pregnancy, chorionic villus sampling, amniocentesis, abdominal trauma during pregnancy, or birth of a Rh-positive infant. Rho(D) immune globulin prevents the development of Rh antibodies that would result in destruction of fetal erythrocytes in subsequent pregnancies.

If the indirect Coombs' test result is positive at any time, indicating sensitization of the pregnant client and the presence of antibodies, Rho(D) immune globulin is not given, and measurement of the antibody titer is repeated at frequent intervals throughout the pregnancy to determine whether the antibody titer is rising. An increase in titer indicates that the process is continuing and that the fetus will be in jeopardy.

Ultrasound examination is used to noninvasively evaluate the condition of the fetus. Doppler studies allow evaluation of cardiac function and blood flow in fetal vessels. The systolic blood flow in the fetal middle cerebral artery is a noninvasive way to assess the degree of fetal anemia. An anemic fetus will increase blood flow to the brain in an effort to maintain oxygenation of the CNS. This increased blood flow is detected by Doppler sonography and can be quantified. Blood flow of 1.5 times the median for the fetal gestational age is predictive of moderate to severe fetal anemia (ACOG, 2018b). Generalized fetal edema, ascites, an enlarged heart, or **polyhydramnios** (excessive amniotic fluid), occurs when the fetus is very anemic. Percutaneous umbilical blood sampling (PUBS), or cordocentesis, allows invasive sampling of fetal blood from cord vessels to determine the degree of erythrocyte destruction. Because it is invasive, PUBS is considered when the fetus is thought to be significantly affected (Cunningham et al., 2022).

Intrauterine transfusion is the direct infusion of O-negative erythrocytes into the umbilical cord by percutaneous umbilical blood transfusion if the fetus is severely affected. Erythrocytes also may be transfused into the fetal abdominal cavity, where they are gradually absorbed into the circulation.

Postpartum Management

If the pregnant client is Rh-negative, umbilical cord blood is taken at delivery to determine blood type, Rh factor, and antibody titer (direct Coombs' test) of the newborn. Rh-negative, unsensitized clients who give birth to Rh-positive infants are given an IM injection of Rho(D) immune globulin within 72 hours after delivery. If Rho(D) immune globulin is given to the client within 72 hours after the birth of a Rh-positive infant, antibodies to the Rh antigen are not produced. If the infant is Rh-negative, Rh antibody formation does not occur and Rho(D) immune globulin is not necessary.

Families often are concerned about the fetus, and nurses should be sensitive to cues that indicate that the family is anxious and should be able to offer honest reassurance. This is especially important if the client is sensitized and fetal testing is necessary throughout pregnancy.

DRUG GUIDE

Rho(D) Immune Globulin (RhoGAM, HypRho-D, BayRho-D, Gamulin Rh, Rhophylac)

Classification

Concentrated immunoglobulins directed toward the red blood cell (RBC) antigen Rho(D). Prepared from the plasma or serum of human donors.

Action

Suppresses the immune reaction of the Rh-negative client to the D antigen in Rh-positive blood; suppresses antibody response and thereby prevents hemolytic disease of the fetus and newborn in Rh-positive fetus; used for both males and females who are Rh-negative but exposed to Rh-positive blood or for immune thrombocytopenic purpura (ITP).

Indications (Pregnancy-Related)

Administered to Rh-negative clients who are not sensitized to the Rho (D) antigen as demonstrated by a negative indirect Coombs' test in the following situations:

- Prophylactically at approximately 28 weeks of gestation
- Following amniocentesis, chorionic villus sampling, fetal blood sampling, external cephalic version, or abdominal trauma during pregnancy
- Spontaneous or induced abortion (miscarriage or pregnancy termination for any reason)
- Ectopic pregnancy, molar pregnancy, fetal death
- Antepartum bleeding: placenta previa, placental abruption, threatened miscarriage
- Delivery of a Rh-positive baby
- Receipt of inadvertent transfusion of Rh-positive blood

Dosage and Route

One standard dose (300 mcg) administered intramuscularly:

- At approximately 28 weeks of gestation and within 72 hours of delivery of a Rh-positive infant.
- When 13 weeks of gestation or more give within 72 hours of
  - Invasive procedures (chorionic villus sampling, amniocentesis) or intraabdominal trauma
  - Spontaneous or induced termination of a pregnancy
  - Antepartum hemorrhage (placenta previa; placental abruption)
  - Fetal death, ectopic pregnancy

One microdose (50 to 120 mcg) when less than 13 weeks gestation give within 72 hours after

- Invasive procedures (chorionic villus sampling, amniocentesis) or intraabdominal trauma
- Spontaneous or induced termination of a pregnancy
- Fetal death, ectopic pregnancy

The dose of Rho(D) immune globulin is calculated based on the volume of fetal-maternal hemorrhage or Rh-positive blood administered in transfusion accidents. A standard dose of 1500 international units (IU) or 300 mcg will protect against 30 mL of Rh-positive whole blood or 15 mL of packed RBCs. Prescribed dosages may be adjusted based on the estimated volume of fetal-maternal hemorrhage. (ACOG, 2021b; Cunningham et al., 2022).

Absorption

Well absorbed from IM sites.

Excretion

Metabolism and excretion unknown.

Contraindications and Precautions

Clients who are Rh-positive or clients previously sensitized to Rho(D) should not receive Rho(D) immune globulin. It is used cautiously for clients with previous hypersensitivity reactions to immune globulins.

Adverse Reactions

Local pain at IM site, fever, or both.

Nursing Implications

Type and antibody screening (indirect Coombs' test) of the client's blood should be performed before administration. For postpartum administration, blood type of the newborn should be performed to determine the need for the medication (if the newborn is Rh-negative, the medication is not necessary). The client must be Rh-negative and negative for Rh antibodies. The newborn must be Rh-positive. If the fetal blood type after termination of pregnancy, invasive procedures, or trauma is uncertain, the medication should be administered. The newborn may have a weakly positive antibody test if the client received Rho(D) immune globulin during pregnancy. The drug is administered to the postpartum client, not the infant. The deltoid muscle is recommended for IM administration.

During labor, the nurse should carefully label the tube of cord blood obtained for analysis of the newborn's blood type and Rh factor. During the postpartum period, nurses are responsible for follow-up to determine whether Rho(D) immune globulin is necessary and for administering the injection within the prescribed time.

ABO INCOMPATIBILITY

ABO incompatibility occurs when the pregnant client is blood type O and the fetus is blood type A, B, or AB. Types A, B, and AB blood contain an antigen that is not present in type O blood.

People with type O blood develop anti-A or anti-B antibodies naturally as a result of exposure to antigens in the foods they eat or to bacterial infections. Some clients with blood type O have developed high serum anti-A and anti-B antibody titers before their first pregnancy. The antibodies may be either IgG or IgM. When the client becomes pregnant, the IgG antibodies cross the placenta and may cause hemolysis of fetal RBCs. However, ABO incompatibility is less severe than Rh incompatibility because the primary antibodies of the ABO system are IgM, which do not readily cross the placenta.

No specific prenatal care is needed; however, the nurse should be aware of the possibility of ABO incompatibility. During the delivery, cord blood is taken to determine the blood type of the newborn and the antibody titer (direct Coombs' test). The newborn is carefully screened for jaundice, which indicates hyperbilirubinemia.

KNOWLEDGE CHECK

22. Why do unsensitized Rh-negative expectant clients receive Rho(D) immune globulin during pregnancy and after an abortion, amniocentesis, and childbirth?
23. What are the fetal effects of Rh sensitization of the pregnant client?
24. Why is the first fetus sometimes affected if ABO incompatibility occurs? Why are the effects of ABO incompatibility milder than those of Rh sensitization?

CONCURRENT CONDITIONS

Pregnancy affects the care of clients with a medical condition in two ways. First, pregnancy may alter the course of the disease. Second, the disease or its treatment may have unwanted effects on the pregnancy. Antepartum care should be adapted to include increased surveillance of the pregnant client and the fetus.

DIABETES MELLITUS

Etiology and Pathophysiology

Diabetes mellitus is a complex disorder of carbohydrate metabolism caused primarily by a partial or complete lack of insulin secretion by the beta cells of the pancreas. Some cells, such as those in skeletal and cardiac muscles and adipose tissue, rely on insulin to carry glucose across the cell membranes. Without insulin, glucose accumulates in blood, resulting in hyperglycemia. The body attempts to dilute the glucose load by any means possible. The first strategy is to increase thirst (**polydipsia**), a classic symptom of diabetes mellitus. Next, fluid from the intracellular spaces is drawn into the vascular bed, resulting in dehydration at the cellular level but fluid volume excess in the vascular compartment. The kidneys attempt to excrete large volumes of this fluid and the heavy solute load of glucose (**osmotic diuresis**). This excretion produces the second hallmark of diabetes, **polyuria**, with **glycosuria** (glucose in urine). Without glucose the cells starve, so weight loss occurs, even though the person ingests large amounts of food (**polyphagia**).

Because the body cannot metabolize glucose, it begins to metabolize protein and fat to meet energy needs. Metabolism of protein produces a negative nitrogen balance, and the metabolism of fat results in the buildup of ketone bodies (e.g., acetone, acetoacetic acid, or beta-hydroxybutyric acid) or **ketosis** (accumulation of acids in the body).

If the disease is not well controlled, serious complications may occur. Hypoglycemia or hyperglycemia can result if the amount of insulin does not match the diet. Fluctuating periods of hyperglycemia and hypoglycemia damage small blood vessels throughout the body. This damage can cause serious impairment, especially in the kidneys, eyes, and heart.

Effect of Pregnancy on Fuel Metabolism

To understand the relationship between diabetes mellitus and pregnancy, an understanding of the way pregnancy and diabetes alter the metabolism of food is necessary.

Early Pregnancy. Metabolic changes can be divided into those that occur early in pregnancy (1 to 20 weeks of gestation) and those that occur late in pregnancy (20 to 40 weeks of gestation). In early pregnancy, metabolic rates and energy needs change little. During this time, however, insulin release in response to serum glucose levels accelerates. As a result, significant hypoglycemia may occur as more glucose is transported into the cells. The nausea, vomiting, and anorexia that often arise during the first weeks of pregnancy may increase the incidence of hypoglycemia.

In an uncomplicated pregnancy, the availability of glucose and insulin favors the development and storage of fat during the first half of pregnancy. Accumulation of fat prepares the pregnant client for the rise in energy use by the growing fetus during the second half of pregnancy.

Late Pregnancy. During the second half of pregnancy, levels of placental hormones rise sharply. These hormones, particularly estrogen, progesterone, and human placental lactogen (hPL), create resistance to insulin in cells. This resistance allows an abundant supply of glucose to be available for transport to the fetus. However, the hormones have a **diabetogenic effect** in that they may leave the client with insufficient insulin and episodes of hyperglycemia.

For most pregnant clients, insulin resistance is not a problem. The pancreas responds by simply increasing the production of insulin. If the pancreas is unable to respond adequately, the client will have periods of hyperglycemia.

Postpartum Period. The need for additional insulin falls during the postpartum period. Breastfeeding is encouraged for the newborn's benefit and because the added calories used for lactation helps lower the amount of insulin needed by the postpartum client with diabetes mellitus. The client with gestational diabetes mellitus (GDM) usually needs no insulin after birth, but the greater risk for later development of type 2 diabetes should be emphasized with teaching before discharge.

Classification

Diabetes that exists before the second trimester of pregnancy is classified as type 1 (insulin deficient) or type 2 (insulin resistant, with a relative deficiency of insulin to metabolize carbohydrate). A third type, GDM, is one in which any degree of glucose intolerance has its onset or first recognition during the second or third trimester of pregnancy (ACOG, 2020b; ADA, 2021a) (Box 10.3).

An additional classification of diabetes is sometimes used for descriptive purposes. White's classification describes the age at onset of diabetes, its duration based on the client's current age, and vascular complications that are present. GDM descriptions in White's classification include A-1 (diet controlled) and A-2 (diet- and medication-controlled). Pregestational diabetes is classified based on the presence of complications that may be found with type 1 or type 2 diabetes (vascular disease, retinopathy, nephropathy, coronary artery disease) (Landon et al., 2021).

Incidence

Diabetes mellitus is a common medical condition that often affects pregnancy. Approximately 37 million Americans have diabetes; the vast majority, 90% to 95%, have type 2 while only about 5% of diabetics have a diagnosis of type 1 (CDC, 2021d). The pregnant client may have preexisting diabetes (type 1 or type 2) or may develop GDM during the second or third trimester of pregnancy. Undiagnosed type 2 diabetes that is discovered during pregnancy screening for GDM continues to be a medical issue after childbirth (Landon et al., 2021).

Although the true incidence of gestational diabetes is unknown, the CDC (2021c) found a prevalence rate of 2% to 10% among different ethnic groups. The higher risk for GDM exists in clients of African American, Hispanic/Latino Americans, American Indian, Alaska Native, Native Hawaiian, and Pacific Islander backgrounds; the lowest prevalence is found in non-Hispanic Whites. Many of the clients with GDM will develop type 2 diabetes later in life (ACOG, 2019a; American Diabetes Association [ADA], 2021a; CDC, 2021b).

Preexisting Diabetes Mellitus

The course of pregnancy for clients with diabetes mellitus has improved greatly as a result of treatments and more effective methods of fetal surveillance. However, the incidence of complications affecting the pregnant client and fetus remains higher than that experienced by those who do not have diabetes.

Effects on the Pregnant Client

Diabetes can adversely affect a pregnant client and the developing baby in several ways. During the first trimester, when major fetal organs are developing, the effects of the abnormal metabolic environment such as hyperglycemia may lead to increased incidence of spontaneous abortion (miscarriage) or major fetal malformations. Hypertension, especially preeclampsia, is more likely to develop if the client has preexisting diabetes (ACOG, 2020b). The development of ketoacidosis is a threat to clients with type 1 diabetes and is most often precipitated by infection or missed insulin doses. In addition, ketoacidosis may develop in these clients at lower thresholds of hyperglycemia than those seen in nonpregnant individuals. Untreated ketoacidosis can progress to death of the pregnant client and fetus. UTIs are more common, possibly because of glucose in the urine, which provides a nutrient-rich medium for bacterial growth.

Other effects include polyhydramnios, which may result from fetal hyperglycemia and consequent fetal diuresis and premature rupture of membranes, which may be caused by overdistention of the uterus by polyhydramnios or a large fetus. Problems that arise during labor and childbirth if the fetus has **macrosomia** (weighs more than 8.8 lb [4000 g]) may include a difficult labor, shoulder **dystocia** (delayed or difficult birth of fetal shoulders after the head is born), and consequent injury to the birth canal or the infant. Large fetal size also increases the likelihood of a cesarean birth and the risk for postpartum hemorrhage (Table 10.5).

Fetal Effects

Fetal and neonatal effects of preexisting diabetes depend on the timing and severity of hyperglycemia in the pregnant client and the degree of vascular impairment that has occurred.

Congenital Malformation. Fewer malformations occur if the client maintains a normal blood glucose level before conception and throughout pregnancy. The risk for a major

TABLE 10.5   Major Effects of Diabetes Mellitus on Pregnancy

Effect	Probable Cause
Increased Risk to the Pregnant Client	
Hypertension, preeclampsia	Unknown but increased even without renal or vascular impairment
Urinary tract infections	Increased bacterial growth in nutrient-rich urine
Ketoacidosis (risk for pregnant client and fetus)	Uncontrolled hyperglycemia or infection; most common in clients with type 1 diabetes
Uterine atony with hemorrhage after birth	Hydramnios secondary to fetal osmotic diuresis caused by hyperglycemia; uterus is overstretched
Labor dystocia, cesarean birth, injury to tissues (hematoma, lacerations)	Fetal macrosomia causing difficult birth
Increased Fetal and Neonatal Risks	
Congenital anomalies	Hyperglycemia in the pregnant client during organ formation in first trimester. Effects clients with preexisting diabetes.
Intrauterine fetal growth restriction; perinatal death	Poor placental perfusion because of vascular impairment, primarily in clients with type 1 diabetes
Macrosomia (>4000 g)	Fetal hyperglycemia stimulating production of insulin to metabolize carbohydrates; excess nutrients transported to fetus
Preterm labor, premature rupture of membranes, preterm birth	Overdistention of uterus caused by hydramnios and large fetal size at preterm gestation
Birth injury	Large fetal size; shoulder dystocia or other difficult delivery
Hypoglycemia	Neonatal hyperinsulinemia after birth when glucose is no longer available from the pregnant client (but insulin production remains high)
Polycythemia	Fetal hypoxemia stimulating erythrocyte production
Hyperbilirubinemia	Breakdown of excessive red blood cells after birth
Hypocalcemia	Relative hyperparathyroidism in the pregnant client or changes in the magnesium–calcium balance
Respiratory distress syndrome	Delayed maturation of fetal lungs; inadequate production of pulmonary surfactant; slowed absorption of fetal lung fluid

congenital malformation is two to six times higher than for the general population if hyperglycemia is not controlled during the first trimester. The most common major congenital malformations associated with preexisting diabetes are neural tube defects (NTDs), **caudal regression syndrome** (failure of sacrum, lumbar spine, and lower extremities to develop), and cardiac defects (Landon et al., 2021).

Variations in Fetal Size. Fetal growth is related to vascular integrity of the pregnant client. In clients without vascular impairment, glucose and oxygen are easily transported to the fetus. If the pregnant client is hyperglycemic, so is the fetus. Although insulin from the pregnant client does not cross the placenta, the fetus produces insulin by the 10th week of gestation. Fetal macrosomia results when elevated levels of blood glucose stimulate excessive production of fetal insulin, which acts as a powerful growth hormone. This is a major neonatal effect with consequent increase in the rate of cesarean birth or birth injury from shoulder dystocia.

Conversely, if vascular impairment is present, placental perfusion may be decreased. Vascular impairment may be caused by complications of the diabetes such as vasoconstriction, which occurs in preeclampsia or as a result of the disease process of diabetes. Impaired placental perfusion decreases supplies of glucose and oxygen delivered to the fetus. As a result, intrauterine growth restriction (IUGR) is likely. Amniotic fluid may be reduced (oligohydramnios) as the fetus conserves oxygen for the heart and brain rather than providing normal circulation to the kidneys.

Neonatal Effects

The four major neonatal complications of preexisting diabetes are hypoglycemia, hypocalcemia, hyperbilirubinemia, and respiratory distress syndrome. Maintaining normal glucose levels in the pregnant client reduces the incidence and severity of neonatal complications.

Hypoglycemia. The neonate is at higher risk for hypoglycemia because fetal insulin production is accelerated during pregnancy to metabolize the excessive glucose received from the pregnant client. The constant stimulation of hyperglycemia leads to hyperplasia and hypertrophy of the islets of Langerhans in the fetal pancreas. When the glucose supply from the pregnant client is abruptly withdrawn at birth, the level of neonatal insulin exceeds the available glucose, and hypoglycemia develops rapidly (Landon et al., 2021).

Hypocalcemia. Neonatal hypocalcemia is defined and a total serum calcium level of less than 7 mg/dL in a preterm infant or less than 8 mg/dL in a term infant (Blackburn, 2018). It is likely due to a relative hyperparathyroidism seen in many diabetic clients (Blackburn, 2018). Other possible causes include changes in the magnesium–calcium balance, asphyxia, or preterm birth (Blackburn, 2018; Cunningham et al., 2022; Landon et al., 2021).

Hyperbilirubinemia. The fetus experiencing recurrent hypoxia, as occurs in the fetus of a client with diabetes, compensates by production of additional erythrocytes (polycythemia) to carry oxygen. (Cunningham et al., 2022). After birth, the excess erythrocytes are broken down, which releases large amounts of bilirubin into the neonate's circulation. Clients with poor glycemic control are more likely to deliver before term. Preterm gestation further reduces the infant's ability to metabolize and excrete excess bilirubin due to immaturity of the liver (Landon et al., 2021).

Respiratory Distress Syndrome. Fetal hyperinsulinemia slows the production of cortisol, which is necessary for the synthesis of surfactant. Surfactant is needed to keep the newborn's alveoli open after birth, thereby increasing the risk for respiratory distress syndrome. Reduced lung fluid clearance and delayed thinning of lung connective tissue also may be a factor. Respiratory distress syndrome is more likely to occur if the pregnant client's glycemic control is poor (Landon et al., 2021).

Stable blood glucose levels in the pregnant client decreases client, fetal, and newborn complications. The objective of the team providing treatment is to devise a plan that allows the client to maintain a level as close to normal as possible.

❓ KNOWLEDGE CHECK

25. What effects do the hormones of pregnancy have on glucose metabolism of the pregnant client?
26. What are the effects of type 1 diabetes mellitus on the pregnant client? What are possible fetal and neonatal effects?
27. How do insulin needs vary from the first trimester through the postpartum period?

Assessment of the Pregnant Client

Preconception care is ideal in a client with preexisting diabetes. If the client's body can be in the best condition before conception, including diabetes management, pregnancy is likely to have fewer or less severe complications than if care is started after conception. When the client with preexisting diabetes initiates care, a thorough evaluation of their health status should be completed. This evaluation includes history, physical examination, and laboratory tests.

Identification of Undiagnosed Diabetes. As the incidence of obesity and type 2 diabetes has increased, the number of persons of childbearing age with undiagnosed preexisting diabetes also has increased. Therefore current recommendations are that all pregnant clients with a body mass index (BMI) greater than 25 (23 in Asian Americans) and one or more of the following risk factors should be screened with laboratory testing for diabetes at the first prenatal visit (ACOG, 2019a; ADA, 2021a):

- Previous birth to an infant weighing 4000 g or more (approximately 9 lb)
- Gestational diabetes in previous pregnancy
- History of abnormal glucose tolerance

- History of diabetes in a close (first-degree) relative
- Member of a high-risk ethnic group (African American, Hispanic or Latino, American Indian, Asian American, or Pacific Islanders)
- History of prediabetes (elevated blood glucose that does not meet the criteria for diabetes)
- History of polycystic ovary syndrome (PCOS)
- Physical inactivity
- Hypertension
- History of cardiovascular disease
- Elevated HDL or triglyceride

History. A detailed history should include the onset and management of the diabetic condition. How long have they had the disease? How do they maintain a normal blood glucose level? Are they familiar with ways to monitor blood glucose level and administer insulin? The degree of glycemic control before pregnancy is of particular interest. Effective management depends on adherence to a plan of care. Therefore knowledge of how diabetes affects pregnancy and how pregnancy affects diabetes should be determined. The support person's knowledge should be assessed, and specific learning needs should be identified. In addition, the client's emotional status should be assessed to determine how they are coping with pregnancy superimposed on preexisting diabetes.

All pregnant clients with diabetes should be seen by a qualified diabetes educator for an individualized assessment to ensure the client can monitor their blood glucose level accurately. Accurate readings depend on performing the test correctly and at the times recommended by the health care team. In addition to home monitoring of blood glucose level, the nurse should observe the client's skill in mixing and self-administering insulin, using a sliding scale for added insulin, or using an insulin pump. Although the use of oral hypoglycemics, such as metformin, for the management of pregestational diabetes are being studied, there are limited data on the long-term effect of these medications on the children. "Thus, insulin is the preferred treatment for pregestational diabetes in pregnancy not controlled by diet and exercise" (ACOG, 2020b, p. e235).

Physical Examination. In addition to routine prenatal examination, specific efforts should be made to assess the effects of diabetes. A baseline electrocardiogram (ECG) should be obtained to determine cardiovascular status. Evaluation for retinopathy should be performed, with referral to an ophthalmologist, if necessary. The client's weight and BP should be monitored because of the increased risk for hypertension, including preeclampsia. Fundal height should be measured, noting any abnormal increase in size that may indicate macrosomia or polyhydramnios. Fundal height less than expected for the gestational age may indicate fetal growth restriction or intrauterine death secondary to poor placental perfusion.

Laboratory Tests. In addition to routine prenatal laboratory examinations, baseline renal function should be assessed with a 24-hour urine collection for total protein excretion and creatinine clearance. A random urine sample should be checked at each prenatal visit for possible UTIs, which are common in clients with diabetes. Urine also should be checked for the presence of glucose, ketones, and protein. Thyroid function tests should be performed in the client with preexisting diabetes because of their risk for coexisting thyroid disease.

Glycemic control should be evaluated on the basis of the level of glycosylated Hgb or hemoglobin A_{1C} (HgbA$_{1C}$). The glycosylated Hgb assay is an accurate measurement of the average glucose concentrations during the preceding 2 to 3 months. Unlike tests that reflect the amount of glucose in the plasma at that moment, the HgbA$_{1C}$ measurement is not affected by recent intake or restriction of food.

Fetal Surveillance

Because of the increased risk for **congenital anomalies** or fetal death, surveillance should begin early for clients with preexisting diabetes. Fetal viability and accurate estimates of the gestational age and due date can be determined by an ultrasound early in the gestation. Testing for anomalies includes multiple-marker screening to identify possible neural tube or other open defects and for possible chromosome abnormalities. Testing also includes performing detailed ultrasonography at 18 to 20 weeks of gestation and fetal echocardiography at 20 to 22 weeks to determine the integrity of the fetal body and cardiac structure (ACOG, 2020b; Landon et al., 2021).

During the third trimester, the goal of fetal surveillance is to identify markers that suggest a worsening intrauterine environment with an increased risk for fetal death. Surveillance may include client assessment of fetal movement ("kick counts"), BPPs, NSTs, and contraction stress tests (ACOG, 2020b; Landon et al., 2021). Serial sonograms are used to document fetal growth rates in an effort to identify fetuses at risk for IUGR, macrosomia, and shoulder dystocia (ACOG, 2020b; Landon et al., 2021). Doppler velocimetry of the umbilical artery may be used to assess vascular complications and poor fetal growth (ACOG, 2020b).

Therapeutic Management

The goals of therapeutic management for a pregnant client with pregestational diabetes are to (1) maintain normal blood glucose levels, (2) facilitate the birth of a healthy baby, and (3) avoid accelerated impairment of blood vessels and other major organs. To achieve this outcome, an intensive, team approach to care is required.

Members of the team often include an endocrinologist who assists in regulation of the client's blood glucose level; an obstetrician or a maternal-fetal medicine specialist (**perinatologist**) who monitors the pregnant client and fetus and determines the optimal time for birth; a registered dietitian (RD) or registered dietary technician (RDT), who provides a balanced meal plan; and a diabetes educator, often a specialized nurse, who provides ongoing education and support as the therapy changes throughout pregnancy. The team is completed by a neonatologist, who will care for the newborn; the family physician or obstetric provider; and the pediatrician, who will provide ongoing care for the postpartum client and infant.

Preconception Care. Ideally, care should begin before conception. If diabetes exists before pregnancy, both prospective parents should participate in care sessions to learn more about the following measures that need to be taken by the health care team:

- Establishing the optimal time to undertake pregnancy, based on maintenance of normal client blood glucose levels, to reduce the risk for major fetal malformations
- Identifying whether diabetes complications exist in other organ systems
- Determining the degree of glycemic control based on client records or laboratory studies
- Instructing a client about how to use a glucometer for blood glucose level measurement and having the client demonstrate a correct technique
- Having the client take a daily prenatal vitamin with folic acid. A higher dose of folic acid is recommended for the client who had a previous child with an NTD

Diet. Diet recommendations are individualized during pregnancy in a client with diabetes. The average recommended caloric intake for the pregnant client with diabetes who is of normal weight is 30 to 35 kilocalories per kilogram of body weight per day (kcal/kg/day). Approximately 40% to 50% of the calories should be from high-fiber complex carbohydrates, 15% to 30% from protein, and up to 20% to 35% from primarily unsaturated fat (ACOG, 2020b). Caloric intake should be distributed among three meals and two or more snacks. The bedtime snack should include a complex carbohydrate and a protein. Clients who are overweight or underweight usually have lower or higher caloric goals.

Self-Monitoring of Blood Glucose Level. The best frequency for self-monitoring of blood glucose level of capillary blood has not yet been established. One common testing regimen requires obtaining fasting and 1 or 2 hours postprandial levels and at bedtime. Another includes testing six times per day: a fasting capillary glucose level, 1 to 2 hours after breakfast, before and after lunch, before dinner, and at bedtime. Normal fasting and postprandial glucose levels have been associated with better outcomes, including a lower risk for fetal macrosomia, neonatal hypoglycemia, and labor dystocia that results in cesarean birth. Preprandial glucose levels may be needed for smoother control if the glucose level is difficult to control. The target capillary blood glucose levels are as follows: fasting—95 mg/dL or less; 1 hour postprandial—140 mg/dL or less; or 2 hour postprandial—120 mg/dL or less. Nighttime levels should be 60 mg/dL or more (ACOG, 2020b). In addition to regular monitoring, the client also should perform a glucose test when symptomatic of hypoglycemia. All test results should be recorded on a log sheet or cell phone app for review by the health care provider at each visit.

Insulin Therapy. The need to maintain rigorous control of metabolism during pregnancy requires more frequent doses of insulin than usual. ACOG (2020b) recommends the use of rapid-acting insulins, such as Lispro or Aspart, before meals and longer-acting insulins, such as NPH, before breakfast (along with the rapid-acting insulin) and at bedtime. Because placental hormones cause insulin needs to change throughout pregnancy, insulin coverage will need to be adjusted as pregnancy progresses.

The use of insulin pumps and continuous glucose monitors (CGM) to manage blood sugar is becoming more common. An insulin pump is a small machine worn outside the body on a belt or in a pocket. The pump delivers a small continuous stream of insulin throughout the day and night through a small needle inserted under the client's skin. The client can self-administer bolus doses as needed and prescribed by their health care provider. With CGM, a small sensor inserted under the skin measures glucose levels every few minutes. This information is transmitted to a monitor, which may be a separate device or integrated into the client's insulin pump. With some systems, the pump adjusts the dose of insulin based on the glucose values. Although finger sticks are still needed to calibrate the CGM, and both systems should be changed out every few days, these devices decrease the number of times the client must stick themselves and may increase the level of glucose control (ACOG, 2020b).

First Trimester. Insulin needs generally decline during the first trimester because the secretion of placental hormones antagonistic to insulin remains low. The client also may experience nausea, vomiting, and anorexia, which result in decreased intake of food; therefore less insulin is required. In addition, the fetus receives its share of glucose, which reduces plasma glucose levels and decreases the need for insulin.

Second and Third Trimesters. Insulin needs increase markedly during the second and third trimesters when placental hormones, which initiate resistance to the effects of insulin, reach their peak. In addition, the nausea of early pregnancy usually resolves, and the diet includes additional calories per day to meet the increased metabolic demands of pregnancy.

During Labor. Maintenance of tight glucose control during birth is desirable to reduce neonatal hypoglycemia. Capillary blood glucose is checked hourly. The initial mainline IV should be normal saline. When active labor begins, or the capillary blood glucose levels drop to less than 70 mg/dL, the mainline is changed to a solution containing 5% dextrose. If glucose levels exceed 100 to 110mg/dL, an IV infusion of regular insulin is begun to maintain blood glucose levels between 80 and 110 mg/dL or according to facility policy (ACOG, 2020b; Landon et al., 2021).

Postpartum Period. Insulin needs should decline rapidly after the delivery of the placenta and abrupt cessation of placental hormones. However, blood glucose levels should be monitored at least four times daily so that the insulin dose can be adjusted to meet individual needs. Clients with type 1 diabetes usually return to their prepregnancy dosages. Those with type 2 diabetes are monitored, as ordered, and insulin is ordered only if needed.

Timing of Delivery. If possible, the pregnancy is allowed to progress to 39 weeks or later to allow the fetal lungs to mature, reducing the risk for neonatal respiratory distress syndrome. With evidence of fetal compromise, such as a low BPP or reduced amniotic fluid, delivery may be required. The decision to deliver before 39 weeks of gestation should be based on evidence of worsening condition of the pregnant client or the fetus. In these cases, evidence of fetal lung maturity is not critical (Landon et al., 2021). Cesarean birth may be considered to avoid traumatic birth injuries if the estimated fetal weight is more than 4500 g (ACOG, 2020b).

Gestational Diabetes Mellitus

Any degree of carbohydrate intolerance first diagnosed during the second or third trimester of pregnancy is classified as GDM (ACOG, 2020b; ADA, 2021a).

Identifying Gestational Diabetes Mellitus

All pregnant clients should be screened for GDM (those with risk for undiagnosed type 2 diabetes should be tested at the first prenatal visit as discussed above). The two-step test method is most often used in the United States. In this method, the client is screened with a 1-hour glucose challenge test followed by a 3-hour oral glucose tolerance test as indicated.

Glucose Challenge Test. A glucose challenge test (GCT) is administered between 24 and 28 weeks of gestation. Fasting is not necessary for a GCT, and the client is not required to follow any pretest dietary instructions. The client should ingest 50 g of oral glucose solution. A blood sample is taken 1 hour later. A positive screen of a 1-hour blood glucose concentration of 130 to 140 mg/dL or greater is followed by a 3-hour oral glucose tolerance test (OGTT). Evidence shows no clear advantage to using a cutoff of 130 or 140 mg/dL. Therefore the provider may use either value based on factors such as prevalence rates in the community (ACOG, 2019a).

Oral Glucose Tolerance Test. The 3-hour OGTT is the gold standard for diagnosing diabetes, but it is a more complex test. The client should have 3 days of unrestricted diet and activity followed by an 8-hour fast prior to the test. They should not smoke or eat throughout the test (Roth, 2021). After a fasting plasma glucose level is determined, the client should ingest 100 g of oral glucose solution. Plasma glucose levels are then determined at 1, 2, and 3 hours. A diagnosis of GDM is made if two or more of the values meet or exceed the threshold (ACOG, 2019a; Landon et al., 2021):

- Fasting 95 mg/dL
- 1 hour, 180 mg/dL
- 2 hours, 155 mg/dL
- 3 hours, 140 mg/dL

Based on client population, available resources, regional practice, and institutional policy, some providers may use thresholds of 105 for fasting, 190 for 1 hour, 165 for 2 hours, and 145 for 3 hours (ACOG, 2019a; ADA, 2021a; Landon et al., 2021).

Effects on the Client, Fetus, and Neonate

The client with GDM has an increased risk for the development of preeclampsia and a cesarean birth. The greatest risk is the increased possibility of development of diabetes later in life. Up to 70% of these clients will develop diabetes, usually type 2, later in life (ACOG, 2019a; Landon, et al., 2021).

With a few important exceptions, the fetal and neonatal effects of GDM are similar to those associated with preexisting diabetes. The exceptions are that GDM is not associated with an increased risk for ketoacidosis or spontaneous abortion, and there is a decreased chance of preexisting vascular and organ damage associated with diabetes. Because GDM develops after the first trimester, the critical period of major fetal organ development (organogenesis), it usually is not associated with an increase in major congenital malformations. Nevertheless, poorly controlled GDM, characterized by hyperglycemia during the third trimester, is associated with increased neonatal morbidity and mortality. The major fetal complications are macrosomia leading to birth injuries or cesarean birth, neonatal hypoglycemia, and hyperbilirubinemia. (See Table 10.5 for a summary of the effects of diabetes during pregnancy for the pregnant client, fetus and newborn.)

Therapeutic Management

Diet. Ideally, an RD, RDT, or diabetes educator develops an individualized nutrition plan with the client with GDM. The diet should provide the calories and nutrients needed for the health of the pregnant client and fetus, result in euglycemia, avoid ketosis, and promote appropriate weight gain. Calories should be distributed similar to clients with preexisting diabetes. Simple sugars, found in concentrated sweets, should be eliminated from the diet. Based on a nonobese prepregnancy weight, an average of 30 to 35 kcal/kg per day is recommended. Calorie restriction to 25 kcal/kg each day may be recommended for clients with obesity (Landon et al., 2021). These clients may be prescribed a diet with a smaller percentage of carbohydrates than for those of normal weight to limit hyperglycemia. An evening snack is usually needed to prevent ketosis at night. Typically, calories are divided among three meals and two to four snacks.

Exercise. Evidence on the effect of exercise and lifestyle changes specific to pregnant clients with GDM is very limited. However, what is available suggests a positive effect on glucose control for these clients (ACOG, 2019a). Based on this information and the demonstrated effect of exercise in the adults who are not pregnant, ACOG (2019a) recommends a goal of 30 minutes per day of moderate-intensity aerobic exercise at least 5 days a week, or 150 minutes per week. A graduated physical exercise program should be recommended by the provider, considering each client's risk factors as part of the treatment plan for clients with GDM.

Blood Glucose Monitoring. Blood glucose levels are used to evaluate the effect of diet and exercise and ensure euglycemia. A common method is measurement of fasting blood glucose level and postprandial blood glucose level (1 or 2 hours after each meal). Frequency of glucose monitoring may be modified once the glucose levels are well controlled by diet and exercise (ACOG, 2019a). If fasting capillary blood glucose levels repeatedly exceed 95 mg/dL or postprandial values exceed 140 mg/dL at 1 hour or 120 mg/dL at 2 hours, pharmacologic therapy may be added (ACOG, 2019a). Additional tests for glucose levels may be performed, as needed.

Pharmacologic Treatment. Pharmacologic treatment may be required for some clients with GDM when diet and exercise do not achieve glycemic targets. Insulin is the preferred medication for treatment of hyperglycemia in GDM (ACOG, 2019a; ADA, 2021b). Insulin is typically started at 0.7 to 1 unit/kg/day given in divided doses (ACOG, 2019a). Intermediate-acting and long-acting insulin may be used alone or in combination. Dosage should be adjusted to the client's blood glucose levels at particular times of the day (ACOG, 2019a).

Although insulin remains the only drug widely accepted for treatment of diabetes during pregnancy because it does not cross the placenta, oral agents are being studied more closely for GDM treatment (Landon et al., 2021). ACOG (2019a) recognizes oral agents may be used in GDM when the client declines insulin, is not able to safely administer, or cannot afford insulin. Glyburide (Micronase) and metformin (Glucophage) have been studied for use with GDM and have demonstrated glucose control comparable to insulin without apparent complications in the pregnant client or neonate (Landon et al., 2021), although adequate data from long-term follow-up studies is not available (ACOG, 2019a; ADA, 2021b). Because further research is needed on the long-term outcomes of oral diabetic therapy with GDM, ACOG (2019a) recommends client counseling with this treatment plan.

Fetal Surveillance. Testing to identify fetal compromise may be of benefit for clients with GDM and poor glycemic control and those who require medication, but there is no consensus regarding antepartum fetal testing for clients with GDM and good glycemic control (ACOG, 2019a). Testing may begin as early as 28 weeks of gestation if the client has poor glycemic control and comorbidities or by 32 weeks of gestation for those without comorbidities. The surveillance testing may include "kick counts," NST, BPP, and CST (Moore et al., 2019).

Postpartum Follow-Up. The client with gestational diabetes has a significant increased risk of developing diabetes later in life. These clients require follow-up with their primary care provider and should be screened for diabetes at between 4 and 12 weeks postpartum and then every 1 to 3 years. Abnormal findings should be treated with appropriate lifestyle changes or medical treatment. Those who plan to have additional pregnancies may benefit from more frequent screening between pregnancies (ACOG, 2019a).

Nursing Considerations

The care of pregnant clients with diabetes mellitus focuses primarily on maintaining normal blood glucose levels. As stated earlier, this maintenance involves a rather rigid schedule of controlling the diet, performing blood glucose tests, administering insulin, and performing regular fetal surveillance. Some clients respond calmly to the intense medical supervision. Others respond with anxiety, fear, denial, or anger and may feel inadequate or unable to control the diabetes to the degree expected by the health care team. These feelings may not be shared spontaneously, but they may affect the client's ability to achieve the desired outcomes. Also, nurses should remember to provide for normal pregnancy care in addition to monitoring the pregnant client's diabetes.

Increasing Effective Communication

A client often does not volunteer information about their feelings and concerns, especially if they have negative feelings about their care. In addition, the client and the nurse both may be unaware of any misunderstanding or conflict regarding the plan of care. Nurses should ask specifically about the feelings and concerns the client and their family have about the pregnancy.

Broad opening questions such as "What are your major concerns?" and "How do you feel about the plan of care?" are helpful. These should be followed by more specific questions such as "How do you feel about the fetal testing?" and "What would you like to change about the diet?" The client's responses may provide valuable information about their emotional response to the care plan. One client remarked, "I can tell you one thing, I don't feel like a person. I feel like an incubator, a faulty incubator." Another client who had a difficult time achieving the desired blood glucose level said, "I feel as though my whole life has been taken over by diabetes. I'm tired of feeling like a sick person."

The nurse should be an active listener and allow time for both the client and family to express concerns and feelings. The nurse should convey acceptance of both negative feelings and positive feelings that are expressed. Many clients are reassured to hear that their feelings of stress or anger are normal and learn that the health care team understands those feelings. Sharing of emotions will help them avoid or diminish unnecessary guilt, anxiety, and frustration and thus promote positive feelings about their ability to participate successfully in their plan of care.

Most clients benefit from praise when diabetes control is well maintained. They feel competent and trusted by the health care team and are motivated to continue their efforts.

Providing Opportunities for Control

Allowing the client to make as many decisions as possible increases the sense of being in control. For instance, selecting foods from the exchange list that provide the necessary nutrients but still allow some choice. A dietitian or dietary technician should be consulted if the list does not include foods they like or that suit their ethnic or cultural preferences. A regular schedule of exercise and sleep that helps keep the blood glucose level under control is important. The client can develop the schedule for rest and exercise that best suits their lifestyle. Nurses should allow as much flexibility as possible when scheduling stressful events such as fetal monitoring tests and amniocentesis.

Some clients resent being "treated as though ill," even when their diabetes control is excellent. They may be capable of making more decisions regarding their care during pregnancy, but they need the support of an understanding team to do this.

Providing Normal Pregnancy Care

Some clients express a need for more attention to the normal aspects of their pregnancies. This can be overlooked because of the intense focus on preventing complications that can occur with diabetes. Clients with diabetes also experience discomforts such as morning sickness, fatigue, backache, and difficulty sleeping during pregnancy. The nurse caring for these clients should therefore provide the usual education and counseling regarding pregnancy.

❓ KNOWLEDGE CHECK

28. What is the importance of the glycosylated hemoglobin (HgbA$_{1c}$) measurement in monitoring diabetes mellitus?
29. How does GDM compare with pregestational type 1 and type 2 diabetes mellitus in terms of onset and treatment?
30. What is the difference between GCT and OGTT? What instructions should be provided to the client for each test?
31. How do the effects of gestational diabetes on the pregnant client, fetus, and neonate differ from those of preexisting diabetes?

APPLICATION OF THE NURSING PROCESS: THE PREGNANT CLIENT WITH DIABETES MELLITUS

Assessment

Determine how well the client understands the prescribed management and how the family plans to carry out the recommended regimen. They may be newly diagnosed and have no experience in the necessary skills and procedures. Those who had diabetes before becoming pregnant may be skilled in monitoring glucose level and administering insulin. However, the client with preexisting diabetes may have no knowledge of how diabetes can affect pregnancy or how pregnancy can affect diabetes. They may have been using premixed insulin exclusively and now must begin mixing insulins of different types. Those with type 2 diabetes may have taken only oral medication and now must learn to mix and inject insulin.

To determine whether the pregnant client's techniques are accurate, ask them to demonstrate how they monitor blood glucose level and observe as the insulin is mixed and injected. Verify that the client and family are aware of the need to select appropriate sites and injection techniques that prevent insulin leakage.

Although diet is developed by a dietitian or diabetes educator, the nurse should assess how well the family understands the diet. Determine whether special problems with food preferences or availability of recommended foods exist. Diet recommendations include a target number of calories, plus targets for grams of carbohydrate, protein, and fat to meet calorie needs. Any of the several methods to count and exchange foods may be used. One method uses exchange lists, in which the listed foods all have about the same number of grams of carbohydrate, protein, and fat. Therefore one food from the list may be substituted, or exchanged, for another in the same list. Another method uses carbohydrate counting, in which foods on the starch, fruit, or milk list supply about 15 g of carbohydrate, or one carbohydrate choice. The diet plan would prescribe the number of carbohydrate choices for each meal and snack. Insulin is often adjusted according to the carbohydrate count for each meal or snack.

Identify special needs related to food preferences, culturally prescribed foods, or the availability of recommended foods. It may be necessary to review an exchange list and ask the client how they plan to substitute and exchange foods to obtain the prescribed number of foods from each list.

Identify the client's knowledge of potential complications such as hypoglycemia and hyperglycemia so that both client and family can be provided with pertinent information to avoid it or treat it.

Determine their knowledge of fetal surveillance techniques and response to the need for frequent tests. Some clients are highly motivated to continue the treatment regimen when test results indicate that the fetus is thriving. Others find the frequent testing stressful and inconvenient.

Identification of Client Problems

A common problem for clients with diabetes during pregnancy is the need for client teaching of (1) measures to maintain normal blood glucose levels, (2) measures to manage abnormal glucose levels, and (3) common fetal surveillance procedures.

Planning: Expected Outcomes

Goals for this problem are that the client and their family will do the following:

- Demonstrate competence in blood glucose monitoring and administration of insulin before home management is initiated.
- Describe a plan for meeting dietary recommendations that fits family lifestyle and food preferences.
- Identify signs and symptoms of hypoglycemia and hyperglycemia and the management required for each.
- Verbalize knowledge of fetal surveillance procedures and keep scheduled appointments for testing.

Interventions

Management of diabetes mellitus during pregnancy is a team effort, and the nurse is responsible to provide or reinforce accurate information about the therapeutic regimen and offer consistent support for the client's efforts to comply with the recommendations. It may be necessary to demonstrate specific skills that the client and their support person should master and to review and reinforce information from other members of the health care team.

Teaching Self-Care Skills

Demonstrations and return demonstrations are effective ways to teach and evaluate psychomotor skills. The client (and family) should learn to (1) use a meter and obtain a small sample of blood, (2) test for glucose level, and (3) mix and inject insulin. The procedures are invasive and cause mild discomfort, which may make the client reluctant to start. Mixing insulins accurately or using a sliding scale may be intimidating at first. Using food exchanges is often unfamiliar to the client who is newly diagnosed, but it is critical to glucose control. Acknowledge these feelings before teaching begins.

Self-Monitoring of Blood Glucose Level. Spring-loaded lancets make home blood glucose monitoring easier. The side of the fingertip is less sensitive than the pad, so using the side reduces discomfort. Teach the client to cleanse the area with warm water before obtaining a sample to prevent infection. If alcohol is used to clean the area, let it dry thoroughly. The first drop of blood is wiped away, and the second drop is placed on the meter's strip. Each home monitoring kit contains specific instructions for use of the meter and the type of reagent strip or cartridge that should be used. Teach the client how to record glucose values in a handwritten log or cell phone app. Teach them that current glucose monitors have a memory option to provide retrieval of previous glucose readings.

Insulin Administration. The client is often prescribed a combination of rapid-acting or short-acting and intermediate-acting insulins. Teach about the difference in onset, peak, and duration of action of each type of insulin in the prescribed combination. The client may also need to learn how to mix insulins in the same syringe. If they will use a sliding scale to keep glucose levels close to normal, they will need teaching about how to determine the additional dose of insulin if they have never used a sliding scale for insulin administration.

Insulin is administered subcutaneously. Common sites include the upper thighs, abdomen, and upper arms. Because the pregnant client is injecting insulin frequently, emphasize the following precautions:

- To prevent hypoglycemia, a meal should be taken 30 minutes after regular insulin is injected. Because of its 10-minute onset of action, lispro (Humalog) insulin is injected just before eating.
- Unless the client is very thin, insulin should be injected with the short needle inserted at a 90-degree angle so that the tip of the needle reaches the fatty tissue layer.
- The needle should be inserted quickly to minimize discomfort.
- The tissue pinch, if used, is released after inserting the needle and before injecting insulin because pressure from the pinch can promote insulin leakage from subcutaneous tissue.
- Aspirating is not necessary when injecting into subcutaneous tissue.
- Insulin is injected slowly (over 2 to 4 seconds) to allow tissue expansion and minimize pressure, which can cause insulin leakage.
- The needle is withdrawn quickly to minimize the formation of a track, which might cause insulin to leak out.

Emphasize the importance of administering the correct dosage at the correct time. Teach the client and family about the function of insulin and the importance of following the directions of the health care provider in regard to coordinating meals with the administration of insulin.

Continuous Glucose Monitors and Subcutaneous Insulin Infusion. Many clients who have preexisting diabetes use CGM and subcutaneous insulin infusion pumps and wish to continue with this method during pregnancy. The use of CGM and programmable insulin infusion pumps allows tailoring of insulin administration to the client's individual lifestyle. The client should know how to change out both systems, how to calibrate the CGM, and what to do in case of monitor or pump problems.

Teaching Dietary Management

Although a dietitian develops the recommended diet, the nurse should be aware of the general requirements and be sensitive to the client's dietary habits and preferences. Often, reviewing and clarifying how exchange lists are used to plan meals and snacks are necessary. Encourage the client to avoid simple sugars (candy, cake, cookies), which raise the blood glucose levels quickly but may result in wide swings between high and low glucose levels.

It may be necessary to help the client select foods that are high in nutrients but low in cost or meet cultural or religious constraints. Animal protein is especially expensive, and alternative sources of protein (beans, peas, corn, grains) can be substituted to meet some of the protein needs, as well as provide high-quality carbohydrate and fiber. A nutrition and dietetic technician can help a pregnant client who is a vegetarian meet their individual needs depending on what foods are acceptable to them.

Allow the expectant client to verbalize their frustrations or problems with the diet, and collaborate with the dietitian if they have a particular problem.

Managing Hypoglycemia and Hyperglycemia

Every client and their family should be aware of signs and symptoms that indicate abnormal glucose levels and what actions to take for these levels. Hypoglycemia and hyperglycemia pose a threat to the client and the fetus if these problems are not identified and corrected quickly.

Hypoglycemia. Treat hypoglycemia at once. The client should take 15 g of carbohydrate if they can swallow food. Examples of foods that supply this are three glucose tablets or glucose gel, ½ cup of fruit juice or regular soft drink, 6 saltine crackers, or 1 tbsp of syrup or honey. Large quantities of high-carbohydrate foods such as candy will increase the blood glucose excessively, making a sudden fall in the level more likely. Retesting should occur 15 minutes after the carbohydrate intake and repeat the treatment if the blood glucose level remains below 70 mg/dL. If it is more than 1 hour until the next meal or snack, test again 60 minutes after treatment; additional carbohydrate may be required.

⚡ SAFETY CHECK

Signs and symptoms of hypoglycemia in the pregnant client include the following:
- Shakiness (tremors)
- Sweating
- Pallor; cold, clammy skin
- Disorientation, irritability
- Headache
- Hunger
- Blurred vision

⚡ SAFETY CHECK

Signs and symptoms of hyperglycemia in the pregnant client include the following:
- Fatigue
- Flushed, hot skin
- Dry mouth, excessive thirst
- Frequent urination
- Rapid, deep respirations; fruity smell to the breath
- Drowsiness, headache
- Depressed reflexes

Teach family members how to inject glucagon if the client cannot swallow or retain food. Notify the provider at once. IV glucose will be administered if they are hospitalized. If untreated, hypoglycemia can progress to seizures and death.

To prevent hypoglycemia, instruct the client to have meals and snacks at a fixed time each day and at bedtime. Suggest that they always carry glucose tablets or gel or some crackers with them.

Hyperglycemia. Because infection is the most common cause of hyperglycemia, pregnant clients should be instructed to notify the provider whenever they have an infection of any type.

Untreated hyperglycemia can lead to ketoacidosis, coma, and client and fetal death. If signs and symptoms occur, notify the provider at once so treatment can be initiated. Hospitalization often is necessary to monitor blood glucose levels, for IV insulin administration to normalize glucose levels, and for treatment of any underlying infection.

Explaining Procedures, Tests, and Plan of Care

Explain the schedule and the reasons for frequent checkups and necessary tests. Encourage the client and family to ask questions if any part of the schedule is confusing. This is particularly important for clients who are aware that their prenatal care differs significantly from that of their friends who do not have diabetes. Knowing that the tests provide information about the condition of the client and fetus reduces frustration and anxiety. Explain why more frequent antepartum surveillance testing is needed when diabetes complicates pregnancy. The client needs to know their diabetic care will require more time and effort than it did before pregnancy but that this care greatly improves their likelihood of having a healthy infant.

Evaluation

After procedures, tests, and plan of care have been explained, evaluation should ensure the following:
- The client and at least one support person can demonstrate competence in home glucose monitoring and administration of insulin.
- The client can develop a weekly meal plan for meeting individual dietary requirements.
- The client and at least one support person can list the signs and symptoms of hypoglycemia and hyperglycemia and describe the initial management of these conditions.
- The client can verbalize knowledge of the reason for fetal surveillance procedures and keeps appointments for tests.

TABLE 10.6	World Health Organization Body Mass Categories
Category	BMI
Underweight	<18.5
Normal weight	18.5–24.9
Overweight	25.0–29.9
Obesity class I	30.0–34.9
Obesity class II	35.0–39.9
Obesity class III	≥40

OBESITY

Obesity is determined by one's BMI defined as weight in kilograms divided by height in meters squared (kg/m²). The WHO (2000) organizes BMI into six categories: underweight, normal weight, overweight, and three classes of obesity. A person is considered to have class I obesity when they have a BMI of 30.0 to 34.9, class II obesity with a BMI of 35.0 to 39.9, and class III obesity (also known as morbid obesity) with a BMI of 40 or greater (Table 10.6).

Obesity in Pregnancy

When planning for pregnancy, clients are encouraged to adopt healthy habits and make positive lifestyle changes such as healthy eating and maintaining a healthy weight. However, many pregnancies are unplanned/unintended, resulting in the loss of opportunity to achieve optimal health prior to conceiving. Obesity in pregnancy has become a global epidemic with as many as one-third of all clients of childbearing age considered overweight or obese (Stubert et al., 2018).

Obesity and Fertility

Obesity can impact all aspects of childbearing, starting with fertility. An increased BMI can inhibit ovulation, prohibiting or making it more difficult to get pregnant (Smid et al., 2019). For those undergoing fertility treatments, such as in vitro fertilization, obesity can decrease the likelihood of a successful pregnancy (Smid et al., 2019). For those who are able to achieve pregnancy, obesity increases the risk of recurrent miscarriage, preterm birth, stillbirth, and neonatal and infant death (ACOG, 2021d; Louis, 2021; Smid et al., 2019).

Obesity and Pregnancy

Obesity during pregnancy significantly increases the risk of pregnancy complications such as, but not limited to, obstructive sleep apnea, gestational hypertension, preeclampsia, GDM, preterm labor, prolonged pregnancy, induction of labor, and cesarean birth (ACOG, 2021d; Louis, 2021). In addition to the increased risk for perinatal death, the fetus/newborn is also at risk for macrosomia, low Apgar score, admission to the neonatal intensive care unit, and congenital malformations (ACOG, 2021d; Louis, 2021; Stubert et al., 2018). Obesity during pregnancy also increases the risk of the child developing obesity in childhood, adolescence, and adult life (Louis, 2021; Smid et al., 2019).

Antenatal Care

At the first prenatal visit, the client's BMI should be determined. Pregnant clients with obesity should be counseled on the risks associated with obesity during pregnancy, and goals for weight gain during pregnancy should be discussed at each prenatal visit (Louis, 2021). The recommended weight gain in pregnancy is 11 to 20 lb in clients with obesity (BMI 30 or greater) and 15 to 25 lb in those who are overweight (BMI 25 to 29.9) (ACOG, 2021d; Institute of Medicine [IOM], 2009). Exercise programs should be individualized and adjusted based on clinical evaluation of the client. For most, an eventual goal of 20 to 30 minutes of moderate activity 5 to 7 days of the week is appropriate (ACOG, 2020d). Referral to a registered dietitian for development of a healthy eating plan may be appropriate. Because there is an association between obesity during pregnancy and psychological and emotional issues such as depression, anxiety, and stress (Louis, 2021), referral to a counselor or mental health provider may be reasonable.

Clients with obesity have an increased risk for undiagnosed type 2 diabetes mellitus. Those with a BMI of 30 or greater or who have additional risk factors such as a previous history of gestational diabetes, physical inactivity, or first-degree relative with diabetes should be screened at the first prenatal visit and again at 24 to 28 weeks of gestation (ACOG, 2018a; ACOG 2021d).

Obesity increases the risk for sleep apnea. If the pregnant client with obesity has symptoms of snoring at night, sleepiness, or chronic fatigue or cannot concentrate, a referral for a sleep study may be appropriate (Louis, 2021). Finally, an ultrasound should be obtained between 18 and 22 weeks to review fetal anatomy; however, the client should be informed that obesity limits the ability to detect fetal anomalies (ACOG, 2021d; Louis, 2021). Serial growth scans may be needed because of difficulty assessing fetal growth by fundal height measurements (Cunningham et al., 2022).

Intrapartum Care

Special equipment for the pregnant client with obesity may be necessary during labor and delivery. These include a bariatric bed, commode or toilet seat; extra-large gowns; correct-size BP cuff; correct-size sequential compression devices; bariatric wheelchairs; and a proper scale to weigh the client. Should the client require a cesarean section, a bariatric operating room table, as well as appropriate extra-long surgical instruments, may be necessary.

Nursing care during labor involves frequent assessment of the FHR and uterine activity. Clients with obesity may necessitate one-to-one or two-to-one nursing care in some cases. External monitoring of the FHR and uterine activity is difficult and may require the use of internal monitoring techniques for assessments of the FHR and uterine contractions.

Due to the increased rates of comorbidities and prolonged pregnancy, clients with obesity are more likely to have an induction of labor and may require higher doses of oxytocin to achieve birth (ACOG, 2021d; Cunningham et al., 2022; Louis, 2021). They also have a slower rate of labor progress and an increased risk for operative vaginal births and cesarean births (Cunningham et al., 2022; Louis, 2021).

Cesarean births are technically more difficult in this population with longer surgery times and greater blood loss (Smid et al., 2019). Postoperatively, obesity increases the risk for respiratory suppression and airway obstruction (Louis, 2021). There is an increased risk for thromboembolism; therefore sequential compression devices should be used, and thromboprophylaxis may be prescribed. Surgical site infections are more likely; higher doses of perioperative antibiotics may be required (ACOG, 2021d; Cunningham et al., 2022; Smid et al., 2019). A vertical skin incision may be performed, and the physician may elect to involve a wound care nurse for follow-up.

Analgesia and anesthesia may be difficult to achieve. Regional anesthesia is difficult because of the decreased ability to identify landmarks and inability to correctly position the client; there is a higher rate of failed epidural placement in this population. Endotracheal intubation is more difficult, and there is an increased risk for failed intubation and aspiration of gastric contents (Louis, 2021; Smid et al., 2019).

Postpartum

Obesity can also cause complication during the postpartum period. Clients with obesity are at an increased risk of developing venous thromboembolism, pulmonary embolism, and postpartum hemorrhage, as well as postpartum depression, breastfeeding difficulties, and postpartum anemia (ACOG, 2021d; Cunningham et al., 2022; Smid et al., 2019). For clients with obesity who required a cesarean birth, there is an increased risk for poor wound healing, and/or postoperative wound infection (ACOG, 2021d).

Breastfeeding is beneficial to the client with obesity and the newborn. However, delayed lactogenesis with decreased breastfeeding initiation rates and decreased continuation of breastfeeding are more likely in this population (Ballesta-Castillejos et al., 2020; Preusting et al., 2017). During the postpartum period, the nurse should encourage and support breastfeeding. At the postpartum office appointment, the client should be reassessed for gestational diabetes and hypertension. Finally, postpartum clients with obesity should be encouraged to optimize their health before another pregnancy.

Pregnancy after Bariatric Surgery

Bariatric surgery is an effective treatment option for morbid obesity in some clients. Although it is not appropriate during pregnancy, some clients with obesity may elect to have weight reduction surgery before conceiving. In these clients, the rates of obstetric complications are lower than in the client with morbid obesity. Following bariatric surgery, pregnancy should be postponed for 12 to 24 months to allow for weight stabilization. During pregnancy, the client should be monitored for vitamin and nutritional deficiency and for signs of intestinal obstruction (ACOG, 2021d; Cunningham et al., 2022).

Nursing Considerations

When caring for the client with obesity it is important to remain respectful and considerate. Evidence shows that clients with obesity experience bias and a lack of proper and comprehensive care when accessing the health care system (ACOG, 2019b). They often hesitate to seek care due to fear of the treatment they will receive. Health care providers should self-assess for any biases and be mindful of the language that is used. For example, ACOG (2019b) recommends that health care providers utilize the term "clients with obesity," as opposed to labeling a client by saying "obese client." Nurses should assess the client's readiness to learn and consider any social determinants of health that may be inhibiting adapting healthier lifestyle choices. For example, recommending that a client from a lower socioeconomic status with limited funds eat all organic food may not be a feasible option. Instead, assess what food establishments are accessible and assist the client to make healthier choices. Pregnancy can also be a great time to start low-impact moderate exercise for those that have not previously exercised (ACOG, 2021c). Activities such as walking and swimming can be enjoyable and provide significant health benefits (ACOG, 2021c). Clients who exercise regularly can continue provided they do not overexert. Exercise should be discussed with and approved by their health care provider to maintain safety (March of Dimes, 2020).

Specialized equipment should be available for the care of clients with obesity. This includes appropriate-sized gowns, BP cuffs, beds, OR tables, wheelchairs, and surgical equipment. In addition, staff should be trained on proper body mechanics and the use of assistive devices with bariatric clients.

> **❓ KNOWLEDGE CHECK**
>
> 32. How much should the client with obesity gain during pregnancy?
> 33. When caring for clients with obesity, what nursing assessments are required during the intrapartum period?

ANEMIAS

Anemia is a condition in which a decline in circulating RBC mass reduces the capacity to carry oxygen to the vital organs of the pregnant client or the fetus. Significant anemia is associated with preterm birth and low birth weight. A pregnant client is usually considered anemic when the Hgb level is less than 10.5 g/dL in the second trimester or less than 11 g/dL in the first and third trimesters (CDC, 1998; Samuels, 2021).

Anemia is one of the most common problems of pregnancy, affecting 36.5% of pregnant clients worldwide and 11.5% of pregnant clients in the United States in 2019 (WHO, 2022b). The incidence varies according to geographic location and socioeconomic group. Anemia may be caused by a variety of factors, including nutritional deficits, hemolysis, and blood loss. The most common type of anemia observed during pregnancy is iron-deficiency anemia; less common causes are megaloblastic anemia due to folic acid or vitamin B_{12} deficiency, sickle cell disease, and thalassemia.

Iron-Deficiency Anemia

The total iron requirement for a typical pregnancy with a single fetus is approximately 1000 mg (Cunningham et al., 2022). Unfortunately, most clients of reproductive age do not have this amount of iron stores because of menstrual blood loss. Furthermore, meeting pregnancy needs by diet alone is difficult, although iron is present in many foods. The primary sources of iron are liver, oysters, lean red meat, tuna, salmon, chicken (dark meat), fortified cereals, dried beans, whole grains, and green leafy vegetables (Raymond & Morrow, 2021).

Effects on the Pregnant Client

Signs and symptoms of iron deficiency anemia include tachycardia, pallor, fatigue, lethargy, and headache. Clinical findings also may include inflammations of the lips and tongue and pica (consuming nonfood substances such as clay, dirt, ice, and starch). Laboratory findings for iron-deficiency anemia include RBCs that are microcytic (small) and hypochromic (pale). Plasma iron and serum ferritin levels are low, whereas the total iron-binding capacity is higher than normal (ACOG, 2021e). Clients who have multifetal pregnancies or bleeding complications are more likely to be anemic during pregnancy. Anemia during pregnancy increases the risk for complications from blood loss during birth and the postpartum period due to lower hemoglobin levels. In addition, there may be an association between perinatal anemia and postpartum depression (ACOG, 2021e).

Fetal and Neonatal Effects

Iron-deficiency anemia may increase the risk for preterm birth, low birth weight, and perinatal mortality. In addition, there may be a negative effect later in life in the mental and psychomotor performance of the child (ACOG, 2021e).

Therapeutic Management

Routine supplemental iron therapy in addition to the amount in prenatal vitamins, rather than therapy based on an indication of anemia, is controversial. Ferrous sulfate 325 mg (which provides 60 to 65 mg of elemental iron), one to three times per day, is commonly prescribed. Many clients experience less gastrointestinal discomfort if iron supplementation is taken with meals, although absorption is less. Taking iron supplementation with vitamin C may enhance absorption. Parenteral therapy may be necessary for the client who cannot or will not take oral iron supplementation and is significantly anemic but does not require a transfusion (Samuels, 2021).

Megaloblastic Anemia (Folic Acid and Vitamin B₁₂ Deficiency)

Folic acid and vitamin B_{12} are essential nutrients for the formation of RBCs. Although inadequate folic acid is the most common cause of megaloblastic anemia during pregnancy, increased rates of bariatric surgery are contributing to the incidences due to a vitamin B_{12} deficiency (ACOG, 2021e; Samuels, 2021).

Effects on the Pregnant Client

The requirement for folic acid doubles during pregnancy in response to the demand for greater production of erythrocytes and fetal and placental growth. A deficiency in either folic acid or vitamin B_{12} results in the presence of large, immature erythrocytes (megaloblasts).

Although prolonged inadequate dietary intake is a significant contributor to folic acid deficiency, nonfood factors include hemolytic anemias with increased RBC turnover, multifetal pregnancies, some medications (such as anticonvulsants), and malabsorption entities. Folic acid deficiency may be present in association with iron-deficiency anemia.

Vitamin B_{12} is found primarily in animal products such as fish, meats, dairy, and eggs. Inadequate intake is usually associated with a history of bariatric surgery, vegan diet, or gastrointestinal diseases such as Crohn's disease. Prolonged deficiency of vitamin B_{12} can result in neuropathy as well as anemia (Samuels, 2021).

Fetal and Neonatal Effects

In addition to the possible increased occurrence of preterm birth and low birth weight, there is a known association between folic acid deficiency and an increase in NTDs.

Therapeutic Management

The recommended daily allowance for folic acid for all clients of childbearing age is 400 mcg, and some clients have difficulty ingesting the amount needed, even though it does occur widely in foods. The best sources of folic acid are fortified grains, beans such as black beans and lentils, peanuts, and fresh, dark-green leafy vegetables.

Most nonprescription prenatal vitamins contain 0.8 to 1 mg of folic acid to ensure sufficient intake. Higher doses of folate may be prescribed according to individual needs. Vitamin B_{12} deficiency is treated with IM injections of the vitamin (Kilpatrick & Kitahara, 2019).

? KNOWLEDGE CHECK

34. Why is supplemental iron needed by most clients who are pregnant?
35. What are the fetal and neonatal effects of iron-deficiency anemia?

Sickle Cell Disease

Sickle cell disease is an autosomal recessive genetic disorder. It occurs when the gene for the production of Hgb S is inherited from both parents. Heterozygosity occurs with inheritance of an affected gene from one parent and an unaffected gene from the other. This results in a carrier status, or sickle cell trait, rather than the disease.

With sickle cell disease, the defect in the Hgb causes erythrocytes to become shaped like a sickle, or crescent, under certain conditions. Low oxygen concentration usually causes the sickling, with acidosis and dehydration worsening the process. At first the erythrocytes regain their normal shape, but eventually they remain permanently sickled. Because of their distorted shape, the erythrocytes cannot pass through small arteries and capillaries and tend to clump together and occlude the blood vessel.

The disease is characterized by chronic anemia because of the short life span of erythrocytes affected with Hgb S, increased susceptibility to infection, and periodic episodes of obstruction of blood vessels by the abnormally shaped erythrocytes. Sickle cell disease occurs most often in people who have ancestors from sub-Saharan Africa, the Caribbean, South and Central America, Saudi Arabia, India, and Mediterranean countries. Sickle cell anemia affects 90,000 to 100,000 people in the United States. Of Black people or African Americans, 1 in 12 to 13 are carriers of the sickle cell trait and may pass the gene on to their children, even though they are not affected (ACOG, 2022a; National Institutes of Health [NIH] & National Heart, Lung, & Blood Institute [NHLBI], 2020; Samuels, 2021).

Effects on the Pregnant Client

Physiologic anemia, increased coagulation factors, and venous stasis, which are normal in pregnancy, may bring on sickle cell crisis, sometimes for the first time. This broad term includes several different conditions, particularly temporary cessation of bone marrow function, hemolytic crisis with massive erythrocyte destruction resulting in jaundice, and severe pain caused by infarctions located in the joints and the major organs. In addition, expectant clients with sickle cell disease are prone to pyelonephritis, bone infection, heart disease, and hypertensive complications of pregnancy (Samuels, 2021). Clients with higher Hgb F (fetal Hgb) levels may have a lower perinatal mortality rate, but safety in pregnancy has not been established for administration of hydroxyurea which increases its production (ACOG, 2022a; Samuels, 2021).

Fetal and Neonatal Effects

Pregnancies complicated by sickle cell disease are associated with increased risk for spontaneous abortion (miscarriage), preterm labor, IUGR, and stillbirth (ACOG, 2022a, NIH & NHLBI, 2020).

Therapeutic Management

Clients with sickle cell disease should seek preconception care or early prenatal care and be informed of the risks associated with the pregnancy. Folic acid supplementation of 4 mg (400 mcg) daily is prescribed, ideally before conception, because of frequent erythrocyte turnover (ACOG, 2022a). Frequent measurements of Hgb, complete blood cell count, serum iron, total iron-binding capacity, and serum folate may be necessary to determine the degree of anemia and iron and folic acid stores. Testing is performed for infections such as hepatitis, human immunodeficiency virus (HIV) infection, tuberculosis, and sexually transmitted infections (STIs). Noninfected clients who are not immune are immunized as appropriate based on pregnancy status. Urinalysis, with culture and sensitivity, if indicated, identifies both clinical and subclinical UTIs that should be treated.

Fetal surveillance studies (ultrasonography, NSTs, and BPPs) assess fetal growth and development and placental function. The use of prophylactic blood transfusion is controversial. The current recommendation is to limit transfusions to clinically indicated situations such as worsening anemia, hemorrhage, and painful crisis (ACOG, 2022a). Risks for prophylactic transfusions are comparable with risks in the client without sickle cell disease. The client with sickle cell disease may have a transfusion reaction and is likely to develop higher levels of antibodies to the cells in the transfused blood. Finding compatible blood for later transfusion might be more difficult. Prenatal supplementation of vitamins without iron may be prescribed for the client who receives multiple transfusions but for whom additional folic acid is indicated (ACOG, 2022a; Cunningham et al., 2022; NIH & NHLBI, 2020; Samuels, 2021).

The goal of nursing management is to help the pregnant client with sickle cell disease maintain a healthy state and avoid hospitalization. Clients should be encouraged to keep all prenatal care appointments, usually every other week and more frequently if needed. Topics in prenatal education include the need for (1) adequate hydration to prevent sickling, (2) adequate nutrition to meet metabolic needs, (3) folic acid supplementation for erythrocyte production, (4) rest periods throughout the day, (5) good hygiene practices and the avoidance of persons with infectious illnesses, and (6) prompt treatment for fever or other signs of infection.

Nurses should be alert for signs of a sickle cell crisis. The most common indications are pain in the abdomen, chest, vertebrae, joints, or extremities; pallor; and signs of cardiac failure. Nurses also should provide comfort measures such as repositioning and good skin care, assisting with ambulation and movement in bed, and assisting the client to splint the abdomen with a pillow for coughing or deep breathing.

Nurses should remember that pain is not always related to the sickling crisis but could be related to a complication of pregnancy. Clients with sickle cell disease can also have ectopic pregnancy, placental abruption, appendicitis, and other painful complications not related to their blood disorder.

Intrapartum care focuses on preventing the development of sickle cell crisis. Oxygen is administered continuously, and fluids should be administered to prevent dehydration because hypoxemia and dehydration, as well as exertion, infection, and acidosis, stimulate the sickling process.

Thalassemia

Like sickle cell anemia, thalassemia is a genetic disorder that involves the abnormal synthesis of alpha or beta chains of Hgb. Thalassemia is named and classified by the type of chain that is abnormal. Beta-thalassemia is most frequently encountered in the United States, often in those of Mediterranean, Middle Eastern, and Asian descent.

Beta-thalassemia minor refers to the heterozygous form that results from the inheritance of one affected gene from either parent. Beta-thalassemia major refers to inheritance of the gene from both parents (homozygous form). Although regular blood transfusions and treatment with chelation therapy has increased the life expectancy and reproductive possibilities for those with Beta-thalassemia major (Cooley's anemia), pregnancy is uncommon (Kilpatrick & Kitahara, 2019; Samuels, 2021).

Effects on the Pregnant Client

Pregnant clients with beta-thalassemia minor often are mildly anemic but otherwise healthy. Laboratory values normally associated with beta-thalassemia minor indicate a mild hypochromic and microcytic anemia. Because persons with beta-thalassemia absorb and store iron in their bodies, supplemental iron should not exceed prophylactic dosage unless iron deficiency is documented

Fetal and Neonatal Effects

Whether the disorders are associated with increased fetal or neonatal morbidity remains unresolved because of the many variants of thalassemia. There appears to be no increase in the rate of prematurity, low-birth-weight infants, or abnormal size for gestation associated with beta-thalassemia minor (Kilpatrick & Kitahara, 2019). The fetus may inherit the serious problem of beta-thalassemia major if both parents have beta-thalassemia minor.

Therapeutic Management

No specific therapy for beta-thalassemia minor during pregnancy exists. Generally, the outcomes for the client and fetus are satisfactory (ACOG, 2022a; Cunningham et al., 2022; Samuels, 2021). Infections that depress the production of RBCs and accelerate erythrocyte destruction should be identified and treated promptly.

KNOWLEDGE CHECK

36. What are the effects of sickle cell disease on the pregnant client?
37. How is sickle cell disease treated during pregnancy?
38. Why is iron supplementation often not recommended for clients with thalassemia?

OTHER MEDICAL CONDITIONS

Clients with a preexisting medical condition should be aware of the effects that pregnancy will have on their conditions as well as the impact of their medical conditions on pregnancy outcome. Some conditions that complicate pregnancy are discussed in this section; others are described in Table 10.7.

Autoimmune Diseases

Autoimmune diseases are conditions characterized by malfunctioning of the immune system. In these conditions, the body is not able to distinguish foreign cells from healthy body cells. The body attacks its own tissues as it would foreign antigens resulting in tissue damage. Autoimmune conditions include systemic lupus erythematosus (SLE), antiphospholipid syndrome, Graves disease, Hashimoto's thyroiditis, and rheumatoid arthritis.

Systemic Lupus Erythematosus

SLE is a chronic inflammatory autoimmune disease that can affect any organ or system in the body. Although the cause is unknown, there is a genetic predisposition that probably is affected by environment and infectious exposures; hormonal factors may also be involved (Benson & Branch, 2021). The most common signs and symptoms of SLE are joint pain, fatigue, malaise, photosensitivity, and rash, including a characteristic "butterfly rash" on the face, which may be less apparent during pregnancy because of the normal pigmentation changes. The disease is marked by episodes of exacerbation (flares), when the symptoms become worse, and quiescence, when the symptoms recede.

The disease tends to affect young clients but may occur in any age group. Females are affected more often than males. It is more common in Black/African American, Hispanic/Latino, Asian, and Native American clients than in White/Caucasians (CDC, 2018).

Pregnant clients with SLE have an increased risk for complications such as hypertensive disorders (including preeclampsia), preterm birth, IUGR, fetal loss, and stillbirth (Benson & Branch, 2021; Cunningham et al., 2022; Sammaritano et al., 2019). The most serious potential complication for the neonate is a complete heart block, which usually is permanent and will require a pacemaker (Benson & Branch, 2021). Pregnancy is most likely to have a favorable outcome in the client whose disease is well controlled prior to pregnancy and who does not have renal involvement. Clients with SLE, especially those with a history of renal involvement, should be advised to seek the advice of a health care provider before becoming pregnant.

Antiphospholipid Syndrome

Antiphospholipid syndrome (APS) is an autoimmune condition characterized by the production of antiphospholipid antibodies combined with certain clinical features. Specific clinical features include thrombosis confirmed by imaging or pathologic studies, recurrent abnormal pregnancy outcomes, and elevated anticardiolipin antibody or presence of lupus anticoagulant. Pregnancy problems may include the following:

- One or more unexplained fetal deaths at or after 10 weeks of gestation
- One or more preterm births of a normal infant at or before 34 weeks of gestation that is related to preeclampsia with severe features or severe placental insufficiency
- Three or more unexplained recurrent spontaneous abortions before 10 weeks of gestation

Although the syndrome occurs most often in clients with other underlying autoimmune diseases such as SLE, it also is diagnosed in clients with no other recognizable autoimmune disease.

Clients with APS should be informed about potential medical and obstetric problems, including a possible risk for stroke, preeclampsia, and placental insufficiency. Combinations of low-dose aspirin and prophylactic heparin or enoxaparin are recommended for pregnant clients with APS (Benson & Branch, 2021).

TABLE 10.7 Other Medical Conditions and Their Effects on Pregnancy

Condition	Effects	Considerations
Appendicitis		
Inflammation of appendix, often with fever.	Is difficult to diagnose during pregnancy. Early symptoms mimic common conditions of pregnancy. Ultrasonography may help rule out other diagnoses such as ectopic pregnancy.	When reasonable doubt exists that the client has appendicitis, appendix should be removed to prevent rupture and consequent complications. Location of appendix often is altered by growing uterus. Fetal hyperthermia may be caused by fever in the pregnant client.
Asthma		
Obstructive lung disease caused by airway inflammation. Characterized by dyspnea, cough, wheezing. Course in pregnancy is variable.	Effective therapy and avoidance of severe attacks are associated with good pregnancy outcome. Severe, uncontrolled disease is associated with increased complications for the pregnant client and fetus. Medications used are well tolerated in pregnancy and appear to be safe for fetus. Oral steroids may be associated with increased risk for cleft lip and palate, but the benefit of disease control outweighs the risk. Breastfeeding is safe for newborn and may reduce risk for allergies.	Medical management is stair stepped based on the persistence and severity of the disease. Short-acting inhaled beta agonists, such as albuterol, are used to manage symptoms in mild intermittent asthma. Low-dose inhaled steroids may be added as prophylaxis in mild persistent cases. If the client's asthma is classified as moderate persistent, long-acting beta agonists will be included in the treatment plan. For severe cases, the dosage of inhaled corticosteroids is increased and in very severe persistent cases, oral corticosteroids are added. The client should be counseled regarding avoidance of triggers and the importance of disease control with prescribed medications.
Phenylketonuria (PKU) in the Pregnant Client		
Inherited autosomal recessive defect leading to inability to metabolize essential amino acid phenylalanine, resulting in high serum levels of phenylalanine. Irreparable physical and intellectual disability occurs in the fetus if pregnant client is not treated prior to conception and in early pregnancy with a diet that provides adequate protein but restricts phenylalanine.	Client must have low-phenylalanine diet before conception and pregnancy. If not, fetal risk for microcephaly, intellectual disability, heart defects, and intrauterine growth restriction increases.	Special low-phenylalanine foods are expensive, but they may be obtained through the state's Supplemental Nutrition Program for Women, Infants, and Children (WIC) or Medicaid or may be covered by private insurance. Newborn screens test for the presence of PKU in the infant. Child either will be a carrier of the gene or will inherit the disease, depending on the presence of the gene in the father of the child. Infant with PKU will require pediatric endocrinologist consult and special formula.

Graves Disease

Graves disease is an autoimmune disorder affecting the thyroid. It is the cause of most cases of hyperthyroidism in pregnancy (ACOG, 2020f; Cunningham et al., 2022). Untreated hyperthyroidism increases the risk for preeclampsia with severe features, heart failure, and thyroid storm in the pregnant client. Effects on the fetus and neonate include medically indicated preterm births, low birth weight, miscarriage, and stillbirth. In addition, the fetus is at risk for fetal thyrotoxicosis, which presents with fetal tachycardia and poor fetal growth (ACOG, 2020f). Thionamide medications, propylthiouracil (PTU) or methimazole, are generally effective for control of the disease. Although both are rare, methimazole is associated with an increased risk for fetal malformation, and PTU is associated with a risk for hepatotoxicity. Therefore methimazole is usually avoided during the first trimester.

PTU is used during this time, but some providers may transition the client to methimazole afterward. However, transitioning may result in a period of poor control of the disease. Risks and benefits of the medications and the disease should be discussed with the client.

Two rare but life-threatening complications of inadequately controlled hyperthyroidism are thyroid storm and thyrotoxic heart failure. Thyroid storm may be precipitated by stress such as labor and birth, infection, preeclampsia, or surgery. Symptoms include fever, tachycardia with cardiac dysrhythmia, vomiting, and stupor. Heart failure and pulmonary hypertension as a result of cardiomyopathy due to excessive thyroxine may also occur in clients with thyrotoxicosis. The cardiac decompensation is usually triggered by preeclampsia, anemia, or sepsis. Management of thyroid storm and thyrotoxic heart failure are the same and should occur in an intensive care area such as a special care unit in the labor suite. The client should receive a high dose of PTU followed by iodine then dexamethasone (ACOG, 2020f; Cunningham et al., 2022). Oxygen, IV fluids, antipyretics, and beta blockers may also be administered.

Hashimoto's Thyroiditis

Hashimoto's thyroiditis, characterized by antithyroid antibodies, causes most cases of hypothyroidism in females. Untreated hypothyroidism in pregnancy increases risk for miscarriage, preterm birth, and preeclampsia and can adversely affect the child's mental development. Thyroid-stimulating hormone (TSH) level should be tested before or in early pregnancy in clients with a personal or family history of thyroid disease, type 1 diabetes mellitus, or clinical indication of thyroid disease. Hypothyroidism is corrected with levothyroxine (ACOG, 2020f; Sullivan et al., 2021).

Rheumatoid Arthritis

Rheumatoid arthritis (RA) is an autoimmune disease with chronic inflammation of the synovial (hinged) joints.

Many clients experience improvement in symptoms of RA during pregnancy. The exact reason is unclear, but improvement is reported to parallel the rise in regulatory T cells during pregnancy, which suppresses inflammatory reactions. Hormonal factors also have been suggested. Unfortunately, a relapse (postpartum flare) typically occurs within 3 months after birth (Benson & Branch, 2021).

The risk for pregnancy complications due to RA are small. There is a slight increased risk of miscarriage, possible preterm birth, small-for-gestational-age (SGA) infant, and gestational hypertension. However, some antirheumatic medications may be contraindicated in pregnancy. A preconception visit to the health care provider allows assessment of risks and appropriate management of medications.

Neurologic Disorders
Seizure Disorders

Seizures are the most common form of epilepsy, which is a recurrent disorder of cerebral function. Epilepsy effects less than 1% of pregnant clients (Douglas & Aminoff, 2019). Most seizures in adults are focal, meaning they originate in a localized area of the brain. Seizure control is a priority of treatment for the pregnant client (Cunningham et al., 2022).

The effect of pregnancy on the course of epilepsy is variable and unpredictable. For most clients, the frequency of seizures remains the same; less than one-third of the clients will have an increase in the frequency, and less than one-fourth will decrease (Bhatia et al., 2021). In general, the longer the client has been seizure-free before pregnancy and the less frequent seizures occur, the less likely is the occurrence of seizures during pregnancy. No seizures for at least 9 months prior to pregnancy is associated with good seizure control during pregnancy (Bhatia et al., 2021; Cunningham et al., 2022; Douglas & Aminoff, 2019).

The effect of epilepsy on pregnancy can be significant. Clients with epilepsy have a slightly increased incidence of miscarriage, antepartum and postpartum hemorrhage, hypertensive disorders, placental abruption, preterm birth, IUGR, labor induction, and cesarean birth (Salman et al., 2018; Viale et al., 2015). There may also be an increased risk for death and postpartum depression (Cunningham et al., 2022). Seizures during pregnancy increase the risk to the client and fetus, yet many anticonvulsants have a teratogenic effect on the fetus. Comprehensive care by an interprofessional health care team with preconception care, close medical supervision, and inclusion of the client and family in the development of the plan of care can minimize the risks associated with seizure disorder allowing most of these clients a successful pregnancy (Bhatia et al., 2021).

A major concern is the teratogenic effects of anticonvulsant drugs on the fetus. Valproic acid is associated with an increase in major congenital malformations such as neural tube defects, cleft lip and cleft palate, cardiac defects, and others. It is also associated with increased rates of cognitive and behavioral deficits. A specific syndrome known as fetal hydantoin syndrome, which includes craniofacial abnormalities, limb reduction defects, growth restriction, and intellectual disability, has been described with use of phenytoin during pregnancy. Other anticonvulsants such as trimethadione, paramethadione, and carbamazepine also are associated with malformation syndromes. Lamotrigine and levetiracetam have lower rates of structural and cognitive effects and are now the most commonly used anticonvulsants during pregnancy (Bhatia et al., 2021).

Despite the risks associated with anticonvulsant medications, the risk of untreated or undertreated epilepsy exceeds the risk of the anticonvulsants. The goal is to control seizures prior to conception and during the pregnancy with the lowest dosage of medication with the lowest risk of fetal effects. It is important to counsel the client on the necessity of continued anticonvulsant therapy during pregnancy and the potential complications associated with abrupt discontinuation. Normal physiologic alterations in pregnancy such as vomiting, reduced gastric motility, use of gastrointestinal medications, and weight gain affect the absorption and distribution of anticonvulsant drugs. Serum levels of anticonvulsants should be monitored before, during, and after pregnancy with adjustment in dosages as indicated.

Some anticonvulsant drugs compete with folate for absorption, which may result in folate deficiency; many interfere with the production of vitamin D. Folic acid supplementation before and during pregnancy is recommended, and some clients may need additional vitamin D. Because of the risk for IUGR, an accurate gestational age should be determined early in the pregnancy. Fetal testing may include an alpha-fetoprotein screen for NTD and a specialized anatomic sonogram for congenital anomalies. After birth, the serum levels of anticonvulsants may drop; therefore continued evaluation with adjustments in dosage is recommended. Although most anticonvulsants are found in breast milk, at this time there is insufficient data to outweigh the known benefits of breast-feeding (Bhatia et al., 2021). However, sleep deprivation may increase the risk for seizures. The partner or other support person should be available to assist with nighttime feedings to allow the client 6 to 8 hours of uninterrupted sleep each night. The client should be taught to pump following daytime feedings to establish and maintain a supply of milk for nighttime feedings. Other safety measures to cover in discharge planning include the need for another adult to be present when the client bathes the baby, change diapers on a pad on the floor instead of a changing table, avoid stairs if possible, and use a stroller rather than an infant carrier strapped to the client's body. Because clients with epilepsy are at increased risk for peripartum mood disorders, signs and symptoms, as well as resources and contact information for health care providers, should be discussed with the client and family (Bhatia et al., 2021).

Bell's Palsy

Bell's palsy is a sudden unilateral neuropathy of the seventh cranial (facial) nerve that causes facial paralysis with weakness of the forehead and lower face. No cause for the neuropathy is often identified, although reactivation of a viral infection and inflammation of the facial nerve are possible causes. It is more common in females and rates increase during pregnancy. The effect of pregnancy on the prognosis for Bell's palsy is unclear (Cunningham et al., 2022).

The face feels stiff and pulled to one side. Closing the eye on the affected side may be difficult or impossible. Difficulty with eating or fine facial movements may occur. The ability to taste also may be disturbed.

Treatment is controversial. Some providers prescribe steroids within the first few days. Supportive care includes applying a patch over the eye and applying ointment or eye drops to prevent dryness or injury to the exposed cornea. Facial massage may be helpful, and the client should be cautioned to chew carefully to avoid biting the inside of the mouth or tongue. Psychological support is necessary to assist the client and family deal with the anxiety they naturally feel when sudden paralysis of the face occurs. They should be reassured that the condition is temporary in the majority of clients who have Bell's palsy.

> **? KNOWLEDGE CHECK**
>
> 39. What are the effects of SLE on the pregnant client and fetus?
> 40. In what ways does pregnancy affect RA?
> 41. How can Hashimoto's thyroiditis affect the newborn?
> 42. What is the major concern about administering anticonvulsant drugs for the pregnant client with epilepsy?
> 43. What is the recommended supportive care for pregnant clients with Bell's palsy?

INFECTIONS DURING PREGNANCY

Some infections acquired during pregnancy can adversely affect the health of the fetus, the pregnant client, or both. Some are mild or even subclinical in the pregnant client and yet may cause severe birth defects or death of the fetus. Other infections may have adverse effects by increasing the risk for other pregnancy complications such as preterm labor. Some infections are transmitted primarily or exclusively by sexual means, whereas others may have different modes of transmission.

The wide variety of infections affecting pregnancy care are divided into those caused by viruses and those caused by other organisms. Table 10.8 presents nursing considerations related to major STIs and vaginal infections and summarizes UTIs and their effects on pregnancy.

Viral Infections

Pregnancy does not worsen the effects of most viral infections. Although viral infections may be mild or even asymptomatic in pregnant clients, fetal and neonatal consequences can be catastrophic. Perinatal infections with cytomegalovirus (CMV), rubella, varicella-zoster virus, herpes simplex, hepatitis B, and HIV have the greatest potential for causing harm to the fetus or newborn. SARS-CoV-2, the virus that causes COVID-19, also has significant implications for the pregnant client, fetus, and newborn.

Cytomegalovirus

CMV, a member of the herpes virus group, is widespread and eventually infects most humans. CMV has been isolated from urine, saliva, blood, cervical mucus, semen, breast milk, and stool (Bernstein & Lee, 2021). Transmission may occur from contamination with any of these fluids, although close personal contact is required. Highest transmission occurs from urine and saliva of infants and children infected with CMV. CMV infection during pregnancy may be primary or recurrent. Symptoms of CMV infection are so vague that the client is often unaware of the infection.

Daycare centers are a common place for transmission of CMV among children, especially toddlers, because they often share objects contaminated with saliva. Parents and caregivers of young children who attend a daycare center should be aware that a child might acquire an infection in the center and transmit it to those who are at risk for infection (Bernstein & Lee, 2021). As puberty approaches, behaviors such as kissing, sexual intercourse, and other close bodily contacts again increase the possibility that CMV infection will be transmitted.

After primary infection the virus becomes latent, but like other herpes virus infections, periodic reactivation and shedding of the virus may occur. **Seroconversion** (change in blood test from negative to positive indicating development of antibodies in response to infection or immunization) and a rise in the specific IgM antibody titer may not differentiate a primary and recurrent infection. Specific CMV IgG avidity testing may be useful for this purpose, as primary infections have low IgG avidity (Cunningham et al., 2022). Most infections are asymptomatic, so they may not be suspected during pregnancy, and testing may not be done. Diagnosis of neonatal infection is by urine culture.

Fetal and Neonatal Effects. While most infants born with CMV are asymptomatic, approximately 5% to 18% of newborns infected with CMV show signs of congenital infection

TABLE 10.8   Sexually Transmitted Infections and Urinary Tract and Vaginal Infections

Impact on Pregnancy

Effects	Nursing Considerations
Sexually Transmitted Infections (STIs)	

Syphilis (Causative Organism: Spirochete Treponema pallidum)

If untreated, infection may cross placenta to fetus and result in miscarriage, stillborn infant, hydrops, congenital anomalies, or congenital syphilis. Major signs of congenital syphilis are enlarged liver and spleen, skin lesions, rashes, osteochondritis, and rhinitis.	Benzathine penicillin G is primary treatment to cure disease in both client and fetus. Clients who are allergic are desensitized and then treated.

Gonorrhea (Causative Organism: Bacterium Neisseria gonorrhoeae)

Transmission from client to newborn most often occurs during birth and may cause ophthalmia neonatorum. Infection during pregnancy may result in amniotic infection syndrome, which is associated with preterm rupture of the fetal membranes and increases the risk for preterm birth and neonatal infection. There is a high rate of coinfection with chlamydia.	Cephalosporins such as ceftriaxone are recommended for gonorrhea during pregnancy. Because 20%–50% of clients with gonorrhea also have chlamydial infection, azithromycin is recommended to accompany gonorrhea treatment. Partner also should be treated to prevent reinfection. Infants are treated with an ophthalmic antibiotic such as erythromycin at birth to prevent ophthalmia neonatorum. Tetracycline should not be used in a pregnant client for chlamydial infection that often accompanies gonorrhea.

Chlamydial Infection (Causative Organism: Bacterium Chlamydia trachomatis)

Chlamydial infection is most common bacterial STI in United States and often accompanies gonorrhea. Fetus may be infected during birth and suffer neonatal conjunctivitis or pneumonitis. Chlamydia may be responsible for premature rupture of membranes, premature birth, low birth weight, and neonatal death.	Education is particularly important because infection is usually asymptomatic. Both partners should be treated to prevent recurrent infection. As with all STIs, use of condoms decreases risk for infection. Azithromycin or amoxicillin is recommended treatment during pregnancy. Tetracycline should not be used during pregnancy.

Trichomoniasis (Causative Organism: Protozoan Trichomonas vaginalis)

Common cause of vaginitis in pregnant clients. Associated with premature rupture of membranes and postpartum endometritis.	Metronidazole (Flagyl), may be given to pregnant client as 2-g single oral dose. Some sources recommend withholding breastfeeding during treatment and 12–24 hours after last dose. Consistent association between fetal abnormalities or injury and metronidazole use has not been upheld.

Condyloma Acuminatum (Causative Organism: Human Papillomavirus [HPV])

Transmission of condyloma acuminatum, also called venereal or genital warts, may occur during vaginal birth and is associated with development of epithelial tumors of mucous membranes of larynx in children. Pregnancy can cause proliferation of lesions, which are associated with cervical dysplasia and cancer.	Common choices for nonpregnant therapy (podophyllin, podofilox, imiquimod) are not recommended during pregnancy. Excision of lesions by cryotherapy or cautery may be done. HPV vaccine is available to protect against the HPV strains that are the most common cause of cervical cancer (and some cancers of the vulva, vagina, anus, and oropharynx) and genital warts. Routine immunization of females should start at 11–12 years but can start as young as 9 years.

| **Vaginal Infections** | |

Candidiasis (Causative Organism: Candida albicans—Yeast)

Oral candidiasis (thrush) may develop in newborns if vaginal infection is present at birth. Thrush is treated with application of nystatin (Mycostatin) over surfaces of oral cavity four times a day for several days. Characteristic "cottage cheese" vaginal discharge with vulvar pruritus, burning, and dyspareunia. Vulva may be red, tender, and edematous.	C. albicans is part of the normal vaginal flora but may become pathogenic if the yeast becomes excessive. Candidiasis is a persistent problem for many clients during pregnancy. Examples of treatment choices include topical nystatin, miconazole, clotrimazole, butoconazole terconazole, and tioconazole. Fluconazole (oral agent) should be avoided in the first trimester.

Effects	Nursing Considerations

TABLE 10.8 Sexually Transmitted Infections and Urinary Tract and Vaginal Infections—cont'd

Bacterial Vaginosis (Causative Organism: Gardnerella vaginalis)

Adverse pregnancy outcomes include preterm rupture of membranes, preterm labor and birth, intraamniotic infection, and postpartum endometritis. Marked by a major shift in vaginal flora from normal predominance of lactobacilli to predominance of anaerobic bacteria. Causes, malodorous, "fishy" vaginal discharge. "Clue cells" may be seen microscopically in a wet mount preparation of vaginal secretions.

Metronidazole vaginal application or clindamycin oral therapy for 7 days is recommended during pregnancy. Clinical trials have shown that clients at high risk for preterm birth may benefit from this medication regimen.

Urinary Tract Infections

Asymptomatic Bacteriuria (Causative Organisms: Escherichia coli, Klebsiella, Proteus)

Ascending bacterial infection can result in cystitis or and pyelonephritis if condition remains untreated. Pyelonephritis can lead to sepsis, ARDS, and preterm birth.

Treated with the same antibiotics as cystitis (see below).

Cystitis (Causative Organisms: E. coli, Klebsiella, Proteus)

Signs and symptoms include dysuria, frequency, urgency, and suprapubic tenderness. Ascending infection may lead to pyelonephritis.

Antibiotics used for both asymptomatic bacteriuria and cystitis may include amoxicillin, ampicillin, trimethoprim-sulfamethoxazole, or nitrofurantoin. Emphasize importance of reporting signs of urinary tract infection. Stress importance of taking all medication prescribed in the treatment course even if symptoms abate. Provide information about hygiene measures such as front-to-back perineal care after urination or bowel movements.

Acute Pyelonephritis (Causative Organisms: E. coli, Klebsiella, Proteus)

Increased risk for preterm labor and premature delivery. Complications include a high fever, flank pain, septic shock, and adult respiratory distress syndrome. Pregnant clients often require hospitalization for acute care.

Inform clients with asymptomatic bacteriuria or cystitis of signs and symptoms, such as sudden onset of fever (often higher than 102.2°F [39°C]), chills, flank pain or tenderness, nausea, and vomiting so that treatment can begin promptly. Skin cooling equipment may be used to lower temperature below 100.4°F (38°C), reducing possible compromise of fetal oxygen level. Client may be hospitalized for intravenous administration of antibiotics. Common combinations include ampicillin or a cephalosporin plus an aminoglycoside. Serum levels of aminoglycosides are often measured to ensure an adequate dose without reaching a toxic level.

Data from Duff, W. (2021). Maternal and perinatal infection in pregnancy: Bacterial. In M. B. Landon, H. L. Galan, R. M. Jauniaux, D. A. Driscoll, et al. (Eds.), *Gabbe's obstetrics: Normal and problem pregnancies* (8th ed., pp. 1124–1144). Elsevier.; Duff, P. (2019). Maternal and fetal infections. In R. Resnik, C. J. Lockwood, T. R. Moore, M. F. Greene, J. A. Copel & R. M. Silver (Eds.), *Creasy & Resnik's maternal-fetal medicine: principles and practice* (8th ed., pp. 862–918). Elsevier; CDC (2020.07.10). Syphilis. https://www.cdc.gov/nchhstp/pregnancy/effects/syphilis.html.

at birth, which may include jaundice, petechiae, thrombocytopenia, growth restriction, and hydrops. Long-term effects include intellectual and physical disability, seizures, and sensorineural deficits. Congenital CMV is the most common cause of hearing loss in children (Bernstein & Lee, 2021).

Therapeutic Management. No effective therapy is currently available for the treatment of congenital CMV infection. Ultrasound scanning may identify manifestations of the infection, such as cranial abnormalities or growth restriction. The best defense against acquisition of CMV for the pregnant client is good hygiene, especially handwashing. This is most important for clients who care for small children (Bernstein & Lee, 2021; Cunningham et al., 2022).

Rubella

Rubella is caused by a virus transmitted from person to person through droplets or through direct contact with articles contaminated by nasopharyngeal secretions. Rubella infection after birth is a mild disease, but congenital rubella could have severe consequences for the newborn. Common rubella signs, and symptoms include fever, general malaise, and a characteristic maculopapular rash that begins on the face and migrates over the body. Fewer than 10% of pregnant clients are nonimmune because infection or vaccination confers permanent immunity.

The overall incidence of rubella has declined since the vaccine became available in 1969. Most cases of rubella occur in unvaccinated persons (Bernstein & Lee, 2021). The decline in adult rubella has virtually eliminated congenital rubella in the United States.

Fetal and Neonatal Effects. Rubella virus from the pregnant client can cross the placenta and infect the fetus at any time during pregnancy. The greatest risk to the fetus is during the first trimester, when miscarriage and congenital rubella syndrome are likely. Most often, the symptoms of congenital rubella syndrome are growth restriction and deafness. Other symptoms include developmental delay, cataracts, cardiac defects, and microcephaly. As pregnancy progresses, the effects on the fetus of and infection in the pregnant client decreases (Bernstein and Lee, 2021). Infants born to clients who had rubella during pregnancy shed the virus for many months and therefore pose a threat to other infants and susceptible adults who come in contact with them.

Therapeutic Management. Prevention is the only effective protection for the fetus. People who are immune do not become infected, so determining the immune status of all childbearing aged clients is critical. Those who are not immune should be vaccinated before they become pregnant, and they should be advised not to become pregnant for 28 days after vaccination because of the possible risk to the fetus from the live-virus vaccine. However, there are no known cases of congenital rubella developing in infants of clients who inadvertently received an immunization during pregnancy (Bernstein & Lee, 2021). Many nonimmune clients are vaccinated during the postpartum period. In most facilities, anyone of childbearing age must read and sign a document indicating they understand the risks to the fetus if they become pregnant within 28 days.

Varicella-Zoster Virus

Varicella infection (chickenpox) is caused by varicella-zoster virus (VZV), a herpes virus transmitted by direct contact or through the respiratory tract. Over 90% of people will have varicella infection before reaching reproductive age. After the primary varicella infection, the virus can become latent in the nerve ganglia. If VZV is reactivated, herpes zoster (shingles) results. Complications of acute varicella infection in the pregnant client may include preterm labor, encephalitis, and varicella pneumonia, which is the most serious complication associated with VZV. Varicella immunization has resulted in a marked decrease in children's varicella, well before they reach the reproductive age.

Fetal and Neonatal Effects. Spontaneous abortion (miscarriage), fetal death, and congenital varicella may result from varicella infection in the pregnant client. The frequency of fetal and neonatal effects depend on the time of infection. If the infection occurs during the first trimester, the fetus has a small risk for congenital varicella syndrome (0.4%). The greatest risk for development of congenital varicella

syndrome occurs during 13 to 20 weeks of gestation (2% of births) (Bernstein & Lee, 2021). Clinical findings include limb hypoplasia, cutaneous scars, chorioretinitis, cataracts, microcephaly, and IUGR.

The infant who is infected during the perinatal period (5 days before through 2 days after birth) will not have the benefit of antibodies from the pregnant client. Five days before birth is not sufficient time for the pregnant client to develop antibodies to VZV and pass them to the fetus, which leaves the infant at risk for life-threatening neonatal varicella infection. Varicella-zoster immune globulin (VZIG or VariZIG) or antiviral agents such as acyclovir or valacyclovir is indicated for the infant infected perinatally.

Therapeutic Management. Immune testing may be recommended for pregnant clients who are presumed to be susceptible. VZIG should be administered to those who have been exposed and whose fetuses are at high risk for congenital varicella syndrome, although this may not prevent primary infection. Clients infected with varicella during pregnancy should be instructed to report pulmonary symptoms immediately. Hospitalization, fetal surveillance, full respiratory support, and hemodynamic monitoring should be available for clients diagnosed with varicella-zoster pneumonia because it may become severe in a short time. Acyclovir is the primary drug used to treat varicella quickly.

For infants born to a client infected with varicella during the perinatal period, immunization with VZIG as soon as possible but within 96 hours of birth provides passive immunity against varicella. Clients and their infants with varicella are highly contagious and should be placed in airborne and contact isolation. Only staff members known to be immune to varicella should come in contact with these clients.

Adult immunization with the live attenuated varicella vaccine (Varivax) is recommended for nonpregnant adults who have no evidence of having had varicella. A pregnant client should not be immunized, but members of the household may be immunized because the vaccine is not transmissible from one person to another. A nonimmune postpartum client should receive the vaccine before discharge and a second dose 4 to 8 weeks postpartum. They should be instructed to avoid pregnancy for 1 month after each of the two injections. Nonimmune health care workers should be immunized (CDC, 2021a).

Herpes Simplex Virus

Genital herpes is one of the most common STIs in the herpes simplex virus (HSV) group. It may be caused by HSV type 1 or 2. Most infections of genital herpes are caused by type 2. HSV infection occurs as a result of direct contact of the skin or mucous membrane with an active lesion. Lesions form at the site of contact and begin as a group of painful papules that progress rapidly to become vesicles, shallow ulcers, pustules, and crusts. The infected person sheds the virus until the lesions are healed. The virus then migrates along the sensory nerves to reside in the sensory ganglion, and the disease enters a latent phase. It can be reactivated later as a recurrent infection. Many clients infected with HSV do not have signs and symptoms of infection and thus may shed the virus unknowingly (ACOG, 2020g; Bernstein & Lee, 2021).

In a pregnant client with active lesions or prodromal symptoms, vertical transmission (from client to infant) generally occurs in one of two ways: (1) after rupture of membranes, when the virus ascends from active lesions or (2) during birth, when the fetus comes in contact with infectious genital secretions.

Fetal and Neonatal Effects. Neonatal herpes infection is uncommon but potentially devastating. The neonate may have lesions limited to skin, eyes, and mouth (SEM), systemic (disseminated) infection, or CNS disease (ACOG, 2020g; Bernstein & Lee, 2021). Symptoms of SEM and disseminated infection usually appear within the first week; CNS disease occurs during the second or third week after birth (Bernstein & Lee, 2021). Disseminated disease is associated with a 30% mortality rate; CNS disease with a 4% rate. However, the majority (83%) of survivors of disseminated disease have normal neurologic development compared with only 31% of the CNS disease survivors (ACOG, 2020g; Bernstein & Lee, 2021). The risk for neonatal infection is greatest if the pregnant client has a primary (rather than recurrent) infection during the perinatal period. This is most likely because the amount of virus shed is higher during a primary infection than during subsequent ones (Bernstein & Lee, 2021).

Therapeutic Management. No known cure for herpes infection exists, although antiviral chemotherapy (acyclovir or valacyclovir) is prescribed at the time of an outbreak to reduce severity and duration of symptoms and shorten the duration of viral shedding. Clients with a clinical history of genital herpes should be offered antiviral therapy beginning and 36 weeks of gestation to decrease the risk of transmission to the fetus/neonate; if a primary outbreak occurs during the third trimester, the medication may be continued until birth (ACOG, 2020g).

For clients with a history of genital herpes, vaginal birth is allowed if there are no genital lesions or prodromal symptoms at the time of labor. Cesarean birth is recommended for clients with active lesions or prodromal symptoms. A cesarean birth is also offered to any client with HSV infection at any time during the third trimester due to the possibility of prolonged viral shedding. Use of fetal scalp electrodes, which cause a break in the skin, is acceptable when clinically indicated if there are no active lesions or prodromal symptoms (ACOG, 2020g).

Expectant clients need information about effective ways to deal with the emotional and physical effects of herpes. Many are concerned about privacy and do not want family members to know why special considerations are necessary. These clients should be assured that their wishes will be respected. Some clients may need an opportunity to discuss their feelings of shame, anger, or anxiety about the possible effects of the virus on their infant.

After delivery, isolation of the client from the infant is not necessary if direct contact with lesions is avoided and careful handwashing techniques are used. Breastfeeding is supported if there are no lesions on the breasts. The infant is observed for signs of infection, including temperature instability, lethargy, poor sucking reflex, jaundice, seizures, and herpetic lesions. Acyclovir therapy is prescribed for neonatal infection (Bernstein and Lee, 2021).

> ### ❓ KNOWLEDGE CHECK
>
> 44. What are the fetal and neonatal effects of CMV infection?
> 45. Why is rubella infection most dangerous in the first trimester?
> 46. How can rubella be prevented?
> 47. How are infants born to clients with varicella at the time of birth treated?
> 48. How does vertical transmission of the herpesvirus occur?

Parvovirus B19

Erythema infectiosum (also called fifth disease), caused by human parvovirus B19, is an acute, communicable disease characterized by a highly distinctive rash. The rash starts on the face with a "slapped-cheeks" appearance, followed by a generalized maculopapular rash. Other symptoms include fever, malaise, and joint pain. Erythema infectiosum is most contagious before the rash is evident. The infection is more common among children and often occurs in community epidemics. The prognosis is usually excellent. However, if the disease occurs in pregnancy, potential fetal and neonatal effects exist (CDC, 2019a). Parvovirus titers can be done if exposure during pregnancy is suspected to determine whether the client is immune. PCR analysis of viral DNA is a more sensitive test than antibodies (Bernstein & Lee, 2021).

Fetal and Neonatal Effects. Although rare, when infection occurs during pregnancy, fetal death can result, usually from failure of fetal RBC production, followed by severe fetal anemia, hydrops (generalized edema), and heart failure. The risk to the fetus is greatest when infections occur in the first 20 weeks of pregnancy. If infection is confirmed, serial sonograms are performed every 1 to 2 weeks for 8 to 12 weeks. The sonograms evaluate middle cerebral artery blood flow (MCA) and for signs of hydrops, both of which indicate fetal anemia (ACOG, 2020a; Bernstein & Lee, 2021; Duff, 2019). If anemia is suspected, fetal blood sampling with cordocentesis is performed for diagnosis. Intrauterine transfusion is an option to treat severe fetal anemia (ACOG, 2020a; Bernstein & Lee, 2021; Duff, 2019). Most infants who survive do very well, although there may be a small risk for developmental delays (Bernstein & Lee, 2021; Cunningham, 2022; Duff, 2019).

Therapeutic Management. Currently, there is no vaccine for parvovirus and no specific treatment exists; antiviral medications are not recommended. Because the virus is contagious before the onset of symptoms, and up to 20% of infected individuals are asymptomatic, it is difficult to limit potential exposure (ACOG, 2020a).

Management of symptoms in the pregnant client including starch baths may help reduce pruritus, and analgesics may be necessary to relieve mild joint pain.

Hepatitis

Multiple serotypes of hepatitis are recognized, but three are common in the United States: A, B, and C. Other serotypes such as D, E, and G require the presence of other hepatitis viruses to exist. Hepatitis A is transmitted primarily by fecal-oral contamination and can be limited by simple hygiene. Hepatitis A is rarely transmitted perinatally, and supportive care is usually sufficient. Hepatitis C is acquired through blood products. Those at higher risk include IV drug users; those with recurrent STIs, including HIV; and persons needing recurrent blood products (such as hemophiliacs). Hepatitis C may remain undiagnosed until the client develops chronic liver disease that often requires liver transplantation. The incidence of hepatitis C in pregnancy or those of childbearing age is approximately 1% to 2% (ACOG, 2021a; Bernstein & Lee, 2021; Schillie, 2018). Currently, there are no treatment options to decrease the risk of transmission of hepatitis C to the fetus or neonate.

Hepatitis B virus (HBV) is transmitted via blood, saliva, vaginal secretions, or semen and readily crosses the placenta. Mortality associated with acute hepatitis B is about 1%, but about 85% to 90% of adults recover. Chronic hepatitis B develops in 10% to 15% of infected clients, who can continue to transmit the disease to others. Persons with chronic hepatitis B also are at greater risk for chronic liver disease, cirrhosis of the liver, and primary hepatocellular carcinoma (ACOG, 2021a; Bernstein & Lee, 2021). Serologic tests confirm the diagnosis of acute and chronic hepatitis B. Persons with acute HBV are positive for the hepatitis B surface antigen (HbSag) and positive for IgM antibody. Those with chronic HBV are positive for the surface antigen (HbSag) and for the IgG antibody (Duff, 2019). Hepatitis B is preventable with a vaccine, which is safe during pregnancy. Newborn vaccination against hepatitis B starts before discharge, with the second dose given 1 to 2 months later and the third dose given at 6 to 18 months (CDC, 2019b).

The incidence of HBV has fallen significantly with screening and immunization of at-risk people, including health care providers. Goals to eliminate HBV in the United States include the following:

- Universal newborn vaccination
- Routine screening of all pregnant clients and provision of immunoprophylaxis to infants born to those infected with HBV or with unknown infection status
- Routine vaccination to unvaccinated children and adolescents
- Vaccination of adults at increased risk for infection, including health care workers, those with STIs, household contacts or sexual partners of those having chronic HBV infection, multiple sex partners, recipients of certain blood products, and dialysis clients

Fetal and Neonatal Effects. Transmission of the infection to the newborn is the greatest risk. Infection of the newborn of the HBsAg-positive client usually can be prevented by administration of hepatitis B immune globulin (HBIG, Hep-B-Gammagee) and hepatitis B vaccine (Recombivax HB, Engerix-B) within 12 hours of birth. The newborn should be carefully bathed before any injections are given to prevent infections from skin surface contamination by the virus. The infant's vaccination should be repeated at 1 to 2 months and 6 to 18 months. Breastfeeding is considered safe as long as the newborn has received HBIG and the hepatitis B vaccine (ACOG, 2021a; Bernstein & Lee, 2021).

Therapeutic Management. Hepatitis B is a preventable infection. Simple hygiene measures such as safe sex and the use of standard precautions with bodily fluids provide primary prevention. Hepatitis B vaccines are available as a series of three IM injections into the deltoid for adults, with the second and third doses given 1 and 6 months after the first. Vaccination is recommended for any population at risk, including nurses and other health care workers who frequently come in contact with body fluids.

All pregnant clients should be screened for HBsAg. Those at high risk for hepatitis should be rescreened in the third trimester if the initial screen is negative. Household members and sexual contacts should be tested and offered vaccination if they are not immune. No specific treatment exists for acute HBV infection. Recommended supportive treatment includes bed rest and a high-protein, low-fat diet.

Human Immunodeficiency Virus

Human immunodeficiency virus (HIV) is a virus that attacks the immune system. Left untreated, it can lead to the development of acquired immunodeficiency syndrome (AIDS), a failure in immune function. The person with AIDS develops opportunistic infections or malignancies that ultimately are fatal. Transmission of HIV infection is predominantly through three modes: (1) sexual exposure to secretions of an infected person, (2) parenteral exposure through IV drug use, and (3) perinatal exposure during pregnancy, birth, or breastfeeding (vertical transmission). Transmission through blood transfusion is exceedingly rare (Duff, 2019). Diagnosis and treatment during pregnancy significantly decreases the risk of perinatal transmission and maximizes the health status of the pregnant client (ACOG, 2018d).

Fetal and Neonatal Effects. When the pregnant client is infected with HIV, the risk to the fetus and neonate is transmission of the disease. Transmission of the infection may occur during pregnancy, during labor and birth, or after birth if the infant is breastfed. Appropriate treatment during the antepartum, intrapartum, and neonatal period can decrease the transmission rate from approximately 25% without treatment to 1% to 2% with treatment (ACOG, 2018d; Duff, 2019).

Therapeutic Management. Prevention remains the only way to control HIV infection. The risk for sexual transmission in sexually active individuals is decreased by a reduced number of sexual partners (mutual monogamy is best) and the use of condoms with each sexual act. IV drug users who refuse rehabilitative treatment should be taught to wash the equipment with water, soap, and bleach before each use to reduce transmission of the virus through a soiled needle.

Prevention of perinatal transmission is accomplished through routine HIV testing of all pregnant clients and combination antiretroviral therapy (ART)—the use of multiple antiretroviral drugs from different classes—for pregnant clients with HIV. In the ideal situation, ART is started before conception and continued through the antepartum, intrapartum, postpartum, and neonatal periods. If the client does not seek care, or the infection is not identified until after conception, the medications should be started as soon as possible, even if that is on arrival to the birth facility (ACOG, 2018d). Guidelines for the latest treatments from the NIH for pregnant as well as nonpregnant clients may be found at https://clinicalinfo.hiv.gov/en/guidelines/perinatal/antiretroviral-management-newborns-perinatal-hiv-exposure-or-hiv-infection.

Vaginal birth is acceptable for those clients with a viral load less than 1000 copies/mL. Cesarean birth is recommended at 38 weeks of gestation (before the onset of labor and rupture of membranes) for clients with higher loads (Bernstein & Lee, 2021; Duff, 2019). During the intrapartum period, care should be taken to minimize the opportunities for perinatal exposure such as routine use of fetal scalp electrodes, episiotomy, and instrumental delivery.

After birth, the newborn and postpartum client should continue with ART. An infected newborn may be asymptomatic at birth, but all newborns exposed to HIV perinatally, should receive ART (NIH, 2021b). Breastfeeding should be avoided in this population (Bernstein & Lee, 2021; NIH, 2021a). The infant should be bathed as soon as possible after birth (Association for Women's Health, Obstetric and Neonatal Nurses [AWHONN], 2018).

Considerations. Learning of HIV infection during pregnancy can have a devastating and immobilizing effect on the entire family. However, the prognosis of and HIV infection has changed significantly in the last 30 years. Identifying and correcting misperceptions about HIV and AIDS with client and family teaching will be important. Many people are not aware of the advances that have been made in managing HIV. Nurses frequently must determine what the family perceives as the most pressing needs and worries. Some of the most common fears are loss of control, loss of support and love, social isolation, and loss of privacy. The nurse's response may involve finding ways for the client to retain control and assisting them to select those within the family or support system who will provide continued love and emotional support. Reassuring the client that their right to privacy will not be violated is necessary.

The nurse should also provide information on routine ongoing health care. Examples are cervical cancer screening, adult immunizations, and mental health or substance abuse treatment. Instruction in signs and symptoms of postpartum depression and providing sources of assistance should be offered before discharge, just as for anyone in the postpartum period.

The client almost certainly will experience a great deal of anxiety about whether their infant will be HIV-positive. Nurses need to respond honestly that testing will be required but that most infants do not contract the virus if the medication regimen is followed carefully.

CRITICAL TO REMEMBER

Facts about Human Immunodeficiency Virus

- HIV is transmitted by sexual contact with an infected person, by sharing IV drug paraphernalia, and perinatally through the placenta at birth or through breast milk.
- During the initial phase of HIV, the person may be unaware of the infection yet highly infectious. Symptoms are vague and "flu-like." Many clients do not have any symptoms.
- There is a latent or "chronic" period from HIV infection to development of acquired immunodeficiency syndrome (AIDS). Antiretroviral therapy and supportive care can extend this phase.
- The third phase, AIDS, the immune system is severely damaged; increasing numbers of opportunistic infections occur.
- A person infected by HIV can pass the virus to another person, even without symptoms.
- There is not yet a cure for the HIV infection or AIDS. Antiretroviral medications are available to slow the replication of the virus and delay the onset of opportunistic diseases and are very effective.
- Antiretroviral treatment should be part of the medication regimen for a pregnant client to reduce the risk for transmission to the fetus. The newborn also should receive antiretroviral treatment after birth.

COVID-19

Coronaviruses are a group of viruses, some of which cause respiratory illness in humans. In December 2019, the first case of COVID-19, a disease caused by the corona virus identified as SARS-CoV-2, was reported. By early 2022, over 450 million cases and over 6 million deaths had been reported worldwide (WHO, n.d.). The pattern of the pandemic has been one of periodic surges as new variants of the virus develop.

Most people with COVID-19 will have a mild to moderate respiratory illness and will not need special care. However, severe, life-threatening disease requiring hospitalization, intensive care, and ventilatory support may develop in some people with risk factors for severe disease. Pregnancy is one of the risk factors for severe disease. Some other risk factors known at this time include most chronic diseases such as cardiovascular diseases (hypertension, cardiac disease, cerebrovascular disease), diabetes (type I, II, and gestational), obesity, respiratory diseases (asthma, COPD, cystic fibrosis), immunocompromised (cancer, HIV), liver disease, mental health conditions (depression, schizophrenia, substance abuse disorders), hemoglobinopathies (sickle cell disease, thalassemia), tuberculosis, and age >65 years (CDC, 2022c). See https://www.cdc.gov/coronavirus/2019-ncov/hcp/clinical-care/underlyingconditions.html for more complete and current information on identified risk factors.

The disease is spread by respiratory droplets. Symptoms vary but may include fever, cough, fatigue, loss of taste or smell, sore throat, headache, and body aches. Symptoms of serious disease include dyspnea, tachypnea, decreased oxygen saturations, chest pain, loss of speech, mobility, or confusion (Cunningham, 2022; WHO, 2022a). Pregnant clients with

COVID-19 are at an increased risk for preterm birth and fetal demise (CDC, 2022d). They may also be at increased risk for hypertensive conditions of pregnancy, including preeclampsia, other infections, heavy postpartum bleeding, and coagulopathies (ACOG, 2022c).

Fetal and Neonatal Effects. Effects of COVID-19 infection on the fetus are being studied. At this time, vertical transmission to the fetus appears to be rare; severity of the disease in the neonate varies from asymptomatic to severe (Cunningham, 2022). Newborns can become infected after birth if exposed to the virus.

Therapeutic Management. Supportive care is appropriate for most pregnant clients with COVID-19. Clients with additional risk factors for severe disease may be offered monoclonal antibodies. Other treatments to decrease the risk of progression to severe disease are under development and may be appropriate for pregnant clients. Current evidence supports rooming in after birth; the risk for the newborn becoming infected from the client is not increased by remaining in the same room. However, the bassinet may be kept 6 feet from the client's bed. The client should thoroughly wash their hands before touching the baby and wear a mask when within 6 feet. Face coverings should not be used on newborns. Studies demonstrate that the virus does not pass into breast milk, but maternal antibodies probably do. Therefore breastfeeding is supported (ACOG, 2022c).

Recommendations for management of pregnant clients with COVID-19 are updated frequently based on evidence from ongoing research. Current recommendations can be found on the ACOG website (https://www.acog.org/womens-health/faqs/coronavirus-covid-19-pregnancy-and-breastfeeding; https://www.acog.org/clinical-information/physician-faqs/covid-19-faqs-for-ob-gyns-obstetrics); the CDC website (https://www.cdc.gov/coronavirus/2019-ncov/need-extra-precautions/pregnant-people.html#anchor_1614967129618); or the NIH website (https://www.covid19treatmentguidelines.nih.gov/special-populations/pregnancy/).

Prevention of infection is the best treatment option. Nonpharmacologic interventions such as wearing a mask, hand hygiene, and distancing of at least 6 feet from others are important techniques to decrease the risk of infection with COVID-19. Vaccination against COVID-19 is strongly recommended by ACOG (2022c) and the CDC (2022b). The evidence continues to increase demonstrating that COVID vaccines are effective in decreasing the risk of severe disease in pregnancy and lactation. The evidence is also demonstrating that the vaccines are not only safe for pregnant and lactating clients and their fetuses and newborns, but they also provide protection to the newborn after birth (ACOG, 2022c; CDC, 2022b).

Considerations. The global COVID-19 pandemic is rapidly evolving with new information available every day. Social media and online resources provide easily accessible information. An important role of all health care providers, especially nurses, is to help clients navigate the information. It is important to direct clients and families to reliable sources for information and to correct misperceptions. Some of the reliable websites include ACOG's client information site at https://www.acog.org/womens-health/resources-for-you?utm_source=redirect&utm_medium=web&utm_campaign=otn#f:@patientportalcontenttype=[faqs] and the CDC page for pregnant and recently pregnant people at https://www.cdc.gov/coronavirus/2019-ncov/need-extra-precautions/pregnant-people.html#anchor_1614967129618. Health care providers are expected to stay up to date with the information for client care as it becomes available. This can be achieved with resources provided by membership in professional organizations such as the American Nurses Association (ANA) and AWHONN.

KNOWLEDGE CHECK

49. What are the fetal and neonatal effects of parvovirus B19 infection?
50. How is HBV transmitted? How are newborns treated?
51. How can HIV infection be prevented?
52. What is the medical management for a pregnant client with HIV infection?
53. What are the benefits of COVID vaccination for the pregnancy client?

Nonviral Infections

Toxoplasmosis

Toxoplasmosis is a protozoan infection caused by *Toxoplasma gondii*. Infection is transmitted through organisms in raw and undercooked meat, through contact with infected cat feces or soil, and across the placenta to the fetus if the expectant client acquires the infection during pregnancy. Poor handwashing and sanitation of surfaces after food preparation increases the risk for toxoplasmosis.

Toxoplasmosis often is subclinical. The pregnant person may experience a few days of fatigue, muscle pains, and swollen glands but may be unaware of the disease. If the infection is suspected, diagnosis can be confirmed by positive results of serologic tests for IgG and IgM or PCR tests (ACOG, 2020a; Duff, 2019). Immune-compromised persons such as clients who received transplants or those infected with HIV are more likely to have severe toxoplasmosis infection.

Fetal and Neonatal Effects. Although toxoplasmosis may remain unnoticed in the pregnant client, it may cause abortion (miscarriage) or result in the birth of an infant with the disease. Approximately 40% of infants born to those who had an acute primary infection during pregnancy have congenital toxoplasmosis. More than 50% of affected infants may be asymptomatic at birth, but others have serious effects such as enlarged liver and spleen, chorioretinitis, ascites, rash, seizures, intellectual disability, periventricular calcifications, and ventriculomegaly. Severe complications may develop several years after birth (Duff, 2021). Early treatment of the pregnant client can reduce the incidence of congenital infection especially in the first two trimesters (CDC, 2022a; Duff, 2021).

Therapeutic Management. All pregnant clients should be advised to do the following to decrease the risk of infection:

- Cook meat, particularly pork, beef, and lamb, thoroughly until the juices run clear.
- Avoid touching the mucous membranes of your mouth and eyes while handling raw meat.
- Avoid eating undercooked or raw clams, mussels, or oysters.
- Wash all surfaces that come in contact with uncooked meat.
- Wash your hands thoroughly after handling raw meat.
- Avoid uncooked eggs and unpasteurized milk.
- Wash fruits and vegetables before consumption.
- Avoid contact with materials that are possibly contaminated with cat feces (such as cat litter boxes, sandboxes, garden soil).

If infection occurs, treatment of toxoplasmosis during pregnancy is essential to reduce the risk for congenital infection of the fetus. Sulfonamides can be used alone but are less effective than combination therapy. Spiramycin is the recommended treatment for toxoplasmosis in pregnancy (ACOG, 2020a; Duff, 2021).

Group B Streptococcus Infection

Group B *Streptococcus* (GBS) is a leading cause of life-threatening perinatal infections in the United States. The Gram-positive bacterium colonizes the rectum, vagina, cervix, and urethra of pregnant as well as nonpregnant clients. Approximately 20% to 25% of pregnant clients are colonized by GBS in the vaginal or rectal area (Duff, 2021), but isolating the organism is often possible only intermittently. Frequently, these clients are asymptomatic, although symptomatic infections, including UTIs and intrauterine infections (chorioamnionitis and endometritis) can occur. GBS is also associated with preterm labor and preterm prelabor rupture of the membranes (PPROM). Most clients respond quickly to antimicrobial therapy which, when given intravenously during labor, is most effective in preventing neonatal infection (ACOG, 2020c; CDC, 2020b; Duff, 2021).

Fetal and Neonatal Effects. Early onset newborn GBS disease occurs during the first week after birth, often within 48 hours. Pregnant clients who have GBS in the rectovaginal area at the time of birth have a 60% chance of transmitting the organism to the newborn, and about 1% to 2% of these infants will develop early-onset GBS disease (ACOG, 2020c). Sepsis, pneumonia, and meningitis are the primary infections in early-onset GBS disease (AAP & ACOG, 2017). Late-onset GBS disease occurs after the first week of life, and meningitis, pneumonia, and bacteremia are the most common clinical manifestations (ACOG, 2020c; Duff, 2021).

Therapeutic Management. Health care providers have difficulty identifying pregnant clients who are asymptomatic GBS carriers because the duration of carrier status is unpredictable. Optimal identification of the GBS carrier status is obtained by vaginal and rectal culture between 36^0 and 37^6 weeks of gestation. Cesarean birth before membrane rupture does not require GBS antibiotic therapy.

Penicillin is the first-line agent for antibiotic treatment of the infected clients during birth. Cephazolin is the alternative for the client with non–life-threatening penicillin allergy. Vancomycin is used for the client at high risk for anaphylaxis; clindamycin may be used if the organism is known to be susceptible (ACOG, 2020c; Duff, 2021). Administration of antibiotic therapy at least 4 hours before birth is ideal.

Tuberculosis

Tuberculosis (TB) results from infection with *Mycobacterium tuberculosis*. It is transmitted by aerosolized droplets of liquid containing the bacterium, which are inhaled by a noninfected individual and taken into the lung. TB can remain inactive or become active. Most pregnant clients diagnosed with TB have inactive, asymptomatic disease and are not contagious. If the TB infection becomes active, there is an increased risk for preterm birth, low birth weight, IUGR, cesarean birth, and perinatal mortality (Pacheco et al., 2021). Clients at risk for active TB should be screened during prenatal care if they are not already known to be positive. This screening involves an intradermal injection of mycobacterial protein (purified protein derivative [PPD]), which is safe and valid for use during pregnancy. If the reaction is positive or the client is already known to have a positive reaction, sputum samples should be collected and a chest radiograph is taken, with the abdomen protected by a lead shield. The client should also be assessed for physical symptoms, which include general malaise, fatigue, loss of appetite, weight loss, and fever. Symptoms occur in the late afternoon and evening and are accompanied by night sweats. As the disease progresses, a chronic cough develops, and mucopurulent sputum is produced; hemoptysis may develop (Pacheco et al., 2021).

Fetal and Neonatal Effects. Although perinatal infection is rare, TB may be transmitted to the fetus in utero or as a result of the fetus swallowing or aspirating infected amniotic fluid or vaginal secretions at birth (Miele et al., 2020). Signs of congenital TB include lethargy, respiratory distress, fever, and enlargement of the spleen and liver (Yeh et al., 2019). If the postpartum client remains untreated, the newborn is at high risk for acquiring TB by inhalation of infectious respiratory droplets from the infected person.

Therapeutic Management. Untreated TB poses a greater hazard to the fetus than its treatment (CDC, 2020c). The preferred treatment for a pregnant client with active TB is isoniazid (INH) and rifampin (RIF) with or without ethambutol (EMB) daily for 2 months, followed by INH and RIF daily or twice weekly for 7 months, for 9 months of total treatment duration. Pyridoxine (vitamin B_6) should be given with isoniazid to prevent fetal neurotoxicity and because pregnancy itself increases the demand for this vitamin (Pacheco et al., 2021; Whitty & Dombrowski, 2019). Drug resistance in the TB organism may require addition of other drugs, although the following drugs are not recommended in pregnancy: streptomycin, kanamycin, capreomycin, ethionamide, cycloserine, pyrazinamide, amikacin, and fluoroquinolones (CDC, 2020c; Pacheco et al., 2021).

Management of the infant born to a client with TB involves preventing the disease and treating the infection early. If the client's sputum is free of organisms, the infant does not need to be isolated. Breastfeeding is safe once the postpartum client is no longer infectious (latent TB or after at least 2 weeks of treatment for active TB). Although small amounts of the medications may be secreted in breast milk, the amount is not adequate for infant treatment. If the infant is also receiving treatment, the infant should not breastfeed (Whitty & Dombrowski, 2019). Drug serum levels in the infant can be measured to identify if levels are too high. Disease prevention focuses on teaching the client and the family how the disease is transmitted so that they can protect the infant and other family members from airborne

organisms. The infant should be skin-tested at birth and may be started on preventive isoniazid therapy immediately. Skin testing is repeated at 3 months. Isoniazid is usually continued for the infant until the postpartum client's TB has been inactive for at least 3 months. Infant TB medication may be stopped if the postpartum client and other family members have received full treatment and show no additional disease. If the skin test result shows conversion to positive, a full course of drug therapy should be given to the infant (AAP & ACOG, 2017; Pacheco et al., 2021).

❓ KNOWLEDGE CHECK

54. How can toxoplasmosis be prevented?
55. How is GBS colonization of the newborn prevented?
56. How is TB treated in the client? How is it diagnosed and treated in the newborn?

■ SUMMARY CONCEPTS

- The most common cause of a spontaneous abortion (miscarriage) is chromosomal abnormalities. Treatment is aimed at preventing complications such as hypovolemic shock and infection and providing emotional support for the grieving client and family.
- A common factor for ectopic pregnancy is scarring of the fallopian tubes due to pelvic infection, inflammation, or surgery. The goals of management are to prevent severe hemorrhage and preserve the fallopian tube so that future fertility is retained.
- Management of gestational trophoblastic disease (hydatidiform mole) involves two phases: (1) evacuation of the molar pregnancy and (2) follow-up for 1 year to rule out development of choriocarcinoma.
- Disorders of the placenta (placenta previa and placental abruption) are responsible for hemorrhagic conditions of the last half of pregnancy. Either condition may result in hemorrhage and death of the pregnant client or fetus.
- The cause of hyperemesis gravidarum remains unclear, but the goals of management are to prevent dehydration, malnutrition, excess weight loss, and electrolyte imbalance. Emotional support is an important responsibility of nurses, in addition to physical care.
- Classifications of hypertension during pregnancy include gestational hypertension, preeclampsia–eclampsia, chronic (preexisting or persistent) hypertension, and chronic hypertension with superimposed preeclampsia.
- Preeclampsia is caused by generalized vasoconstriction and vasospasm, which decreases circulation to all organs of the body, including the placenta. Major organs affected include the liver, kidneys, heart, and brain.
- Treatment of preeclampsia includes reduced activity, reduction of environmental stimuli, and administration of medications to prevent generalized seizures and, when necessary, administration of antihypertensive agents.

- Magnesium sulfate, used to prevent preeclampsia from progressing to generalized eclamptic seizures, may have adverse effects. Adverse effects such as respiratory depression or absent deep tendon reflexes are more likely to occur if the blood level of magnesium rises over the therapeutic range.
- Nurses monitor the client with preeclampsia to evaluate the effectiveness of medical therapy and identify signs the condition is worsening, such as increasing hyperreflexia. Nurses also control external stimuli and initiate protective measures during eclamptic seizures.
- Pregnant clients who have chronic hypertension are at increased risk for preeclampsia and should be monitored for worsening hypertension, proteinuria, change in laboratory values, or development of signs and symptoms of preeclampsia. Antihypertensive medication should be continued or initiated if blood pressure is consistently elevated above 160 mm Hg systolic and 90 to 100 mm Hg diastolic.
- Rh incompatibility can occur if an Rh-negative client conceives a child who is Rh-positive. As a result of exposure to the Rh-positive antigen, the pregnant or postpartum client may develop antibodies that cause hemolysis of fetal Rh-positive RBCs in subsequent pregnancies.
- Administration of Rho(D) immune globulin prevents production of anti-Rh antibodies, thereby preventing destruction of Rh-positive red blood cells in subsequent pregnancies.
- ABO incompatibility usually occurs when the pregnant client has type O blood and naturally occurring anti-A and anti-B antibodies, which cause hemolysis if the fetus's blood is not type O. ABO incompatibility may result in hyperbilirubinemia of the infant, but it usually presents no serious threat to the health of the child.

- The release of insulin accelerates during early pregnancy, which may result in episodes of hypoglycemia. The availability of glucose and insulin favors the development and storage of fat that the pregnant client will need later.
- Placental hormones, which reach their peak during the second and third trimesters, create resistance to insulin, resulting in increased insulin needs throughout the rest of pregnancy.
- Diabetes during pregnancy is classified according to onset preexisting the pregnancy or gestational diabetes. Gestational diabetes is diagnosed in the second or third trimester.
- Pregnant clients with risk factors for preexisting type 2 diabetes should be screened at the first prenatal visit.
- Because hyperglycemia during the first trimester increases the risk for congenital anomalies in the fetus, a major goal of management for the client with preexisting diabetes is to establish normal blood glucose levels before conception.
- In addition to having an increased risk for congenital anomalies, the infant of a client with preexisting diabetes has an increased risk for hypoglycemia, hypocalcemia, hyperbilirubinemia, and respiratory distress syndrome, IUGR, or fetal macrosomia.
- Adverse effects of gestational diabetes for the pregnant client include increased urinary tract infections, polyhydramnios, premature rupture of membranes, and the development of preeclampsia.
- Gestational diabetes increases the risk for fetal macrosomia and neonatal hypoglycemia.
- Iron supplementation often is needed during pregnancy because most pregnant clients do not have sufficient iron stores to meet the demands of pregnancy with diet alone.
- Folic acid deficiency is associated with increased risk for spontaneous abortion, placental abruption, and fetal anomalies such as neural tube defects. Folic acid supplementation of 400 mcg (0.4 mg) daily is recommended for all clients of childbearing age to reduce the risk for neural tube defects.
- Sickle cell disease often is worsened by pregnancy, and a primary goal is to prevent sickle cell crisis during pregnancy.
- Laboratory values for thalassemia are similar to those for iron deficiency. However, administration of iron is risky because increased iron absorption and storage makes the client susceptible to iron overload.
- Although the client with systemic lupus erythematosus can have a normal pregnancy and give birth to a normal newborn, the pregnancy should be treated as high-risk because of the increased incidence of abortion, fetal death during the first trimester, and possible exacerbation of the disease.
- Antiphospholipid syndrome is an autoimmune disorder associated with an increased risk for thrombosis, fetal loss, and decreased platelets. Preeclampsia is more common in the client with antiphospholipid syndrome.
- Marked improvement in rheumatoid arthritis often occurs during pregnancy, possibly as a result of pregnancy-specific hormonal factors. However, most clients relapse soon after childbirth.
- Management of epilepsy is complex because of the teratogenic effects of many anticonvulsant medications coupled with the importance of preventing seizures. Changes in anticonvulsant therapy that reduce the risks for adverse effects may be possible for the client who wants to become pregnant.
- Although Bell's palsy usually is temporary, the client may be anxious. Supportive care and emotional support are essential.
- Viral infections that occur during pregnancy can be transmitted to the fetus in two ways: across the placenta or by exposure to organisms during birth. Although they may be mild or even subclinical in the pregnant client, viral infections can have serious effects on the fetus and neonate.
- The health care team is responsible for teaching how infectious diseases can be prevented and that early treatment may reduce fetal and neonatal exposure to infections.
- Human immunodeficiency virus is a retrovirus that gradually allows a decline in the effectiveness of the client's immune response. Treatment with ART can substantially reduce transmission of the infection to the fetus and maximize the health of the pregnant client.
- Specific pregnancy and postbirth treatment of nonviral infections such as toxoplasmosis, group B *Streptococcus* infection, and tuberculosis reduce long-term complications for the client and newborn.
- Pregnancy is a risk factor for severe disease with COVID-19.

Clinical Judgment and Next-Generation NCLEX® Examination-Style Questions

Case 1

A 23-year-old, gravida 1 para 0 at 38.4 weeks' gestation presents to Labor and Delivery to rule out labor. The client denies any significant medical history. The client's obstetric history includes bed rest for the last 6 weeks due to preterm labor. Weight gain of 36 lb, current weight 163, BMI 27.1. The cervical examination on admission reveals cervical dilation of 4 cm, 90% effaced, at -1 station. Admission vital signs (VS): blood pressure (BP) 167/120, heart rate 102, respiratory rate 20, temperature 98.4°F. Repeat BP taken 15 minutes after the initial BP 143/93. Provider ordered the client to be admitted for labor, serial BPs every 15 minutes, notify the provider if BP increased above 160 systolic or 110 diastolic, and preeclampsia laboratories (comprehensive metabolic profile and urine protein creatinine ratio).

1. **For each assessment finding, use an X to indicate whether it requires nursing follow-up or is an expected (no follow-up required) finding at this time.**

Lab Results or Other Symptoms	Requires Nursing Follow-Up	Expected Finding
Platelets 90,000/μL		
Urine protein-to-creatinine ratio 0.2 mg		
Headache or visual disturbances (blurred vision, seeing spots)		
Bilateral breath sounds clear to auscultation		
Deep tendon reflexes 4+ in lower extremities		
Right-sided epigastric pain		
Bilateral lower extremity edema 1+		
Hemoglobin 8 g/dL		

Almost 8 hours after admission, the client's cervix was completely dilated. After pushing for 2 hours with no progress the provider decided a cesarean section was needed. During surgery, the client's BP increased 156/101, then 162/108. The provider ordered magnesium sulfate 4-g loading dose to be administered over a 20-minute period, followed by 2 g an hour maintenance dosing.

2. **Choose the most likely options for the information missing from the statement below by selecting from the lists of options provided.**

   Magnesium sulfate is an anticonvulsant that ____1_____ irritability in the ____2_____ and relaxes smooth muscle. Magnesium is administered either ____3_____ or ____4_____.

Option 1	Option 2	Option 3	Option 4
Depresses	Heart	Intravenously	Intravenously
Increases	Central nervous system	Intramuscularly	Intramuscularly
Does not impact	Lymphatic system	By mouth	By mouth

3. **Almost 24 hours later, the postpartum nurse performs a shift assessment. Place a check mark next to the assessment findings that require follow-up by the nurse.**
   - Complaint of shortness of breath
   - Blood pressure = 167/115 mm Hg
   - Heart rate = 138 beats/min
   - Respirations = 32 breaths/min
   - Oxygen saturation = 90% (room air)
   - Temp. 98.9°F; 37.1°C
   - Skin clammy and cool to touch
   - Mild wheezing noted to bilateral lower lung fields
   - Deep tendon reflexes = 2+ bilateral lower extremities
   - Mild edema noted in lower extremities
   - Urine output = 35 mL/hour for the past 2 hours
   - Magnesium sulfate infusing at 2 g/hour per IV pump

Case 2

A client, G_1P_0 at 32 weeks' gestation arrives to Labor and Delivery with the report of sudden onset of bright red vaginal bleeding. Assessment findings include: BP 110/62, RR 22, P 98. The nurse weighs the peripad that the client was wearing and quantifies the blood loss as 80 mL. The client is crying and fearful but denies contractions or abdominal pain.

4. **Use an X for the nursing actions below that are appropriate, contraindicated, or nonessential (makes no difference; is not necessary) for the client's care at this time.**

Nursing Action	Appropriate	Contraindicated	Nonessential
Assess fetal heart rate			
Perform vaginal examination to assess for cervical change			
Initiate IV			
Monitor output			
Assess DTRs			
Access or request prenatal record			

Case 3

A 25-year-old G_0P_0 with a 10-year history of IDDM is being seen by the nurse during an annual checkup. The client expresses a desire to have a baby and asks the nurse if the diabetes will affect pregnancy.

5. **Choose the best option for the information missing from the statement by selecting from the lists of options provided.**

   The nurse teaches the client that preexisting diabetes increases the risk for ____1_____, ____2_____, ____3_____ and ____4_____ in the pregnant client, ____5_____, ____6_____ and ____7_____ in the fetus and ____8_____, ____9_____, ____10_____ and ____11_____, in the neonate.
   In addition, during the first trimester of pregnancy, insulin requirements usually ____12_____, while in the second and third trimesters, the insulin need ____13_____.

Options for 1, 2, 3 and 4	Options for 5, 6 and 7	Options for 8, 9, 10 and 11	Options for 12	Options for 13
Cardiac decompensation	Congenital anomalies	Hypoglycemia	Increase	Increase
Miscarriage	Macrosomia (large body)	Hypocalcemia	Decrease	Decrease
Ketoacidosis	Anemia	Hyperbilirubinemia	Stay the same	Stay the same
Thromboembolism	Postterm birth	Hyperglycemia		
Anemia	Birth injury	Hypokalemia		
Birth trauma	Chromosomal abnormalities	Cold stress		
Preeclampsia		Respiratory distress syndrome		

REFERENCES

American Academy of Pediatrics (AAP) & American College of Obstetricians and Gynecologists (ACOG). (2017). *Guidelines for perinatal care* (8th ed.). American Academy of Pediatrics & American College of Obstetricians and Gynecologists.

American College of Obstetricians and Gynecologists. (2018a). Practice Bulletin No. 190: Gestational diabetes mellitus. *Obstetrics & Gynecology, 131*(2), e49–e64. https://doi.org/10.1097/AOG.0000000000002501.

American College of Obstetricians and Gynecologists (ACOG). (2018b). Practice Bulletin No. 192: Management of alloimmunization during pregnancy. *Obstetrics & Gynecology, 131*(3), e82–e90. https://doi.org/10.1097/AOG.0000000000002528.

American College of Obstetricians and Gynecologists (ACOG). (2018c). Committee Opinion No. 743: Low-Dose aspirin use during pregnancy. *Obstetrics & Gynecology, 132*(1), e44–e52. https://doi.org/10.1097/AOG.0000000000002708.

American College of Obstetricians and Gynecologists (ACOG). (2018d). Committee Opinion No. 752: Prenatal and perinatal human immunodeficiency virus testing. *Obstetrics & Gynecology, 132*, e138–e142. https://doi.org/10.1097/AOG.0000000000002825ACOG.

American College of Obstetricians and Gynecologists (ACOG). (2019a). Practice Bulletin No. 190: Gestational diabetes mellitus. *Obstetrics & Gynecology, 131*(2), e49–e64. https://doi.org/10.1097/AOG.0000000000002501. Published 2018, reaffirmed 2019.

American College of Obstetricians and Gynecologists (ACOG). (2019b). Committee Opinion No. 763: Ethical considerations for the care of patients with obesity. *Obstetrics & Gynecology, 133*(1), e90–e96. https://doi.org/10.1097/AOG.0000000000003015.

American College of Obstetricians and Gynecologists (ACOG). (2019c). Practice Bulletin No. 203: Chronic hypertension in pregnancy. *Obstetrics & Gynecology, 133*(1), e26–e50. https://doi.org/10.1097/AOG.0000000000003020.

American College of Obstetricians and Gynecologists (ACOG). (2020a). Practice Bulletin no. 151: Cytomegalovirus, parvovirus B19, varicella zoster, and toxoplasmosis in pregnancy. 2015 *Obstetrics & Gynecology, 125*(6), 1510–1525. https://doi.org/10.1097/01.AOG.0000466430.19823.53. published 2015, reaffirmed 2020.

American College of Obstetricians and Gynecologists (ACOG). (2020b). Practice Bulletin No. 201: Pregestational diabetes mellitus. *Obstetrics & Gynecology, 132*(6), e228–e248. https://doi.org/10.1097/AOG.0000000000002960. Published 2018, reaffirmed 2020.

American College of Obstetricians and Gynecologists (ACOG). (2020c). Committee Opinion No. 797: Prevention of Group B streptococcal early-onset disease in newborns. *Obstetrics & Gynecology, 135*(2), e51–e72. https://doi.org/10.1097/AOG.0000000000003668.

American College of Obstetricians and Gynecologists (ACOG). (2020d). Committee Opinion No. 804: Physical activity and exercise during pregnancy and the postpartum period. *Obstetrics & Gynecology, 135*(4), e178–e188. https://doi.org/10.1097/AOG.0000000000003772.

American College of Obstetricians and Gynecologists (ACOG). (2020e). Practice Bulletin No. 222: Gestational hypertension and preeclampsia. *Obstetrics & Gynecology, 135*(6), e237–e260. https://doi.org/10.1097/AOG.0000000000003891.

American College of Obstetricians and Gynecologists (ACOG). (2020f). Practice Bulletin No. 223: Thyroid disease in pregnancy. *Obstetrics & Gynecology, 135*(6), e261–e274. https://doi.org/10.1097/AOG.0000000000003893.

American College of Obstetricians and Gynecologists (ACOG). (2020g). Practice Bulletin No. 220: Management of genital herpes in pregnancy. *Obstetrics & Gynecology, 136*(4), 850–851. https://doi.org/10.1097/AOG.0000000000004115.

American College of Obstetricians and Gynecologists (ACOG). (2021a). Practice Bulletin No. 86: Viral hepatitis in pregnancy. *Obstetrics & Gynecology, 110*(4), 941–956. https://doi.org/10.1097/01.AOG.0000263930.28382.2a. Published 2007, reaffirmed 2021.

American College of Obstetricians and Gynecologists (ACOG). (2021b). Practice Bulletin No. 181: Prevention of Rh D alloimmunization. *Obstetrics & Gynecology, 130*(2), e57–e70. https://doi.org/10.1097/AOG.0000000000002232. Published 2017, reaffirmed 2021.

American College of Obstetricians and Gynecologists (ACOG). (2021c). *FAQ Obesity and pregnancy*. https://www.acog.org/womens-health/faqs/obesity-and-pregnancy#:~:text=Birth%20defects%E2%80%94Babies%20born%20to,anatomy%20on%20an%20ultrasound%20exam.

American College of Obstetricians and Gynecologists (ACOG). (2021d). Practice Bulletin No. 230: Obesity in pregnancy. *Obstetrics & Gynecology, 137*(6), e128–e144. https://doi.org/10.1097/AOG.0000000000004395.

American College of Obstetricians and Gynecologists (ACOG). (2021e). Practice Bulletin No. 233: Anemia in pregnancy. *Obstetrics & Gynecology, 138*(2), e55–e64. https://doi.org/10.1097/AOG.0000000000004477.

American College of Obstetricians and Gynecologists (ACOG). (2022a). Practice Bulletin No. 78: Hemoglobinopathies in pregnancy. *Obstetrics & Gynecology, 109*(1), 229–237. https://doi.org/10.1097/00006250-200701000-00055. Published 2007, reaffirmed 2022.

American College of Obstetricians and Gynecologists (ACOG). (2022b). Practice Bulletin No. 189: Nausea and vomiting of pregnancy. *Obstetrics & Gynecology, 131*(1), e15–e30. https://doi.org/10.1097/AOG.0000000000002456.

American College of Obstetricians and Gynecologists (ACOG). (2022c). *FAQ COVID-19, pregnancy, childbirth and breastfeeding: Answers from Ob-Gyns*. https://www.acog.org/womens-health/faqs/coronavirus-covid-19-pregnancy-and-breastfeeding.

American Diabetes Association (ADA). (2021a). 2. Classification and diagnosis of diabetes: Standards of medical care in diabetes-2021. *Diabetes Care, 44*(Suppl. 1), S15–S33.

American Diabetes Association (ADA). (2021b). 14. Management of diabetes in pregnancy: Standards of medical care in diabetes-2021. *Diabetes Care, 44*(Suppl. 1), S200–S210.

Association of Women's Health, Obstetrics and Neonatology. (2018). *Neonatal skin care: Evidence-based clinical practice guidelines* (4th ed.).

Ballesta-Castillejos, A., Gomez-Salgado, J., Rodriguez-Almagro, J., Ortiz-Esquinas, I., & Hernandez-Martinez, A. (2020). Relationship between maternal body mass index with the onset of breastfeeding and its associated problems: An online survey. *International Breastfeeding Journal, 15*(1), 55. https://doi.org/10.1186/s13006-020-00298-5.

Benson, A. E., & Branch, D. W. (2021). Collagen vascular diseases. In M. B. Landon, H. L. Galan, E. R. M. Jauniaux, D. A. Driscoll, V. Berghella, W. A. Grobman, et al. (Eds.), *Gabbe's obstetrics: Normal and problem pregnancies* (8th ed., pp. 987–1002). Elsevier.

Bernstein, H., & Lee, M. (2021). Maternal and perinatal infection: Viral. In M. B. Landon, H. L. Galan, R. M. Jauniaux, D. A. Driscoll, et al. (Eds.), *Gabbe's obstetrics: Normal and problem pregnancies* (8th ed., pp. 1092–1121). Elsevier.

Bhatia, R., Bevan, C., & Gerard, E. E. (2021). Neurologic disorders in pregnancy. In M. B. Landon, H. L. Galan, E. R. M. Jauniaux, D. A. Driscoll, V. Berghella, W. A. Grobman, et al. (Eds.), *Gabbe's obstetrics: Normal and problem pregnancies* (8th ed., pp. 1038–1061). Elsevier.

Blackburn, S. T. (2018). *Maternal, fetal, & neonatal physiology: A clinical perspective* (5th ed.). Elsevier.

Burgess, A. (2021). Hypertensive disorders of pregnancy. In K. R. Simpson, P. A. Creehan, N. O'Brien-Abel, C. K. Roth, & A. J. Rohan (Eds.), *Perinatal nursing* (5th ed., pp. 99–123). Wolters Kluwer.

Centers for Disease Control and Prevention (CDC). (1998). *Recommendations to prevent and control iron deficiency in the United States.* https://www.cdc.gov/mmwr/preview/mmwrhtml/00051880.htm.

Centers for Disease Control and Prevention (CDC). (2018). *Systemic lupus erythematosus.* https://www.cdc.gov/lupus/facts/detailed.html.

Centers for Disease Control and Prevention (CDC). (2019a). *Pregnancy and fifth disease.* https://www.cdc.gov/parvovirusb19/pregnancy.html.

Centers for Disease Control and Prevention (CDC). (2019b). *Hepatitis B vaccine.* https://www.cdc.gov/hepatitis/hbv/pdfs/hepbperinatal-protecthepbyourbaby.pdf.

Centers for Disease Control and Prevention (CDC). (2020a). *Hypertension: Know your risk for high blood pressure.* https://www.cdc.gov/bloodpressure/risk_factors.htm.

Centers for Disease Control and Prevention (CDC). (2020b). *Group B Strep (GBS).* https://www.cdc.gov/groupbstrep/index.html.

Centers for Disease Control and Prevention (CDC). (2020c). *Treatment of TB & pregnancy. Tuberculosis (TB).* https://www.cdc.gov/tb/topic/treatment/pregnancy.htm.

Centers for Disease Control and Prevention (CDC). (2021a). *Chickenpox (varicella).* https://www.cdc.gov/chickenpox/hcp/index.html.

Centers for Disease Control and Prevention (CDC). (2021b). *Diabetes risk factors.* https://www.cdc.gov/diabetes/basics/risk-factors.html.

Centers for Disease Control and Prevention (CDC). (2021c). *Gestational diabetes.* https://www.cdc.gov/diabetes/basics/gestational.html.

Centers for Disease Control and Prevention (CDC). (2021d). *Type 2 diabetes.* https://www.cdc.gov/diabetes/basics/type2.html.

Centers for Disease Control and Prevention (CDC). (2022a). *Parasites-toxoplasmosis (Toxoplasma infection).* https://www.cdc.gov/parasites/toxoplasmosis/health_professionals/index.html.

Centers for Disease Control and Prevention (CDC). (2022b). *Covid-19 vaccines while pregnant or breastfeeding. COVID-19.* https://www.cdc.gov/coronavirus/2019-ncov/hcp/clinical-care/underlyingconditions.html.

Centers for Disease Control and Prevention (CDC). (2022c). *Underlying medical conditions associated with higher risk for severe COVID-19: Information for healthcare professionals.* https://www.cdc.gov/coronavirus/2019-ncov/hcp/clinical-care/underlyingconditions.html.

Centers for Disease Control and Prevention (CDC). (2022d). *Investigating the impact of COVID-19 during pregnancy. Covid-19.* https://www.cdc.gov/coronavirus/2019-ncov/cases-updates/special-populations/pregnancy-data-on-covid-19/what-cdc-is-doing.html.

Cohn, D., Ramaswamy, B., Christian, B., & Bixel, K. (2019). Malignancy and pregnancy. In R. Resnik, J. D., C. J. Lockwood, T. R. Moore, et al. (Eds.), *Creasy & Resnik's maternal-fetal medicine: Principles and practice* (8th ed., pp. 1007–1024). Elsevier.

Cunningham, F. G., Leveno, K. J., Dashe, J. S., Hoffman, B. L., Spong, C. Y., & Casey, B. M. (2022). *Williams' obstetrics* (26th ed.). McGraw-Hill.

Dean, C., Bannigan, K., & Marsden, J. (2018). Reviewing the effect of hyperemesis gravidarum on women's lives and mental health. *British Journal of Midwifery, 26*(2), 109–119. https://www.magonlinelibrary.com/doi/full/10.12968/bjom.2018.26.2.109.

Dekkers, G. W. F., Broeren, M. A. C., Truijens, S. E. M., Kop, W. J., & Pop, V. J. M. (2020). Hormonal and psychological factors in nausea and vomiting during pregnancy. *Psychological Medicine, 50,* 229–236. org/10.1017/S0033291718004105.

Douglas, V. C., & Aminoff, M. J. (2019). Neurologic disorders. In R. Resnik, C. J. Lockwood, T. R. Moore, M. F. Greene, J. A. Copel, & R. M. Silver (Eds.), *Creasy & Resnik's maternal-fetal medicine: Principles and practice* (8th ed., pp. 1208–1231). Elsevier.

Druzin, M. L., Shields, L. E., Peterson, N. L., & Cape, V. (2013). *Preeclampsia toolkit: Improving health care response to preeclampsia: A California toolkit to transform maternity care. Developed under contract #11-10006 with the California Department of Public Health; Maternal, Child and Adolescent Health Division; published by the California Maternal Quality Care Collaborative.* https://pqcnc-documents.s3.amazonaws.com/cmop/cmopresources/CMQCC_Preeclampsia_Toolkit_1.17.14.pdf.

Duff, P. (2019). Maternal and fetal infections. In R. Resnik, C. J. Lockwood, T. R. Moore, M. F. Greene, J. A. Copel, & R. M. Silver (Eds.), *Creasy & Resnik's maternal-fetal medicine: Principles and practice* (8th ed., pp. 862–918). Elsevier.

Duff, W. (2021). Maternal and perinatal infection in pregnancy: Bacterial. In M. B. Landon, H. L. Galan, R. M. Jauniaux, D. A. Driscoll, et al. (Eds.), *Gabbe's obstetrics: Normal and problem pregnancies* (8th ed., pp. 1124–1144). Elsevier.

Fiaschi, L., Nelson-Piercy, C., Deb, S., King, R., & Tata, L. J. (2019). Clinical management of nausea and vomiting in pregnancy and hyperemesis gravidarum across primary and secondary care: A population-based study. *BJOG: An International Journal of Obstetrics and Gynaecology, 126*(10), 1201–1211. https://doi.org/10.1111/1471-0528.15662.

Francois, K. E., & Foley, M. R. (2021). Antepartum and postpartum hemorrhage. In M. B. Landon, H. L. Galan, E. R. M. Jauniaux, D. A. Driscoll, V. Berghella, W. A. Grobman, et al. (Eds.), *Gabbe's obstetrics: Normal and problem pregnancies* (8th ed., pp. 343–374). Elsevier.

Gregory, K. D., Ramos, D. E., & Jauniaux, E. R. M. (2021). Preconception and prenatal care. In M. B. Landon, H. L. Galan, E. R. M. Jauniaux, D. A. Driscoll, V. Berghella, W. A. Grobman, et al. (Eds.), *Gabbe's obstetrics: Normal and problem pregnancies* (8th ed., pp. 88–107). Elsevier.

Gyamfi-Bannerman, C. (2018). Society for Maternal-Fetal Medicine (SMFM) Consult series #44: Management of bleeding in the late preterm period. *American Journal of Obstetrics and Gynecology, 218*(1), B2–B8. https://doi.org/10.1016/j.ajog.2017.10.019.

Harper, L. M., Tita, A., & Ananth Karumanchi, S. (2019). Pregnancy-related hypertension. In R. Resnik, C. Lockwood, T. Moore, M. Greene, J. A. Copel, & R. M. Silver (Eds.), *Creasy & Resnik's maternal-fetal medicine: Principles and practice* (8th ed., pp. 810–838). Elsevier.

Hsiao, H. F., Thomas, A., Kay-Smith, C., & Grzeskowiak, L. E. (2021). Pregnant women report being denied medications to treat severe nausea and vomiting of pregnancy or hyperemesis gravidarum - findings from an Australian online survey. *The Australian and New Zealand Journal of Obstetrics and Gynaecology*, *61*(4), 616–620. https://doi.org/10.1111/ajo.13359.

Hu, Y., Amoah, A. N., Zhan, H., Fu, R., Qui, Y., Cao, Y., et al. (2022). Effect of finger in the treatment of nausea and vomiting compared with vitamin B_6 and placebo during pregnancy: A meta-analysis. *Journal of Maternal-Fetal and Neonatal Medicine*, *35*(1), 187–196. https://doi.org/10.1080/14767058.2020.1712714.

Hull, A. D., Resnik, R., & Silver, R. M. (2019). Placenta previa and accreta, vasa previa, subchorionic hemorrhage and abruptio placentae. In R. Resnik, C. J. Lockwood, T. R. Moore, et al. (Eds.), *Creasy & Resnik's maternal-fetal medicine: Principles and practice* (8th ed., pp. 786–797). Elsevier.

Institute of Medicine Committee to Reexamine IOM Pregnancy Weight Guidelines. (2009). *Weight gain during pregnancy: Reexamining the guidelines.* https://doi.org/10.17226/12584. https://www.nap.edu/read/12584/chapter/1.

Institute for Safe Medication Practices. (2018). *ISMP List of high alert medications in the acute care setting.* https://www.ismp.org/sites/default/files/attachments/2018-08/highAlert2018-Acute-Final.pdf.

Jacobson, J. C., & Connolly, S. (2019). First-trimester bleeding. In J. R. Butler, A. N. Amin, L. E. Fitmaurice, & C. M. Kim (Eds.), *OB/GYN hospital medicine: Principles and practice.* McGraw Hill.

Jauniaux, E. R. M., & Simpson, J. L. (2021). Pregnancy loss. In M. B. Landon, H. L. Galan, E. R. M. Jauniaux, D. A. Driscoll, V. Berghella, W. A. Grobman, et al. (Eds.), *Gabbe's obstetrics: Normal and problem pregnancies* (8th ed., pp. 615–632). Elsevier.

Kelly, T. F., & Savides, T. J. (2019). Gastrointestinal disease in pregnancy. In R. Resnik, C. J. Lockwood, T. R. Moore, M. F. Greene, J. A. Copel, & R. M. Silver (Eds.), *Creasy & Resnik's maternal-fetal medicine: Principles and practice* (8th ed., p. 1158–1072). Elsevier.

Khorasani, F., Hossein, A., Sobhi, A., Aryan, R., Abavi-Sani, A., Ghazanfarpour, M., et al. (2020). A systematic review of the efficacy of alternative medicine in the treatment of nausea and vomiting of pregnancy. *Journal of Obstetrics and Gynecology*, *40*(1), 10–19. https://doi.org/10.1080/01443615.2019.1587392.

Kilpatrick, S. J., & Kitahara, S. (2019). Anemia and pregnancy. In R. Resnik, C. J. Lockwood, T. R. Moore, M. F. Greene, J. A. Copel, & R. M. Silver (Eds.), *Creasy & Resnik's maternal-fetal medicine: Principles and practice* (8th ed., pp. 991–1006). Elsevier.

Landon, M. B., Catalano, P. M., & Gabbe, S. G. (2021). Diabetes mellitus complicating pregnancy. In M. B. Landon, H. L. Galan, E. R. M. Jauniaux, D. A. Driscoll, V. Berghella, W. A. Grobman, et al. (Eds.), *Gabbe's obstetrics: Normal and problem pregnancies* (8th ed., pp. 871–907). Elsevier.

Lee, R. H., Chung, R. T., & Pringle, P. (2019). Diseases of the liver, biliary system, and pancreas. In R. Resnik, C. Lockwood, T. Moore, M. Greene, J. A. Copel, & R. M. Silver (Eds.), *Creasy & Resnik's maternal-fetal medicine: Principles and practice* (8th ed., pp. 1173–1191). Elsevier.

Linnakaari, R., Helle, N., Mentula, M., Bloigu, A., Gissler, M., Heikinheimo, O., et al. (2019). Trends in the incidence, rate and treatment of miscarriage—nationwide register-study in Finland, 1998–2016. *Human Reproduction*, *34*(11), 2120–2128.

Louis, J. (2021). Obesity in pregnancy. In M. B. Landon, H. L. Galan, E. R. M. Jauniaux, D. A. Driscoll, V. Berghella, W. A. Grobman, et al. (Eds.), *Gabbe's obstetrics: Normal and problem pregnancies* (8th ed., pp. 908–918). Elsevier.

Magnesium Sulfate: Drug Information. (2021). www.uptodate.com/contents/magnesium-sulfate-drug-information?source=search_result&search=magnesium+sulfate&selectedTitle=1%7E147.

March of Dimes. (2020). *Exercise during pregnancy.* https://www.marchofdimes.org/pregnancy/exercise-during-pregnancy.aspx.

Miele, K., Bamrah Morris, S., & Tepper, N. (2020). Tuberculosis in pregnancy. *Obstetrics & Gynecology*, *135*(6), 1444–1453. https://doi.org/10.1097/AOG.0000000000003890.

Mobarakabadi, S. S., Shahbazzadegan, S., & Ozgoli, G. (2020). The effect of P6 acupressure on nausea and vomiting of pregnancy: A randomized, single-blind, placebo-controlled trial. *Advances in Integrative Medicine*, *7*(2), 67–72. https://doi.org/10.1016/j.aimed.2019.07.002.

Moore, T. R., Hauguel-DeMouzon, S., & Catalano, P. (2019). Diabetes in pregnancy. In R. Resnik, C. J. Lockwood, T. R. Moore, M. F. Greene, J. A. Copel, & R. M. Silver (Eds.), *Creasy & Resnik's maternal-fetal medicine: Principles and practice* (8th ed., pp. 1067–1098). Elsevier.

National Institutes of Health (2021a). HIV and AIDS: The basics. *HIV info.* https://hivinfo.nih.gov/understanding-hiv/fact-sheets/hiv-and-aids-basics.

National Institutes of Health. (2021b). *Recommendations for the use of antiretroviral drugs during pregnancy and interventions to reduce perinatal HIV transmission in the United States.* https://clinicalinfo.hiv.gov/en/guidelines/perinatal/antiretroviral-management-newborns-perinatal-hiv-exposure-or-hiv-infection.

National Institutes of Health & National Heart, Lung, & Blood Institute. (2020). *Sickle cell disease.* https://www.nhlbi.nih.gov/health-topics/sickle-cell-disease.

Ngan, H. Y. S., Seckl, M. J., Berkowitz, R. S., Xiang, Y., Golfier, F., Sekharan, P. K., et al. (2018). FIGO cancer report 2018. Update on the diagnosis and management of gestational trophoblastic disease. *International Journal of Gynecology & Obstetrics*, *143*(S2), 79–85. https://doi.org/10.1002/ijgo.12615.

Pacheco, L., Saad, A., La Rosa De Los Rios, M., & Webb, C. (2021). Respiratory diseases in pregnancy. In M. B. Landon, H. L. Galan, R. M. Jauniaux, D. A. Driscoll, et al. (Eds.), *Gabbe's obstetrics: Normal and problem pregnancies* (8th ed., pp. 844–846). Elsevier.

Preusting, I., Brumley, J., Odibo, L., Spatz, D. L., & Louis, J. M. (2017). Obesity as a predictor of delayed Lactogenesis II. *Journal of Human Lactation*, *33*(4), 684–691.

Raymond, J. L., & Morrow, K. (2021). *Krause and Mahan's food & the nutrition care process* (15th ed.). Elsevier.

Roth, C. K. (2021). Diabetes in pregnancy. In K. R. Simpson, P. A. Creehan, N. O'Brien-Abel, C. K. Roth, & A. J. Rohan (Eds.), *Perinatal nursing* (5th ed., pp. 182–199). Wolters Kluwer.

Salera-Vieira, J. (2021). Bleeding in pregnancy. In K. R. Simpson, P. A. Creehan, N. O'Brien-Abel, C. K. Roth, & A. J. Rohan (Eds.), *Perinatal nursing* (5th ed., pp. 124–141). Wolters Kluwer.

Salman, L., Shmueli, A., Ashwal, E., Hiershc, L., Hadar, E., Yogev, Y., et al. (2018). The impact of maternal epilepsy on perinatal outcome in singleton gestations. *Journal of Maternal-Fetal and Neonatal Medicine, 31*(24), 3283–3286. https://doi.org/10.1080/14767058.2017.1368483.

Sammaritano, L. R., Salmon, J. E., & Branch, D. W. (2019). Pregnancy and rheumatic diseases. In R. Resnik, C. J. Lockwood, T. R. Moore, M. F. Greene, J. A. Copel, & R. M. Silver (Eds.), *Creasy & Resnik's maternal-fetal medicine: Principles and practice* (8th ed., pp. 1192–1207). Elsevier.

Samuels, P. (2021). Hematologic complications of pregnancy. In M. B. Landon, H. L. Galan, E. R. M. Jauniaux, D. A. Driscoll, V. Berghella, W. A. Grobman, et al. (Eds.), *Gabbe's obstetrics: Normal and problem pregnancies* (8th ed., pp. 954–971). Elsevier.

Schillie, S., Vellozzi, C., Reingold, A., Harris, A., Haber, P., Ward, J. W., et al. (2018). Prevention of hepatitis B virus infection in the United States: Recommendation of the advisory committee on immunization practices. *Morbidity and Mortality Weekly Report Recommendations and Reports, 67*(1), 1–31. https://doi.org/10.15585/mmwr.rr6701a1.

Sharifzadeh, F., Kashanian, M., Koohpayehzadeh, J., Rezaian, F., Sheikhansari, N., & Eshraghi, N. (2018). A comparison between the effects of ginger, pyridoxine (vitamin B6) and placebo for the treatment of the first trimester nausea and vomiting of pregnancy (NVP). *Journal of Maternal-Fetal and Neonatal Medicine, 31*(19), 2509–2514. https://doi.org/10.1080/14767058.2017.1344965.

Shepherd, E., Salam, R. A., Middleton, P., Makrides, M., McIntyre, S., Badawi, N., et al. (2017). Antenatal and intrapartum interventions for preventing cerebral palsy: An overview of Cochrane systematic reviews (Review). *Cochrane Database of Systematic Reviews, 2017*(8), CD012077. https://doi.org/10.1002/14651858.CD012077.pub2.

Sibai, B. M. (2021). Preeclampsia and hypertensive disorders. In M. Landon, H. Galan, E. Jauniaux, D. Driscoll, V. Berghella, W. Grobman, et al. (Eds.), *Gabbe's obstetrics: Normal and problem pregnancies* (8th ed., pp. 709–751). Elsevier.

Smid, M., Kelly, T. F., & Lacoursiere, D. Y. (2019). Obesity in pregnancy. In R. Resnik, R., C. J. Lockwood, T. R. Moore, et al. (Eds.), *Creasy & Resnik's maternal-fetal medicine: Principles and practice* (8th ed., pp. 1099–1115). Elsevier.

Soper, J. T. (2021). Gestational trophoblastic disease: Current evaluation and management. *Obstetrics & Gynecology, 137*(2), 355–370.

Storry, J. R., Clausen, F. B., Castilho, L., Chen, Q., Daniels, G., Denomme, G., et al. (2019). International society of blood transfusion working party on red cell immunogenetics and blood group terminology: Report of the Dubai, Copenhagen and Toronto meetings. *Vox Sanguinis, 114*(1), 95–102. https://doi.org/10.1111/vox.12717.

Stubert, J., Reister, F., Hartmann, S., & Janni, W. (2018). The risks associated with obesity in pregnancy. *Deutsches Arzteblatt International, 115*(16), 276–283. https://doi.org/10.3238/arztebl.2018.0276.

Sullivan, S. A., Goodier, C., & Cuff, R. D. (2021). Thyroid and parathyroid diseases in pregnancy. In M. B. Landon, H. L. Galan, E. R. M. Jauniaux, D. A. Driscoll, V. Berghella, W. A. Grobman, et al. (Eds.), *Gabbe's obstetrics: Normal and problem pregnancies* (8th ed., pp. 919–944). Elsevier.

U.S. Preventive Services Task Force. (2021). *Aspirin use to prevent morbidity and mortality from preeclampsia: Preventive medication.* https://www.uspreventiveservicestaskforce.org/uspstf/Document/draft-evidence-review/aspirin-use-to-prevent-preeclampsia-and-related-morbidity-and-mortality-preventive-medication1.

Viale, L., Allotey, J., Cheong-See, F., Arroyo-Manzano, D., Mccorry, D., Bagary, M., et al. (2015). Epilepsy in pregnancy and reproductive outcomes: A systemic review and meta-analysis. *Lancet, 386*, 1845–1852. https://doi.org/10.1016/S0140-6736(15)00045-8.

Whitty, J. E., & Dombrowski, M. P. (2019). Respiratory diseases in pregnancy. In R. Resnik, C. J. Lockwood, T. R. Moore, M. F. Greene, J. A. Copel, & R. M. Silver (Eds.), *Creasy & Resnik's maternal-fetal medicine: Principles and practice* (8th ed., pp. 1043–1066). Elsevier.

Williams, Z., & Scott, J. R. (2019). Recurrent pregnancy loss. In R. Resnik, C. J. Lockwood, T. R. Moore, M. F. Greene, J. A. Copel, & R. M Silver (Eds.), *Creasy & Resnik's maternal-fetal medicine: Principles and practice* (8th ed., pp. 758–768). Elsevier.

Witcher, P. M., & Shah, S. S. (2019). Hypertension in pregnancy. In N. A. Troiano, P. M. Witcher, & S. M. Baird (Eds.), *High-risk & critical care obstetrics* (4th ed., pp. 113–133). Wolters Kluwer.

World Health Organization. (n.d.). *WHO coronavirus (Covid-19) dashboard.* https://covid19.who.int/.

World Health Organization. (2018). *WHO recommendations: Drug treatment for severe hypertension in pregnancy.* https://apps.who.int/iris/handle/10665/277234.

World Health Organization. (2000). *Obesity: Preventing and managing the global epidemic: Report of a WHO consultation.* WHO Technical Report Series, 894. https://apps.who.int/iris/handle/10665/42330.

World Health Organization. (2022a). *Coronavirus disease (COVID-19): Symptoms.* https://www.who.int/health-topics/coronavirus#tab=tab_3.

World Health Organization. (2022b). *WHO global anaemia estimates, 2021 Edition.* https://www.who.int/data/gho/data/themes/topics/anaemia_in_women_and_children#:~:text=In%202019%2C%20global%20anaemia%20prevalence,39.1%25)%20in%20pregnant%20women.

Yeh, J. J., Lin, S. C., & Lin, W. C. (2019). Congenital tuberculosis in a neonate: A case report and literature review. *Frontiers in Pediatrics, 7*, 255. https://doi.org/10.3389/fped.2019.00255. 1–256.

The Childbearing Family with Special Needs

Jessica L. McNeil-Santiel

All families must make major changes as they adapt to pregnancy and childbirth. For some families, however, the changes are particularly difficult. Families may have special needs such as young or advanced parental age, substance use disorders (SUDs), birth of an infant with a congenital anomaly, perinatal loss, adoption, surrogacy, or a perinatal mood disorder. Through specialized care and therapeutic communication, perinatal nurses can make a difference in the lives of these families.

ADOLESCENT PREGNANCY

Throughout the years, many public health interventions have been aimed at reducing teenage pregnancy rates. From 2016 to 2017, the teenage pregnancy rate decreased 7% (Centers for Disease Control and Prevention [CDC], 2019). The overall birth rate among teens ages 15 and below has steadily decreased every year since 1992 (Maddow-Zimet & Kost, 2021). The CDC and the U.S. Department of Health and Human Services have partnered to fund programs that focus on developing interventions and focusing on social determinants of health to prevent teenage pregnancy for teenage mothers and fathers (CDC, 2019). Research shows adequate access to contraceptive services plays an important role in decreasing teenage pregnancy rates. According to data from the Guttmacher Institute (2019), almost 1 million teenage clients use services from publicly funded clinics to access contraception options annually. Some of the decline in rates can be contributed to more comprehensive sex education programs and/or greater access to contraceptives and higher rate of abstinence among teenage individuals (CDC, 2019; Guttmacher, 2019). Although the decline is encouraging, teenage pregnancy rates in the United States are still substantially higher than in other Western countries, and there are significant racial disparities.

Factors Associated with Teenage Pregnancy

Many factors may contribute to one becoming a teenage parent. Teenage clients are at an increased risk of developing complications during and after pregnancy, such as preterm labor, eclampsia, and endometritis (World Health Organization [WHO], 2020). Adolescents tend to engage in more frequent high-risk sexual behaviors because there may be a lack of consideration of the consequences that accompany their actions. Many adolescents believe teenage pregnancy will never happen to them. Increased abstinence, education, and more effective contraceptive practices have assisted in the recent decline of teenage pregnancies.

Some adolescents chance pregnancy and parenthood as a means of maintaining a relationship and/or having someone to love them, whereas others see it as a means to gain independence. Factors contributing to teenage pregnancy are listed in Box 11.1.

BOX 11.1 Factors Contributing to Teenage Pregnancy

Peer pressure to begin sexual activity
High rate of sexual activity
Limited access to contraceptive options/services
Lack of accurate information about how to use contraceptives correctly
Incorrect or lack of use of contraceptives
Fear of reporting sexual activity to parents
Ambivalence toward sexuality; intercourse not planned
Feelings of invincibility
Low self-esteem and associated inability to set limits on sexual activity
Desire to attain love or escape present situation
Lack of appropriate role models

Sex Education

Sex education for teens should focus on helping teens clarify their own values and beliefs regarding sexual behavior, recognize consequences associated with risky sexual behaviors, understand how to set appropriate boundaries regarding their own sexual behaviors, and learn effective measures to prevent pregnancy and sexually transmitted infections (STIs). It is especially important for teens to learn the importance of setting limits on sexual behavior and equipping them with the tools to know how to say, "Not now," "Not yet," and "Not you." Many teenagers may find themselves feeling pressured by peers into engaging in sexual activities when they lack the emotional maturity to deal responsibly with intercourse, contraception, or an unplanned pregnancy.

When providing sex education, nurses should keep in mind adolescent males and females mature at different rates and may be more comfortable learning and discussing topics in separate groups. In talking with teenagers, nurses should use simple but correct language such as, "uterus," "testicles," "penis," and "vagina."

Socioeconomic Implications

Teenage pregnancy can prove to be an economic burden because often the teen is still in school and unable to work and make enough money to sufficiently provide for the child. Often it is necessary for the teen to receive government assistance to have the basic resources needed to provide food and shelter. Other contributing factors toward teenage pregnancies include lack of access to contraception and lack of proper sexual education and knowledge of how their bodies work (WHO, 2020).

Although the financial cost of teenage pregnancy is huge, there is also a psychosocial cost to the teen and a cost to society. The developmental tasks of adolescence, such as achieving independence from parents and establishing a personally satisfying lifestyle, may be interrupted when a pregnancy increases the need for financial and emotional support from parents (Table 11.1). Instead of becoming independent, they often become more dependent on their parents or their partners because of pregnancy. Education goals may be curtailed for some young parents, limiting employment opportunities and resulting in reliance on the welfare system.

Positive outcomes from the pregnancy also may occur. For some adolescents, pregnancy provides them with a motivation to further their education and provide a better life for their child. Pregnancy and birth may have a stabilizing and maturing effect on adolescents who use the experience as an opportunity to change past poor lifestyle choices and become more goal-directed.

Implications for Client Health

Statistics show teen pregnancies increase the risk of significant hardships such as lower socioeconomic status and increased risk of STIs (Guttmacher, 2019). In fact, individuals between the ages of 15 and 24 account for half of all newly diagnosed STIs (Guttmacher, 2019). When teenage clients become pregnant, they experience higher rates of preeclampsia or gestational hypertension and preterm labor. These health conditions may be attributed to inadequate or no prenatal care. Teenage clients may delay seeking prenatal care due to lack of knowledge, limited access, and fear or stigma associated with their pregnancy (Karatasli et al., 2019; Leftwich & Alves, 2017). While the overall rates of elective abortions have continued to steadily decrease, evidence shows in areas where there is limited access to contraceptive services, and among those of lower income levels, there appears to be higher abortion rates (Bearak et al., 2020). These statistics further highlight the importance of safe and comprehensive contraceptive education and services across socioeconomic demographics.

Implications for Fetal and Neonatal Health

The lower the socioeconomic status of the teenage client, the higher the neonatal mortality risk. Compared with older clients, teenage pregnant individuals have an increased risk of delivering low-birth-weight or growth-restricted infants and lower 5-minute Apgar score associated with care in the neonatal intensive care unit (Adams, 2021; Karatasli et al., 2019).

Impact of Teenage Pregnancy on Parenting

Evidence shows that 50% of teenage pregnancies are unintended, and these unintended pregnancies occur more frequently between adolescents, minorities, and those with lower socioeconomic and education levels (CDC, 2018). This unexpected and unwanted life event can lead to difficulties in the client establishing a bond with the child and embracing the new role as parent. Teenage parents often need substantial resources to adequately provide for their children. Policy initiatives such as increasing funding for community-wide programs that support at-need parents, as well as increasing availability and access to long-acting reversible contraceptives (LARCs), are beneficial in preventing unintended teenage pregnancies and preparing teenage parents to adequately care for themselves and their child (CDC, 2018).

TABLE 11.1 Impact of Pregnancy on the Developmental Tasks of Adolescence

Developmental Task	Impact of Pregnancy	Nursing Considerations
Achievement of a Stable Identity: How the person sees themselves and how the person perceives others see them. Peer group approval provides confirmation and is a major component of identity development.	The ability to adapt and respond to stress is a good indicator of identity development. Adolescents who become pregnant before a stable identity is developed may not be able to accept the responsibilities of parenthood and to plan for the future.	Explore the availability of a school-based parents' program that provides peer support. Emphasize the importance of prenatal classes and the effect of prenatal care on pregnancy. Encourage both parents to attend parenting classes and describe the expected growth and development of infants. Focus on the infant's need to develop trust and on the parenting behaviors that promote this.
Achievement of Comfort with Body Image: Requires internalization of mature body size, contour, and function.	The adolescent must learn to cope with body changes of pregnancy (increasing size, contour, pigmentation changes, and striae) before they have learned to accept the body changes of puberty. May deny pregnancy or severely restrict calories to avoid gaining weight. May be disgusted with the physical changes of pregnancy, which makes the client look different from peers.	Allow time for the teenager to verbalize their feelings about the body changes of pregnancy. Emphasize dieting is harmful to the infant and will not stop the changes in body size and contour. Provide exercises that help the client maintain a healthy weight and lifestyle.
Acceptance of Sexual Role and Identity: Requires internalization of strong sexual urges and achievement of intimacy with others.	Adolescents may need to achieve an intimate relationship with another person and form an exclusive relationship before they are ready. Pregnant teenagers will also need to cope with changes in relationships with friends. They often have difficulty seeing themselves as a sexual being or as a parent.	Allow the teenager to express feelings about sexuality and about parenthood. Initiate groups designed specifically for adolescents (e.g., childbirth education, parenting classes, groups focused on nutrition). This will help the client deal with changing relationships with their peers and move toward a parenting role.
Development of a Personal Value System: Able to consider the rights and feelings of others.	Pregnancy may occur before the adolescent is able to move from following rules to considering the rights and feelings of others and developing ethical standards. The adolescent may experience conflict when adjusting to the responsibilities of premature parenthood.	Initiate a discussion of the teenager's feelings of conflict about the role as a parent versus the role as student. Explore the teenager's views about parenthood: What are the expected life changes and future plans? Present options and assist in exploring goals.
Preparation for Vocation or Career: Completing educational or vocational goals; youths living in poverty may not have the means or encouragement to accomplish this.	Pregnancy often interrupts school for both parents. This may be a major frustration, and it may result in permanent withdrawal from school and limited access to jobs that pay more than the minimum wage.	Discuss the importance of continued education, and elicit the teenager's feelings and plans to accomplish this. Determine the amount and availability of support from their parents. Refer client to social services for needed assistance.
Achievement of Independence from Parents: Competent in the social environment and able to function without parental guidance.	Must adjust to the need for continued financial assistance and dependence on parents at a time when achieving independence is a major priority.	Assist the teenager to verbalize feelings about continued dependence on parents. Discuss the reality of the situation and the need for financial support and help with the care of the infant. Determine the reaction of the parents to the pregnancy and whether they will continue to live at home. How much support will they provide? What are the conditions for remaining in the parents' home with the infant?

Modified from Mercer, R. T. (1990). *Parents at risk*. Springer.

APPLICATION OF THE NURSING PROCESS: THE PREGNANT TEENAGER

Assessment

Physical Assessment

Assessment of pregnant teenagers is similar to assessment of older clients in many respects. At the initial visit, obtain a thorough health and family history to determine whether conditions such as diabetes or infectious diseases increase the risk for the client and the fetus. Monitor closely for signs of iron-deficiency anemia, preeclampsia, or STIs. Attempt to identify behavioral risk factors such as poor nutrition, smoking, alcohol or drug use, or unprotected sex, which could harm the client or the fetus. Screen for physical or sexual abuse, which is more common in pregnant teenagers.

Teenagers are sometimes defensive and inconsistent in their responses. They may not volunteer information about nutrition, exercise, and the use of alcohol or other drugs; therefore, the nurse may need to ask for more details. The teenager's statement "I eat okay, and I'm pretty active" requires follow-up questions worded to obtain specific information: "What foods do you especially like? What did you eat yesterday?" "What kind of things do you like to do?"

Structure the interview so questions can be interspersed in a more general conversation that explores the teenager's likes and concerns. For example, a question such as, "Will you be able to continue the swim team after the baby is born?" may help the nurse establish rapport, gain a better understanding of the teenager, and determine whether they are making plans for the future.

Cognitive Development

Determine the teenager's level of cognitive development and ability to absorb health counseling. The three most important areas of cognitive development are as follows:

1. Egocentrism (interest centered on the self), which involves the ability to defer personal satisfaction to respond to the needs of the infant: "What will you do when the baby gets sick?" "How will you help the baby get better?"
2. Present–future orientation, which involves the ability to make long-term plans: "What are your plans for finishing high school?" "What will you and the infant need in the first year of the infant's life?"
3. Abstract thinking, which involves identifying cause and effect: "Why is it important to keep clinic appointments?" "Why should condoms be used during sex even though you're pregnant?"

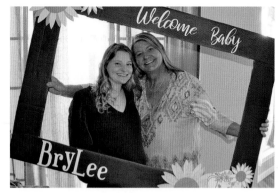

Fig. 11.1 Pregnant Adolescent. Approximately 23% of pregnant adolescents will have a second teenage pregnancy.

Knowledge of Infant Needs

Assess knowledge of infant needs and parenting skills. How does the teenager plan to feed the infant? What will they do when the infant cries? How will they know when the infant is ill and should be taken to a pediatrician? Do they know how much the infant should sleep? What plans have been made to provide for the safety needs of the infant?

Family Assessment

Begin assessment of the family unit by determining the degree of participation by the infant's other parent. The significant other may deny responsibility for the pregnancy, be married to or plan to marry the expectant client, participate in the pregnancy and rearing of the child without marriage, or be totally uninvolved.

Assessing the adolescent without the presence of their parents is important, yet it is crucial to determine the availability and amount of family support (Fig. 11.1). Will the pregnant teenager live with their parents? How do their parents feel about the pregnancy? How will they incorporate the client and infant into the family?

Families generally respond in one of the following three ways:

1. A family member (often the adolescent's parent) assumes the caregiver role, which the teenager may abdicate willingly.
2. All care and responsibilities are left to the adolescent parent, although shelter and food are provided.
3. The family shares care and responsibilities, which allows the teenager to grow in the parenting role while completing the developmental tasks of adolescence.

It is particularly important to assess the perceptions of the pregnant teenager's parents. How do they feel about becoming a grandparent? Many parents feel embarrassed and disgraced. They may feel they have "failed" as parents, or they may resent the new cycle of child care. Is communication with their child open? Are they aware of the difficult role conflict (as adolescent and parent) their child will experience? Many pregnant adolescents live with their parents, who provide various levels of support.

If the pregnant client's family is unable or unwilling to provide care for an adolescent with an infant, what other social support can be identified? In some situations, the family of the infant's other parent may be of assistance.

Identification of Client Problems

Many adolescents wait until the second or third trimester to seek prenatal care because they either do not realize they are pregnant, continue to deny they are pregnant, or want to hide the pregnancy. They may not know where to go for care and may fear the effects of pregnancy on their lives and relationships. In addition, many teenagers have little information about physiologic demands such as the increased need for nutrients that pregnancy imposes on their bodies. As a result, they may have a pattern of sporadic prenatal care and missed appointments. Many adolescents are unaware of ways to promote health during pregnancy and therefore need health teaching. Increased family stress as a result of inadequate coping strategies is another common problem.

Planning: Expected Outcomes

The expected outcomes for the need for health teaching are as follows:
1. The expectant client will keep prenatal appointments and follow health care instructions throughout pregnancy.
2. The expectant client will communicate concerns throughout pregnancy and participate in learning about infant care.
3. The family will verbalize emotions and concerns and maintain functional support of the expectant client and the infant.

Interventions

Eliminating Barriers to Health Care

The two major barriers to health care are (1) scheduling conflicts and (2) negative attitudes of some health care workers. Help adolescents locate the clinic closest to them that offers appointments when they (and their partner, if they wish) are available. Provide information about public transportation to the location, if necessary. Some clinics are open in the evening or on Saturday.

Communicating with adolescents requires special skills. Nurses should match their teaching with the teenager's cognitive development. Those who are 15 years old or younger need concrete explanations because their ability to understand abstract reasoning is not yet developed. Nurses should avoid seeming authoritarian because teens may see this behavior as interfering with their independence and may not return for care. When nurses work with adolescents as partners in care, adolescents are more likely to follow nursing recommendations.

Applying Teaching and Learning Principles

The lives of adolescents change greatly during pregnancy and even more after the infant is born. They often feel isolated from peers, who may not understand the responsibilities of parenthood. They may not be able to participate in activities with their friends because of child care obligations.

Teens often are hesitant to ask questions. Discuss concerns that are common to pregnant adolescents and ask if they have

> **BOX 11.2 Recommended Methods for Teaching Pregnant Adolescents**
>
> Identify and correct barriers to prenatal care
> Consider social determinants of health
> Communicate with kindness and respect
> Form small groups with similar concerns
> Allow ample time for clarification and discussion
> Use audiovisual materials
> Consider use of social media or mobile phone applications
> Provide information in appropriate language easily understood by teens
> Convey empathetic concern by using nonverbal communication skills
> Include other family members or support persons when appropriate

other questions. Because peers are important to adolescents, arrange for them to participate in small groups with common concerns. Being with peers may make them feel more comfortable asking questions and voicing concerns about needs such as the benefits of prenatal care or help eliminating unhealthy habits such as smoking, drug use, or alcohol consumption. Find common goals that may be discussed in groups in which the teens can assist each other to have a healthier pregnancy. As pregnancy progresses, needs and group focus change, and preparation for labor and delivery and infant care become priorities.

Repetition is an important method of teaching and clarifying misinformation. Allow ample time for discussions. Although teenagers may not read or benefit from printed materials to the same degree that older parents do, material that is prepared with adolescents in mind may be helpful. Information regarding reliable internet sites may be well-received. Teens often respond well to audiovisual aids. Numerous well-made videos are available that deal with all aspects of prenatal and infant care.

It is particularly important the nurse does not sound like a parent when working with adolescents. Avoid using the words "should" and "ought," offering unwanted advice, and making decisions for the teenagers. Maintain an open, friendly posture and convey empathy by using attending behaviors such as eye contact, frequent nodding, and leaning toward the speaker. Box 11.2 summarizes additional recommended methods for teaching adolescents.

Counseling

Allow time to counsel teenagers about their specific concerns such as nutrition, stress reduction, and infant care.

Nutrition. Nutrition counseling is one way to help reduce the incidence of low-birth-weight infants. Determine the adolescent's general nutritional status and assess for eating disorders that would reduce caloric intake and possibly affect fetal growth. Emphasize that the adolescent is still growing and intake should be adequate for personal growth as well as the baby's needs. Ask whether the adolescent prepares their own meals, whether someone else prepares them, or whether eating out is common for most meals. Discuss nutrition during lactation, pointing out the advantages for both parent and baby.

Tailor information to suit the individual adolescent's likes and peer group habits. Teach adolescents how to prepare simple meals and how to make the most nutritious selection from fast-food menus or select and plan for healthy snacks when away from home. Nutrition education should be socially and culturally appropriate (see Chapter 8).

Refer the teen to food stamp providers; the Special Supplemental Food Program for Women, Infants, and Children (WIC); surplus food distributors; and food banks, if necessary. Many teenagers have limited access to food and lack the ability to store or prepare it.

Self-Care. Provide the same teaching about self-care that would be given to an older client. In addition, emphasize the importance of using a condom for prevention of STIs while pregnant. Counsel the adolescent about lifestyle changes such as cessation of smoking or substance use, which will benefit both the client and the fetus, and refer the adolescent to resources that offer help with these problems.

Stress Reduction. Identify the stressors in the adolescent's life. Stress may be related to basic needs such as food, shelter, and health care. Fear of labor and delivery and fear of being single, alone, and unsupported all create stress. Meeting the developmental tasks of adolescence while working on the tasks of pregnancy is another stressor.

A variety of measures may be used to reduce stress, depending on the teenager's age, situation, and available support. Refer adolescents with chronic life stress to a social worker for help achieving stability. If the client is very young or the pregnancy is a result of rape or incest, social services and law enforcement agencies should become involved to provide protection and assistance.

Pregnant teenagers often experience stress because they have not told their parents or their significant other about the pregnancy. Explore their reluctance to do this, and role-play the encounter with them to work out a plan for breaking the news. Although there is strain on the relationship when many teens first tells their parents, their relationship may improve over time if their parents are supportive. If appropriate, encourage them to tell the other expectant parent so they can work out their role.

Teens who experience high levels of stress during pregnancy and the postpartum period may spend less time on infant care activities, feel less competent as parents, and have a more difficult time adjusting to being parents compared with teens with lower levels of stress during pregnancy and postpartum. Therefore, interventions to reduce stress in pregnant adolescents have an impact on the infant as well as the parents.

Help teens think ahead to how their life will change because of the pregnancy and what may interfere with the parenting role. Help them identify possible solutions to the problems presented. Other important interventions include identifying new sources of support to help resolve conflict.

Attachment to the Fetus. Because attachment begins during pregnancy, helping the adolescent begin this process

is important. Seeing the fetus move during an ultrasound often changes the pregnant client's perceptions about the fetus. Hearing the fetal heartbeat and feeling the baby move may increase attachment. Looking at illustrations of the fetus at different gestational ages increases the client's interest. A heightened awareness of the fetus may make the adolescent more likely to follow suggestions that will enhance fetal well-being. Discussion of the fetal changes month to month may lead to discussion of the capabilities and needs of the neonate.

Infant Care. The priorities for teaching gradually change from parent needs to infant needs, with emphasis on infant care and normal growth and development. Discuss common early developmental changes to help the young client understand the normal progression of infant abilities.

Explain and demonstrate infant cues (using behaviors of the infants in videos or in the group as examples) in terms of gaze, vocalization, facial expression, body position, and limb movement. Describe the way infants use these behaviors to "talk" without words and ways in which parents can use the behaviors to respond to their infants. Emphasize eye contact, holding, cuddling, and verbal stimulation are important for the child's development.

Adolescents tend to have a more rigid and punitive approach to child care and may need help understanding how infants develop a sense of trust when their needs are met promptly and gently. In addition, their future development depends on attaining a sense of trust during infancy. Emphasize crying does not indicate the infant is spoiled but simply the infant has a need for food, warmth, comfort, and love.

If a support person will be involved in helping care for the infant, include that person in teaching, especially if the support person has limited experience with babies. Having a support person learn with them may help the teenager remember the information better.

Breastfeeding. Adolescents who decide to breastfeed their infants need support in their endeavor. They should be praised for their decision to do what is best for the baby. The nurse should adapt teaching to the client's level of understanding. Encourage questions because the young parent may have much misinformation. Privacy is important to adolescents; they often feel embarrassed to breastfeed in front of others. Provide help with correct positioning and latching-on of the infant. Show them how to drape a blanket to cover their breast and the nursing infant.

Check on adolescent clients frequently during feedings to identify any problems and intervene appropriately and in a timely manner. Discuss problems that may occur so they have a realistic understanding of challenges and know when and where to seek help, if necessary. Offer praise liberally. Success in the baby latching-on to the breast and seeing the infant gain weight may be very rewarding for the parent.

Promoting Family Support

Pregnant teenagers need encouragement to include their family in their decision-making and problem solving. The involvement of their parents, older siblings, or other close relatives is particularly important in terms of future plans. Discuss topics such as who will care for the infant, whether the teenager will return to school, and what financial assistance is available from the family and the infant's other parent. Adolescent parents who have adequate emotional support are more likely to learn appropriate parenting techniques.

However, if the family has multiple problems such as substance use or family violence, involving family members may be inappropriate. In such situations, the teenager should be encouraged to communicate with a family friend or another trusted adult.

Providing Support during Labor

The needs of pregnant adolescents during labor are similar to those of the older client. Nursing support at this time is especially important in helping them feel safe and cared for so they can have a successful childbirth experience.

Providing Referrals

Make referrals to conveniently located national and community resources for pregnant adolescents. Include well-baby clinics offered by the public health service and assistance programs offered by state social services agencies. Church and community organizations also may provide needed assistance. Childbirth education classes specifically for teenagers are often available.

Programs for school-age parents are offered by many school districts and provide an opportunity to complete high school education and take the much-needed classes in childbearing and parenting. Some schools include pregnant adolescents in regular classes and add other classes to meet their special needs.

Evaluation

Nursing care has been effective if the pregnant adolescent keeps prenatal appointments and participates actively in their plan of care, as demonstrated by asking questions, sharing concerns, and adhering to the recommended program of care. They should demonstrate basic knowledge of the infant's needs and care of the infant. Family support should be available, but if it is not, refer adolescents to agencies that can provide assistance.

> **❓ KNOWLEDGE CHECK**
>
> 3. What methods are effective for teaching pregnant teenagers?
> 4. What should prospective teenage parents be taught about infant growth and development?

DELAYED PREGNANCY

It has become increasingly common for individuals to delay childbearing to further their careers, marry later, or establish financial security. However, delaying childbearing is not without risk. With advanced maternal age comes an increased risk for several reproductive and pregnancy complications,

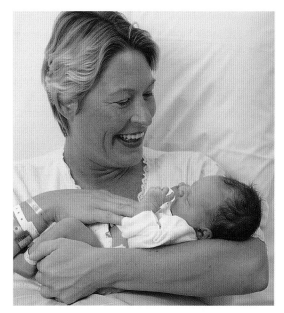

Fig. 11.2 Older primigravidas bring maturity and problem-solving skills to the maternal role, but they are at somewhat increased risk for physiologic problems related to pregnancy and birth.

such as but not limited to congenital anomalies, ectopic pregnancy, preeclampsia, gestational diabetes, placenta previa, and spontaneous abortion (Fretts et al., 2021). Although advances in contraception and fertility management have provided options to clients who choose to delay childbearing and the ability to still conceive, there are physical and financial constraints they may face. A client is considered to be at an advanced maternal age at the age of 35 (Fig. 11.2). While in general most clients still have many childbearing years ahead of them at 35, research shows fertility begins to decline around this age (CHU Sainte-Justine Mother and Child University Hospital Center, 2021).

Maternal and Fetal Implications

Some of the risks associated with advanced maternal age, aside from infertility, include miscarriage, chromosome disorders such as Down's syndrome, preterm labor, and increased risk for cesarean delivery (Fretts et al., 2021). Older clients are also at an increased risk for preexisting chronic conditions such as hypertension, diabetes mellitus, and uterine myomas (fibroids). One should also consider the psychological implications that may come with infertility struggles. Clients may experience a wide array of emotions such as depression, anxiety, and guilt for delaying childbearing (Rooney & Domar, 2018).

Advantages of Delayed Childbirth

Some significant advantages also are found with delayed childbirth. Clients who have delayed childbirth tend to be more mature and of higher education and socioeconomic status (Fretts et al., 2021). These traits result in them often being better equipped to deal with the emotional and financial demands of parenthood.

Nursing Considerations

All clients of advanced maternal age (older than 35 years at estimated due date) should receive honest and clear preconception education so a plan can be identified with their health care provider before trying to conceive. Chronic conditions should be treated before conception. Clients should be counseled on all diagnostic tests available to detect chromosomal abnormalities early in the pregnancy so they can make educated decisions. For some clients, these tests may result in the choice to terminate the pregnancy should an abnormality be detected. As a nurse it is important to recognize any bias regarding the client's decision-making and remain nonjudgmental and respectful to the client during this difficult time. Other clients may choose to undergo genetic testing to make necessary arrangements should the child be affected with a disorder.

There are also emotional difficulties for the client who has chosen to delay childbearing. The more mature client may have had an imagined plan and picture of what pregnancy and parenthood should look like and may find it difficult to cope when things do not go exactly as planned. This new journey to parenthood may mean the client has to give up or alter career plans. For the more accomplished client this may be a difficult and unexpected transition. Nurses should be prepared to address both the physical and emotional needs of a client experiencing delayed childbirth. Although these clients may have some unique needs throughout their journey to parenthood, many go on to have healthy, enjoyable pregnancies.

Facilitating Expression of Emotions

Several days or weeks may pass between performance of some diagnostic studies and receipt of the results. This is a particularly difficult time for many expectant parents, and nurses often assist the couple to express their concerns and emotions.

A broad statement such as "Many couples find it difficult to wait for the results" will often elicit free expression of the parents' feelings. Follow-up questions such as "What concerns you most?" may reveal anxiety about the procedure itself or about the possible effects of the procedure on the fetus. Simply acknowledging it is a stressful time helps the couple cope with their emotions.

Clients who have undergone many tests and procedures for infertility may be especially anxious. Once pregnancy is achieved, they worry about their ability to carry the fetus to term and may see themselves as being at higher risk than they actually are. If they have had unsuccessful pregnancies in the past, they may fear the present pregnancy may also be lost, making it hard for them to be optimistic about success.

Mature gravidas also worry about complications that may affect the fetus or their own health. They are aware they may not have another opportunity for pregnancy because of their age. They may be concerned about their ability to balance their careers with increased family responsibilities.

Providing Parenting Information

Nurses often help the mature client prepare for effective parenting by pointing out their individual strengths and advantages. Anticipatory guidance about measures that will help conserve energy after childbirth is very useful. These include meal planning and setting realistic housekeeping goals. In addition, many older clients need to mobilize all available support so they can reserve their energy for care of the infant.

When giving suggestions about conserving energy and obtaining support, avoid using terms like "elderly primipara" when referring to the expectant client. It is important not to make them feel abnormal because of their age. Unless they have complications, they should know their prenatal course will be the same as any other pregnant client.

During the first weeks after childbirth the client may experience feelings of social isolation, particularly if their friends have children who are much older. They may miss the mental stimulation of a job while staying at home. If they elect to return to work, they are likely to experience guilt and grief because they must leave their infant. Balancing the needs of the infant and the challenges of a career or occupation may be difficult.

Older clients are likely to seek information they need from a variety of sources. They are particularly interested in learning how the infant grows and develops and what they can do to provide nurturing care for the infant. Meeting other older expectant parents in classes may provide friendships that can continue after the birth and help clients provide support for each other. Play groups are another source of support where clients can compare notes on parenting.

Older parents may interview care providers before choosing one. They may have special concerns and ask many questions. They often adopt health-promoting activities such as improving nutrition and eliminating harmful substances. Printed materials can be used to reinforce teaching.

> **❓ KNOWLEDGE CHECK**
>
> 5. What special resources do mature gravidas often have?
> 6. Why is it important to offer prenatal testing to the mature gravida?
> 7. What anticipatory guidance should the nurse provide the older client for the first weeks at home after childbirth?

SUBSTANCE USE

Chemical dependence is the physical and psychological dependence on a substance such as alcohol, tobacco, or drugs, either legal or illicit. When present during pregnancy, it can pose serious risk to both the parent and infant.

Incidence

Current research shows polysubstance use in pregnancy is common and continues to increase (CDC, 2020a). The true scope of the problem is not fully known because many clients are afraid to disclose their substance use out of fear of stigma or losing their parental rights (CDC, 2020a). In particular, alcohol, tobacco, marijuana, and opioids are all substances that are frequently used during pregnancy (CDC, 2020a).

TABLE 11.2 Maternal and Fetal or Neonatal Effects of Commonly Used Substances

Substance	Client Effects	Fetal or Neonatal Effects
Caffeine (coffee, tea, cola, chocolate, cold remedies, analgesics)	Metabolism of caffeine slows as pregnancy progresses, stimulates CNS and cardiac function, causes vasoconstriction of cerebral and cardiac vessels, causes diuresis, respiratory bronchodilation and gastrointestinal acid secretion, stimulates secretion of the catecholamine stress hormones (epinephrine and norepinephrine), physical dependence, increased risk of miscarriage or having a small for gestational age infant	Crosses placental barrier and stimulates fetus; elevated catecholamine levels have the potential to increase placental vasoconstriction and increase fetal heart rate; increased risk of childhood acute leukemia and childhood overweight and obesity
Tobacco	Decreased placental perfusion, abruptio placentae, anemia, PROM, preterm labor, spontaneous abortion	Prematurity, LBW, neurodevelopmental problems, increased incidence of SIDS, perinatal mortality
Alcohol (beer, wine, mixed drinks, after-dinner drinks)	Spontaneous abortion, abruptio placentae	Fetal demise, IUGR, fetal alcohol spectrum disorders, FAS (facial and cranial anomalies, developmental delay, cognitive impairment, short attention span)
Marijuana ("pot" or "grass")	Often used with other drugs: tobacco, alcohol, cocaine; physical dependence	Unclear; more study needed; may be related to problems in motor development; increased risk for anomalies or mortality unproven
Cocaine ("crack")	Hyperarousal state, euphoria, generalized vasoconstriction, hypertension, tachycardia, STIs, spontaneous abortion, abruptio placentae, preeclampsia, PROM, preterm labor, precipitous delivery	Fetal hypoxia, tachycardia, meconium staining, stillbirth, prematurity, irritability, sleep followed by agitation, poor response to comforting or interaction, possible attention and language problems
Amphetamines and methamphetamines ("speed," "crystal," "glass," "ice," "ecstasy")	Malnutrition, vasoconstriction, tachycardia, hypertension, spontaneous abortion, preterm labor, abruptio placentae, preeclampsia, retroplacental hemorrhage	Increased risk for IUGR, prematurity, abnormal sleep patterns, agitation, poor feeding, vomiting
Opioids (heroin, methadone, morphine)	Malnutrition, anemia, increased incidence of STIs, thrombosis, cardiac disease, spontaneous abortion, preterm labor; physical dependence	IUGR, LBW, NAS, meconium aspiration syndrome, fetal or neonatal death, SIDS, child abuse and neglect; long-term developmental effects unclear
Antidepressants (e.g., selective serotonin reuptake inhibitors)	Relief of anxiety and depression, risk for anomalies with paroxetine, small risk for anomalies with other antidepressants	Transient respiratory problems, irritability, poor tone, persistent pulmonary hypertension

CNS, Central nervous system; FAS, fetal alcohol syndrome; IUGR, intrauterine growth restriction; HIV, human immunodeficiency virus; LBW, low birth weight; NAS, neonatal abstinence syndrome; PROM, premature rupture of membranes; SIDS, sudden infant death syndrome; STIs, sexually transmitted infections.
James, J. (2021). Maternal caffeine consumption and pregnancy outcomes: A narrative review with implications for advice to mothers and mothers-to-be. BMJ Evidence-Based Medicine, 26:114–115. https://ebm.bmj.com/content/26/3/114.

Maternal and Fetal Effects

When a pregnant client uses an illicit or harmful substance by drinking, smoking, snorting, or injecting it, the fetus experiences the same systemic effects as the expectant client but often more severely and for a longer time. The fetus is unable to metabolize drugs efficiently; therefore, a drug that causes intoxication in the client causes it for prolonged periods in the fetus. Substances taken by the client can have a great impact on the fetus and interfere with normal fetal development and health. Maternal, fetal, and neonatal effects of commonly used substances are summarized in Table 11.2.

Tobacco

Tobacco use can impact fertility, pregnancy, and the developing fetus both during and after pregnancy (CDC, 2020b).

Tobacco use during pregnancy increases the risk of miscarriage, can cause damage to fetal brain and lungs, and can result in fetal low birth weight as a result of the vasoconstrictive effects of nicotine, which reduces placental blood flow (CDC, 2020b). In addition, clients who smoke have an increased risk of preterm labor, and the babies of these clients have an increased risk for sudden infant death syndrome (SIDS) (CDC, 2020b).

Maternal and Fetal Effects. Some specific effects of cigarette smoking on the pregnant client include decreased appetite, poor weight gain, and poor nutritional status.

Childhood Effects. Childhood effects include increased risk of respiratory infections, asthma, colic, bone fractures, and childhood obesity (American College of Obstetricians and Gynecologists [ACOG], 2020).

Alcohol

Alcohol use is a common occurrence during pregnancy. Alcohol is a teratogen known to have the potential to cause both mental delays and birth malformations in the developing fetus. There is a direct correlation between the amount and timing of alcohol ingested and the degree of impact to the fetus. Although alcohol intake during the first trimester appears to have the largest negative impact on cell growth and division, alcohol use during any point in the pregnancy can have harmful effects on the fetus. It is important for clients to know there is no safe level of alcohol in pregnancy (ACOG, 2018).

Pregnant Client and Fetal Effects. The use of alcohol in pregnancy can increase the risk for preterm labor and birth, birth defects, and fetal alcohol syndrome.

Neonatal Effects. Alcohol use during pregnancy is one of the primary causes of preventable birth defects and developmental delays (Dejong et al., 2019).

The teratogenic impacts of alcohol can lead to fetal alcohol spectrum disorders, the most severe of which is fetal alcohol syndrome (FAS) (ACOG, 2018). FAS is characterized by three distinct features: prenatal and postnatal growth restriction, central nervous system (CNS) impairment, and an identifiable grouping of facial abnormalities (American Academy of Pediatrics [AAP] & ACOG, 2017). Growth restriction is evident in length, weight, and head circumference. CNS deficits include intellectual incapacities, learning disabilities, attention deficit disorder, and reduced short-term memory. Facial features frequently associated with FAS include microcephaly, short palpebral fissures (the openings between the eyelids), epicanthal folds, flat midface with a low nasal bridge, indistinct philtrum (groove between the nose and upper lip), and a thin upper lip. Although not all infants exposed to alcohol during pregnancy will have signs or symptoms of FAS, it is important to educate clients that there is no safe level of alcohol during pregnancy.

Marijuana

Marijuana is the most commonly used illegal substance during pregnancy, with rates continuing to increase among all demographics (Substance Abuse and Mental Health Services Administration [SAMHSA], 2021b).

Maternal and Fetal Effects. While many clients attempt to use marijuana to assist with nausea and vomiting in pregnancy, there is no safe amount of marijuana consumption in pregnancy, and in fact, it can be harmful to both the client and developing fetus (SAMHSA, 2021b). Some potential risk factors with marijuana use during pregnancy include intrauterine growth restriction (IUGR), preterm birth, and an increased risk for neonatal stillbirth (SAMHSA, 2021b). Marijuana is also found in breast milk when consumed while breastfeeding, and evidence shows it can impact infant brain development (SAMHSA, 2021b).

Cocaine

Cocaine is a powerful short-acting CNS stimulant. It blocks the reuptake of the neurotransmitters *norepinephrine* and *dopamine* at the nerve terminals, producing a hyperarousal state that results in euphoria, sexual excitement, increased alertness, and a heightened sense of well-being. Physical effects of cocaine use are related to cardiovascular stimulation and vasoconstriction. Hypertension, tachycardia, arrhythmias, tremors, anemia, anorexia, and even death to both the client and/or fetus can occur.

When the initial euphoria wears off, a period of irritability, exhaustion, lethargy, depression, and anxiety occurs. This state elicits a strong desire for additional cocaine so the initial feelings can be recaptured.

Maternal and Fetal Effects. It is difficult to define the exact effects of cocaine on the fetus because many clients who use cocaine also use other drugs, such as alcohol, tranquilizers, heroin, or marijuana, to "come down" from the hyperarousal state that cocaine produces. Clients who use cocaine are less likely to seek prenatal care or eat a diet containing adequate nutrition. Sex may be exchanged for drugs, increasing the risk for STIs.

Placental abruption is a known risk due to the vasoconstriction of placental vessels caused by cocaine use. Cocaine also stimulates uterine contractions, resulting in increased incidence of spontaneous abortion, premature rupture of membranes, preterm labor, and precipitous delivery.

Neonatal Effects. Like other illegal drugs, cocaine use during pregnancy can result in serious harm to the developing fetus. Potential neonatal risk factors seen with cocaine include miscarriage, IUGR, neonatal abstinence syndrome (NAS), childhood learning difficulties, childhood behavior issues, and vision problems (March of Dimes, 2020a).

Bath Salts

A new class of drugs known as psychoactive bath salts have become increasingly popular in recent years and, like other illegal drugs, pose a significant threat to both clients and babies. Bath salts are synthetic cathinones that come from the khat plant and are analogs of amphetamines (Schloemerkemper, 2018). Although little is known of the effect psychoactive bath salts have on pregnancy, the serious maternal impact can lead one to infer they would be harmful to a developing fetus.

Amphetamines and Methamphetamines

Amphetamines and methamphetamines are CNS stimulants that produce feelings of immense pleasure.

Maternal and Fetal Effects. Amphetamine and methamphetamine use in pregnancy causes increases in blood pressure and an increased risk for placental abruption. Evidence shows methamphetamine use in pregnancy has the potential to cause significant birth deformities, as well as low birth weight (ACOG, 2021a).

Neonatal Effects. Infants exposed to amphetamines or methamphetamines have been shown to have lower 1- and 5-minute Apgar scores, as well as difficulty with memory and concentration on tasks during childhood (ACOG, 2021a).

Antidepressants

Antidepressants such as selective serotonin reuptake inhibitors (SSRIs) are frequently prescribed during pregnancy for clients with depression and anxiety. Although negative side effects and risk to the baby can occur when taking these medications, in many cases the benefits and safety to the client outweigh the risk.

Maternal, Fetal, and Neonatal Effects. SSRIs can cause infants to show signs of medication withdrawal such as jitteriness, respiratory depression, poor feeding, and irritability (Mayo Clinic, 2020).

Opiates

Opioid use in pregnancy has been steadily increasing over the last several years. Opiates include drugs such as morphine, methadone, meperidine (Demerol), oxycodone (OxyContin), hydromorphone hydrochloride (Dilaudid), and heroin. Many opiates are frequently used and prescribed by providers to treat chronic pain; however, they are very addictive. As prescription opioid use has increased, the use of heroin has increased as well, as it is easier to access than opioid pills (Titus-Glover et al., 2021). Opiates are CNS depressants, and they generally leave individuals experiencing feelings of drowsiness, mental dullness, and stupor. Unlike many other substances, there are medications that can be used to treat the addiction and withdrawal symptoms of opioid use. Methadone and buprenorphine are both medications for opioid use disorder (MOUDs) and have been shown to significantly increase the success of recovery and decrease rates of overdose in those with opioid use disorder (Titus-Glover et al, 2021). Pregnant clients who use opiates have an increased risk for maternal death, preterm birth, still birth, and birth defects (CDC, 2021).

Maternal and Fetal Effects. Due to the addictive nature of opiates such as heroin, clients will typically alternate between periods of overdose and periods of withdrawal. These episodes expose the neonate to intermittent hypoxia, which increases the risk for meconium aspiration syndrome. Heroin is extremely addictive, and its use can lead to multiple serious health issues in clients such as increased risk of STIs, chronic respiratory distress, kidney and liver disease, heart and lung infections, and coma (March of Dimes, 2020b). As a result of the highly addictive nature of heroin and other opiates, these medications cannot be immediately stopped. The sudden discontinuation of opioids can cause dangerous complications for both client and baby, the most serious of which is overdose death (March of Dimes, 2020b).

Neonatal Effects. Opiates such as heroin frequently cause NAS. This syndrome occurs when an infant has been exposed to opioids in utero and begins to experience severe withdrawal symptoms after birth. Symptoms of NAS include irritability with high-pitched cry, poor feeding and sucking, loose stools, sweating, seizures, tremors, yawning and sneezing, hyperactive reflexes, and sleeping difficulty (CDC, 2021).

Diagnosis and Management of Substance Use

It is not uncommon for clients with SUDs to have inconsistent prenatal care or no prenatal care at all (Prince & Ayers, 2021). The client may fear the baby will be taken away if a health care provider finds out they have an SUD. Statistics show mental illness often accompanies SUDs in pregnancy (Prince & Ayers, 2021). For these reasons, it is important for nurses to carefully assess their clients for any signs or symptoms of substance use and/or mental illness and report their findings to the proper members of the health care team so the client can get access to needed care and treatment. Medications such as methadone and buprenorphine can assist in reducing symptoms of withdrawal and addiction and assist clients in being able to live full, productive lives that are not dominated by opioid addiction (Caritis & Panigrahy, 2019). Methadone can be taken orally and is long-acting, providing consistent blood levels to decrease the adverse fetal effects of wide swings in blood level found with heroin use. The daily dose can be gradually decreased to wean the client off the drug. However, if the baby is born before the drug is discontinued, the newborn must withdraw from methadone after birth. Buprenorphine may be used instead of methadone. Although neonatal withdrawal still occurs, it is shorter and less severe than with methadone.

Ensuring the client has access to treatment resources is important because research has shown the greatest risk for substance use relapse is within the first 6 to 12 months after delivery because clients think they no longer run the risk for causing harm to the baby (Prince & Ayers, 2021). Parents who are actively seeking or receiving medication-assisted therapy (MAT) with methadone or buprenorphine can and should be encouraged to breastfeed (SAMHSA, 2021a). In several states any substance use during pregnancy is considered a crime and recognized as child neglect and abuse. The client can be criminally prosecuted, leaving the client at risk for losing their parental rights (Guttmacher, 2021). Many states also require nurses to report any type of substance use in pregnancy; however, it is important to note this action can impede clients from accessing the health care system and/or coming forward and admitting they are using drugs or alcohol out of fear of incarceration. Many professional health organizations advocate against the criminalization of pregnant clients with SUD and instead recommend universal substance use screening for all clients, as well as priority access to substance use treatment centers for those who are pregnant (Coleman, 2019). Nurses should be able to identify clients who need help in relation to substance use and ensure the appropriate care for both the client and their infant.

> ### ? KNOWLEDGE CHECK
>
> 8. How does smoking affect the neonate? What are the long-term effects on the child?
> 9. What problems are associated with fetal alcohol syndrome?
> 10. What are the effects of maternal cocaine use on the infant?
> 11. Why are clients who use heroin encouraged to use methadone or buprenorphine during pregnancy?

APPLICATION OF THE NURSING PROCESS: MATERNAL SUBSTANCE USE

Nursing care related to substance use may occur during the antepartum, intrapartum, or postpartum period.

ANTEPARTUM PERIOD

Assessment

Polysubstance use appears to be the most common substance use problem, and all clients should be screened at the first prenatal visit for tobacco, alcohol, and other drug use. Because substance use occurs in all populations, the nurse should not make assumptions based on class, race, or economic status.

Certain behaviors are strongly associated with substance use: seeking prenatal care late in the pregnancy, failing to keep appointments, and following recommended regimens inconsistently.

⚡ SAFETY CHECK

Signs of Possible Drug Use

Seeking prenatal care late in pregnancy
Failure to keep prenatal appointments
Inconsistent follow-through with recommended care
Poor grooming, inadequate weight gain
Needle punctures, thrombosed veins, cellulitis
Defensive or hostile reactions
Anger or apathy regarding pregnancy
Severe mood swings

Clients who use drugs may have low self-esteem. They are dealing with conflicting issues: the physical and psychological need for the substance, denying the substance is harming the fetus, and guilt that they may be responsible for harming the fetus. Fear of prosecution for use of illegal drugs may prevent the client from seeking prenatal care, increasing risk for the client and the fetus. In addition, many clients with substance use problems face discrimination and resentment from health care professionals who direct their frustration at the client rather than the problem.

Given the powerful deterrents to self-disclosure, extensive history taking provides the best opportunity to determine current and past substance use. The nurse taking the health history should maintain a nonjudgmental attitude, exhibit patience and empathy, and display an attitude of concern for the client and infant.

Medical History

Determine whether the client has medical conditions that are prevalent among clients who use drugs—for example, seizures, hepatitis, cellulitis, STIs, hypertension, depression, and suicide attempts. Current problems may include insomnia, panic attacks, exhaustion, heart palpitations, depression, and suicidal ideation.

BOX 11.3 Techniques for Interviewing a Client about Substance Use

To determine whether the client uses substances:
- Display an accepting and nonjudgmental attitude
- Explain why it is important to know about substance use: "We need to know about anything that might affect you or your baby during the pregnancy."
- Let them know these questions are asked of all pregnant clients
- Acknowledge that parents may be reluctant to disclose information: "I know it's difficult to talk to us about this, but we need to know so we can give you and your baby the best care possible."
- Begin with questions about over-the-counter or prescription drugs and lead up to use of tobacco, alcohol, and, finally, illicit drugs
- Demonstrate knowledge of types and forms of drugs commonly used in the community: "Do you have friends who are using ecstasy?"

When substance use is acknowledged, the important points in the drug history include the following:
- The type of drug used
- The amount used
- The frequency of use
- The time of last dose
- Any polysubstance use

Ask specific questions:
- How often have you taken over-the-counter medications?
- What drugs did you take last month? Were they prescribed?
- How many cigarettes do you smoke on a daily basis? Are there times when you smoke more?
- How many times a week do you drink alcoholic beverages (beer, wine, mixed drinks)?
- How many in a day? Are there times when you have more drinks?
- How often did you use [drug used] before becoming pregnant? How often do you use it now? What is your preferred method/route of use (snort, smoke, inhale, IV injection)?

Obstetric History

Evaluate for past and current complications of pregnancy. Spontaneous abortions, premature deliveries, placental abruption, and stillbirths are associated with substance use. Current complications may include STIs, vaginal bleeding, and an inactive or hyperactive fetus. Fundal height may be inconsistent with gestational age, suggesting IUGR.

Investigate emotional responses such as anger or apathy regarding the pregnancy. These feelings are particularly significant during the latter half of the pregnancy, when the normal feelings of ambivalence are usually resolved. Negative feelings toward the pregnancy may interfere with prenatal compliance with recommended care.

History of Substance Use

Obtaining an accurate history of substance use is difficult and depends in large part on the way the health care worker approaches the client. A sincere, nonjudgmental, and empathic approach promotes open exchange of information (Box 11.3).

Ask about all forms of drug use, including cigarettes, e-cigarettes, over-the-counter drugs, prescription medications, alcohol, and illicit drugs. Examine patterns of drug use, which can range from occasional, recreational use to weekly binges to daily dependence on a particular drug or group of drugs.

Identification of Client Problems

Some clients acknowledge the use of harmful substances but do not fully understand the adverse effects. Other clients are aware of the risks but are unable to stop using these substances. Common client problems include lack of knowledge of the effects of substance use on themselves and the fetus and inability to manage stress without the use of drugs. Both of these problems can result in the need for health teaching.

Planning: Expected Outcomes

Expected outcomes include the following:
1. Identify the harmful effects of substances on themselves and their infant.
2. Verbalize feelings related to continued use of harmful substances.
3. Identify personal strengths and accept resources offered by the health care delivery system to stop using drugs.

Interventions

Effective interventions for substance use require the combined efforts of nurses, health care providers, social workers, and numerous community and federal agencies. Nurses should realize progress is slow and frustrating. The major priority is to protect the fetus and the expectant parent from the harmful effects of drugs.

Examining Attitudes

When working with pregnant clients with substance use problems, nurses should identify their own knowledge level, feelings, and prejudices. They may have limited knowledge about perinatal substance use and negative attitudes toward clients who use substances. Nurses may be angry at the client who not only engages in self-destructive behavior but also may be inflicting harm on their fetus. Maintaining feelings of empathy or concern without becoming judgmental or even unknowingly punitive to the pregnant client may be difficult. Nurses also may feel helpless and discouraged when the pregnant client continues to use drugs despite the best efforts of the health care team.

In-service education, professional consultation, and peer support are all helpful for professionals working with pregnant clients who use drugs. These processes can allow opportunities for discussion and sharing of feelings, problems, and particularly troublesome treatment issues.

Preventing Substance Use

Participate in campaigns to prevent substance use throughout the community. Provide accurate information in terms the parents can easily understand. Use posters, diagrams, pamphlets, and other visual aids to describe the effects of tobacco, alcohol, and other drugs on the fetus. Post visual aids in schools, groceries stores, shopping centers, and other areas where clients of childbearing age will be exposed to them.

Focus on the benefits of remaining drug-free, which include a decrease in maternal and neonatal complications. For example, the effects of smoking tobacco are dose-related and cumulative, and nurses should encourage and support cessation at any point during pregnancy.

Clients who use alcohol during pregnancy may not realize the effect on the fetus. Social drinkers will often stop drinking once they know about the dangers. Those with heavy alcohol use need counseling and referral for further treatment.

Communicating with the Parent

Ask the expectant parent about stressors in their life that may be contributing to their substance use. Additional stressors may include inadequate housing, economic predicaments, intimate partner violence, and emotional or physical illness.

Be honest at all times, while displaying a patient, nonjudgmental attitude and genuine interest and concern. This is especially important when the client relapses into substance-use patterns. Allow the client to express guilt, and provide reassurance that abstinence is possible and they can and must begin again.

Helping the Client Identify Strengths

Pregnant clients with substance use problems may need assistance in identifying personal strengths due to a poor self-image. Acknowledge their actions when they abstain from drugs or alcohol for even a short time. Praise for maintaining an adequate weight gain and attending prenatal classes may increase their confidence and compliance with the recommended regimen of care.

Providing Ongoing Care

At each antepartum visit, consider the current status of substance use, social service needs, education needs, and compliance with treatment referrals. Address current drug use because clients may change their pattern of drug use during pregnancy. For example, they may stop using cocaine but may increase their use of heroin or alcohol.

Verify compliance with recommended treatment regimens such as antepartum clinics and chemical-dependence referral programs. Coordinate care among various service providers such as group therapy and prenatal classes. Establish communication with all agencies that provide care, and facilitate communication that helps the client with a chaotic lifestyle meet treatment objectives.

Provide continuing prenatal education about the anatomy and physiology of pregnancy and consequences of prenatal substance use. Describe how the newborn benefits when the client abstains from using drugs, tobacco, and alcohol. Drug screens will be performed periodically throughout the pregnancy. Praise any attempts at abstinence and encourage the expectant client to try again if relapse occurs.

Assess signs of maternal attachment to the fetus because it may help reduce or eliminate the substance use. Fetal movement often increases the client's awareness of the fetus and may lead to a discussion about the plans for the infant and lifestyle changes that have occurred and will occur. Help make realistic plans for care of the baby. Include support persons if possible.

When the client's partner uses substances, the client is more likely to continue to use them or to stop during the pregnancy but start again after birth. Explain to the partner the importance of avoiding use to enhance the outcome of the pregnancy and avoid exposure of children to the adverse effects of substances.

When clients use substances during pregnancy, child welfare services may be involved to ensure the safety of the infant after discharge. The infant may become a ward of the courts and be placed in foster care until the client is in rehabilitation. Use therapeutic communication techniques to help the client express feelings about this loss. Help the client make plans for implementing changes that will allow custody of or visitation with the infant.

Evaluation

Interventions have been successful if expectant clients identify the harmful effects of substance use on themselves and on the fetus, discuss their strengths and feelings about continued use of substances, and are receptive to assistance to stop using drugs.

INTRAPARTUM PERIOD

Assessment

Nurses who work in labor and delivery units should become skilled at identifying drug-induced signs and symptoms.

Cocaine

Behaviors associated with frequent or recent use of cocaine include profuse sweating, hypertension, tachycardia, and irregular respirations combined with a lethargic response to labor and apparent lack of interest in the necessary interventions. Additional signs include dilated pupils, increased body temperature, and sudden onset of severely painful contractions. Fetal signs often include tachycardia and excessive fetal activity. Fetal bradycardia and late decelerations may occur (see Chapter 14).

Emotional signs of recent cocaine use may include angry, caustic, or abusive reactions to those attempting to provide care. Emotional lability and paranoia are signs of cocaine intoxication.

Heroin

The pregnant client dependent on heroin may come to the labor and delivery unit intoxicated from recent drug use. When the effects of the drug begin to wear off, withdrawal symptoms may be observed. These include yawning, diaphoresis, rhinorrhea, restlessness, excessive tearing of the eyes, nausea, vomiting, and abdominal cramping.

Identification of Client Problems

One of the most immediate client problems during the intrapartum period is potential injury of the client, fetus, and newborn because of physiologic and psychological effects of recent drug use.

Planning: Expected Outcomes

The major goal or expected outcome is the client and the fetus will remain free from injury during labor and childbirth.

Interventions
Preventing Injury

When a laboring client has recently used a substance, the nurse should intervene to meet the needs of the client and the fetus for safety, oxygen, and comfort.

Admitting Procedure. Two nurses may be needed to admit the client into the labor unit. One nurse helps the client into bed and initiates electronic fetal monitoring. The other nurse acts as the communicator.

Clients who have recently used a drug may have difficulty following directions; therefore, only one nurse should be communicating to the client. This nurse states firmly what is happening and exactly what the client should do: "Lie on your left side." "This helps us watch how the baby is doing." Maintain eye contact with the client while giving instructions.

Setting Limits. It is essential to set limits to protect the safety of the client and the fetus. For instance, the client cannot smoke. The nurse may say, "It's difficult not to smoke, but there is real danger to everyone if you smoke where oxygen is being used." The client who must remain in bed may become agitated. The nurse may say, "I know it's hard to stay in bed, but we can't take good care of the baby when you walk." If walking is safe for the client, the nurse should set limits about where walking is allowed (in the labor room, not to the cafeteria).

Initiating Seizure Precautions. The laboring client who recently used cocaine is at risk for seizures. Take the following seizure precautions:

- Keep the bed in a low, locked position.
- Pad the side rails and keep them up at all times.
- Check the oxygen and oxygen administration equipment.
- Make sure the suction equipment functions properly to prevent aspiration.
- Reduce environmental stimuli (lights, noise) as much as possible.

Maintaining Effective Communication

Establishing a therapeutic pattern of communication is essential. Avoid confrontation. Instead, acknowledge feelings: "I know you hurt and are frightened. I'll do everything I can to make you comfortable." When the client is abusive, be careful not to take the abuse personally or react in a defensive manner. Inform the client inappropriate words or actions will not be tolerated. Discuss the situation with the charge nurse and provider and incorporate facility security staff if necessary to help deescalate dangerous situations.

Examine your own feelings when clients are abusive and acknowledge when anger is getting in the way of providing care. Another nurse may need to assume care of the client for a time to allow some relief from being the target of unrelenting abusive comments or actions.

Providing Pain Control

Pain control for clients who are substance users poses a difficult problem because it is often challenging to determine the type or combination of drugs that were used before admission. If pain medication can be administered safely, do not withhold it under the false assumption that the client does not need it or that medication will contribute to chemical dependence. Include nonpharmacologic comfort measures such as sacral pressure, back rubs, a cool cloth on the forehead, and continual support and encouragement as for any other client in labor.

Preventing Heroin Withdrawal

To prevent heroin withdrawal during labor, give methadone or buprenorphine as ordered to the client who usually receives a daily dose. It is important to avoid the use of opioid agonist–antagonist drugs such as butorphanol (Stadol) and nalbuphine (Nubain) in clients who are opiate-dependent because acute withdrawal signs and symptoms will occur in the client and the fetus.

Evaluation

Both the expectant client and the fetus may have experienced the harmful effects of drugs throughout pregnancy. However, the interventions for this client problem can be considered effective if neither the client nor the fetus sustain additional injury during labor and childbirth.

POSTPARTUM PERIOD

During the postpartum period, nursing care is focused on helping the client with bonding, providing infant care, and planning to provide self-care and infant care after discharge. Observe for signs of recent drug use and continue to assess the vital signs and level of consciousness of the client.

Observe the client–infant interaction and assess whether bonding and attachment are occurring. Encourage the client to continue efforts to stop taking substances. Clients who stop or reduce use during pregnancy may return to using at previous levels after pregnancy and need support to continue abstinence. Referral to social services and child protective agencies may be necessary for the follow-up care of the client and the infant.

KNOWLEDGE CHECK

12. What prenatal behaviors may indicate substance use?
13. What signs and symptoms indicate recent cocaine use?
14. How does nursing care differ during the intrapartum period when the client has recently taken illicit drugs?

BIRTH OF AN INFANT WITH CONGENITAL ANOMALIES

Even when everything goes according to plan, childbirth is a time of stress for parents. Their anxiety about the condition of the infant is obvious as they carefully trace the features and count the fingers and toes of their newborn. When the infant is not perfect but is born with anomalies, the parents are often overwhelmed with shock and grief. What may appear to be a minor malformation to some individuals or health care providers may manifest itself as a severe impairment to the parents. Nurses have an opportunity to help the family adjust and cope with their feelings.

Factors Influencing Emotional Responses of Parents

Timing and Manner of Being Told

At one time, common practice was to remove the infant from the delivery area before parents could see a congenital anomaly and to tell them about it later. This practice changed, however, when it was realized parents experienced less stress if they were told at once and were permitted to hold their baby if the physical status of the infant allowed. The manner of presenting information also changed. Providers and nurses became aware of the importance of helping the parents accept and bond with the newborn.

Prior Knowledge of the Birth Malformation

Although ultrasonography does not identify all fetal anomalies, many parents become aware of congenital anomalies during ultrasound examinations performed during pregnancy. These parents have time for anticipatory grieving before the birth. They may not demonstrate the shock and disbelief at birth that may be seen in parents who are unprepared. Their reactions should not be interpreted to mean they do not experience grief but rather they have completed some of the early phases of grieving before the birth. Their grief is real and profound, even though it is expressed differently.

One couple was aware from 18 weeks' gestation the fetus had hydrocephalus and protrusion of brain tissue from the skull. The client elected to carry the fetus to term so the infant would have "every chance at life." When the infant died within minutes after birth, the parents calmly held their child and called the infant by the name they had selected several weeks previously. The only overt signs of grief were silent tears and a request to see their clergy.

Once the anomaly is discovered by ultrasound, the pregnancy is no longer seen as normal, and the focus may be on specialized care for the client in preparation for the birth. Parents may feel isolated from those with normal pregnancies. Some parents seek information from others who have a child with a similar anomaly. The full extent of the problem may not be known until after the birth. There may be a long period of worry and fear between the ultrasound diagnosis and the birth.

Type of Malformation

Although any malformation in a newborn produces extreme concern and anxiety, certain malformations are associated with long-term parenting problems. Accepting an infant with facial or genital anomalies is particularly difficult for the family and the community.

The face is visible to everyone, and parents are fearful about whether the child will be accepted. If the congenital malformation is cleft lip and palate, the parents are concerned about surgical repair. They are often anxious about how grandparents and siblings will accept the child. With time and support, parents often work out unique methods to help the family develop strong feelings of attachment.

Gender is associated with a person's identity, and any malformation of the genitals, however slight or correctable, arouses deep concern in both parents. Some anomalies such as hypospadias (opening of the urethra on the underside of the penis) are repaired in early childhood. Other genital anomalies such as ambiguous genitalia (when assignment of gender is in doubt) cause extreme concern in the family and affect such basic issues as what to name the infant, how to dress the infant, and how to respond to questions about the infant's gender.

Irreparable Congenital Malformation

Although the initial impact of any birth malformation is profound disappointment and concern, when the malformation is irreparable, the parents must grapple with the knowledge the infant will have a lifelong disability. Examples of irreparable congenital malformation include Down's syndrome, microcephaly, and amelia (absence of an entire limb).

Grief and Mourning

Grief describes the emotional response to loss. Mourning is the process of going through the phases of grief until the loss can be accepted and resolved. Birth of an infant with a birth malformation evokes a grief response. The family must mourn the loss of the perfect infant they imagined during pregnancy. Early emotions include denial, anger, and guilt.

Denial and disbelief are the initial reactions of most parents to the birth of an infant with a congenital malformation, asking "How could this happen?" Anger is often a pervasive response and may take the form of fault-finding or resentment. Anger may be directed toward the family, the medical personnel, or themselves, but it is seldom directed toward the infant. Guilt may be expressed as a question of responsibility for the malformation as many parents search for a cause.

Other emotions include fear, which may be expressed as concern about what must be done in the immediate or distant future (surgical procedures, complicated care, the infant's potential for a normal life). Sadness and depression, manifested by crying, withdrawal from relationships, lack of energy, inability to sleep, and decreased appetite, may precede acceptance and resolution. Gradually—often after a prolonged time—the feelings of sadness abate, and the family is able to adapt to the loss and resolve its grief.

KNOWLEDGE CHECK

15. When should parents be told the infant has anomalies?
16. What types of malformations most affect parenting?
17. How can the reaction of parents to birth anomalies be described?

Nursing Considerations
Assisting with the Grieving Process

Whenever possible, both parents should be present when they are told about the infant's condition. The nurse should use therapeutic communication techniques to help them discuss their feelings and fears. They should be given as much information as possible about the anomaly before the birth. If the infant will go to the neonatal intensive care unit (NICU), a tour before the birth may help them understand the type of care their infant will receive.

At birth, the parents continue to grieve the loss of the perfect infant they expected and form an attachment with this newborn. Whether the parents learned about the problem before or after the birth, it is helpful if the nurse remains with them as they go through the initial phase of shock and disbelief. The nurse maintains an atmosphere that encourages them to express their feelings by listening carefully to what the parents say and reflecting the content and feelings they express.

For example, the parent of an infant with cleft palate says, "How could this happen? I should have gone to the doctor earlier." A helpful response might be, "It sounds like you feel responsible for this problem. Actually, we don't know the exact causes of cleft palate, but let's talk about how you are feeling." This offers reassurance but keeps the interaction open to explore the underlying feelings of guilt the client may be expressing.

Nurses should recognize grief responses vary among individuals, and cultural and religious beliefs affect the expression of grief. Some people express grief openly by crying, becoming angry, or seeking comfort from a support group. Those in other cultures (e.g., Asian and Native American) may appear stoic and may not reveal the depths of their grief. In some cultures (such as Hispanic), it is acceptable for females, but not for males, to grieve publicly. The couple should be offered a private room, if possible. The infant should be examined in front of the parents so they can ask questions. Information about normal needs of the newborn should be given at the same time as information about the anomaly.

Promoting Bonding and Attachment

A priority nursing intervention is to promote bonding and attachment, which may be disrupted when the infant is born with an abnormality. The process is facilitated when the nurse communicates acceptance of the infant.

To promote bonding, the nurse handles the newborn gently and presents the infant as someone precious. Parents are particularly sensitive to facial expressions of shock or distress. The infant should be called by name. Many nurses emphasize the normal aspects of the infant's body: "Look at how alert your baby is, and those beautiful eyes." Perhaps it is most important to help the parents hold their infant as soon as possible. Touching and cuddling are essential to caring (Fig. 11.3).

Providing Accurate Information

Nurses who work in perinatal settings should be aware of follow-up treatment and timing of surgical procedures for common anomalies so they can clarify and reinforce the

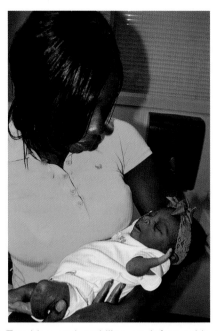

Fig. 11.3 Touching and cuddling an infant with congenital anomalies fosters attachment and helps client's cope with the grieving process. This infant has anomalies of the hand and arm. (Courtesy Cheryl Briggs, RNC, Annapolis, MD.)

information given by the provider. This involves discussing the plan of care with the provider as well as researching the nursing care that will be required. Parents develop trust in the health care team when consistent information is presented clearly and explained fully.

If possible, one primary nurse or a team of nurses should work with the family throughout the hospital stay. The nurse should assess the parents' understanding of the condition and the treatment plan. Parents often need information repeated frequently because it is difficult for them to absorb all they are told at this time of intense emotions.

Facilitating Communication

Nurses are sometimes fearful of being asked questions they are unable to answer, or they fear they will say the wrong thing.

The most helpful course of action is to answer questions as honestly as possible. If uncertain about information, say so: "I'm not sure, but I'll find out for you." In addition to answers, parents need kindness, support, and genuine concern.

It is crucial family members communicate with one another as well as with the health care professionals. Information and empathy should be offered consistently to both parents. Both parents should be included in all discussions, demonstrations, and care of the infant. Without this attention, the partner cannot be expected to support the client, explain the infant's condition to relatives and friends, or cope with their own shock and sadness.

The nurse should assess the client for signs of postpartum depression. The partner should be made aware of the client's increased risk for prolonged depression. The signs of depression and the differences among normal

"baby blues," normal grieving, and postpartum depression should be explained.

Participating in Infant Care

Parents should be involved in giving care to the infant as soon as possible to increase bonding and help them feel they can parent the infant. Providing care for the infant can also elicit feelings of anxiety for some parents, so it is important to frequently ask and assess their comfort level when incorporating parents in the care of their infant (Haward et al., 2020).

Planning for Discharge

Teach parents the special feeding, holding, and positioning techniques their infant needs. Early participation in infant care fosters feelings of attachment and responsibility for the infant, as well as increasing feelings of confidence. They should also know what type of follow-up care with the health care provider is necessary and what other services may be needed.

Provide other anticipatory guidance that may help prevent problems when the infant is discharged. The reaction and behavior of siblings depends on their ages and abilities to understand the needs of the infant. Young children, who are often jealous of the attention and care the infant requires, may regress to infantile behaviors such as bedwetting and thumb sucking. Remind parents this indicates a need for attention rather than naughtiness.

Although grandparents can be a great source of strength and support, they also may have difficulty adjusting to the infant with an abnormality. When appropriate and if the parents are willing, include grandparents when teaching the special care the infant will need.

Providing Referrals

Initiate referrals to national and community resources, as needed. Parents may benefit from a referral to the social worker or grief counselor in the hospital. Parents may also benefit from information about the Easterseals Disability Services, the March of Dimes, or the disabled children's services of the public health department. In addition, organizations such as Shriners International provide funds for the care of children. Support groups vary among communities, and perinatal nurses may wish to provide a list of the names, addresses, and telephone numbers of these organizations.

> **KNOWLEDGE CHECK**
>
> 18. How do nurses promote bonding in families of an infant with congenital anomalies?
> 19. What should be included in discharge planning for the family of an infant with congenital anomalies?

PERINATAL LOSS

Perinatal death can occur at any time. Early spontaneous abortion, ectopic pregnancy, fetal demise at any point in pregnancy, stillbirth, or neonatal death when the infant survives for a few days or weeks can be equally devastating for the parents. The death may occur after a complicated pregnancy or one in which all seemed well until the baby died. Parents may have a short time with their baby while it still lives or none at all.

Parents experiencing perinatal death often feel alone in their grief. Friends and family members may be hesitant to discuss the loss for fear of saying the wrong thing. They may be uncomfortable with the topic and change the subject when parents want to talk.

Early Pregnancy Loss

Early pregnancy loss from spontaneous abortion or ectopic pregnancy may precipitate intense grief in the parents. The parents may not yet have told family and friends about the pregnancy. Those who do know may minimize the grief that occurs at this time. Comments such as "You shouldn't have any problems getting pregnant again" discount the intensity of the parents' feelings. Frequently, the health care of a client experiencing early pregnancy loss focuses on the physical needs with little attention given to the emotional needs of the client and family.

Concurrent Death and Survival in Multifetal Pregnancy

Parents experience conflicting and complex feelings of joy and grief when one or more infants in a multifetal pregnancy live and one or more infants in the same gestation die. Parents do not grieve less for the dead infant because of the joy they experience in the surviving child.

For parents experiencing survival of one infant and death of another, the grieving process may be more complicated. They may have fears about the health of the surviving infant, especially if the infant is preterm or ill. They may be unable to grieve for the dead child because of their concerns and responsibilities for the surviving child. They also may experience problems with attachment to the surviving infant because of grieving or fear of losing this infant as well. In addition, they may receive less support from others compared with parents who have lost their child in a single gestation.

Parents who experience the death of one infant and the survival of another need the same interventions as those offered for parents who lose the child in a single gestation. These interventions include allowing the parents to hold the dead infant and gathering mementos. In addition, nurses should be prepared to confirm the cause of death, if known, and the health status of the surviving infant.

Perinatal Palliative or Hospice Care Services

When parents learn the fetus has a terminal condition, they may choose to continue the pregnancy and deliver at term, knowing the infant will survive only a short time. Perinatal palliative or hospice care services provide care by nurses experienced in hospice or palliative care. These nurses assist the family through the processes of birth, death, and grief. The emphasis of care is on promoting quality of life, minimizing suffering, and supporting parents in their grief. It allows parents to plan for the birth and death of their baby. They support the parents in navigating through the pregnancy and making end-of-life decisions in the most therapeutic way possible (ACOG, 2021b).

Previous Pregnancy Loss

Clients who have experienced previous pregnancy losses, regardless of the gestational age at the time of the loss, can experience a range of emotions such as anxiety, grief, depression, and posttraumatic stress (Tiemeyer et al., 2020).

Having other, healthy children does not reduce the degree of anxiety during a pregnancy following a perinatal loss. Parents may delay telling family and friends about the pregnancy until they feel confident about the outcome. They may not tell those who do not already know about the loss of the previous pregnancy. Some do not prepare the baby's room at all during the pregnancy. Others wait until near the end of pregnancy to make preparations to bring an infant into the home. Conflicting emotions of excitement, fear, and doubt occur as the pregnancy progresses normally.

Early prenatal care is especially important during a pregnancy after a loss. Both parents may be more comfortable with more frequent contact with the health care provider. Clients tend to be extra careful to do what is recommended in pregnancy and hypervigilant about signs that might indicate something is wrong. Less fetal activity than usual is very worrying, and feeling the baby move is reassuring. They need frequent reassurance about the status of the fetus and emotional support throughout the pregnancy.

Although parents may request extra diagnostic testing to help relieve their anxiety, they may not always feel as reassured by normal test results as they had hoped. It is important for nurses to provide an opportunity for parents to express their distress and fears. Referrals to support groups or mental health providers may be appropriate.

APPLICATION OF THE NURSING PROCESS: PREGNANCY LOSS

Assessment

Nursing assessment of the family that has experienced the loss of a fetus or infant requires sensitivity. Collect as much information as possible before meeting the client and family for the first time so hurtful mistakes can be avoided. Knowing the child's gender, weight, length, and gestational age, and whether any abnormalities were noted will help the nurse communicate effectively.

Many perinatal units design a sticker or symbol to place on the door and chart so all staff who encounter the family will be alerted the infant has not survived. This visual symbol diminishes the chance an uninformed person will make inadvertent comments that cause pain.

Nurses are often unsure about how to interact with a family that has experienced the loss of an infant. It is helpful to acknowledge the situation and clarify the nurse's role at once: "I'm Dawn, and I'll be your nurse today. I'm so sorry for your loss. What can I do today that would be most helpful to you?"

This is not an appropriate time for self-disclosure or for false reassurance. Keep the focus on the family's response and their ability to support one another.

Initial grief responses are similar to those expressed by parents of infants with anomalies. Crying and expressions of anger often occur during the client's stay in the birth facility. Guilt is often an underlying feeling as the parents search for a reason for their child's death.

Nurses who provide home care or make follow-up telephone calls should be aware of subtle cues of grief such as sighing, excessive sleeping, apathy, poor hygiene, and loss of appetite. These signs are especially important when assessing members of cultural groups who do not display grief publicly. In addition, nurses should observe for signs of postpartum depression, posttraumatic stress disorder, and panic disorder, which may occur after perinatal loss.

Evaluate the availability of a support system, which includes family members or faith leaders. Ask whether the family would like a spiritual advisor called. The family may want the infant baptized or blessed.

Assess the partner's needs as well because they are sometimes perceived as needing less support than the client.

Identification of Client Problems

Perinatal loss affects the entire family. Many families experience changes in their relationships and family processes because of grief.

Planning: Expected Outcomes

Expected outcomes for changes in family processes are the parents will do the following:
1. Acknowledge their grief and express the meaning of the loss.
2. Share their grief with significant others.
3. Provide support to each family member.

Interventions
Allowing Expression of Feelings

Stay with the parents as they express their feelings. Allow them to cry or respond as they wish. Parents may want to have some time alone but may also appreciate having the nurse sit quietly nearby. When they are ready to talk, listen attentively.

Acknowledging the Infant

It was once believed when an infant was stillborn or died shortly after birth, the less parents knew of the infant, the less they would grieve. The infant often was whisked away so the parents never saw their newborn. Relatives disposed of the clothes and infant equipment before the parents returned home, and they were left with very few memories of the infant's birth.

Allow the parents to talk about the baby as much as they wish. Refer to the infant by name. If the infant lived for a time, talk about what happened during that time and answer any questions the parents have. If the infant is dying, allow parents to hold and care for their baby. Take pictures of the infant if the parents wish.

Presenting the Infant to the Parents

When the baby dies, the way in which the infant is presented to the parents is extremely important because these are the memories they will retain. Parents should be prepared for the appearance of the infant, especially if maceration (peeling) of the skin is present or there are disfigured areas. If necessary, wash the infant and apply baby lotion. The sense of smell is very powerful. Applying baby lotion provides olfactory stimulation. Wrap the infant in a soft, warm blanket. Some parents may wish to participate in bathing and dressing the baby.

If possible, bring the parents and the infant together while the infant is still warm and soft. Keeping the infant in a warmed incubator may be necessary if some time elapses before the parents have contact with the infant. If this is not possible, rewarm the infant under a radiant warmer. Wrap the infant in warmed blankets. Allow the parents to keep the infant as long as they wish, and tell them to feel free to unwrap the infant if they wish.

When the stillborn infant has severe deformities, explain the malformations briefly and gently. Wrap the infant to expose the most normal aspects. When the infant has deformities of the head and face, wrap the infant with the blanket draped loosely over the most severely affected areas so the parents do not see those areas first. Use diapers to cover genital malformations and booties and mittens to cover abnormalities of the hands and feet.

It is not advisable to try to hide the malformations completely. Allow parents to progress at their own speed in inspecting the infant. Parents may look at the abnormality or choose to leave the infant wrapped. They may quietly discuss positive features of the infant: "The baby has your ears." "Look at those long fingers."

Some parents may provide care before their baby dies. If death is near, ventilators and other equipment may be removed so the parents can feel closer to the infant. They may hold the infant during the dying process. Many feel this is very helpful to them, as it provides a chance to say goodbye and is the only opportunity they will have to parent their baby. Other family members also may be present at this time.

Allow as much privacy and time as the parents and other family members need to be together. Remain sensitive to cues—some members of the family want to talk and some prefer silence. A sympathetic smile or a promise to return at a certain time and then returning as promised are equally important. It is all right to say, "Do you want to talk?" Then listening quietly and provide reflection on the client's or partner's feelings. If the parents request privacy, check intermittently to see if they need assistance.

Although many parents want to spend time caring for or holding their baby before or after death, others may not. It is important not to make the parents feel guilty or that they should behave in a certain way. Nurses should accept each family needs to go through this difficult experience in their own way.

Preparing a Memory Packet

Mourning requires memories. Nurses help the family create memories of the infant so the existence of the child is confirmed and the parents can complete the grieving process.

Most parents treasure a memory packet. Prepare one that includes a photograph; a birth identification band with the date and time of birth; the crib card with the infant's name, weight, and length; a tape measure; and a blanket and cap used for the baby. If the baby has enough hair, ask the parents for permission to cut a lock of hair from the nape of the neck where it will not be noticeable. Some hospitals offer commercial remembrance materials to parents. The packets or boxes may contain clothing for the baby to wear and provide a place to keep baby items. Make paper handprints or soft modeling material impressions of the infant's hands and feet.

Take photographs of the infant to help parents remember the baby's features, and assist them through the grieving process. Take photographs of the infant dressed and undressed, wrapped and unwrapped, and of the parents and other family members with the infant. The infant should be positioned in natural newborn positions for the photos such as lying on the stomach with the knees tucked under and the head turned to one side. Professional photographers may be available from the Now I Lay Me Down To Sleep foundation, a nonprofit organization that provides bereavement photos to families. A list of photographers and their locations is available at https://www.nowilaymedowntosleep.org. Keep the memory packet and photographs on file if the parents do not wish to take them home because they may want them at a later time. Many couples feel these concrete forms of remembrance are invaluable in helping them remember the baby as a person who really existed when they have no other signs of life.

Respecting Cultural Practices

In some cultures, seeing or holding the baby after death is not acceptable. Cutting a lock of hair may not be permissible. It is culturally unacceptable in certain groups to take photographs of a person after death. Pictures taken before death occurs may be more acceptable. Therefore, ask permission before doing any memento preparation. Expression of grief may be loud and open, or parents may appear stoic, depending on cultural expectations. The nurse should be accepting of the family's method of coping with their loss.

Assisting with Other Needs

If the family includes other children, help the parents plan how to tell them about the death of the expected infant. Give them information about sibling responses and needs based on the ages of their other children. Provide the parents with written information about perinatal loss, grieving, and children's responses to death for later use. Other family members and close friends may be important in helping care for siblings as the parents cope with their own grief.

Offer to call clergy or other faith leaders, and discuss plans for a funeral or memorial service, if the family wishes. Parents may want to discuss this with their own faith leader, or a hospital chaplain may assist them. Discuss the normal grieving process, and explain a considerable amount of time is involved. Describe common reactions family members and friends might have. For example, some family members or friends may minimize the loss, whereas others, in a misguided attempt to offer comfort, may urge the couple to have another baby. Let them know grandparents also go through grief because of the loss of their grandchild, as well as the pain their children must endure.

Providing Follow-Up Care

Parents may find friends and relatives expect them to recover quickly from perinatal loss and cannot understand their continued grief. Suggest they allow the parents to "tell the story" of the infant as often as they want because this helps them in the grief process. Suggest they help parents collect and talk about mementos to help establish memories of the infant.

Siblings are often expecting to be a "big brother" or "big sister" and need help understanding why that will not occur. Help the parents explore how they will tell their other children the new baby will not be coming home. Explain some young children think they have done something to cause the death and need reassurance. They may have questions (such as "Is the baby still dead?" or "Is the baby alive?"), which should be answered simply but truthfully. Because the parents may experience grief in different ways, they may not understand each other's responses. Clients who want to talk about the loss repeatedly may have partners who deal with their grief by being stoic and brooding or by focusing their energy on work. Emphasize the individuality of grief and no single method or duration of grieving is right for everyone.

Couples usually want to know the cause of their infant's death. An autopsy may be recommended even if the cause of death is obvious. This gives parents the most accurate diagnosis and possibility of recurrence in a future pregnancy. In some cases, the cause may never be found. Referral for genetic counseling may be appropriate for some parents. Future pregnancies will be stressful, and the client will need closer follow-up than usual to identify any problems as soon as possible. The anxiety may continue in the neonatal period, and parents may need education and emotional support during this time.

Providing Referrals

Many birth agencies offer bereavement programs or counselors to provide ongoing help for parents. A social services referral is important. Telephone calls made during the first week, 1 to 2 weeks later, at the time of the postpartum checkup, and at the 1-year anniversary are helpful. Sympathy cards may be sent by agency staff with a list of resources that may be helpful. The greatest help often comes from contact with people who have experienced a similar loss, and a variety of support groups have been formed.

Refer parents to resources at the birth facility or in the community designed to help parents cope with loss. Many internet resources are available. Examples are the MISS Foundation at https://www.missfoundation.org and Helping After Neonatal Death (HAND) at https://www.handonline.org.

Some families join internet perinatal loss support groups. Such groups may be particularly helpful after the immediate period surrounding the death. Extended family and friends may no longer be as supportive at this time and do not realize the length of time involved in grieving. As parents move toward healing, they gradually develop a feeling of control over their lives and being able to make decisions.

Evaluation

Nursing care has been successful if the family members share their feelings of loss and grief, communicate them to their significant others, and are supportive of one another.

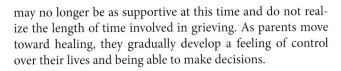

> **KNOWLEDGE CHECK**
>
> 20. How should the stillborn infant be presented to the parents? Why?
> 21. What is a memory packet, and what should it include?

ADOPTION

Although pregnancy is a planned and exciting time for some, it can be a time of great strife and distress for others. For some clients, pregnancy can be unexpected, and for a variety of reasons they may find themselves choosing adoption for their child. Caring for a client deciding on adoption can present interesting challenges for nurses. Making a choice for adoption can be both a difficult and rewarding experience for a birth parent (Adoption & Surrogacy Choices of Colorado, 2021). Although the pregnant birth parent may find a great sense of joy in knowing they could give their child a better life through making a decision for adoption, they may also struggle with intense feelings of guilt, depression, and regret.

Adoption has changed greatly in recent years and now offers birth parents the option of choosing how involved they would like to be in their child's life. The decision for adoption is a very personal one and will look different for each person. For some individuals, it is very important to them that they have a relationship with their child and they have an opportunity to be a part of the child's life, whereas for others, having a relationship may prove too emotionally difficult, and they choose to not maintain any relationship or communication with the child or adopted parents. For this reason, many adoption agencies now offer a variety of choices to the birthing person, ranging from having an open adoption that permits the birthing person to have regular contact with the child and adoptive family, to partially open or to closed adoptions. The relationship between birth parents and adoptive parents may vary greatly among clients. Some birth parents can interview and pick which family they would like to adopt their child. They may have had time to develop a close relationship throughout the pregnancy, with the adoptive family attending doctor appointments and, in some cases, even attending the birth. In other circumstances, the birthing person may choose to let an adoption agency make the decision on where to best place the child and not know or have any contact with the adoptive family at all.

It is important that health care providers are equipped to deal with the physical and emotional needs of clients deciding on adoption, as well as the adopting family. Knowing whether the client has made a decision for adoption, whether an adoptive family has been chosen, and who will be a part of the delivery are vital pieces of information a nurse should have to best support the client. Health care providers should be sensitive and nonjudgmental in their speech and care of the client deciding on adoption. It is important nurses withhold any personal biases they may have and remember that making a decision for adoption is a courageous act of love by the birthing person, not abandonment. Nurses should make every effort to respect and meet any special needs or requests the client may have during the birth experience. Most birth parents make a plan for how much contact they would like with the infant, how involved in the infant's care they would like to be, and how involved they would like the adoptive parents to be during the hospital stay. It is common for birth parents to want as much information as possible about the infant and have some time alone with the infant. The birthing person should be encouraged to take as much time as necessary with the infant, and hospital mementos such as keepsake footprints, baby bands, and infant blankets should be given to the birthing person if so desired. Such actions provide memories of the infant and help the client through the grieving process that may occur with adoption.

It is important the nurse is able to form a rapport and trusting relationship with the birthing person. Therapeutic communication techniques are useful in helping the client explore feelings. Although the client has made a choice for adoption, the grief felt may be similar to experiencing death. This grief may not be shared with family or friends, and those close to the client may not understand those feelings. It is imperative the nurse acknowledge any feelings the client may have, while avoiding offering advice or coming across as judgmental. The nurse plays a vital role in helping the client transition through a very emotional and difficult experience by serving as an advocate for the client's feelings and well-being.

In the event the adoptive parents have been chosen, the nurse should acknowledge their needs and emotions as well. All efforts should be made to give adoptive parents a private room to process through emotions and adapt to their new role as parents. Nurses should teach adoptive parents how to care for their newborn and what to expect in growth and development. Adoptive parents may experience an array of emotions such as joy, anxiety, fear, shame, and feeling overwhelmed (Child Welfare Information Gateway, 2019). Demonstrations, as well as return demonstrations, may be helpful in assisting them in learning to care for their newborn.

SURROGACY

Families are made in a variety of ways. For the client unable to conceive by natural means, surrogacy may be an option they choose to start their family. There are different types of surrogates, and it is important for nurses to have an understanding of the different types.

Traditional Surrogacy

With traditional surrogacy, surrogates (individuals carrying the pregnancy) use their own egg that is inseminated with sperm from one of the intended legal parents. With traditional surrogacy, the surrogate and one of the child's parents are genetically linked to the pregnancy, and the other parent has no genetic link to the pregnancy (Patel et al., 2018). These types of surrogacy cases have historically caused a myriad of legal and ethical issues. Traditional surrogacies are no longer allowed in the United States (Adoption & Surrogacy Choices of Colorado, 2021).

Gestational Surrogate

With gestational surrogacy an egg from the intended legal parents or a donated egg is artificially inseminated with sperm from one of the intended parents or from donor sperm. The inseminated egg is then transferred into the uterus of the surrogate. With gestational surrogacy the surrogate has no genetic link to the pregnancy (Patel et al., 2018).

Altruistic versus Commercial Surrogacy

When altruistic surrogacy takes place, the surrogate receives no financial compensation for carrying the pregnancy, other than coverage of medical expenses directly related to the pregnancy (Patel et al., 2018). Alternatively, with commercial surrogacy, the surrogate receives an agreed upon, legally binding, financial compensation, in addition to the cost of their medical expenses related to the pregnancy (Patel et al., 2018). Laws related to surrogacy and compensation vary by state.

Emotional Impact of Surrogacy

Similar to adoption, the client utilizing surrogacy may experience a wide array of emotions. The intended parents may have a surrogate who is someone close to them and has agreed to carry the pregnancy, or they may select a surrogate through an agency. Despite what method is selected, surrogacy can be very expensive and forces both the intended parents and the surrogate to trust and rely on each other in a manner that may feel unnatural and frightening. The intended parents may have difficulty bonding with the pregnancy since they are unable to carry the infant, physically feel the infant grow, and experience the changes that accompany pregnancy. Likewise, the surrogate may experience a sense of loss and mourning when the pregnancy ends and they have to relinquish the child (Patel et al., 2018). Surrogacy can also be a time of great joy and excitement, as it can provide the intended parents with hope and happiness that they can finally grow their family, and provide the surrogate with a deep sense of meaning and self-fulfillment, helping a family in this way (Patel et al., 2018).

Nursing Care with Surrogacy

Nursing care of the surrogate and the intended parents should start with clear and detailed communication and include both parties. Care of the surrogate should follow standard of care for any pregnant client. Often, the surrogate and the intended parents predetermine how in-depth their involvement will be prior to and during delivery. Decisions regarding whether or not the intended parents can be in the birthing suite, or if the surrogate will just have their partner present at delivery are typically outlined in legal documents; however these questions should be asked and clarified when the surrogate presents to the hospital. After delivery, the intended parents should receive the infant security bands and their own room. Intended parents should be taught how to care for the infant and incorporated into care and assessments of the infant, as well as be the legal and designated decision makers regarding infant medical decisions. It is important to assess whether the surrogate and intended parents have agreed for the surrogate to breastfeed and/or provide breast milk. If the parents do not want the surrogate to breastfeed, then instruction should be provided to the surrogate regarding appropriate breast care following delivery. It is imperative to address the emotional needs of both the surrogate and the intended parents as the infant's birth signals a transition in their relationship life roles, with the surrogate preparing to resume a presurrogacy lifestyle and the intended parents adjusting to their new role as parents.

❓ KNOWLEDGE CHECK

22. What is meant by the phrase, "Adoption is an act of love"?
23. What are the nurse's responsibilities to the adoptive parents?
24. What are the nurse's responsibilities to the surrogate?
25. What are the nurse's responsibilities to the intended parents?

PERINATAL PSYCHOLOGICAL COMPLICATIONS

Although pregnancy and birth are a time of great joy and excitement for many clients, for others it can be a time of great stress and sadness and bring to the forefront underlying psychological disorders. Psychological disorders during pregnancy can have several causes ranging from genetic predisposition to stressful life events (Postpartum Depression, 2021). Left untreated, perinatal psychological complications can result in serious harm to both the client and infant.

Perinatal Mood and Anxiety Disorders

Perinatal mood and anxiety disorders are feelings of depression and anxiety that occur during pregnancy or after the first year of childbirth (Children's Hospital of Philadelphia, 2021). Signs and symptoms of a mood disorder include anxiety, mood swings, agitation, consistently sad mood, feelings of worthlessness, difficulty thinking or concentrating, loss of energy, crying fits, fatigue, headache, and loss of appetite (Mayo Clinic, 2018). Psychosis-associated mood disorders are rare; however, they do occur. Symptoms include thoughts of delusions, auditory hallucinations, cognitive impairment, disorganized thinking, inability to discern delusions from reality, rapidly changing moods, and actions and behaviors that are out of the ordinary for the individual (Postpartum Depression, 2021). Although the disorders occur more often during the postpartum period, prenatal episodes are also possible.

BOX 11.4 Risk Factors for Postpartum Depression

Prior history of depression

Depression during pregnancy or previous postpartum depression (strong predictors)

First pregnancy

Hormonal fluctuations following childbirth

Medical problems during pregnancy or after birth, such as preeclampsia, preexisting diabetes mellitus, anemia, or postpartum thyroid dysfunction

Personal or family history of depression, mental illness, or alcoholism

Personality characteristics, such as immaturity and low self-esteem

Marital dysfunction or difficult relationship with the significant other, resulting in lack of support

Anger or ambivalence about the pregnancy

Single status

Young client age

Feelings of isolation, lack of social support, or inadequate support

Fatigue, lack of sleep

Financial worries

Child care stress (infant who is ill, has anomalies, or has a difficult temperament)

Multifetal pregnancy

Chronic stressors

Unwanted or unplanned pregnancy

⚡ SAFETY CHECK

Signs and symptoms of postpartum depression include the following:

Anxiety

Feelings of guilt

Agitation

Fatigue, sleeplessness

Feeling unwell

Irritability

Difficulty concentrating or making decisions, confusion

Appetite changes

Loss of pleasure in normal activities

Lack of energy

Crying

Sadness

Depression (may not be present at first)

Suicidal thoughts

Less responsive to infant

Postpartum Depression

Postpartum depression is defined as depression that takes place after childbirth and persists longer than 2 weeks. In contrast, postpartum blues (*baby blues, maternity blues*) is a mild, transient condition that typically resolves within 2 weeks. Postpartum depression can present within days or weeks of childbirth and has the potential to last up to a year (Cleveland Clinic, 2018). Postpartum depression is a common complication of childbirth, as 1 in 1000 clients experience postpartum depression during one of their pregnancies (Cleveland Clinic, 2018). Although postpartum depression can affect anyone after giving birth, some individuals are at an increased risk (Box 11.4). Clients with a history of depression or sexual abuse, clients experiencing an unexpected or unwanted pregnancy, or those who experienced a pregnancy complication or traumatic childbirth and lack social support are all at increased risk for this disorder (March of Dimes, 2019). As medical professionals, it is imperative to remember each client's experience is different, and care and treatment options should be individualized to the client. It is also important to acknowledge that depressive symptoms, screening, and treatment vary throughout different countries and regions. Depression may be accepted differently based on the client's culture (Ahmad et al., 2021).

Postpartum Psychosis

Postpartum psychosis is an intense form of postpartum depression that is rare and typically occurs shortly after birth (Massachusetts General Hospital Postpartum Psychosis Project [MGHP3], 2021). Postpartum psychosis is characterized by serious mood instabilities, which peak from 48 hours to 2 weeks postpartum. To truly be characterized as a postpartum psychosis episode, clients must experience a depressive episode (either manic or major depressive episode), with accompanying psychotic symptoms (MGHP3, 2021). Postpartum psychosis is a serious medical emergency that requires immediate intervention, usually hospitalization, psychotherapy, and appropriate medication. There is an increased risk for development of postpartum psychosis in first-time parents, as well as those with bipolar I disorder (MGHP3, 2021).

Bipolar Disorder

Bipolar disorder is a combination of depressive and manic symptoms. There are three types of bipolar disorder: bipolar I, bipolar II, and cyclothymic. A diagnosis of bipolar I requires manic episodes and depressive episodes, and a bipolar II diagnosis requires depressive episodes and hypomania, while a cyclothymic diagnosis requires recurrent mood changes of both depressive episodes and hypomania lasting 2 years (National Institute of Mental Health, 2020). Pregnancy often intensifies symptoms for the client with bipolar disorder and can send them into a depressive or manic episode; however, many clients stop taking their medications during pregnancy out of fear they will cause harm to the baby. It is imperative medical professionals work with these clients to establish risk versus benefit regarding medications during pregnancy. The client may have to continue to take medications, despite the known risk to the baby, to ensure their own safety and well-being.

Postpartum Anxiety Disorders

Postpartum anxiety is a condition in which a person experiences intense feelings of fear and constant worry after giving birth (Toler et al., 2018). The signs and symptoms of an anxiety disorder include inability to relax, intrusive thoughts, restlessness, dread, difficulty concentrating, irritability, insomnia, anguish about making decisions, panic, phobias, and constant worrying (Toler et. al, 2018). It is estimated between 11% and 21% of clients experience perinatal anxiety disorders (Zappas et al., 2020).

APPLICATION OF THE NURSING PROCESS: PERINATAL PSYCHOLOGICAL COMPLICATIONS

Assessment

Clients should be assessed for depression during pregnancy, at the birth facility, and during follow-up visits after birth. Early identification is paramount. The client should be reassessed at each contact with health care providers (including follow-up telephone calls). Clients whose infants are in a NICU should be assessed for postpartum depression during visits to their infants.

Assessment tools such as the Postpartum Depression Predictors Inventory–Revised may be helpful. This inventory identifies prenatal depression, current life stress, social support, prenatal anxiety, satisfaction with marital relationship, history of depression, self-esteem, unwanted or unplanned pregnancy, marital status, socioeconomic status, child care stress, infant temperament, and maternity blues as factors that may predict the likelihood of a client developing postpartum depression (Alves et al., 2019). In addition, screening for excessive fatigue in the first 2 weeks after childbirth may help identify clients who will later develop postpartum depression and enable them to get early treatment.

Some examples of other screening tools include the Edinburgh Postnatal Depression Scale and the Postpartum Depression Checklist (James & Suplee, 2021). Ask the clients if they are often sad or depressed or if they have felt a loss of pleasure or interest in things they once enjoyed. These questions may enable early identification and treatment of depression.

Observe for subjective symptoms, such as apathy, lack of interest or energy, anorexia, or sleeplessness. The client's verbalizations of failure, sadness, loneliness, anxiety, or vague confusion are important cues. Focus on the frequency, duration, and intensity of the client's feelings to determine their severity.

Assess for objective data, such as crying, sleeplessness, poor personal hygiene, or inability to follow directions or concentrate. Determine what, if any, support is available. Clients with an absent or unavailable support system may feel increasingly isolated, leading to stress and feeling unable to manage pregnancy or being a parent. Inappropriate expressions of blame or anger toward the partner and unmet expectations of the baby or the parenting role are sometimes present.

Identification of Client Problem

Clients with psychological disorders during the perinatal period lack effective coping techniques to manage the stressors associated with childbirth and parenting.

Planning: Expected Outcomes

To achieve the expected outcomes, the client will do the following:
- Verbalize feelings with the health care provider and significant other throughout the postpartum period.
- Discuss challenges and strengths in dealing with emotions/feelings.
- Identify available resources for the postpartum period.

Interventions
Providing Anticipatory Guidance

Because of short hospital stays for new parents, and timing of the usual onset of affective disorders, most incidences of postpartum depression (and postpartum psychosis) occur after the client has gone home. Anticipatory guidance of the client and family is the most critical nursing intervention. Success of treatment is largely affected by early diagnosis. During the prenatal period, initiate a discussion with all pregnant clients and their partners to provide anticipatory guidance about the early weeks at home. Explain the importance of seeking early help to decrease the length of time the condition lasts.

Discuss the need for frequent contact with other adults so the client does not become isolated. Emphasize the importance of continued communication with the partner or a close friend who can provide support when loneliness or anxiety becomes a problem.

Explain that adequate rest and nutrition can help the client maintain energy and a feeling of health and well-being. Teach clients and their support persons the signs of postpartum depression and other postpartum psychological disorders, including when they should seek help.

Demonstrating Caring

Conveying a caring attitude is an important nursing strategy to help clients decrease their emotional distress and guide them in regaining their well-being during the peripartum period. Acknowledge something is wrong and the client seems depressed. Spend time with clients and reassure them this condition is not their fault.

Explain to the client these feelings are a common experience after childbirth. Encourage the client to talk about their feelings and provide reassurance that help is available.

Helping the Client Verbalize Feelings

Because clients are expected to be happy after giving birth, many clients do not discuss their negative feelings with others. They may feel ashamed and believe a social stigma is attached to admitting to depression at any time and especially after giving birth. They may fear their infant may be taken away from them if they disclose their problem. If they do discuss their feelings, their friends or even health care workers may trivialize the problem by making comments such as, "You'll get over it. After all, you have a beautiful baby." Clients and their families minimize depression because they cannot find the exact cause.

Discuss some feelings may seem "unreasonable" (anger, guilt, shame); however, the client should acknowledge negative feelings and insist others recognize them, too. Discuss the realities of parenting and how it can be exhausting.

Enhancing Sensitivity to Infant Cues

Point out infant cues and explain their meaning. Model behavior to show the client how to respond to the infant's cues. Measures to help the client relax may help improve the mood and response to the infant.

Assess the infant's growth and development. Depressed clients may not give the care and nurturing needed. Determine the infant's weight gain or loss and observe the client's response to the infant's crying. If the client is breastfeeding, suggest continuing because it may increase feelings of closeness to the infant. If the client is taking medication, be sure it is recommended for use during lactation.

Helping Family Members

Include the partner in discussions about depression, before and after the birth. Acknowledge their feelings and those of the client. Offer practical suggestions of ways the partner can help manage the changes in their lives. Discuss ways to help, such as arranging for the client to get more sleep and to eat better, which may help decrease irritability and anxiety. Determine the partner's need for additional support and explain the impact of postpartum depression on each family member. Emphasize the importance of the client taking medications as ordered. Discuss signs that indicate the client's depression is worsening and when to call the health care provider.

Providing Help

Explore with the family practical suggestions on how to help the client. Explain the importance of sleep and suggest another family member care for the infant at night, if possible, to allow the client to sleep. Depressed clients do not interact with their infants well; therefore, emphasize the importance of other family members holding and interacting with the infant.

Discussing Options and Resources

Ask the client about stressors that may be contributing to the depression. Help plan ways to reduce common areas of stress. Assist the client and partner to identify people who are available to provide support. In addition, provide telephone numbers for local postpartum depression support groups. Internet sources are another place to find help. Examples are Postpartum Support International (https://www.postpartum.net) and the National Women's Health Information Center (https://www.womenshealth.gov).

Evaluation

The interventions are successful if the client does the following:
- Talks about feelings to staff and family members.
- Identifies personal strengths and ways to overcome challenges.
- Discusses community and family resources and makes plans to use them.

? KNOWLEDGE CHECK

26. What are the symptoms of postpartum depression, and how does it differ from postpartum blues?
27. How can nurses intervene for postpartum depression?
28. What screening tools are appropriate for use prior to discharge from the facility?
29. What is the therapeutic management for postpartum psychosis?

SUMMARY CONCEPTS

- Teenage pregnancy is a major health problem in the United States. Adolescents need to receive accurate information about contraceptives and how to set limits on sexual behavior.
- Adolescent pregnancy imposes serious physiologic risks, which result in a higher incidence of complications for the client and the fetus.
- Teenage pregnancy interrupts the developmental tasks of adolescence and may result in childbirth before the parents are capable of providing a nurturing home for the infant without a great deal of assistance.
- The mature gravida often has financial and emotional resources that younger clients do not have. The older client may experience anxiety, however, about recommended antepartum testing and the ability to parent effectively.
- Polysubstance use is a widespread problem that can have devastating fetal and neonatal effects, which may persist and become long-term developmental problems for the child.
- The lifestyle associated with illicit drug use includes inadequate nutrition, inadequate prenatal care, and increased incidence of sexually transmitted infections. It requires interdisciplinary interventions to prevent injury to the expectant client and the fetus.
- The birth of an infant with congenital anomalies produces strong emotions of shock and grief in the family. It calls for a sensitive response from the health care team to help the family grieve for the loss of the perfect or "fantasy" infant and form an attachment to the newborn.
- Pregnancy loss at any stage produces grief, which should be acknowledged and expressed before it can be resolved. Mourning requires memories, and nurses intervene to arrange unlimited contact between the family and the stillborn infant and gather a memento packet for the family.
- Nursing care for the client who is placing the infant for adoption is based on the knowledge that adoption is an act of love, not abandonment.
- There are four types of surrogacies: traditional, gestational, altruistic, and commercial. Knowledge of the different types and how to support the surrogate and intended parents is integral to providing thorough nursing care.

- Mood disorders include postpartum blues, postpartum depression, and postpartum psychosis.
- Postpartum depression is a disabling affective disorder that has an impact on the entire family. Nurses help the client acknowledge feelings and assist in identifying measures that will help the client cope with the condition.
- Anxiety disorders include panic disorder, postpartum obsessive-compulsive disorder, and posttraumatic stress disorder.

Clinical Judgment And Next-Generation NCLEX® Examination-Style Questions

Case 1

During a postpartum follow-up telephone call, a nurse evaluates a 22-year-old single client who identifies as female, 16 days after the cesarean-section birth of a healthy 7-lb son. The client is crying and states she just can't seem to stop crying, "I cry about everything, and I cry about nothing." Client reports minimal light pink lochia, surgical wound tender, pinkish red on the right side without any drainage. Client reports normal bowel and bladder functioning for self and newborn and reports that the baby weighs 2 oz more than he did at birth. Client lives alone with newborn son, and a relative has been coming to visit for an hour or so every day. The church community has provided food a couple of times, although the client states, "Eating is the last thing I want to do." The client is the first in the family to breastfeed but states the baby is hungry all the time: "I feel exhausted, I never sleep!" The client requests information about formula supplementation. Client reports adherence to medications, daily prenatal vitamins, stool softener, and occasional acetaminophen for abdominal cramps. She states she hasn't taken Lexapro since she got pregnant. Reports oral fluid intake daily, about three glasses of water, and two diet cokes daily. Relative present with client reports, "This is the cutest baby boy; I don't know why these baby blues are such a big deal. After my baby, I just got up every day and loved on them and went back to work as soon as I could. I was just so happy." Client reports plans to return to parttime desk job at 4 weeks postpartum to be able to pay the bills.

1. **Highlight or place a check mark next to the assessment findings that require follow-up by the nurse.**

   Single female
   Crying
   Lives alone
   Vaginal discharge
   Urine output
   Abdominal cramps
   Sleep pattern
   Surgical wound
   Medications
   Family support
   Return to work

2. **Use an X to indicate whether the nursing actions listed below are indicated (appropriate or necessary), contraindicated (could be harmful), or nonessential (make no difference or are not necessary) for the client's care at this time.**

Nursing Action	Indicated	Contraindicated	Nonessential
Educate client regarding diet for breastfeeding mothers.			
Discuss outside support resources such as WIC, La Leche League, church community.			
Encourage client to spend time alone to foster a restful environment.			
Teach family ways to support client at this stage of her postpartum period.			
Encourage resting when infant sleeps.			
Discuss routine cesarean section, newborn care, and follow-up.			
Congratulate client on breastfeeding success thus far and provide formula supplementation information as requested.			
Contact health care provider to discuss current assessment of client.			
Provide consult to a lactation consultant to assist client.			

3. **For each client or family response, use an X to indicate whether the nurse's teaching was effective (helped the client understand how to manage postpartum depression), ineffective (did not help the client**

understand how to manage postpartum depression), or unrelated (not related to the health teaching about postpartum depression).

Client Response	Effective	Ineffective	Unrelated
"Going for a walk with my baby each day will help me get out of the house and get some fresh air."			
"So, crying all the time is a sign I might need some extra help, letting my health care provider know I feel overwhelmed is important."			
"Because of this condition, I should limit my visitors so my baby and I can get to know each other better."			
"I need to rest when my baby rests and let my family help with laundry, cooking, and even baby care if it helps me get some sleep."			
"I should discuss with my health care provider restarting my Lexapro since it was so effective before I was pregnant."			
"I cannot take Lexapro or any medications like these while I am breastfeeding."			
"Baby blues will go away, waiting it out is the best thing to do."			
"If I develop any drainage or redness from my C-section scar, I will clean it with peroxide and tell my doctor when I go back to the office in 6 weeks."			

Case 2

The nurse assesses a 28-year-old G1P0 client on admission to L & D in active labor. The client is 35 weeks' gestation, screaming the baby is coming, will not follow directions, is verbally abusive to labor partner, and is resistant to nurses' physical assessment. With much encouragement from the nurse, low lights, and decreased stimulation in the room, the client allows physical assessment, IV start, and routine laboratory work to be collected. Vital signs are heart rate 132, respiratory rate 22, temperature 97.2°F, oxygen saturation 92%. Fetal heart rate (FHR) 162 with decreased variability and late decelerations. Cervical examination indicates client is 8 cm dilated, completely effaced, and +2, contractions are every 90 seconds lasting 90 seconds. Membranes are ruptured with dark meconium staining. Client states contractions began about 20 to 30 minutes ago. Client's pupils are pinpoint,

speech is clear, denies use of medications, smoking, or alcohol, although partner indicates client smokes pot a couple times a day. Client is screaming for pain medication and shouts, "This baby is coming!"

Fetal head is visible at vaginal os, and client delivers male infant in the bed, Apgars 4/6/8. Neonatal team notes at 20-minute assessment infant HR 206 with oxygen saturation of 89.

Maternal laboratory values are pending.

1. **Highlight or place a check mark next to the assessment findings that require follow-up by the nurse.**

   28-year-old G1P0

   Heart rate 132

   Respiratory rate 22

   Temperature 97.2°F

   Oxygen saturation 92%

   35 weeks' gestation

   Rupture of membranes

   Contractions

   Pupils

   Agitation

   Fetal monitoring

   Cervical examination

   Medications

   Apgars

   Infant heart rate 206

   Infant oxygen saturation 89%

   Maternal laboratories

2. **Use an X to indicate whether the nursing actions listed below are indicated (appropriate or necessary), contraindicated (could be harmful), or nonessential (make no difference or are not necessary) for the client's care at this time.**

Nursing Action	Indicated	Contraindicated	Nonessential
Obtain orders for additional laboratory work beyond routine admission screen.			
Provide immediate postpartum care for client in multibed recovery room.			
Encourage skin-to-skin contact with client and infant.			
Transfer infant to the NICU.			
Encourage labor partner to stay with client during recovery period.			
Explain procedures and prepare client for transfer to the postpartum unit.			

Continued

Nursing Action	Indicated	Contraindicated	Nonessential
Congratulate client on delivery and birth of infant.			
Assess infant for irritability, signs of drug withdrawal.			
Provide quiet environment with low stimulation for infant in NICU.			

REFERENCES & READINGS

Adams, E. D. (2021). Antenatal care. In K. Simpson, P. Creehan, N. O'Brien-Abel, C. Roth, & A. Rohan (Eds.), *AWHONN's perinatal nursing* (5th ed., pp. 66–97). Wolters Kluwer.

Adoption & Surrogacy Choices of Colorado. (2021). *Types of surrogacy and definitions*. https://www.adoptionchoices.org/types-of-surrogacy-definitions/.

Ahmad, H. A., Alkhatib, A., & Luo, J. (2021). *Prevalence and risk factors of postpartum depression in the Middle East: A systematic review and meta-analysis*. https://bmcpregnancychildbirth.biomedcentral.com/articles/10.1186/s12884-021-04016-9.

Alves, S., Fonseca, A., Canavarro, M. C., & Pereira, M. (2019). *Predictive validity of the Postpartum Depression Predictors Inventory-Revised (PDPI-R): A longitudinal study with Portuguese women*. https://www.sciencedirect.com/science/article/abs/pii/S026661381830336X.

American Academy of Pediatrics & American College of Obstetricians and Gynecologists (AAP & ACOG). (2017). *Guidelines for perinatal care* (8th ed.).

American College of Obstetricians and Gynecologists (ACOG). (2018). *Alcohol and pregnancy*. https://www.acog.org/-/media/project/acog/acogorg/womens-health/files/infographics/alcohol-and-pregnancy.pdf?la=en&hash=2ECD5B519C26F0DF52DFA449D062EBE1.

American College of Obstetricians and Gynecologists (ACOG). (2020). *Tobacco and nicotine cessation during pregnancy*. ACOG Committee Opinion. (807). Published 2017, reaffirmed 2020.

American College of Obstetricians and Gynecologists (ACOG). (2021a). *Methamphetamine abuse in women of reproductive age*. ACOG Committee Opinion. (479). Published 2011, reaffirmed 2021.

American College of Obstetricians and Gynecologists (ACOG). (2021b). *Perinatal palliative care*. ACOG Committee Opinion. (786). Published 2019, reaffirmed 2021.

Bearak, J., Popinchalk, A., Ganatra, B., Moller, A.-B., Tuncalp, O., & Beavin, C. (2020). *Unintended pregnancy and abortion by income, region, and the legal status of abortion: estimates from a comprehensive model for 1990–2019*. https://www.thelancet.com/journals/langlo/article/PIIS2214-109X(20)30315-6/fulltext.

Caritis, S., & Panigrahy, A. (2019). *Opioids affect the fetal brain: reframing the detoxification debate*. https://www.ajog.org/article/S0002-9378(19)30906-8/fulltext.

Centers for Disease Control and Prevention (CDC). (2018). *Prevent unintended pregnancy*. Centers for Disease Control and Prevention. https://www.cdc.gov/sixeighteen/pregnancy/index.htm.

Centers for Disease Control and Prevention (CDC). (2019). *Social Determinants and Eliminating Disparities in Teen Pregnancy*. Centers for Disease Control and Prevention. https://www.cdc.gov/teenpregnancy/about/social-determinants-disparities-teen-pregnancy.htm#action.

Centers for Disease Control and Prevention (CDC). (2020a). *Polysubstance use in pregnancy*. https://www.cdc.gov/pregnancy/polysubstance-use-in-pregnancy.html.

Centers For Disease Control and Prevention (CDC). (2020b). *Smoking during pregnancy*. https://www.cdc.gov/tobacco/basic_information/health_effects/pregnancy/index.htm.

Centers for Disease Control and Prevention (CDC). (2021). *About opioid use during pregnancy*. https://www.cdc.gov/pregnancy/opioids/basics.html.

Child Welfare Information Gateway. (2019). *The Impact of Adoption*. Washington, DC: U.S. Department of Health and Human Services, Administration for Children and Families, Children's Bureau.

Children's Hospital of Philadelphia. (2021). *Perinatal or postpartum mood and anxiety disorders*. https://www.chop.edu/conditions-diseases/perinatal-or-postpartum-mood-and-anxiety-disorders.

CHU Sainte-Justine Mother and Child University Hospital Center. (2021). *Advanced maternal age: Maternal pregnancy complications*. https://www.chusj.org/en/soins-services/C/complications-de-grossesse/complications-mere/Complications/age-avance.

Cleveland Clinic (2018). *Postpartum depression: Types, symptoms, treatment & prevention*. https://my.clevelandclinic.org/health/diseases/9312-postpartum-depression.

Coleman, E. (2019). *Many states prosecute pregnant women for drug use. New research says that's a bad idea*. https://www.vumc.org/childhealthpolicy/news-events/many-states-prosecute-pregnant-women-drug-use-new-research-says-thats-bad-idea.

Dejong, K., Olyaei, A., & Lo, J. O. (2019). Alcohol use in pregnancy. *Clin Obstet Gynecol*, 62(1), 142–155. https://www.ncbi.nlm.nih.gov/pmc/articles/PMC7061927/.

Fretts, R., Wilkins-Haug, L., Simpson, L., & Chakrabarti, A. (2021). *Management of pregnancy in women of advanced age*. https://www.uptodate.com/contents/management-of-pregnancy-in-women-of-advanced-age#.

Guttmacher Institute. (2019). *Adolescent sexual and reproductive health in the United States*. https://www.guttmacher.org/fact-sheet/american-teens-sexual-and-reproductive-health.

Guttmacher Institute. (2021). *Substance use during pregnancy*. https://www.guttmacher.org/state-policy/explore/substance-use-during-pregnancy#.

Haward, M. F., Lantos, J., Janvier, A., & Group, for the P. O. S. T. (2020). *Helping parents cope in the NICU*. https://pediatrics.aappublications.org/content/145/6/e20193567.

James, D. C., & Suplee, P. D. (2021). Postpartum care. In K. Simpson, P. Creehan, N. O'Brien-Abel, C. Roth, & A. Rohan (Eds.), *AWHONN's perinatal nursing* (5th ed., pp. 509–563). Wolters Kluwer.

James, J. (2021). *Maternal caffeine consumption and pregnancy outcomes: A narrative review with implications for advice to mothers and mothers-to-be*. https://ebm.bmj.com/content/26/3/114.

Karatasli, V., Kanmaz, A. G., Inan, A. H., Budak, A., & Beyan, E. (2019). Maternal and neonatal outcomes of adolescent pregnancy. *Journal of Gynecology Obstetrics and Human*

Reproduction, 48, 347–350. https://doi.org/10.1016/j.jogoh.2019.02.011.

Leftwich, H. K., & Alves, M. V. (2017). Adolescent pregnancy. *Pediatric Clinics of North America, 64*(2), 381–388. https://doi.org/10.1016/j.pcl.2016.11.007.

Maddow-Zimet, I., & Kost, K. (2021). *Pregnancies, births and abortions in the United States, 1973–2017: National and state trends by age.* Guttmacher Institute. https://www.guttmacher.org/report/pregnancies-births-abortions-in-united-states-1973-2017#.

March of Dimes. (2019). *Postpartum depression.* https://www.marchofdimes.org/pregnancy/postpartum-depression.aspx.

March of Dimes. (2020a). *Cocaine and pregnancy.* https://www.marchofdimes.org/pregnancy/cocaine.aspx.

March of Dimes. (2020b). *Heroin and pregnancy.* https://www.marchofdimes.org/pregnancy/heroin-and-pregnancy.aspx.

Massachusetts General Hospital Postpartum Psychosis Project (MGHP3). (2021). *A review of postpartum psychosis.* https://www.mghp3.org/post/a-review-of-postpartum-psychosis-2021.

Mayo Clinic. (2018). *Postpartum depression.* https://www.mayoclinic.org/diseases-conditions/postpartum-depression/symptoms-causes/syc-20376617.

Mayo Clinic. (2020). *Antidepressants: Safe during pregnancy?* https://www.mayoclinic.org/healthy-lifestyle/pregnancy-week-by-week/in-depth/antidepressants/art-20046420#:~:text=SSRIs%20are%20generally%20considered%20an,t%20associated%20with%20birth%20defects.

Mercer, R. T. (1990). *Parents at risk.* Springer.

National Institute of Mental Health (NIMH). (2020). *Bipolar disorder.* https://www.nimh.nih.gov/health/topics/bipolar-disorder/.

Patel, N. H., Jadeja, Y. D., Bhadarka, H. K., Patel, M. N., Patel, N. H., & Sodagar, N. R. (2018). *Insight into different aspects of surrogacy practices.* https://www.ncbi.nlm.nih.gov/pmc/articles/PMC6262674/.

Postpartum Depression. (2021). *Postpartum depression causes & risk factors.* https://www.postpartumdepression.org/postpartum-depression/causes/.

Prince, M. K., & Ayers, D. (2021). *Substance use in pregnancy.* https://www.ncbi.nlm.nih.gov/books/NBK542330/.

Rooney, K. L., & Domar, A. D. (2018). *The relationship between stress and infertility.* https://www.ncbi.nlm.nih.gov/pmc/articles/PMC6016043/.

Schloemerkemper, N. (2018). *Psychotic due to bath salts and methamphetamines: Emergency cesarean section under general anesthesia.* https://pubmed.ncbi.nlm.nih.gov/29970622/.

Substance Abuse and Mental Health Services Administration (SAMHSA). (2021a). Buprenorphine. https://www.samhsa.gov/medication-assisted-treatment/medications-counseling-related-conditions/buprenorphine.

Substance Abuse and Mental Health Services Administration (SAMHSA). (2021b). *Marijuana and pregnancy.* https://www.samhsa.gov/marijuana/marijuana-pregnancy.

Tiemeyer, S., Shreffler, K., & McQuillan, J. (2020). *Pregnancy happiness: Implications of prior loss and pregnancy intendedness.* https://www.ncbi.nlm.nih.gov/pmc/articles/PMC6942239/.

Titus-Glover, D., Shaya, T., Welsh, C., Qato, D., Shah, S., Gresssler, L., & Vivrette, R. (2021). *Opioid use disorder in pregnancy: Leveraging provider perceptions to inform comprehensive treatment.* https://bmchealthservres.biomedcentral.com/track/pdf/10.1186/s12913-021-06182-0.pdf.

Toler, S., Stapleton, S., Kertsburg, K., Callahan, T. J., & Hastings-Tolsma, M. (2018). *Screening for postpartum anxiety: A quality improvement project to promote the screening of women suffering in silence.* https://www.ncbi.nlm.nih.gov/pmc/articles/PMC8040026/.

World Health Organization (WHO). (2020). *Adolescent pregnancy.* https://www.who.int/news-room/fact-sheets/detail/adolescent-pregnancy.

Zappas, M. P., Becker, K., & Walton-Moss, B. (2020). *Postpartum anxiety.* https://www.npjournal.org/article/S1555-4155(20)30452-9/fulltext.

12

Processes of Birth

Kristine DeButy, Kristin L. Scheffer

OBJECTIVES

After studying this chapter, you should be able to:
1. Describe the client's physiologic and psychological responses to labor.
2. Describe fetal responses to labor.
3. Explain how each component of the birth process affects the course of labor and birth and the interrelation of these components.
4. Relate the mechanisms of labor to the process of vaginal birth.
5. Explain early signs of labor.
6. Differentiate true and false labor.
7. Compare the labors of nulliparous and parous clients.
8. Compare the stages of labor.

Understanding the physiologic and psychological components of the birth process helps the nurse provide safe, effective care for the childbearing family. Awareness of expected changes allows the nurse to support the laboring client when these occur and provides a basis for identifying abnormal occurrences. This chapter focuses on the process of birth.

PHYSIOLOGIC EFFECTS OF THE LABOR PROCESS

The birth process affects the physiologic systems of both the client and fetus.

Client Response

The most obvious changes of pregnancy and birth occur in the reproductive system; however, significant changes also occur during labor in the cardiovascular, respiratory, gastrointestinal, urinary, and hematopoietic systems.

Reproductive System

Characteristics of Contractions. Normal labor contractions are coordinated, involuntary, and intermittent.

Coordinated. The uterus can contract and relax in a coordinated way like the heart and other smooth muscles. Contractions during pregnancy are of low intensity and uncoordinated. As the client approaches full term, contractions become organized and gradually assume a regular pattern of increasing **frequency** (*period from the beginning of one uterine contraction to the beginning of the next*), **duration** (*period from the beginning of a uterine contraction to the end of the*

same contraction), and **intensity** (*strength of a contraction*) during labor. Coordinated labor contractions begin in the uterine fundus and spread downward toward the cervix to propel the fetus through the pelvis.

Involuntary. Uterine contractions are involuntary and are not under conscious control. The client cannot cause labor to start and stop by conscious effort. Walking and other activities, however, may stimulate early labor contractions. Anxiety and excessive stress can diminish contractions because of elevated catecholamine levels that may cause uterine relaxation and dysfunctional labor patterns (Simpson & O'Brien-Abel, 2021). Relaxation and coping strategies can facilitate the labor processes.

Intermittent. Labor contractions are intermittent rather than sustained, allowing relaxation of the uterine muscle and resumption of blood flow to and from the placenta.

Contraction Cycle. Each contraction consists of three phases (Fig. 12.1). The **increment,** *period of increasing strength*, occurs as the contraction begins in the fundus and spreads throughout the uterus. The **peak,** or acme, is *the period during which the contraction is most intense.* The **decrement** is *the period of decreasing intensity as the uterus relaxes.*

The contraction cycle and pattern of contractions are also described in terms of frequency, duration, and intensity. Frequency may be expressed in minutes and fractions of minutes (e.g., contractions are 3½–4 minutes apart). The 2008 National Institute of Child Health and Human Development (NICHD) Workshop's report on electronic fetal monitoring (Macones et al., 2008) recommends that frequency be assessed as the number of contractions in 10 minutes, averaged over

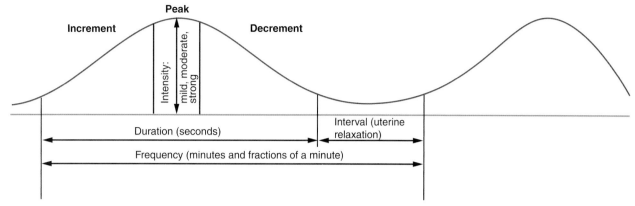

FIG. 12.1 Contraction cycle.

30 minutes (e.g., three contractions in 10 minutes). Duration is usually expressed in seconds (e.g., contractions last 55–65 seconds). The terms *mild, moderate,* and *strong* describe contraction intensity as palpated by the nurse. Different descriptions of intensity apply when an internal pressure catheter is used to record contractions (see Chapter 14).

The **interval**, or relaxation time, is *the period between the end of one contraction and the beginning of the next.* The uterine resting tone is also assessed during this timeframe. **Resting tone** is *the degree of uterine tension between contractions* and is described as either soft/relaxed or firm (Miller et al., 2022). The uterus should palpate soft during this time. Most fetal exchange of oxygen, nutrients, and waste products occurs in the placenta at this time.

Uterine Muscle. Uterine activity during labor is characterized by opposing features. The upper two-thirds of the uterus contracts actively to push the fetus down. The lower third of the uterus remains less active, promoting downward passage of the fetus. The cervix is passive. The net effect of labor contractions is enhanced because the downward push from the upper uterus is accompanied by reduced resistance to fetal descent in the lower uterus (Cunningham et al., 2022).

Myometrial (pertaining to the uterine muscle) cells in the upper uterus remain shorter at the end of each contraction rather than returning to their original length; myometrial cells in the lower uterus become longer with each contraction. These two characteristics enable the upper uterus to maintain tension between contractions to preserve the cervical changes and downward fetal progress made with each contraction (Norwitz et al., 2019).

The opposing characteristics of myometrial contraction in the upper and lower uterine segments cause changes in the thickness of the uterine wall during labor. The upper uterus becomes thicker, and the lower uterus becomes thinner and is pulled upward during labor. The physiologic retraction ring marks the division between the upper and lower segments of the uterus (Fig. 12.2).

The upper and lower uterine segments work opposite of each other, causing the uterine cavity to change shape, becoming more elongated and narrow as labor progresses. This change in uterine shape straightens the fetal body and efficiently directs the fetus downward in the pelvis.

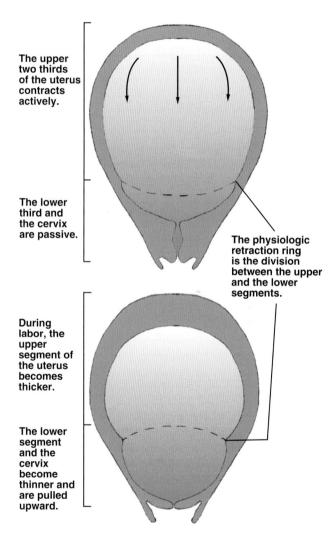

FIG. 12.2 Opposing characteristics of uterine contraction in the upper and lower segments of the uterus.

Cervical Changes. **Effacement** (*thinning and shortening*) and **dilation** (*opening*) are the major cervical changes during labor. Effacement and dilation occur concurrently during labor. The **nullipara** (*a client who has not completed a pregnancy of at least 20 weeks of gestation*) completes most cervical effacement early in the process of cervical dilation. In contrast, the cervix of a parous client (a **para** is *a client who*

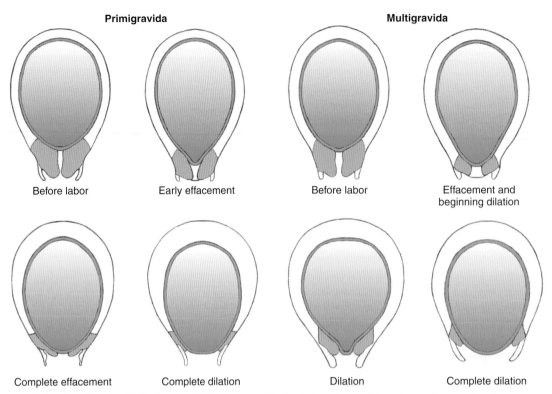

Primigravida

Before labor   Early effacement

Complete effacement   Complete dilation

Multigravida

Before labor   Effacement and beginning dilation

Dilation   Complete dilation

FIG. 12.3 Cervical Dilation and Effacement. During labor, the multipara's cervix remains thicker than the nullipara's cervix.

has given birth after a pregnancy of at least 20 weeks' gestation; it also designates the number of pregnancies that end after at least 20 weeks of gestation) is usually thicker than that of a nullipara at any point during labor (Fig. 12.3).

Effacement. Before labor the cervix is a cylindrical structure about 3 to 4 cm long at the lower end of the uterus (Jafari-Dehkordi et al., 2015; Simhan et al., 2019). Toward the end of pregnancy, the cervix becomes softer and more pliable to prepare for labor. Labor contractions push the fetus downward against the cervix while pulling the cervix upward. If the membranes are intact, **hydrostatic** (fluid) pressure of the amniotic sac adds to the force of the **presenting part** (the part of the fetal body that enters the pelvis first) on the cervix. The cervix becomes shorter and thinner as it is drawn over the fetus and amniotic sac. The cervix merges with the thinning lower uterine segment rather than remaining a distinct structure. Effacement is estimated as a percentage of the original cervical length. A fully thinned cervix is 100% effaced.

Dilation. As the cervix is pulled upward and the fetus is pushed downward, the cervix dilates. Dilation is expressed in centimeters. Full dilation is approximately 10 cm, sufficient to allow passage of the average-size, full-term fetus. At 10 cm, the cervix cannot be felt by an examiner. The action during effacement and dilation can be likened to pushing a ball out through the cuff of a sock.

Cardiovascular System

During each uterine contraction, the muscle fibers of the uterus constrict around the spiral arteries that supply the placenta. This temporarily shunts 300 to 500 mL of blood back into systemic circulation, thereby causing a relative increase in the client's blood volume (Mastrobattista & Monga, 2019). This temporary change increases the blood pressure slightly and slows the client's pulse rate. Therefore the client's vital signs are best assessed during the interval between contractions. Hypotension may occur during labor if the client is supine, as a result of aortocaval compression. The supine position can result in a decrease in cardiac output by 25% to 30% (Mastrobattista & Monga, 2019). The client should be encouraged to rest in lateral positions to promote blood return to the heart and thus enhance blood flow to the placenta and promote fetal oxygenation.

Respiratory System

The depth and rate of respirations increase during labor, especially if the client is anxious or in pain. A client who breathes rapidly and deeply may experience symptoms of hyperventilation. Respiratory alkalosis occurs as the client exhales too much carbon dioxide (Izakson et al., 2020). The client may feel numbness, dizziness and/or tingling of hands and feet. The nurse should help the client slow breathing through nonpharmacologic or pharmacologic pain control measures (See Chapter 13).

Gastrointestinal System

Gastric motility is reduced during labor, which can result in nausea and vomiting. Controversy exists on whether laboring clients should be allowed to eat or drink during labor. Concerns surround the risk for vomiting and aspiration of gastric contents in the event general anesthesia is required for an emergent cesarean delivery. The need for calories to perform the work of labor is underappreciated. Increased glucose utilization and oxygen consumption occur during labor, resulting in the need for additional nutrition (American College of Nurse-Midwives [ACNM], 2016). The American Society of Anesthesiologists' (ASA, 2016) *Practice Guidelines for Obstetrical Anesthesia* position statement on aspiration prevention states that oral intake of clear liquids is appropriate in low-risk laboring clients; however, solid foods should be avoided. Ice chips, juices, broth, and popsicles in moderate amounts are reasonable options for clients during labor.

Urinary System

The most common change in the urinary system during labor is a reduced sensation of a full bladder. Because of intense contractions and the effects of regional anesthesia, the client may be unaware that the bladder is full, yet it may contribute to discomfort. A full bladder can inhibit fetal descent of the presenting part because it occupies space in the pelvis. A distended bladder may increase the risk of bladder hypotonia and infection (Cunningham et al., 2022). Bladder status should be evaluated throughout labor for distention.

Hematopoietic System

Most authorities recognize 500 to 1000 mL as the normal blood loss during childbirth (ACOG, 2019). Clients usually tolerate this loss well because the blood volume increases during pregnancy by 40% to 45% (Blackburn, 2018; Cunningham et al., 2022; Troiano et al., 2019). A client who is anemic at the beginning of labor has less reserve for normal blood loss and a poor tolerance for excess bleeding. A hemoglobin (Hgb) level of 11 grams per deciliter (g/dL) and a hematocrit (Hct) of 33% or higher before birth give most clients an adequate margin of safety for blood loss associated with normal birth (Cunningham et al., 2022). The leukocyte count may be 20,000 to 30,000/mm³ during active labor, with no other evidence of infection (Antony et al., 2021).

Levels of several clotting factors, especially fibrinogen, are elevated during pregnancy and continue to be higher during labor and after birth. This increase provides protection from hemorrhage but also increases the client's risk for a venous thrombosis during pregnancy and after birth (Antony et al., 2021).

Fetal Response
Placental Circulation

The exchange of oxygen, nutrients, and waste products between the client and fetus occurs in the intervillous spaces of the placenta without mixing of maternal and fetal blood. During strong labor contractions, the blood supply to the placenta decreases as the spiral arteries supplying the intervillous spaces are compressed by the uterine muscle. Therefore most placental exchange occurs during the interval between contractions. The placental circulation usually has enough reserve compared with fetal basal needs to tolerate the periodic interruption of blood flow.

Fetal protective mechanisms include the following (Ross & Ervin, 2021):
- Fetal Hgb (Hgb F), which more readily takes on oxygen and releases carbon dioxide compared with adult Hgb

- High Hgb and Hct levels, which can carry more oxygen than adult Hgb
- A high cardiac output

The fetus may not tolerate labor contractions well in conditions associated with reduced placental function, such as diabetes and hypertension, and conditions associated with reduced fetal oxygen-carrying capacity, such as fetal anemia.

Cardiovascular System

The fetal cardiovascular system reacts quickly to events during labor. Alterations in the rate and rhythm of the fetal heart may result from normal labor effects or suggest fetal intolerance to the stress of labor. The fetal heart rate (FHR) is rapid and ranges from 110 to 160 beats per minute (Macones et al., 2008). The preterm fetus often has a heart rate in the higher end of this range because of an immature parasympathetic nervous system (O'Brien-Abel & Simpson, 2021).

Pulmonary System

The fetal lungs produce fluid to allow for normal development of the airways. The fetus also has breathing motions in utero when breathing in amniotic fluid. Lung fluid must be cleared to allow normal air breathing after birth. As term gestation nears, production of fetal lung fluid decreases to approximately 65% of its maximum production, and its absorption into the interstitium of the lungs increases. Labor speeds the absorption of lung fluid. Approximately 35% of the maximum amount remains in the airways at birth (Kamath-Rayne & Jobe, 2019). Some fluid is expelled from the upper airways as the fetal head and thorax are compressed during passage through the birth canal. Most remaining lung fluid is absorbed into the interstitial spaces of the newborn's lungs and then into the circulatory system. A small amount is cleared by the lymphatic circulation (Blackburn, 2018).

Catecholamines (primarily epinephrine and norepinephrine) produced by the fetal adrenal glands in response to the stress of labor appear to contribute to the infant's adaptation to extrauterine life. These hormones stimulate cardiac contraction and breathing, quicken the clearance of remaining lung fluid, and aid in temperature regulation. Infants born by cesarean birth not preceded by labor are more likely to have transient breathing difficulty (Fraser, 2021).

❓ KNOWLEDGE CHECK

1. How do labor contractions cause the cervix to efface and dilate? How do labor contractions cause fetal descent?
2. What differences in effacement are expected in the parous client compared with the client who has not previously given birth?
3. What changes occur in the cardiovascular, respiratory, gastrointestinal, urinary, and hematopoietic systems during labor?
4. Why are intermittent rather than sustained uterine contractions important?
5. How does the normal process of vaginal birth benefit the newborn after birth?

COMPONENTS OF THE BIRTH PROCESS

Four major factors interact during normal childbirth. These factors are often called the *four Ps:* powers, passage, passenger, and psyche.

Powers

Uterine Contractions

During the first stage of labor (onset to full cervical dilation), uterine contractions are the primary force moving the fetus through the pelvis.

Pushing Efforts

During the **second stage of labor** (*full cervical dilation to birth of the baby*), uterine contractions continue to propel the fetus through the pelvis. In addition, the client feels an urge to push and bears down as the fetus distends the vagina and puts pressure on the rectum. The client's voluntary pushing efforts add to the force of uterine contractions in second-stage labor.

Passage

The birth passage consists of the pelvis and soft tissues. The bony pelvis is usually more important to the outcome of labor than the soft tissue because the bones and joints do not readily yield to the forces of labor. However, softening of the cartilage linking the pelvic bones occurs near term because of increased levels of the hormone relaxin.

The linea terminalis (pelvic brim) divides the bony pelvis into the false pelvis (top) and true pelvis (bottom). The true pelvis is most important in childbirth. The true pelvis has three subdivisions: (1) the inlet, or upper pelvic opening; (2) the midpelvis, or pelvic cavity; and (3) the outlet, or lower pelvic opening. During birth, the true pelvis functions as a curved cylinder with different dimensions at different levels (Fig. 12.4).

Passenger

The passenger is the fetus, membranes, and placenta. Several fetal anatomic and positional variables influence the course of labor.

Fetal Head

The fetus enters the birth canal in the cephalic **presentation** (*the fetal part that enters the pelvic inlet first*) 96% to 97% of the time (Thorp & Grantz, 2019). The fetal shoulders are also important because of their width, but they usually can be moved to adapt to the diameter of the pelvis.

Bones, Sutures, and Fontanels. The bones of the fetal head involved in the birth process are the two frontal bones on the forehead, two parietal bones at the crown of the head, and one occipital bone at the back of the head (Fig. 12.5). The five major bones are not fused but are connected by **sutures**, which are *narrow areas of flexible tissue that connect fetal skull bones,* permitting slight movement during labor. The **fontanels** are *wider spaces at the intersections of the sutures connecting fetal or infant skull bones.*

The anterior fontanel has a diamond shape formed by the intersection of four sutures: the one frontal, one sagittal, and two coronal sutures, which connect the two frontal and two parietal bones. The posterior fontanel has a triangular shape formed by the intersection of three sutures: one sagittal and two lambdoid sutures, which connect the two parietal bones and occipital bone. The posterior fontanel is very small and often looks or feels more like a slight indentation in the skull. The sutures and fontanels allow the bones to move slightly, changing the shape of the fetal head so it can adapt to the size and shape of the pelvis by **molding** (*shaping of the fetal head during movement through the birth canal).* The sutures and different shapes of the fontanels provide important landmarks to determine fetal **position** (*relation of a fixed reference point on the fetus to the quadrants of the maternal pelvis)* and head flexion during vaginal examination.

Fetal Head Diameters. Most fetuses enter the pelvis in the cephalic presentation, but several variations are possible. The major transverse diameter of the fetal head is the biparietal diameter, measured between the two parietal bones. The biparietal diameter averages 9.5 cm in a term fetus.

The anteroposterior diameter of the head varies with the degree of flexion. In the most favorable situation, the head becomes fully flexed during labor and the anteroposterior diameter is suboccipitobregmatic, averaging 9.5 cm (see Fig. 12.5).

Fetal Lie

The orientation of the long axis (spine) of the fetus to the long axis (spine) of the client is called the **fetal lie** (Fig. 12.6). In more than 99% of pregnancies, the lie is longitudinal and parallel to the long axis of the pregnant client (Cunningham et al., 2022). In the longitudinal lie, either the head or the buttocks of the fetus enter the pelvis first. A transverse lie exists when the long axis of the fetus is at a right angle to the client's long axis. This occurs in approximately 1 of every 300 deliveries (Thorp & Grantz, 2019). An oblique lie is at some angle between the longitudinal lie and the transverse lie.

Attitude

The relation of fetal body parts to one another is the **attitude** of the fetus (Fig. 12.7). The normal fetal attitude is one of flexion, with the head flexed toward the chest and the arms and legs flexed over the thorax. The back is curved in a convex C shape. Extension is an abnormal attitude in which the head is extended away from the fetal chest, resulting in a face or brow presentation. Flexion remains a characteristic feature of the term *newborn.*

Presentation

The fetal part that first enters the pelvis is termed the *presenting part.* Presentation falls into three categories: (1) cephalic, (2) breech, and (3) shoulder. The cephalic presentation with the fetal head flexed is the most common. Other presentations are associated with prolonged labor and are more likely to require cesarean birth.

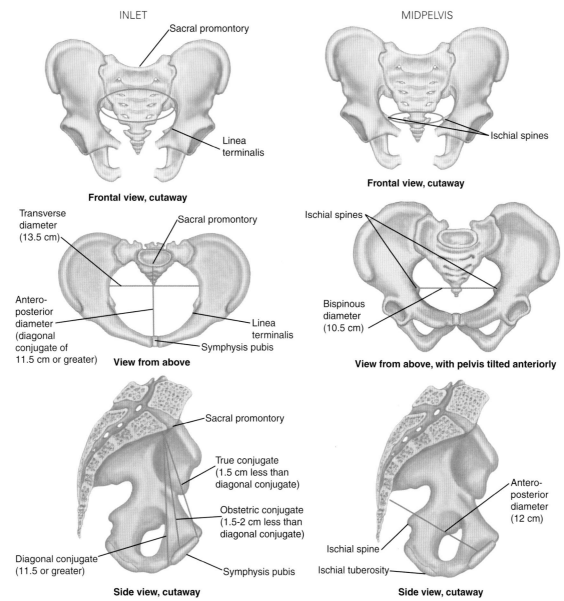

INLET

Frontal view, cutaway

View from above

Side view, cutaway

MIDPELVIS

Frontal view, cutaway

View from above, with pelvis tilted anteriorly

Side view, cutaway

The boundaries of the inlet are the symphysis pubis anteriorly, the sacral promontory posteriorly, and the linea terminalis on the sides. The inlet is slightly wider in its transverse diameter (13.5 cm) than in its anteroposterior (diagonal conjugate) diameter (11.5 cm or greater).

The diagonal conjugate is slightly larger than both the obstetric and true conjugates. The obstetric conjugate is the narrowest of the three conjugate diameters but cannot be measured directly. The obstetric conjugate is estimated by first measuring the diagonal conjugate and then subtracting 1.5 to 2 cm.

If the inlet is small, the fetal head may not be able to enter it. Because it is almost entirely surrounded by bone, except for cartilage at the sacroiliac joint and symphysis pubis, the inlet cannot enlarge much to accommodate the fetus. The bony measurements are essentially fixed.

The midpelvis, or pelvic cavity, is the narrowest part of the pelvis through which the fetus must pass during birth. Midpelvic diameters are measured at the level of the ischial spines. The anteroposterior diameter averages 12 cm.

The transverse diameter (bispinous or interspinous) averages 10.5 cm. Prominent ischial spines that project into the midpelvis can reduce the bispinous diameter.

FIG. 12.4 Pelvic Divisions and Measurements.

OUTLET

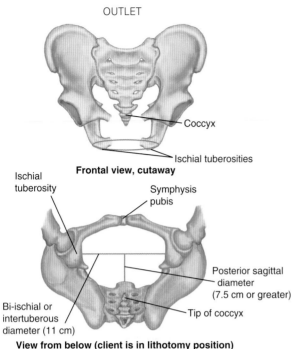

Frontal view, cutaway

View from below (client is in lithotomy position)

Side view, cutaway

Three important diameters of the pelvic outlet are (1) the anteroposterior, (2) the transverse (bi-ischial or intertuberous), and (3) the posterior sagittal. The angle of the pubic arch also is an important pelvic outlet measure.

The anteroposterior diameter ranges from 9.5 to 11.5 cm, varying with the curve between the sacrococcygeal joint and the tip of the coccyx. The anteroposterior diameter can increase if the coccyx is easily movable.

The transverse diameter is the bi-ischial, or intertuberous, diameter. This is the distance between the ischial tuberosities ("sit bones"). It averages 11 cm. The posterior sagittal diameter is normally at least 7.5 cm. It is a measure of the posterior pelvis.

The posterior sagittal diameter measures the distance from the sacrococcygeal joint to the middle of the transverse (bi-ischial) diameter. The angle of the pubic arch is important because it must be wide enough for the fetus to pass under it.

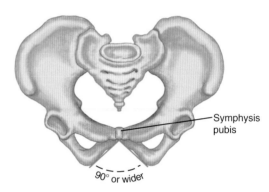

Frontal view, with pelvis tilted anteriorly

The angle of the pubic arch should be at least 90 degrees. A narrow pubic arch displaces the fetus posteriorly toward the coccyx as it tries to pass under the arch.

FIG. 12.4, cont'd

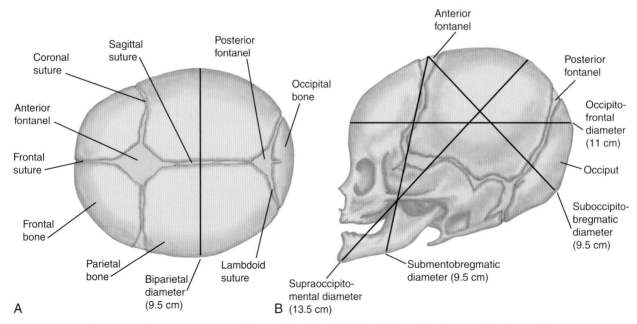

FIG. 12.5 A, Bones, sutures, and fontanels of the fetal head. Note that the anterior fontanel has a diamond shape, whereas the posterior fontanel is triangular. B, Lateral view of the fetal head demonstrating that anteroposterior diameters vary with the amount of flexion or extension.

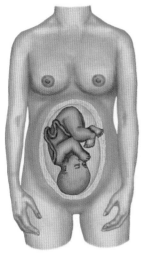
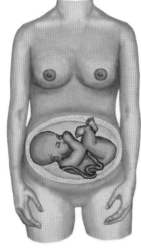

A Longitudinal lie   B Transverse lie

FIG. 12.6 **Fetal Lie.** A, In a longitudinal lie, the long axis of the fetus is parallel to the long axis of the client. B, In a transverse lie, the long axis of the fetus is at right angles to the long axis of the client. The client's abdomen has a wide, short appearance.

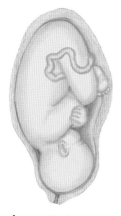
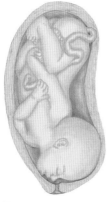

A Flexion   B Extension

FIG. 12.7 **Attitude.** A, The fetus is in the normal attitude of flexion, with the head, arms, and legs flexed tightly against the trunk. B, The fetus is in an abnormal attitude of extension. The head is extended, and the right arm is extended. A face presentation is illustrated.

Cephalic Presentation. The cephalic presentation is more favorable than others for the following reasons:
- The fetal head is the largest single fetal part, although the breech (buttocks), with the legs and feet flexed on the abdomen, is collectively larger than the head. After the head is born, the smaller parts follow easily as the extremities unfold.
- During labor, the fetal head can gradually change shape, molding to adapt to the size and shape of the pelvis.
- The fetal head is smooth, round, and hard, making it a more effective part to dilate the cervix, which is also round.

Cephalic presentation has the following four variations (Fig. 12.8):

- Vertex—The most common type of cephalic presentation, in which the fetal head is fully flexed. It is called a *vertex* or *occiput presentation* and is the most favorable for normal progress of labor because the smallest suboccipitobregmatic diameter is presenting.
- Military—The head is in a neutral position, neither flexed nor extended. The longer occipitofrontal diameter is presenting.
- Brow—The fetal head is partly extended. The brow presentation is unstable, usually converting to a vertex presentation if the head flexes or to a face presentation if it extends. The longest supraoccipitomental diameter is presenting.
- Face—The head is extended, and the fetal occiput is near the fetal spine. The submentobregmatic diameter is presenting.

Breech Presentation. A breech presentation occurs when the fetal buttocks or legs enter the pelvis first, which happens in approximately 3% to 4% of births (Thorp & Grantz, 2019). Breech presentation is more common in preterm births, **hydrocephaly** (enlargement of the head with fluid), multiple gestations, abnormalities of the uterus and pelvis, prior breech delivery, and with **placenta previa** (placenta in the lower uterus) (Cunningham et al., 2022).

Breech presentations are associated with the following disadvantages:
- The buttocks are not smooth and firm like the head and are less effective at dilating the cervix.
- The fetal head is the last part to be born. By the time the fetal head is deep in the pelvis, the umbilical cord is outside the mother's body and is subject to compression between the fetal head and the maternal pelvis.
- Because the umbilical cord can be compressed after the fetal chest is born, the head should be delivered quickly to allow the infant to breathe. This does not permit gradual molding of the fetal head as it passes through the pelvis.

The breech presentation has the following three variations, depending on the relationship of the legs to the body (Fig. 12.9):
- Frank breech—The most common variation, occurring when the fetal legs are extended across the abdomen toward the shoulders.
- Complete breech—Reversal of the usual cephalic presentation. The head, knees, and hips are flexed, but the buttocks are presenting.
- Footling breech—Occurs when one or both feet are presenting.

Shoulder Presentation. The shoulder is typically presenting in a transverse lie and accounts for only 0.3% of births (Thorp & Grantz, 2019). It occurs more often with preterm gestation, high parity, hydramnios, placenta previa, and abnormal uterine anatomy (Cunningham et al., 2022). A cesarean birth is necessary when the fetus is **viable** (one of a gestational age that might survive).

KNOWLEDGE CHECK
6. What are the two powers of labor?
7. What are the three divisions of the true pelvis?
8. Why is the vertex presentation best during birth?

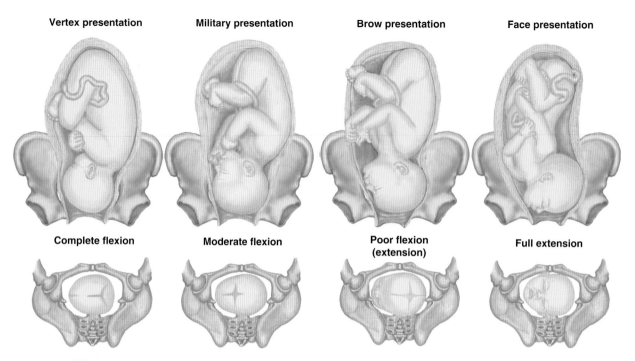

FIG. 12.8 Four Variations of Cephalic Presentation. The vertex presentation is normal. Note positional changes of the anterior and posterior fontanels in relation to the maternal pelvis.

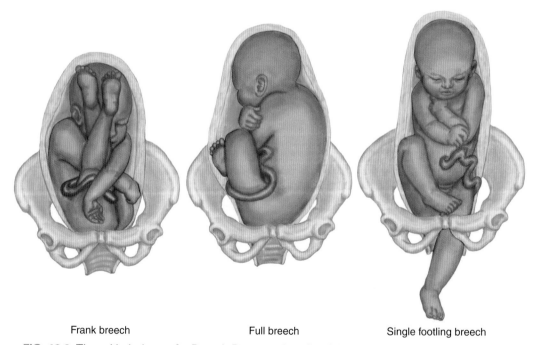

FIG. 12.9 Three Variations of a Breech Presentation. Frank breech is the most common variation. Footling breeches may be single or double.

Position

Fetal position describes the location of a fixed reference point on the presenting part in relation to the four quadrants of the maternal pelvis (Fig. 12.10). The four quadrants are the right and left anterior and right and left posterior. The fetal position is not fixed but changes during labor as the fetus moves downward and adapts to the pelvic contours. Abbreviations indicate the relationship between the fetal presenting part and pelvis.

Right (R) or Left (L). The first letter of the abbreviation describes whether the fetal reference point is to the right or left of the client's pelvis. If the fetal reference point is neither to the right nor to the left of the pelvis, this letter is omitted.

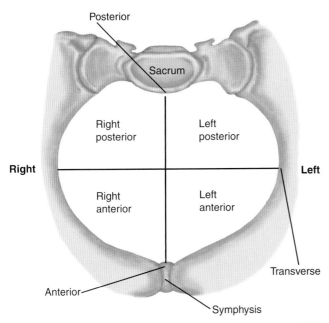

FIG. 12.10 Four quadrants of the pelvis from above, which are used to describe fetal position.

Occiput (O), Mentum (M), or Sacrum (S). The second letter of the abbreviation refers to the fixed fetal reference point, which varies with the presentation. The occiput is used in a vertex presentation. The chin, or mentum, is the reference point in a face presentation. The sacrum is used for breech presentations. Letters may also designate the less common brow (F for fronto) and shoulder (Sc for scapula) presentations.

Anterior (A), Posterior (P), or Transverse (T). A, P, and T describe whether the fetal reference point is in the anterior or posterior quadrant of the client's pelvis. If the fetal reference point is in neither an anterior nor a posterior quadrant, it is described as transverse. If the fetal occiput is in the left anterior quadrant of the pelvis, the position is described as left occiput anterior (LOA). If the occiput is in the client's anterior pelvis, neither to the right nor to the left, it is described as occiput anterior (OA). If the fetal sacrum is in the client's right posterior pelvis, the abbreviation is R (right) S (sacrum) P (posterior) (Fig. 12.11).

❓ KNOWLEDGE CHECK

9. For each fetal position listed, describe the fetal landmark. Where is this landmark located in relation to the client's pelvis: ROP? OA? RSA? LMA?
10. If the fetus is in the face presentation, why is using the occiput to determine position within the pelvis not possible?

Psyche

A client's psychological response to labor and birth are influenced by anxiety, culture, expectations, life experiences, and support.

Anxiety

Marked anxiety and fear may decrease a client's ability to cope with pain in labor. Catecholamines secreted in response to anxiety and fear can inhibit uterine contractility and placental blood flow (Simpson & O'Brien-Abel, 2021; Hawkins & Bucklin, 2021). In contrast, relaxation augments the natural process of labor. Prenatal education or childbirth classes can increase a client's knowledge, enhancing their ability to work with the body's efforts rather than resist natural forces. Much of the nurse's care during labor involves reducing anxiety and fear and assisting with coping strategies. Information, a positive sense of control, and labor support increase the client's sense of satisfaction with the birth experience (AWHONN, 2018; Bohren et al., 2017).

Culture and Expectations

A client's culture affects values and expectations for and responses to birth and the practices surrounding it. The nurse's familiarity with a group's cultural values and practices provides a framework to care for the client and family as individuals. The nurse should assess the personal expectations and values of each client and support person related to birth within this general framework. Questions for the intrapartum period might include the following:

- Are there any cultural practices or beliefs that are important for the health care team to know?
- What is the primary language used? Do the client and support person speak the same language? Are they comfortable communicating in the nurse's language if that is not their usual language? How does a client with hearing impairment communicate with people who can hear? If an interpreter is needed, what people would the client or family consider unacceptable interpreters (e.g., men or members of certain religious groups)?
- Who is the client's primary support person for labor? What is that person's role? Will that person actively support the laboring client (e.g., by coaching breathing techniques), or will they take a less active role? Who will be present at the birth?
- Who is the decision maker, or who should be consulted about important decisions?
- Will another relative (such as a grandmother) assume primary care for the infant?
- Is a professional caregiver (such as a nurse or physician) of the same gender and cultural group essential?
- What are the client's feelings about touch? Is the client comfortable telling the nurse when touch is not welcomed?
- How is pain perceived? What are acceptable pain levels and appropriate pain reduction strategies?
- Are specific symbols, practices, and ceremonies used during the birth period? Who will conduct any ceremonies?

Birth as an Experience

Childbirth is a physical and an emotional experience. It is an irrevocable event that forever changes a client and a family. Families describe the births of their children as they describe

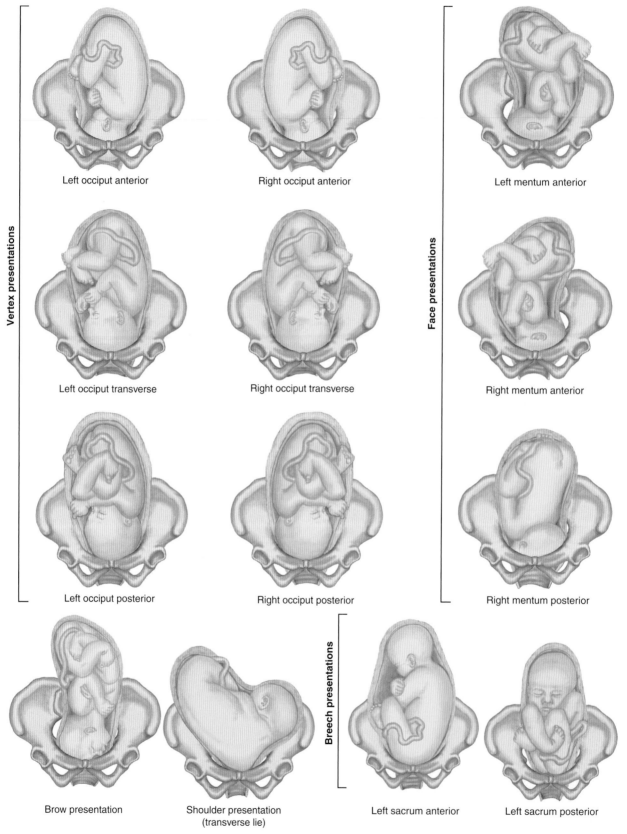

Vertex presentations

Left occiput anterior

Right occiput anterior

Left occiput transverse

Right occiput transverse

Left occiput posterior

Right occiput posterior

Face presentations

Left mentum anterior

Right mentum anterior

Right mentum posterior

Brow presentation

Shoulder presentation
(transverse lie)

Breech presentations

Left sacrum anterior

Left sacrum posterior

FIG. 12.11 Fetal Presentations and Positions.

other pivotal events in life such as marriages, anniversaries, religious events, and even deaths. A client who has realistic expectations about birth is more likely to have a positive experience. Nursing measures that increase the client's sense of control and mastery during birth help clients perceive the birth as a positive event. The client's past experiences with childbirth, pain, and personal success and failure will influence expectations for this birth.

Support

The positive effects of continuous labor support are well documented (AWHONN, 2018; Bohren et al., 2017; California Maternal Quality Care Collaborative [CMQCC], 2017). Support includes physical comfort measures, providing information, advocacy, praise and reassurance, presence, and the maintenance of a calm and comfortable environment.

Interrelationships of Components

The four Ps have been described separately but are actually an interrelated whole. For instance, a client with a small pelvis (passage) and a large fetus (passenger) may be able to have a normal labor and birth if the fetus is ideally positioned and the uterine contractions and bearing-down efforts (powers) are vigorous. The nurse's supportive attitude strengthens positive psychological elements (psyche) and enhances the processes of birth. The nurse can act as an advocate for the laboring client and support person to increase their sense of control and mastery of labor, which often reduces anxiety and fear and helps them achieve their desired birth experience.

NORMAL LABOR

Theories of Onset

Despite continuing research, the exact mechanisms that initiate labor remain unknown (Kilpatrick et al., 2021). Labor normally starts when the fetus is mature enough to adjust easily to extrauterine life but before it grows so large that vaginal birth is impossible. This stage (term gestation) occurs between 37 and 42 weeks after the first day of the client's last menstrual period (Norwitz et al., 2019).

Natural labor begins when forces favoring continuation of pregnancy are offset by forces favoring its end. Factors that appear to have a role in starting labor include the following (Cunningham et al., 2022; Kilpatrick et al., 2021):

- Changes in the ratio of estrogen to progesterone so that estrogen levels are higher than progesterone levels. Progesterone promotes smooth muscle relaxation of the uterus during most of pregnancy. Estrogen levels tend to increase as progesterone levels fall near the onset of labor. This process enhances uterine sensitivity to substances that stimulate uterine contractions: prostaglandins from the fetal membranes and oxytocin from the client's posterior pituitary gland. Estrogens increase the number of gap junctions—connections that allow the individual uterine muscle cells to contract as a coordinated unit.

- Prostaglandins produced by the decidua (the modified endometrium during pregnancy) and fetal membranes may have a role in preparing the uterus for oxytocin stimulation at term. Prostaglandins are secreted from the lower area of the fetal membranes (forebag) during labor and may reflect inflammation caused by contact with microorganisms from the client's vagina.

- Increased secretion of natural oxytocin appears to maintain labor once it has begun. Oxytocin alone does not appear to start labor but may play a part in labor's initiation in conjunction with other substances. Evidence of fetal oxytocin secretion also exists.

- Oxytocin receptors in the uterus increase markedly as labor begins, and the increase continues during labor and peaks at delivery. Oxytocin has little effect on the uterine muscle if the receptors have not developed.

- A fetal role in the initiation of labor appears likely. The fetal membranes release prostaglandin in high concentrations during labor. In addition to fetal oxytocin secretion, large quantities of cortisol are secreted by the fetal adrenal glands, possibly acting as a uterine stimulant.

- Stretching, pressure, and irritation of the uterus and cervix increase as the fetus reaches term size. During early pregnancy the uterus has not reacted to stretching by contracting as smooth muscle normally does. A feedback loop is likely responsible for labor contractions at term: the fetal head stretches the cervix, causing the fundus of the uterus to contract, pushing the fetal head against the cervix, and causing more fundal contractions. Cervical stretching also causes secretion of oxytocin.

Premonitory Signs
Braxton Hicks Contractions

As term gestation approaches, **Braxton Hicks contractions** *(irregular, mild uterine contractions that occur throughout pregnancy and become stronger in the last trimester)* become more noticeable and even painful. Parous clients often describe more uterine activity preceding labor than do nulliparous clients.

Increased perception of Braxton Hicks contractions often makes sleep difficult at the end of pregnancy. The contractions may become regular at times, only to decrease spontaneously. These contractions are often uncomfortable and sometimes regular, which can cause clients to be confused about whether labor has begun.

Lightening

As the fetus descends toward the pelvic inlet ("dropping"), the client notices that breathing becomes easier because upward pressure on the diaphragm is reduced. However, increased pressure on the bladder causes more frequent urination. Pressure of the fetal head in the pelvis also may cause leg cramps and edema. **Lightening** *(descent of the fetus toward the pelvic inlet before labor)* is most noticeable in nulliparas and occurs about 2 to 3 weeks before the natural onset of labor.

Increased Vaginal Mucous Secretions

An increase in clear and nonirritating vaginal secretions occurs as fetal pressure causes congestion of the vaginal mucosa.

Cervical Ripening and Bloody Show

As full term nears, the cervix *softens because of the effects of the hormone relaxin.* These changes (**ripening**) allow the cervix to yield more easily to the forces of labor contractions. As the fetal head descends with lightening, it puts pressure on the cervix, starting the process of effacement and dilation. Effacement and dilation cause expulsion of the mucus plug that sealed the cervix during pregnancy, rupturing small cervical capillaries in the process. **Bloody show** *(a mixture of cervical mucus and pink or brown blood from ruptured capillaries in the cervix; often precedes labor and increases with cervical dilation)* may begin several days to a few weeks before the onset of labor, especially in the nulliparous client, or it may not begin until labor starts. Bloody show increases during labor as the cervix completes dilation and effacement. Clients who have previously had a vaginal birth often have less bloody show than nulliparas.

Energy Spurt

Some clients have a sudden increase in energy, which is called "nesting." They should be cautioned to conserve their energy so that they are not exhausted when labor begins.

Weight Loss

A small weight loss of 2.2 to 6.6 kg (1 to 3 lb) may occur because the altered estrogen-to-progesterone ratio causes excretion of some of the extra fluid that accumulates during pregnancy.

True Labor and False Labor

False labor, also called *prodromal labor* or *prelabor,* is a common occurrence as the client approaches full term. The onset of labor can be a gradual process with contractions occurring intermittently over the weeks or days leading up to the onset of labor. False labor can be defined as uterine contractions in the absence of cervical change. False labor may cause clients to go to the birth center, thinking that labor has started. Clients may be observed in the labor unit for enough time to establish maternal/fetal well-being and to have two cervical examinations to evaluate cervical change (American Academy of Pediatrics [AAP] & ACOG, 2017). Clients in latent labor should be offered supportive techniques and education on self-care activities related to pain, nutrition, and rest. The term *false labor* may be discouraging to clients if they do not realize that these "false" contractions are preparation for true labor.

Several characteristics distinguish true labor from false labor: contractions, discomfort, and cervical change. The best distinction between true and false labor is that contractions of true labor cause progressive change in the cervix. A more rapid increase in effacement and dilation occurs with true labor contractions.

Approximately 8% of clients may experience premature rupture of membranes, or PROM, when membrane rupture occurs before the onset of labor (AAP & ACOG, 2017). If this occurs, the client should go to the birth center for evaluation. Infection and compression of the fetal umbilical cord are possible complications.

CLIENT EDUCATION

How to Know Whether Labor Is "Real"

True labor differs from false labor in three categories.

False Labor	True Labor
Contractions	
Are inconsistent in frequency, duration, and intensity	Usually have a consistent or regular pattern of increasing frequency, duration, and intensity
Do not change or may decrease with activity (such as walking)	Tend to increase with walking
Discomfort	
Is felt in the abdomen and groin	Begins in the lower back and gradually sweeps around to lower abdomen
May be more annoying than truly painful	May persist as back pain in some clients
	Can often resemble menstrual cramps during early labor
Cervix	
Does not significantly change effacement or dilation	Includes progressive effacement and dilation (most important characteristic)

LABOR MECHANISMS

The mechanisms (cardinal movements) of labor occur as the fetus is moved through the pelvis during birth. The fetus undergoes several positional changes to adapt to the size and shape of the client's pelvis at different levels (Fig. 12.12). Although the mechanisms of labor are described separately in Fig. 12.12, some occur concurrently. In a vertex presentation, the mechanisms include the following:

- Descent of the fetal presenting part through the true pelvis
- **Engagement** of the fetal presenting part as its widest diameter reaches the level of the ischial spines of the client's pelvis (0 station)
- Flexion of the fetal head, allowing the smallest head diameters to align with the smaller diameters of the midpelvis as the fetus descends
- Internal rotation to allow the largest fetal head diameter to align with the largest pelvic diameter
- Extension of the fetal head as the neck pivots on the inner margin of the symphysis pubis, allowing the head to align with the curves of the pelvic outlet
- External rotation of the fetal head, aligning the head with the shoulders during expulsion
- Expulsion of the fetal shoulders and fetal body

The mechanisms of labor are different in presentations other than the vertex, but the reason is the same: to effectively use the available space in the maternal pelvis.

DESCENT, ENGAGEMENT, AND FLEXION

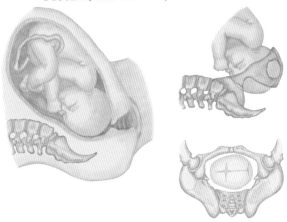

Descent of the fetus is a mechanism of labor that accompanies all the others. Without descent, none of the mechanisms will occur.

Station

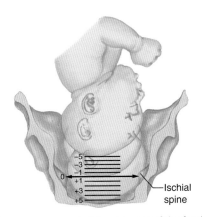

Station is a measurement of the descent of the fetal presenting part in relation to the level of the ischial spines of the maternal pelvis. The level of the ischial spines is a zero station. Other stations are described with numbers representing the approximate number of centimeters above (negative numbers) or below (positive numbers) the ischial spines. As the fetus descends through the pelvis, the station changes from higher negative numbers (−5, −3. −4, −2, −1) to zero to higher positive numbers (+1, +2, +3, +4 +5, etc.). Sometimes the terms *floating* or *ballotable* may describe a fetal presenting part that is so high that it is easily displaced upward during abdominal or vaginal examination, similar to tossing a ball upward.

Engagement

Engagement occurs when the largest diameter of the fetal presenting part (normally the head) has passed the pelvic inlet and entered the pelvic cavity. Engagement is presumed to have occurred when the station of the presenting part is zero or lower. Engagement often takes place before onset of labor in nulliparous clients. In many parous clients and in some nulliparas, it does not occur until after labor begins.

Flexion

As the fetus descends, the fetal head is flexed farther as it meets resistance from the soft tissues of the pelvis. Head flexion presents the smallest anteroposterior diameter (suboccipitobregmatic) to the pelvis.

Internal Rotation

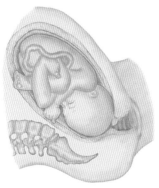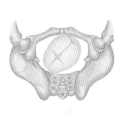

The fetus enters the pelvic inlet with the sagittal suture in a transverse or oblique orientation to the maternal pelvis because that is the widest inlet diameter. Internal rotation allows the longest fetal head diameter (the anteroposterior) to conform to the longest diameter of the maternal pelvis. The longest pelvic outlet diameter is the anteroposterior. As the head descends to the level of the ischial spines, it gradually turns so that the fetal occiput is in the anterior of the pelvis (OA position, directly under the maternal symphysis pubis). When internal rotation is complete, the sagittal suture is oriented in the anteroposterior pelvic diameter (OA). Less commonly, the head may turn posteriorly so that the occiput is directed toward the mother's sacrum (OP).

FIG. 12.12 Mechanisms (Cardinal Movements) of Labor.

EXTENSION

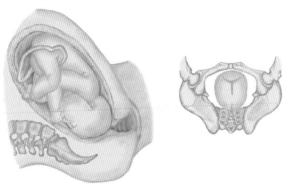

Extension beginning (internal rotation complete)

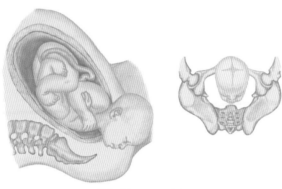

Extension complete

Because the true pelvis is shaped like a curved cylinder, the fetal face is directed posteriorly toward the rectum as it begins its rotation and descent. To negotiate the curve of the pelvis, the fetal head must change from an attitude of flexion to one of extension.

While still in flexion, the fetal head meets resistance from the tissues of the pelvic floor. At the same time, the fetal neck stops under the symphysis, which acts as a pivot. The combination of resistance from the pelvic floor and the pivoting action of the symphysis causes the fetal head to swing anteriorly, or extend, with each maternal pushing effort. The head is born in extension, with the occiput sliding under the symphysis and the face directed toward the rectum. The fetal brow, nose, and chin slide over the perineum as the head is born.

EXTERNAL ROTATION

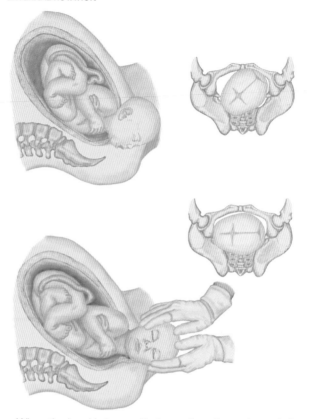

When the head is born with the occiput directed anteriorly, the shoulders must rotate internally so that they align with the anteroposterior diameter of the pelvis.

After the head is born, it spontaneously turns to the same side as it was in utero as it realigns with the shoulders and back (through a process called *restitution*). The head then turns farther to that side in external rotation as the shoulders internally rotate and are positioned with their transverse diameter in the anteroposterior diameter of the pelvic outlet. External rotation of the head accompanies internal rotation of the shoulders.

EXPULSION

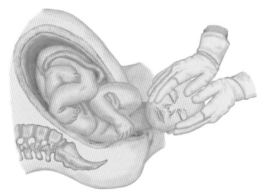

Expulsion occurs first as the anterior, then the posterior, shoulder passes under the symphysis. After the shoulders are born, the rest of body follows.

FIG. 12.12, cont'd

TABLE 12.1	Characteristics of Normal Labor			
Characteristics	**First Stage**	**Second Stage**	**Third Stage**	**Fourth Stage**
Work accomplished	Effacement and dilation of cervix	Expulsion of fetus	Separation of placenta	Physical recovery and bonding with newborn
Forces	Uterine contractions	Uterine contractions and voluntary bearing-down efforts	Uterine contractions	Uterine contraction to control bleeding from placental site
Cervical dilation	*Latent phase[a]:* 0 cm–5 cm *Active phase[a]:* 6 cm–10 cm	10 cm (complete dilation)	Not applicable	Not applicable
Uterine contractions	Initially mild and infrequent; gradually progress to strong intensity, with 3–5 contractions in a 10-minute period	Strong, 5–6 contractions in a 10 min period; may be slightly less intense than during late first stage; may pause briefly as second stage begins	Firmly contracted	Firmly contracted
Discomfort[b]	Often begins with a low backache and sensations similar to those of menstrual cramps; back discomfort gradually sweeps to lower abdomen in a girdle-like fashion; discomfort intensifies as labor progresses	Urge to push or bear down with contractions, which becomes stronger as fetus descends; distention of vagina and vulva may cause a stretching or splitting sensation	Little discomfort; sometimes slight cramp is felt as placenta is passed	Discomfort varies; some clients have afterpains, more common in multigravidas or those who have had a large baby; as anesthesia wears off, perineal discomfort may become noticeable
Client behaviors[b]	Sociable, excited, and somewhat anxious during early labor; becomes more inwardly focused as labor intensifies; may lose control during late active phase	Intense concentration on pushing with contractions; often oblivious to surroundings and appears to doze between contractions	Excited and relieved after baby's birth; usually very tired; often cries	Tired but may find it difficult to rest because of excitement; eager to become acquainted with the newborn

[a]Contemporary cervical dilatation for latent and active phase are shown here. Historical definition of the phases of first-stage labor: Latent—0 cm to 4 cm; Active—5 cm to 7 cm; Transition—8 cm to 10 cm.
[b]Client discomfort and behaviors often vary with pain-relief method chosen.

KNOWLEDGE CHECK

11. What are some signs and symptoms that a client might experience before labor begins?
12. What are the differences between true and false labor? Which difference is the most significant?
13. Why does the fetus enter the pelvis with the sagittal suture aligned with the transverse diameter of the client's pelvic inlet?
14. Why does the fetal head turn during labor until the sagittal suture aligns with the anteroposterior diameter of the client's pelvic outlet?

Stages and Phases of Labor

Labor is divided into four stages. Each stage has unique qualities (Table 12.1). This chapter describes typical physiologic characteristics and behaviors in the average client. Clients vary in their labor patterns and responses to this process. Regional anesthesia may alter some of the behaviors.

First Stage

Cervical effacement and dilation occur in the first stage, or the stage of dilation. It begins with the onset of true labor contractions and ends with complete dilation (10 cm) and effacement (100%) of the cervix. The first stage of labor is the longest for both nulliparous and parous clients. Historically, three phases were described in the first stage of labor: latent, active, and transition. However, the transition phase is rarely identifiable, especially for clients with epidurals. Each phase is characterized by changing behaviors. These behaviors vary with the client's preparation, use of coping skills, and use of medication.

Latent Phase. The latent phase can be described as the onset of regular, painful contractions resulting in the beginning of cervical effacement and dilation, preparing for more rapid changes. Historically, the latent phase has been defined as 0 to 3 cm dilated. However, contemporary research describes the latent phase as lasting until 5 to 6 cm dilated (ACOG & Society for Maternal-Fetal Medicine (SMFM), 2019; Spong et al., 2012; Zhang et al., 2010). Its length varies among clients but may be longer for the nullipara than for the multipara. Latent labor may be quite long, and much of it may pass unnoticed by the pregnant client as latent labor gradually merges into active labor.

Contractions gradually increase in frequency, duration, and intensity. The interval between contractions shortens until they are about 5 minutes apart as the client progresses to

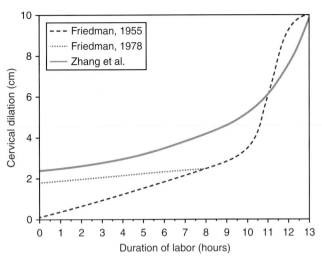

FIG. 12.13 Comparison of historical and contemporary patterns of cervical dilation. (From Zhang, J., Troendle, J. F., & Yancey, M. K. [2002]. Reassessing the labor curve in nulliparous women. *American Journal of Obstetrics & Gynecology, 187*[4], 824–828.)

the active phase. Initially, the contractions are mild, and the contracting uterus can be easily indented with the fingertips. They then progress to moderate intensity, during which the uterine muscle is indented with more difficulty. The contractions gradually build to their peak intensity and remain at the peak briefly before diminishing.

During latent labor, the client may notice discomfort in the back. As labor progresses, back discomfort encircles the lower abdomen with each contraction. Many clients compare the discomfort to menstrual cramps, especially during early labor.

The client is usually sociable, excited, and cooperative. Anxiety may occur as the client realizes that these contractions are not Braxton Hicks contractions but the "real thing." The client is usually relieved that the birth of the baby is close.

Active Phase. When the rate of cervical change accelerates, the client has progressed to active phase (Kilpatrick et al., 2021).

For nearly 70 years, our understanding of the progress of normal labor has been based on the classic research of Dr. Emanuel Friedman in the 1950s (Friedman, 1955). The Friedman labor curve has been used to assess labor progress in the clinical setting. Per Friedman's work, the active phase of first stage labor begins at 4 cm dilation. After this point, the cervical change is much faster.

More current research indicates that for various reasons, modern women progress through labor at a slower rate (Fig. 12.13) (Thorp & Grantz, 2019; Laughon et al., 2012; Spong et al., 2012; Zhang et al., 2010). Per these findings, the active phase of first-stage labor begins at 5 to 6 cm dilation. These findings are supported by the American College of Obstetricians and Gynecologists (ACOG) and the Society for Maternal-Fetal Medicine (SMFM) (ACOG & SMFM, 2019).

In the active phase, the frequency of contractions gradually increases from about three contractions in a 10-minute period to five contractions in that same period. Duration of the contractions is steady at 60 to 80 seconds with an intensity that ranges from moderate to strong. (Bakker, 2007; Caldeyro-Barcia, 1960; Cunningham et al., 2022). Active labor contractions resist indenting, reach their peak intensity quickly, and stay at the peak longer than during the latent phase. As contractions intensify, discomfort also increases if the client has not had analgesia, such as an epidural block. Strong contractions combined with fetal descent may cause the client to have an urge to push and bear down during contractions. Leg tremors, nausea, and vomiting are common near the end of the first stage of labor.

The client's behavior changes. They become more anxious and may feel helpless as the contractions intensify. The sociability that characterized early labor is gone and is replaced by a serious, inward focus. The client is unlikely to initiate interactions unless they have specific requests. These behaviors are typical of a person concentrating intently on a demanding task. Clients who choose to take pain medication and regional analgesia usually do so during this phase. The nurse helps the client maintain concentration, supports coping techniques, and helps find alternatives for coping methods that are not working. As the labor progresses, the client who does not choose epidural analgesia may become irritable and lose control. The partner may be confused because actions that were helpful just a short time ago are now irritating. The nurse can encourage the client and support person that the end of labor is near and help them use coping techniques most effectively. If premature bearing down is a problem, the nurse can help the client blow outward with each breath until the urge passes.

Second Stage

The second stage (expulsion) begins with complete (10 cm) dilation and full (100%) effacement of the cervix and ends with the birth of the baby. Duration of the second stage for the nullipara with no epidural averages 2.8 hours, whereas the average duration is 3.6 hours with an epidural. Duration of the second stage for the multipara with no epidural ranges from 1.1 to 1.3 hours, and the average duration is 1.6 to 2 hours with an epidural (Zhang et al., 2010).

Contractions may diminish slightly or even pause briefly as the second stage begins. They are strong and about 2 to 3 minutes apart, with a duration of 60 to 80 seconds.

As the fetus descends, pressure of the presenting part on the rectum and the pelvic floor causes an involuntary pushing response. The client may verbalize that they need to have a bowel movement or say "the baby's coming" or "I have to push." Voluntary pushing efforts augment involuntary uterine contractions. As the fetus descends low in the pelvis and the vulva distends with the crowning of the fetal head, the client may feel a sensation of stretching or splitting even if no trauma occurs. The urge to push does not always occur the moment full dilatation occurs. Allowing the client to "labor down" is beneficial in most cases (see Chapter 15).

The client often regains a feeling of control during the second stage of labor. Contractions are strong, but the client may feel more in control and know that they are doing something

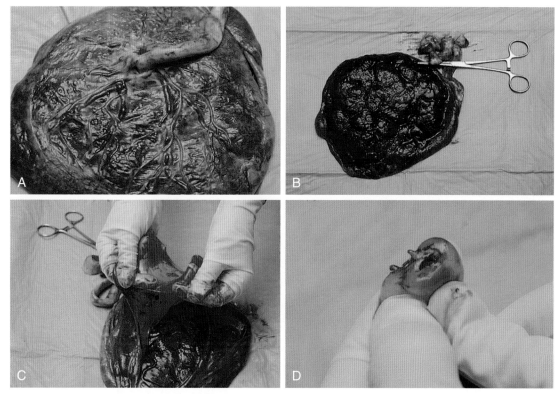

FIG. 12.14 (A) Fetal side of the placenta. (B) Maternal side of the placenta. (C) Separating membranes. (D) Umbilical cord vessels: two arteries and one vein.

to complete the process by pushing with the contractions. The word *labor* aptly describes the second stage. The client exerts intense physical effort to push the baby out. Between contractions, clients may be oblivious to the surroundings and appear to be asleep. The client feels tremendous relief and excitement as the second stage ends with the birth of the baby.

Third Stage

The third (placental) stage begins with the birth of the baby and ends with the expulsion of the placenta (Fig. 12.14). This stage is the shortest, with an average length of 6 minutes (Kilpatrick et. al, 2021). No difference in duration exists between nulliparas and parous clients.

When the infant is born, the uterine cavity becomes much smaller. The reduced size decreases the size of the placenta site, causing it to separate from the uterine wall. The following four signs suggest placenta separation:

- The uterus has a spherical shape.
- The uterus rises upward in the abdomen as the placenta descends into the vagina and pushes the fundus upward.
- The cord descends further from the vagina.
- A gush of blood appears as blood trapped behind the placenta is released.

The uterus must contract firmly and remain contracted after the placenta is expelled to compress open vessels at the implantation site. Inadequate uterine contraction after birth may result in hemorrhage.

Pain during the third stage of labor results from uterine contractions and brief stretching of the cervix as the placenta passes through it.

Fourth Stage

The fourth stage of labor is the stage of physical recovery for the client and infant. It lasts from the delivery of the placenta through 1 to 4 hours after birth.

Immediately after birth, the firmly contracted uterus can be palpated through the abdominal wall as a firm, rounded mass approximately 10 to 15 cm (4 to 6 inches) in diameter at or below the level of the umbilicus. Uterine size varies with the size of the infant and parity of the client and is larger when the infant is large or the client is a multipara. A full bladder or blood clot in the uterus interferes with uterine contraction, increasing blood loss. A soft (boggy) uterus and increasing uterine size are associated with postpartum hemorrhage because large blood vessels at the placenta site are not compressed (see Chapter 18).

The *vaginal drainage after childbirth* is called **lochia**. The three stages are lochia rubra, lochia serosa, and lochia alba (see Chapter 17). Lochia rubra, consisting mostly of blood, is present in the fourth stage of labor and may continue for 3 to 4 days.

Many clients feel chilled after birth. The cause of this reaction is unknown but may be because of the sudden decrease in effort, loss of the heat produced by the fetus, decrease in intraabdominal pressure, and fetal blood cells entering the client's circulation. The chill lasts for about 20 minutes and subsides spontaneously. A warm blanket, a hot drink, or soup may help shorten the chill and make the client more comfortable.

Discomfort during the fourth stage usually results from birth trauma and afterpains. Localized discomfort from birth trauma such as lacerations, an **episiotomy** (surgical incision of the perineum to enlarge the vaginal opening), edema, or a hematoma is evident as the effects of local and regional anesthetics diminish. Ice packs on the perineum limit this edema and hematoma formation.

Afterpains are intermittent uterine contractions occurring after birth as the uterus begins to return to the prepregnancy state. The discomfort is like menstrual cramps. Afterpains are more common in multiparas, clients who breastfeed, clients who have large babies, cases of uterine overdistention during pregnancy, and in those involving interference with uterine contraction because of a full bladder or blood clot that remains in the uterus.

Clients are simultaneously excited and tired after birth. They may be exhausted but too excited to rest. The fourth stage of labor is an ideal time for bonding of the new family because the interest of both the parents and the newborn is high. It is the best time to initiate breastfeeding. The baby is alert and seeks eye contact with the new parents, giving powerful reinforcement for the parents' attachment to their newborn.

KNOWLEDGE CHECK

15. How do client behaviors change during each phase of first-stage labor and the second stage?
16. What are typical characteristics of contractions during each phase of first-stage and second-stage labor?
17. What four signs may indicate that the placenta has separated?
18. What complication may occur if the uterus does not contract firmly and remain contracted after the placenta is expelled?

Duration of Labor

The total duration of labor is significantly different for clients who have never given birth and those who have previously given birth vaginally. However, some nulliparas progress through labor quickly, whereas labor for some parous clients resembles that of someone who has never given birth.

Because of the high cesarean birth rate and fewer **vaginal births after cesarean** (**VBAC**), a parous client may have had no vaginal births. In this situation, the client is likely to have a labor more like that of the nullipara, particularly if they did not labor before the previous cesarean birth.

THE IMPACT OF TECHNOLOGY

The goal of maternity care is to protect the health of the client, fetus, and newborn and to support and enrich the family's birth experience. Technology helps caregivers identify problems and intervene quickly to promote maternal and fetal well-being. However, extensive use of sophisticated technology may make maternity care seem impersonal. Clients may think their feelings are less important than the data from the monitors and infusion pumps attached to them. The nurse should guard against "nursing the machines" or internal feelings of being unnecessary to the client's birth experience. If the nurse focuses on the client as the child bearer and the machine as a tool, frustration for all concerned is less likely.

Although normal labor and birth do not require routine use of sophisticated technology, clients may quickly agree to suggested interventions and not voice their desire for a low-intervention birth. Other clients simply have not thought of a low-technology birth, possibly because many friends and relatives have had a high-technology birth. Communication on the indications and risks and benefits to the use of technology is important in planning each individual's care. The intrapartum nurse can be the bridge between the technology and humanity of the birth experience by keeping the focus on the clients, the fetus, and the support person rather than on the technology.

SUMMARY CONCEPTS

- Labor contractions are intermittent, which allows oxygen, nutrients, and waste products to be exchanged between maternal and fetal circulations during the interval between contractions.
- The upper uterus contracts actively during labor, maintaining tension to pull the more passive lower uterus and cervix over the fetal presenting part. These actions result in cervical effacement and dilation.
- Vital signs are best assessed between contractions because alterations in the client's blood pressure and pulse rate may occur during a contraction.
- Hyperventilation may occur if the client breathes deeply and rapidly. Its manifestations include tingling of the hands and feet, numbness, and dizziness.
- The fetal heart rate and rhythm respond rapidly to events occurring during labor.
- Several occurrences during late pregnancy and labor aid the newborn in making adaptations to extrauterine life: reduced production of fetal lung fluid and increased absorption of lung fluid into the interstitium of the fetal lungs; expulsion of fluid from upper airways during the compression forces of labor; and increased catecholamine secretion by the fetal adrenal glands to stimulate cardiac contraction and breathing, speed clearance of remaining lung fluid, and aid in temperature regulation.
- Four interrelated components affecting the process of birth are the powers, passage, passenger, and psyche. Presentation and position further describe the relation of the fetus (passenger) to the maternal pelvis (passage).
- The exact reasons for the beginning of labor are unknown, but several factors seem to have a role. These include fetal adrenal gland production of cortisol; an increase in the ratio of estrogen to progesterone; increased uterine oxytocin receptors and gap junctions; and stretching of the uterus and cervix.
- As labor approaches, the client may notice one or more premonitory signs preceding its onset: increase in frequency and intensity of Braxton Hicks contractions,

lightening, increased vaginal secretions, bloody show, a spurt of energy, and weight loss.

- The conclusive difference between true labor and false labor is that progressive effacement and dilation of the cervix occur with true labor.
- The four stages and phases of labor are characterized by different physiologic events and client behaviors: first

stage, cervical dilation and effacement; second stage, expulsion of the fetus; third stage, expulsion of the placenta; and fourth stage, physiologic stabilization and parent–infant bonding.

- Normal labor is characterized by consistent progression of uterine contractions, cervical dilation and effacement, and fetal descent.

Clinical Judgment and Next-Generation NCLEX® Examination-Style Questions

1. **Choose the most likely options for the information missing from the statement below by selecting from the lists of options provided.**

When palpating the fetal head to determine position during an admission vaginal exam, the nurse identifies a "Y" shaped juncture of three bones with a small soft area that is triangle shaped, known as the ____**1**_____. From this landmark, the nurse follows the ____**2**_____ to a larger, diamond-shaped soft area known as the ____**3**_____.

Options for 1, 2 and 3
Anterior fontanel
Lambdoid suture
Occipito-frontal diameter
Posterior fontanel
Sagittal suture
Supraoccipitomental diameter

2. **Choose the most likely options for the information missing from the statement below by selecting from the lists of options provided.**

The provider performs a vaginal exam to determine a client's progress in labor and documents that the cervix is 3 cm; 80%; –1. The nurse understands the presenting part of the fetus is located ____**1**_____, and the cervix is dilated (opened) ____**2**_____ and effaced (thinned out) ____**3**_____ .

Options for 1	Options for 2	Options for 3
1 cm below the ischial spines	1 cm	1 cm thick
1 cm above the ischial spines	3 cm	3 cm thick
3 cm above the ischial spines	80%	80%
3 cm below the ischial spines		
80% of the way from the pelvic inlet to the ischial spines		
80% of the way from the ischial spines to the symphysis pubis		

REFERENCES

American Academy of Pediatrics & American College of Obstetricians and Gynecologists (AAP & ACOG). (2017). *Guidelines for perinatal care* (8th ed.).

American College of Nurse-Midwives (ACNM). (2016). Clinical bulletin no. 16. Providing oral nutrition to women in labor. *Journal of Midwifery and Women's Health, 61*(4), 528–534.

American College of Obstetricians and Gynecologists (ACOG). (2019). *Postpartum Hemorrhage.* ACOG Practice Bulletin No. 183. Published 2017, reaffirmed 2019.

American College of Obstetricians and Gynecologists & Society for Maternal-Fetal Medicine (ACOG & SMFM). (2019). Safe Prevention of the Primary Cesarean Delivery. *Obstetric Care Consensus* (No. 1). Published 2014, reaffirmed, 2019. https://doi.org/10.1097/01AOG.0000444441.04111.1d.

American Society of Anesthesiologists (ASA). (2016). Practice guidelines for obstetric anesthesia: An updated report by the American Society of Anesthesiologists Task Force on Obstetric Anesthesia and Perinatology. *Anesthesiology, 124*(2), 270–300. https://doi.org/10.1097/ALN.0000000000000935.

Antony, K. M., Pacusin, D. A., Aagaard, K., & Dildy, G. A. (2021). Maternal physiology. In M. B. Landon, H. L. Galan, E. R. M. Jauniaux, D. A. Driscoll, V. Berghella, W. A. Grobman, S. J. Kilpatrick, & A. G. Cahill (Eds.), *Gabbe's obstetrics: Normal and problem pregnancies* (8th ed., pp. 43–67). Elsevier.

Association of Women's Health, Obstetric and Neonatal Nurses (AWHONN). (2018). Continuous labor support for every woman: AWHONN position statement. *Journal of Obstetric, Gynecologic, and Neonatal Nurses, 47*(1), 73–74. https://doi: 10.1016/j.jogn.2017.11.010.

Bakker, P. C. A., Kurver, P. H. J., Kuik, D. J., & Van Geijn, H. P. (2007). Elevated uterine activity increases the risk of fetal acidosis at birth. *American Journal of Obstetrics & Gynecology, 196*(4), 313–315. https://doi-org.ezproxy.baylor.edu/10.1016/j.ajog.2006.11.035.

Blackburn, S. T. (2018). *Maternal, fetal, and neonatal physiology: A clinical perspective* (5th ed.). Elsevier.

Bohren, M. A., Hofmeyr, G. J., Sakala, C., Fukuzawa, R. K., & Cuthbert, A. (2017). Continuous support for women during childbirth. *Cochrane Database of Systematic Reviews, 2017*(7), CD003766. https://doi.org/10.1002/14651858.CD003766.pub6.

Caldeyro-Barcia, R. & Poseiro, J. J. (1960). Physiology of the uterine contraction. *Clinical Obstetrics & Gynecology, 3*(2), 386–410.

California Maternal Quality Care Collaborative (CMQCC). (2017). Toolkit to support vaginal birth and reduce primary cesareans. https://www.cmqcc.org/VBirthToolkitResource.

Cunningham, F. G., Leveno, K. J., Bloom, S. L., Dashe, J. S., Hoffman, B. L., Casey, B. M., & Spong, C. Y. (2022). *Williams obstetrics* (26th ed.). McGraw-Hill Companies.

Fraser, D. (2021). Newborn adaptation to extrauterine life. In K. R. Simpson & P. A. Creehan (Eds.), *AWHONN's perinatal nursing* (5th ed., pp. 564–578). Wolters Kluwer.

Friedman, E. A. (1955). Primigravid labor: A graphicostatistical analysis. *Obstetrics and Gynecology, 6*(6), 567–589.

Hawkins, J. L., & Bucklin, B. A. (2021). Obstetric anesthesia. In M. B. Landon, H. L. Galan, E. R. M. Jauniaux, D. A. Driscoll, V. Berghella, W. A. Grobman, S. J. Kilpatrick, & A. G. Cahill (Eds.), *Gabbe's obstetrics: Normal and problem pregnancies* (8th ed., pp. 295–318). Elsevier.

Izakson, A., Cohen, Y., & Landau, R. (2020). Physiologic changes in the airway and the respiratory system affecting management in pregnancy. In S. Einav, C. F. Weiniger, & R. Landau (Eds.), *Principles and practice of maternal critical care.* Springer Cham. https://doi.org/10.1007/978-3-030-43477-9_20.

Jafari-Dehkordi, E., Adibi, A., & Sirus, M. (2015). Reference range of the weekly uterine cervical length at 8 to 38 weeks of gestation in the center of Iran. *Advanced Biomedical Research, 4*(115). https://doi.org/10.4103/2277-9175.157839.

Kamath-Rayne, B. D., & Jobe, A. H. (2019). Fetal lung development and surfactant. In R. Resnik, C. Lockwood, T. Moore, M. Greene, J. Copel, & R. Silver (Eds.), *Creasy & Resnik's maternal-fetal medicine: Principles and practice* (8th ed., pp. 223–234. e2–1). Elsevier.

Kilpatrick, S. J., Garrison, E., & Fairbrother, E. (2021). Normal labor and delivery. In M. B. Landon, H. L. Galan, E. R. M. Jauniaux, D. A. Driscoll, V. Berghella, W. A. Grobman, S. J. Kilpatrick, & A. G. Cahill (Eds.), *Gabbe's obstetrics: Normal and problem pregnancies* (8th ed., pp. 204–225). Elsevier.

Laughon, S. K., Branch, D. W., Beaver, J., & Zhang, J. (2012). Changes in labor patterns over 50 years. *American Journal of Obstetrics and Gynecology, 205*(5), 419.e1–419.e9.

Macones, G. A., Hankins, G. D., Spong, C. Y., Hauth, J., & Moore, T. (2008). The 2008 National Institute of Child Health and Human Development workshop report on electronic fetal monitoring: Update on definitions, interpretation and research guidelines. *Journal Obstetric, Gynecologic, and Neonatal Nursing, 37*(5), 510–515. https://doi.org/10.1111/j.1552-6909-2008.00284.x.

Mastrobattista, J., & Monga, M. (2019). Maternal cardiovascular, respiratory, and renal adaptation to pregnancy. In R. Resnik, C. Lockwood, T. Moore, M. Greene, J. Copel, & R. Silver (Eds.), *Creasy & Resnik's maternal-fetal medicine: Principles and practice* (8th ed., pp. 141–147.e3). Elsevier. https://www.clinicalkey.com/#!/content/book/3-s2.0-B9780323479103000097.

Miller, L. A., Miller, D. A., & Cypher, R. L. (2022). *Mosby's pocket guide to fetal monitoring: A multidisciplinary approach* (9th ed.). Elsevier.

Norwitz, E. R., Mahendroo, M., & Lye, S. J. (2019). Physiology of parturition. In R. Resnik, C. J. Lockwood, T. R. Moore, M. F

Greene, J. A. Copel, & R. M. Silver (Eds.), *Creasy & Resnik's maternal-fetal medicine: Principles and practice* (8th ed., pp. 81–95e6). Elsevier.

O'Brien-Abel, N., & Simpson, K. R. (2021). Fetal assessment in labor. In K. R. Simpson & P. A. Creehan (Eds.), *AWHONN's perinatal nursing* (5th ed., pp. 413–465). Wolters Kluwer.

Ross, M. G., & Ervin, M. G. (2021). Fetal development, physiology, and effects on long-term health. In M. B. Landon, H. L. Galan, E. R. M. Jauniaux, D. A. Driscoll, V. Berghella, W. A. Grobman, S. J. Kilpatrick, & A. G. Cahill (Eds.), *Gabbe's obstetrics: Normal and problem pregnancies* (8th ed., pp. 26–42). Elsevier.

Simhan, H. N., Berghella, V., & Iams, J. D. (2019). Prevention and management of preterm parturition. In R. Resnik, C. J. Lockwood, T. R. Moore, M. F. Greene, J. A. Copel, & R. M. Silver (Eds.), *Creasy & Resnik's maternal-fetal medicine: Principles and practice* (8th ed., pp. 679–711.e10). Elsevier.

Simpson, K. R., & O'Brien-Abel, N. (2021). Labor and birth. In K. R. Simpson, & P. A. Creehan (Eds.), *AWHONN's perinatal nursing* (5th ed., pp. 326–412). Wolters Kluwer.

Singata, M., Tranmer, J., & Gyte, G. M. L. (2013). Restricting oral fluid and food intake during labour. *Cochrane Database of Systematic Reviews,* (1), CD003930.

Spong, C. Y., Berghella, V., Wenstrom, K. D., Mercer, B. M., & Saade, G. R. (2012). Preventing the first cesarean delivery: Summary of a joint Eunice Kennedy Shriver National Institute of Child Health and Human Development, Society for Maternal-Fetal Medicine, and American College of Obstetricians and Gynecologists Workshop. *Obstetrics and Gynecology, 120*(5), 1181–1193. https://doi.org/10.1097/aog.0b013e3182704880.

Thorp, J. M., & Grantz, K. L. (2019). Clinical aspects of normal and abnormal labor. In R. Resnik, C. Lockwood, T. Moore, M. Greene, J. Copel, & R. Silver (Eds.), *Creasy & Resnik's maternal-fetal medicine: Principles and practice* (8th ed., pp. 723–757.e7). Elsevier.

Troiano, N. H., Witcher, P. M., & Baird, S. M. (2019). *High-risk & critical care obstetrics* (4th ed.). Wolters Kluwer.

Zhang, J., Landy, H. J., Branch, D. W., Burkman, R., Haberman, S., Gregory, K. D., et al. (2010). Contemporary patterns of spontaneous labor with normal neonatal outcomes. Consortium on Safe Labor. *Obstetrics and Gynecology, 116,* 1281–1287.

Zhang, J., Troendle, J. F., & Yancey, M. K. (2002). Reassessing the labor curve in nulliparous women. *American Journal of Obstetrics & Gynecology, 187*(4), 824–828. https://doi-org.ezproxy.baylor.edu/10.1067/mob.2002.127142.

Pain Management During Childbirth

Jane Lin Chien, Melissa R. Espey-Mueller

OBJECTIVES

After studying this chapter, you should be able to:

1. Compare childbirth pain with other types of pain.
2. Describe how excessive pain affects the laboring client and the fetus.
3. Examine how physical and psychological forces interact in the laboring client's pain experience.
4. Describe use of nonpharmacologic pain management techniques in labor.
5. Describe the way medications may affect both the client and the fetus.
6. Explain benefits and risks of specific pharmacologic pain control methods.
7. Explain nursing care related to nonpharmacologic and pharmacologic care during the different stages of labor.

Each client has unique expectations about birth, including assumptions regarding the pain of labor and their ability to manage it. The client who successfully copes with the pain of labor is more likely to view their experience as a positive life event. The experience with labor pain varies with several physical and psychological elements, and each client responds differently. Nonpharmacologic and pharmacologic methods offer a selection of pain management techniques from which clients may choose.

UNIQUE NATURE OF PAIN DURING BIRTH

Pain is a universal experience that can be difficult to define. It is a generalized or localized sensation of distress resulting from stimulation of sensory nerves.

Pain involves two components:

- A physiologic component that includes reception by sensory nerves and transmission to the central nervous system (CNS)
- A psychological component that involves recognizing the sensation, interpreting it as painful, and reacting to the interpretation

Pain is subjective and personal. No one can feel another's pain, and no two people will manage it the same. Childbirth pain is unique and differs from other types of pain in the following important aspects:

- Childbirth pain is part of a normal process—other types of pain relate to injury or illness.
- Childbirth pain is purposeful and may lead a client to assume different positions that assist in labor progression and/or descent of the fetus.
- The pain of labor is anticipated and expected, which allows the client and the partner to prepare for labor, helping to promote realistic expectations about birth and helping them to develop skills to cope with labor and birth.
- It is self-limiting, meaning it is confined to a given period of time. It is not infinite; labor pain will end.
- Labor pain is not constant, but rather intermittent—a client may describe little to no discomfort when contractions end. They may even sleep or rest between contractions. Even during late labor, a client may be relatively comfortable and experience complete relief between contractions.
- Labor ends with the birth of the baby—the emotional significance of the child's birth impacts a client's response to pain. Care about the fetus often motivates clients to tolerate more pain during labor than they otherwise might be willing to endure.

ADVERSE EFFECTS OF EXCESSIVE PAIN

Although expected during labor, pain that exceeds a client's tolerance can have distressing effects on both the client and the fetus. It can cause clients to feel the experience is "happening" to them, rather than being in control and actively participating in their labor.

Physiologic Effects

Fear of the unknown may cause a client who is uninformed or unsupported to make fear-driven decisions that may later cause regret. Excessive pain can heighten a client's fear and anxiety, which stimulates sympathetic nervous system activity and results in increased secretion of catecholamines (epinephrine and norepinephrine). Catecholamines stimulate alpha and beta receptors, causing effects on the blood vessels and uterine muscles.

Stimulation of the alpha receptors causes uterine and generalized vasoconstriction and an increase in the uterine muscle tone. These effects reduce uterine blood flow as they raise the client's blood pressure.

Stimulation of the beta receptors relaxes the uterine muscle and causes systemic vasodilation. However, uterine vessels are already dilated in pregnancy, so dilation of other vessels allows the client's blood to pool in them. The pooling of blood reduces the amount of blood available to perfuse the placenta.

The combined effects of excessive catecholamine secretion are as follows:

- Reduced blood flow to and from the placenta, restricting fetal oxygen supply and waste removal.
- Reduced effectiveness of uterine contractions, slowing labor progress.

Labor increases a client's metabolic rate and demand for oxygen. Pain and anxiety increase the already high metabolic rate. The client breathes fast to obtain more oxygen, exhaling excessive amounts of carbon dioxide in the process. Significant changes, more than anticipated during labor, can occur in the client's partial pressure of oxygen (PaO_2), partial pressure of carbon dioxide ($PaCO_2$) levels, and arterial pH. If persistent, these respiratory and metabolic changes alter placental exchange significantly. The fetus may have less oxygen available and have less ability to expel carbon dioxide. The net result is the fetus shifts to anaerobic metabolism, with buildup of hydrogen ions (acidosis). This can lead to metabolic acidosis, which does not resolve as quickly after birth as respiratory acidosis (Blackburn, 2018; Cunningham et al., 2022).

Psychological Effects

Clients have a remarkable threshold for labor pain. However, poorly managed pain lessens the pleasure of this extraordinary life event for both partners. The client may find it difficult to interact with the infant because of exhaustion from painful labor and may report the labor as traumatizing. Unpleasant memories of the birth may affect the client's response to sexual activity or future pregnancies and labor. The support person may feel inadequate during birth, often feeling helpless and frustrated when the client's pain is unrelieved.

It is helpful to remember some clients will manage the pain and not categorize it as suffering and utilize many learned and instinctual tactics to cope with labor pain.

> ### KNOWLEDGE CHECK
> 1. How does the pain of childbirth differ from other kinds of pain?
> 2. How can excessive pain adversely affect a laboring client and the fetus?

VARIABLES IN CHILDBIRTH PAIN

A variety of physical and psychosocial factors contribute to a client's pain perception and response during labor. These factors provide possibilities for nursing interventions for pain relief.

Physical Factors

Childbirth pain is of two types: visceral and somatic. Visceral pain is a slow, deep, poorly localized pain that is often described as dull or aching. Visceral pain dominates during first-stage labor as the uterus contracts and the cervix dilates.

Somatic pain is a quick, sharp pain that can be precisely localized. Somatic pain is most prominent during late first-stage labor and during second-stage labor as the descending fetus puts direct pressure on the client's tissues.

Sources of Pain

There are four sources of labor pain: tissue ischemia, cervical dilation, pressure and pulling on pelvic structures, and distention of the vagina and perineum. Other physical factors may modify labor pain, increasing or decreasing it.

Tissue Ischemia. The blood supply to the uterus decreases during contractions, leading to tissue hypoxia and anaerobic metabolism. Ischemic uterine pain has been likened to ischemic heart pain.

Cervical Dilation. Dilation and stretching of the cervix and lower uterus are a major source of pain. Pain stimuli from cervical dilation travel through the hypogastric plexus, entering the spinal cord at the T10, T11, T12, and L1 levels (Fig. 13.1).

Pressure and Pulling on Pelvic Structures. Some pain results from pressure and pulling on pelvic structures such as ligaments, fallopian tubes, ovaries, bladder, and perineum. This type of pain is visceral pain; a client may feel it as referred pain in the back and legs.

Distention of the Vagina and Perineum. Marked distention of the vagina and perineum occurs with fetal descent, especially during the second stage. The client may describe a sensation of burning, tearing, or splitting (somatic pain). Pain from vaginal and perineal distention and pressure and pulling on adjacent structures enters the spinal cord at the S2, S3, and S4 levels (see Fig. 13.1) (Cunningham et al., 2022).

Factors Influencing Perception or Tolerance of Pain

Although physiologic processes are responsible for labor pain, a client's perception and tolerance of pain is affected by other physical and psychosocial influences.

Labor Intensity. The client who has precipitous labor may complain of severe pain with a more rapid onset because each contraction does so much work (effacement, dilation, and fetal descent). A rapid labor may limit the client's ability to cope due to shorter recovery times. Precipitous labor may also decrease options for adequate pharmacologic pain relief.

Cervical Readiness. If cervical changes such as thinning, shortening, and softening prior to labor are minimal, the cervix does not open, or dilate, as easily or efficiently once labor begins. This can increase the duration of labor and result in greater fatigue of the laboring client.

Fetal Position. Labor is likely to be longer and more uncomfortable when the fetus is in an unfavorable position in relationship to the birthing pelvis. An occiput posterior

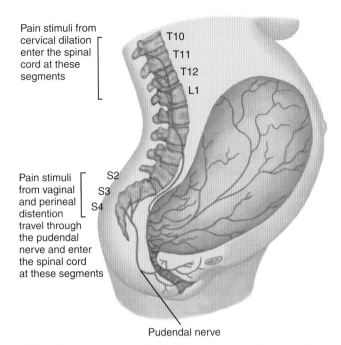

Pain stimuli from cervical dilation enter the spinal cord at these segments

T10
T11
T12
L1

Pain stimuli from vaginal and perineal distention travel through the pudendal nerve and enter the spinal cord at these segments

S2
S3
S4

Pudendal nerve

FIG. 13.1 Pathways of Pain Transmission during Labor.

(OP) position is a common variant seen in otherwise normal labors. In this position, each contraction pushes the fetal occiput against the client's sacrum. The client may experience intense back discomfort (**back labor**), which persists between contractions. It is important to remember that pelvic anatomy, specifically the inlet and outlet, varies in shape and size. Some clients can deliver their fetus "straight" OP without difficulty; however, in other cases, the client may not be able to deliver the fetus until it rotates to the occiput anterior (OA) position. The fetal head must therefore rotate a wider arc before the mechanisms of extension and expulsion occur, increasing the duration of labor and pushing in some instances (see Fig. 12.12).

Back pain may decrease dramatically when a fetus rotates into the OA position. Additionally, contractions may become more regular, and labor may progress more efficiently. A client who has an asynclitic fetus, meaning the head is tilted toward the shoulder and not in alignment with the birth canal, may also experience an insufficient labor pattern with increased discomfort with little to no cervical progress. Pain without progress is often more difficult to manage physically and mentally.

Pelvic Anatomy. The size and shape of a client's pelvis influences the course and length of labor. Abnormalities and unique pelvic structure, such as a high pelvic arch or a narrow pelvic brim, may contribute to fetal malpresentation or malposition, resulting in a longer, more difficult labor.

Fatigue. Fatigue reduces a client's ability to tolerate pain and to use learned coping skills. Therefore, it is not only the pain of labor but the duration of labor that causes clients to lose their ability to manage pain effectively. They may be unable to focus on techniques that would otherwise help them cope with increasing contraction intensity. An extremely fatigued client may have an exaggerated response to contractions or may be unable to respond to sensations of labor such as the urge to push. The client's energy reserves are likely to be depleted in a long labor.

Caregiver Interventions. Although they may be appropriate for the well-being of a client and fetus, common interventions often add discomfort to the natural pain of labor.

Intravenous (IV) lines cause pain when inserted. Fetal monitoring equipment is uncomfortable to some clients, while others may find comfort in fetal heart rate sounds. Both may limit a client's mobility, which could increase pain and the length of labor. A client may expect routine electronic fetal monitoring (EFM) and ignore personal comfort for reassurance of the baby's well-being.

A client whose labor is induced or augmented often reports more pain and discomfort. Perhaps the client wished to spend early labor in the comfort of the home and now feels more anxious in an unfamiliar environment. The client may also feel contractions become more intense sooner, making it harder to cope with the pain.

When a labor is synthetically driven, whether induction or augmentation, it will incorporate more interventions, often adding to client discomforts. Interventions such as vaginal examinations, amniotomy (rupture of the amniotic membranes), or insertion of internal fetal or uterine monitoring devices also increase a client's discomfort and perceptions of pain during the birth experience.

It is important to remember that while many of these interventions are necessary, a client may report a more painful or traumatic experience in the absence of adequate education and informed consent from staff.

Psychosocial Factors

Several psychosocial variables influence a client's experience of pain.

Culture

A client's sociocultural roots influence the perception, interpretation, and response to pain during childbirth. Some cultures encourage loud and vigorous expression of pain, whereas others value self-control. However, clients are individuals within their cultural groups. The experience of pain is personal, and caregivers should not make assumptions about how a client will behave during labor.

Clients should be encouraged to express themselves in any way they find comforting, and the diversity of their expressions should be respected. Loud and vigorous expression may be a client's personal pain coping mechanism, whereas a quiet client may need medication relief but feels the need to remain stoic. Accepting a client's individual response to labor and pain promotes a therapeutic relationship. The nurse should avoid praising behaviors (such as stoicism) and belittling others (such as noisy expression).

The unique nature of childbirth pain and the diverse responses to it make nursing management complex. The nurse can miss important cues if the client is either stoic or outspoken about the pain. With either extreme, the nurse may not readily identify critical information such as impending birth or symptoms of a complication.

Race

Racial and ethnic bias in health care, as well as disparities relating to maternal and infant mortality rates, may cause more fear and anxiety in clients of color. This can lead to higher levels of fight-or-flight response in labor, increasing heart rate and blood pressure. Exposure to structural racism and dismissal by medical professionals can cause the inability to cope with the labor pain or avoidance of pharmacologic pain relief due to loss of sensation and feeling out of control.

Anxiety and Fear

Mild or moderate anxiety can enhance attention and learning. However, high anxiety and fear magnify sensitivity to pain and impair a client's ability to tolerate pain. Anxiety and fear consume energy the client needs to cope with the birth process, including its painful aspects.

Anxiety and fear increase muscle tension, diverting oxygenated blood to the brain and skeletal muscles. Tension in pelvic muscles counters the expulsive forces of uterine contractions and the laboring client's pushing. Prolonged tension results in general fatigue, increased **pain perception** or decreased pain **threshold** (lowest stimulus level perceived as painful), and reduced ability to cope with pain. If a previous pregnancy had a poor outcome such as a stillborn infant or one with abnormalities, a client is probably more anxious during labor and for a time after birth.

Previous Experiences with Pain

Early in life a child learns pain means bodily injury. Consequently, fear and withdrawal are natural reactions to pain during labor. Learning about the normal sensations of labor, including pain, helps a client suppress natural reactions of fear and withdrawal, allowing the body to do the work of birth.

A client who has given birth previously has a different perspective. If it was a vaginal birth, the client is probably aware of normal labor sensations and is less likely to associate them with injury or abnormality. A client who had a previous long and difficult labor may be anxious about the outcome of the present one and may be surprised the second labor moves more quickly than the first. The client having a second (or third) vaginal birth may find late first-stage and second-stage labor to be more painful because the fetus descends faster.

A client who plans a trial of labor after cesarean section (TOLAC) but has never experienced labor may be particularly anxious. The experience of cesarean birth is known, whereas labor is unknown. A repeat cesarean birth may seem to be the quicker and less painful option, and yet, clients may prefer a vaginal birth. These clients may have a difficult time yielding to the normal forces of birth.

Previous experiences may positively affect a client's ability to deal with pain. They may have learned ways to cope with pain during other episodes of pain or during other births and may use these skills adaptively during labor.

If clients have experienced molestation and/or sexual assault, they may associate vaginal, pelvic, or rectal pain and/or pressure with a past traumatic experience; triggering unbearable pain and emotional anguish. They may be unable to relax during pelvic examinations or react negatively to any unsolicited touch or repositioning.

Preparation for Childbirth

Preparation for childbirth does not ensure a pain-free labor, but it can encourage a positive perception and an enhanced ability to manage the pain. Labor is unpredictable, and it is ideal when the client has realistic expectations about pain management and options, such as analgesia and anesthesia.

Preparation reduces anxiety and fear of the unknown. It allows a client to rehearse for labor and learn a variety of skills to cope with pain as labor progresses. If the client and partner learn about expected behavioral changes during labor, and how to navigate the unexpected, their knowledge may help decrease their fear and anxiety.

Support System

An anxious partner may have difficulty providing the objective and subjective support and reassurance a client needs during labor. In addition, anxiety in others can be contagious, increasing the client's anxiety and worry. The client may assume if others are worried, then something must be wrong.

The birth experiences and shared recollections of a client's family and friends can bring fear or reassurance to a client, depending on the circumstances and outcome. No two labors are alike, even in the same client.

A doula is a professional labor support person and may be hired by the client as a source of support during pregnancy, labor, birth, and postpartum. Doulas are trained to offer evidence-based information, education, and emotional and physical support to parents before, during, and after the birth of an infant. A doula does not perform clinical tasks.

Clients who have continuous labor support have less interventions, have a decreased desire for pain medications, and are less likely to have an instrumental birth or a cesarean section. They are also less likely to be dissatisfied with their birth experience, no matter the outcome (Bohren et al., 2017; Minehart & Minnich, 2020; Simkin & Rohs, 2018).

? KNOWLEDGE CHECK

3. How may physical and psychological factors interact in a client's labor pain experience?
4. What four sources of pain are present in most labors?
5. How can each of the following physical factors influence the pain a client experiences during childbirth: Labor intensity? Cervical readiness? Fetal position? Pelvic anatomy? Fatigue?
6. What psychosocial factors influence a client's experience with labor pain?

STANDARDS FOR PAIN MANAGEMENT

The Joint Commission (TJC) (2019) has recognized that pain management is an essential part of the care provided in health care settings, and the client should be involved in the assessment and management of pain through nonpharmacologic and pharmacologic strategies.

NONPHARMACOLOGIC PAIN MANAGEMENT

The key word is management. Some clients will do well managing their pain using positional changes, breathing techniques, hydrotherapy, and other techniques, while others will not. The nurse who cares for clients in labor and birth can offer many nonpharmacologic options to help a client feel supported. However, if a client feels they can no longer manage or tolerate the pain, pharmacologic pain management methods should be discussed.

Education about nonpharmacologic pain management is the foundation of most prepared childbirth classes, although today's classes contain significant content on pharmacologic pain management options as well.

To be most helpful to clients and their labor partners, the intrapartum nurse should review the unique nature of labor pain (Table 13.1) and learn methods taught in local childbirth classes. Recommending techniques during labor that conflict with what the client has learned and practiced may cause confusion and anxiety.

Advantages

When nonpharmacologic pain control is effective, it has several advantages over pharmacologic methods. Many clients prefer to be mobile during labor, and to have more control over their bodies and positioning. Some clients fear losing sensation and the ability to move, often associated with the use of epidural anesthesia, more than the pain itself.

Unlike pharmacologic methods, nonpharmacologic methods have no side effects or risk for allergy. Unmedicated clients may also feel the benefits of endorphin release resulting from movement and frequent position changes.

The client who chooses analgesia may need to utilize alternative pain management techniques until they receive medication. Once medicated, the pharmacologic method may not completely eliminate labor pain. Therefore, nonpharmacologic techniques may be needed for the remaining discomfort.

Nonpharmacologic methods may be the only realistic option for the client who arrives in advanced, rapid labor. Medications might not have enough time to take effect, or there may not be adequate time to administer an epidural block before birth. In addition, the time of peak drug action in terms of newborn respiratory effort should be considered if an **analgesic** (systemic agent to relieve pain) medication is given.

Limitations

Nonpharmacologic methods also have limitations, especially as the sole method of pain control. Clients do not always

TABLE 13.1	**PAIN Acronym**
Many childbirth educators use the acronym PAIN when discussing and teaching about the pain of labor, describing it as:	
P	Purposeful
A	Anticipated
I	Intermittent
N	Normal

achieve their desired level of pain control using these methods alone. Even a well-prepared and highly motivated client may have a difficult labor and may request analgesia or anesthesia.

Gate-Control Theory

A discussion of nonpharmacologic pain management techniques would not be complete without discussion of the **gate-control theory**. Per this theory, transmission of nerve impulses is controlled by a neural mechanism in the dorsal horn of the spinal cord that acts like a gate to control impulses transmitted to the brain. Transmission is affected by stimulation of sensory nerve fibers and descending impulses from the brain. This mechanism opens or closes the "gate" to pain sensation by allowing or preventing some impulses from reaching the brain, where they are recognized as pain (Peter & Booth, 2020).

Pain is transmitted through small-diameter sensory nerve fibers. Stimulation of large-diameter fibers in the skin blocks pain conduction through the small-diameter fibers, thereby "closing the gate" and decreasing the amount of pain felt. Examples of this stimulation include tactile stimulation such as massage, thermal stimulation, or hydrotherapy (Blackburn, 2018).

Impulses from the brain have a similar ability to impede transmission through the dorsal horn using visual and auditory stimulation techniques. Examples of this stimulation include use of a focal point or breathing techniques.

Memory and cognitive processes affect the perception of stimuli as painful. Education and support during labor are used to increase the client's relaxation, confidence, self-efficacy, and feeling of control. Although these methods may not completely prevent pain, they may decrease the severity of perceived pain (Cunningham et al., 2022).

Preparation for Pain Management

The ideal time to prepare for nonpharmacologic pain control is before labor. During the last trimester of pregnancy, the client learns about physiologic birth, including its painful aspects. Childbirth classes allow the opportunity to learn about a variety of coping mechanisms and prepare for the pain of labor. The support person learns specific methods to encourage and support the client. After admission, the nurse can review and reinforce what the partners learned in class.

The nurse can teach the unprepared client and the support person nonpharmacologic techniques. The latent phase of labor is the best time for intrapartum teaching because the

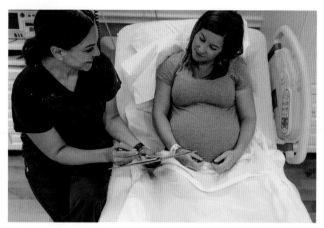

FIG. 13.2 The nurse explains coping techniques while the client is in early labor, allowing for greater client engagement and understanding.

client is usually still relatively comfortable and able to engage, listen, and understand (Fig. 13.2). The nurse should attempt to teach between contractions as labor progresses because the client's focus becomes very narrow during contractions.

No one method or combination of methods helps every client. Most methods may become less comforting and effective (**habituation**) after prolonged use, and changing techniques counters this problem. Knowing a variety of methods gives the nurse options and allows the client to feel more productive in managing the discomfort.

Application of Nonpharmacologic Techniques

Techniques utilized during labor include relaxation, cutaneous stimulation, hydrotherapy, mental stimulation, and breathing techniques. Many studies have assessed nonpharmacologic methods of labor analgesia; however, they are often criticized for not being scientific in their methods (Minehart & Minnich, 2020).

Relaxation

Promoting relaxation is a basis for all other methods, both nonpharmacologic and pharmacologic, because it achieves the following:

- Promotes uterine blood flow, improving fetal oxygenation
- Promotes efficient uterine contractions
- Reduces tension, which decreases pain perception and increases **pain tolerance** (maximum pain one is willing to endure)
- Reduces tension, which can facilitate fetal descent

Environmental Comfort. Comfortable surroundings support relaxation, trust, and hormone release. A client needs an environment that exhibits feelings of safety and intimacy in order to suppress the fight-or-flight hormones, known as catecholamines.

The nurse can reduce irritants such as bright lights. Dim lighting increases the release of endogenous oxytocin. The nurse should also practice speaking quietly and with intention, limiting questions and unnecessary chatter. This type of communication will allow the client to move from a thinking

brain to a more primal brain, increasing the ability to cope with pain. Most importantly, nursing staff should maintain awareness of the client's coping and focus on supporting their labor progress.

Music masks outside noise and encourages positive feelings and soothing imagery, which can be a distraction from pain preceptors. The use of television and blue lights can increase stress hormones (catecholamines), which can slow labor progress.

Aromatherapy may provide multiple benefits: decreased anxiety, pain relief, and nausea and vomiting relief and aid in labor progression. Lavender, for example, has shown to decrease cortisol secretion while increasing serotonin secretion, helping decrease pain and improving the client's mood (Burke, 2021). Although studies for aromatherapy during labor are lacking, most would agree aromas provide a more pleasant and relaxing environment. Creating this type of atmosphere helps everyone in the labor room to relax, including hospital personnel (Simkin & Rohs, 2018).

General Comfort and Dignity. Promoting personal comfort and dignity for clients helps them focus on using pain management techniques during labor. This includes actions to increase comfort and reduce the effects of irritants. When possible, a client should be allowed to wear whatever feels comfortable or nothing at all. The nurse should work diligently to protect the client's privacy and dignity at all times, keeping clients covered, maintaining clean linens, and respecting cultural and religious boundaries and expectations.

Reducing Anxiety and Fear. The nurse may reduce a client's anxiety and increase the pain threshold and self-efficacy by providing accurate information and focusing on the normality of the labor. Hospitals are typically associated with illness or injury, situations that provoke anxiety. However, in North America, hospitals are the most common site for physiologic birth.

Simple nursing practices help remind the client that birth is normal, natural, and healthy (Lamaze International, 2021). Empowerment in childbirth comes from providing informed consent to clients and giving them the ability to make choices that feel safe and necessary. Working to establish trust by listening to a client's hopes and expectations in relation to the birth experience will help the nurse to establish trust and lessen fear-driven decision-making by the client.

Specific Relaxation Techniques. Relaxation techniques work best if they are practiced prior to labor. During practice sessions at home, couples may practice *progressive relaxation,* in which the client contracts and then releases specific muscle groups until all muscles are released. *Neuromuscular dissociation* helps the client learn to release all muscles except those that are working (e.g., the uterus or the abdominal muscles when pushing). The client can learn *touch relaxation* in response to a partner's touch, and *relaxation against pain* as the partner deliberately causes mild pain and the client learns to release and relax despite the pain.

Even if the client did not practice these relaxation techniques at home, the nurse can teach the client how to consciously relax as labor progresses. The partner can learn to watch for signs of tension, touching the area, and direct the client to release the tense muscles.

It is important to note the word "relax" can be perceived as a trigger word to a client who has been victim to abuse or sexual assault. Exchanging the word "relax" for "release" can be helpful in protecting the mental and emotional comfort of your client. For example, the nurse may see the client clenching fists. Instead of saying, "Relax your fists," the nurse could say, "Release the tension in your hands."

Cutaneous Stimulation

Cutaneous stimulation has several variations that are often combined with each other or with other techniques.

Massage. Massage increases the release of endorphins, promotes circulation, and reduces muscle tension. Clients may rub their abdomen or legs during labor (**effleurage**) to counteract discomfort. Some find abdominal touch irritating, especially near the umbilicus. With permission, the support person or nurse can rub the client's back, shoulders, legs, or any area where massage is helpful.

Clients in labor may find firm stroking more helpful than light stroking. They may hold another person's hand tightly during a contraction. The nurse should determine whether these actions indicate excess pain or whether they are a client's way of coping.

Counterpressure. Counterpressure, through sacral pressure, hip squeeze, or knee press, may help when the client has back pain. Sacral pressure may be applied using the palm of the hand or a firm object, such as two tennis balls in a sock. A double hip squeeze is performed by placing palms on the client's hips and pressing up and inward toward the symphysis (Fig. 13.3) (Burke, 2021). If the client is sitting upright, counterpressure can be executed by using the palms of the hands to press the knees straight back, causing the client's lower back to press firmly against the chair or bed providing relief. When pressure is used, the client should guide the support person regarding the amount of pressure.

Touch. Nonclinical touch by the nurse or support person can be a powerful tool if the client does not object. Eye-to-eye contact, holding the client's hand, stroking hair, or similar actions convey caring, comfort, affirmation, and reassurance during this vulnerable time (Fig. 13.4). It is important to make certain contact is welcomed; always ask for permission before touching the client.

Thermal Stimulation. Many clients appreciate warmth applied to the back, abdomen, or perineum during labor. Warmth increases oxytocin release and local blood flow, relaxes muscles, and raises the pain threshold. Massage is often more comfortable to a tense client after the skin is warmed. Heating pads provide gentle warmth and can be used to apply warm pressure to the sacral area. When using external heating devices, care should be taken to avoid burning the client's skin.

Cool, damp washcloths placed on the head, throat, or lower abdomen can provide comforting coolness if the client feels hot. If the provider has ordered nothing by mouth (NPO), the

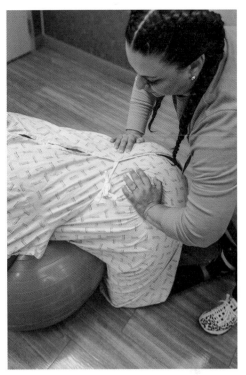

FIG. 13.3 **Double-Hip Squeeze.** Support person provides counter pressure, which counteracts the painful perception of labor.

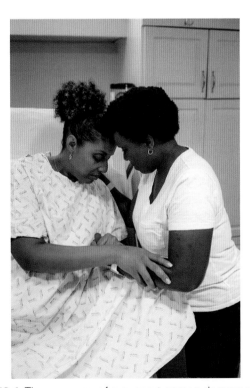

FIG. 13.4 The presence of a support person decreases anxiety and fear.

client also may want the washcloth in their mouth to relieve dryness. Ice chips cool the mouth and provide hydration.

Acupressure. Acupressure is a directed form of massage in which the support person applies pressure to specific points using hands, rollers, balls, or other equipment. It is related to its invasive counterpart, acupuncture, in which tiny needles are inserted into similar points. Acupuncture and acupressure have data to support effectiveness to relieve nausea and vomiting, including morning sickness of pregnancy, pain, anxiety, stress, headaches, and so on (Burke, 2021). Few controlled studies exist on acupressure's usefulness during birth. For updated objective information on acupressure and other complementary and alternative medicine (CAM) techniques, visit the website for the National Center for Complementary and Integrative Health (https://www.nccih.nih.gov/), which is part of the National Institutes of Health (NIH) (NIH, 2019).

Hydrotherapy

Water therapy can supplement any relaxation technique. A shower, tub bath, or whirlpool bath is relaxing and provides thermal stimulation. Several studies have shown benefits of water therapy during labor, including immersion in a tub or whirlpool (Burke, 2021).

The buoyancy afforded by immersion supports and equalizes pressure on the body and aids muscle relaxation. In addition, fluid shifts from the extravascular space to the intravascular space, reducing edema as the excess fluid is excreted by the kidneys. Clients who used water therapy effectively during the first stage of labor had decreased use of anesthesia, analgesia, decreased duration of labor, and improved satisfaction (American Academy of Pediatrics [AAP] & American College of Obstetricians and Gynecologists [ACOG], 2014; ACOG, 2019; Davies et al., 2015; Mallen-Perez et al, 2018).

The major concern about immersion therapy has been newborn and postpartum infections. The 2018 Cochrane Database review *Immersion in Water during Labour and Birth* looked at 15 studies involving approximately 3600 women in both first- and second-stage labor. The review found that clients who utilized hydrotherapy were not at increased risk for infection, blood loss, operative vaginal or cesarean section delivery, or perineal trauma. They did note decreased use of regional anesthesia (Cluett et al., 2018). Facility policies should be written to outline specific guidelines based on most recent evidence for use of hydrotherapy.

Mental Stimulation

Mental techniques occupy the client's mind and compete with pain stimuli. They also aid relaxation by providing a tranquil imaginary atmosphere. These techniques use the CNS control method, also known as "power of the mind." A client will rely on information and education to help control what they are thinking while they are experiencing labor discomfort. Hypnobirthing classes or practicing guided meditations help them cope with labor. Clients may repeat a mantra, or series of words, to help them stay focused and in control.

Imagery. If the client has not practiced a specific imagery technique, the nurse can help them create a relaxing mental scene. Most clients find images of warmth, softness, security, and total relaxation comforting. Imagery can help the client dissociate from the painful aspects of labor (Burke, 2021).

> ### KNOWLEDGE CHECK
>
> 7. How does the gate-control theory of pain relate to non-pharmacologic methods of pain control?
> 8. What are some nursing actions to encourage relaxation during labor?
> 9. How can the nurse reduce a laboring client's anxiety or fear?
> 10. How might each of these cutaneous stimulation techniques be used to aid relaxation during labor: Massage? Counterpressure? Warmth or cold?

Breathing Techniques

Often clients will forget to breathe when they are experiencing pain. Holding your breath typically happens in tandem with pain, muscle tension, and fear. Breathing techniques give a client a different focus during contractions, interfering with pain sensory transmission and activating the parasympathetic nervous system. The parasympathetic nervous system releases antistress hormones, such as acetylcholine, prolactin, oxytocin, and vasopressin, helping a client to stay calm and relaxed. When a client is intentional about breathing, relaxation will more than likely follow.

First-Stage Breathing. Breathing in the first stage of labor consists of a deep cleansing breath in through the nose and out through the mouth.

Taking a Cleansing Breath. Each contraction begins and ends with a deep inspiration and expiration known as the *cleansing breath.* Like a sigh, a cleansing breath helps the client release tension. It provides oxygen to help reduce myometrial hypoxia, one cause of labor pain. The cleansing breath also helps clients clear their mind to focus on relaxing and signals their labor partner the contraction is beginning or ending. "Sigh" breathing is not learned and comes naturally as a way to release distress and let go of tension. When we teach deep breathing and model it as "sigh" breathing, clients will engage their muscle memory of using this breath previously to relieve tension, fear, stress, or discomfort.

Slow-Paced Breathing. Slow, deep breathing increases relaxation. Clients should concentrate on relaxing their body rather than regulating the rate of their breathing. This type of breathing lowers their heart rate and blood pressure, and redirects blood flow away from the locomotive muscles and toward digestive and reproductive organs. It also works to increase the release of endorphins, activating the immune system and creating sleepiness or a "dream-like" state in clients. Slow-paced breathing is usually about half of the client's normal respiratory rate (in-2-3-4; out-2-3-4). Slow-paced breathing should be used as long as possible during labor because it promotes relaxation and oxygenation.

As the intensity of the contractions increase, the client may need to increase the rate of breathing and breathe in and out through the mouth. As the contraction strength decreases, the rate of breathing should decrease and return to slow paced breathing—in through the nose and out through the mouth, ending with a cleansing breath.

Breathing to Prevent Pushing. If a client begins pushing before the cervix is completely dilated, it increases risk of cervical edema and injury to the cervix and fetal head. Blowing prevents the closure of the glottis and breath holding, creating pressure on the pelvic floor. When the urge to push is strong, encourage the client to take a deep breath in and blow out through loose, vibrating lips or to blow like they are blowing out a candle.

Overcoming Common Problems. Hyperventilation and mouth dryness are common when breathing techniques are used. Hyperventilation results from rapid deep breathing, which causes excessive loss of carbon dioxide and therefore respiratory alkalosis. The client may feel dizzy or lightheaded and may have impaired thinking. Vasoconstriction leads to tingling and numbness in the fingers and lips. If hyperventilation continues, tetany occurring from decreased levels of calcium in tissues and blood may result in stiffness of the face and lips and carpopedal spasm. If this happens, clients should be encouraged to slow down their breathing in order to normalize carbon dioxide levels.

Eye-to-eye contact and modeled deep breathing can help clients regain control over their breathing patterns. When the partner hugs or holds the client and takes slow, deep breaths, the client will often regulate their own breathing with that of the support person.

Second-Stage Breathing. Care in the second stage of labor encourages a physiologic completion of labor, assisting the client to respond to their urge to push rather than directing them to push as soon as the cervix is completely dilated. Lengthy pushing in second stage has been shown to result in greater fatigue, more operative births, and indeterminate or abnormal fetal heart rate (FHR) patterns and does not significantly shorten the second stage (Association of Women's Health, Obstetric and Neonatal Nurses [AWHONN], 2019).

Research has shown strenuous directed pushing increases risk for structural and neurogenic injury to a client's pelvic floor. Closed-glottis pushing (Valsalva pushing) causes recurrent increases in intrathoracic pressure with a resulting fall in cardiac output and blood pressure (AWHONN, 2019). The client's lower blood pressure then causes less blood to be delivered to the placenta, resulting in fetal hypoxia, which is reflected in indeterminate or abnormal fetal heart patterns.

Promoting a physiologic second stage uses nondirected, open-glottis pushing. The client makes the decision with the nurse about when it is time to start pushing. Pushing three to four times for 6 to 8 seconds is likely to be effective in aiding descent and is safe for the baby. Adjust the pushing process depending on the fetal status.

With lighter concentrations of local anesthetics, clients with epidural analgesia may still feel the urge to push, although not as strongly as the urge felt by clients who do not have an epidural. Using their natural urge to push, even if reduced, helps them push with contractions most effectively. Delaying pushing for up to 1 to 2 hours after complete dilation has shown benefits similar to those in clients who do not have epidural analgesia (AWHONN, 2019).

Activating the vagus nerve, the largest nerve in the parasympathetic nervous system during labor, especially during pushing, can be beneficial to help the client stay focused. When a client is completely dilated and feels the need to push, low, deep sounds that vibrate the vocal cords and open the throat in the client's neck will send a message through the vagus nerve relaxing and releasing the pelvic floor and neck of the uterus (cervix). High-pitched sounds work to do the opposite and cause a clinching or tension within the pelvic floor making pushing efforts and station change more difficult.

> ### ❓ KNOWLEDGE CHECK
>
> 11. Why is it important to avoid hyperventilation in labor?
> 12. What is the purpose of a cleansing breath?
> 13. Is there a valid reason why a client should push as soon as the cervix is completely dilated? Why, or why not?

PHARMACOLOGIC PAIN MANAGEMENT

As mentioned previously, each client's labor is unique, and each client experiences labor differently. The way a contraction feels varies for each client and might even feel different from one pregnancy to the next. Along with nonpharmacologic methods for managing pain, some clients choose pharmacologic pain relief during their labor. Before medicating the client with oral or IV pain medications, they should be informed of the different pain management options available to them at the different stages of labor.

Pharmacologic methods for pain management include systemic medications, **regional** pain management techniques (blockage of pain in localized area without loss of consciousness; includes **neuraxial** anesthesia—epidural and spinal blocks), and **general** anesthesia (the loss of consciousness and protective reflexes). When offering a certain method, one should assess the risk versus benefit to both client and fetus.

Special Considerations for Medicating a Pregnant Client

When medicating a pregnant client, consider the following:

- Any medication taken by the client may affect the fetus. Special consideration should be made for the gestation of the fetus and the expected delivery time.
- Physiologic changes that take place in the client during pregnancy. This includes anatomic as well as hormonal changes. Obesity and advanced client age can effect the physiologic changes of pregnancy and should also be considered.
- Certain medications may affect the course and length of labor.
- Pregnancy complications may limit the choice of pharmacologic pain management methods.
- Clients who require other therapeutic drugs, use herbal or botanical preparations, or practice substance abuse may have fewer safe choices for labor pain relief.

Effects on the Fetus

Before administering medications to a pregnant client, it is important to be prepared for the effects the medicine may have on the fetus. Such effects to the fetus may be direct, resulting from passage of the medication or its metabolites across the placenta to the fetus. An example of a direct effect on the fetus is decreased FHR variability after administration of an analgesic to the client.

Effects on the fetus may also be indirect, or secondary to medication effects in the client. For example, if a medication causes hypotension in the pregnant client, blood flow to the placenta is reduced. Fetal hypoxia and acidosis may result.

Physiologic Changes

There are six body changes in the pregnant client that have the greatest implications for pharmacologic pain management methods. The effect of obesity and advanced client age should also be considered.

Cardiovascular Changes. Compression of the aorta and inferior vena cava by the uterus can occur when a client lies in the supine position (aortocaval compression). If the client must be in the supine position temporarily, the uterus should be displaced to one side with either a pillow or a towel roll under one hip.

During cesarean delivery, operating room tables are often tilted slightly to one side for a cesarean birth to provide the uterine displacement. Proper uterine displacement requires a hard wedge. It is important to position the client to ensure aortocaval compression does not occur.

Respiratory Changes. A pregnant client's full uterus reduces the functional residual respiratory capacity of the lungs. To compensate, the client breathes more rapidly and therefore is more vulnerable to reduced arterial oxygenation. This condition makes the client even more sensitive to the inhalational anesthetic agents given for general anesthesia. Edema caused by pregnancy may also present in the upper airway, causing difficulty if the client must be intubated (ACOG, 2020).

Gastrointestinal Changes. A pregnant client's stomach is displaced upward by the large uterus. During pregnancy, the normal release of progesterone slows peristalsis and reduces the tone of the sphincter at the junction of the stomach and esophagus. These changes make a pregnant client vulnerable to regurgitation and aspiration (inhalation) of gastric contents during general anesthesia. Previous practice restricted clients from having any oral intake during labor. More recent data suggests modest amounts of clear liquids are allowed in uncomplicated laboring clients (American Society of Anesthesiologists [ASA], 2016; AWHONN, 2020a; Cunningham et al., 2022). If a cesarean birth is planned, a light meal may be consumed up to 6 hours before surgery (Wilson et al., 2018).

Nervous System Changes. During pregnancy and labor, circulating levels of **endorphins** and **enkephalins**, natural substances with analgesic properties, are high. These substances modify pain perception and should reduce requirements for analgesia and anesthesia.

The epidural and **subarachnoid spaces** between the arachnoid mater and pia mater are smaller during pregnancy, enhancing the spread of anesthetic agents used for epidural blocks or subarachnoid blocks (SABs).

Cerebrospinal fluid (CSF) pressure is higher during contractions and when the client is pushing. Nerve fibers are more sensitive to local anesthetic agents during pregnancy. High intraabdominal pressure causes engorgement of the epidural veins, increasing the risk for intravascular injection of anesthetic agents. Due to these changes, a reduced amount of analgesics and local anesthetics is needed to achieve satisfactory pain management with either an epidural block or SAB (Wong, 2020).

Obesity. Obesity affects all body systems mentioned above. Special considerations should be made for the obese client. Obesity is often defined as a body mass index (BMI) above 30. These clients are at increased risk for obstetric, anesthetic, neonatal, surgical, and postoperative complications.

Cardiovascular changes may become even more pronounced, and an increased incidence of hypertension may occur (Dalton & Strehlow, 2019). Special consideration should be made on how to properly apply blood pressure cuffs so accurate pressures are being taken. The care team should be vigilant about preventing aortocaval compression.

The increased weight poses a challenge for pain management for several reasons. Proper dosing of narcotics may be more difficult to determine. Breathing may be more difficult due to the decrease in chest wall and lung compliance. Obese clients are at an increased risk of developing sleep apnea. Combined with the decrease in lung functional residual capacity, these clients will experience oxygen desaturation quickly if they develop respiratory depression from narcotics and sedatives. It is important to monitor these clients closely whenever any sedative or opioid narcotic is administered. Pulse oximetry should be continuously monitored for any client with sleep apnea.

Obese pregnant clients are at increased risk of pulmonary aspiration. Research findings indicate obese laboring clients have increased gastric volumes, a higher incidence of gastroesophageal reflux (GERD), and hiatal hernias. These findings make management of the airway more challenging for anesthesia providers if an emergency cesarean section is needed and an epidural is not in place (Habib & D'Angelo, 2020).

Advanced Age of the Pregnant Client. Another challenge in pain management during childbirth is advanced age of the pregnant client. With increasing age additional risk factors are noted. For each 5-year increase in client age beyond 34 there is a linear upward trend in the potential complications. According to the researchers, the increased risks associated between age and mortality persisted after data was controlled for parity, prenatal care, and education. The increased risks were often related to cardiac compromises, vascular issues, coagulopathies, and other medical conditions (Mhyre, 2020).

Effects on the Course of Labor

Ideally, analgesics are given when labor is well established. However, regardless of the cervical dilation, caregivers should consider the adverse effects of excessive pain on labor progress. It was once believed regional blocks could slow progress during the second stage by reducing a client's spontaneous urge to push. Epidurals may actually help labor progress in the second stage by relaxing the client's muscles. Studies suggest the early onset of severe pain and the need for more analgesia are a better predictor of abnormal labor and delivery by cesarean section (ACOG, 2020; Wong, 2020).

Effects of Complications

Complications during pregnancy may limit the choices of analgesia or anesthesia. In order to receive a regional anesthetic, the pregnant client should be healthy enough to handle potential hemodynamic instability and have normal blood clotting function. Local anesthetics may cause antisympathetic effects, which lead to vasodilation once the medication starts to take effect. In order to offset the hypotension that is often experienced, a large volume of intravenous fluid is infused prior to or with initiation of epidural placement. With certain medical conditions, such as preeclampsia or cardiac disease, large fluid boluses are contraindicated and may cause pulmonary edema (Cunningham et al., 2022).

Although coagulation laboratories and platelet counts are not always ordered before neuraxial anesthesia, it is important to remember thrombocytopenia does develop in 5% to 10% of the pregnant population. If the coagulation values are low, the client may develop a hematoma at the site of the introducer needle, thus leading to possible paralysis if not identified timely (Wong, 2020).

Interactions with Other Substances

Clients on certain medications, illicit drugs, or herbal supplements may have fewer pain management options because of interactions between these substances and analgesics or anesthetics.

Recent alcohol, marijuana, or narcotic use increases the depressant effects of some analgesics and sedatives, making both the client and the newborn susceptible to respiratory depression. Clients taking pain medications may require a higher dose of opioid analgesics, and this can make postoperative pain management challenging (Wong, 2020).

Illicit drugs, such as cocaine, may cause cardiac collapse once the local anesthetics take effect. Another challenge is clients taking anticoagulant drug therapies. Clients may need to wait a certain amount of time before they are eligible for a regional anesthetic.

KNOWLEDGE CHECK

14. How can medications taken by the pregnant client affect the fetus?
15. How do changes in the following body systems affect pharmacologic pain management: Cardiovascular system? Respiratory system? Gastrointestinal system? Nervous system?
16. Why is it important to know about a client's intake of prescribed or over-the-counter medications, herbal medicines, legal substances (such as alcohol), and illegal drugs?

Systemic Medications for Labor

Systemic medications, such as opioids or inhaled analgesics, have effects on multiple systems because they are distributed throughout the body.

Nitrous Oxide

Nitrous oxide use is gaining popularity in the United States for laboring clients. This inhaled analgesic known as "laughing gas" helps increase the feeling of well-being, decreasing pain and anxiety, making labor easier to manage. It may be used independently for pain management or administered before the client gets a regional anesthetic. It is sometimes used in combination with the neuraxial anesthesia if the client complains of a "hot spot" (a specific region without pain relief) but does not wish additional epidural medication. Nitrous is an odorless and tasteless gas which does not enter the bloodstream and is excreted through the lungs when the mask is removed. For labor pain, the gas is delivered as a 50% nitrous oxide and 50% oxygen mix. The gases are connected to a breathing circuit that opens only during inspiration. Nitrous oxide in labor is self-administered; this helps assure the client does not over medicate. For maximal effectiveness, the client should start to inhale 30 seconds before the start of a contraction (ACOG, 2020; Burke, 2021; Cunningham et al., 2022; Hellams et al., 2018; Wong, 2020).

When preparing to use nitrous for the client it is important to outline both the benefits and potential risks. Nausea, vomiting, and dizziness are the most common side effects. Explain to both the client and family that only the client may apply the mask over their face. In many institutions, labor and delivery nurses set up the nitrous machines. Special training should be given on how to properly set up the machine and to check if the nitrous cylinders are full and functioning. Before nitrous can be used, a scavenger system (a means of removing excess gas) should be available in the room in order to provide a safe environment for the client's support team.

Parenteral Analgesia

Opioid analgesics are the most common parenteral medications given to reduce perception of pain and can be used to promote therapeutic rest during an unusually long labor. Parenteral analgesics often used for labor include morphine, fentanyl (Sublimaze), butorphanol (Stadol), remifentanil, and nalbuphine (Nubain) (Table 13.2) (ACOG, 2020; AWHONN, 2020a; Cunningham et al., 2022; Hawkins & Bucklin, 2021).

Fentanyl, morphine and remifentanil are opioid **agonists**, acting directly on the pain receptors, while butorphanol and nalbuphine have mixed opioid agonist and **antagonist** effects (blocking another substance or brain receptor). A client who is dependent on opiates, such as narcotics and heroin, should avoid agonist–antagonist medications because they may cause withdrawal effects for the client and newborn. Agonist–antagonist drugs have a "ceiling effect" on the amount of analgesia they provide and may not be suitable for the increasing pain of labor. Remifentanil is administered through patient-controlled analgesia (PCA) in clients who are not candidates for neuraxial analgesia (ACOG, 2020; AWHONN, 2020a; Wong, 2020).

TABLE 13.2   Drugs Commonly Used for Intrapartum Pain Management

Drug/Dose	Comments
Opioid Analgesics	
Fentanyl (Sublimaze)	Onset is quick (5 minutes for IV administration), but duration of action is short.
50–100 mcg; may be repeated every hour; may be given by PCA	Less nausea, vomiting, and respiratory depression occurs than with meperidine.
Adjunct to epidural analgesia during labor (dose individualized)	Epidural use may cause pruritus.
Butorphanol (Stadol)	Has some narcotic antagonist effects; should not be given to the opiate-dependent client (may precipitate withdrawal) or after other narcotics such as meperidine (may reverse their analgesic effects); also a respiratory depressant. 1–3 mg IV may be given to relieve pruritus associated with epidural narcotics.
1–2 mg every 3–4 hour; range 0.5–2 mg IV; may be given by PCA	
Nalbuphine (Nubain)	Same as butorphanol.
10 mg every 3 hours IV	2.5–10 mg may be given to relieve pruritus associated with epidural narcotics.
Adjunctive Drugs	
Ondansetron (Zofran)	4–8 mg to relieve pruritus associated with epidural narcotics.
4 mg to prevent or treat nausea from opioid administration	
Metoclopramide (Reglan)	Before or during cesarean birth for aspiration prophylaxis.
10 mg IV	Antiemetic, with sedative properties. Enhances analgesics.
Promethazine (Pheneragan)	
6.25 mg IV up to 25 mg	
Diphenhydramine (Benadryl)	Given to relieve pruritus from epidural narcotics.
10–50 mg every 4–6 hour IV	
Narcotic Antagonists	
Naloxone (Narcan)	Action shorter than most narcotics it reverses; observe for recurrent respiratory depression and be prepared to give additional doses.
To reduce respiratory depression induced by opioids: 0.4–2 mg IV (adult)	
To reverse pruritus from epidural opioids: 40–80 mcg IV or IV infusion 0.25–2 mcg/kg/hour	
Vasopressor	
Phenylephrine 50–100 mcg or **ephedrine** 5–10 mg IV	Corrects hypotension related to epidural or subarachnoid block.

IM, Intramuscularly; *IV,* intravenously; *PCA,* patient-controlled analgesia; *PO,* orally.
Bujedo, B. M. (2016). An update on neuraxial opioid induced pruritus prevention. *J Anesth Crit Care Open Access 6*(2): 00226. https://doi.org/10.15406/jaccoa.2016.06.00226; Cunningham, F. G., Leveno, K. J., Bloom, S. L., Dashe, J. S., Hoffman, B. L., Casey, B. M., & Spong, C. Y. (2018). *Williams obstetrics* (25th ed.). McGraw-Hill Education; Hawkins, J. L., & Bucklin, B. A. (2021). Obstetric anesthesia. In S. Gabbe, J. Niebyl, J. Simpson, M. Landon, H. Galan, R. Jauniaux, D. Driscollet, et al. (Eds.), *Obstetrics: Normal and problem pregnancies* (8th ed., pp. 295–318). Elsevier; Wong, C. A. (2020). Epidural and spinal analgesia/anesthesia for labor and vaginal delivery. In D. Chestnut, C. Wong, L. Tsen, D. Warwick, Y. Beilin, J. Mhyre, & B. Bateman (Eds.), *Chestnut's obstetric anesthesia: Principles and practice* (6th ed.). Elsevier.

The primary side effect concern for opioids is respiratory depression. All opioids cross the placenta, which is likely to affect the newborn. Timing of administration is important to reduce neonatal respiratory depression. An infant who is born at the peak of the drug's action is more likely to have respiratory depression than if born earlier or later. In addition to respiratory depression risk, Remifentanil has been associated with breastfeeding problems (AWHONN, 2020a). Opioid agonist–antagonists such as butorphanol (Stadol) and nalbuphine (Nubain) are also used for OB analgesia. They produce a lower incidence of nausea, vomiting, dysphoria, and respiratory depression than other medications.

Due to the potential for respiratory depression in both client and newborn, opioid analgesics are given in small, frequent doses by IV route during labor to provide a rapid onset of analgesia. If the client is within 1 to 2 hours of delivering, additional parenteral analgesics may no longer be administered. Although opioids promote rest, they do not completely eliminate labor pain or pain experienced during delivery. Narcotics can affect the baby at birth and cause client drowsiness, nausea, and vomiting.

Opioid Antagonists. Naloxone (Narcan) is a pure opioid antagonist; it reverses opioid-induced respiratory depression. However, it does not reverse respiratory depression from other causes such as normeperidine, benzodiazepines, nonopioid drugs, anesthetics or pathologic conditions. Naloxone has a shorter duration of action (30 to 90 minutes) than most of the opioids it reverses, and respiratory depression may reoccur.

Naloxone can cause an opiate-dependent client or newborn to have withdrawal symptoms, such as seizures (Wong, 2020). Airway management (e.g., bag-and-mask ventilation) takes precedence over use of naloxone for the newborn experiencing respiratory depression (AAP & ACOG, 2017).

Adjunctive Medications. Adjunctive medications during the intrapartum period include those with tranquilizing effects, sedatives, and antiemetics. Examples include ondansetron (Zofran), promethazine (Phenergan), and metoclopramide (Reglan). These medications are given to reduce nausea and anxiety and to promote rest (see Table 13.2). It is important to know potential side effects of medications administered. Although they are frequently given, both promethazine and metoclopramide may cause both psychological effects and decreased cardiac output. Metoclopramide (Reglan) increases gastric motility, reducing nausea and vomiting. However, it may also cause hypotension, drowsiness, and the feeling of impending doom.

Sedatives. Sedatives such as benzodiazepines, most commonly diazepam (Valium), midazolam (Versed) or lorazepam (Ativan), are not routinely given because they have prolonged depressant effects on the neonate. However, a small dose of a short-acting benzodiazepine may be given to promote rest if a client is fatigued from false labor or a prolonged latent phase.

🏷 DRUG GUIDE

Butorphanol (Stadol)

Classification
Opioid analgesic.

Action
Opioid analgesic with some agonist–antagonist effects; exact mechanism of action unknown; produces respiratory depression that does not increase markedly with larger doses.

Indications
Systemic pain relief during labor.

Dosage and Route
Intravenous or Intramuscular
1 mg every 3 to 4 hours; range 0.5 to 2 mg; may be given undiluted.

Absorption
Onset of analgesia almost immediate with intravenous or intramuscular administration, peaks after approximately 30 minutes, and lasts 3 to 4 hours; faster onset and shorter duration of action than meperidine or morphine.

Excretion
Excreted in urine; crosses placental barrier; secreted in breast milk.

Contraindications and Precautions
Contraindicated in persons who are hypersensitive; not used in opiate-dependent persons because antagonist activity of the drug may cause withdrawal symptoms in the client or newborn; drug actions potentiated (enhanced) by barbiturates, phenothiazines, cimetidine, and other tranquilizers.

Adverse Reactions
Respiratory depression or apnea (client or newborn), anaphylaxis; dizziness, lightheadedness, sedation, lethargy, headache, euphoria, mental clouding, fainting, restlessness, excitement, tremors, delirium, insomnia; nausea, vomiting, constipation, increased biliary pressure, dry mouth, anorexia; flushing, altered heart rate and blood pressure, circulatory collapse; urinary retention; sensitivity to cold.

Nursing Considerations
Assess for allergies and opiate dependence. Observe vital signs and respiratory function in client (respiratory rate of at least 12 breaths per minute) and newborn (respiratory rate of at least 30 breaths per minute). May use naloxone for respiratory depression in the client. Have resuscitation equipment available. Report nausea or vomiting to the provider for a possible order for an antiemetic. Antiemetics or other CNS depressants may enhance the respiratory depressant effects of butorphanol.

❓ KNOWLEDGE CHECK

17. What is the primary adverse effect of opioid administration during labor? How can this effect be reduced?
18. What is the preferred order of resuscitation for the newborn who has respiratory depression? Does naloxone have any use in an adult?

Birth Analgesics
Local Infiltration Anesthesia
Infiltration of the perineum with a local anesthetic is done by the provider before an episiotomy or perineal repair if the client doesn't have an effective epidural (Fig. 13.5). Local infiltration does not alter pain from uterine contractions or distention of the vagina. The local agent provides anesthesia in the immediate area of the episiotomy or laceration. A short delay occurs between anesthetic injection and onset of numbness. The drug burns as it is injected, but the local infiltration rarely has adverse effects on either client or infant.

Regional Pain Management Techniques
Regional pain management includes pudendal blocks, epidurals, spinals (SABs), combined spinal–epidurals, and continuous spinals. These forms of analgesia are the safest form of analgesia for both the client and fetus. Regional anesthesia may be used for intrapartum analgesia, surgical anesthesia, or both. These methods provide pain relief without loss of consciousness in the client, therefore allowing the client to be fully present for the birth experience. The client may feel some pressure and discomfort; however, these sensations are greatly reduced. Disadvantages depend on the specific technique. The effects on the fetus depend primarily on how the client responds, rather than on direct drug effects.

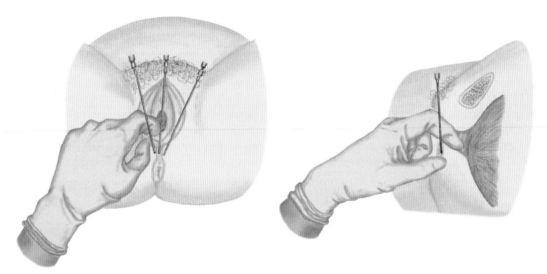

FIG. 13.5 Local infiltration anesthesia numbs the perineum just before birth for an episiotomy or after birth for suturing of a laceration. The obstetric provider protects the fetal head by placing a finger inside the vagina while injecting the perineum in a fan-like pattern or as needed.

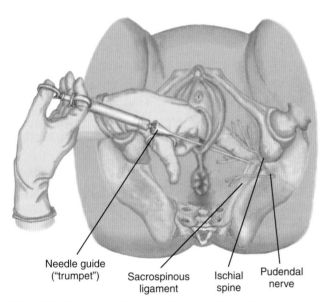

Needle guide
("trumpet")   Sacrospinous   Ischial   Pudendal
                 ligament   spine   nerve

FIG. 13.6 Pudendal block provides anesthesia for an episiotomy and use of low forceps. A needle guide ("trumpet") protects the client and fetal tissues from the long needle needed to reach the pudendal nerve. Only about 1.25 cm (½ inch) of the long needle protrudes from the guide.

Pudendal Block

A pudendal block anesthetizes the lower vagina and part of the perineum. It is often used to provide anesthesia for an episiotomy and vaginal birth, especially one that requires using low forceps. A pudendal block does not block pain from uterine contractions, and the client feels pressure. The pudendal block is a highly localized type of regional block, like a dental anesthetic provides numbness for dental procedures.

The provider injects the pudendal nerves near each ischial spine with a local anesthetic (Fig. 13.6). The perineum is infiltrated with local anesthetic because the pudendal block does not fully anesthetize this area. As in local infiltration, a brief delay occurs between injection and onset of numbness. Possible complications include a toxic reaction to the anesthetic, rectal puncture, hematoma, and sciatic nerve block. If toxicity is avoided, the fetus usually is not affected (ACOG, 2020).

Neuraxial Anesthesia

Epidural blocks, SABs or spinals, continuous spinals, and combined spinal–epidurals (CSE) are all placed and managed by an anesthesia provider, either an anesthesiologist or a certified registered nurse anesthetist (CRNA). Both AWHONN and the American Association of Nurse Anesthetists (AANA) support regional analgesia/anesthesia being monitored by the nonanesthetist nurse (AANA, 2017; AWHONN, 2020a).

Epidural Block

The lumbar epidural block is a popular regional block that provides analgesia and anesthesia for labor and birth without sedation of the client and fetus. It is used for both vaginal and cesarean section births. An epidural block is performed by injecting a local anesthetic agent, often combined with an opioid, into the small epidural space. The **epidural space** lays just outside the dura mater, between the dura and the spinal canal. It is loosely filled with fat, connective tissue, and epidural veins, which are dilated during pregnancy (Fig. 13.7). The level of the epidural block can be extended to provide anesthesia for a cesarean birth or a tubal ligation after birth.

Analgesia, rather than full loss of movement and sensation, is preferred for the labor epidural. Lower concentrations of the local anesthetic agent and an epidural opioid often provide adequate pain relief without complete **motor block** (loss of voluntary movement) for most clients. Higher concentrations of the local anesthetic agent result in greater loss of both motor and sensory functions (ACOG, 2020; Wong, 2020).

The exact time to begin an epidural block is individualized. If the client is in early labor and needs pain relief, nitrous or parenteral opioids may be given until their labor is more

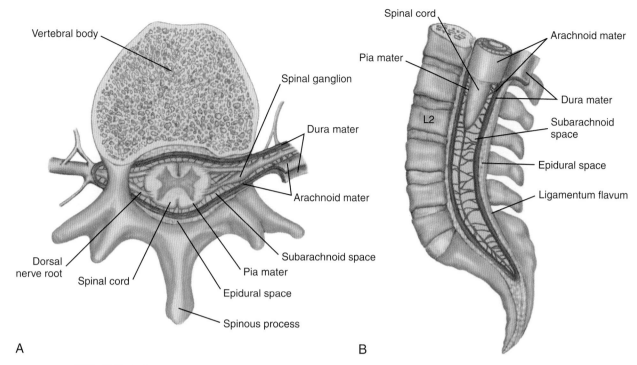

FIG. 13.7 (A) Cross-section of spinal cord, meninges, and protective vertebrae. The dura mater and arachnoid mater lie close together. The pia mater is the innermost of the meninges and covers the brain and spinal cord. The subarachnoid space is between the arachnoid mater and pia mater. (B) Sagittal section of spinal cord, meninges, and vertebrae. The epidural and subarachnoid spaces are illustrated. Note the spinal cord ends at the L2 vertebra.

active. Studies show there is no greater incidence of cesarean birth, forceps delivery, or fetal malposition if the client receives an epidural during the latent phase of labor. Lower concentrations of local anesthetics and the avoidance of aortocaval compression have been linked to fewer cesarean sections (Cunningham et al., 2022; Wong, 2020).

Technique. The client's back should be curved outward (like an angry cat) for epidural placement. This is achieved in a sitting or side-lying position, based on the preference of the anesthesia provider. In the sitting position, hugging a pillow or small birth ball helps the client hold the correct position. The client is told to notify the provider if a contraction occurs during the procedure and warned that a brief "electric shock" sensation may be felt as the epidural catheter is passed.

The epidural space is created at the L3–L4 interspace (below the end of the spinal cord), and a catheter is passed through the needle into the epidural space (Fig. 13.8). The catheter allows for continuous or intermittent injection of medication to maintain pain relief during labor and vaginal or cesarean birth. The infusion of epidural medication during labor may be regulated by a patient-controlled epidural analgesia (PCEA) pump (Hawkins & Bucklin, 2021; Tsen & Bateman, 2020; Wong, 2020).

Potential Epidural Complications.

Intravascular Injections. Epidural blocks may require a large volume of local anesthetic because the catheter lays outside the meninges. Before injecting any epidural medications, a small test dose of lidocaine with epinephrine should be injected by the anesthesia provider, to determine whether the epidural catheter has inadvertently punctured a blood vessel or the dura (Hawkins & Bucklin, 2021; Wong, 2020).

If the test dose reaches the bloodstream, an immediate elevation in the client's heart rate is noted. An increase of 20 beats per minute within 45 seconds indicates the epidural is intravascular (AANA, 2017). However, increased heart rates may also be in relation to experiencing an excessive amount of pain. Other signs of an intravascular injection include numbness of the tongue and lips, a metallic taste in the mouth, lightheadedness, dizziness, tinnitus, or a feeling of impending doom may occur with intravascular injection, although these symptoms usually only occur if a large volume of local anesthesia reaches the client's bloodstream.

If the test dose reaches the subarachnoid space instead of the epidural space, the client experiences rapid, intense motor and sensory block (loss of sensation). This blockade may cause the client to experience the sensation of not breathing. Thus it may become necessary to administer oxygen and monitor pulse oximeter readings. Reassurance may help the client become less anxious; however, it may become necessary to medicate the client to help relaxation.

Dural Puncture. Because the tough dura and the fragile web-like arachnoid membranes lie closely together, dural puncture also punctures the arachnoid. If the dura is unintentionally punctured with the needle used to introduce the epidural catheter, leakage of CSF will most likely occur, which may result in a postdural puncture (PDPH or "spinal") headache. Dural puncture and headache can occur without obvious CSF leakage.

These headaches differ from most headaches. The client typically reports the headache is worse when they sit up or

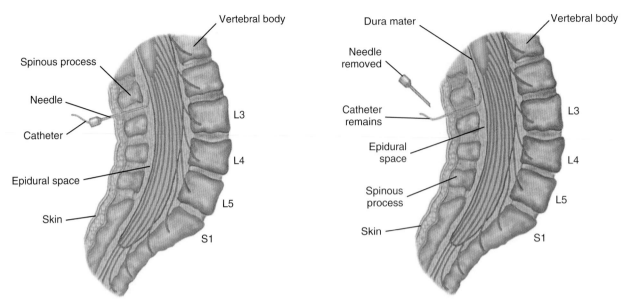

FIG. 13.8 Technique for Epidural Block. The epidural space is entered with a needle below where the spinal cord ends. A fine catheter is threaded through the needle. After the catheter is threaded into the epidural space, the needle is removed. Medication can then be injected into the epidural space intermittently or by continuous infusion for pain relief during labor and birth.

stand or if they are in a brightly lit room. The only reliable treatment for these headaches is the epidural blood patch. It was once thought an increase in either PO or IV fluids, caffeinated beverages or analgesics, and time should help correct the headaches. Research does not support such measures, and with the birth of a new baby, most clients prefer the more reliable and quicker treatment, the blood patch.

A blood patch is when autologous blood is obtained from the client under sterile conditions and then injected into the client's epidural space. The blood causes a tamponade effect and forms a gelatinous seal over the hole in the dura, therefore stopping spinal fluid leakage (Fig. 13.9). The client is then encouraged to lay flat for a period of 2 hours (Chestnut, 2020; Peralta & Macarthur, 2020).

Contraindications and Precautions for Regional Anesthesia. The regional block is not suitable for all laboring clients. Contraindications include increased intracranial pressure secondary to a mass lesion, client refusal or inability to cooperate during the regional placement, uncorrected coagulation conditions, uncorrected hypovolemia, an infection in the area of insertion, a severe systemic infection (sepsis), or a fetal condition that demands immediate birth.

Clients who have had spinal surgery, such as for an injury or correction of scoliosis (spinal curvature), are evaluated individually. The anesthesia provider may request previous scans of the client's spinal column if the client has a history of spine surgery for any reason (ACOG, 2020; Chestnut, 2020).

Adverse Effects of Regional Anesthesia

Hypotension. Sympathetic nerves are blocked along with pain nerves, which may result in vasodilation and

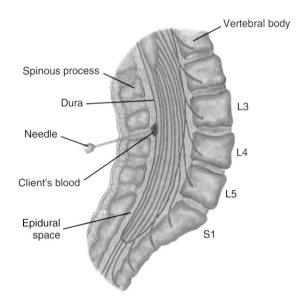

FIG. 13.9 Blood Patch for Relief of Spinal Headache. To seal a dural puncture, a small amount of the client's blood is injected into the epidural space. Other fluids such as normal saline or dextran may be injected using a similar technique.

hypotension. This is most likely to occur within the first 15 minutes of an epidural's initial infusion. However, a significant percentage of clients may have hypotension, which occurs within 1 hour of initiation or repeat bolus doses with the epidural (AWHONN, 2019; Chestnut, 2020; Hawkins & Bucklin, 2021). This hypotensive state has the potential to interrupt the fetal oxygenation pathway by reducing placental perfusion causing indeterminate or abnormal FHR tracings (see Chapter 14) (ACOG, 2020; AWHONN, 2020a).

Rapid infusion of an isotonic IV solution, such as lactated ringers or normal saline, 15 to 30 minutes before initiation of the neuraxial block or administered concurrently with block initiation fills the vascular system to offset vasodilation. Typically, pre- or co-load IV quantities are 500 to 1000 mL infused rapidly (ACOG, 2020; ASA, 2016; AWHONN, 2020a; Chestnut, 2020; Hawkins & Bucklin, 2021). If hypotension occurs and techniques such as fluid bolus, client repositioning with uterine displacement, and oxygen administration are ineffective, then IV phenylephrine in increments of 50 to 100 mcg or ephedrine in increments of 5 to 10 mg may be given to counteract the decrease in blood pressure (ASA, 2016; AWHONN, 2020a; Cunningham et al., 2022; Hawkins & Bucklin, 2021).

It is important to inform the anesthesia provider of the client's pertinent health history if asked to dose the client in addition to the PCEA. Some clients may have heart conditions requiring a slower dosing of local anesthetics to offset sensitivity to the antisympathetic effects of the local anesthetic.

Bladder Distention. A client's bladder fills quickly because of the large quantity of IV solution, but the sensation to void is reduced by regional anesthesia. Bladder distention may cause pain that remains after initiation of the block and may interfere with fetal descent in labor. It is important to monitor urine output after a regional block is placed. Bladder management should be individualized and includes voiding on a bedpan, in and out (I&O) catheters, or indwelling catheter placement (AWHONN, 2020a).

Prolonged Second Stage. Delayed pushing is often intentional for second-stage labor, and the urge to push may be less intense for the client who has an epidural block, particularly if the motor block is dense. The pelvic muscles may be relaxed, which can interfere with the mechanism of internal rotation. The frequency and intensity of uterine contractions may also decrease during second stage due to regional anesthesia. These factors may increase the chance for the need for either a vacuum extractor or a forceps-assisted delivery. Studies show the second stage of labor is only prolonged in clients with an anesthesia-induced dense motor block that do not have interventions, like use of a peanut ball, to assist with positioning and facilitating fetal rotation (AWHONN, 2020a; Cunningham et al., 2022).

Fever. For reasons not completely clear, 20% to 30% of clients with neuraxial anesthesia develop fever compared with 5% to 7% of clients without neuraxial anesthesia (AWHONN, 2020a; Wong, 2020). The fever associated with epidural analgesia is usually not caused by infection but may result from the reduced hyperventilation and decreased heat dissipation, for example, reduced sweating, which can occur when the client's pain is relieved.

Fever is a marker for infection. To avoid needless administration of antibiotics and sepsis evaluations in the newborn, other indicators for infection, for example, fetal tachycardia or amniotic fluid with a cloudy or yellow color and a foul or strong odor, should be assessed for as well. The nurse should remember fever in the pregnant client elevates fetal temperature, resulting in tachycardia and oxygen demand for both. Medical and nursing personnel should try to lower the client's temperature to a normal level and identify and treat any suspected infection. Possible signals to the hypothalamus may result in fever after epidural block include the following (Cunningham et al., 2022; Hawkins & Bucklin, 2021):

1. Decreased hyperventilation, sweating, and activity after onset of pain relief reduces heat production and signal the hypothalamus to raise the client's temperature.
2. Vasodilation redistributes heat from the core to the periphery of the body, where it is lost to the environment. The lower core temperature then signals the hypothalamus to increase heat production.
3. Shivering often occurs with sympathetic blockade accompanied by a dissociation between warm and cold sensations. In effect, the body believes the temperature is lower than the true temperature and raises the "thermostat" to produce heat by shivering, thus increasing the core temperature.

Shivering. Shivering is common in labor and sometimes is associated with neuraxial anesthesia. Warmed fluids and distraction are helpful interventions to decrease shivering (AWHONN, 2020b). If the shivering becomes excessive and uncomfortable, and the delivery is not eminent, the client may be given IV meperidine (Demerol) in small doses to the desired effect. Demerol doses of 10 mg to a total of 25 mg may be safely given if delivery is not projected for 2 to 3 hours.

Catheter Migration. Due to epidural venous engorgement, the epidural catheter may move out of the original space after placement. The client may have symptoms of intravascular injection, intense block or one that is too high, increase in pain sensation, a unilateral block, or absence of anesthesia in a particular region ("a hot spot"). The anesthesia provider should be notified if the client presents with any of these symptoms. Interventions may include a bolus dose, client repositioning, or readjusting the epidural catheter. If these interventions fail, the epidural catheter may need to be replaced.

Neuraxial Opioid Analgesics

Epidural injection of an opioid analgesic provides another option for pain management. The drugs bind to opiate receptors, allowing much smaller doses than would be adequate if given systemically. Clients can feel tightening from their contractions but not pain.

A single dose of a long-acting epidural analgesic, such as morphine (Duramorph), is often given after cesarean birth before removal of the epidural catheter. The client may be comfortable for up to 24 hours or may only require small doses of oral medications. The client's respiratory status should be monitored for 24 hours based on the duration of the action for the specific drug. All drugs injected into the epidural or subarachnoid spaces should be preservative-free (Wong, 2020).

Advantages of neuraxial analgesics include the following:

- Rapid onset of pain relief
- Less potential risk of the fetus being affected by the narcotics because of the slow absorption of these medications by the meninges
- Decreased dose of local anesthetics, decreasing risk of local anesthetic toxicity or a very dense block
- A sedating effect may help the client to relax and allow labor to progress

Adverse Effects of Neuraxial Opioids. Adverse effects associated with neuraxial opioids may include nausea, vomiting, pruritus, and delayed respiratory depression in the pregnant or postpartum client.

Nausea and Vomiting. Nausea and vomiting occur during labor. Hormonal changes slow the gastrointestinal (GI) system. However, sometimes it is related to either IV or epidural opioid administration. Opiates cause vasodilatory effects, which can result in hypotension. Medications such as ephedrine or phenylephrine may be needed to increase the client's blood pressure. Adjunctive medications used for treatment of nausea and vomiting include ondansetron (Zofran) and metoclopramide (Reglan).

Pruritus. Itching of the face and neck may occur with epidural opioids. Although clients may not specifically complain of itching, they may rub or scratch their face and neck. Diphenhydramine (Benadryl), naloxone (Narcan), or nalbuphine (Nubain) may relieve pruritus (see Table 13.2) (Wong, 2020).

Delayed Respiratory Depression. The possibility of late respiratory depression in the client exists for up to 18 hours after the administration of an intrathecal opioid, depending on the duration of action of the medication used (Wong, 2020). Usually, the longer-acting narcotics are only given to clients who have had cesarean deliveries or who have required additional epidural dosing for a postdelivery vaginal repair.

Nursing Care. Nurses with proper education who have demonstrated current competence should be able to participate in labor pain management with neuraxial anesthesia (ACOG, 2020; AWHONN, 2020b; ASA, 2016). The nurse should record baseline vital signs and FHR patterns for comparison with prenatal levels and those after the block. IV access is ensured, and the prescribed pre- or co-load of fluid is given. The nurse helps to support the client in the correct position and notifies the anesthesia provider when the client is having a contraction. The client may feel a brief "electric shock" sensation as the catheter is passed into the epidural space. The nurse should assist the client in remaining still while the block is completed. After the medication is injected, the nurse observes for signs of subarachnoid puncture or intravascular injection.

Evidence-based practice guidelines from AWHONN (2019) and ACOG (2020) suggest assessing the client's blood pressure (BP) and FHR every 5 minutes during the first 15 minutes after initiation of the epidural or any additional bolus doses of epidural medication. Repeat assessment of BP and FHR at 30 minutes and 1 hour after the procedure. Individual facilities may use these recommendations or develop their own guidelines. The anesthesia provider may request more frequent monitoring of vital signs if the client is bleeding, has indeterminate or abnormal (category II or III) FHR pattern, has gestational hypertension, or seems to be extra sensitive to the effects of the local anesthetic.

The client's bladder should be assessed frequently because of the large IV fluid load and the reduced sensation to void. Clients given low-concentration bupivacaine and opiate should still be able to sense the need to void (Wong, 2020). The nurse should observe for signs associated with catheter migration from the epidural space and for adverse effects from epidural opioids, such as nausea, vomiting, and pruritus.

Intrathecal Opioid Analgesics

Intrathecal (Subarachnoid) injection of an opioid analgesic provides another option for pain management without sedation. The medications bind to opiate receptors, allowing much smaller doses than would be adequate if given systemically or through the epidural.

Advantages of intrathecal analgesics include the following:
- Rapid onset of pain relief without sedation
- No increase in motor block, enabling the client to ambulate soon after
- No sympathetic block, with its hypotensive effects
- Less potential risk of the fetus being affected by the narcotics

Disadvantages may include the following:
- Limited duration of action, possibly requiring another medication for continued pain relief
- Inadequate pain relief for late labor and birth, requiring additional measures to manage pain at these times

Adverse Effects of Intrathecal Opioids. As with IV and epidural opioids, nausea, vomiting, and pruritus may occur. Delayed respiratory depression may occur, depending on the duration of action of the medication used.

Nursing Care. Vital signs and FHR are taken at the usual intervals for the client's stage of labor. Side effects, such as nausea, vomiting, or pruritus, are reported and managed similarly to those occurring with the intravenous doses. Reduced effectiveness suggests the medication's duration of action is ending or the client is in late labor. Other pain management interventions may be needed for the remainder of labor and birth (George et al., 2020).

Subarachnoid (Spinal) Block

The SAB, or spinal, is a much quicker procedure than the epidural block and may be performed when a quick cesarean birth is necessary and an epidural catheter is not in place. The anesthesia provider injects local anesthetic with or without opioids into the subarachnoid space in a single dose. The client loses both sensory and motor function below the level of the SAB, with relief of pain from contractions. Loss of motor function is dependent on the concentration of the local anesthetic used.

Technique. The L3–L4 interspace is located, and a spinal needle (25 to 27 gauge in diameter) is inserted. Appearance of CSF fluid at the needle hub ensures correct placement,

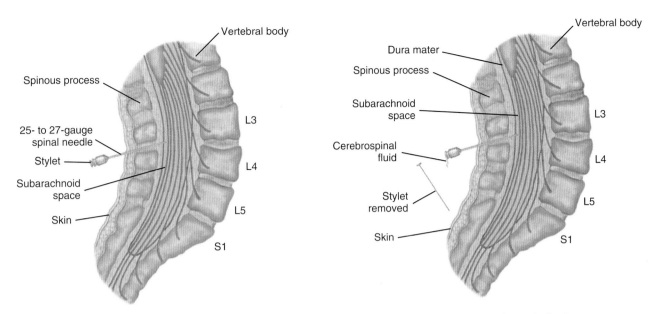

FIG. 13.10 Technique for Subarachnoid Block. A 25- to 27-gauge spinal needle with a stylet occluding its lumen is passed into the subarachnoid space below where the spinal cord ends. The stylet is removed, and one or more drops of clear cerebrospinal fluid at the needle hub confirm correct needle placement. Medication is then injected, and the needle is removed.

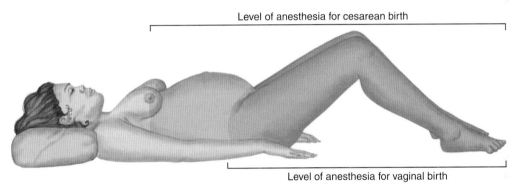

FIG. 13.11 Levels of Anesthesia for Epidural and Subarachnoid Blocks. A level of T10 through S5 is adequate for vaginal birth. A higher level of T4 to T6 is needed for cesarean birth.

and a preservative-free opioid and local anesthetic is injected (Fig. 13.10). No test dose is given because the placement of the needle is confirmed by the flow of the CSF. The level of anesthesia is determined by the volume, concentration, and density of the medication (Fig. 13.11).

Contraindications and Precautions. Contraindications and precautions are similar to those for the epidural block: increased intracranial pressure secondary to a mass lesion, client refusal or inability to cooperate during the regional placement, uncorrected coagulation conditions, uncorrected hypovolemia, an infection in the area of needle insertion, a severe systemic infection (sepsis), or a fetal condition that demands immediate birth.

Nursing considerations are similar to the ones for the epidural placement, except sympathetic blockade occurs more rapidly. Anesthesia providers may try to offset the possible

hypotension by administering vasopressors such as ephedrine or phenylephrine prior to injecting the spinal medication. Adequate IV hydration prior to initiation of the SAB is important.

Vital signs should be assessed every 5 minutes for 30 minutes or per facilities guidelines. During a cesarean birth, the client's vital signs are assessed every 5 minutes until the end of the surgery.

Although spinal needles are much smaller than those used for epidural placement, postdural spinal headaches may still occur. They are treated as they would be for a PDPH caused by an epidural catheter (Wong, 2020).

Combined Spinal–Epidural Blocks

A combined spinal–epidural (CSE) allows for rapid pain relief and the ability to provide ongoing pain relief with additional anesthetics, which can be injected through the epidural catheter. Benefits of CSE include a quick onset of medication administered and access to the epidural catheter to provide additional anesthesia if the need arises for either further pain relief or cesarean delivery.

Technique. The same technique is used to place a CSE and an epidural. Once the epidural space is found, a spinal needle is inserted. CSF fluid observed at the needle hub indicates correct placement, and preservative-free opioid and local anesthetic is injected. After removal of the spinal needle, the epidural catheter is then threaded into the epidural space. A test dose is not administered until the catheter is ready to be used for additional medications.

Care of and side effects experienced by the client undergoing a CSE block are the same as caring for clients receiving an epidural block. Potential complications are similar to the ones for the epidural placement. Refer to the facilities guidelines for guidance on monitoring clients receiving neuraxial analgesia.

Reduced effectiveness suggests the medication's duration of action is ending or the client is in late labor. Other pain management methods may be needed for the remainder of labor. Additional medications may be given via the epidural catheter. A test dose should be given prior to infusion of any medications through the epidural catheter. The test dose is to assess whether the catheter is still in the epidural space and has not migrated into either a blood vessel or into the subarachnoid space.

Continuous Spinals

Today more anesthesia providers are opting for continuous spinals because they are assured the client will continue to remain comfortable. Unlike continuous epidurals, the catheter tip is less likely to migrate from the subarachnoid area. With epidurals, catheter migration may occur, and "hot spots" are more common. The continuous spinal catheter is placed similar to the CSE. Risks are similar to the risks for spinals.

General Anesthesia

General anesthesia is a systemic pain control method involving both loss of consciousness and loss of protective reflexes. It is the method of anesthesia sometimes used for cesarean births. Some clients either refuse or are not good candidates for either the epidural block or SAB for cesarean birth, and, occasionally, a planned epidural block or SAB proves to be inadequate for surgical anesthesia. General anesthesia may be needed unexpectedly and quickly for emergency procedures at any stage of pregnancy, such as to repair injury resulting from an accident or domestic violence or to perform an appendectomy or in times of fetal distress.

Technique

Before induction of general anesthesia, anesthesia providers ensure monitors are applied to the client and administer 100% oxygen for 3 to 5 minutes, or at least four deep breaths. This increases oxygen stores for both the client and the fetus for the short period of apnea that occurs during rapid anesthesia induction. The client has a wedge under one side or the operating table is tilted to reduce aortocaval compression and increase placental blood flow (ASA, 2016).

Adverse Effects

Major adverse effects are possible with the use of general anesthesia.

Failed intubation. Pregnancy increases circulating blood volume, which often leads to blood vessel engorgement throughout the client's circulatory system. This increase in blood volume may lead to edema throughout the body, including the airway. The edema in the airway may make intubation more challenging. The failed intubation rate in pregnancy is 10 times higher than in the nonpregnant population (Hawkins, 2019). If failed intubation occurs, the anesthesia team must find another means of managing the airway prior to the start of surgery (AANA, 2017; ASA, 2016). Staff members in the operating room should be prepared for the need for possible additional staff or equipment.

Aspiration of Gastric Contents. Regurgitation with aspiration of acidic gastric contents is a potentially fatal complication of general anesthesia. Aspiration of food particles may result in chemical injury to the airways resulting in **aspiration pneumonitis**. Infection often occurs after the initial lung injury.

Adverse Reaction to Anesthetic Medications. There are several different medications administered in order to perform a general anesthetic. Many obstetric clients are young and healthy and do not have significant medical histories, such as surgical interventions.

Anaphylaxis. Muscle relaxants are known to be the root cause of many anaphylactic reactions under general anesthesia. This predominantly young, healthy population may not know whether they are allergic to certain anesthetic agents. An anaphylactic reaction, although rare, may occur, and everyone in the operating room should be prepared.

Malignant Hyperthermia. Malignant hyperthermia (MH) is very rare but produces a severe reaction to inhalational gases and succinylcholine, a muscle relaxant used for general anesthesia. When clients have a familial history of MH, the anesthesia provider will choose different induction agents. Nursing personnel need to be prepared for MH crisis, knowing the location of MH treatment carts and how to administer the primary treatment drug, dantrolene (Douglas, 2020).

Respiratory Depression. Fetal respiratory depression may occur due to the anesthetic agents used. This is more likely to occur if the interval between induction of anesthesia and cord clamping is long. Given this risk, induction of general anesthesia will not begin until the surgeon and the neonatal resuscitation team are present.

Magnesium Sulfate. If the client has been on or needs to continue magnesium sulfate, a prolonged duration of the muscle relaxant may be seen. Although not strictly an anesthesia-related concern, magnesium sulfate promotes uterine relaxation. A client on a magnesium sulfate is at risk of increased bleeding postdelivery.

Uterine Relaxation. Inhalational anesthetics (gases) cause uterine relaxation. This characteristic is desirable for treating some complications, for example, replacing an inverted uterus. However, severe postpartum hemorrhage may occur if the uterus relaxation after birth is not quickly treated (Setty & Fernando, 2020).

Methods to Minimize Adverse Effects

General anesthesia may be needed unexpectedly and quickly for emergency procedures at any stage of pregnancy. Measures to reduce the risk for adverse reactions should be taken.

- Obtain accurate medical history including a review of family history for anesthesia complications.
- Restrict intake to clear fluids. If the client is scheduled for a cesarean birth, nothing by mouth (NPO) should be maintained. The ASA (2016) recommends no solid foods be consumed 6 hours prior to the start of anesthesia and clear liquids not be consumed for at least 2 hours, thereby decreasing the risk for aspiration.
- Administer medications to raise the gastric pH and make secretions less acidic—for example, sodium citrate (Bicitra), ranitidine (Zantac), or famotidine (Pepcid).
- Administer medications to increase gastric emptying—for example, metoclopramide (Reglan).
- Make certain the anesthesia provider has a resource to administer cricoid pressure (Sellick's maneuver) to block the esophagus by pressing the rigid trachea against it (Fig. 13.12).

Neonatal respiratory depression may be minimized by doing the following:

- Reducing the time from induction of anesthesia to clamping of the umbilical cord.
- Minimize administration of sedating medications and anesthetics until the cord is clamped.

To reduce the time from induction of anesthesia to cord clamping, the client is prepared and draped, and the surgeons are ready before anesthesia is induced. Anesthesia is kept light until the infant is born. The anesthesia level is deepened as soon as the cord is clamped.

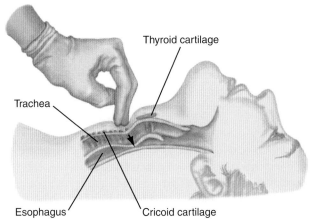

FIG. 13.12 Cricoid pressure, or Sellick's maneuver, is used to prevent vomitus from entering the trachea during intubation for general anesthesia. An assistant applies pressure to the cricoid cartilage to obstruct the esophagus. Once the client is successfully intubated with a cuffed endotracheal tube, gastric secretions cannot enter the trachea.

expected and has a purpose in labor. The nurse's role is to teach about various pain management methods, support the client's choices, evaluate the effectiveness, and monitor for complications. Clients vary in their responses to labor pain and choices for pain management. Providing pain management options and supporting the client's choices allows an increased sense of control over the birth experience. The client who successfully manages pain and other physical demands of labor is more likely to view the experience as positive. Most clients will use a combination of nonpharmacologic, pharmacologic, and regional block methods of pain management over the course of labor and birth. Nursing care related to pain management should be combined with support for normal labor and any complications that arise.

Assessment

Pain assessment begins at admission and continues throughout labor and postpartum.

When assessing pain, clarify the words a client uses. When asked if they have "pain," the client may deny it. Yet changing the word used to "discomfort," "cramping," "aching," "pressure," or other words may elicit a different response. Pain is an individual experience, and so is the expression of pain. Ask the client about the need for additional assistance with pain management. A stoic client may give little evidence of pain yet may want pain assistance.

Asking a client to rate the pain on a scale of 0 to 10 helps clarify the intensity of the pain. A zero represents no pain, whereas 10 is the worst possible pain. Ask the client to rate pain on this scale before and after pain-relief measures to evaluate their effectiveness. Multilingual and picture scales are available for those who do not speak the dominant language.

❓ KNOWLEDGE CHECK

19. What are two major advantages of using regional pain management techniques during childbirth?
20. What is the major adverse effect of the epidural block or SAB? How can the fetus be affected? How may this effect be reduced?
21. What are common side effects of epidural or intrathecal opioid analgesics, and how are these managed?
22. What are the major adverse effects of general anesthesia? How can the fetus be affected? What measures reduce the risks?

APPLICATION OF THE NURSING PROCESS: PAIN MANAGEMENT

Working with people in pain is difficult, and most nurses feel compelled to relieve pain promptly, yet pain is

A surprising number of clients have difficulty using a pain scale because they have little experience with pain. They may underrate current pain, expecting an increase in the amount of pain (and therefore pain number) later in labor, or they may say they have no idea what the "worst pain imaginable" is and therefore cannot guess how a pain rating of 10 feels. However, a scale or description by the client does provide one measure of how pain feels before and after relief measures.

Body language gives a clue to comfort level. Moaning, crying, thrashing, and loss of effectiveness of previously effective nonpharmacologic techniques are indications of inadequate pain management and the need for additional interventions, including different nonpharmacologic techniques as well as pharmacologic pain management methods. More subtle clues such as remaining tense between contractions also suggest difficulty coping with pain.

Evaluate the client's labor status to help them choose the most appropriate method of pain management. When discussing pharmacologic methods, be aware that options are not restricted based only on time or cervical dilatation. Multiple factors including the estimated time of birth, amount of time needed to establish a specific method, and the pharmacology of the drug or drugs are considered.

Avoid making assumptions about a client's pain based on their rate of labor progress, cervical dilation, or apparent intensity of contractions. Do not assume a client whose cervix is 2 cm dilated has little pain and a client whose cervix is dilated 8 cm has intense pain. An obese client's contractions may be strong, but they may seem mild if they are assessed by palpation or an external monitor because of a thick abdominal fat pad. *Labor progress or contraction intensity cannot be equated with a client's pain perception or tolerance.*

Observe for and report pain that is not typical of normal labor. Although labor pain is often intense, it should come and go with each contraction. The uterus should not be tender or board-like between contractions and should not cause constant intense pain.

Because multiple pain management techniques may be used throughout the course of labor, the nursing assessment should be comprehensive. Even if the client does not plan to use pharmacologic techniques, plans frequently change as labor progresses, and an unplanned cesarean birth is always a possibility. A database that includes pertinent information provides the best foundation for assisting the client throughout labor and birth. This information should be included in any handoff report.

The nurse collects and analyzes critical assessments related to:

- Evidence of pain—verbal statement, requests for pain-relief measures, crying, moaning, and nonverbal evidence such as tense, guarded posture or facial expression
- Pain scale
- Birth plan with preferences for pain management
- Identification of support person(s)
- Preparation for childbirth
- If applicable, pain management used in previous births and client's satisfaction with the method(s)
- Pain management methods that have been used before arrival at birth facility and the effectiveness of the methods
- FHR and uterine activity patterns; cervical examination results
- Vital signs
- Previous surgeries, type of anesthesia, and any anesthesia-associated problems
- Allergies, focusing especially on allergy to opioid analgesics, dental anesthetics, and iodine (used in some skin preparation solutions)
- Skin assessment of lower back (potential site for epidural or spinal)
- Oral intake—time and type of last intake

Identification of Client Problems

Analysis of the data collected enables the nurse to identify actual and potential client problems and to develop an individualized plan of care. Pain is expected in normal childbirth, and elimination of pain is not always possible or desirable. Most laboring clients have nursing needs relating to effective management of pain. Actual and potential problems related to pain management may be general, related to ineffective coping with pain, or due to effects of specific strategies such as an epidural. "Pain due to ineffective use of pain management techniques" may be an appropriate problem for pain management in general. "Fetal hypoxemia related to decreased placental perfusion secondary to epidural" and "client injury resulting from reduced sensation and movement secondary to epidural" may be additional problems for a client with an epidural.

Coping/Pain Management
Planning: Expected Outcomes

Because pain is a subjective experience and expected in labor, realistic outcomes include:

1. During labor, the client will state the chosen pain management method or methods are satisfactory and will communicate if others are needed.
2. During labor, the client will demonstrate relaxation between contractions as evidenced by a relaxed facial expression and body posture.
3. By discharge, the client and support person will express satisfaction with pain management and describe the birth experience as positive.

Interventions

Nursing care related to intrapartum pain management focuses on reducing factors that hinder the client's pain control and enhancing those that benefit it. Although epidurals are very common in North American hospitals, do not make the assumption every client will want one for birth. Most clients will use some nonpharmacologic techniques for pain management prior to receiving an epidural; some will also use pharmacologic methods before or instead of an epidural. Caring contact with a nurse enhances pain management and the overall experience of giving birth. Nursing interventions for pain in labor include promoting relaxation, reducing anxiety and fear, assisting with nonpharmacologic methods, encouragement, and incorporating pharmacologic methods as needed and desired. Caring for the birth partner is also an important nursing intervention that promotes pain management and a positive birth experience.

Promoting Relaxation. Simple attention to details promotes relaxation. If noise is a problem, suggest music to mask it. A warm blanket, a cool cloth, or a warm pack provides tangible comfort and conveys the nurse's caring attitude. Reduce intrusions as much as possible. For example, wait until a contraction is over before asking questions or performing a procedure. Longer assessments and procedures may span several contractions, but whenever possible, pause during each contraction.

In addition to specific relaxation techniques, environmental control, hygiene, positioning, and assistance with voiding affect the client's ability to relax, which enhances the effectiveness of all pain management techniques.

Relaxation Techniques. Assist the client and labor partner with their preferred relaxation techniques (see "Application of Nonpharmacologic Techniques" earlier in this chapter). Teach and support different techniques as needed.

Environment. Soft, indirect lighting is soothing, whereas a bright overhead light is irritating. Bright lights imply a hospital ("sick") atmosphere rather than a normal event such as birth. A bright, overhead light should be used only when needed. Labor is hard work, and the client in labor is often hot and perspiring. Cool, damp washcloths on the client's face and neck can promote comfort. Other interventions include placing socks when the client's feet are cold or using a fan to circulate air in the labor room. After birth, remove the fan to protect the newborn from the air currents which could contribute to neonatal hypothermia.

Hygiene. Bloody show and amniotic fluid leak from the client's vagina during labor. Change the gown, linens, and underpads as needed to keep the client clean and dry and to reduce microorganisms that might ascend into the vagina. Offer the client a warm shower or bath, especially if the client is tense (Box 13.1). In addition to promoting relaxation, mild nipple stimulation, which occurs in a whirlpool or shower, may intensify contractions in a client whose labor has slowed, causing the posterior pituitary gland to secrete oxytocin.

Ice chips, frozen juice bars, and hard candy on a stick reduce dry mouth. Brushing the teeth and rinsing the mouth are often helpful. Lip balm can relieve dry lips.

Bladder. A full bladder intensifies pain during labor and can delay fetal descent. It may cause pain that remains after an epidural is started. Assess the suprapubic area for distention hourly and encourage voiding every 2 hours or more if the client has received a large quantity of IV fluids. Catheterization may be required for some clients. Most intrapartum order sets include an order for catheterization if the client cannot void and the bladder is full.

Positioning. Client preferences and cultural background may influence the positions they choose when laboring. Encourage the client to assume any position that is comfortable (other than supine) and change positions frequently (see Fig. 15.5).

BOX 13.1 Use of Water Therapy during Labor

Use of water therapy has accompanied trends toward a low-intervention approach to intrapartum care. Water therapy can be delivered in the following ways:
- Shower
- Standard tub
- Whirlpool

Benefits
- Associated with a more natural, home-like atmosphere, which decreases anxiety
- Upright position facilitates progress of labor
- Buoyancy relieves tired muscles, reduces pressure, and facilitates client movement
- Facilitates fetal rotation from occiput posterior or transverse positions to the occiput anterior position
- Reduces the need for epidural and other pharmacologic options
- Increases client satisfaction with the birth experience

Disadvantages
- May reduce frequency of contractions and progress of dilation if used during the latent phase of labor
- Fetal assessment may need to be intermittent rather than continuous
- Requires 1:1 nursing care
- Client should exit the water for cleaning/water replacement if excess debris accumulates during labor

Contraindications and Precautions
- Fetal gestation less than 37 weeks
- Thick meconium in the amniotic fluid is an indication for continuous electronic fetal monitoring in most birth facilities and would preclude use of water therapy if wireless monitoring unavailable
- Bleeding
- Oxytocin induction or augmentation—use of both oxytocin and water therapy could cause excessive uterine activity
- Maintain water temperature at 36°C to 37°C (96.8°F to 98.6°F) to avoid hyperthermia in the pregnant client and fetus which increases oxygen demand
- Encourage fluids to prevent dehydration related to greater fluid excretion by the kidneys

American College of Obstetricians and Gynecologists (ACOG). (2021). *Immersion in water during labor and delivery.* ACOG Committee Opinion No. 679, November 2016, reaffirmed 2021. Author; Burke, C. (2021). Pain in labor: Nonpharmacologic and pharmacologic management. In K. Simpson, P. Creehan, N. O'Brien-Abel, C. Roth, & A. Rohan (Eds.), *AWHONN's perinatal nursing* (5th ed., pp. 466–508). Wolters Kluwer.

Movement and frequent position changes in labor decrease pain, improve circulation between the pregnant client and the fetus, improve the strength and effectiveness of contractions, decrease the length of labor, facilitate fetal descent, and decrease perineal trauma and episiotomies (AWHONN, 2019; CMQCC, 2017). Support the client with pillows as needed.

"Back labor" is common when the back of the fetal head puts pressure on the client's sacral promontory (OP position).

The discomfort of back labor is difficult to relieve with medication alone. Positions that encourage the fetus to move away from the sacral promontory and increase the pelvic diameter may help reduce back pain and enhance the internal rotation mechanism of labor. Such positions include the hands-and-knees position or leaning forward over a birthing ball. Side-lying release is another option: The client assumes a side-lying position on a firm surface, keeping the hips aligned and allowing the top leg to hang down in front of the client (Spinning Babies, 2021). Smaller versions of the birthing ball are available for use when the client is sitting and leaning forward.

Reducing Anxiety and Fear. Accurate information reduces the negative psychological impact and fear of the unknown. Tell the client about the labor and its progress. You cannot predict when the client will give birth but tell the client if labor progress is or is not on course. Sometimes, they need only the reassurance from an experienced nurse that their intense contractions are indeed normal. Clients may be willing to endure more discomfort than they otherwise would if they are making progress.

Be honest if problems do occur. A client usually knows if a problem exists and is more anxious if they do not know what it is. Explain all measures taken to correct the problem and inform the client of the results.

Helping the Client Use Nonpharmacologic Techniques. If the nonpharmacologic method is safe for the client and fetus and if it is effective, do not interfere with its use. Try not to distract clients from whatever technique they are using (see "Application of Nonpharmacologic Techniques" earlier in this chapter).

Massage. If fetal monitor belts hinder abdominal effleurage, encourage the client to do effleurage on uncovered areas of the abdomen or to stroke the thighs. Consider using intermittent auscultation or intermittent EFM (see Chapter 14).

Seek feedback from the client about the best location and amount of pressure to use for sacral pressure or other massage. Because this information may change during labor or massage may become uncomfortable rather than helpful, seek the client's feedback regularly.

Mental Stimulation. Use a low, soothing voice when helping a client use imagery. Speaking close to their ear is often helpful when trying to create a tranquil imaginary scene or to calm them. Use of a low, soothing voice during an emergency has a calming effect as well. Music can enhance mental stimulation techniques.

Breathing. Clients often modify the techniques they learn in class or invent some of their own during labor. Encourage clients to follow their instincts and change techniques when they feel it is necessary. If they have trouble maintaining their concentration, the nurse or the support person may try to make eye contact (if culturally appropriate) and breathe with clients.

Symptoms of hyperventilation (dizziness, tingling and numbness of the fingers and lips, carpopedal spasm) are likely if the client breathes fast and deep. If hyperventilating, the client should breathe into cupped hands, a paper bag, or a washcloth placed over the nose and mouth. Talk gently to slow the client's breathing.

Teach breathing techniques to the unprepared client and coach when the client is admitted. Review them when they seem to need a different method. If they make up a breathing technique that works, leave it alone.

When teaching pain management techniques to the unprepared client who is in advanced labor, follow these guidelines:
- Teach one method at a time.
- Demonstrate the method between contractions.
- Use breathing techniques with the client while maintaining eye contact.
- Give the client control over the labor (e.g., who is present or what technique is used).
- Speak in a soft, calm tone of voice.

Encouragement. Clients who receive continuous support in labor have improved outcomes compared with clients who do not have support (AWHONN, 2019). Clients need the nurse to tell them when labor is progressing. When clients see their efforts are effective, they have more courage to continue. Help the client touch or see the baby's head with a mirror as crowning occurs. Praise the client and the support person when they use breathing and other coping techniques effectively. This reinforces their actions, gives them a sense of control, and conveys the respect and support of the nurse. If one technique is not helpful after a reasonable trial (three to five contractions), encourage them to try other techniques.

Although the client and support person may have prepared for childbirth, they often welcome suggestions and affirmation from the nurse. They are more likely to use the techniques they learned if the nurse helps them. The nurse's presence, gentle coaching, and encouragement help clients have confidence in their own bodies' ability to give birth.

Incorporating Pharmacologic Methods. Childbirth is a normal process; however, many clients desire pharmacologic pain management. The nurse should be informative but neutral when explaining available pain medication.

Some clients may have a firm goal to avoid pain medication during labor. Careful review of the client's birth plan and specific teaching or review of available options establish a therapeutic relationship with the client, support person, and the nurse. This should be done as early in the labor as possible while the client is still in control and can think critically. The discussion should include the option for clients to change their minds and how that will be communicated. Other clients may plan to use a specific method such as epidural analgesia.

All pharmacologic methods require collaboration with medical personnel for orders. Tell the client soon after admission what medication is available if they need it. This is intended not to undermine their self-confidence but to allow them to make an informed choice about medication. Analgesia is most effective if it is given before pain is severe.

Tell clients that their preferences about pain-relief methods will be honored, if possible, but predicting the course of their labor is impossible. Their preferred method of pain management may be inappropriate if labor has unexpected developments. Assure them no pharmacologic method will

CLIENT TEACHING

How Will This Medicine Affect Our Baby?

Clients and their partners often ask whether pain medication or anesthesia will harm their baby. The nurse can help them choose wisely from available options by providing honest, evidence-based information, as follows:

- Pain that you cannot tolerate is not good for you or your baby, and it reduces the joy of this special event.
- Some risk is associated with every type of pain medication or anesthesia, but careful selection and the use of preventive measures minimize this risk. If complications occur, corrective measures can reduce the risk to you and your baby.
- Some pain relievers can cause your baby to be slow to breathe at birth, but carefully controlling the timing and dose of the medication reduces the likelihood this will occur.
- Epidurals can be beneficial because we can control the level of painful pressure you may feel without causing sedation. The epidural is also beneficial because it would be available in case of an emergency, such as an unplanned cesarean delivery.

be used without their understanding and consent (see Client Teaching: How Will This Medicine Affect Our Baby?).

When contacting the obstetric provider for medication orders, report the status of the pregnant client and the fetus including fetal heart rate patterns, client vital signs, labor status, pain management techniques in use and their effectiveness as well as the client's request for medication. If the client has a continuous epidural block, contact the anesthesia provider. Observe special nursing considerations associated with the method used (Table 13.3).

Care for the Birth Partner. The client's support person is an integral part of the labor care. A labor partner can provide care and comfort that support the client's ability to give birth. Some partners are coaches in the true sense of the word, actively assisting the client through labor. Others want the client and nurse to lead them and tell them how to help. They are eager to do what they can but expect instructions about methods and timing. Caring for the support person includes respect for the couple's wishes about partner involvement in the birth process. The nurse should provide support that the partner cannot and should consider the partner's physical needs for food and rest.

Evaluation

Achievement of the goals or expected outcomes occurs if the following conditions are met:

The client indicates satisfaction with the method of pain management or requests nursing assistance to find other, more satisfactory methods.

Between contractions, the client's body posture and facial expression are relaxed.

The client and support person express satisfaction with pain management and describe the birth experience as positive.

The first two goals regarding satisfaction with pain management are continually reevaluated throughout labor. If either of the goals is not met, the nurse reassesses, provides additional support, and reviews information about other pain management techniques and methods as appropriate. The last goal, describing the birth experience as positive, is evaluated after the client and significant other have had time to begin putting the birth experience into perspective.

Epidural

Planning: Expected Outcomes

The possible client problems specific to epidurals are "fetal hypoxemia related to decreased placental perfusion secondary to epidural" and "client injury resulting from reduced sensation and movement secondary to epidural." Goals or expected outcomes that may be appropriate for the client with an epidural include the following:

1. After epidural administration, the fetus will remain oxygenated as evidenced by FHR baseline rate 110 to 160 and moderate variability, and client BP will remain consistent with preepidural values.
2. The client is free from treatment-related injuries while sensation and mobility are reduced.

Interventions

Hypotension. Hypotension in the pregnant client interrupts the fetal oxygenation pathway by reducing blood supply to the placenta. Birth facilities have protocols or standing orders providing specific guidelines for care when clients receive an epidural block. Infuse the prescribed IV solution, typically 500 to 1000 mL, before or during the block's initiation. If the client has not received the full amount when the block is begun, notify the anesthesia provider.

Assess the client's blood pressure and pulse rate (often an automatic cuff is used) every 3 to 5 minutes or per the facility's protocol for 15 to 30 minutes after the initial injection of medication, comparing findings with baseline values. Maintain continuous EFM. A significant blood pressure decrease is a 20% fall from baseline or a drop to 100 mm Hg or lower systolic. Hypotension of any degree accompanied by FHR decelerations or loss of variability is significant. If hypotension occurs, increase the rate of IV fluid infusion and reposition the client, avoiding aortocaval compression. If the hypotension is significant and does not improve with additional fluid and repositioning, administer phenylephrine or ephedrine per protocol. When the blood pressure is stable, reassess it every 15 minutes. Hypotension following epidural placement should be reported to the anesthesia provider for definitive treatment.

Continue observing the FHR. Signs of reduced placental perfusion may be evident before the client shows signs of hypotension. These include fetal tachycardia (more than 160 beats per minute [bpm]) or bradycardia (less than 110 bpm), prolonged decelerations, and late decelerations (see Chapter 14). Monitor the client's temperature to identify

TABLE 13.3   Pharmacologic Methods of Intrapartum Pain Management

Method and Uses	Nursing Considerations
Opioid Analgesics Systemic analgesia during labor and for postoperative pain after cesarean birth. May be combined with an adjunctive drug to reduce nausea and vomiting, which sometimes occur with narcotic use and after surgery. Often delivered by PCA pump in postoperative period.	1. Assess the client for drug use at admission. 2. Clients who are opiate-dependent should not receive analgesics having mixed agonist-antagonist actions (butorphanol and nalbuphine). 3. Observe neonate for respiratory depression, especially if client had opioid narcotics within 4 hours of birth or delivery occurs at the peak medication action, or if client received multiple opioid doses during labor: • Delay in initiating or sustaining normal depth and rate of respirations • Respiratory rate <30/min • Poor muscle tone: Limp, floppy 4. Use of adjunctive drugs for nausea, such as promethazine and metoclopramide, enhances respiratory depressant effects. 5. Respiratory (bag-and-mask) and cardiac support precede medication administration in neonatal resuscitation. If naloxone is given, observe for recurrent respiratory depression.
Epidural Opioids *Labor:* Mixed with a local anesthetic agent to give better pain relief with less motor block. *Postoperatively:* Gives long-acting analgesia without sedation, allowing client and infant to interact more easily.	1. Monitor for same nursing implications as with epidural block. 2. Do not give additional opioids or other CNS depressants except as ordered by anesthesia provider. Nonsteroidal antiinflammatory medications or oral analgesics are often prescribed in routine orders. 3. Respiratory depression in the pregnant or postpartum client may be delayed for up to 24 hours and varies with medication given. Observe respiratory rate and depth, oxygen saturation, and arousability hourly for 24 hours or as ordered. Notify the anesthesia provider of respiratory rate of <12/min, persistent oxygen saturation of <95% on pulse oximetry, reduced respiratory effort, or difficulty arousing. Cyanosis is a late sign of respiratory depression. 4. Have naloxone 0.4 mg, an oral airway, and an Ambu bag and mask immediately available, such as on a "crash cart." 5. Observe for pruritus or rubbing of face and neck. Routine postoperative orders to relieve pruritus are usually provided. Notify the anesthesia provider if these are inadequate. 6. Urinary retention may occur after indwelling catheter removal. Observe for adequacy of voiding, as in all postpartum clients. 7. Notify the anesthesia provider for relief of nausea or vomiting. 8. Assess sensation and mobility before allowing ambulation.
Intrathecal Opioid Analgesics Provides analgesia for most of first-stage labor without sedation. A very small dose of the drug is needed because it is injected near spinal cord where sensory fibers enter. Usually not adequate for late labor or birth itself. Often combined with epidural block for CSE technique for labor.	1. Observe for common side effects of nausea, vomiting, and pruritus. Notify the anesthesia provider if these effects occur, and have an antagonist such as naloxone available. 2. Observe for delayed respiratory depression, depending on drug given. Use a pulse oximeter, as indicated. 3. Observe for indeterminate or abnormal FHR patterns, which may be associated with reduced oxygenation of the pregnant client.
Local Infiltration Anesthesia Numbs perineum for episiotomy or repair of laceration at vaginal birth. No relief of labor pain. Not adequate for instrument-assisted birth.	1. Assess for drug allergies, especially to dental anesthetics because they are related to those used in obstetric care. 2. Apply ice to perineum after birth to reduce edema and hematoma formation and to increase comfort.

TABLE 13.3 Pharmacologic Methods of Intrapartum Pain Management—cont'd

Method and Uses	Nursing Considerations
Pudendal Block Numbs lower vagina and perineum for vaginal birth. No relief of labor pain because it is done just before birth. Provides adequate anesthesia for many instrument-assisted births.	1. Use same interventions as for local infiltration. A client or partner may be alarmed if the long needle is noticed (about 15 cm [6 inches]). Educate client that in order to reach the pudendal nerve through the vagina a longer needle is used. The needle is inserted only about 1.25 cm (½ inch) near the location of the nerve. A guide ("trumpet") will be used to avoid injuring vaginal tissue or the baby.
Epidural Block *Labor:* Insertion of catheter provides pain relief for labor and vaginal birth (T10–S5 levels). *Cesarean birth:* If epidural was used during labor, level of block can be extended upward (T4–T6 level). Also used for cesarean birth, which is not preceded by labor.	1. Pre- or co-load client with 500–1000 mL crystalloid solution such as lactated Ringer's or normal saline solution. 2. Displace uterus manually or with a wedge placed under client's side to enhance placental perfusion. 3. Assess for hypotension at least every 3 to 5 minutes for 15 to 30 minutes after block is begun and with each new dose until vital signs are stable. Report following to anesthesia provider: Systolic BP of <100 mm Hg or a fall of 20% or more from baseline levels, pallor, or diaphoresis. Facility protocols give further guidance. 4. Assess FHR for signs of impaired placental perfusion, and report the following to the anesthesia and obstetric providers: tachycardia (>160 bpm for 10 min), bradycardia (<110 bpm for 10 min), late decelerations, absent variability (see Chapter 14). 5. If hypotension or signs of impaired placental perfusion occur, increase IV fluid rate, reposition client laterally, and administer oxygen by face mask (10 L/min) as indicated. Have phenylephrine or ephedrine available. 6. Observe for a full bladder, and catheterize client if unable to void. 7. Leg movement and strength vary after an epidural block. Transfer with help avoid muscle strains to the nurse or the client. 8. Have the client ambulate only if adequate sensation and movement are present and with another person's assistance with first ambulation.

Subarachnoid Block
Cesarean birth: Can be established slightly faster than epidural block.
Rarely used for complicated vaginal birth.
Does not provide pain relief for labor because it is done just before birth.
May be combined with an epidural block in a CSE.
	1. See "Epidural Block" for these interventions:
	  • IV pre- or co-load
	  • Uterine displacement
	  • Observation of BP and FHR
	  • Care for hypotension or signs of impaired placental perfusion
	  • Observation and intervention for bladder distention
	  • Transfer and ambulation precautions
	2. Observe for postdural puncture headache—a headache that is worse when the client is upright and may disappear when lying flat. Notify the anesthesia provider if it occurs (a blood patch may be done).
	3. Nursing interventions for postdural puncture headache: Encourage bed rest, increase oral fluids if not contraindicated, give oral caffeine, and give analgesics, as ordered.

General Anesthesia Cesarean birth if epidural or spinal block is not possible or if client refuses regional anesthesia. May be required for emergency procedures.	1. Determine type and time of last food intake on admission. 2. Restrict oral intake to clear liquids or as ordered. Consult with the obstetric provider if surgical intervention is likely. 3. Report to anesthesia provider: pertinent medical history, reason for the cesarean section, and oral intake before and during labor, vomiting. 4. Displace uterus (see "Epidural Block"). 5. Give preoperative medications such as sodium citrate (Bicitra). 6. Apply cricoid pressure (Sellick's maneuver) during intubation as indicated. 7. Client will remain intubated until the effects of the muscle relaxant, such as the protective (gag) reflexes have returned. Have oral airway and suction immediately available. 8. Oxygen by face tent or face mask should be given after extubation. 9. Interventions for postoperative respiratory depression: be prepared to give positive-pressure oxygen by face mask; observe oxygen saturation with pulse oximetry until client is awake and alert; have client take several deep breaths if oxygen saturation falls below 95%. Notify the anesthesia provider.

BP, blood pressure; *CNS*, central nervous system; *CSE*, combined spinal–epidural; *FHR*, fetal heart rate; *IV*, intravenous; *PCA*, patient-controlled analgesia.

elevations that may also contribute to fetal tachycardia. Pulse oximetry values below 95% identify a decrease in client oxygenation, which may also contribute to FHR changes.

Avoidance of Injury. Epidural block reduces lower extremity sensation and movement to varying degrees. Assess the degree of motor block and sensation hourly. If a distinct increase or change is noted, report it to the anesthesia provider as this may indicate catheter migration or another complication.

A client who has reduced mobility and sensation should be repositioned frequently (every 20 to 30 minutes in labor) to avoid prolonged pressure on one area and promote labor progress. When positioning a pregnant client with decreased sensation and motor control, it is important to avoid aortocaval compression, maintain correct alignment, and provide any support needed to maintain the position with small pillows or folded blankets. Also, check for and remove any small items such as plastic needle covers and IV tubing covers that may have fallen into the bed. Verify IV tubing is not kinked or caught under the client. Ensuring the linens are clean and smooth and that the call button is easily accessible are the final steps of repositioning any client.

Evaluation

Achievement of the goals or expected outcomes occurs if the following conditions are met:
1. FHR remains stable with a baseline rate 110 to 160 and moderate variability; client BP remains within 20% of preepidural values.
2. The client is free from injuries related to altered sensation and mobility.

APPLICATION OF THE NURSING PROCESS: RESPIRATORY COMPROMISE

Assessment

General anesthesia may be needed at any time during birth, most often for an emergency cesarean birth when a client does not have an epidural in place. Document the type (solids or liquids) and time of the client's last oral intake. Anesthesia providers can anticipate and prevent problems better if they know the actual oral intake, although most assume every birthing person has food in their stomach and induce general anesthesia accordingly.

Identification of Client Problems

Analysis of the data collected enables the nurse to identify actual and potential client problems and to develop an individualized plan of care. The client is at risk for respiratory compromise as a result of aspiration.

Planning: Expected Outcomes

The expected outcome is the client will not experience respiratory compromise from aspiration of gastric contents during the perioperative period.

Interventions

Nursing interventions relate to identifying factors that increase a client's risk for aspiration as well as collaborative and nursing measures to reduce the risk for aspiration or lung injury.

Identifying Risk Factors

Report oral intake both before and after admission to the anesthesia provider. Oral intake during labor may be restricted to medications, clear liquids such as water and ice, clear fruit juices, carbonated drinks, clear tea and coffee, sports drinks, or ice pops.

Vomiting is a common occurrence during normal labor, regardless of the client's oral intake. If vomiting occurs, document the time, quantity, and character (amount, color, and presence of undigested food).

Perioperative Care

Restrict oral intake, as ordered, if surgery is expected. Give ordered medications such as sodium citrate (Bicitra). Depending on when the medications are needed, either the nurse or the anesthesia provider may administer parenteral drugs such as famotidine (Pepcid) and metoclopramide (Reglan).

An experienced nurse or a trained anesthesia assistant may provide cricoid pressure (Sellick's maneuver) to block the esophagus until the client is intubated and the cuff of the endotracheal tube is inflated. Successful intubation with the cuffed endotracheal tube blocks passage of any gastric contents into the trachea. However, the value of cricoid pressure has not been thoroughly researched (ASA, 2016; Tsen & Bateman, 2020).

Postoperative Care

Facility protocols guide postoperative care, including pre-extubation and postextubation care for the client who has had general anesthesia. Clients are extubated when their protective laryngeal reflexes have returned and they are able to respond to verbal commands. Suction equipment and an Ambu bag with an appropriate-sized mask should be immediately available. Administer oxygen by mask or face tent until the client is awake and alert because the agents used for general anesthesia are respiratory depressants. Monitor oxygen saturation with a pulse oximeter. If oxygen saturation falls below 95%, have the client take several deep breaths. Deep breathing also helps to eliminate inhalational anesthetics and reduces stasis of pulmonary secretions.

Assess the client's pulse rate, respiration, and blood pressure every 15 minutes for 1 hour or until stable, then continue per policy. In addition to using pulse oximetry, observe the client's color for pallor or cyanosis, which suggest shock or hypoventilation, respectively (ASA, 2016).

Evaluation

Interventions for this client problem are preventive and short-term because it is a temporary high-risk situation. The goal is met if the client does not aspirate gastric contents during the perioperative period.

SUMMARY CONCEPTS

- Childbirth pain is unique because it is normal and self-limiting, the pregnant client has time to prepare for the pain, and the pain ends with the baby's birth.
- Excess or poorly relieved pain may be harmful to the client and fetus.
- Pain is a complex physical and psychological experience. It is subjective and personal.
- Four sources of pain are present in most labors, but other physical and psychological factors may increase or decrease the pain felt from these sources. These sources are cervical dilation, uterine ischemia, pressure and pulling on pelvic structures, and distention of the vagina and perineum.
- Relaxation enhances all other pain management techniques.
- Several nonpharmacologic pain management techniques supplement relaxation—cutaneous stimulation, hydrotherapy, mental stimulation, and breathing techniques.
- Physiologic alterations of pregnancy may affect a client's response to medications.
- Any medication the pregnant client takes, whether therapeutic or abused, including herbal or botanical preparations, also may affect the fetus. Fetal effects may be direct or indirect, and their durations of action may be different from those in an adult.
- The nurse should observe for respiratory depression, primarily in the newborn, if the client has received opioid analgesics during labor.
- The major advantages of regional pain management methods are the client can participate in the birth without pain and retain protective airway reflexes.
- The nurse should monitor and take actions to prevent hypotension, which may result from an epidural or subarachnoid block.
- If the client receives a regional pain management technique that carries the risk for hypotension, the nurse should observe for fetal heart rate changes associated with impaired placental perfusion.
- The primary adverse effects that should be monitored in the client who receives epidural or intrathecal opioids are nausea and vomiting, pruritus, and delayed respiratory depression.
- Regurgitation with aspiration of acidic gastric contents is the greatest risk for a client who receives general anesthesia.

Clinical Judgment And Next-Generation NCLEX® Examination-Style Questions

1. A Vietnamese–American client, G_1P_0, is in labor. Cervical dilation is 6 cm, effacement is 100%, and the fetus is at a +1 station. Contractions occur every 3 minutes, last 50 to 60 seconds, and are firm to palpation. FHR is auscultated at 145 bpm and regular. The client's support person is resting in the recliner next to the bed. The client smiles at the nurse each time the nurse asks questions but does not talk much. During contractions, the client's body stiffens, and there is minimal interaction with the support person or the nurse.

Review of the admission database reveals the client did not participate in any childbirth preparation program, does not have a specific birth plan, and does not have any known allergies. The client indicated only the partner should use touch for comfort and pain management techniques.

What nursing actions are appropriate for the client at this time? Select all that apply.

_____ A. Suggest additional pain management techniques be used due to indicators of pain.

_____ B. Congratulate the client and partner for their effective use of pain management techniques.

_____ C. Teach basic breathing and relaxation techniques to the client and partner between contractions.

_____ D. Notify the provider that the client is progressing and managing pain effectively at this time.

_____ E. If agreeable to the client, notify the anesthesia provider of the client's need for an epidural.

_____ F. Teach the partner "touch and relax" technique to use when the client demonstrates tension.

2. A client in labor has just received an epidural and is repositioned to semi-Fowler's with a left tilt. Vital signs before the epidural were:
- Blood pressure 117/68
- Heart rate 72
- Respiratory rate 22

The client begins complaining of ringing in the ears, a metallic taste in the mouth, and shortness of breath. The following vital sign changes were noted:
- Blood pressure 96/48
- Heart rate 105
- Respiratory rate 30

Which of the following actions should the nurse take? Select all that apply.

_____ A. Reassure client and change vital sign frequency to every hour

_____ B. Notify anesthesia provider

_____ C. Apply pulse oximeter

_____ D. Assess lung sounds

_____ E. Raise head of bed to a 90-degree angle

_____ F. Administer 50 mcg phenylephrine subcutaneously

_____ G. Continuously monitor the fetal heart rate tracing

_____ H. Administer 500 mL lactated Ringer's fluid bolus

_____ I. Turn off epidural infusion pump

3. **Highlight the findings that would require follow-up.**
A 41-year-old (G_4P_{3003}) at 37 1/7 weeks presented to labor and delivery with spontaneous rupture of membranes and active labor. The cervical examination was 6 cm, 50% effaced, and a fetal vertex at a +1 station. Vital signs between contractions:

Blood pressure: 125/70; pulse: 96, respiratory rate:18. The client reported pain that was 7 out of 10 and requested an epidural. A certified registered nurse anesthetist placed the epidural following a rapid infusion of 1000ml bolus of lactated Ringer's 30 minutes prior to the procedure.

Five minutes after the procedure, the client states "My pain is 2 out of 10 but I'm feeling lightheaded." Vital signs: blood pressure 90/44, pulse rate 124, respiratory rate 20, and oxygen saturation 99%. Repeat blood pressures taken every 5 minutes 88/50, 90/48, and 89/50. External monitoring: category II FHR tracing with baseline rate 145 bpm, minimal variability, and recurrent late decelerations; contractions every 2 to 3.5 minutes, 50 to 100 seconds, firm on palpation and resting tone soft between contractions. Maintenance IV fluid of lactated Ringer's infusing at 125 ml/hour.

4. **Use an X to indicate which actions listed in the left column would be implemented.**

Potential Steps	Plan of Care
Notify anesthesia provider.	
Increase maintenance IV fluid infusion rate	
Administer intravenous phenylephrine as per protocol or standing orders	
Perform a cervical examination	
Reposition the client to a lateral position	
Continue blood pressures every 5 minutes	
Administer terbutaline 0.25 mg intravenously	
Discontinue the epidural infusion	

The nurse assesses the client 1 hour later. **For each finding, place an "X" to specify whether the finding indicates the nursing interventions were effective, ineffective, or unrelated.**

Assessment Finding	Effective	Ineffective	Unrelated
FHR BL rate 135 bpm			
Blood pressure 118/78 and 122/76			
Cervical examination 7 cm/60%/ 0 station			
Moderate variability			
FHR accelerations			

REFERENCES

American Academy of Pediatrics & American College of Obstetricians and Gynecologists (AAP & ACOG). (2014). Clinical report: Immersion in water during labor and delivery. *Pediatrics, 133*(4), 758–761.

American Academy of Pediatrics & American College of Obstetricians and Gynecologists (AAP & ACOG). (2017). *Guidelines for perinatal care* (8th ed.).

American Association of Nurse Anesthetists (AANA). (2017). *Analgesia and anesthesia for the obstetric patient: Practice guidelines.* www.aana.com/docs/default-source/practice-aana-com-web-documents-(all)/professional-practice-manual/analgesia-and-anesthesia-for-the-obstetric-patient.pdf?sfvrsn=be7446b1_8.

American College of Obstetricians and Gynecologists (ACOG). (2019). *Approaches to limit intervention during labor and birth.* ACOG Committee Opinion No. 766.

American College of Obstetricians and Gynecologists (ACOG). (2020). *Obstetric analgesia and anesthesia.* ACOG Practice Bulletin No. 209. April 2017, reaffirmed 2020.

American College of Obstetricians and Gynecologists (ACOG). (2021). *Immersion in water during labor and delivery.* ACOG Committee Opinion No. 679. November 2016, reaffirmed 2021.

American Society of Anesthesiologists (ASA). (2016). Practice guidelines for obstetric anesthesia: An updated report by the American Society of Anesthesiologists Task Force on Obstetric Anesthesia and the Society for Obstetric Anesthesia and Perinatology. *Anesthesiology, 124*(2), 270–300.

Association of Women's Health, Obstetric and Neonatal Nurses (AWHONN). (2019). *Nursing care and management of the second stage of labor: Evidence-based clinical practice guidelines* (3rd ed.).

Association of Women's Health, Obstetric and Neonatal Nurses (AWHONN). (2020a). *Analgesia and anesthesia in the intrapartum period: Evidence-based clinical practice guideline.*

Association of Women's Health, Obstetric and Neonatal Nurses (AWHONN). (2020b). Role of the registered nurse in the care of the pregnant woman receiving analgesia and anesthesia by catheter technique: AWHONN position statement. *Journal of Obstetric, Gynecologic, and Neonatal Nurses, 49*(3), 327–329. https://doi.org/10.1016/j.jogn.2020.02.002.

Blackburn, S. T. (2018). *Maternal, fetal, & neonatal physiology: A clinical perspective* (5th ed.). Elsevier.

Bohren, M.A., Hofmeyr, G.J., Sakala, C., Fukuzawa, R.K., & Cuthbert, A. (2017). Continuous support for women during childbirth. *Cochrane Database of Systematic Reviews, 2017*(7), CD003766. https://doi.org/10.1002/14651858.CD003766.pub6.

Bujedo, B. M. (2016). An update on neuraxial opioid induced pruritus prevention. *J Anesth Crit Care Open Access, 6*(2). https://doi.org/10.15406/jaccoa.2016.06.00226.

Burke, C. (2021). Pain in labor: Nonpharmacologic and pharmacologic management. In K. Simpson, P. Creehan, N.

O'Brien-Abel, C. Roth, & A. Rohan (Eds.), *AWHONN's perinatal nursing* (5th ed., pp. 466–508). Wolters Kluwer.

California Maternal Quality Care Collaborative (CMQCC). (2017). *Toolkit to support vaginal birth and reduce primary cesareans.* https://www.cmqcc.org/VBirthToolkitResource.

Chestnut, D. (2020). Alternative regional analgesic techniques for labor and vaginal delivery. In D. Chestnut, C. Wong, L. Tsen, D. Warwick, Y. Beilin, J. Mhyre, & B. Bateman (Eds.), *Chestnut's obstetric anesthesia: Principles and practice* (6th ed.). Elsevier.

Cluett, E. R., Burns, E., & Cuthbert, A. (2018). Immersion in water during labour and birth. *Cochrane Database of Systematic Reviews* (5), CD000111. https://doi.org/10.1002/14651858. CD000111.pub4.

Cunningham, F., Leveno, K. J., Dashe, J. S., Hoffman, B. L., Spong, C. Y., & Casey, B. M. (2022) *Williams Obstetrics*, 26e. McGraw Hill.

Dalton, J., & Strehlow, S. (2019). Maternal Obesity. In N. Troiano, C. Harvey, & B. Chez (Eds.), *AWHONN high-risk & critical care obstetrics* (4th ed., pp. 232–243). Wolters Kluwer.

Davies, R., Davis, D., Peace, M., & Wong, N. (2015). *The effect of waterbirth on neonatal mortality and morbidity: A systematic review and meta-analysis* https://pubmed.ncbi.nlm.nih.gov.

Douglas, M. J. (2020). Malignant hyperthermia. In D. Chestnut, C. Wong, L. Tsen, D. Warwick, Y. Beilin, J. Mhyre, & B. Bateman (Eds.), *Chestnut's obstetric anesthesia: Principles and practice* (6th ed.). Elsevier.

George, R. B., Carvalho, B., Butwick, A., & Flood, P. (2020). Postoperative Analgesia. In D. Chestnut, C. Wong, L. Tsen, D. Warwick, Y. Beilin, J. Mhyre, & B. Bateman (Eds.), *Chestnut's obstetric anesthesia: Principles and practice* (6th ed.). Elsevier.

Habib, A. S., & D'Angelo, R. (2020). Obesity. In D. Chestnut, C. Wong, L. Tsen, D. Warwick, Y. Beilin, J. Mhyre, & B. Bateman (Eds.), *Chestnut's obstetric anesthesia: Principles and practice* (6th ed.). Elsevier.

Hawkins, J. L. (2019). Anesthesia Considerations for Complicated Pregnancies. In R. Resnik, C. Lockwood, T. Moore, M. Greene, J. Copel, & R. Silver (Eds.), *Creasy and Resnik's maternal-fetal medicine: Principles and practice* (8th ed.). Elsevier.

Hawkins, J. L., & Bucklin, B. A. (2021). Obstetric anesthesia. In S. Gabbe, J. Niebyl, J. Simpson, M. Landon, H. Galan, R. Jauniaux, D. Driscollet, et al. (Eds.), *Obstetrics: Normal and problem pregnancies* (8th ed., pp. 295–318). Elsevier.

Hellams, A., Sprague, T., Saldanha, C., & Archambault, M. (2018). Nitrous oxide for labor analgesia. *Official Journal of the American Academy of Physician Assistants*, 31(1), 41–44. https://doi.org/10.1097/01.jaa.0000527700.00698.8c.

Joint Commission Online. (2019). *R3 Report Issue 24: Provision of care, treatment, and services standards for maternal safety effective July 1, 2020.* www.jointcommission.org/-/medica/tjc/documents/standards/r3-reports/r3_24_maternal_safety_hap_9_6_19_final1.pdf.

Lamaze International. (2021). *Lamaze healthy birth practices.* https://www.lamaze.org/childbirth-practices.

Mallen-Perez, L., Roé-Justiniano, M. T., Colomé Ochoa, N., Ferre Colomat, A., Palacio, M., & Terré-Rull, C. (2018). Use of hydrotherapy during labour: Assessment of pain, use of analgesia and neonatal safety. *Enfermerica Clinica*, 28(5), 309–315. Retrieved from https://pubmed.ncbi.nlm.nih.gov/29239794/.

Mhyre, J. M. (2020). Maternal Mortality. In D. Chestnut, C. Wong, L. Tsen, D. Warwick, Y. Beilin, J. Mhyre, & B. Bateman (Eds.), *Chestnut's obstetric anesthesia: Principles and practice* (6th ed.). Elsevier.

Minehart, R. D., & Minnich, M. E. (2020). Childbirth preparation and nonpharmacologic analgesia. In D. Chestnut, C. Wong, L. Tsen, D. Warwick, Y. Beilin, J. Mhyre, & B. Bateman (Eds.), *Chestnut's obstetric anesthesia: Principles and practice* (6th ed.). Elsevier.

National Institutes of Health (NIH). (2019). *National center for complementary and integrative health.* https://www.nih.gov/about-nih/what-we-do/nih-almanac/national-center-complementary-integrative-health-nccih.

Peralta, F. P., & Macarthur, A. (2020). Postpartum Headache. In D. Chestnut, C. Wong, L. Tsen, D. Warwick, Y. Beilin, J. Mhyre, & B. Bateman (Eds.), *Chestnut's obstetric anesthesia: Principles and practice* (6th ed.). Elsevier.

Peter, P. H., & Booth, J. L. (2020). The pain of childbirth and its effect on the mother and the fetus. In D. Chestnut, C. Wong, L. Tsen, D. Warwick, Y. Beilin, J. Mhyre, & B. Bateman (Eds.), *Chestnut's obstetric anesthesia: Principles and practice* (6th ed.). Elsevier.

Setty, T., & Fernando, R. (2020). Systemic analgesia: Parenteral and inhalation agents. In D. Chestnut, C. Wong, L. Tsen, D. Warwick, Y. Beilin, J. Mhyre, & B. Bateman (Eds.), *Chestnut's obstetric anesthesia: Principles and practice* (6th ed.). Elsevier.

Simkin, P., & Rohs, K. (2018). *The birth partner: A complete guide to childbirth for dads, partners, doulas, and other labor companions* (5th ed.). Harvard Common Press.

Spinning Babies (2021). *Side-lying-release.* https://www.spinningbabies.com/pregnancy-birth/techniques/side-lying-release/.

Tsen, L. C., & Bateman, B. T. (2020). Anesthesia for cesarean delivery. In D. Chestnut, C. Wong, L. Tsen, D. Warwick, Y. Beilin, J. Mhyre, & B. Bateman (Eds.), *Chestnut's obstetric anesthesia: Principles and practice* (6th ed.). Elsevier.

Wilson, R. D., Caughey, A. B., Wood, S. L., Metcalfe, A., Gramlich, L., & Nelson, G. (2018). Guidelines for antenatal and preoperative care in cesarean delivery: Enhanced recovery after surgery society recommendations (part 1). *American Journal of Obstetrics & Gynecology*, 219(6) 523.E1-513.E15. 10.1016/j.ajog.2018.09.015.

Wong, C. A. (2020). Epidural and spinal analgesia/anesthesia for labor and vaginal delivery. In D. Chestnut, C. Wong, L. Tsen, D. Warwick, Y. Beilin, J. Mhyre, & B. Bateman (Eds.), *Chestnut's obstetric anesthesia: Principles and practice* (6th ed.). Elsevier.

Intrapartum Fetal Surveillance

Rebecca L. Cypher

OBJECTIVES

After studying this chapter, you should be able to:

1. Identify key physiologic principles related to fetal oxygenation.
2. Analyze methods and instrumentation used for intrapartum nonelectronic and electronic fetal monitoring (EFM) surveillance.
3. Recognize critical elements of fetal heart rate (FHR) and uterine activity (UA) interpretation using a standardized approach.
4. Describe conservative corrective measures used in management of indeterminate and abnormal FHR patterns.
5. Recall fundamental concepts in fetal monitoring documentation that are the basis for client care and communication.
6. Summarize the rationale for shared decision making when fetal surveillance is applied in the intrapartum period.

Intrapartum fetal surveillance is a critical component of labor management. Over several decades, indirect assessment of fetal oxygenation and interpretation of uterine activity (UA) has transitioned primarily from "low-technology" auscultation and palpation to "high-technology" electronic fetal monitoring (EFM). Today's modern equipment functions as a window into the oxygenation status of the fetal brain. In pregnancy, a sophisticated pathway carries oxygen from an external environment to maternal-fetal blood (Cypher, 2018a). The oxygenation pathway leads from the maternal environment to the fetal environment. When there is an interruption along this pathway, a fetus will respond with specific fetal heart rate (FHR) characteristic patterns that reflect changes in fetal oxygenation. A primary goal in EFM is preventing fetal injury resulting from an interruption of normal oxygenation.

Fetal surveillance using a low-technology method, also known as nonelectronic or intermittent auscultation (IA) of the fetal heart rate, requires a clinician to count the FHR with a fetoscope or Doppler device in relation to UA. Counting and palpation occur at specified intervals for a predetermined amount of time depending on the stage of labor and risk status. Uterine palpation provides general information such as frequency, duration, intensity, and resting tone. Unlike IA and palpation, EFM incorporates a complex electronic device, which acquires, processes, and displays FHR and UA data (Ayers-de-Campos & Noguiera-Reis, 2015). Electronic monitoring can either be external or internal to the client's body and uses different pieces of equipment to collect FHR and UA information.

Each method of fetal surveillance has advantages and limitations. Both nonelectronic and electronic approaches may be interchanged depending on pregnancy risk factors, current clinical situation, health care team and client preference, nurse-to-client ratio, and hospital policy. When necessary, timely and appropriate corrective measures are taken to improve fetal oxygenation so that unnecessary interventions, like cesarean birth, may be avoided. Regardless of which method of surveillance is used, information gathered at the bedside during the intrapartum period can assist nurses with the following:

1. Evaluating fetal oxygenation based on bedside assessments and accurate interpretation of data.
2. Deciding when physiologically based conservative corrective measures are implemented to correct interruptions in the oxygenation pathway.
3. Providing a continuing mechanism to optimize communication between health care team members and clients.
4. Supporting clinical decision making in a shared decision-making model, which promotes an environment that improves communication, client safety, and health care quality.

FETAL OXYGENATION

Understanding the dynamics of uteroplacental exchange and maternal-fetal circulation is essential to recognizing how fetuses respond to labor stressors (e.g., uterine contractions). Oxygen is carried from the environment to the fetus by a maternal and fetal circulation pathway, which includes maternal lungs, heart, vasculature, uterus, placenta, and umbilical cord (Miller et al., 2022; Fig. 14.1). Interruption along this oxygen pathway at one or more points can cause physiologic changes resulting in distinctive FHR characteristics, such as a change in the FHR baseline or decelerations. At each point

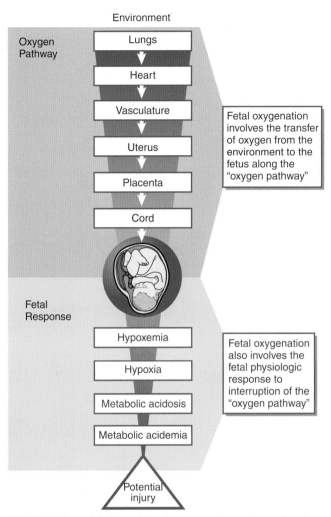

FIG. 14.1 A sophisticated fetal oxygenation pathway involves transfer of oxygen from the environment to the fetus. If there is an interruption of this pathway, there is a physiologic response (i.e., decelerations) by the fetus. (Courtesy David A. Miller, MD.)

along this pathway, conservative corrective measures, sometimes referred to as physiologic interventions or intrauterine resuscitation, may become necessary to optimize fetal oxygenation. An example of a corrective measure is lateral positioning. If there is no fetal response to these interventions, normoxia may gradually evolve into hypoxemia, hypoxia, metabolic acidosis, and finally metabolic acidemia resulting in a potential neurologic injury. Adequate fetal oxygenation requires the following:

1. Sufficient blood flow and volume to the uterus and placenta.
2. Normal oxygen saturation of the pregnant client's blood.
3. Adequate placental exchange of oxygen and carbon dioxide.
4. An open circulatory path from a placenta to a fetus through the umbilical cord.
5. Normal fetal circulatory and oxygen-carrying functions.

Uteroplacental Circulation

The placenta is a unique vascular organ that receives blood from the circulatory systems of both the pregnant client and the fetus. In other words, there are two separate circulatory systems, maternal–placental (i.e., uteroplacental) blood circulation and fetal–placental blood circulation (Wang & Zhao, 2010). Placentas are responsible for gas, nutrient, and substance exchange for fetal growth, development, and oxygenation. These organs also play a vital role in metabolism, endocrine secretion, immunologic safeguards, and protection of the fetus against certain substances in the client's circulation, such as viruses and medications, which may be harmful (Blackburn, 2018; Heuser, 2020; O'Brien-Abel, 2020).

Blood flow to the uterus and placenta originates primarily in the uterine, internal iliac, and ovarian arteries (Blackburn, 2018; Nageotte, 2015). Uterine blood flow progressively increases with each trimester from 50 mL per minute to approximately 500 to 800 mL per minute at term, which represents 10% to 15% of the pregnant client's cardiac output (Blackburn, 2018; O'Brien-Abel, 2021). About 70% to 90% of this blood flow supplies volume for uteroplacental circulation, and the remaining percentage circulates blood to uterine musculature (O'Brien-Abel, 2021; Thaler et al., 1990). A marked increase in cardiac output and changes in arterial blood pressure maintain the flow of oxygen- and nutrient-rich blood to the uterus, placenta, and intervillous spaces of the placenta via spiral arteries. These spiral arteries nourish the intervillous space where maternal-fetal blood exchange occurs throughout pregnancy (Nageotte, 2015). In the nonpregnant state, spiral arteries are small vessels supplying blood to the uterine endometrium. In the first few weeks of pregnancy, spiral arteries are remodeled from a prepregnancy state by changing from high-resistance low capacity to low-resistance high capacity vessels to meet a developing fetus's growth demands (Brosens et al., 2019; Pijnenborg et al., 2006; Wang & Zhao, 2010).

Fetal chorionic villi are protrusions of tissue located in the intervillous space (Fig. 14.2). These microscopic branches are immersed in maternal blood from the newly remodeled spiral arteries. In this intervillous space, substances, such as oxygen, are exchanged without the mixing of maternal and fetal blood. Simultaneously, maternal blood that is carrying away carbon dioxide and fetal waste products drains from the intervillous space through endometrial veins and returns to the client's circulation for elimination (Blackburn, 2018; O'Brien-Abel, 2020).

Interruptions in the oxygenation pathway can alter blood flow through the spiral arteries. For example, during uterine contractions, myometrial pressures can exceed intraarterial pressure within the spiral arteries (Nageotte, 2015). This results in a temporary cessation of maternal blood flow into the intervillous space. Over time, if contractions are too frequent or have inadequate relaxation time, a fetus will respond to these interruptions with FHR changes, which reflect acute or chronic episodes of decreased oxygen. These may progressively worsen over time unless corrective interventions (e.g., titrate oxytocin to a lower dose combined with an intravenous [IV] fluid bolus)

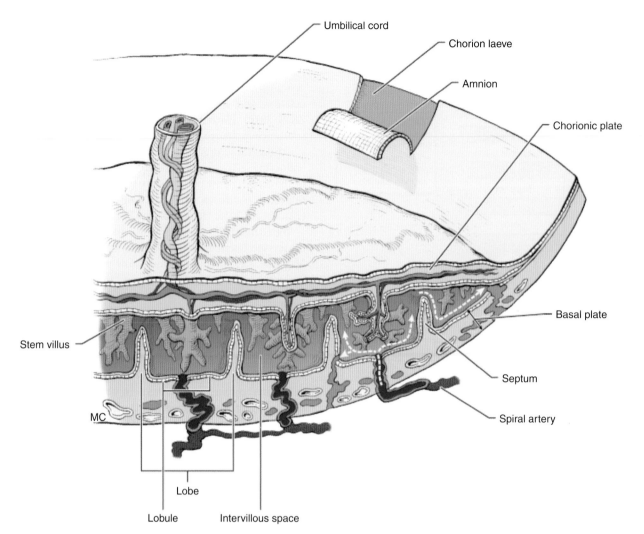

FIG. 14.2 Schematic image of transverse section of a placenta showing maternal–placental (uteroplacental) blood circulation and fetal-placental blood circulation. (From Burton, G. J., Sibly, C. P., Jauniaux, E. R. M. [2021]. Placental anatomy and physiology. In M. B. Landon, H. L. Galan, E. R. M. Jauniaux, D. A. Driscoll, V. Berghella, W. A. Grobman, S. J. Kilpatrick, & A. G. Cahill. [Eds.]. *Gabbe's Obstetrics: Normal and problem pregnancies.* [8th ed., pp. 2–25]. Elsevier.)

are performed. A fetus may also react to these changes in oxygenation by redistributing or "shunting" blood flow to the vital organs (heart, brain, and adrenal glands) and decreasing blood flow to the nonvital organs (lungs, kidneys, liver, gastrointestinal tract, and periphery). Persistent redistribution of blood flow may cause a loss of fetal cerebral autoregulation, resulting in decreased fetal cardiac output. If this physiologic process continues, a reduction of cerebral blood flow could potentially result in fetal neurologic injury or death.

Fetal Placental Circulation

The umbilical cord links the fetal umbilicus to the placenta's fetal surface (Wang & Zhao, 2010). Protected by Wharton's jelly, an umbilical cord has three vessels: two arteries and one vein. Oxygenated nutrient-rich blood is carried to a fetus by the umbilical vein and is distributed by the fetal heart throughout the body (Fig. 14.3). Deoxygenated blood and waste products circulate back to a placenta via two umbilical arteries. Three anatomic shunts, ductus venosus, foramen

ovale, and ductus arteriosus, allow fetal blood to bypass the fetal liver and lungs. The fetal heart circulates oxygenated blood throughout the fetal body (Moore et al., 2021).

? KNOWLEDGE CHECK

1. Describe how oxygen is carried from the environment to the fetus.
2. How much blood perfuses the uterus at 40 weeks' gestation?
3. Which umbilical cord vessel/vessels is/are responsible for carrying deoxygenated blood back from the fetus to the placenta?

FACTORS INFLUENCING FETAL HEART RATE REGULATION

From a physiologic perspective, FHR modulation is representative of the effects of extrinsic and intrinsic factors. Extrinsic

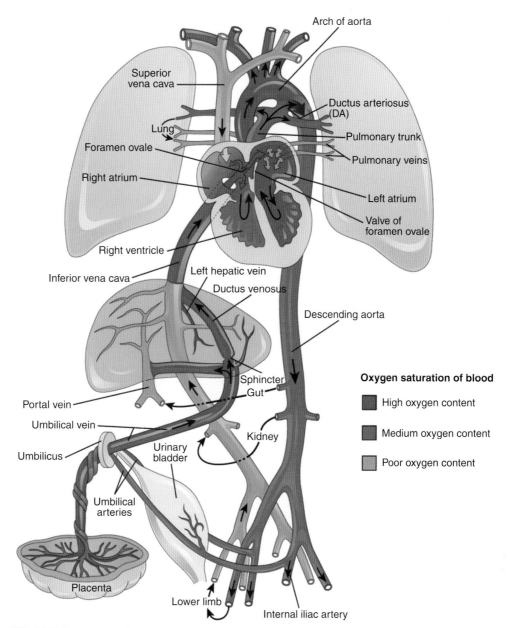

FIG. 14.3 Fetal Circulation. Red, purple, and blue colors in blood vessels depict the oxygen saturation of the blood. Arrows represent blood flow from the placenta to the fetal heart. A small amount of highly oxygenated blood from the inferior vena cava remains in the right atrium and mixes with poorly oxygenated blood from the superior vena cava. Blood with medium oxygenation then passes into the right ventricle. Three shunts (ductus venosus, foramen ovale, and ductus arteriosus) allow the majority of the blood to bypass the fetal liver and lungs. The poorly oxygenated blood returns to the placenta for oxygenation and nutrients through the umbilical arteries. (From Moore, K. L., Persaud, T. V. N., Persaud, M. D., Torchia, M. G. [2021]. Cardiovascular system. In K. Moore, M. Persaud, M. Torchia [Eds.]. *The developing human: Clinically oriented embryology.* [11th ed., pp. 263–314]. Elsevier.)

or "outside" influences are characteristics that affect blood flow. These include maternal, uteroplacental, umbilical circulation, and amniotic fluid features, which may potentially cause an interruption in fetal oxygenation. Intrinsic or an "inside" influence, such as the autonomic nervous system (ANS), assists with maintaining fetal homeostasis.

In the fetal medulla oblongata, the cardioregulatory center (CRC) is responsible for maintaining homeostasis and optimizing oxygen delivery to a fetus (Heuser, 2020; Fig. 14.4). Changes in fetal oxygen, carbon dioxide, or blood pressure

affect the CRC's ability to control FHR baseline, variability (irregular fluctuations of the baseline FHR), and other characteristics. The CRC coordinates input from intrinsic influences from the ANS, the parasympathetic and sympathetic branches, baroreceptors, chemoreceptors, hormonal influences, and other miscellaneous factors such as fetal sleep-wake cycles (Heuser, 2020; Miller et al., 2022; O'Brien-Abel, 2020). For instance, if a CRC detects hypoxic episodes related to tachysystole (more than 5 contractions in 10 minutes, averaged over 30 minutes) and recurrent FHR decelerations,

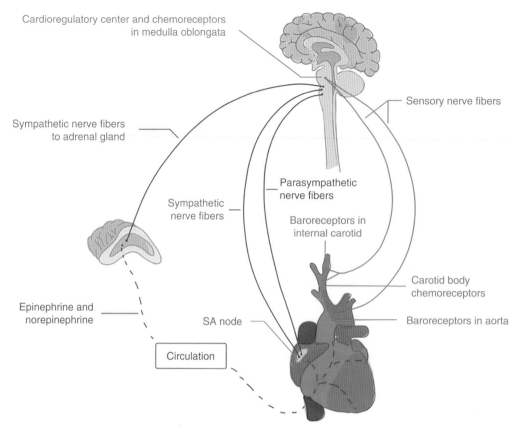

FIG. 14.4 Fetal Heart Rate Regulation. *SA*, Sinoatrial node. (From Heuser, C. C. [2020]. Physiology of fetal heart rate monitoring. *Clinical Obstetrics and Gynecology, 63*[3], 607–615.)

a signal will be sent to alter cardiac output and redistribute blood flow primarily to the vital organs described previously. Thus the FHR pattern represents the final product of the interplay between intrinsic and extrinsic factors.

Autonomic Nervous System

A human's greater nervous system is made up of four distinct structures: the central nervous system, peripheral nervous system, somatic nervous system, and autonomic nervous system (Bordelon et al., 2018). This neural network is complex because this set of connections communicates with other structures of the body, such as the cardiovascular system. Referred to as homeostasis, the neural network assists with maintaining physiologic stability when challenged by circumstances that can interrupt normal function.

The ANS is divided into two branches, parasympathetic and sympathetic, which are balancing forces influencing FHR characteristics (Heuser, 2020; O'Brien-Abel, 2020). The parasympathetic branch is an important mechanism in controlling FHR baseline and variability. Parasympathetic impulses originate in the CRC and are vagal in origin. Both branches of the vagus nerve innervate the sinoatrial and atrioventricular nodes within a fetal heart. When the vagus nerve is stimulated, the parasympathetic branch triggers a slowing of the FHR. The vagus nerve is also significantly involved with FHR variability, which is a direct result of sympathetic and parasympathetic effects on the heart. By the second and third trimesters, the parasympathetic nervous system has a greater

influence on variability. Variability is considered a critical predictor of adequate fetal oxygenation during labor for two reasons (Clark et al., 2013):

1. Adequate oxygenation promotes the normal function of the ANS and helps a fetus maintain homeostasis during labor.
2. Variability evaluates the function of the fetal ANS.

The sympathetic system assists with maintaining brain perfusion during interruptions in the oxygenation pathway, such as maternal hypotension or hemorrhage from a placenta previa (Heuser, 2020; O'Brien-Abel, 2020). This process of sympathetic impulses from the fetal myocardium and vasculature leads to vasoconstriction, hypertension, and increased cardiac output. The result is an increased FHR baseline. Sympathetic nerve terminals are also found in adrenal glands. When fetal oxygenation is inadequate, these glands will release catecholamines (epinephrine and norepinephrine), which also consequently leads to an increased FHR baseline.

Baroreceptors and Chemoreceptors

Furthermore, the CRC receives signals from other nerves and receptor types in the peripheral nervous system. These receptor types are referred to as baroreceptors and chemoreceptors (Heuser, 2020; O'Brien-Abel, 2020). Located in the carotid arch and aortic sinus, baroreceptors are pressure-sensitive stretch receptors that respond to subtle changes in fetal arterial blood pressure. Baroreceptors perceive these blood pressure alterations and send a signal to the brain. An

TABLE 14.1	Benefits and Limitations of Nonelectronic Fetal Monitoring	
	BENEFITS	**LIMITATIONS**
AUSCULTATION	Noninvasive: Does not require ruptured membranes or cervical examinations	Certain conditions may reduce ability to hear fetal heart rate (FHR; e.g., obesity, hydramnios, and client or fetal movement)
	Promotes "high-touch, low-tech" approach to care	Uterine tension during contraction may disrupt FHR assessment
	Capable of widespread application in antepartum and intrapartum settings with appropriate training	Cannot detect specific FHR characteristics (e.g., variability and deceleration types)
	Increased freedom of movement and ambulation for client	Clients may consider intermittent auscultation (IA) intrusive or disruptive
	Allows for FHR assessment during ambulation or alternative birthing locations (e.g., hydrotherapy)	No permanent record on paper tracing or computer archive system for review
	One-to-one nursing care that promotes an optimal environment that elevates the level of care	Creates a potential need to increase or realign staff to meet recommended 1:1 nurse to client ratio
	Inexpensive equipment compared with adjunct devices (e.g., fetal monitor)	Requires competency education, ongoing practice, and skill in auditory assessment
		Counting is intermittent, resulting in the potential to miss events that are a result of an interrupted oxygenation pathway (e.g., prolonged deceleration)
		Not recommended for high-risk pregnancies
PALPATION	Noninvasive: Does not require ruptured membranes or cervical examinations	Real-time intrauterine pressures cannot be detected
	Promotes the "high-touch, low-tech" approach to care	Certain conditions may limit ability to palpate contractions (e.g., obesity)
	Capable of having widespread application in antepartum and intrapartum settings	Subjective assessment; varies from examiner to examiner
	Increased freedom of movement and ambulation for client	Clients may consider palpation painful, intrusive, or disruptive
	Allows for FHR assessment during ambulation or alternative birthing locations (e.g., hydrotherapy)	No permanent record on paper tracing or computer archive system for review
	Inexpensive equipment compared with adjunct devices (e.g., intrauterine pressure catheter [IUPC])	

Adapted from Drummond, S. & Rust, C. (2021). Techniques for fetal heart and uterine activity assessment. In A. Lyndon & K. Wisner (Eds.), *Fetal heart rate monitoring: Principles and practices* (6th ed., pp. 83–116). Kendall-Hunt Publications; Miller, L.A., Miller, D. A., & Cypher, R. L. (2022). *Mosby's pocket guide to fetal monitoring: A multidisciplinary approach* (9th ed.). Elsevier; Wisner, K., & Holschuh, C. (2018). Fetal heart rate auscultation, 3rd ed. *Nursing for Women's Health, 22*(6), e1–e32.

increase in fetal blood pressure typically results in a decreased baseline rate. A falling blood pressure results in an increased FHR baseline that assists in resolving fetal hypotension. Chemoreceptors are located in the medulla oblongata and in the aortic and carotid bodies. Chemoreceptors are cells that are stimulated by changes in oxygen levels that lead to hypoxemia, acidosis, and hypercarbia. These receptor types also respond to physiologic changes by eliciting a sympathetic response. This response results in an increased sympathetic output, fetal tachycardia, and hypertension to improve fetal oxygenation.

Hormonal Influences

Hormones are circulated into the bloodstream by organs such as the adrenal glands, hypothalamus, pituitary gland, and other structures (Lagercrantz & Slotkin, 1986; O'Brien-Abel, 2021). Stressors, like uterine tachysystole, result in a release of hormones that assist with FHR regulation and perfusion of vital organs. Once the adrenal glands secrete

epinephrine and norepinephrine, there will be an increase in myocardial contraction force, an accelerated FHR, and improved arterial blood pressure, comparable to sympathetic branch stimulation. Decreases in fetal blood pressure cause the adrenal cortex to respond by releasing aldosterone and retaining sodium and water, which will increase circulating fetal blood volume.

FETAL HEART MONITORING AND UTERINE ACTIVITY INSTRUMENTATION

Historically, IA of the FHR and palpation of UA were the sole methods of intrapartum surveillance until the introduction of EFM in the late 1960s and early 1970s. Although IA and palpation continue to be a reasonable global approach to assessing fetal status in a low-risk laboring client, EFM technology has predominantly changed the approach to fetal surveillance in the United States. Each mode of monitoring has benefits and limitations, as outlined in Tables 14.1 and 14.2.

TABLE 14.2   Benefits and Limitations of External and Internal Electronic Fetal Monitoring

	BENEFITS	LIMITATIONS
Ultrasound Transducer	Noninvasive; does not require ruptured membranes or cervical examinations	Limits client mobility
	Easy to apply	Frequent repositioning of transducers is often needed to maintain an accurate tracing
	Provides continuous FHR recording	May double-count a slow FHR
		<60 bpm, resulting in an apparently normal FHR during a bradycardia or may half-count a FHR >180 bpm, resulting in an apparently normal FHR during tachycardia
	May be used during both the antepartum and intrapartum periods and with telemetry devices	Client's heart rate may be counted if transducer is placed over arterial vessels, such as the aorta
	No known risks to client or fetus	
	Provides a permanent record on a paper tracing or computer archive system for review	
Toco	Noninvasive; does not require ruptured membranes or cervical examinations	Provides information limited to frequency and duration of UA and does not assess strength or intensity
	Easy to apply	Obesity and preterm or multifetal gestations may be difficult to monitor
	Provides continuous UA recording	Location-sensitive; poor placement may lead to an absence or inadequate data
	May be used during both the antepartum and intrapartum periods and with telemetry devices	Sensitive to client or fetal movement that may be superimposed on the tracing
	No known risks to client or fetus	
	Provides a permanent record on a paper tracing or computer archive system for review	
FSE	Provides continuous FHR detection between 30 and 240 bpm when clinically required and not achievable by US transducer	Invasive: requires intrapartum cervical dilation, ruptured membranes, and an accessible and appropriate presenting part
	Positional changes do not usually affect FHR tracing quality	Contraindicated in placenta previa, herpes infection, HIV, and suspected or confirmed fetal hemophilia
	Provides a permanent record on paper tracing or computer archive system for review	Generally contraindicated in extreme prematurity or when infection such as hepatitis, group B hemolytic *Streptococcus*, syphilis, or gonorrhea are present
	Does not require repositioning to maintain accurate tracing	No opportunity for ambulation because telemetry is not available
		Expensive equipment compared with auscultation
		The pregnant client's heart rate may be recorded instead of FHR in the presence of an intrauterine fetal demise
		Fetal arrhythmias may not be evident if logic or ECG software is engaged
		Improper insertion may cause trauma to the pregnant client such as vaginal lacerations
		May increase risk for infection
IUPC	Provides continuous objective UA data (frequency, duration, intensity, resting tone, and relaxation time) when clinically required and not achievable by a toco	Invasive: requires adequate cervical dilation and ruptured membranes
	Provides a permanent record on paper tracing or computer archive system for review	May be contraindicated with infection where ruptured membranes is discouraged to prevent infection transmission (e.g., herpes, HIV) from the pregnant client to the fetus
	Provides ability to perform amnioinfusion or withdraw fluid for testing	Contraindicated with placenta previa or unknown vaginal bleeding
		No opportunity for ambulation as telemetry is not available
		Positional changes may affect quality of UA data
		Expensive equipment compared with palpation
		Improper insertion may cause trauma to the pregnant client or placenta

ECG, Electrocardiogram; *FHR,* fetal heart rate; *FSE,* fetal spiral electrode; *HIV,* human immunodeficiency virus; *IUPC,* intrauterine pressure catheter; *UA,* uterine activity; *US,* ultrasound.

Adapted from Drummond, S. & Rust, C. (2021). Techniques for fetal heart and uterine activity assessment. In A. Lyndon & K. Wisner (Eds.), *Fetal heart rate monitoring: Principles and practices* (6th ed., pp. 83-116). Kendall-Hunt Publications; Miller, L.A., Miller, D. A., & Cypher, R. L. (2022). *Mosby's pocket guide to fetal monitoring: A multidisciplinary approach* (9th ed.). Elsevier.

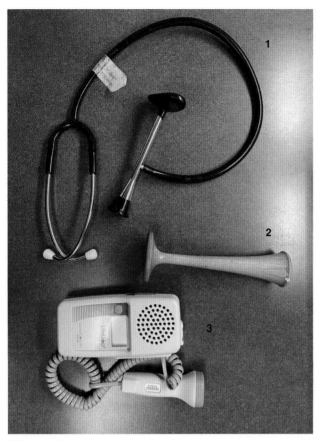

FIG. 14.5 Intermittent fetal heart rate auscultation devices shown top to bottom: 1. DeLee-Hillis fetoscope; 2. Pinard stethoscope; 3. Ultrasound Doppler with fetal heart rate *(FHR)* display. (Courtesy Michelle Hughes, MSN, APRN, CNM.)

Non-Electronic Monitoring
Intermittent Auscultation

Intermittent auscultation in conjunction with palpation is an effective method of surveillance if performed in a consistent manner in accordance with professional and hospital guidelines. This method of assessing FHR and rhythm is done with a Delee-Hillis fetoscope, Pinard stethoscope, or hand-held Doppler ultrasound (Drummond & Rust, 2021; Larry-Osman, 2021; Martis et al., 2017; Maude et al., 2010; Fig. 14.5). A DeLee-Hillis is a binaural (both ears) device with a stethoscope on one end, a head plate which allows for bone conduction to maximize FHR sounds, and a fetoscope at the opposite end. A Pinard stethoscope, sometimes referred to as a Pinard horn, is a monaural trumpet-shaped device. The large end is placed against the fetal back and a small end is placed adjacent to a clinician's ear (Fig. 14.6). Both devices auscultate the opening and closing of the fetal heart valves. A Doppler ultrasound emits sound waves to the level of the fetal heart and then bounces back to convert into sound. Doppler devices are often selected for IA.

Auscultation occurs at selected intervals based on a client's risk status and an obstetric unit's guidelines and policies. There is a lack of evidence of which IA method and counting intervals are best during labor (Blix et al., 2019). Procedure 14.1 describes a step-by-step approach to IA and includes

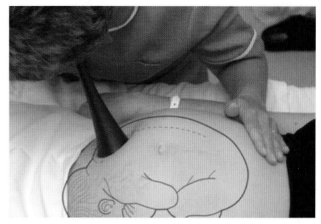

FIG. 14.6 After using Leopold's maneuver to identify the fetal part, a clinician auscultates the fetal heart rate with a Pinard stethoscope. (From Baston, H., & Hall, J. [2018]. Monitoring fetal well-being during routine antenatal care. In H. Baston, J. Hall [Eds.]. *Midwifery essentials: Antenatal.* [2nd ed., Vol. 2, pp. 142–159]. Elsevier.)

several examples of counting methods. Optimally, IA is performed between contractions and when a fetus is not actively moving (American College of Nurse-Midwives [ACNM], 2015; Wisner & Holschuh, 2018). Assessment can also be performed in the latter portion of a contraction and after a contraction for at least 15 to 30 seconds to detect increases or decreases. Generally, nurses listen and count for a set period of time, usually 15 to 60 seconds, to establish a rate. A radial pulse is simultaneously palpated to distinguish between the pregnant client's heart rate and FHR during auscultation.

In conjunction with calculating a FHR, a clinician will establish whether an auscultated rate is regular or irregular (ACNM, 2015; Wisner & Holschuh, 2018). An irregular rhythm is often distinguished as a pattern of skipped beats or pauses between heartbeats. Audible increases or decreases may be detected once a baseline rate has been established. More extended periods of counting may be required depending on the clinical situation. For example, suppose the FHR baseline is within normal limits but has changed significantly from the previous assessment. In that case, a longer listening period or more frequent assessments may clarify whether there is a change in baseline rate or a temporary increase or decrease. Additionally, EFM placement may be necessary to clarify an auscultated pattern, especially if there are fetal condition concerns.

Palpation

Palpation is a subjective method of assessing UA compared with external and internal UA monitoring. The uterus is a complex, smooth muscle organ that contracts and relaxes. During labor, this muscle rhythmically contracts, resulting in an increase in frequency, duration, and strength as labor progresses. Palpation uses light abdominal touch with the fingertips in a location where the uterus rises upward as a contraction develops. This area is generally over the fundal portion of the uterus, where maximal changes occur.

NURSING PROCEDURE 14.1　Fetal Heart Rate Auscultation

Explain the procedure to the client and assist them into a semi-Fowler's or wedged lateral position. Wash your hands with warm water to reduce microorganism transmission and to make your hands more comfortable for the client when touching their abdomen.

1. Use Leopold's maneuvers to identify the fetal lie (fetal long axis or back) (see Procedure 15.1).
   a. Assess FHR with a fetoscope or Doppler device. This is accomplished by moving the fetoscope until you locate where the FHR is loudest.
2. Fetoscope
   a. Delee-Hillis fetoscope: Place the bell over the fetal back with the head plate pressed against the nurse's forehead. The head plate and forehead maintain pressure during auscultation. The stethoscope section is placed in the nurse's ears.
   b. Pinard fetoscope: Place the larger end over the fetal back and the opposite smaller end to a nurse's ear.
3. Doppler device: Review manufacturer's instructions for directions on how to operate the Doppler device. Apply a small amount of water-soluble ultrasound transmission gel on the transducer end. Place the transducer over the fetal back, and reposition until audible clear sounds are located.
4. Palpate the client's radial pulse to verify the palpated heart rate is different from the auscultated FHR. If the pulse is synchronized with the sounds from the fetoscope or Doppler transducer, move the instrument to another location where there is maximum intensity of the fetal heart sounds. Other sounds that may be represented by the Doppler are the uterine souffle (blood flowing through the uterine vessels). This rate is synchronous with the client's pulse.
5. One suggested counting method to determine rate is to listen for at 30 seconds between uterine contractions and multiply by two. For example, if the detected rate in 30 seconds is 72, which is then multiplied by two, the rate for that time frame is 144 beats per minute (bpm). Another auscultation technique is to count for 15 seconds and multiply by 4. In other words, if 43 beats are counted in 15 seconds and multiplied by 4, the documented rate would be 172 bpm.
6. Determine whether the rate is regular or irregular.
7. Increases and decreases from the rate are by calculated with a multiple count strategy. One example is to count in consecutive 6-second intervals during audible changes and multiplying the rate by 10 to estimate FHR in beats per minute (bpm). Counting at 6-second intervals and multiplying each result by 10 give a sequence of numbers that can be averaged. Another option is to count in several 5- to 15-second increments. This method also provides a better picture of the depth and duration of a decrease in FHR while counting.
8. If there are distinct discrepancies during listening periods, auscultate for a longer period of time during, after, and between contractions.

RSA 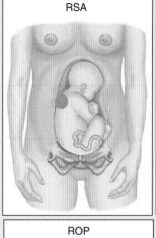　LSA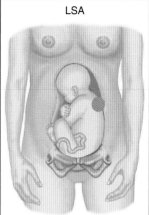

ROP 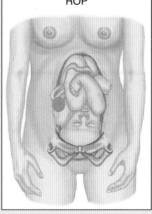　LOP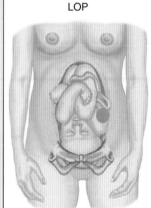

ROA 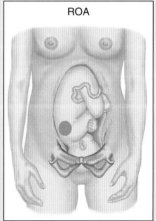　LOA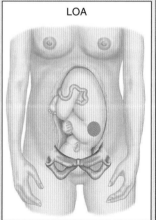

FHR, Fetal heart rate; *RSA,* right sacrum anterior; *LSA,* left sacrum anterior; *ROP,* right occiput posterior; *LOP,* left occiput posterior; *ROA,* right occiput anterior; *LOA,* left occiput anterior.

Adapted from American College of Nurse-Midwives. (2015). Clinical bulletin. No. 60. Intermittent auscultation for intrapartum fetal heart rate surveillance. *Journal of Nurse Midwifery & Women's Health, 61*(1), 626–632. https://doi.org/10.1111/jmwh.12372; Miller, L. A., Miller, D. A., & Cypher, R. L. (2022). *Mosby's pocket guide to fetal monitoring: A multidisciplinary approach* (9th ed.). Elsevier; Wisner, K., & Holschuh, C. (2018). Fetal heart rate auscultation, 3rd ed. *Nursing for Women's Health, 22*(6), e1–e32.

NURSING PROCEDURE 14.2   Palpating Contractions

1. Explain the procedure to the client and support person, and wash your hands with warm water. Assess at least three sequential contractions at the time the fetal heart rate (FHR) is checked (See Chapter 15 for recommended frequency of assessments).
2. Place fingertips of one hand on the uterine fundus, using light pressure. Keep fingertips relatively still rather than moving them over the uterus.
3. Note the time when each contraction begins and ends.
   a. Determine frequency: the time in minutes from the beginning of one contraction to the beginning of the next one. Normal frequency is less than or equal to five contractions in 10 minutes, averaged over 30 minutes.
   b. Determine duration: the time in seconds from the beginning to the end of each contraction.
   c. Determine relaxation time interval: the time in seconds between the end of one contraction and the beginning of the next one.
4. Estimate the average intensity of contractions by noting how easily the uterus can be indented during the peak of the contraction:
   a. With mild contractions, the uterus can be easily indented with the fingertips. The contractions feel similar to the tip of the nose.
   b. With moderate contractions, the uterus is firm and is indented with more difficulty. The contractions feel similar to the chin.

c. With strong contractions, the uterus feels rigid or board-like and cannot be readily indented. The contractions feel similar to the forehead.
5. Estimate the resting tone of the uterus in the absence of contractions or between contractions:
   a. Palpation or Toco: soft or relaxed and firm are used to describe resting tone.
   b. Intrauterine pressure catheter (IUPC): recorded in mm Hg. Palpation is used to confirm the mm Hg reading. Normal resting tone with an IUPC is approximately 10 mm Hg and generally not greater than 20 to 25 mm Hg.
6. Report excessive uterine activity. Excessive uterine activity reduces placental blood flow by prolonged compression of the vessels that supply the intervillous spaces.
   a. Tachysystole—More than five contractions in 10 minutes, averaged over 30 minutes.
   b. Tetanic contractions—Series of single contractions with durations longer than 120 seconds.
   c. Inadequate relaxation time—Intervals shorter than 60 seconds between contractions in first-stage labor; less than 45 to 50 seconds between contractions in second stage.
   d. Hypertonus—Incomplete relaxation of the uterus between contractions; resting tone greater than 20 to 25 mm Hg with an IUPC or a uterus that does not return to soft on palpation.

Palpation allows for an assessment of UA characteristics, especially strength (Procedure 14.2). Comparative differences between client perception, manual palpation, and internal monitoring are illustrated in Fig. 14.7.

Descriptive terms such as soft, mild, moderate, and strong or firm are used in clinical practice (Miller et al., 2022). Soft is described as a uterus that is not taut. Mild is the terminology used to describe a uterine fundus that is tense but easily indented, similar to the tip of a soft nose. Moderate contractions palpate as firm and are difficult to indent, comparable to touching a chin. Strong contractions often feel rigid and are challenging to indent, similar to palpating a forehead.

Electronic Monitoring

This monitoring mode can recognize, analyze, and display specific information regarding FHR, UA, and the pregnant client's vital signs. Electronic monitoring may be external, internal, or a combination of both methods. External FHR and UA monitoring collects data via transducers applied to a client's abdomen. Internal monitoring uses devices placed on a fetal presenting part (i.e., vertex or buttock) to monitor FHR or within the uterine cavity to measure intrauterine pressure.

Equipment

Typical instrumentation for EFM includes a bedside monitor, transducers with or without cables, blood pressure cuff, pulse oximeter sensor to measure oxygen saturation, and other equipment to attach internal monitoring devices or measure

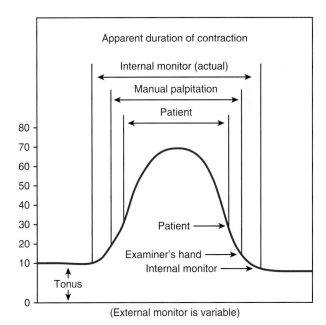

FIG. 14.7 Comparison of uterine contraction sensitivity by client perception, palpation, and internal monitoring with an intrauterine pressure catheter. Contraction sensitivity. (From Freeman, R. K., Garite, T. J., Nageotte, M. P., & Miller, L. A. [2012]. *Fetal heart rate monitoring*. [4th ed.] Lippincott Williams & Wilkins.)

the pregnant client's electrocardiographic status (Fig. 14.8). Data are collected and converted to a visual display in the form of numerical values (Fig. 14.9). A graphic strip of the

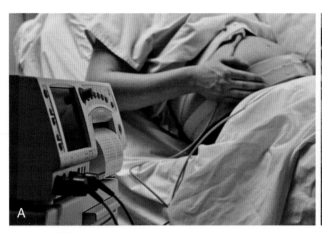
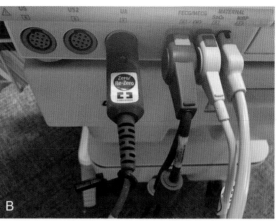

FIG. 14.8 (A) Bedside electronic fetal monitor printing a paper tracing. The external ultrasound transducer is secured with the pink belt, and the tocotransducer is held in place with the blue belt. (B) The front panel display and cable inputs for an electronic fetal monitor. In this example, cables plugged into UA and FECG are measuring uterine activity and fetal heart rate with internal devices. Ultrasound 1 and ultrasound 2 are not in use. Cables inserted into SpO_2 and NIBP are collecting oxygen saturation and blood pressure data. (A–B, Courtesy GE Healthcare)

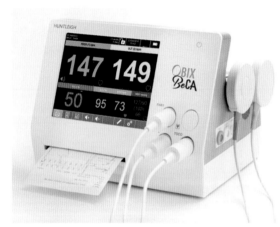

FIG. 14.9 Electronic fetal monitor with a visual monitor display of maternal and fetal data that can be transmitted to a central monitoring system. A paper printout of fetal surveillance information is also shown. Regardless of whether the tracing is on paper or a computer screen, both methods allow clinicians to collaborate together to problem solve, make clinical decisions, and set priorities depending on fetal heart rate *(FHR)* and uterine activity *(UA)* interpretation and the stage of labor. (Courtesy OBIX by Clinical Computer Systems, Inc.)

data is displayed at the bedside on either a paper tracing, computer screen, or both. Modern monitoring systems can simultaneously record twin and triplet heart rates. State-of-the-art obstetric units may also have wireless monitoring equipment that collects continuous data to be transmitted to a base station for interpretation. Wireless systems allow clients to ambulate in labor and may also be used during hydrotherapy (e.g., labor tub).

Integrated fetal surveillance systems are alternatives to traditional external monitoring. Newer equipment can incorporate fetal electrocardiogram (ECG) and uterine electrohysterography into a singular piece of technology (Fig. 14.10). Integrated monitoring systems do not replace traditional internal FHR or UA monitoring when clinically indicated, such as when intrauterine pressure measurements are required to calculate Montevideo units for oxytocin management. Wireless, adhesive patches, similar to adult electrocardiogram pads, are placed on the client's abdomen in several locations. These patches collect electrical activity emitted from the client's heart rate, fetal R-R heart rate intervals, and uterine contraction activity (Monson et al., 2020). Next, the monitor filters and converts the abdominal signals to electrophysiologic data. The client's heart rate, FHR, and UA is then transmitted wirelessly in a digital format, via Bluetooth technology, to a monitor interface (Monica Healthcare, 2018). Data are then displayed on the fetal monitor and central display. These monitoring systems have been found to be beneficial in the obese population when signal loss is problematic with Doppler technology (Monson et al., 2020; Vlemminx et al., 2018).

Computer screens allow remote surveillance from centralized locations like a nursing station or an office in an outpatient clinic. Audible and visual alerts are adjusted for upper and lower limit values of client vital signs and baseline FHR and for signal quality. Contemporary systems may also have clinical support tools that assist health care team members. For example, one perinatal software solution program can assess UA frequency to determine the presence or absence of tachysystole. Another electronic tool uses visual cues to highlight specific FHR characteristics like fetal bradycardia or tachycardia.

An external FHR is obtained by Doppler transducer ("ultrasound"), and UA is acquired by a tocodynamometer or tocotransducer ("toco"). External monitoring, also

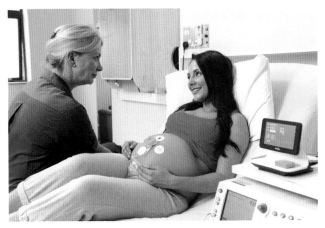

FIG. 14.10 Wireless patch system that collects electrical activity emitted from maternal and fetal heart rate and uterine contraction activity. (Courtesy GE Healthcare.)

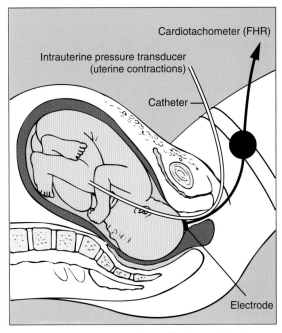

FIG. 14.11 Internal mode of monitoring with intrauterine pressure catheter and spiral electrode attached to the fetal scalp. (From Perry, S. E., Hockenberry, M. J., Cashion, M. C., Alden, K. R., Olshansky, & E., Lowdermilk, D. L. [2023]. Maternal Child Nursing Care, [7th ed.] Elsevier.)

called indirect or noninvasive monitoring, can be used at any time because cervical dilation and ruptured membranes are not necessary for placement (Drummond & Rust, 2021; Miller et al., 2022). Both devices are held in place with either an elastic abdominal belt, an abdominal belly band, or adhesive patches attached to the transducer when wireless monitoring is used for fetal surveillance. Recording FHR requires a small amount of ultrasound conduction gel to be applied on the Doppler surface. Gel assists in transmission of high-frequency sound waves to the fetal heart level where motion is detected. Sound waves then bounce back and are recorded by a monitor's microprocessors. Applying a small amount is an important consideration because too much gel causes a transducer to frequently slide on the client's abdomen, making signal contact difficult. Additionally, excessive gel use is messy, a source of skin irritation, and wasteful.

Before monitor placement, Leopold's maneuver (See Procedure 15.1) can be used to confirm the location of the fetal back. The ultrasound transducer is placed where the point of maximum intensity of the FHR can be heard. Throughout labor, the transducer may need to be readjusted to optimize signal contact. Nurses are also responsible for ensuring the signal being received is the FHR and not the pregnant client's pulse rate. Unfortunately, when Doppler technology is used with EFM transducer, it is susceptible to more periods of inadequate signal quality and to maternal-fetal heart rate misidentification and artifact compared with internal monitoring (Cypher, 2019b). In other words, current EFM equipment can and will monitor and record a maternal heart rate that appears as an FHR pattern.

A toco is required to detect UA. This device is usually placed on the fundus or in a location where contraction intensity is easily palpable. Similar to the ultrasound device, a toco may need to be readjusted during the intrapartum period. Furthermore, a toco does not require ultrasound conduction gel because a pressure-sensitive button identifies changes in uterine shape during contractions or with movement of the pregnant client or fetus.

Internal fetal monitoring requires a fetal spiral electrode (FSE) to record FHR and an intrauterine pressure catheter (IUPC) to document UA (Fig. 14.11). Internal monitoring is referred to as direct or invasive fetal monitoring because this method requires adequate cervical dilation and ruptured membranes (Drummond & Rust, 2021; Miller et al., 2022). Electrodes are applied directly to a fetal presenting part (head or buttocks) and never placed intentionally on the fetal genitalia, face, fontanels, or an unidentified presenting part. Furthermore, a FSE is not deliberately placed in the presence of a known placenta previa, suspected or confirmed hemophilia, human immunodeficiency virus (HIV), and herpes infections. Fetal benefit versus fetal risk is taken into consideration when electrode placement is being contemplated in cases of extreme prematurity or in the presence of an infection such as hepatitis, group B hemolytic *Streptococcus* infection, syphilis, or gonorrhea. Each electrode measures, processes, and records the R-to-R interval in a QRS complex of the FHR. The opposite end of the electrode is attached to a pad and secured on the thigh or lower abdomen. A cable is attached to the pad and plugged into a fetal monitor.

When a tracing warrants better assessment of frequency, duration, intensity, resting tone, and relaxation time, an IUPC may be inserted transcervically into the uterus. There are two IUPC types: transducer-tipped and air-coupled sensor–tipped. These flexible catheters provide an objective measurement of UA by calculating intrauterine pressure in millimeters of mercury (mm Hg). These pressures are displayed on the fetal monitor.

Fetal Monitoring Tracing

As mentioned previously, FHR and UA data are either printed on a paper tracing or displayed on a computer screen. Regardless of the mode, each tracing has an x-axis and y-axis with an upper and lower graph (Fig. 14.12). FHR data are traced on an upper graph, which is vertically scaled in beats per minute (bpm). UA information is recorded on the lower graph and is scaled in mm Hg. The x-axis on the upper and lower graphs reveals thin, light, vertical lines representing 10-second intervals. Every 60 seconds, a thick, dark vertical line is printed, indicating each 1-minute interval. The y-axis on the upper graph has thin, light horizontal lines, which signify FHR in increments of 10 bpm ranging from 30 to 240 bpm. Similarly, the y-axis on the lower graph records uterine pressure in increments of 5 mm Hg, spanning from 0 to 100 mm Hg (Miller et al., 2022).

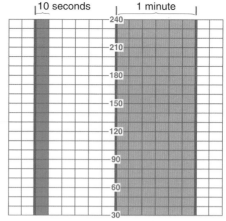
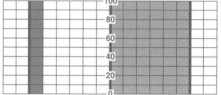

FIG. 14.12 Electronic fetal monitoring data that is displayed on paper, a computer screen, or both. (From Miller, L. A., Miller, D. A., & Cypher, R. L. [2022]. *Mosby's pocket guide to fetal monitoring: A multidisciplinary approach.* [9th ed.]. Elsevier.)

KNOWLEDGE CHECK

4. Name three advantages and limitations of external and internal electronic fetal monitoring (EFM).
5. What are five descriptive terms used to characterize uterine activity (UA) resting tone and strength when palpation is used?
6. Which grid on a paper tracing or computer monitor is used to record fetal heart rate (FHR) and which is used to record uterine activity (UA) data?
7. Which EFM sensor uses heart motion to measure FHR?
8. What are two factors that may affect tocodynamometry accuracy?

FETAL HEART RATE INTERPRETATION

EFM was introduced several decades ago without a nationally agreed on statement regarding standardized definitions and interpretation. Lack of standardization is a key obstacle in effective communication and has the potential to lead to adverse perinatal and neonatal outcomes. Today's clinicians use the National Institute of Child Health and Development (NICHD) consensus statement, which standardizes FHR and UA nomenclature and describes a three-tier system for categorization of FHR patterns (Macones et al., 2008). Multiple professional organizations have endorsed this document. In addition, three fundamental elements of a systematic approach to EFM can be used to facilitate effective communication, promote client safety, and allow health care professionals to strive for optimal outcomes (Miller et al., 2022). These include: (1) *standardized definitions* or nomenclature to define FHR and UA characteristics; (2)

interpretation or the physiologic significance of FHR and UA characteristics; and (3) *management* or clinical response to FHR and UA characteristics.

Baseline Fetal Heart Rate

A baseline FHR is the approximate mean FHR rounded to 5-bpm increments during a 10-minute period (Macones et al., 2008). In this 10-minute assessment, accelerations, decelerations, and periods of marked variability are excluded. Furthermore, a minimum of 2 minutes of identifiable baseline segments that do not need to be contiguous must be present. If a 2-minute period is uninterpretable, the FHR baseline is considered indeterminate. The previous 10-minute period may need to be reviewed to establish a baseline. Baseline (BL) rates are defined as follows:

- Normal: BL rate 110 to 160 bpm (Fig. 14.13)
- Bradycardia: BL rate less than 110 bpm (Fig. 14.14)
- Tachycardia: BL rate greater than 160 bpm (Fig. 14.15)

BL FHR is an integration of several physiologic influences, including cardiac pacemakers and conduction pathways, the ANS, and intrinsic and extrinsic factors (Blackburn, 2018; Lyndon & O-Brien-Abel, 2021; Miller et al., 2022). The fetal heart's sinoatrial node and intrinsic pacemaker generate the actual BL rate. Physiologic control of a FHR baseline and subsequent features interpreted on a tracing are different in a preterm fetus than a term or postterm fetus (Afors & Chandraharan, 2011). Preterm fetuses often average a rate at the upper end of normal (e.g., 155 bpm)

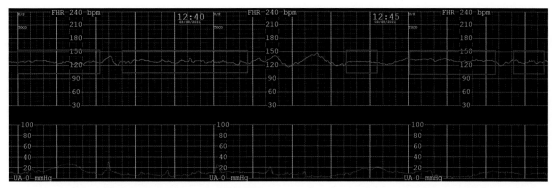

FIG. 14.13 Normal Fetal Heart Rate Baseline. Blue squares represent the identifiable sections of the tracing that represent the fetal heart rate *(FHR)* baseline *(BL)*. In this example, the FHR BL is 130 beats per minute *(bpm)*. (Courtesy OBIX by Clinical Computer Systems, Inc.)

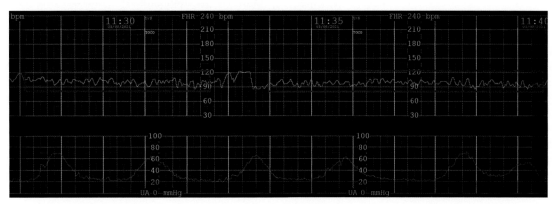

FIG. 14.14 Bradycardia. Blue squares represent the identifiable sections of the tracing that represent the fetal heart rate *(FHR)* baseline *(BL)*. In this example, the FHR BL is 100 beats per minute *(bpm)*. (Courtesy OBIX by Clinical Computer Systems, Inc.)

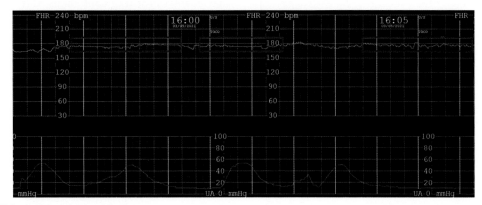

FIG. 14.15 Tachycardia. Blue squares represent the identifiable sections of the tracing that represent the fetal heart rate *(FHR)* baseline *(BL)*. In this example, the FHR BL is 175 beats per minute *(bpm)*. (Courtesy OBIX by Clinical Computer Systems, Inc.)

because the sympathetic branch of the ANS is more dominant. Term fetuses can have a parasympathetic branch that is more dominant. These fetuses may have a FHR baseline at the lower end of normal (e.g., 120 bpm). Potential causes of FHR bradycardia and tachycardia are presented in Boxes 14.1 and 14.2.

Baseline Fetal Heart Rate Variability

BL FHR variability is determined in a 10-minute window, excluding periodic and episodic changes (Macones et al.,

2008). Variability is defined as fluctuations in the BL rate, which are *irregular* in amplitude and frequency. These fluctuations are visually quantitated as the amplitude of the peak-to-trough in bpm. Variability is classified as follows:

- Absent: Amplitude range visually undetectable (Fig. 14.16A)
- Minimal: Amplitude range visually detectable but 5 bpm or less (see Fig. 14.16B)
- Moderate: Amplitude range 6 bpm to 25 bpm (see Fig. 14.16C)

BOX 14.1 Potential Causes of Fetal Heart Rate Bradycardia

Client
  Sympatholytic medications (methyldopa)
  Beta blockers (labetalol [Normodyne], propranolol)
  Sjögren's antibodies
  Hypoglycemia
  Hypothermia
  Viral infection (cytomegalovirus)
Fetal
  Cardiac conduction abnormalities
  Heart block
  Fetal heart failure (hydrops)
  Structural cardiac defects
  Heterotaxia
  Hypothyroidism
  Interrupted fetal oxygenation pathway (umbilical cord prolapse)

BOX 14.2 Potential Cause of Fetal Heart Rate Tachycardia

Client
  Beta-sympathomimetic drugs (terbutaline, epinephrine)
  Parasympatholytic drugs
  Dehydration
  Fever
  Hyperthyroidism
  Infection (chorioamnionitis, appendicitis)
  Cocaine
Fetal
  Acute blood loss
  Fetal anemia
  Heart failure
  Hyperthyroidism
  Hypoxia/hypoxemia
  Increased metabolic rate
  Infection and fetal sepsis
  Tachyarrhythmias

• Marked: Amplitude range greater than 25 bpm (see Fig. 14.16D)

Absent variability with a normal BL rate and an absence of decelerations may represent a preexisting neurologic injury in a fetus (American College of Obstetricians and Gynecologists [ACOG] & American Academy of Pediatrics [AAP], 2014). Both absent and minimal variability can be a sensitive indicator of abnormal fetal acid–base status when found in conjunction with recurrent variable or late decelerations or bradycardia (ACOG, 2019; Esplin, 2020; Parer et al., 2006). On the other hand, the continuum of FHR variability often includes periods of minimal and moderate cycles throughout the labor process (ACOG, 2019). Minimal variability without concomitant decelerations does not reliably predict fetal hypoxemia or metabolic acidemia because there may be other pathologic and nonpathologic causes. These include, but are not limited to, prematurity; medications such as opioids,

magnesium sulfate, and other analgesics; quiet sleep in fetal sleep–wake cycles; congenital anomalies; fetal anemia; fetal cardiac arrhythmias; infection; and preexisting antepartum neurologic injury (ACOG, 2019; ACOG & AAP, 2014; Miller et al., 2022; Timor-Tritsch et al., 1978). Moderate variability reliably predicts the absence of fetal metabolic acidemia at the time it is observed (Macones et al., 2008). This type of variability represents adequate FHR neuromodulation, normal cardiac responsiveness, and normal acid–base status (Parer et al., 2006). In fact, moderate variability in the presence of decelerations has a 98% association with an umbilical pH greater than 7.15 or an Apgar score of at least 7 at 5 minutes. Marked variability is a rare pattern and may be a normal variant or autonomic response to transient interruptions in the oxygenation pathway (Polnaszek et al., 2020). Marked variability is associated with increased respiratory distress. Therefore this type of variability is interpreted in conjunction with other observed FHR characteristics.

Sinusoidal patterns are described as a visually apparent, smooth, sine wave–like undulating pattern in a FHR baseline (Macones et al., 2008) (Fig. 14.17). This wavy pattern occurs with a frequency of three to five cycles per minute that persist for at least 20 minutes. Sinusoidal patterns are excluded from variability definitions because this pattern is characterized by FHR fluctuations that are *regular* in amplitude and frequency. Clinicians sometimes find this pattern difficult to differentiate from other types of variability. A reasonable approach in this situation is to remember variability is irregular in amplitude and frequency, whereas a sinusoidal pattern is more regular in appearance (Miller et al., 2022). The particular type of pattern may be intermittent or continuous with an absence of accelerations, UA responses, and fetal movement with or without stimulation (Modanlou & Freeman, 1982). True sinusoidal patterns are extremely rare and are indicative of a compromised fetus that requires immediate attention to optimize perinatal outcomes (Lyndon & O'Brien-Abel, 2021; Macones et al., 2008; Modanlou & Freeman, 1982; Mondanlou & Murata, 2004). Several potential etiologies for this unique pattern have been identified (Mondanlou & Murata, 2004; Reddy et al., 2009) (Box 14.3).

Sinusoidal *appearing* patterns are different than *true sinusoidal* patterns because the characteristic undulating pattern is observed with opioid administration, fetal sleep cycles, thumb sucking, or rhythmic fetal mouth movements (Lyndon & O'Brien-Abel, 2021; Mondanlou & Murata, 2004). This type of pattern is typically short in duration and resolves as the medication is excreted, when the fetus awakens, or when the fetus stops sucking. More importantly, sinusoidal *appearing* patterns are preceded and followed by normal FHR characteristics, such as moderate variability or accelerations compared with a *true* sinusoidal pattern. Common medications associated with sinusoidal *appearing* patterns include fentanyl, butorphanol, and meperidine. The term *pseudosinusoidal* has been used historically to describe a sinusoidal-appearing pattern after medication administration. This term is not defined in standardized EFM nomenclature and has been abandoned for documentation and communication purposes.

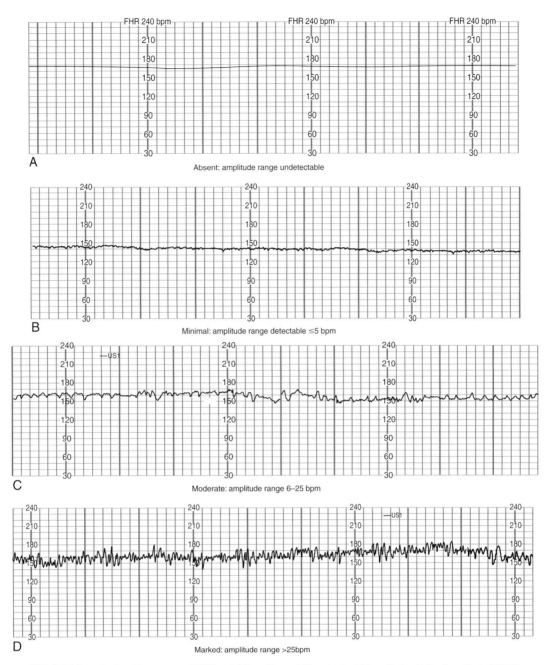

FIG 14.16 A–D, Fetal heart rate *(FHR)* variability. (From Miller, L. A., Miller, D. A., & Cypher, R. L. [2022]. *Mosby's pocket guide to fetal monitoring: A multidisciplinary approach.* [9th ed.]. Elsevier.)

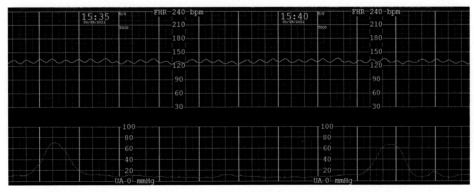

FIG. 14.17 Sinusoidal Pattern. (Courtesy OBIX by Clinical Computer Systems, Inc.)

Periodic and Episodic Fetal Heart Rate Patterns

FHR patterns are classified as BL, periodic, or episodic (Macones et al., 2008). Periodic and episodic patterns are characterized by a relationship to uterine contractions. Periodic patterns are associated with uterine contractions, whereas episodic patterns occur independently of contractions. Periodic patterns are further differentiated from each other based on whether the onset is "abrupt" or "gradual." Abrupt waveforms are quantified as having an onset to a deceleration nadir (lowest point) or onset to acceleration peak in less than 30 seconds. Gradual waveforms take 30 seconds or more from onset to a deceleration nadir. Furthermore, decelerations are defined as recurrent patterns that occur with 50% or more of uterine contractions in any 20-minute period.

Accelerations

Accelerations are defined as visually apparent abrupt increases, for less than 30 seconds, in the FHR from onset to peak and are generally determined in reference to the adjacent BL (Macones et al., 2008). An acceleration peak must be at least 15 bpm above BL, with the entire acceleration lasting at least 15 seconds from onset to return to BL. An acceleration peak does not need to last 15 seconds (Fig. 14.18). In gestations that are less than 32 weeks, an acceleration peak must be at least 10 bpm above the baseline and last at least 10 seconds from onset to return. The acceleration peak is not required to last 10 seconds in the preterm gestation. Accelerations may be periodic or episodic. A prolonged acceleration is 2 or more minutes but less than 10 minutes in duration. Anything greater than 10 minutes is a change in BL. The physiologic mechanism of accelerations is related to stimulation of peripheral nerves, increased catecholamine release, and autonomic stimulation of the fetal heart (Heuser, 2020). Accelerations are also primarily mediated by the sympathetic nervous system and are often a result of fetal movement, vibroacoustic stimulation, or fetal scalp stimulation during a vaginal examination. The goal of scalp stimulation is to elicit an FHR acceleration, which is suggestive of adequate oxygenation and normal acid–base balance. Scalp stimulation is used to evaluate fetal response to gentle tactile stimulation through a dilated cervix and is performed in baseline segments and not during decelerations or bradycardia (Cypher, 2021; Harvey, 1987; Miller, 2016; Miller et al., 2022). This procedure is not a corrective intervention and is only executed when an indeterminate FHR tracing is observed. An absence of an acceleratory response is an indeterminate finding and does not rule out a previous neurologic injury (Ahn et al., 1998; Clark et al., 1984; Cypher, 2021; Skupski et al., 2002).

Accelerations, spontaneous or induced, are predictive of adequate central fetal oxygenation and reliably predict the absence of acidemia at the time of observation (ACOG & AAP, 2014; Heuser, 2020; Macones et al., 2008). Accelerations are predictive of a fetal pH of at least 7.19, which rules out acidemia at the time of observation (Clark et al., 1982; Clark et al., 1984; Lyndon & O'Brien-Abel, 2021; Williams & Galerneau, 2003). An absence of accelerations does not reliably predict fetal acidemia (Macones et al., 2008).

Early Decelerations

Early decelerations (Fig. 14.19A–C) are defined as visually apparent decelerations that are usually symmetric in shape

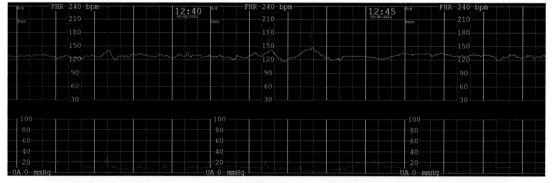

FIG. 14.18 Acceleration of the Fetal Heart Rate. The blue arrows point to each acceleration. Note the peak of the acceleration is at least 15 beats per minute (bpm) above the baseline rate of 125 bpm, lasting at least 15 seconds or more from the onset to return. (Courtesy OBIX by Clinical Computer Systems, Inc.)

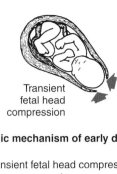

Transient
fetal head
compression

Physiologic mechanism of early deceleration

Transient fetal head compression
↓
Altered intracranial pressure and/or cerebral blood flow
↓
Reflex parasympathetic outflow
↓
Gradual slowing of the FHR
↓
Early deceleration
↓
A   When head compression is relieved, autonomic reflexes subside   B

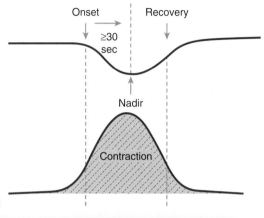

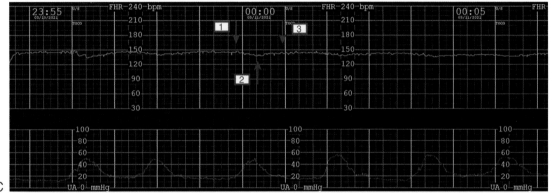

FIG. 14.19 Early Decelerations. (A) The physiologic mechanism of early decelerations is attributed to transient head compression that occurs with uterine contractions. (B) Schematic drawing of an early deceleration. (C) Early deceleration showing blue arrows that represent onset (1) to nadir (2) in more than 30 seconds, with both onset and recovery coincident with the onset and recovery (3) of the contraction. (A, From Miller, L. A., Miller, D. A., & Cypher, R. L. [2022]. *Mosby's pocket guide to fetal monitoring: A multidisciplinary approach.* [9th ed.]. Elsevier; B, From Intrapartum assessment. [2018]. In F. Cunningham, K. J. Leveno, S. L. Bloom, J. S. Dashe, B. L. Hoffman, B. M. Casey, C. Y. Spong [Eds.], *William's obstetrics.* [24th ed., pp. 473–503]. McGraw-Hill; C, Courtesy OBIX by Clinical Computer Systems, Inc.)

(Macones et al., 2008). There is a *gradual* decrease of 30 seconds or more from onset to nadir. Deceleration onset, nadir, and recovery *coincide with,* or mirror, the beginning, peak, and ending of a contraction. Early decelerations are thought to represent a vagal response during fetal head compression and are clinically benign with no known relationship to fetal oxygenation (ACOG & AAP, 2014; Heyborne, 2017; Lyndon & O'Brien-Abel, 2021). The exact physiologic mechanism is unknown but is thought to represent a fetal autonomic response to changes in intracranial pressure or cerebral blood flow during uterine contractions. Corrective measures are not indicated for this type of deceleration, but a complete assessment of deceleration timing is warranted because clinicians may confuse this pattern with late decelerations.

Late Decelerations

Similar to early decelerations, late decelerations (Fig. 14.20, A–C) have a visually apparent *gradual* decrease of 30 seconds

or more from onset to nadir (Macones et al., 2008). Late decelerations are also symmetric in shape and are considered a periodic pattern. In most cases, the onset, nadir, and recovery of the deceleration occur *after* the beginning, peak, and end of a uterine contraction.

Physiologically, late decelerations are representative of a fetal reflex response to transient hypoxemia during uterine contractions (Miller et al., 2022). There is a decreased delivery of oxygenated blood into the intervillous space because uteroplacental vessels are compressed during uterine activity. This results in reduced oxygen diffusion into fetal capillary blood and chorionic villi, leading to decreased fetal Po_2. Chemoreceptors detect this change and signal the brainstem to initiate a protective reflex response. A sympathetic outflow causes peripheral vasoconstriction and shunting of blood volume to vital organs (heart, brain, and adrenal glands). Increased peripheral resistance leads to higher mean arterial blood pressure, which results in a baroreceptor-mediated

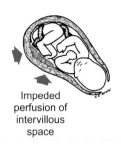

Impeded
perfusion of
intervillous
space

Physiologic mechanism of late deceleration

Uterine contraction impedes
maternal perfusion of the
placental intervillous space
↓
Transient fetal hypoxemia ———→
↓
Chemoreceptor stimulation
↓
Reflex sympathetic outflow
↓
Peripheral vasoconstriction, preferentially
shunting oxygenated blood away from the
peripheral tissues and toward central vital
organs: brain, heart, adrenal glands
↓
Increase in fetal peripheral resistance
and blood pressure
↓
Baroreceptor stimulation
↓
Reflex parasympathetic outflow
↓
Gradual slowing of the FHR
↓
Late deceleration ←——————
↓
After the contraction, these reflexes subside

Note: In the presence
of fetal metabolic
acidemia, transient
hypoxemia may result
in myocardial hypoxia
and a late deceleration
secondary to direct
myocardial depression

A

B

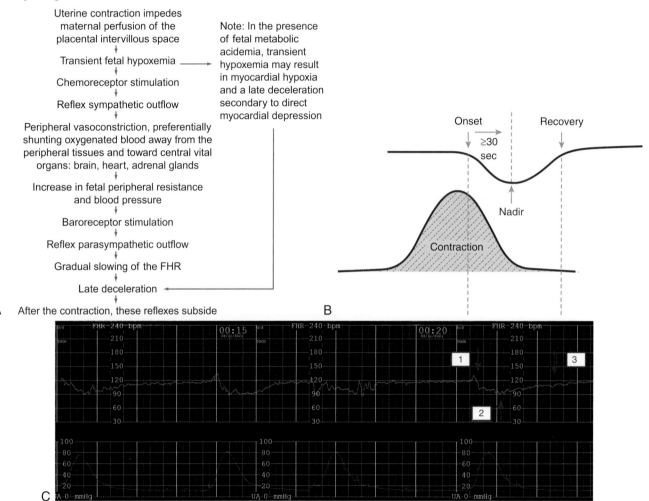

C

FIG. 14.20 Late Decelerations. (A) The physiologic mechanism of late decelerations is attributed to a reflex response to transient hypoxemia during a uterine contraction (uteroplacental). (B) Schematic drawing of a late deceleration. (C) Late deceleration showing blue arrows that represent gradual onset (30 seconds or more) (1) to nadir (2) occurring after the contraction peak, and recovery (3). Onset, nadir, and recovery occur after the beginning, peak, and ending of the contraction. (A, From Miller, L. A., Miller, D. A., & Cypher, R. L. [2022]. *Mosby's pocket guide to fetal monitoring: A multidisciplinary approach.* [9th ed.]. Elsevier; B, From *Intrapartum assessment.* [2018]. In F. Cunningham, K. J. Leveno, S. L. Bloom, J. S. Dashe, B. L. Hoffman, B. M. Casey, C. Y. Spong [Eds.], *William's obstetrics.* [24th ed., pp. 473–503]. McGraw-Hill; C, Courtesy OBIX by Clinical Computer Systems, Inc.)

reflex. The FHR decreases to reduce cardiac output and return fetal blood pressure to a normal range. The FHR returns to a BL rate after a contraction ends. Other potential factors associated with late decelerations in the context of uterine contractions include (Blackburn, 2018; Lyndon & O'Brien-Abel, 2021; Miller et al., 2022):
- Maternal hypertension (chronic or pregnancy-related)

- Maternal hypotension (e.g., supine positioning, hypovolemia, regional anesthesia, or medication administration such as antihypertensives)
- Illicit drug use, which results in tachysystole (e.g., amphetamines or cocaine)
- Placental changes: postmaturity (calcification), abruption, tobacco use by the pregnant client

- Chronic maternal disease processes (e.g., cardiopulmonary disease, diabetes, anemia)

A late deceleration reflects an interruption of the oxygen pathway from the environment to the fetus during uterine contractions, resulting in transient fetal hypoxemia (Miller et al., 2022). Late decelerations with moderate variability do not suggest significant fetal acidemia at the time of observation. Most will resolve when the source of hypoxemia, such as maternal hypotension or tachysystole, is corrected. In contrast, late decelerations with minimal or absent variability are associated with a higher probability of abnormal fetal acid–base balance (Parer et al., 2006). Over time, recurrent or sustained oxygen pathway interruptions may progress to metabolic acidemia (Esplin, 2020; Miller et al., 2022; Parer et al., 2006). FHR patterns with late decelerations warrant further evaluation, taking into account the entire clinical situation, targeted corrective measures with continued surveillance, and reevaluation for a potential expedited birth (Clark et al., 2013; Eller & Esplin, 2020; Raghuraman, 2020).

Variable Decelerations

Variable decelerations (Fig. 14.21A–C) are visually apparent, *abrupt* decreases from onset to nadir of a deceleration (Macones et al., 2008). Onset to deceleration nadir is less than 30 seconds. This type of deceleration drops at least 15 bpm below the BL rate. The entire deceleration lasts at least 15 seconds and no longer than 2 minutes from onset to return to baseline rate. Variable decelerations are suggestive of an interruption of oxygenation at the level of the umbilical cord where cord vessels are compressed. These patterns may be periodic or episodic. The shape, depth, duration, and timing in relation to uterine contractions may vary. Variable decelerations are the most frequent type of deceleration during the intrapartum period (ACOG, 2019).

The physiologic mechanism of variable decelerations is based on the premise of partial or complete occlusion of an umbilical cord related to an interruption of the oxygenation pathway, such as cord compression related to low amniotic fluid volume (Blackburn, 2018; Lyndon & O'Brien, 2021; Miller et al., 2022). Initially, compression of the umbilical cord results in the occlusion of the umbilical vein, which is a thin-walled vessel. Subsequently, there is a reduction in blood flow from the placenta to the fetus. The consequences of this change are decreased cardiac output and hypotension manifesting in a compensatory FHR increase. Further compression leads to occlusion of the umbilical arteries, resulting in increased peripheral vascular resistance, fetal hypertension, and vagal nerve stimulation, which triggers a baroreceptor response. Next, an abrupt FHR decrease can be observed. After cord compression abates, umbilical arteries open, fetal BP decreases, and the FHR returns to BL. Occasionally, a compensatory FHR increase may occur before returning to the BL rate.

Intermittent variable decelerations usually have little clinical significance, especially if accompanied by a normal FHR BL range and moderate variability. In this setting, variable decelerations are generally not associated with significant hypoxia (Miller et al., 2022; Parer et al., 2006). Similar to late decelerations, variable decelerations that become recurrent and are observed with minimal or absent variability may lead to a cascade of progressive physiologic changes, including hypoxemia, hypoxia, metabolic acidosis, and eventually metabolic acidemia. In this setting, associated FHR changes may include a rising BL rate, decreasing variability, absent accelerations, and a slower return to a BL rate as a deceleration ends. These types of variable decelerations necessitate further evaluation, taking into account the entire clinical situation, targeted corrective measures with continued surveillance, and reevaluation for a potential expedited birth (Clark et al., 2013; Eller & Esplin, 2020; Raghuraman, 2020).

Prolonged Decelerations

Prolonged decelerations (Fig. 14.22) are defined as a decrease in the FHR, which lasts a minimum of 2 minutes and no longer than 10 minutes from onset to return to BL (Macones et al., 2008). After 10 minutes, this type of deceleration is considered a BL change, although this new range warrants close evaluation. A prolonged deceleration reflects an interruption of oxygen transfer from the environment to the fetus at one or more points along the pathway. Umbilical cord compression, client seizures, and uterine tachysystole or hypertonus are examples of clinical situations in which a prolonged deceleration may be identified. From a physiologic standpoint, a proposed mechanism of action is a sudden and prolonged reduction in oxygen delivery. The initial stages are vagal in origin, similar to variable and late deceleration (Heuser, 2020). As oxygen exchange further diminishes, direct myocardial depression may evolve into a prolonged deceleration. If possible, the etiology of a prolonged deceleration is identified, and targeted corrective measures are performed. Further clinical management decisions need to be individualized based on gestational age, etiology, stage of labor if applicable, and other obstetric factors.

Categorization of Fetal Heart Rate Patterns

The NICHD consensus statement incorporates a three-tiered categorization system, which uses BL rate, variability, accelerations, and decelerations to determine a specific category during the intrapartum period. Patterns associated with Category I, Category II, and Category III are presented in Box 14.4. The NICHD category system is based on the premise that the FHR tracing provides vital information related to the status of a fetus in terms of those with a normal acid–base status versus those moving along a continuum to abnormal fetal acid–base status. Categories of FHR interpretation include the following (Macones et al., 2008):

- Category I—Normal and are strongly predictive of normal fetal acid–base status at the time of observation
- Category II—Indeterminate and fetal acid–base status is uncertain
- Category III FHR—Abnormal and predictive of abnormal fetal acid–base status at the time of observation.

For example, the continuum starts with FHR characteristics considered normal for an oxygenated fetus (e.g., moderate variability and accelerations). When interruptions in oxygenation

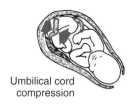

Umbilical cord
compression

Physiologic mechanism of variable deceleration

Umbilical cord compression
↓
Initial compression of umbilical vein
↓
Transient decreased fetal venous return
↓
Transient reduction in fetal cardiac output and blood pressure
↓
Baroreceptor stimulation
↓
Transient reflex rise in FHR
↓
Umbilical artery compression
↓
Abrupt rise in fetal peripheral resistance and blood pressure
↓
Baroreceptor stimulation
↓
Reflex parasympathetic outflow
↓
Abrupt slowing of the FHR
↓
Variable deceleration
↓
When umbilical cord compression is relieved, this process
occurs in reverse

A

B

Variable onset   <30 sec

Contraction

Nadir

C

FIG. 14.21 Variable Decelerations. (A) The physiologic mechanism of variable decelerations is attributed to transient mechanical compression of umbilical blood vessels within the umbilical cord. (B) Schematic drawing of a variable deceleration. (C) Variable deceleration showing blue arrows that represent abrupt onset (1) to nadir (2) that is greater than 15 beats per minute *(bpm)* below a baseline, and recovery (3) with deceleration lasting less than 2 minutes. (A, From Miller, L. A., Miller, D. A., & Cypher, R. L. [2022]. *Mosby's pocket guide to fetal monitoring: A multidisciplinary approach.* [9th ed.]. Elsevier; B, From Intrapartum assessment. [2018]. In F. Cunningham, K. J. Leveno, S. L. Bloom, J. S. Dashe, B. L. Hoffman, B. M. Casey, C. Y. Spong [Eds.], *William's obstetrics.* [24th ed., pp. 473–503]. McGraw-Hill; C, Courtesy OBIX by Clinical Computer Systems, Inc.)

occur, the continuum may move from normal to an "indeterminate" pattern, which suggests hypoxemia or hypoxia. One example may include a normal FHR BL, moderate variability, and intermittent variable decelerations. Finally, if uncorrected, these indeterminate patterns may evolve to a tachycardic FHR BL, absent variability, and recurrent variable decelerations, which are more predictive of inadequate tissue oxygenation and abnormal fetal acid–base balance. Using a three-tiered category system provides a meaningful way to communicate with other team members because each category has specific inclusion criteria. The terms *reassuring* and *nonreassuring* should be abandoned in documentation and communication because each term is imprecise, ill-defined, and not included in the NICHD consensus statement (Miller et al., 2022).

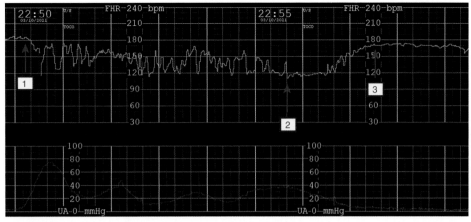

FIG. 14.22 Prolonged Decelerations. Prolonged decelerations showing blue arrows that represent onset (1) and recovery (3) with entire deceleration lasting greater than 2 minutes but less than 10 minutes. (Courtesy OBIX by Clinical Computer Systems Inc.)

BOX 14.4 Categories of Fetal Heart Rate Interpretation

Category I—Normal
  Fetal heart rate (FHR) baseline: 110 to 160 beats per minute (bpm)
  Moderate variability
  Accelerations present or absent
  Variable or late decelerations absent
  Early decelerations present or absent
Category II—Indeterminate
  Tracings not categorized as category I or III
Category III—Abnormal
  Absent variability *AND*
      Recurrent late decelerations
          or
      Recurrent variable decelerations
          or
      Bradycardia
  Sinusoidal pattern

UTERINE ACTIVITY

Standardized definitions are used to describe UA, which is quantified as the number of contractions in a 10-minute window of time, averaged over 30 minutes (Macones et al., 2008). Components of a complete assessment and documentation of UA include frequency, duration, intensity, and resting tone (Drummond & Rust, 2021; Miller et al., 2022) (Fig. 14.23).

Relaxation time is another assessment of UA and is calculated as the amount of time from the end of one contraction to the beginning of the next contraction described in seconds. This is generally 60 seconds or more in first-stage labor and 45 to 50 seconds or more in second-stage labor (Miller et al., 2022). Although relaxation time is not generally documented, assessment of this parameter will assist in managing clients undergoing cervical ripening and labor induction. Once assessment is complete, the following terminology is used to describe UA (Macones et al., 2008):

- Normal: Five or fewer contractions in 10 minutes, averaged over 30 minutes
- Tachysystole: More than five contractions in 10 minutes, averaged over 30 minutes regardless of whether FHR decelerations are present or absent (Fig. 14.24)
  - *Hyperstimulation* and *hypercontractility* are not defined and are no longer used to define UA

Tetany is sometimes referred to in communication among clinicians. There is no standardized definition in fetal monitoring literature, but tetany has been used to describe excessive contraction duration, such as a series of single contractions lasting 2 minutes or more (Miller et al., 2022). Terms such as skewed contractions and polysystole are vague and not included in the NICHD consensus statement. These terms are not used in clinical practice, communication, documentation, or EFM education.

Montevideo units (MVUs) are sometimes used to describe contraction intensity over a 10-minute period when an IUPC is in place. An MVU is calculated by noting each contraction's intensity in mm Hg and subtracting the resting tone. Numbers are added together to report MVUs during that time frame (Caldyero-Barcia & Poseiro, 1959; Caldyero-Barcia & Poseito, 1960). For example, four contractions occur in 10 minutes, each having an intensity of 45, 80, 65, and 75 mm Hg, and a uterine resting tone of 15 mm Hg. This would be calculated as $(45 - 15) + (80 - 15) + (65 - 15) + (75 - 15)$, which results in a total MVUs of 205 during this 10-minute period.

❓ KNOWLEDGE CHECK

9. What is the significance of fetal heart rate (FHR) accelerations and the correlation to fetal acid–base status?
10. Describe the differences between early, late, and variable decelerations in relationship to contractions and onset to nadir.
11. Define uterine contraction frequency, duration, intensity, resting tone, and relaxation time.
12. Which category is interpreted as being predictive of normal fetal acid–base status?

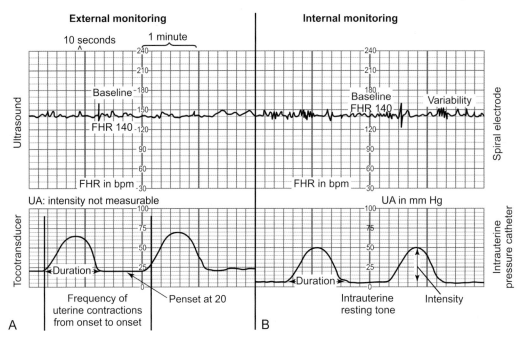

FIG. 14.23 Uterine activity reflecting frequency, duration, and intensity for external and internal monitoring. (From Miller, L. A., Miller, D. A., & Cypher, R. L. [2022]. *Mosby's pocket guide to fetal monitoring: A multidisciplinary approach.* [9th ed.]. Elsevier.)

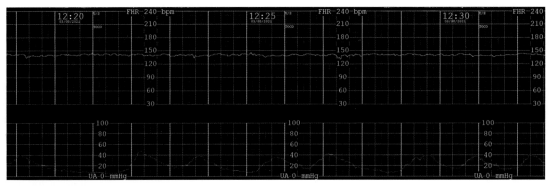

FIG. 14.24 Uterine Tachysystole. From 12:20 to 12:30, there are a total of six contractions. (Courtesy OBIX by Clinical Computer Systems Inc.)

STANDARDIZED INTRAPARTUM INTERPRETATION AND MANAGEMENT

A standardized, evidence-based approach to intrapartum FHR interpretation and management necessitates a shared mental model. A shared mental model implies a team of two or more people will improve from a clinical decision-making and performance perspective if everyone understands each individual's roles and responsibilities. In other words, teams that think similarly, complete tasks together, and perform at a level in which there is overlap or co-understanding of everyone's roles, skill level, and education will work together more effectively (Gisick et al., 2018; Jonker, 2011). For example, a nurse interprets the FHR tracing as a Category II pattern based on fetal tachycardia, minimal variability, and variable decelerations, which are now recurrent in the second stage of labor. The nurse conveys these findings to a midwife, who reports to the bedside to review the tracing. In turn, a physician is consulted because there is

a potential for an operative vaginal birth. The nurse, midwife, and physician use a systematic approach to discuss the client's intrapartum labor course and review the tracing and current clinical situation as a team. Informed consent for a forceps birth is obtained. Because team members used a shared mental model, urgent tasks were performed together with a common goal of optimizing perinatal outcomes. In other words, standardized interpretation and management are critical to the well-being of the client and fetus as long as effective teamwork and meaningful communication occur.

Intrapartum EFM is meant to assess the adequacy of oxygen transfer during labor from the environment to the fetus. The following two evidence-based principles can be inferred when nurses review an intrapartum FHR tracing (Miller et al., 2022):

- Principle 1—Variable, late, and/or prolonged decelerations indicate interruption of oxygen transfer from the environment to the fetus at one or more points.

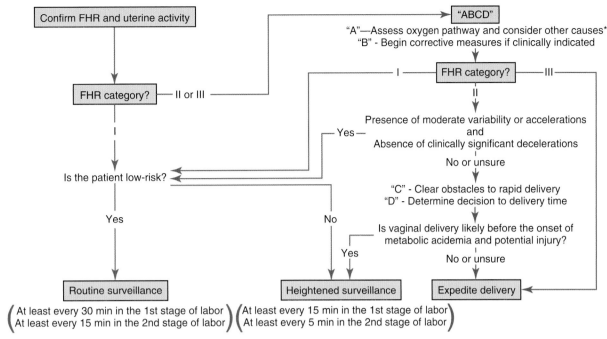

FIG. 14.25 Intrapartum fetal heart rate (*FHR*) management decision model demonstrating an algorithm for management of electronic fetal monitoring tracings during the intrapartum period. (From Miller, L. A., Miller, D. A., & Cypher, R. L. [2022]. *Mosby's pocket guide to fetal monitoring: A multidisciplinary approach.* [9th ed.]. Elsevier.)

- Principle 2—Moderate variability and/or accelerations reliably exclude ongoing hypoxic injury at the time of observation.

Intrapartum Management Decision Model

These evidence-based principles create the groundwork for an intrapartum FHR management decision model (Fig. 14.25). This straightforward algorithm is accurate, logical, and consistent, acting as a safeguard in both low- and high-risk clients to ensure FHR characteristics are not overlooked and management decisions are prompt (Cypher, 2018a; Miller et al., 2022; Table 14.3):

A—Assess oxygen pathway in both the pregnant client and fetus and identify the cause of FHR changes

B—Begin corrective measures

C—Clear obstacles to delivery

D—Delivery plan

This process incorporates the NICHD definitions and principles of interpretation. FHR and UA interpretation require the availability of reliable and useful data. Nurses identify and minimize potential sources of error, so data are recorded satisfactorily for interpretation and management. For example, if an external ultrasound transducer and toco are not able to transmit a continuous tracing in an obese client undergoing labor augmentation, placement of a FSE and IUPC may be required. Once reliable data are confirmed, a systematic approach is performed to evaluate five FHR characteristics: BL rate, variability, accelerations, decelerations, and changes or trends over time. Tracing assessments are completed periodically at reasonable intervals in accordance with professional organization guidance and institutional

policies and procedures. If a category I pattern is identified, a tracing is considered normal because this pattern is reflective of a well-oxygenated fetus. On the other hand, if a category II or category III pattern is identified, further evaluation using the ABCD approach to FHR management is initiated.

A: Assess Oxygenation Pathway

When a Category II or III FHR tracing is present, a rapid, systematic assessment of oxygen transfer along a pathway from the environment to the fetus can identify potential sources of interrupted oxygenation (Miller, 2011; Miller et al., 2022). For example, if a client is having difficulty breathing, counting a respiratory rate, auscultating the breath sounds, and placing a pulse oximeter can uncover much needed data. In this scenario, a respiratory rate of 32 breaths per minute, clear breath sounds, and oxygen saturation readings of 88% to 90% may explain minimal variability. In the presence of late decelerations, maternal vasculature can be assessed with a simple blood pressure evaluation. Late decelerations may accompany a hypotensive reading. A number of factors can influence the appearance of the FHR tracing by mechanisms other than interruptions in fetal oxygenation (Lyndon & O'Brien-Abel, 2021; Miller, 2011). These include but are not limited to fetal sleep cycles, anemia, congenital anomalies, maternal fever, or medication use. In these cases, individualized management is directed at the specific etiology. For instance, administration of an antipyretic for maternal fever may lower the FHR baseline in a tachycardic fetus.

B: Begin Corrective Measures

Once an assessment of FHR and UA information is completed, data obtained will guide physiologically appropriate

TABLE 14.3   ABCD FHR Management

	"A" Assess Oxygen Pathway	**"B"** Begin Corrective Measures[a]		**"C"** Clear Obstacles to Rapid Delivery	**"D"** Determine Decision to Delivery Time
Lungs	Respiration	Oxygen	Facility	Consider: OR availability Equipment	Facility response time
Heart	Heart rate	Position changes	Staff	Consider notifying: *Obstetrician* *Surgical assistant* *Anesthesiologist* *Neonatologist* *Pediatrician* *Nursing staff*	Consider staff: *Availability* *Training* *Experience*
Vasculature	Blood pressure	Fluid bolus Correct hypotension	Client	Consider: *Informed consent* *Anesthesia options* *Laboratory tests* *Blood products* *Intravenous access* *Urinary catheter* *Abdominal prep* *Transfer to OR*	Surgical considerations *(prior surgery)* Medical considerations *(obesity, diabetes)* Obstetric considerations *(parity, pelvimetry)*
Uterus	Contraction strength Contraction frequency Contraction duration Baseline uterine tone Exclude uterine rupture	Reduce stimulant Uterine relaxant	Fetus	Consider: *Fetal number* *Fetal weight* *Gestational age* *Presentation* *Position* *Anomalies*	Consider: *Fetal number* *Fetal weight* *Gestational age* *Presentation* *Position* *Anomalies*
Placenta	Check for bleeding				
Cord	Exclude cord prolapse	Amnioinfusion	Labor	*Confirm that contraction monitoring is adequate to allow appropriately informed management decisions*	Consider factors such as: *Protracted labor* *Previous uterine relaxant* *Remote from delivery* *Poor expulsive efforts*

Examples of clinical factors to be considered in a systematic fashion. Institutions may modify to individual circumstances.
FHR, Fetal heart rate; *OR,* operating room.
[a]Conservative corrective measures should be guided by clinical circumstances. For example, amnioinfusion may be appropriate in the presence of variable decelerations but would not be expected to result in resolution of late decelerations.
From Miller, L.A., Miller, D. A., & Cypher, R. L. (2022). *Mosby's pocket guide to fetal monitoring: A multidisciplinary approach* (9th ed.). Elsevier.

corrective measures. The goal of these conservative interventions is to improve uterine blood flow, umbilical circulation, and maternal-fetal oxygenation (Society of Obstetricians and Gynaecologists Canada [SOGC], 2020). This requires nurses to take action to implement tasks that may maximize oxygen delivery to a fetus. Each intervention is centered on observed FHR characteristics, such as minimal variability or recurrent variable decelerations. A systematic approach is one safety measure that identifies indeterminant or abnormal FHR patterns and allows decisions to be made promptly. Occasionally, more than one corrective measure may be implemented to resolve a category II or III pattern, and not all interventions are used in every clinical scenario. Corrective measures

commonly performed include but are not limited to the following:

- Lateral positioning or change in position
- IV fluid boluses
- Oxygen supplementation
- Reduction in UA
- Correction of blood pressure extremes (hypertension or hypotension)
- Amnioinfusion
- Modification of second-stage pushing efforts

Lateral positioning or a change in position is considered a corrective measure. Two situations exist in which a position change of the pregnant client may improve fetal oxygenation and maximize uteroplacental perfusion (Garite & Simpson, 2011; Raghuraman, 2020; Simpson, 2021). First, repositioning to lateral or hands and knees alters the relationship between an umbilical cord and fetal parts or uterine wall. In this case, umbilical cord compression, which is causing variable or prolonged decelerations, may be minimized. Second, supine positioning is associated with an undesirable impact on the hemodynamics of the pregnant client. Specifically, a decrease in venous return and cardiac output occurs because the gravid uterus, which contains the amniotic fluid, placenta, and fetus or fetuses, compresses the aorta and inferior vena cava. Compression decreases uteroplacental perfusion, which inhibits delivery of oxygenated blood to the fetus. Therefore lateral positioning is a low-risk technique that can increase uteroplacental perfusion.

IV fluid administration can maximize cardiac output, intravascular volume, and uteroplacental perfusion, resulting in improved fetal oxygenation (Garite & Simpson, 2011; Raghuraman, 2020). An IV fluid bolus of 500 to 1000 mL of isotonic fluid, such as lactated Ringer's solution, can improve cardiac output by increasing circulating volume, venous return, left ventricular end-diastolic pressure, ventricular preload, and stroke volume (Miller et al., 2022). Fluid amounts in clients at risk for volume overload and pulmonary edema, such as preeclampsia, are carefully considered. Boluses of solutions containing dextrose are avoided as a corrective measure for indeterminate or abnormal FHR tracings because of potential complications, such as increased fetal lactate, decreased pH, and hyperglycemia (Riegel et al., 2018; Simpson, 2021). However, dextrose IV fluid therapy can be used during labor as a carbohydrate replacement that enhances uterine function during labor and potentially reduces first-stage labor length (Riegel et al., 2018).

Administration of supplemental oxygen has traditionally been used for Category II and III FHR patterns. Fetal oxygenation is dependent on the pregnant client's blood's oxygen content. Theoretically, maternal hyperoxia may increase the transfer of oxygen to the intervillous space, which improves fetal oxygenation and prevents fetal hypoxia from transitioning to acidemia (Raghuraman, 2020). Administering *supplemental oxygen* can improve the client's Po_2. This increases the partial pressure of oxygen, which is dissolved in the client's blood, and the amount of oxygen bound to hemoglobin. In turn, this may increase the oxygen concentration gradient across the placenta, which eventually leads to improved fetal Po_2 and oxygen content (Miller et al., 2022). In contrast, contemporary data suggest there is no association between the practice of oxygen supplementation and improved neonatal outcomes, such as umbilical cord gas results, when supplemental oxygen is used for Category II and III FHR tracings (Raghuraman et al., 2021). Therefore, in the absence of reasonable data demonstrating fetal benefit and potential risk of harm (e.g., harmful oxygen-free radicals), routine and prolonged use of oxygen supplementation in the absence of maternal hypoxia is discouraged. Oxygen can be considered when maternal hypoxia, hypovolemia, or both are suspected

or confirmed (SOGC, 2020). If other corrective measures are performed, and a clinical team deems oxygen is necessary for resolution of a particular FHR pattern, a more judicious approach to supplementation is considered. Oxygen at 10 L/min via nonrebreather face mask for approximately 15 to 30 minutes may be used in these situations (Simpson, 2021). Once moderate variability returns to the tracing, fetal hypoxemia is typically ruled out, and oxygen is no longer indicated.

Decreasing UA is a crucial intervention for improving fetal oxygenation and uteroplacental perfusion. The peak of a uterine contraction produces a temporary cessation of uterine blood flow and oxygen delivery into the intervillous space (Garite & Simpson, 2011; Lyndon & O'Brien-Abel, 2021; Simpson & Miller, 2011). Uterine hypertonus also may affect oxygen delivery. Typically, residual oxygen in the intervillous space is adequate for the fetus to tolerate these changes. Tachysystole, prolonged contractions, hypertonus, or inadequate relaxation time between contractions may result in FHR changes that are the result of decreased oxygen delivery. Corrective measures to reduce UA include the following (Simpson & Miller, 2011; Simpson, 2021):

- Remove dinoprostone insert or withhold next misoprostol dose
- Decrease or discontinue oxytocin (See Chapter 15)
- Lateral positioning
- IV fluid bolus
- Assessment to rule out conditions such as chorioamnionitis or placental abruption
- Administration of beta-sympathomimetic agent or nitroglycerin

The most commonly used medication to reduce UA is off-label use of terbutaline. Typical dosing is a single dose of 0.25 mg subcutaneously (SQ). Safety concerns related to potential client-adverse effects include cardiac arrhythmias, pulmonary edema, myocardial ischemia, hypotension, and tachycardia (Griggs et al., 2020; Parfitt, 2021). Fetal side effects include tachycardia and hyperglycemia. Nurses will verify the client's heart rate before administration. The medication is generally held for a pulse rate greater than 120 bpm or FHR greater than 160 bpm, and a physician or midwife is contacted for further orders. Clients with underlying cardiac conditions may require alternative medication, ECG monitoring during administration, or both. Another less common medication is nitroglycerin 400 µg IV, which may result in decreased mean arterial blood pressure (Pullen et al., 2007).

Correcting client hypotension is another measure that has been found to increase uteroplacental perfusion and fetal oxygenation. Hypotension is caused by inadequate client hydration, insensible fluid losses, supine positioning resulting in decreased venous return and reduced cardiac output, and peripheral vasodilation secondary to sympathetic blockade during regional anesthesia (Miller et al., 2022). Contemporary data have shown narrow pulse pressures (<45) are associated with FHR abnormalities like late decelerations (Lappen et al., 2018; Miller et al., 2013). Therefore a complete assessment of vital signs and judicious fluid management is warranted. Interventions include:

- Lateral repositioning, including Trendelenburg
- IV fluid bolus or increased IV fluid rate
- Possible administration of a vasopressor such as ephedrine or phenylephrine (Association of Women's Health, Obstetric, and Neonatal Nursing [AWHONN], 2020)
  - Ephedrine has a delayed onset and a 60-minute duration of action
  - Phenylephrine has an immediate onset and 5- to 10-minute duration of action; it is the preferred vasopressor treatment for neuraxial-anesthesia–induced or spinal-anesthesia–induced hypotension

Amnioinfusion requires instillation of isotonic fluid, such as lactated Ringer's solution or normal saline, through an IUPC into the amniotic cavity to restore fluid volume to normal or near-normal levels and alleviate cord compression (Miller et al., 2022; Raghuraman, 2020). In the setting of decreased amniotic fluid (oligohydramnios), an oxygen pathway interruption at the level of the umbilical cord can result in variable or prolonged decelerations. By replacing fluid, umbilical cord compression may be relieved, resulting in optimal blood flow through the umbilical cord with oxygenated blood. Hospital policy directs amnioinfusion rates and amounts. One suggested guideline includes an initial bolus of 250 to 500 mL over a 20- to 30-minute time frame via an infusion pump or gravity flow (Miller et al., 2022). A continuous infusion of 120 to 180 mL/hr also may be considered. Fluid return may be assessed by weighing the underpads (1 mL of fluid is equivalent to 1 gram of weight) as a method to avoid uterine overdistention. Uterine resting tone may be elevated, so palpation is key in this situation. If there are concerns related to intrauterine pressure, an amnioinfusion is discontinued for a more accurate assessment.

Modification of second stage pushing efforts is an additional corrective measure. Expulsive pushing efforts with a closed glottis (Valsalva technique) are associated with hemodynamic changes, increases in intrathoracic and intrauterine pressure, and reduction in continuous oxygen delivery because of breath-holding (AWHONN, 2019b; Caldeyro-Barcia, 1979; Eller, 2020). Closed-glottis pushing requires a client to take a deep breath, hold for a count of 10, and repeat three or four times with each contraction. This is sometimes done in a supine position, leading to aortocaval compression. Consequences to the pregnant client and fetus include the following:

- Decrease in venous return to the heart
- Decrease in cardiac output
- Reduction in arterial pressure
- Decline in blood perfusion in the intervillous space, resulting in decreased oxygen supply to the fetus as evidenced by a lower pH and Po_2 of the umbilical arterial blood

Active pushing in the second stage of labor is the most physiologically demanding phase for a fetus, especially when interruptions in the oxygenation pathway are present (Simpson, 2021). Therefore one suggested approach is to modify pushing with an open-glottis technique. This type of effort requires clients to push for 6 to 8 seconds, repeating three to four times per contraction (AWHONN, 2019b; Caldeyro-Barcia, 1979). Open-glottis pushing may result

in expiratory grunting or vocalization, which is normal. Alternative pushing strategies to optimize fetal oxygenation include side-lying or squatting positions, reduced duration of breath holding, and pushing with every other or every third contraction (AWHONN, 2019b; Eller, 2020).

Category II patterns require continued surveillance and further evaluation. In situations where there is moderate variability, accelerations, or both in conjunction with the absence of significant decelerations, heightened observation is appropriate. In other clinical circumstances, category II patterns are more challenging. Despite using a shared mental model, a health care team may disagree on interpretation or level of risk. In these cases, a standardized approach to Category II FHR management is implemented (Clark et al., 2013; Shields et al., 2018). The other extreme in the fetal monitoring spectrum are abnormal patterns, or a category III. Whether vaginally or operatively, an expedited birth may be considered for these patterns, depending on the entire clinical situation and whether corrective measures are effective.

C: Clear Obstacles to Rapid Delivery

When health care team members are uncertain about a clinical situation, the ABCD management model guides everyone to the next step, "C," clear obstacles for delivery. Moderate variability, accelerations and resolution of decelerations may not be observed in a Category II tracing despite corrective measures (Miller et al., 2022). Therefore clinicians need to plan for a possible expedited birth. When moving to this step, there is no obligation to make critical decisions about time or mode of delivery. This part of the management model encourages nurses, midwives, and physicians to focus methodically on potential areas of delays so important factors and tasks are not overlooked. In turn, decisions are made in a timely manner. Five potential sources of unnecessary delays include the hospital facility, staff, client, fetus, and labor. For example, an operative birth could be delayed because an anesthesiologist is not readily available in the hospital.

D: Delivery Plan

The last step in the ABCD approach, "D," is to estimate the time required to accomplish birth in the event of further deterioration of the FHR tracing (Miller et al., 2022). This portion of the management plan - the decision to expedite birth via cesarean or an operative vaginal approach instead of expectant management (e.g., waiting for a spontaneous vaginal birth)- is made by a physician or midwife. Discussing the risks and benefits with a client is an integral part of this decision-making process. Further choices about timing and mode of birth are based on a midwife or physician's clinical judgment.

Umbilical Cord Blood Gas Sampling. After birth, umbilical cord blood gas sampling is used as a direct objective method of quantifying fetal acid–base and oxygenation at the time of cord clamping (Cypher, 2021; Nursing Procedure 14.3). There is a lack of consensus on when umbilical cord blood gas sampling is performed. A suggested indication is when fetal metabolic status is questioned (ACOG & AAP,

NURSING PROCEDURE 14.3 Umbilical Cord Blood Gas Sampling Collection

- Gather two 1-mL heparinized syringes with short, small-gauge needles.
  - Small-gauge needles allow for better control causing minimal injury to the umbilical vessels.
- Create labels ensuring each sample is labeled with client identification and whether the sample is an artery or vein.
- A double-clamped cord segment is obtained after birth.
- Obtain a blood sample from the umbilical artery first.
  - Umbilical arteries are often more difficult to acquire.
  - The umbilical vein may help support the umbilical artery.
- Avoid air bubbles or carefully expel excess air from each syringe.
- Label each sample before transporting it to the laboratory for analysis.

From Cypher, R.L. (2021). Assessment of fetal oxygenation and acid–base status. In A. Lyndon & K. Wisner (Eds.), *Fetal heart monitoring: Principles and practices.* (6th ed., pp. 185–212). Kendall Hunt; Riley, R. J., & Johnson, J. W. (1993). Collecting and analyzing cord blood gases. *Clinical Obstetrics and Gynecology, 36*(1), 13–23. https://doi.org/10.1097/00003081-199303000-00005; Scheans, P. (2011). Umbilical cord blood gases: New clinical relevance for an age-old practice. *Neonatal Network, 30*(2), 123–126. https:/doi.org/10.1891/0730-0832.30.2.123; Wallman, C. M. (1997). Interpretation of fetal cord blood gases. *Neonatal Network, 16*(1), 72–75.

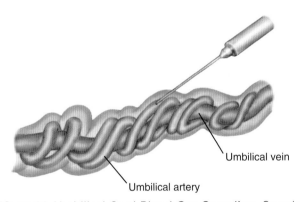

FIG. 14.26 Umbilical Cord Blood Gas Sampling. Samples are drawn from both the umbilical artery and umbilical vein.

2014). If indicated, a double-clamped umbilical cord segment is obtained at birth. Two heparinized syringes (prevent coagulation) with small-gauge needles are used to draw samples from the umbilical artery (deoxygenated) and umbilical vein (oxygenated; Fig. 14.26). Segments and samples in a heparinized syringe are stable for a maximum of 60 minutes at room temperature and do not need to be placed on ice (Cypher, 2021; Manor et al., 1998; SOGC, 2020).

Arterial cord blood is collected first. This blood is typically more challenging to obtain because arterial vessels are small and thick-walled. Additionally, the umbilical vein helps support umbilical arteries to make access easier. Something to remember during sampling is that arteries cross over the vein. An arterial sample best reflects information on blood returning from the fetus to the placenta and describes fetal status at

birth. A sample from the umbilical vein, which is large and thin-walled, reflects placental function and the level of oxygenation at the intervillous space going to a fetus. Collection and analysis of arterial and venous samples confirm the accuracy of the results that are obtained. Analysis for pH, partial pressure of carbon dioxide (P_{CO_2}), bicarbonate (HCO_3) levels, and base deficit or excess will determine the presence or absence of fetal acidosis (Table 14.4). If acidosis is present, respiratory (short-term) acidosis can be distinguished from metabolic (prolonged) or mixed acidosis using the sample algorithm in Box 14.5.

TABLE 14.4 Single-Digit Value Guideline for Umbilical Cord Blood Acid–Base Interpretation

	Normal Values	Metabolic Acidemia	Respiratory Acidemia
pH	≥7.20	<7.20	<7.20
P_{O_2} (mm Hg)	>20	<20	Variable
P_{CO_2} (mm Hg)	<60	<60	>60
Bicarbonate (mEq/L)	>22	<22	≥22
Base deficit (mEq/L)	≤12	>12	<12
Base excess (mEq/L)	≥−12	<−12	>−12

KNOWLEDGE CHECK

13. Describe the standardized intrapartum "ABCD" approach to fetal heart rate (FHR) management.
14. List conservative corrective measures that may be considered to correct a category II or III FHR pattern.
15. How does an IV bolus of fluids benefit fetal oxygenation?
16. What response is elicited when performing fetal scalp stimulation?
17. What is the purpose of umbilical cord blood gas sampling? Which umbilical cord vessels reflect oxygenated and deoxygenated blood?
18. What are potential obstacles that may be encountered during the "C" portion of the ABCD approach?

ASSESSMENT FREQUENCY AND DOCUMENTATION

Documentation that is contemporaneous, logical, explicit, accurate, and readable is the foundation for continuity of client care and communication between clinicians (Cypher, 2018b; Miller et al., 2022). *Contemporaneous* is charting near the time of an assessment, procedure, or occurrence. *Logical* is information that is easily understood and clear. A SOAP (subjective, objective, assessment, plan) progress note is one example. *Explicit* simply refers to using standardized FHR and UA terminology. Avoid vague or ambiguous terms, such as reassuring or nonreassuring. *Accurate* reflects correct times and sequence of events because a record must be truthful.

BOX 14.5   Algorithm for Determining the Presence or Absence of Fetal Acidosis

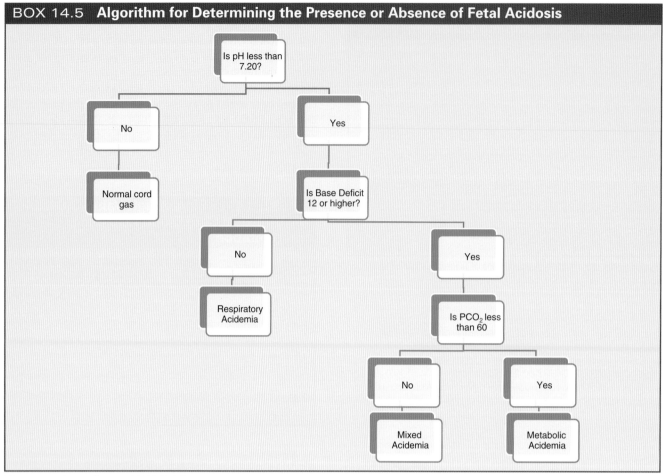

(Courtesy Rebecca Cypher, MSN, PNNP.)

Finally, all entries in a paper chart are required to be *readable* and legible.

Documentation throughout the intrapartum period promotes improved quality of care by encouraging assessment and reevaluation of progress and clinical management plans while meeting professional and legal standards. Contemporary electronic medical records allow a higher level of charting precision incorporating technology, which integrates a variety of features. Medical records validate a clinician's performance to document certain aspects of health care, such as communication with a clinical team and client education, thus promoting client safety (Malane et al., 2019).

A hospital and unit documentation policy will often highlight the charting platform that is used and the style, format, and frequency intervals. Additionally, nursing professional organizations and other entities may have documentation resources that can be used as the basis for hospital policies. For example, AWHONN's position statement has suggested frequency of assessment and documentation parameters for auscultation, palpation, and EFM during the intrapartum period (AWHONN, 2019a; Tables 14.5 and 14.6). At a minimum, documentation includes but is not limited to the following:

- A systematic admission assessment of the client and fetus
- Ongoing assessments of the client and fetus to include FHR and UA data
- Corrective measures and other interventions provided and evaluation of responses
- Communication with the client and family or primary support person
- Interactions and communication with health care team members, including response and actions taken
- Communication related to escalation of concerns

HEALTH INFORMATION TECHNOLOGY IN OBSTETRICS

Nurses play an integral role in health information technology (HIT) as obstetrics continues in a journey to further improve client-centered care and safety. Fetal monitoring systems are more comprehensive and include point-of-care charting, FHR and UA pattern interpretation, clinical decision support software, and archiving capabilities. At the most basic level, HIT measures, consolidates, and analyzes FHR and UA information. Once analyzed, data are interpreted in conjunction with a nurse's clinical knowledge, which has been accumulated through hands-on experience and education (Cypher, 2017). This type of computer technology allows nurses to ask the right questions at an appropriate time, complete structured nursing assessments, accurately determine a correct diagnosis from a multidisciplinary

TABLE 14.5   Frequency of Intermittent Auscultation Assessment and Documentation

	Latent Phase (<4 cm)	Latent Phase (4–5 cm)	Active Phase (≥6 cm)	Second Stage (Passive fetal descent)	Second Stage (Active pushing)
Low-risk without oxytocin	Insufficient evidence to make a recommendation. Frequency at discretion of midwife or physician	Every 15–30 minutes	Every 15–30 minutes	Every 15 minutes	Every 5–15 minutes

Frequency of assessment is determined based on the status of the client and fetus and at times will need to occur more often based on clinical needs (e.g., in response to a temporary or ongoing change).
Summary documentation is acceptable, and individual hospital policy is followed.
From Wisner, K., & Holschuh, C. (2018). Fetal heart rate auscultation, 3rd edition. *Nursing for Women's Health, 22*(6), e1–e32. https://doi.org/10.1016/j.nwh.2018.10.001.

TABLE 14.6   Assessment of Fetal Status Using Electronic Fetal Monitoring

	Latent Phase (<4 cm)	Latent Phase (4–5 cm)	Active Phase (≥ 6 cm)	Second Stage (Passive fetal descent)	Second Stage (Active pushing)
Low risk without oxytocin	Insufficient evidence to make a recommendation Frequency at the discretion of the midwife or physician	Every 30 minutes	Every 30 minutes	Every 30 minutes	Every 15 minutes
With oxytocin or risk factors	Every 15 minutes with oxytocin, every 30 minutes without	Every 15 minutes	Every 15 minutes	Every 15 minutes	Every 5 minutes

Frequency of assessment should always be determined based on the status of the client and fetus and at times will need to occur more often based on clinical needs (e.g., in response to a temporary or ongoing change).
Summary documentation is acceptable, and individual hospital policy should be followed.
From Association of Women's Health, Obstetric and Neonatal Nurses (AWHONN). (2019a). Fetal heart monitoring. (Position Statement). *Journal of Obstetric, Gynecologic, & Neonatal Nursing, 47*(6), 874–877.

approach, and execute interventions along a decision-making process.

FETAL MONITORING EDUCATION AND COMPETENCY

Obstetric nurses are typically the primary team members responsible for fetal surveillance and also provide the majority of client care in an intrapartum setting. Therefore fetal assessment requires skilled nurses to be able to interpret, FHR and UA patterns and make clinical decisions based on these findings. Comprehensive fetal monitoring education may include didactic information, like FHR and UA physiology, and psychomotor skills, such as FSE placement (AWHONN, 2019a). Moreover, education that includes the implications of labor support and interprofessional communication strategies is recommended. Ongoing education and periodic validation of knowledge and clinical competency is recommended.

INTRAPARTUM FETAL SURVEILLANCE AND SHARED DECISION-MAKING

Clients are more involved in today's health care climate where education about diseases or conditions and choices

about options for treatment are a priority. Building relationships with obstetric clients has become an essential part of a shared decision-making environment (Dore & Ehman, 2020). Clients now have the right and responsibility to be more involved with health care choices based on accurate information and consideration of risk factors (Dore & Ehman, 2020; Royal Australian and New Zealand College of Obstetricians and Gynaecologists, 2019). Three components are necessary for a shared decision-making setting (Cypher, 2019a). First, accurate, impartial, and comprehensible information to include no intervention or a right to refuse are relayed to a client. Second, a health care team member needs to be present and proficient in communication for care to be individualized. Last, an individual's values, goals, informed preferences, and concerns are incorporated into the communications. Therefore a client, nurse, and midwife or physician can partner together to use shared decision making to discuss intrapartum fetal surveillance, labor management, pharmacologic and nonpharmacologic methods for pain relief, and other topics to make an informed decision about management of labor and birth. This is facilitated with accurate and up-to-date information, which is evidence-based, culturally appropriate, and tailored to a client's needs.

APPLICATION OF THE NURSING PROCESS: CLIENT TEACHING WITH LACK OF KNOWLEDGE

Clinicians may identify any number of client care challenges when fetal surveillance is used during the intrapartum period. Clients may become anxious if EFM is initiated for oxytocin augmentation when, in the birth plan, they preferred IA and palpation for FHR and UA assessment. Pain that was once relieved with ambulation and hydrotherapy may become intolerable if continuous fetal monitoring is necessary. FHR interpretation may be challenging if narcotics are given in the latent phase of labor. Therefore two nursing care responsibilities related to fetal assessment should be considered: assessing the client's (and support person's) learning needs and expanding nursing care related to fetal oxygenation and potential interruptions along the oxygenation pathway.

Assessment

Identify what the client and support person already know about EFM, IA, and palpation. Clients who have attended prepared childbirth classes or have given birth before may have a basic understanding of the purpose, benefits, and limitations of fetal surveillance. Identifying what clients already know allows clinicians to build on preexisting knowledge and correct any inaccurate information.

If the client is not familiar with either technique of intrapartum fetal assessment, assess their perception and understanding of each method. For example, does the client believe EFM will signal the development of a complication? Does the client expect wireless fetal monitoring will be available during the first stage of labor? Is the client comfortable with IA for fetal assessment, or do they worry that something important will be missed?

Lack of knowledge can contribute to anxiety. Note the anxiety level of the client when the monitor is used. For example, is the client afraid to change positions because the FHR becomes intermittent? Do they frequently question why the monitor is not showing how strong the contractions are? Questions should be answered to the best of the clinician's ability, and then the clinician should assess the client's level of understanding.

Identification of Problems

With increased usage of EFM for labor, one common problem is the need for client education regarding EFM. If IA and palpation are being used, there may also be a need for client education regarding fetal surveillance.

Planning: Expected Outcomes

An expected outcome criteria is for the client (and support person) to express an understanding about equipment, procedures, benefits, limitations, and expected data after receiving education about fetal surveillance.

Interventions

Education should be delivered in a method understood by the client. This includes but is not limited to the purpose and equipment chosen for monitoring, frequency of assessment, and a brief explanation about what is shown on the tracing. Sometimes clarification about how the equipment functions is necessary.

When EFM is used during the intrapartum period, clients may have questions that should be answered. The following are frequently asked questions and suggested answers:

- "Can I move around with all these straps on?"
  "Of course, you can move or reposition yourself in bed as long as your baby tolerates the position change. I will be monitoring your FHR tracing and will adjust the monitors and your position as needed. In fact, repositioning yourself frequently will help your labor progress. Staying in the same position is not only uncomfortable but doesn't promote normal labor. Sometimes the monitor will be unable to record the FHR continuously or record contractions very well. Most of the time it is because the monitor on your belly has shifted out of place and needs to be readjusted. Use your call bell to reach me, and I'll come in to help you. If we continue to have difficulties recording the FHR or contractions, we may discuss other alternatives."
- "What if I need to go to the bathroom?"
  "If you need to go to the bathroom, we'll unplug the cords from the monitor."
- "Why is the baby's heart beating so fast? It sounds like a galloping horse!"
  "A baby's heartbeat is faster than an adult's heartbeat. The normal heart rate for these little ones is about 110 to 160 bpm. If the rate is lower or higher than normal, we'll review the tracing to see what the potential cause is and then make decisions about interventions that may need to be performed."
- "My contractions don't look very strong, but they sure feel strong to me!"
  "I know you're discouraged because the contractions on the tracing are not recording as strong as you feel them. Sometimes contractions appear stronger or weaker than they really are because of the position you're in, how big or small your baby may be, the position of the baby, and how much tissue is between the uterus and the transducer. Remember you have an external monitor that has a pressure sensor button. Because it is external and not internal, the monitor records the contraction frequency and duration but not the actual strength. I'll be feeling your belly to determine how strong your contractions are. If we need to record the actual uterine pressure, we'll talk to you about placing an internal monitor called an IUPC."
- "What do those numbers for contractions mean? They change all the time."
  "The IUPC we placed earlier is recording the pressure inside your uterus. The numbers change when you are contracting. The numbers will also fluctuate when you are breathing heavily, coughing, laughing, or readjusting your position."
- "Will the FSE hurt my baby?"
  "The electrode attaches to the first couple of layers of the baby's skin similar to the thickness of a dime, which is

about 1 mm. We already know your baby is head-down so we're very careful to avoid sensitive areas on the head such as the fontanels (soft spots) or the face."

- "The alarms on the monitor are really annoying. Can you turn down the volume?"

"Thanks for letting me know this information. I know alarms can be distracting to you because I know you want to have a quiet, calming environment for labor. Alarms beep for a variety of reasons. They let me know things like a transducer has slipped out of place and is unable to record the FHR, your blood pressure is too high, or if the FHR becomes too low. Let me lower the volume for you. If it's still too loud, let me know and I can mute the sound in the room. I'll still be able to monitor for problems by visually reviewing the tracing."

Evaluation

Evaluation of knowledge is ongoing because clients may think of questions after initial explanations and as clinical conditions change. Achievement of the goal or expected outcome is evident if a client and support person indicate an understanding after each explanation. This may be accompanied by a decrease in signs of anxiety.

APPLICATION OF THE NURSING PROCESS: OXYGENATION

Assessment

Assessment of the FHR and UA using standardized definitions and a consistent management approach is critical to intrapartum fetal surveillance. Standardized definitions allow clinicians to answer three questions: what we call it, what it means, and what we do about it (Miller et al., 2022). In answering the first question, clinicians are able to interpret FHR and UA data to determine whether a tracing is normal, indeterminate, or abnormal. The second question can be answered by simply applying two principles: whether there is presence or absence of interrupted oxygenation and whether hypoxic injury can be ruled out based on the existence of moderate variability or accelerations. Assessment of client and fetus is continuous during the dynamic process of labor. Comparing BL data with ongoing assessments of FHR patterns and UA will provide an opportunity to observe subtle trends in the data and distinguish between patterns that have similar appearances, such as early and late decelerations. Once these questions are answered, a standardized management approach using corrective measures to improve oxygenation can be applied to the clinical situation.

The nurse collects and analyzes critical assessments related to fetal well-being:

- FHR evaluation: BL rate and variability; periodic and episodic patterns; NICHD category
- UA: Frequency, duration and intensity of contractions; resting tone of the uterus between contractions
- Client vital signs
- Amount and character of amniotic fluid and time of rupture
- Client obstetric history (e.g., preeclampsia, abruption)
- Client medical–surgical history (e.g., asthma, chronic hypertension, cardiac disease)

Identification of Problems

Interruption of oxygen transfer can occur at any or all of the points in the pathway from client to fetus. Hypotension and hypertension, excessively strong and long contractions, and compression of the umbilical cord are examples of client conditions that can affect the oxygen transfer pathway. This interruption can interfere with fetal homeostasis, leading to a deterioration in oxygenation. Eventually, if left uncorrected, fetal oxygenation progresses from hypoxia to metabolic acidemia. Multiple organs and systems, such as the brain, can experience hypoperfusion, reduced oxygenation, lowered pH, and reduced delivery of fuel for metabolism. These changes cause the fetal system to cascade through multiple cellular events that lead to cellular and tissue dysfunction, neurologic injury, and potentially death. Therefore an appropriate patient problem during pregnancy and especially during labor and birth is possible fetal injury because of an interrupted fetal oxygenation pathway.

Planning: Expected Outcome

The nursing plan of care will prioritize the maintenance of fetal oxygenation by promoting placental perfusion for all clients and providing corrective actions and notification of the provider when a category II or III pattern is observed. The expected outcome is that the FHR pattern will maintain evidence of adequate fetal oxygenation, such as a normal BL rate and variability.

Interventions

Once a thorough assessment of BL FHR, variability, accelerations, decelerations, UA, and changes or trends over time has been completed, the standardized management model, "ABCD" is implemented. Using this method will provide a safeguard to ensure important steps in the intervention phase are not overlooked and are accomplished in a timely manner.

If the FHR pattern is related to an interruption in the oxygenation pathway and requires corrective measures, the nurse's priority is to identify the cause and take steps to improve fetal oxygenation. Implementing corrective measures in response to FHR and UA data is within the scope of practice of nurses (AWHONN, 2019a). Most facilities have protocols to give nurses a framework for these steps. Corrective measures may include both independent nursing actions and implementation of standing medical orders. Regardless of the situation, the delivering provider should be notified. Clients may understandably become anxious when the ABCD approach is implemented. Nurses should remain calm at the bedside to avoid increasing a client's fear and anxiety, which can reduce the client's ability to grasp what is occurring. Another way to decrease fear and anxiety is to explain the clinical situation and reason for corrective measures in succinct, simple language that the client will understand.

Evaluation

Ongoing evaluation of the clinical situation is necessary to evaluate the effects of interventions on the condition of the client and fetus. This allows clinicians to determine whether corrective measures were successful. Evaluation will also determine whether the plan was effective and whether an alternative plan should be in place. The outcome is met if the FHR pattern demonstrates adequate fetal oxygenation with a Category I pattern.

SUMMARY CONCEPTS

- A goal of intrapartum fetal heart rate (FHR) surveillance is to assess the adequacy of fetal oxygenation so timely and appropriate steps are taken when necessary to optimize perinatal outcomes.
- Adequate fetal oxygenation depends on an absence of an oxygenation pathway interruption because oxygenated blood must flow from the environment to a fetus via the pregnant client's lungs, heart, vasculature, uterus, placenta, and umbilical cord.
- Two approaches to intrapartum fetal heart rate surveillance include intermittent auscultation (IA) and palpation or electronic fetal monitoring (EFM). Each type has advantages and limitations.
- Intrapartum fetal surveillance consists of an assessment and evaluation of fetal status during labor using standardized definitions.
- The role of intrapartum EFM in assessing fetal physiologic changes caused by interrupted oxygenation includes two principles: (1) Fetal oxygenation involves oxygen transfer from the environment to the fetus and the fetal response to any interruption of oxygen transfer. (2) Certain FHR patterns provide reliable information regarding both of the basic elements of fetal oxygenation.
- A standardized method to FHR management is referred to as the ABCD approach. This includes: "A" to assess the oxygen pathway and identify the cause of FHR pattern changes, "B" to begin corrective measures, "C" to clear obstacles to delivery, and "D" to determine a delivery plan.
- A direct method of assessing the level of fetal oxygenation during the intrapartum period at the time of birth is to perform umbilical cord blood gas sampling at the time of cord clamping.
- Suggested frequency of assessment and documentation of FHR and uterine activity (UA) during the intrapartum period is directed by professional organizations and institutional policies. At a minimum, documentation includes admission evaluation of the maternal-fetal dyad, ongoing systematic assessments using standardized definitions for FHR and UA, corrective measures and response to these interventions, and communication with the health care team and client.

Clinical Judgment and Next-Generation NCLEX® Examination-Style Questions

A 41-year-old client, (G3P2002), is admitted for cervical ripening and labor induction at 39 2/7 weeks for gestational diabetes well controlled with insulin. The past medical–surgical history was unremarkable; gestational diabetes was the only obstetric complication of the pregnancy. After cervical ripening, the cervical exam was 3 cm dilated, 75% effaced, −2 station; oxytocin was initiated via an intravenous (IV) pump. Membranes were artificially ruptured by a midwife. Maintenance IV fluids of lactated Ringer's solution was infusing at 125 mL/hr. Four hours later, the client received an epidural for uterine contractions that were becoming more painful. Cervical examination before epidural placement was 4 cm dilated, 90% effaced, with the fetal vertex at a −2 station. Vital signs: blood pressure (BP): 128/72, temperature (T): 99.1°F (37.2°C), pulse (P): 98, respiration (R): 22. The following electronic fetal monitoring (EFM) tracing is observed by the nurse:

1. **Complete the following sentences by choosing from the list of options:**

The nurse recognizes that the fetal heart rate (FHR) baseline (BL) is ____1____. The FHR pattern is reflective of a ____2____, which is predictive of ____3____ .

Options for 1	Options for 2	Options for 3
Bradycardia	Category I	Abnormal fetal acid–base status at the time of observation
Normal Range	Category II	Indeterminate fetal acid–base status at the time of observation
Tachycardia	Category III	Normal fetal acid–base status at the time of observation

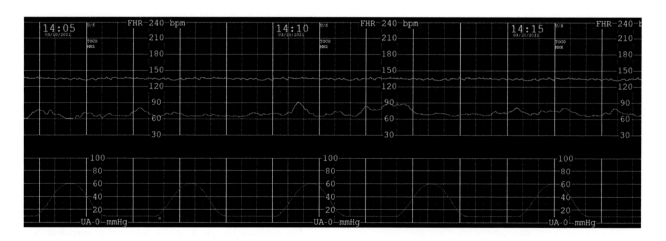

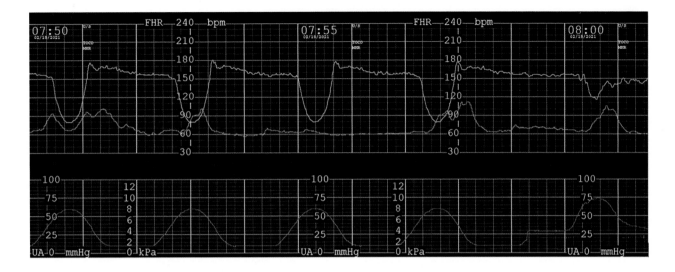

Approximately 5 hours later, the following FHR tracing was observed. The last cervical examination was performed 1.5 hours ago, and the client was 7 cm dilated, 100% effaced, with the fetal vertex at a +1 station. Vital signs: BP: 134/80, P: 96 , R: 22, and T: 100.2°F (37.8°C).

2. **Choose words from the choices below to fill in each blank found in the following sentence:**

The nurse interprets the FHR pattern as having a FHR BL of 155 beats per minute (bpm) with ___1___ variability and ___2___, which is a periodic pattern. This qualifies as a ___3___ in the three-tiered categorization system.

Options for 1	Options for 2	Options for 3
Absent	Intermittent late decelerations	Category I
Minimal	Recurrent early decelerations	Category II
Moderate	Recurrent variable decelerations	Category III
Marked		

3. **Use an X to indicate which actions listed in the left column should be implemented.**

Potential Steps	Implemented
Increase maintenance IV fluid infusion rate.	
Call physician to perform a forceps delivery.	
Prepare for a potential amnioinfusion.	
Perform a cervical examination.	
Reposition the client to a lateral position.	
Initiate blood pressures every 5 minutes.	
Decrease oxytocin infusion.	
Discontinue the epidural infusion.	

REFERENCES

Afors, K., & Chandraharan, E. (2011). Use of continuous electronic fetal monitoring in a preterm fetus: Clinical dilemmas and recommendations for practice. *Journal of Pregnancy*, 1–7. https://doi.org/10.1155/2011/848794.

Ahn, M. O., Korst, L. M., Phelan, J. P., & Martin, G. I. (1998). Does the onset of neonatal seizures correlate with the timing of fetal neurologic injury? *Clinical Pediatrics*, *37*(11), 673–676. https://doi.org/10.1177/000992289803701105.

American College of Nurse-Midwives (ACNM). (2015). Clinical bulletin. No. 60. Intermittent auscultation for intrapartum fetal heart rate surveillance. *Journal of Nurse Midwifery & Women's Health*, *61*(1), 626–632. https://doi.org/10.1111/jmwh.12372.

American College of Obstetricians and Gynecologists (ACOG). (2019). *Management of intrapartum fetal heart rate tracing*. ACOG Practice Bulletin 116. Published 2010, reaffirmed 2019.

American College of Obstetricians and Gynecologists & American Academy of Pediatrics (ACOG & AAP). (2014). *Neonatal encephalopathy and neurologic outcome* (2nd ed.).

Association of Women's Health, Obstetric and Neonatal Nurses (AWHONN). (2019a). Fetal heart monitoring. (Position Statement). *Journal of Obstetric, Gynecologic, & Neonatal Nursing*, *47*(6), 874–877. https://doi.org/10.1016/j.jogn.2018.09.007.

Association of Women's Health, Obstetric and Neonatal Nurses (AWHONN). (2019b). *Nursing management of the second stage of labor: Evidence-based clinical practice guideline* (3rd ed.).

Association of Women's Health, Obstetric and Neonatal Nurses (AWHONN). (2020). *Analgesia and anesthesia in the intrapartum period: Evidence-based clinical practice guideline*.

Ayers-de-Campos, D., & Nogueira-Reis, Z. (2015). Technical characteristics of current cardiotocographic monitors. *Best Practice & Research: Clinical Obstetrics and Gynaecology*, *30*(1), 22–32. https://doi.org/10.1016/j.bpobgyn.2015.05.005.

Baston, H., & Hall, J. (2018). Monitoring fetal well-being during routine antenatal care. In H. Baston, & J. Hall (Eds.), *Midwifery essentials: Antenatal* (2nd ed., Vol. 2, pp. 142–159). Elsevier.

Blackburn, S. T. (2018). *Maternal, fetal & neonatal physiology: A clinical perspective* (5th ed.). Elsevier.

Blix, E., Maude, R., Hals, E., Kisa, S., Karlsen, E., Nohr, E. A., de Jonge, A., Lindgren, H., Down, S., Reinar, L.M., Faureur, M., Pay, A.S.D., & Kaasen, A. (2019). Intermittent auscultation fetal monitoring during labour: A systematic scoping review to identify methods, effects, and accuracy. *PloS one, 14*(7), e0219573. https://doi.org/10.1371/journal.pone.0219573.

Bordelon, C. ,B., Fanning, B., Meredith, J., & Jnah, A. J. (2018). The nervous system. In A. Jnah, & A. Trembath (Eds.), *Fetal and neonatal physiology for the advanced practice nurse* (pp. 43–81). Springer.

Brosens, I., Puttemans, P., & Benagiano, G. (2019). Placental bed research: I. The placental bed: From spiral arteries remodeling to the great obstetrical syndromes. *American Journal of Obstetrics and Gynecology, 221*(5), 437–456. https://doi.org/10.1016/j.ajog.2019.05.044.

Burton, G. J., Sibly, C. P., & Jauniaux, E. R. M. (2021). Placental anatomy and physiology. In M. B. Landon, H. L. Galan, E. R. M. Jauniaux, D. A. Driscoll, V. Berghella, W. A. Grobman, S. J. Kilpatrick, & A. G. Cahill (Eds.), *Obstetrics: Normal and problem pregnancies* (8th ed., pp. 2–25). Elsevier.

Caldeyro-Barcia, R. (1979). The influence of maternal bearing-down efforts during second stage on fetal well-being. *Birth, 6*(1), 17–21. https://doi.org/10.1111/j.1523- 536X.1979.tb01298.x.

Caldeyro-Barcia, R., & Poseiro, J. J. (1959). Oxytocin and contractility of the pregnant human uterus. *Annals of the New York Academy of Sciences, 75*(2), 813–830. https://doi.org/10.1111/j.1749-6632.1959.tb44593.x.

Caldeyro-Barcia, R., & Poseiro, J. J. (1960). Physiology of the uterine contraction. *Clinical Obstetrics and Gynecology, 3*(2), 386–410.

Cashion, K. (2020). Fetal assessment during labor. In D. L. Lowdermilk, S. E. Perry, K. Cashion, K. R. Alden, & E. F. Olshansky (Eds.), *Maternity & women's health care* (12th ed., pp. 358–375). Mosby.

Clark, S. L., Gimovsky, M. L., & Miller, F. C. (1982). Fetal heart rate response to scalp blood sampling. *American Journal of Obstetrics and Gynecology, 144*(6), 706–708. https://doi.org/10.1016/0002-9378(82)90441-0.

Clark, S. L., Gimovsky, M. L., & Miller, F. C. (1984). The scalp stimulation test: A clinical alternative to fetal scalp blood sampling. *American Journal of Obstetrics and Gynecology, 148*(3), 274–277. https://doi.org/10.1016/s0002-9378(84)80067-8.

Clark, S. L., Nageotte, M. P., Garite, T. J., Freeman, R. K., Miller, D. A., Simpson, K. R., Belfort, A., Dildy, G. A., Parer, J. T., Berkowitz, R. L., D'Alton, M., Rouse, D. J., Gilstrap, L. C., Vintzileos, A. M., van Dorsten, P., Boehm, F. H., Miller, L. A., & Hankins, G. D. (2013). Intrapartum management of category II fetal heart rate tracings: Towards standardization of care. *American Journal of Obstetrics and Gynecology, 209*(2), 89–97. https://doi.org/10.1016/j.ajog.2013.04.030.

Cypher, R. L. (2017, October). *Technologies in perinatal nursing: Time to accept and embrace the challenge.* Perigen. https://perigen.com/wpcontent/uploads/2017/10/TechnologyAndPerinatalNursingbyRebeccaCypher.pdf.

Cypher, R. L. (2018a). A standardized approach to electronic fetal monitoring in critical care obstetrics. *Journal of Perinatal & Neonatal Nursing, 32*(3), 212–221. https://doi.org/10.1097/JPN.0000000000000343.

Cypher, R. L. (2018b). Electronic fetal monitoring documentation: Connecting points for quality care and communication. *The Journal of Perinatal & Neonatal Nursing, 32*(1), 24–33. https://doi.org/10.1097/JPN.0000000000000299.

Cypher, R. L. (2019a). Shared decision-making: A model for effective communication and patient satisfaction. *The Journal of Perinatal & Neonatal Nursing, 33*(4), 285–287. https://doi.org/10.1097/JPN.0000000000000441

Cypher, R. L. (2019b). When signals become crossed: Maternal-Fetal signal ambiguity. *The Journal of Perinatal & Neonatal Nursing, 33*(2), 105–107. https://doi.org/doi:10.1097/JPN.0000000000000404.

Cypher, R. L. (2021). Assessment of fetal oxygenation and acid–base status. In A. Lyndon, & K. Wisner (Eds.), *Fetal heart monitoring: Principles and practices* (6th ed., pp. 185–212). Kendall Hunt.

Dore, S., & Ehman, W. (2020). No. 396-Fetal health surveillance: Intrapartum consensus guideline. *Journal of Obstetrics and Gynaecology Canada, 42*(3), 316–348. https://doi.org/10.1016/j.jogc.2019.05.007.

Drummond, S., & Rust, C. (2021). Techniques for fetal heart and uterine activity assessment. In A. Lyndon, & K. Wisner (Eds.), *Fetal heart rate monitoring: Principles and practices* (6th ed., pp. 83–116). Kendall-Hunt.

Eller, A. G. (2020). Interventions for intrapartum fetal heart rate abnormalities. *Clinical Obstetrics and Gynecology, 63*(3), 635–644. https://doi.org/10.1097/GRF.0000000000000552.

Eller, A. G., & Esplin, M. (2020). Management of the category II fetal heart rate tracing. *Clinical Obstetrics and Gynecology, 63*(3), 659–667. https://doi.org/10.1097/GRF.0000000000000551.

Esplin, M. S. (2020). Identification of the fetus at risk for metabolic acidemia using continuous fetal heart rate monitoring. *Clinical Obstetrics and Gynecology, 63*(3), 616–624. https://doi.org/10.1097/GRF.0000000000000546.

Freeman, R. K., Garite, T. J., Nageotte, M. P., & Miller, L. A. (2012). *Fetal heart rate monitoring* (4th ed.). Lippincott Williams & Wilkins.

Garite, T. J., & Simpson, K. R. (2011). Intrauterine resuscitation during labor. *Clinical Obstetrics and Gynecology, 54*(1), 28–39. https://doi.org/10.1097/GRF.0b013e31820a062b.

Gisick, L. M., Webster, K. L., Keebler, J. R., Lazzara, E. H., Fouquet, S., Fletcher, K., Fagerlund, A., Lew, V., & Chan, R. (2018). Measuring shared mental models in healthcare. *Journal of Patient Safety and Risk Management, 23*(5), 207–219. https://doi.org/10.1177%2F2516043518796442.

Griggs, K. M., Hrelic, D. A., Williams, N., McEwen-Campbell, M., & Cypher, R. (2020). Preterm labor and birth: A clinical review. *MCN: The American Journal of Maternal/Child Nursing, 45*(6), 328–337. https://doi.org/10.1097/NMC.0000000000000656.

Harvey, C. J. (1987). Fetal scalp stimulation: Enhancing the interpretation of fetal monitor tracings. *Journal of Perinatal and Neonatal Nursing, 1*(1), 13–21. https://doi.org/10.1097/00005237-198707000-00006.

Heuser, C. C. (2020). Physiology of fetal heart rate monitoring. *Clinical Obstetrics and Gynecology, 63*(3), 607–615. https://doi.org/10.1097/GRF.0000000000000553.

Heyborne, K. D. (2017). A systematic review of intrapartum fetal head compression: What is the impact on the fetal brain? *American Journal of Perinatology Reports, 7*(2), e79. https://doi.org/10.1055%2Fs-0037-1602658.

Intrapartum Assessment. (2018). In F. Cunningham, K. J. Leveno, S. L. Bloom, J. Dashe, B. L. Hoffman, B. M Casey, & C. Y. Spong (Eds.), *William's obstetrics* (24th ed., pp. 473–503). McGraw-Hill.

Jonker, C. M., Van Riemsdijk, M. B., & Vermeulen, B. (2011). Shared mental models. In *Coordination, organizations, institutions, and norms in agent systems* (pp. 132–151). Springer.

Lappen, J. R., Chien, E. K., & Mercer, B. M. (2018). Contraction-associated maternal heart rate decelerations: A pragmatic marker of intrapartum volume status. *Obstetrics & Gynecology, 132*(4), 1011–1017. https://doi.org/10.1097/AOG.0000000000002808.

Lagercrantz, H., & Slotkin, T. A. (1986). The "stress" of being born. *Scientific American*, *254*(4), 100–107. https://doi.org/10.1038/scientificamerican0486-100.

Larry-Osman, C. (2021). Intrapartum fetal monitoring: A historical perspective. In A. Lyndon, & K. Wisner (Eds.), *Fetal heart rate monitoring: Principles and practices* (6th ed., pp. 3–22). Kendall-Hunt Publications.

Lyndon, A., & O'Brien-Abel (2021). Fetal heart rate interpretation. In A. Lyndon, & K. Wisner (Eds.), *Fetal heart rate monitoring: Principles and practices* (6th ed., pp. 117–154). Kendall-Hunt Publications.

Macones, G. A., Hankins, G. D., Spong, C. Y., Hauth, J., & Moore, T. (2008). The 2008 National Institute of Child Health and Human Development workshop report on electronic fetal monitoring: Update on definitions, interpretation, and research guidelines. *Obstetrics and Gynecology*, *112*(3), 661–666. https://doi.org/10.1097/aog.0b013e3181841395.

Malane, E. A., Richardson, C., & Burke, K. G. (2019). A novel approach to electronic nursing documentation education: Ambassador of learning program. *Journal For Nurses in Professional Development*, *35*(6), 324–329. https://doi.org/10.1097/NND.0000000000000587.

Manor, M., Blickstein, I., Hazan, Y., Flidel-Rimon, O., & Hagay, Z. J. (1998). Postpartum determination of umbilical artery blood gases: Effect of time and temperature. *Clinical Chemistry*, *44*(3), 681–683.

Martis, R., Emilia, O., Nurdiati, D. S., & Brown, J. (2017). Intermittent auscultation (IA) of fetal heart rate in labour for fetal well-being. *Cochrane Database of Systematic Reviews*, (2). https://doi.org/10.1002/14651858.CD008680.pub2.

Maude, R., Lawson, J., & Foureur, M. (2010). Auscultation: The action of listening. *New Zealand College of Midwives Journal*, *43*(1), 13–18.

Miller, D. A. (2011). Intrapartum fetal heart rate monitoring: A standardized approach to management. *Clinical obstetrics and gynecology*, *54*(1), 22–27. https://doi.org/10.1097/GRF.0b013e31820a0564.

Miller, L. A. (2016). The more things change, the more they stay the same: Thirty years of fetal monitoring in perspective. *The Journal of Perinatal & Neonatal nursing*, *30*(3), 255–258. https://doi.org/10.1097/JPN.0000000000000180.

Miller, L. A., Miller, D. A., & Cypher, R. L. (2022). *Mosby's pocket guide to fetal monitoring: A multidisciplinary approach* (9th ed.). Elsevier.

Miller, N. R., Cypher, R. L., Nielsen, P. E., & Foglia, L. M. (2013). Maternal pulse pressure at admission is a risk factor for fetal heart rate changes after initial dosing of a labor epidural: A retrospective cohort study. *American Journal of Obstetrics and Gynecology*, *209*(4), 382-e1. https://doi.org/10.1016/j.ajog.2013.05.049.

Modanlou, H. D., & Freeman, R. K. (1982). Sinusoidal fetal heart rate pattern: Its definition and clinical significance. *American Journal of Obstetrics and Gynecology*, *142*(8), 1033–1038. https://doi.org/10.1016/0002-9378(82)90789-X.

Modanlou, H. D., & Murata, Y. (2004). Sinusoidal heart rate pattern: Reappraisal of its definition and clinical significance. *Journal of Obstetrics & Gynaecology Research*, *30*(3), 169–180. https://doi.org/10.1111/j.1447-0756.2004.00186.x

Monica Healthcare. (2018). *Novii™ Wireless patch system clinical application guide*. https://www.womens-health.net/data/files/mic-eu-novii-wireless-patch-system-clinical-application-guide-english-06-2018-jb52979xxb.pdf.2017.

Monson, M., Heuser, C., Einerson, B. D., Esplin, I., Snow, G., Varner, M., & Esplin, M. S. (2020). Evaluation of an external fetal electrocardiogram monitoring system: A randomized controlled trial. *American journal of obstetrics and gynecology*, *223*(2), 244.e1. https://doi.org/10.1016/j.ajog.2020.02.012.

Moore, K. L., Persaud, T. V. N., Persaud, M. D., & Torchia, M. G. (2021). Cardiovascular system. In K. Moore, M. Persaud, & M. Torchia (Eds.), *The developing human: Clinically oriented embryology* (11th ed., pp. 263–314). Elsevier.

Nageotte, M. P. (2015). Fetal heart rate monitoring. *Seminars in Fetal and Neonatal Medicine*, *20*(3), 144–148. https://doi.org/10.1016/j.siny.2015.02.002.

O'Brien-Abel, N. (2020). Clinical implications of fetal heart rate interpretation based on underlying physiology. *MCN: The American Journal of Maternal/Child Nursing*, *45*(2), 82–91. https://doi.org/10.1097/NMC.0000000000000596.

O'Brien-Abel, N. (2021). Physiologic basis for fetal monitoring. In A. Lyndon, & K. Wisner (Eds.), *Fetal heart monitoring: Principles and practices* (6th ed., pp. 23–50). Kendall Hunt.

Parer, J. T., King, T., Flanders, S., Fox, M., & Kilpatrick, S. (2006). Fetal acidemia and electronic fetal heart rate patterns: Is there evidence of an association? *Journal of Maternal, Fetal, & Neonatal Medicine*, *19*(5), 289–294.

Parfitt, S. E. (2021). Preterm labor and birth. In K. R. Simpson, P. A. Creehan, N. O'Brien-Abel, C. K. Roth, & A. J. Rohan (Eds.), *Perinatal Nursing* (5th ed., pp. 142–181). Wolters Kluwer.

Pijnenborg, R., Vercruysse, L., & Hanssens, M. (2006). The uterine spiral arteries in human pregnancy: Facts and controversies. *Placenta*, *27*(9), 939–958. https://doi.org/10.1016/j.placenta.2005.12.006.

Polnaszek, B., López, J. D., Clark, R., Raghuraman, N., Macones, G. A., & Cahill, A. G. (2020). Marked variability in intrapartum electronic fetal heart rate patterns: Association with neonatal morbidity and abnormal arterial cord gas. *Journal of Perinatology*, *40*, 56–62. https://doi.org/10.1038/s41372-019-0520-9.

Pullen, K. M., Riley, E. T., Waller, S. A., Taylor, L., Caughey, A. B., Druzin, M. L., & El-Sayed, Y. Y., (2007). Randomized comparison of intravenous terbutaline vs nitroglycerin for acute intrapartum fetal resuscitation. *American Journal of Obstetrics and Gynecology*, *197*(4), 414.e1. https://doi.org/10.1016/j.ajog.2007.06.063.

Raghuraman, N. (2020). Response to category II tracings: Does anything help? *Seminars in Perinatology*, *44*(2), 1–4. https://doi.org/10.1016/j.semperi.2019.151217.

Raghuraman, N., Temming, L. A., Doering, M. M., Stoll, C. R., Palanisamy, A., Stout, M. J., et al. (2021). Maternal oxygen supplementation compared with room air for intrauterine resuscitation: A systematic review and meta-analysis. *JAMA Pediatrics*, *174*(4), 368–376. https://doi.org/10.1001/jamapediatrics.2020.5351.

Reddy, A., Moulden, M., & Redman, C. W. G. (2009). Antepartum high-frequency fetal heart rate sinusoidal rhythm: Computerized detection and fetal anemia. *American Journal of Obstetrics and Gynecology*, *200*(4), 407.e1–407.e6. https://doi.org/10.1016/j.ajog.2008.10.026.

Riegel, M., Saccone, G., Locci, M., Salim, R., Fisher, A., Repke, J., et al. (2018). Dextrose intravenous fluid therapy in labor reduces the length of the first stage of labor. *European Journal of Obstetrics & Gynecology and Reproductive Biology*, *228*. https://doi.org/10.1016/j.ejogrb.2018.07.019.

Riley, R. J., & Johnson, J. W. (1993). Collecting and analyzing cord blood gases. *Clinical Obstetrics and Gynecology, 36*(1), 13–23. https://doi.org/10.1097/00003081-199303000- 00005.

Royal Australian and New Zealand College of Obstetricians and Gynaecologists. (2019). *Intrapartum fetal surveillance clinical guidelines* (4th ed.). https://ranzcog.edu.au/RANZCOG_SITE/media/RANZCOG- MEDIA/Women%27s%20Health/Statement%20and%20guide lines/Clinical- Obstetrics/IFS-Guideline-4thEdition-2019.pdf?ext=. pdf.

Scheans, P. (2011). Umbilical cord blood gases: New clinical relevance for an age-old practice. *Neonatal Network, 30*(2), 123–126. https:/doi.org/10.1891/0730-0832.30.2.123.

Shields, L. E., Wiesner, S., Klein, C., Pelletreau, B., & Hedriana, H. L. (2018). A standardized approach for category II fetal heart rate with significant decelerations: Maternal and neonatal outcomes. *American Journal of Perinatology, 35*(14), 1405–1410.

Simpson, K. R. (2021). Physiologic interventions for fetal heart rate patterns. In A. Lyndon, & K. Wisner (Eds.), *Fetal heart rate monitoring: Principles and practices* (6th ed, pp. 155–184). Kendall-Hunt Publications.

Simpson, K. R., & Miller, L. (2011). Assessment and optimization of uterine activity during labor. *Clinical Obstetrics and Gynecology, 54*(1), 40–49. https://doi.org/10.1097/GRF.0b013e31820a06aa.

Skupski, D. W., Rosenberg, C. R., & Eglinton, G. S. (2002). Intrapartum fetal stimulation tests: A meta-analysis. *Obstetrics and Gynecology, 99*(1), 129–134. https://doi.org/10.1016/s00297844(01)01645-3.

Society of Obstetricians and Gynaecologists Canada. (2020). Fetal health surveillance: Intrapartum consensus guideline (No. 396). *Journal of Obstetrics and Gynaecology Canada, 42*(3), 316–348. https://doi.org/10.1016/j.jogc.2019.05.007.

Thaler, I., Manor, D., Itskovitz, J., Rottem, S., Levit, N., Timor-Tritsch, I., & Brandes, J. M. (1990). Changes in uterine blood flow during human pregnancy. *American Journal of Obstetrics and Gynecology, 162*(1), 121–125. https://doi.org/10.1016/0002-9378(90)90834-T.

Timor-Tritsch, I. E., Dierker, L. J., Hertz, R. H., Deagan, N. C., & Rosen, M. G. (1978). Studies of antepartum behavioral state in the human fetus at term. *American Journal of Obstetrics and Gynecology, 132*(5), 524–528.

Vlemminx, M. W., Rabotti, C., van der Hout–van der Jagt, M. B., & Oei, S. G. (2018). Clinical use of electrohysterography during term labor: A systematic review on diagnostic value, advantages, and limitations. *Obstetrical & Gynecological Survey, 73*(5), 303–324. https://doi.org.10.1097/OGX.0000000000000560.

Wallman, C. M. (1997). Interpretation of fetal cord blood gases. *Neonatal Network, 16*(1), 72–75.

Wang, Y., & Zhao, S. (2010). *Vascular biology of the placenta.* Morgan & Claypool Life Sciences.

Williams, K. P., & Galerneau, F. (2003). Intrapartum fetal heart rate patterns in the prediction of neonatal acidemia. *American Journal of Obstetrics and Gynecology, 188*(3), 820–823. https://doi.org/10.1067/mob.2003.183.

Wisner, K., & Holschuh, C. (2018). Fetal heart rate auscultation, 3rd ed. *Nursing for Women's Health, 22*(6), e1–e32. https://doi.org/10.1016/j.nwh.2018.10.001.

Nursing Care During Labor and Birth

Kristin L. Scheffer, Kristine DeButy

OBJECTIVES

After studying this chapter, you should be able to:

1. Teach the client and family when to go to the birth facility.
2. Communicate therapeutically with the intrapartum client and significant other.
3. Contrast true and false labor.
4. Describe admission and continuing intrapartum nursing assessments.
5. Apply the nursing process to care of the client and significant other during the intrapartum period.
6. Describe common nursing procedures used when caring for clients during the intrapartum period including indications, contraindications, risks, and nursing considerations.
7. Prioritize nursing care of the intrapartum client in emergent situations.
8. Apply the nursing process to care for the client having a cesarean birth.

Care of clients and their families during labor and birth is a rewarding yet demanding specialty within nursing. Birth is more than a physical event. It is a powerful, life-changing event that leaves a lasting impact on the childbearing client and family. Every culture recognizes that birth has deep personal and social significance. Roles and relationships are forever altered by this event.

Intrapartum nurse responsibilities include assessing, supporting, and facilitating normal physiologic labor; documenting; and communicating labor progress to clients, their families, and providers (Association of Women's Health, Obstetric, and Neonatal Nurses [AWHONN], 2018). The nurse must support natural physical processes, promote a meaningful experience for the family, and be alert for complications. Additionally, the nurse cares for two clients, one of whom—the fetus—cannot be observed directly.

Although labor is a normal process, some clients require special procedures to help them and their fetuses. This chapter will also address the nursing considerations for some of these procedures.

ADMISSION TO THE BIRTH FACILITY

The Decision to Go to the Birth Facility

During the last trimester of pregnancy, the client needs to know when to go to the hospital or birth center. Factors to consider include the following:

- Number and duration of any previous labors
- Distance from the hospital
- Available transportation
- Childcare needs
- Risk status

During prenatal care, nurses teach clients to distinguish between false (prodromal) and true labor. Nurses teach guidelines for going to the birth center and reinforce those given by the provider (see Client Teaching: When to Go to the Hospital or Birth Center). Not everyone has a typical labor, so clients should be encouraged to go to the birth center if they have any concerns.

CLIENT TEACHING

When to Go to the Hospital or Birth Center

These are guidelines for providing individualized instruction to clients about when to go to the hospital or birth center.

- Contractions: A pattern of increasing regularity, frequency, duration, and intensity.
  - Regular contractions: The general recommendation is when contractions are 5 minutes apart, lasting 1 minute, for 1 hour.
- Ruptured membranes: A gush or trickle of fluid from the vagina should be evaluated, regardless of whether contractions are occurring.
- Bleeding: Bright-red bleeding should be evaluated promptly. Normal bloody show is thicker, pink or dark red, and mixed with mucus.
- Decreased fetal movement: A decrease in the baby's normal activity requires evaluation; the provider should be notified, and/or the client should come to the labor unit.
- Other concerns: These guidelines cannot cover all situations and do not replace specific instructions given by the provider. Therefore go to the hospital for evaluation of any concerns and feelings that something may be wrong.

Nursing Responsibilities During Admission

Developing rapport and assessment of the family, including maternal-fetal status and birth expectations, are key components of the initial interaction during admission.

Establish a Therapeutic Relationship (Developing Rapport)

The nurse should quickly establish a therapeutic relationship with the client and significant other. First impressions can influence the client's entire birth experience. Even when the unit is busy, the nurse should communicate interest, friendliness, caring, and competence.

Providing culturally competent care is essential to maintain the safety and well-being of clients. When the client's native language is not spoken by the health care team, arranging for a culturally acceptable interpreter makes the client and family feel welcome, promotes safety through enhanced understanding, and meets regulatory standards (The Joint Commission [TJC], 2019). Hospitals offer interpreters via telephone, online device, or in person when available.

Convey confidence. From the first encounter, the nurse should convey confidence and optimism in the client's ability to give birth. Whether it is a client's first baby or they have had many children, labor can be overwhelming. The nurse provides reassurance that intense contractions are normal in active labor while helping them manage the pain and simultaneously watching for complications.

Assign a primary nurse. Having one nurse provide all care during labor is ideal but often unrealistic. Changes in caregivers should be limited as much as possible.

Use touch for comfort. Touch can communicate acceptance, offer reassurance, and provide physical and emotional comfort to many laboring clients. Clients who usually do not welcome touch may appreciate it during labor. Cultural norms and personal history influence a client's acceptance of touch from an unrelated person. The nurse should not assume the client desires touch but instead ask if touch is welcomed or beneficial. As labor progresses, the client's desire for touch may change; it may become irritating rather than comforting.

Respect cultural values. Cultural beliefs and practices give structure, meaning, and richness to the birth experience. Many cultural groups have specific practices related to childbearing. Incorporating cultural beliefs and individualizing care is important and requires ongoing dialogue with the client about preferred practices because beliefs may change from generation to generation (Callister, 2021).

Determine family expectations about birth. Regardless of their number of children, clients and their partners have expectations about their birth experience. Some clients use birth plans describing what they desire, whereas others may not have specific plans but have expectations shaped by contact with relatives, friends, previous birth experiences, and the media. Individualized birth plans serve as a communication tool to help the team meet the client's birth expectations. If the client does not have a specific birth plan, the nurse should use open-ended questions to identify the expectations of the client and support people.

KNOWLEDGE CHECK

1. What communication skills can the nurse use to establish a therapeutic relationship when the client and family enter the hospital or birth center?
2. How can the nurse incorporate a couple's cultural practices into intrapartum care?

Assessment

Assessment of the obstetric client is an ongoing, multidimensional process that begins with admission and continues throughout the hospital stay. The admission process includes reviewing the client's medical, surgical, and obstetric history; performing a physical examination; performing a psychosocial assessment; and asking about personal preferences and expectations for labor and birth. This inquiry includes both the client's perspective and that of their support system. Assessment does not end with completion of the admission intake process. The obstetric registered nurse (RN) continually assesses maternal-fetal status while supporting the client and family throughout the antenatal, birth, and postpartum periods.

The prenatal record serves as a communication tool between the provider and the birth facility. During admission, information obtained from the prenatal record is verified or updated as needed. Clients who have not had prenatal care or have no prenatal record available upon admission require more extensive assessments by the nurse and provider.

Focused assessment. On admission, a focused assessment is performed before the broader database assessment is completed. Assessment priorities are set by the condition of the client and fetus and whether birth is imminent (see Box 15.1 for assisting with an imminent birth). This assessment includes, at a minimum, the client's chief complaint; assessment of the fetal heart rate (FHR), vital signs, and uterine contractions; labor progress; client's perception of fetal movement; and evaluation of any high-risk condition (American Academy of Pediatrics & American College of Obstetricians and Gynecologists [AAP & ACOG], 2017; Simpson & O'Brien-Abel, 2021).

Fetal heart rate. FHR is an important aspect of assessing oxygenation and fetal status. On admission and throughout labor, the nurse assesses the FHR for category and fetal tolerance of labor (see Table 15.1 and Chapter 14).

Vital signs. Vital signs provide insight into the well-being of both the client and the fetus. They identify complications such as hypertension or infection. Hypertension during pregnancy is defined as a sustained blood pressure of 140 mm Hg systolic or 90 mm Hg diastolic or higher. Hypertension may be transient, related to pregnancy, or chronic (AAP & ACOG, 2017; ACOG, 2020b). A temperature of 38°C (100.4°F) or higher suggests infection. Tachypnea, hypotension, and tachycardia also can be associated with varying degrees of complications, such as infection/sepsis, respiratory distress, or blood loss.

Impending birth. Grunting sounds, bearing down, sitting on one buttock, and saying urgently, "The baby's coming" suggest imminent birth. In this situation, the nurse abbreviates the initial assessment and collects other information after birth. While the nurse cares for the client, pertinent/critical information can be quickly gathered if birth is imminent:

- Names of client and support person(s)
- Obstetric provider name
- Number of pregnancies and prior births, including whether the births were vaginal or cesarean
- Status of membranes
- Estimated due date (EDD)

BOX 15.1 Assisting With an Imminent Birth

Delivery of infants may occur rapidly, and the nurse must be prepared to respond to the urgent needs of the client and newborn.

Nursing Priorities for an Imminent Birth in any Setting
Prevent or reduce injury to the client and infant.
Maintain the infant's airway and temperature after birth.

Preparing for an Imminent Birth
Study the delivery sequence in Fig. 15.6, "Vaginal Birth."
Locate the emergency delivery pack ("precip" tray) on the unit.

During the Birth
Remain with the client to provide support during birth. Use the call light, emergency cord or ask the partner to call for help. Stay calm to reduce the couple's anxiety.
Put on gloves to prevent contact with blood and other secretions. Sterile gloves reduce transmission of environmental organisms to the client and the infant. However, the nurse will be "catching" the infant in this situation. No invasive procedure is expected, so clean gloves are adequate.

After the Birth
Observe the infant's color and respirations for distress. Wipe excess secretions from the infant's face and mouth with a clean cloth. Suction the mouth and nose with a bulb syringe if necessary.
Dry the infant and place skin-to-skin with the client. Cover the client and baby with warmed blankets to maintain warmth.
Put the infant to the client's breast and encourage suckling to promote uterine contraction, which will facilitate placental expulsion and control bleeding and initiate lactation.

- Complications during this or other pregnancies
- Significant medical and surgical history
- Allergies to medications, foods, or other substances
- Time and type of last oral intake
- Vital signs and FHR
- Pain: Location, intensity, factors that intensify or relieve, duration, whether constant or intermittent, whether the pain is acceptable to the client, and effectiveness of current coping techniques

The provider is notified promptly if any of the following are identified or suspected (AAP & ACOG, 2017; Simpson & O'Brien-Abel, 2021; Wisner & Larry-Osman, 2021):

- Imminent birth
- Indeterminate (category II) or abnormal (category III) FHR (see Chapter 14)
- Abnormal vital signs
- Vaginal bleeding (more than bloody show)
- Preterm labor
- Preterm premature rupture of membranes (PPROM)
- Acute abdominal pain

KNOWLEDGE CHECK

3. What are the three assessment priorities when a client comes to the intrapartum unit?
4. What observations suggest a client is going to give birth very soon? What should the nurse do in that case?

Database assessment. If focused assessments of client and fetus are normal and birth is not imminent, a more complete admission assessment is performed to further evaluate the client, fetus, and available support persons (see Table 15.1).

Basic assessment. Regulatory agencies and defined standards of care require certain elements to be assessed on admission to the hospital. Intrapartum admission forms guide the nurse to obtain required information.

The client may be accompanied by their significant other or support system during admission. Use caution when asking sensitive information, such as about prior pregnancies, sexually transmitted infections (STIs), and potential abuse,

TABLE 15.1 Intrapartum Assessment Guide[a]

Assessment, Method (Selected Rationales)	Common Findings	Significant Findings and Nursing Action
Interview *Purpose:* To obtain information about the client's pregnancy, labor, and conditions that may affect care. The interview is curtailed if delivery is imminent. *Introduction:* Introduce yourself and ask the client how they prefer to be addressed. Ask if the partner and/or family can remain during the interview and assessment. *(Shows respect for the client and allows control over who remains at the bedside.)*	Many clients prefer to be addressed by their first names during labor. Some clients will prefer certain pronouns (her/she/they/them) to be used.	The surname (family name) precedes the given name in some cultures. Clarify which name is used to properly address the client and to properly identify both client and newborn. Verify accuracy of identification bands before placing them on the client and baby.

Continued

TABLE 15.1   Intrapartum Assessment Guide[a]—cont'd

Assessment, Method (Selected Rationales)	Common Findings	Significant Findings and Nursing Action
Culture and language: If the client is from another culture, ask what language is preferred and what language(s) are spoken, read, or verbally understood. *(Identifies the need for an interpreter and enables the most accurate data collection.)*	Common non-English languages of clients in the United States are Spanish and some Asian dialects. The most common non-English languages vary with location.	Secure an interpreter fluent in the client's primary language. Ask if there are people who are not acceptable as interpreters (e.g., males or members of a group in conflict with their culture). Family members are not acceptable as interpreters because they may interpret selectively, adding or subtracting information as they see fit. Online or phone interpreters are available in many facilities. Hearing-impaired clients may read lips well, or they may need sign-language interpreters or other assistance.
Communication: Ask the client to tell you when they are experiencing contractions or pain and pause during the interview and physical assessment. *(Shows sensitivity and allows the client to concentrate more fully on the information the nurse requests.)*	Clients in active labor have difficulty answering questions or cooperating with a physical examination while they are having a contraction.	If contractions are very frequent, assess the client's labor status promptly rather than continuing the interview. Ask only the most critical questions.
Nonverbal cues: Observe the client's behaviors and interactions with family and the nurse. *(Permits estimation of anxiety level. Identifies behaviors indicating a prompt vaginal examination is necessary to determine whether birth is imminent.)*	*Latent phase:* Client is sociable and mildly anxious. *Active phase:* Client concentrates intently during contractions; often uses prepared childbirth techniques.	The unprepared or extremely anxious client may breathe deeply and rapidly, displaying a tense facial and body posture during and between contractions. Euphoria, combativeness, or sedation suggests recent illicit drug ingestion.
Reason for admission (Chief complaint): "What brings you to the hospital/birth center today?" *(Open-ended question promotes more complete answer.)*	Labor contractions at term, induction of labor, or observation for false labor are common reasons for admission.	Bleeding, preterm labor, pain other than labor contractions. Report these findings to the physician or nurse-midwife promptly.
Prenatal care: "Did you see a doctor or nurse-midwife during your pregnancy?" "Who is your doctor or nurse-midwife?" "How far along were you in your pregnancy when you saw the physician or nurse-midwife?" "Have you ever been admitted here before during this pregnancy?" *(Enables location of prenatal record and prior visit records.)*	Early and regular prenatal care promotes client and fetal health.	No prenatal care or care that was irregular or begun in late pregnancy may suggest complications may not have been identified.
Estimated due date (EDD): "When is your baby due?" *(Determines whether gestation is term.)* "When did your last menstrual period begin?" *(For estimation of EDD if client did not have prenatal care.)*	Term gestation: 37–42 wk. The client's gestation may have been confirmed or adjusted during pregnancy with an ultrasound or other clinical examination.	Gestations earlier than the beginning of the 37th wk (preterm) or later than the end of the 42nd wk (postterm) are associated with more fetal or neonatal problems. The provider may try to stop labor that occurs earlier than 36 wks if there are no contraindications for client or fetus.
Gravidity, parity, abortions: "How many times have you been pregnant?" "How many babies have you had? Were they full term or premature?" "How many children are now living?" "Have you had any miscarriages or abortions?" "Were there any problems with your babies after they were born?" *(Helps estimate probable speed of labor and anticipate neonatal problems.)* Note: These questions should be asked when the client is alone to protect privacy.	Labor may be faster for the client who has given birth before. Miscarriage is used to describe a spontaneous abortion because many lay people associate the term *abortion* with only induced abortions.	Parity of 5 or more (grand multiparity) is associated with placenta previa (see Chapter 10) and postpartum hemorrhage (see Chapter 18). Clients who have had several spontaneous abortions or who have given birth to infants with abnormalities may face a higher risk for an infant with a birth defect.

TABLE 15.1 Intrapartum Assessment Guide^a—cont'd

Assessment, Method (Selected Rationales)	Common Findings	Significant Findings and Nursing Action
Medical/Surgical History: Do you have a history of any medical or surgical procedures? Any diabetes, asthma, high blood pressure, kidney or thyroid disease, liver problems, etc.? Any surgeries other than the previous delivery information you shared?	Clients who have other medical/surgical history may have further complications during hospitalization/labor.	Although complications may not be anticipated, the nurse should be aware of the client's medical and surgical history, which could lead to possible complications during labor or postpartum stay.
Allergies: "Are you allergic to any foods, medicines, or other substances?" "Do you have an allergy to latex?" "What kind of reaction do you have?" "Have you ever had a problem with anesthesia?" *(Determines possible sensitivity to drugs that may be used or history of malignant hyperthermia.)*	Record any known allergies to food, medication, or other substances. As needed, describe how they affected the client.	Allergy to seafood, iodized salt, or imaging contrast media may indicate iodine allergy. Because iodine is used in many "prep" solutions, alternative ones should be used. Allergy to latex is more common. Allergy to anesthetics may indicate possible allergy to the drugs used for local or regional anesthetics. These drugs usually end in the suffix *-caine.* Anesthetics also can cause severe changes in temperature and muscle contraction, which can be fatal.

Pregnancy History (identifies problems that may affect this birth)

Present pregnancy: "Have you had any problems during this pregnancy, such as high blood pressure, diabetes, infections, or bleeding?"	Complications are not expected.	Clients who have diabetes or hypertension may have poor placental blood flow, possibly resulting in fetal compromise. Some complications of past pregnancies, such as gestational diabetes, may recur in another pregnancy.
Past pregnancies: "Were there any problems with your other pregnancy(ies)?" "Were your other babies born vaginally or by cesarean birth?"	Clients who had previous cesarean birth(s) may have a trial of labor (TOLAC) and vaginal birth (VBAC). A client who previously had a difficult labor or a cesarean birth may be more anxious than one who had an uncomplicated labor and birth.	Although VBAC is less common, it may be chosen for a variety of reasons. The nurse should be aware of the need for support and for complications that may be more likely in the current pregnancy.
Other: "Is there anything else you think we should know so we can better care for you?"	This open-ended question gives the client a chance to share information that may not be elicited by other questions.	
Labor status: "When did your contractions become regular?" "What time did you begin to think you might really be in labor?" *(Facilitates a more accurate estimation of the time labor began.)*	Varies among clients. Many clients go to the birth facility when contractions first begin. Others wait until they are reasonably sure they are really in labor.	Clients who say they have been "in labor" for an unusual length of time (e.g., "for 2 days") have probably had false (prodromal) labor. These clients may be very tired from the annoying and apparently nonproductive contractions.
Contractions: "How often are your contractions coming?" "How long do they last?" "Are they getting stronger?" "Tell me if you have a contraction while we are talking." *(Obtains the client's subjective evaluation of the contractions. Alerts the nurse to palpate contractions that occur during the interview.)*	Varies according to the stage and phase of labor. Labor contractions are usually regular and show a pattern of increasing frequency, duration, and intensity.	Irregular contractions or those that do not increase in frequency, duration, or intensity are more likely to represent false labor. Contractions that are too frequent or too long can reduce placental blood flow. Incomplete uterine relaxation between contractions also can reduce placental blood flow.
Membrane status: "Has your water broken?" "What time did it break?" "What did the fluid look like?" "About how much fluid did you lose—was it a big gush or a trickle?" *(Alerts the nurse of the need to verify whether the membranes have ruptured if it is not obvious. Identifies possible prolonged rupture of membranes, preterm rupture, or meconium-stained fluid.)*	Most clients go to the birth facility for evaluation soon after their membranes rupture. If a client is not already in labor, contractions usually begin within a few hours after the membranes rupture at term.	If the membranes have ruptured and the client is not in labor or is preterm, a vaginal examination is often deferred. A speculum examination may be done by the physician or nurse-midwife to identify the client's admission status. Labor may be induced if the client is at term with ruptured membranes.

Continued

TABLE 15.1   Intrapartum Assessment Guide[a]—cont'd

Assessment, Method (Selected Rationales)	Common Findings	Significant Findings and Nursing Action
Oral intake: "When was the last time you had something to eat or drink?" "What did you have?" (*Provides information needed to most safely administer general anesthesia if required. Identifies possible fluid or energy deficit.*)	Record the time of the client's last food intake and what was consumed. Include both liquids and solids.	If the client denies any intake for an unusual length of time, question more specifically: "Is there any food you may have forgotten, such as a snack or a drink of water or other liquid?"
Recent illness: "Have you been ill recently?" "What was the problem?" "What did you do for it?" "Have you been around anyone with a contagious illness recently?"	Most pregnant clients are healthy.	Urinary tract infections are associated with preterm labor. The client who has had contact with someone having a communicable disease may become ill and possibly infect others in the facility.
Medications/illicit drug use: "What medications do you take that your doctor or nurse-midwife has prescribed?" "Are there any over-the-counter or herbal drugs you use?" "I know this may be uncomfortable to discuss, but we need to know about any illegal or abused substances that you use, to more safely care for you and your baby." (*Permits evaluation of the client's drug intake and encourages disclosure of nonprescribed use.*)	Prenatal vitamins and iron are commonly prescribed. Record all medications the client takes, including time and amount of last ingestion. Clients often do not consider botanical preparations to be drugs. Clients who use illegal substances often conceal or diminish the extent of their use because they fear reprisals.	Drugs may interact with other medications given during labor, especially analgesics and anesthetics. Substance use is associated with complications for the client and infant (see Chapter 11). If the client discloses illegal drug use, ask what kind and the last time taken. A nonjudgmental approach in private is more likely to result in honest information.
Tobacco or alcohol: "Do you smoke or use tobacco in any other form? How many cigarettes a day?" "Do you use alcohol? How many drinks do you have each day (or week)?" (*Evaluates use of these legal substances.*)	As in substance use, clients may underreport the extent of their use of tobacco or alcohol.	Infants of heavy smokers are often smaller and may have reduced placental blood flow during labor. Infants of clients who use alcohol may show fetal alcohol effects at birth or later.
Birth Plans (Shows respect for the client and family as individuals and promotes achievement of their expectations; enables more culturally appropriate care.)		
Coach or primary support person: "Who is the main person you want to be with you during labor?" Ask that person how they want to be addressed, such as by their first name or as Mr. or Miss/Mrs. or if there are specific pronouns they prefer.	This may be the client's significant other, the baby's father, or it may also be other family members, like a mother, sister, or a friend.	The client who has little or no support from significant others probably needs more intense nursing support during labor and after the birth.
Other support: "Is there anyone else you would like to be present during labor?" "Do you have a doula?"	Clients may want another support person present.	
Preparation for childbirth: "Did you attend prepared childbirth classes?" "Did someone attend class with you?"	Ideally, the client and a partner have had some preparation in classes (in person or virtually) or self-study. Clients who attended classes during previous pregnancies do not always repeat the classes during subsequent pregnancies.	The unprepared client may need more support with simple relaxation and breathing techniques during labor. The partner may need to learn techniques to assist the client.
Preferences: "Are there any special plans you have for this birth?" "Is there anything you want to avoid?" "Did you plan to record the birth with pictures or video?"	Some clients or couples have strong feelings regarding certain interventions. Common ones are (1) analgesia or anesthesia; (2) intravenous lines; (3) fetal monitoring; (4) use of episiotomy or forceps.	Conflict may arise if the client has not previously discussed preferences with the physician or nurse-midwife or if the client is unaware of what services are available at the birth facility.
Cultural needs: "Are there any special cultural practices that you plan when you have your baby?" "How can we best help you to fulfill these practices?"	Clients from Asian and Hispanic cultures may subscribe to the "hot-and-cold" theory of illness and want specific foods after birth, such as soft-boiled eggs. They may not want their water or other fluids iced.	Try to incorporate all positive or neutral cultural practices. If a practice is harmful, explain why and try to find a way to work around it if the family does not want to give it up.

TABLE 15.1 Intrapartum Assessment Guide[a]—cont'd

Assessment, Method (Selected Rationales)	Common Findings	Significant Findings and Nursing Action
Fetal Evaluation		
Purpose: To determine whether the fetus seems to be healthy and tolerating labor well.		
Fetal heart rate (FHR): Assess by intermittent auscultation or apply an external fetal monitor if that is the facility's policy (most common in the United States). Document FHR according to the risk status, stage of labor, and facility policy.	Average rate at term is 110–160 bpm. Rate usually increases when the fetus moves.	These signs may indicate fetal stress and should be reported to the physician or nurse-midwife: 1. Rate outside the normal limits 2. Slowing of the rate, which persists after the contraction ends 3. No increase in rate when the fetus moves 4. Irregular rhythm More frequent assessments should be made of the FHR and contractions if any finding is questionable.
Labor Status		
Purpose: To identify whether the client is in labor and if birth is imminent. If the client displays signs of imminent birth, this assessment is done as soon as possible during admission.		
Contractions (yields objective information about labor status): In addition to asking the client about the contraction pattern, assess the contractions by palpation with the fingertips of one hand. Contractions should be assessed each time the FHR is assessed.	See Interview section earlier in table.	See Interview section earlier in table. Clients who have intense contractions or who are making rapid progress should be assessed more frequently.
Vaginal examination *(Determines cervical dilation and effacement; fetal presentation, position, and station; bloody show; and status of the membranes.)*	Varies according to the stage and phase of labor. It may not be possible to determine the fetal position by vaginal examination when membranes are intact and bulging over the presenting part.	A vaginal examination is not performed if the client reports or has evidence of active bleeding (heavier and more red than bloody show) and may not be done if the gestation is 36 wks or less and the client does not seem to be in active labor. Report reasons for omitting a vaginal examination to the physician or nurse-midwife.
Status of membranes: During a vaginal examination, a flow of fluid suggests ruptured membranes. A **pH test** and/or **fern test** may be done, often using a sterile speculum examination. The presence of amniotic fluid will turn pH paper blue. The fern test involves collecting fluid from the vagina during a speculum exam, smearing it on a microscope slide and examining the slide under the microscope. Amniotic fluid will form a fern pattern on the slide when it dries. *(Test is not needed if it is obvious the membranes have ruptured.)*	Amniotic fluid should be clear, possibly containing flecks of white vernix. Its odor is distinctive but not offensive. The test with a color change of blue–green to dark blue (pH >6.5) suggests true rupture of the membranes but is not conclusive. The fern test is more diagnostic of true rupture of membranes because it is less likely to be affected by vaginal infections, recent intercourse, or other factors.	A greenish color indicates meconium staining, which may be associated with fetal compromise or postterm gestation and puts the infant at risk for meconium aspiration syndrome (see Chapter 25). Thick green–black meconium may be passed by the fetus in a breech presentation and is not necessarily associated with fetal compromise. Cloudy, yellowish, strong-smelling, or foul-smelling fluid suggests infection. Bloody fluid may indicate partial placental separation (see Chapter 10).
Leopold's maneuvers (See Nursing Procedure 15.1): Often done before assessing the FHR to locate the best place for assessment. *(Identifies fetal presentation and position. Most accurate when combined with information from vaginal examination.)*	A cephalic presentation with the head well flexed (vertex) is normal. The fetal head is often easily displaced upward ("floating") if the client is not in labor. When the head is engaged, it cannot be displaced upward with Leopold's maneuvers.	A hard, round, freely movable object in the fundus suggests a fetal head, meaning the fetus is in a breech presentation. Less commonly, the fetus may be crosswise in the uterus—a transverse lie.

Continued

TABLE 15.1 **Intrapartum Assessment Guide[a]—cont'd**

Assessment, Method (Selected Rationales)	Common Findings	Significant Findings and Nursing Action
Pain: Note discomfort during and between contractions. Note tenderness when palpating contractions. (*Distinguishes between normal labor pain and abnormal pain, which may be associated with a complication.*)	There may be verbal or nonverbal evidence of pain with contractions, but the client should be relatively comfortable between contractions. The skin around the umbilicus is often sensitive.	Constant pain or a tender, rigid uterus suggests a complication, such as placental abruption (separated placenta) or, less commonly, uterine rupture.

Risk Screening (Identifies possible complications and areas of vulnerability or safety concerns)

Use facility-approved tools to identify increased risk for complications of labor and birth, including shoulder dystocia, postpartum hemorrhage, thromboembolic disease, sepsis, domestic violence, human trafficking, anxiety, depression, and suicide risk.	When screening psychosocial characteristics, domestic violence, or trafficking, ask only when the client is alone. Risk screening is performed to identify clients at risk for increased morbidity and mortality.	Clients may not disclose they are not safe when the abuser is present. Providing a safe environment when asking these questions helps establish rapport and trust. High-risk screening scores allow for measures aimed at prevention and/or early recognition of potential complications.
Other admission screenings: Nutritional status Resources at home Level of education and learning style		

Physical Examination

Purpose: To evaluate the client's general health and identify conditions that may affect intrapartum and postpartum care. *General appearance:* Observe skin color and texture, nutritional state, and appearance of rest or fatigue. Examine the client's face, fingers, and lower extremities for edema.	Clients are often fatigued if their sleep has been interrupted by Braxton Hicks contractions, fetal activity, or frequent urination. Mild edema of the lower extremities is common in late pregnancy.	Pallor suggests anemia. Substantial edema of the face and fingers or extreme (pitting) edema of the lower extremities is associated with preeclampsia, although it may occur in the absence of this hypertensive disorder (see Chapter 10).
Vital signs: Take the client's temperature, pulse rate, respirations, and blood pressure. Reassess the temperature every 2–4 hr (every hour after membranes rupture or if temperature is elevated); reassess blood pressure, pulse, and respirations every hour.	*Temperature:* 35.8–37.3°C (96.4–99.1°F) *Pulse rate:* 60–100 bpm *Respirations:* 12–20/min, even and unlabored Blood pressure near baseline levels established during pregnancy. Transient elevations of blood pressure are common when the client is first admitted, but they return to baseline levels within about 30 min.	Report abnormalities to physician or nurse-midwife. Temperature of 38°C (100.4°F) or higher suggests infection. Pulse rate and blood pressure may be elevated if the client is extremely anxious or in pain. A blood pressure ≥140 mm Hg systolic or ≥90 mm Hg diastolic or higher is considered hypertensive. For clients who did not have prenatal care, there is no baseline for comparison.
Heart and lung sounds: Auscultate all areas with a stethoscope.	Heart sounds should be clear with a distinct S_1 and S_2. A physiologic murmur is common because of the increased blood volume and cardiac output. Breath sounds should be clear, with respirations even and unlabored.	The client who is breathing rapidly and deeply may have symptoms of hyperventilation: tingling and spasm of the fingers, numbness around the lips.
Abdomen: Observe for scars at the same time Leopold's maneuvers and the FHR are assessed. It is usually sufficient to assess the fundal height by observing its relation to the xiphoid process.	Striae (stretch marks) are common. If scars are noted, ask the client what surgery occurred and when. The fundus at term is usually slightly below the xiphoid process but varies with client height and fetal size and number.	Report a previous cesarean birth to the physician or nurse-midwife. Transverse uterine scars are least likely to rupture if the client is in labor. Measure the fundal height (see Chapter 7) if the fetus seems small or if the gestation is questionable.

TABLE 15.1 Intrapartum Assessment Guide^a—cont'd

Assessment, Method (Selected Rationales)	Common Findings	Significant Findings and Nursing Action
Deep tendon reflexes (DTRs): Assess patellar reflex (see Chapter 10). Upper extremity DTRs also should be evaluated at admission if epidural block analgesia is planned because they are normally not as strong as the patellar reflex.	A brisk jerk without spasm or sustained muscle contraction is normal. Some clients normally have hypoactive reflexes, but at least a slight twitch is expected. Obese clients may appear to have diminished reflexes because of the adipose tissue over the tendon.	Report absent (uncommon unless the client is receiving magnesium sulfate) or hyperactive reflexes. Hyperactive reflexes and clonus (repeated tapping when the foot is dorsiflexed) are associated with preeclampsia and hypertension and often precede a seizure (see Chapter 10).
Midstream urine specimen: Assess protein and glucose levels. Check for ketones if the client has not eaten for a prolonged period or has been vomiting. Send a separate specimen for urinalysis, if ordered.	Negative or trace protein and glucose; negative ketones.	Proteinuria is associated with preeclampsia but also may be associated with urinary tract infections or a specimen contaminated with vaginal secretions. Glycosuria is associated with diabetes. Ketonuria is common in poorly controlled diabetes or if the client does not eat adequate carbohydrates to meet energy needs or is experiencing dehydration.
Laboratory tests: Clients who have had prenatal care may not need as many admission tests. Common tests include the following: 1. Complete blood cell count (or hematocrit done on unit) 2. Blood type and Rh factor	1. Hemoglobin at least 11 g/dL (grams per deciliter); hematocrit at least 33%. 2. The client who is Rh-negative and has had regular prenatal care receives Rh immune globulin at 28 wks of gestation to prevent formation of anti-Rh antibodies.	1. Values lower than these reduce reserve for normal blood loss at birth. 2. Rh-negative clients need Rh immune globulin after birth if the infant is Rh-positive.
3. Venereal disease research laboratory (VDRL) or rapid plasma regain (RPR) tests for syphilis. Other routine admission tests include serum HIV, Hepatitis B surface antigen, and rubella titer. Vaginal GBS tests may be performed, if unknown at admission. Drug screens may also be ordered.	3. Negative on all. GBS screening may have been done recently during a prenatal visit late in pregnancy.	3. A positive test indicates the baby could be infected and needs treatment after birth. The client should be treated if not previously treated. Antibiotics are given for positive GBS to reduce newborn infection from organisms within the vagina.

bpm, Beats per minute; *GBS,* group B *Streptococcus; HIV,* human immunodeficiency virus; *VBAC,* vaginal birth after cesarean.
^aClients who have had prenatal care have much of this information available on their prenatal record. The nurse need only verify it or update it, as needed.

when others are present. The client's partner and other visitors may be unaware of the medical or obstetric history. Delay asking intimate information until the client is alone for confidentiality, safety, and accuracy.

Physical examination. A physical examination evaluates the client's overall health and covers important observations relating to pregnancy, including the presence and location of edema, abdominal scars, and the height of the fundus.

Fetal assessments. The fetal presentation and position are assessed using a combination of vaginal examination and Leopold's maneuvers (Procedure 15.1). The FHR is assessed by intermittent auscultation or electronic monitoring (see Chapter 14).

Labor status. The client's labor status is determined by assessing the FHR and contraction pattern, performing vaginal examination, and determining whether the membranes have

ruptured. Contractions are assessed by palpation (Procedure 14.2). Cervical dilation, effacement, station, fetal presentation, and position are evaluated by vaginal examination (Fig. 15.1). The vaginal examination may also reveal whether the membranes have ruptured if fluid is not obviously leaking from the vagina. The nurse documents the time of rupture, color, amount, and odor of the amniotic fluid. Vaginal examination is not performed if the client has active bleeding (other than bloody show). Speculum rather than vaginal examination may be done if the gestation is preterm or if active bleeding is present.

KNOWLEDGE CHECK

5. Why would the nurse defer asking a client about a history of domestic violence?
6. What data are collected to determine the current status of the client's labor?

Leopold's Maneuvers use four distinct maneuvers systematically to determine presentation and position of the fetus and aid in location of fetal heart sounds. The maneuvers also provide assessment of uterine tone, irritability, tenderness, and presence or absence of contractions. Possible challenges when completing Leopold's Maneuvers include abdominal muscle tension or guarding, obesity, anterior placenta implantation, or polyhydramnios (Cunningham et al., 2022; Simpson & O'Brien-Abel, 2021).

1. Explain procedure and rationale to the client.
2. Ensure the bladder is empty, position client supine with knees slightly flexed and a small pillow or folded towel under one hip.
3. Wash your hands. Wear gloves if contact with secretions is likely.
4. Stand facing the client's head with your dominant hand nearest the client. *The first three maneuvers are most easily performed in this position.*
5. First maneuver—Assesses the uterine fundus and helps identify fetal lie and presentation. Using the flat palmar surface of hands, with fingers together, apply gentle but firm pressure to the uterine fundus. The breech (buttocks) is softer and more irregular in shape than the head. Moving the breech also moves the fetal trunk. The head is harder and has a round, uniform shape. The head can be moved without moving the entire fetal trunk.

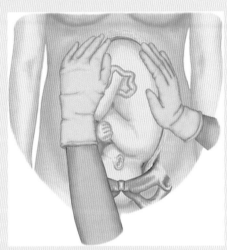

6. Second maneuver—Place palms on either side of the abdomen. Hold left hand steady on one side of the uterus while palpating the opposite side of the uterus with the right hand. Start palpating at the uterine fundus and progress downward toward the symphysis pubis. Then hold the right hand steady while palpating the opposite side of the uterus with the left hand. The fetal back is a smooth, convex surface. The fetal arms and legs feel nodular, irregular, or protruding.

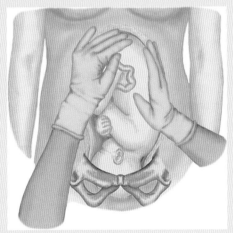

7. Third maneuver (Pallach's maneuver or grip)—Palpate the suprapubic area. Attempt to grasp the presenting part gently between the thumb and middle finger. If the presenting part is not engaged, the grasping movement moves it upward in the uterus. If the presenting part is engaged, it remains fixed and difficult to move.
8. Omit the fourth maneuver if the fetus is in a breech presentation. This maneuver helps determine whether the fetal head is flexed.

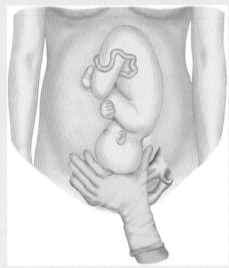

9. Fourth maneuver—Turn facing the client's feet. This maneuver may be uncomfortable for the client; therefore thorough explanation of the process should be done before completing this step.
10. Place your hands on each side of the uterus with fingers pointed toward the pelvic inlet. Simultaneously slide hands down each side of the uterus. On one side, your fingers easily slide to the upper edge of the symphysis. On the other side, your fingers meet an obstruction, the cephalic prominence. If the head is flexed (vertex), the cephalic prominence (the forehead) is felt on the opposite side from the fetal back. If the head is extended (face), the cephalic prominence (the occiput) is felt on the same side as the fetal back.

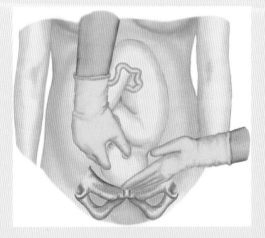

Admission Procedures

Notify the provider. After assessment, the nurse notifies the obstetric provider to report the client's status and obtain orders. The following data are provided:

- The client's name and age
- Gravidity, parity, term and preterm births, abortions (spontaneous and elective), and living children
- EDD and fundal height if it conflicts with the date (see Chapter 7)
- Contraction pattern
- Results of vaginal examination:
  - Cervical dilation and effacement
  - Fetal presentation and position
  - Station of the presenting part
  - Membrane status
  - FHR and uterine activity (UA) pattern
  - Vital signs
  - Relevant history, including medical, surgical, and obstetric findings
  - Any identified abnormalities and concerns about the client's or fetus' condition
  - Pain, anxiety, or other reactions to labor
  - Birth plans

Consent forms. The client signs consent for care during labor, such as anesthesia, vaginal birth and/or cesarean birth, induction (oxytocin, cervical ripening), and blood transfusion. Even when cesarean birth, induction, and blood transfusion are not anticipated, many facilities include these procedures in admission consents because of the potential emergent nature of complications during labor or birth. If the client requests postpartum sterilization, consent may be required before labor and verified at the time of birth with the emphasis that permanent sterility is expected after bilateral tubal ligation. Consent for newborn care and circumcision are often completed on the client's admission to the birth facility.

Laboratory tests. Common laboratory results are needed on admission to the labor and delivery unit (see Table 15.1). Clients who receive prenatal care may have laboratory results available on the prenatal record. Guidelines for STI testing are recommended by the state health department in collaboration with the Centers for Disease Control and Prevention (CDC). The obstetric provider may order additional tests pertinent to the client's presenting complaint and medical history. When there is no prenatal record available on admission, more extensive testing may be required.

Intravenous access. If ordered, intravenous (IV) access is started with a large-bore (18-gauge or larger) catheter. A saline lock may be used, or the client may receive a continuous infusion of fluids. The saline lock allows freedom of movement when walking during early labor but provides quick access if fluids or medications are needed. Continuous fluid infusion reduces dehydration and is necessary if epidural analgesia is used. IV solutions containing electrolytes, such as lactated Ringer's solution, are the most common fluids administered (Simpson & O'Brien-Abel, 2021).

APPLICATION OF THE NURSING PROCESS: FALSE OR EARLY LABOR

Assessment

After observation, the nurse may realize the client is not in true active labor. If cervical dilation and effacement remains unchanged and the membranes are intact, the client is usually discharged to await active labor.

Identification of Client Problems

At times, it can be difficult to differentiate between true and false labor, leading to client frustration. This frustration may lead to resistance to returning to the birth center, possibly causing a needless delay of care. There is often a need for client teaching regarding the characteristics of true labor.

Planning: Expected Outcomes

An expected outcome for this problem is: Before discharge, the client and support person will describe reasons for returning to the birth center for evaluation.

Interventions
Reassurance

Clients sent home after observation may feel foolish and frustrated. They may want to have labor induced simply to "get it over with." Reassure the client of the difficulty in distinguishing true from false labor. Educate the client about cervical changes in early labor, such as softening of the cervix, even if obvious progress, such as cervical dilation, has not yet occurred. Early latent labor may gradually intensify as it merges into the active phase of first stage. Other clients may notice a more abrupt intensity and frequency change as the latent phase becomes active labor.

Teaching

Review guidelines for returning to the birth center (see Client Teaching: When to Go to the Hospital or Birth Center). Explain that these are only guidelines and the client should return if concerns occur. Returning with false labor is better than entering in advanced labor or developing complications at home. Remind the client early labor is the first step in making the final preparations for birth.

Evaluation

The client and support person should describe guidelines for returning to the birth center. These include regular contractions, leaking of amniotic fluid, bleeding other than bloody show, and decreased fetal movement.

APPLICATION OF THE NURSING PROCESS: TRUE LABOR

The admission assessment may confirm the client is in true labor, or labor may be evident after an observation period. Nursing care of the client during labor and birth includes ongoing assessments, pain management as covered in Chapter 13, promotion of fetal oxygenation as covered in Chapter 14, promotion of labor progress, and prevention of injury.

PURPOSES

To determine whether membranes have ruptured.
To determine cervical effacement and dilation.
To determine fetal presentation, position, and station.

METHOD

Vaginal examination is not usually performed by the inexperienced nurse except when training for graduate nursing practice in the intrapartum area.

EQUIPMENT

Sterile gloves, sterile lubricant. If a pH swab or nitrazine paper is being used to test for ruptured membranes, lubricant is not used to avoid altering the test paper.

HAND POSITION

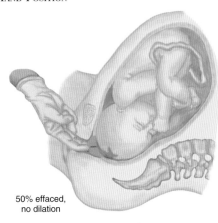

50% effaced,
no dilation

The nurse usually uses the index and middle fingers of the dominant hand for vaginal examination. The thumb and other fingers are kept out of the way to avoid carrying microorganisms into the vagina.

DETERMINING WHETHER MEMBRANES HAVE RUPTURED

Intact membranes feel like a slippery membrane over the fetal presenting part. No leakage of amniotic fluid can be detected.
Bulging membranes feel like a slippery, fluid-filled balloon over the presenting part. It may be difficult to feel the presenting part clearly if the membranes are bulging tensely.
Ruptured membranes show drainage of fluid from the vagina as the nurse manipulates the cervix and presenting part.

DETERMINING CERVICAL EFFACEMENT AND DILATION

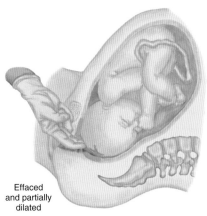

Effaced
and partially
dilated

The nurse determines *effacement* by estimating the thickness of the cervix. The uneffaced cervix is about 2 cm long. If it is 50% effaced, it is about 1 cm long. Effacement is expressed as a percentage (0% to 100%), or it may be described as the length in centimeters.
Dilation is determined by sweeping the fingertips across the cervical opening. Dilation is expressed as closed, fingertip, or 1-10cm.

DETERMINING THE PRESENTING PART

The fetal skull feels smooth, hard, and rounded in a cephalic presentation. The fetal buttocks are softer and more irregular in a breech presentation. If the membranes are ruptured, the fetus in a breech presentation may expel thick, green-black meconium. (Presence of meconium in a breech presentation is *not* necessarily a sign of fetal compromise. The nurse must evaluate other signs of fetal condition.)

DETERMINING THE FETAL POSITION

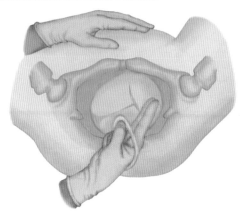

In a cephalic presentation, the nurse feels for the distinctive features of the fetal skull. The posterior fontanel is usually felt in a vertex presentation and is triangular with three suture lines (two lambdoid and one sagittal) leading into it. The anterior fontanel is not felt unless the head is poorly flexed or is in the mechanism of extension in late labor. It feels like a diamond-shaped depression with four suture lines (one frontal, two coronal, and one sagittal) leading into it.

DETERMINING THE STATION

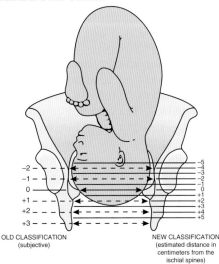

−2	−5
	−4
	−3
−1	−2
	−1
0	0
	+1
+1	+2
	+3
+2	+4
	+5
+3	

OLD CLASSIFICATION
(subjective)

NEW CLASSIFICATION
(estimated distance in
centimeters from the
ischial spines)

Fig. 15.1 Vaginal examination during labor.

Assessment

If it is unclear after the initial assessment whether the client is in true labor, the client may be observed. After 1 or 2 hours, progressive cervical change (effacement, dilation, or both) strongly suggests true labor.

After the admission assessment, ongoing evaluations based on risk status promote client and fetal well-being, minimize risks, and avoid unnecessary interventions.

Client Assessments

Labor progress. The frequency of vaginal examinations depends on the client's parity, membrane status, and overall labor speed. Vaginal examinations are limited to minimize the introduction of microorganisms from the perineal area into the uterus, which could lead to infection.

Pressure of the fetal head on the rectum in late labor is frequently perceived as the need to have a bowel movement. The nurse should look at the perineum for **crowning** (appearance of the fetal scalp or presenting part at the vaginal opening) and perform a sterile vaginal examination if the client suddenly expresses an urge to push or to have a bowel movement during a contraction.

Contractions. Contractions can be assessed by palpation or with the electronic fetal monitor (EFM; see Chapter 14). Normal uterine activity (UA) during labor is less than or equal to five contractions in 10 minutes, averaged over a 30-minute time frame. As defined by National Institute of Child Health and Human Development, excessive UA leads to progressive fetal decompensation secondary to inadequate blood flow to the intervillous spaces of the placenta. Decreased blood flow to the intervillous spaces compromises fetal gas exchange and results in an increased risk for development of fetal acidemia (Bakker et al., 2007; Macones et al., 2008; Miller et al., 2022; O'Brien-Abel & Simpson, 2021). The goal is to maintain normal UA by intervening for any cases of excessive UA. Assessment frequency is based on standards published by professional organizations (e.g., ACOG, AWHONN).

Guidelines for minimal frequency of assessments for low-risk clients are (Wisner & Ivory, 2021):

a. Latent phase: Less than 4 cm, at least hourly; 4 to 5 cm, every 30 minutes
b. Every 30 minutes during active phase
c. Every 30 minutes during second-stage passive descent (laboring down)
d. Every 15 minutes during active second stage

When using the EFM to assess contractions, palpate to validate intensity and resting tone. External monitors are often not accurate because of the thickness of the abdominal fat pad, maternal position, and fetal position.

Intake and output. Oral and IV intake and each void are recorded. Labor may reduce a client's urge to void; therefore suprapubic palpation should occur every 2 hours or more frequently to identify bladder distention.

Response to labor. The client's behavioral responses change as labor intensifies, especially without epidural analgesia. This response may be determined by cultural expectations, anxiety, loss of control, loss of self-confidence, and coping and support mechanisms. The client may withdraw from interactions but need more nursing presence and reassurance. The client may also experience anxiety for any number of reasons: pain and fear of bodily injury, unknown outcome, loss of control, unresolved psychological issues that influence readiness to give birth (e.g., sexual abuse, previous birth experiences), or unexpected occurrences during labor. Anxiety has been associated with increased catecholamine release, which can cause dysfunctional labor or ineffective UA (Simpson & O'Brien-Abel, 2021).

Clients experience a broad range of emotions that can affect their ability to cope with labor. Interventions to assist the client include both nonpharmacologic and pharmacologic measures. The goal of nursing care is to support the client's desires and provide pain management, while not interfering with labor progress or causing adverse outcomes for the client or fetus. Assessing a client's ability to cope with labor is an alternative to the traditional pain scale of 0 to 10 (AWHONN, 2018; AWHONN, 2019; California Maternal Quality Care Collaborative (CMQCC), 2017; Fairchild et al., 2017; Roberts et al., 2010). Signs of coping include the following:

- Client states they are coping
- Inward focus
- Rhythmic motion and breathing patterns
- Ability to relax between contractions

Behaviors that suggest the client may not be coping with labor include the following:

- Specific requests for medication and other pain control measures such as epidural analgesia
- Statements that current measures are ineffective
- Tension of muscles and arching of back or panicked activity during contractions
- Crying, tearfulness, tremulous voice
- A tense facial expression, rolling in the bed
- Client states they are not coping; may use expressions such as "I can't take it anymore"

Labor support plays an integral role in perinatal outcomes. The 2017 Cochrane Database review on continuous labor support during childbirth looked at 26 studies involving over 15,000 women. They found clients who had continuous labor support were more likely to have shorter labors without analgesia, which resulted in spontaneous vaginal delivery. They were less likely to have operative vaginal births or infants with low 5-minute Apgar status or to report dissatisfaction with the birth experience. This review also stated support was most effective when it was delivered by someone who could provide continuous support without having additional responsibilities. It was recommended that the support person was experienced and/or had a modest amount of training in labor support. Authors found an increase in client's satisfaction when it was a friend or family member (Bohren et al., 2017). Therefore the inclusion of the client's support system is integral to labor progress.

Support Person's Response

Labor can be stressful for the client's partner/support person. Often, the person may become anxious, fearful, or tired. The

CRITICAL TO REMEMBER

Conditions Associated with Fetal Compromise

Fetal heart rate (FHR) outside the normal range of 110 to 160 bpm or loss of FHR variability with electronic FHR monitoring

Meconium-stained (greenish) amniotic fluid

Cloudy, yellowish, or foul-smelling amniotic fluid (suggests infection)

Excessive frequency or duration of contractions (reduces placental blood flow)

Incomplete uterine relaxation and intervals shorter than 45 to 60 seconds between contractions (reduces placental blood flow)

Hypotension (may divert blood flow away from the placenta to ensure adequate perfusion of the client's brain and heart)

Hypertension (may be associated with vasospasm in spiral arteries, which supply the intervillous spaces of the placenta)

Fever (38°C [100.4°F] or higher)

person may feel a responsibility to protect and support the client but may have limited resources for doing so. Watching the client in pain is difficult, even if the pain is normal. The support person may respond to stress in many ways, including by being quiet, suffering silently, or reacting with pacing and anger. At times, the person may respond by leaving the room frequently or for long periods, whereas others resist even short breaks.

Cultural norms may dictate that the partner or support person's presence during labor and birth is strictly prohibited. The partner may be pulled in two directions, wanting to be included but hesitating because cultural norms do not customarily include involvement in birth. The nurse should respect the values of each couple and their wishes about the partner's involvement.

The nurse should remember that anyone who assists the client during labor may have feelings of anxiety and helplessness at times. Reassurance and care for the labor partner strengthens the person's ability to support the client and enhances the likelihood that both will view the birth experience as positive.

Fetal Assessments

Assessments are performed to identify signs of well-being and signs that suggest compromise. The principal assessments include FHR patterns and character of the amniotic fluid. Abnormalities revealed in these assessments may be associated with impaired fetal gas exchange and infection (see Chapter 14 and Critical to Remember: Conditions Associated with Fetal Compromise).

Fetal Heart Rate. FHR is assessed using either intermittent auscultation or EFM. Frequency of assessment and documentation depends on the risk status of the client and fetus, the stage of labor, and is at least as frequent as assessment of contractions. In addition, FHR assessments are recommended before and after procedures or interventions that might change the intrauterine environment or the relationship of the fetus to its environment. Some examples include rupture of membranes (spontaneous or artificial), ambulation of the client, administration of analgesia or anesthesia, administrations of induction agents, or vaginal examinations. This assessment and documentation of fetal status allows the clinician to demonstrate the response of the fetus to procedures/interventions.

Fetal membranes and amniotic fluid. Spontaneous rupture of membranes (SROM) may occur, or the provider may perform an amniotomy. **Amniotomy** (artificial rupture of the membranes or AROM) is usually performed in conjunction with **induction** (artificial initiation of uterine contractions) and **augmentation** of labor (artificial stimulation of uterine contractions) and to allow internal EFM.

The time of rupture, FHR, color, odor, and quantity of the amniotic fluid are noted and charted. Assessment of the FHR is the first priority to rule out a prolapsed umbilical cord. The time of rupture and assessment of the amniotic fluid is the second priority. The fluid should be clear and may include bits of vernix, the creamy white fetal skin lubricant, and have a mild, musty smell. A large amount of vernix in the fluid suggests the fetus may be preterm. Greenish, meconium-stained fluid may be seen in response to transient fetal hypoxia, term and postterm gestation, or placental insufficiency (Rohan, 2021). Fluid with a foul or strong odor, cloudy appearance, or yellow color suggests **chorioamnionitis** (inflammation of the amniotic sac, usually caused by bacterial and viral infections).

Quantity of fluid should be described in approximate terms; for example, at term, a "large" amount is more than 1000 mL, a "moderate" amount is approximately 500 to 1000 mL, and "scant" amniotic fluid is a trickle, barely enough to detect. If the fetus is engaged in the pelvis when the membranes rupture, a small amount of fluid in front of the fetal presenting part may be discharged (forewaters or forebag), with the rest lost at birth. **Polyhydramnios** (amniotic fluid index greater than or equal to 24 cm) is associated with some fetal abnormalities. **Oligohydramnios** (amniotic fluid index less than or equal to 5 cm) may be associated with placental insufficiency or fetal urinary tract abnormalities (ACOG, 2020e).

AROM and SROM are associated with risks for which the nurse must observe, including prolapse of the umbilical cord, infection, and placental abruption.

Prolapse of the umbilical cord. The primary risk at the time of rupture is that the umbilical cord will slip down with the gush of fluid. The cord can be compressed between the fetal presenting part and the client's pelvis, obstructing blood flow to and from the placenta and reducing fetal gas exchange. The FHR is assessed for at least one full minute after amniotomy or SROM. Indeterminate or abnormal patterns or significant changes from previous assessments are reported promptly to the provider. Cord compression is usually accompanied by variable or prolonged decelerations or a bradycardic FHR.

Infection. With interruption of the membrane barrier, vaginal organisms have free access to the intrauterine cavity and may cause chorioamnionitis. The risk is low at first but increases as the amount of time between membrane rupture and birth increases. When ruptured 24 hours or longer, 24% of clients will develop chorioamnionitis. Rates of up to 77% incidence are noted in pregnancies that are remote from term (Mercer & Chien, 2019). Birth within 24 hours of membrane rupture is desirable, although infection does not occur at any absolute time.

Abruptio placentae. Abruptio placentae, also known as placental abruption (see Chapter 10), can occur if the uterus is distended with excessive amniotic fluid when the membranes rupture. As the uterus collapses with discharge of the amniotic fluid, the area of placental attachment shrinks. The placenta then no longer fits its implantation site and partially separates. A large area of placental disruption can significantly reduce fetal oxygenation, nutrition, and waste disposal. The client is at risk for disseminated intravascular coagulation, shock, need for blood replacement, hysterectomy, organ failure, or death as a result of placental abruption (Cunningham et al., 2022).

Nursing considerations: Assisting with an amniotomy. Obtain a baseline FHR via EFM or auscultation before amniotomy is performed. The initial fetal assessment provides a baseline to compare with later assessments.

Before amniotomy, two or three underpads should be placed under the client's buttocks to absorb the fluid; the underpads should be overlapped to extend from the client's waist to knees. A folded bath towel under the buttocks absorbs more amniotic fluid. Explain amniotomy is no more painful than a vaginal examination because there are no sensory nerves in the amniotic sac.

Other supplies needed are a sterile, disposable plastic membrane perforator, sterile gloves for the provider, and sterile lubricant. The nurse should partly open the package containing the plastic hook at the handle end and hold back the package until the provider takes the hook (Fig. 15.2).

The provider performs the amniotomy after a vaginal examination to determine cervical dilation, effacement, station, and fetal presenting part. Amniotomy is often deferred if the fetal presenting part is high or the presentation is not cephalic. The risk for a prolapsed cord is increased in these situations. The hook is passed through the cervical opening, snagging the membranes. The opening in the membranes is enlarged with the finger, allowing fluid to drain.

KNOWLEDGE CHECK

9. What factors are considered in determining the frequency of assessment of FHR?
10. What are three risks associated with AROM and SROM?
11. Describe the significance of each of the following types of amniotic fluid: greenish, cloudy, yellowish, foul-smelling.

Identification of Client Problems

Many factors affect the progress of normal labor (see Chapter 12). The potential problem of prolonged labor requires collaboration of medical and nursing staffs with the client and the support persons. The nursing role is largely proactive, providing education and support to promote labor progress.

Planning: Expected Outcomes

The expected outcome is that the client will use positioning, movement, pain management, breathing and pushing techniques to promote labor progress.

Interventions: Promotion of Labor Progress

The nurse supports labor progress by using client positions which promote progress, as well as frequent changes in client positions. Adequate pain management and client teaching

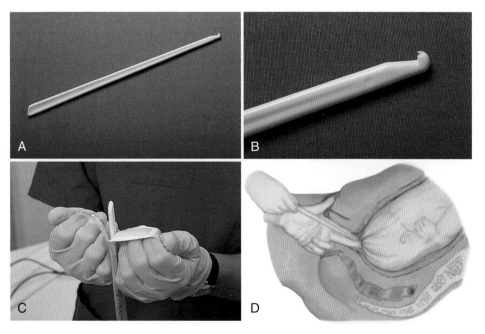

Fig. 15.2 (A) Disposable plastic membrane perforator. (B) Close-up of hook end of plastic membrane perforator. (C) Correct method to open the package. (D) Technique for artificial rupture of membranes.

also contribute to cervical changes and descent of the fetus in labor.

Positioning and Movement

Encourage the client to assume any position that is comfortable (other than supine) and change positions frequently (Figs. 15.3–15.5). Movement and frequent position changes in labor decrease pain, improve maternal-fetal circulation, improve the strength and effectiveness of contractions, decrease the length of labor, facilitate fetal descent, and decrease perineal trauma and episiotomies (AWHONN, 2019; CMQCC, 2017). Less dystocia and shortened second-stage labor were noted when nurses follow the six physiologic principles related to client positioning in labor proposed by Fenwick and Simkin (1987): promote spinal flexion (client curved around baby, body aligned like a "C"), promote an increase in the utero-spinal drive angle (C-curve directs the baby toward the posterior part of the pelvis), facilitate stronger expulsive forces, promote a good fit, increase pelvic diameter, and facilitate occiput posterior rotation (AWHONN, 2019; Berta et al., 2019; Gupta et al., 2017).

Although ambulation and some positions may not be safe for clients with an epidural, many options are available by using the flexibility of modern birthing beds with leg supports, squatting bars, and multiple positions of the head and foot sections. Use of the peanut ball to assist with positioning has been shown to decrease the time of first- and second-stage labor in primiparous clients with epidurals and decrease the incidence of cesarean section in these clients (AWHONN, 2019; CMQCC, 2017; Hickey & Savage, 2019; Roth et al., 2016; Tussey et al., 2015). Nursing care of the client with an epidural includes assisting with position changes every 20 to 30 minutes (AWONN, 2019; CMQCC, 2017).

Teaching

Teaching the client in labor is a continuously changing task based on the labor progress, preferred pain management methods, and their effectiveness.

First stage. First-stage and second-stages of labor are divided into two categories: latent and active (see Chapter 12). Many clients become discouraged because the latent phase of the first stage can last from hours to days. From a time standpoint, 5 cm is approximately two-thirds of the way through first-stage labor because the rate of dilation increases during the active phase. Client teaching during the first stage includes keeping them informed of the progress of labor and the status of the fetus. The nurse also should teach the client about alternative pain management options if the chosen methods do not meet the client's expectations.

A client's urge to push can occur on complete dilation and effacement with the fetus at +1 station or lower. However, as the client nears the second stage, the fetus may descend enough to elicit the urge to push before full cervical dilation. This urge is triggered by the presenting part stretching the pelvic floor muscles and is commonly referred to as Ferguson's reflex. This process releases endogenous oxytocin, stimulating an urge to push (AWHONN, 2019; CMQCC, 2017; Simpson & O'Brien-Abel, 2021). The timing of pushing should be individualized to the client's response.

Pushing against a cervix that is not completely dilated may result in cervical lacerations or cervical edema, which can block labor progress. If the client has a strong urge to push but pushing is likely to injure the cervix or cause cervical edema, teach the client to exhale in short breaths.

Second stage. Second stage begins with complete dilation and ends with birth of the baby (see Chapter 12). The client may need help to trust the sensations felt and push most effectively. Client teaching for this stage of labor includes when to start pushing, positions for pushing, and the method for pushing.

Laboring down. Allowing passive descent of the fetus while waiting for the client to feel the urge to push provides benefit to the client and fetus. Clients push most effectively

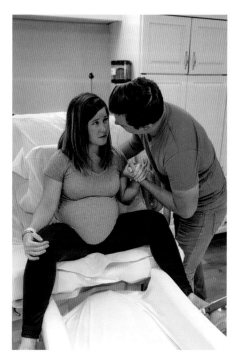

Fig. 15.3 Eye-to-eye contact and being reminded to take deep cleansing breaths by a nurse or support person can be helpful in supporting the laboring client.

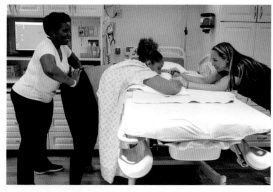

Fig. 15.4 Providing reassurance and nonclinical touch can offer client support, decreasing fear and anxiety.

when they feel the reflex urge to do so as the fetus descends. Clients with regional analgesia may not have an urge to push. Many times, the urge to push is not felt immediately when the cervix is fully dilated, even if no regional analgesia, such as an epidural, is administered. A brief slowing of contractions often occurs at the beginning of the second stage. Pushing as soon as complete dilation is achieved with no regard to client readiness can lead to issues such as client exhaustion and pelvic floor injuries (AWHONN, 2019; CMQCC, 2017; Simpson & O'Brien-Abel, 2021).

The technique of delaying pushing until the reflex urge to push occurs may be called *delayed pushing, laboring down, rest and descend,* or *passive descent.* Active pushing is the most physiologically stressful part of labor for the fetus. Delayed pushing has been shown to result in less client fatigue, decreased pushing time, decreased risk for instrument-assisted and cesarean births, decreased third- and fourth-degree lacerations, decreased injuries to the pelvic floor, and blood loss/rates of hemorrhage equivalent to those of clients who pushed immediately on full cervical dilation (AWHONN, 2019; CMQCC, 2017; Simpson & O'Brien-Abel, 2021).

Simply put, laboring down means allowing uterine contractions to cause most of the fetal internal rotation and descent after full dilation. The client rests before actively pushing the baby out. The use of protocols to evaluate client and fetal status have shown success with laboring down. When no fetal descent has occurred after 2 hours, an evaluation by the provider is necessary.

Positions. Although vertical client positions enhance fetal descent and shorten labor, often the client is placed in a recumbent position for provider convenience (Simpson & O'Brien-Abel, 2021). Squatting is an ideal position for pushing because it enlarges the pelvic outlet slightly and adds the force of gravity to the client's efforts, which is an advantage if the pelvis appears small and/ or the fetus is large. If the client is too tired to squat, the toilet can be used for support while maintaining an upright, open pelvis position (AWHONN, 2019; Simpson & O'Brien-Abel, 2021). Pushing while sitting on a birthing ball, pulling against a squatting bar on the bed, or playing "tug of war" with another person provides a similar gravitational advantage. Clients may find pulling on something from above is efficient. The upper torso should be

POSITIONS FOR FIRST-STAGE LABOR

Standing

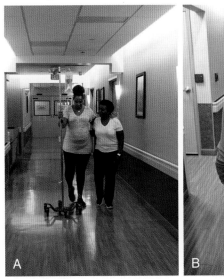 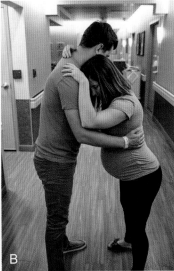

Advantages
Walking/standing increases endorphin release.
Gravity assists with fetal descent.
Makes contractions less uncomfortable and more efficient.
Allows client to feel less confined and more productive.

Disadvantages
Tiring over long periods.
Continuous fetal monitoring is not possible without telemetry if the
    client is walking in the hall.

Nursing Implications
It is important to balance activity and rest, especially during long labors.
If the client has intravenous (IV) fluid running, give them a rolling IV pole.
Remind the client and support person when to return for evaluation of
    the fetal heart rate and labor status.

Fig. 15.5 Common Positions for Labor. Many labor positions can be adapted for the first and second stage of labor.

POSITIONS FOR FIRST-STAGE LABOR

Lunge

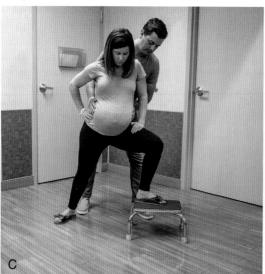
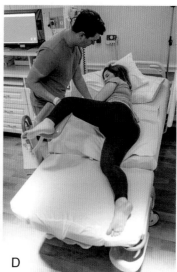

Advantages
Allows one side of the pelvis to open more than the other, which facilitates cardinal
   fetal movements through the pelvis.
Able to do it in standing position or when client is lying in bed (epiduralized).
Assists with descent and fetal rotation.

Disadvantages
May make labor more uncomfortable as the fetus descends.
Monitoring may be challenging in these positions.

Nursing Implications
May use stirrup, peanut ball, or stacked pillows.
May cause rapid descent in epiduralized client; prepare for delivery.
Epiduralized client may be unable to feel if this position is stretching nerves or contributing
   to a lower extremity nerve injury; therefore reposition client every 20 minutes.

Fig. 15.5 cont'd

in front of the client's pelvis to allow the coccyx to move backward as the fetus descends deeply into the pelvis (AWHONN, 2019). Epidural analgesia may limit the positions a client can assume for pushing; however, with modern birthing beds, many modified positions are safe and effective with or without epidural analgesia.

If clients push in the sitting or semisitting position, teach them to curve their body around their uterus in a C shape rather than arching their back. For greatest effectiveness, clients should pull on their knees, handholds, or a squat bar while pushing. Clients should maintain a similar C shape to their upper body if they push on their side. Evidence has demonstrated injury is possible to the peroneal nerve, also termed lower extremity nerve injury (LENI), while pushing for extended periods of time. This injury is noted to occur in the following situations: deep tissue pressure on the posterior aspect of thigh directly under the client's knee, placing the client in stirrups or supporting the leg against a hard surface while pushing, or when the client's thighs are forcibly pushed against their abdomen (greater than a 90-degree angle) for an extended period of time. Therefore grasping the knee, placing the feet flat on the bed or against foot pedals while pushing, and frequent position changes should be used during the

second stage to decrease incidence of injury (AWHONN, 2020; Simpson & O'Brien-Abel, 2021).

Method and breathing pattern. Support the client's spontaneous pushing techniques if they are effective. The client should push with abdominal muscles while relaxing the perineum. When coaching the client, teach to begin by taking a breath and exhaling and then taking another breath and exhaling while pushing for 6 to 8 seconds at a time. Sustained pushing while holding a breath (Valsalva maneuver or "purple pushing") or pushing more than four times per contraction reduces blood flow to the placenta, increases intrathoracic pressure, is fatiguing, and should be discouraged (AWHONN, 2019; Simpson & O'Brien-Abel, 2021). Another deep breath that is more like a sigh helps to relax after the contraction.

Pushing efforts may be inhibited by a client who is modest or fears losing control if instructed to push similar to having a bowel movement, particularly if the client is in a bed or chair.

Evaluation

Because labor progress is a collaborative process, the goal is evaluated by the client's use of a variety of techniques to promote progression rather than the actual length of the labor.

POSITIONS FOR FIRST-STAGE LABOR

Abdominal Lift and Tuck

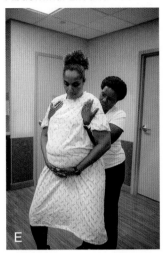

Advantages
Maintains the C-curve positioning, which aids/facilitates fetal engagement and descent.

Disadvantages
May be tiring for client during long labors

Nursing Implications
While standing, bend knees, lift belly, and tuck pelvis in (flattening the lower back angle).
Use this maneuver when the fetus is not in the pelvis or when client is experiencing back labor.
May perform up to 10 contractions in a row.
May cause rapid descent; prepare for delivery as indicated.

Counterpressure

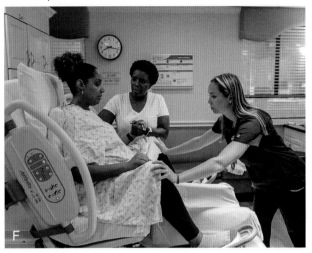

Advantages
May use this when client is unable to get out of bed (epidural, continuous monitoring).
Provides distraction from and relief of labor pain (see Chapter 13 for gate-control theory).
Allows therapeutic touch from support person or nurse.

Disadvantages
Tiring for support person and may not be sustainable.

Nursing Implications
Different counterpressure techniques may need to be used throughout labor (hip squeezes, knee press, and sacral pressure).
Varying techniques allow for relief and rest of both client and support person.

Sitting/Squatting

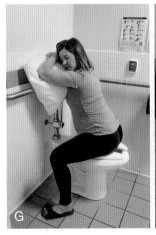 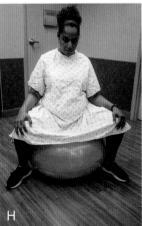

Fig. 15.5 cont'd

POSITIONS FOR FIRST-STAGE LABOR

Sitting/Squatting (Cont)

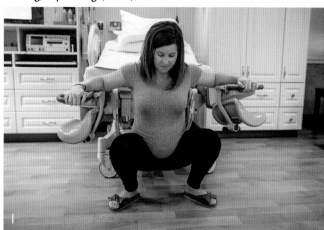

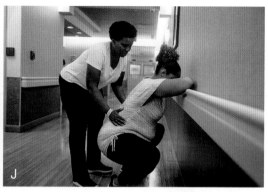

Nursing Implications
Need client to continue to change positions frequently
   to promote good circulation.
Ensure client is stable on the birthing ball; provide
   support as needed.
Continuous monitoring may be difficult in the bathroom,
   but the birthing ball would allow proximity to monitor.
Sitting on the ball can mimic squatting, which opens
   the pelvic diameter.

Advantages
Increases pelvic diameter.
Decreases forceps/vacuum, episiotomy/tears.
Natural way to stretch perineum.
Gravity assists with fetal descent.
Shortens and aligns birth canal.
Toilet "dilation station" relaxes pelvic floor.
A birthing ball loosens pelvic floor when sitting on a softer
   surface.

Disadvantages
Toilet—hard to monitor.
May not tolerate one position for an extended period because
   of the discomfort, exhaustion, and possible insufficient
   circulation of lower extremities.

Side-Lying or Lateral Position

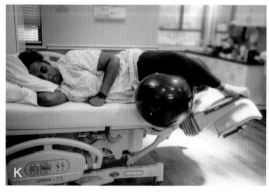

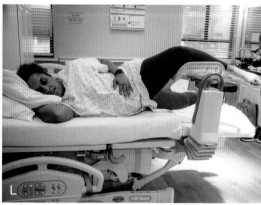

Advantages
It is a restful position.
Side-lying increases uteroplacental perfusion.
Allows for continuous fetal monitoring.

Disadvantages
Does not use gravity to aid in fetal descent.

Nursing Implications
This position offers a break from more tiring positions.
Use of the peanut ball, pillows, or stirrups help open
   the pelvic inlet or outlet as needed.
Use pillows for support.
Alternate side to side every 20 minutes.

Fig. 15.5 cont'd

POSITIONS FOR FIRST-STAGE LABOR

Flying Cowgirl (Spinning Babies, 2021a)

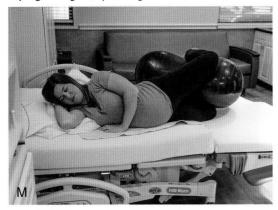

Advantages
Same as side-lying/lateral position.
Opens the pelvic inlet (provides more space from the anterior to posterior diameter at the top of the pelvis) and promotes engagement within the pelvis and fetal descent.

Disadvantages
It should only be done during 3 to 6 contractions, then reposition to other side and repeat.
Fetal heart rate may experience decelerations during rapid descent.

Nursing Implications
This offers a break from more tiring positions.
Use pillows for support.
Alternate side to side every 20 minutes.

Side-Lying Release (Spinning Babies, 2021b)

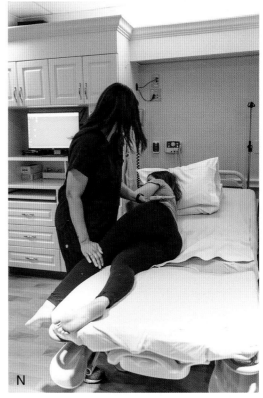

Advantages
Dangling the upper leg stretches and releases the psoas muscle, which allows more pelvic mobility and labor progress.
Decreases pain.
Helps asynclitic or malpositioned fetus realign and engage in the pelvis.

Disadvantages
The benefits of this maneuver are temporary and may need to be repeated.

Nursing Implications
Cannot use this position on clients with hypermobility (very loose joints) or with previous back injuries.
Shoulders need to be positioned evenly with the hips.
Nurse must provide support when the client is in this position. Fall risk increases with side rail down and leg dangling off the bed.
May repeat throughout labor every 4 to 6 hours.

Fig. 15.5 cont'd

KNOWLEDGE CHECK

12. What are three ways nurses can promote labor progress?
13. What is "laboring down"? What are the benefits?
14. When pushing in a sitting or semisitting position, how should the client's body be shaped?

APPLICATION OF THE NURSING PROCESS: PREVENT INJURY

Client problems change during labor because the intrapartum period is an active process. Problems related to fetal oxygenation are covered in Chapter 14. Problems related to pain management are covered in Chapter 13. During the second stage of labor (full dilation to birth), the client is at risk for injury.

Assessment

Nursing assessments of the client and fetus continue throughout birth. During the second stage, observe the client's perineum to determine when to make final birth preparations.

The exact time for final birth preparations varies according to the client's parity, overall speed of labor, and fetal

POSITIONS FOR FIRST-STAGE LABOR

Hands/Knees

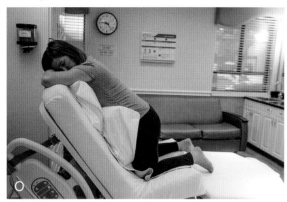

Advantages
Reduces back pain.
Helps with realignment of the occiput posterior (OP) fetal presentation.
Gravity assists with fetal descent.
Used with continuous fetal monitoring.
Access to client's back for counterpressure and massage.
Decreases tearing.
Provides more biofeedback—more natural position and empowers the client with a stronger mind–body connection.
May use this position for first- or second-stage labor. Promotes a stronger response to Ferguson's reflex.

Disadvantages
Tired legs/knees.
Caregivers must reorient themselves because the landmarks are upside-down from their usual perspective.

Nursing Implications
Clients with a history of abuse or sexual assault/trauma may be triggered when caregivers are behind them and they cannot see who is supporting/touching them.
Facilitates moving into Gaskin maneuver to assist with shoulder dystocia.

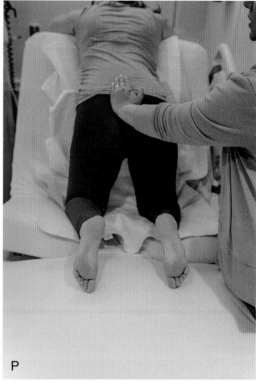

Application of sacral pressure helps provide relief of contraction discomfort.

Fig. 15.5 cont'd

station. Preparations are usually completed when fetal head begins to crown in the nullipara. The multipara is prepared sooner, usually when the cervix is fully dilated and the fetal head is engaged in the pelvis, typically before crowning has occurred.

Identification of Client Problems

The client is vulnerable to injury immediately before and after birth for several reasons: (1) altered physical sensations such as intense pressure and effects of medication, (2) positional changes for birth, and (3) unexpectedly rapid progress.

Planning: Expected Outcomes

The nurse's primary objective is to prevent and minimize potential injuries. The goal or expected outcome for this problem is that the client does not have a preventable injury, such as muscle strains, thrombosis, nerve injury, and lacerations during birth.

Interventions

Positioning the client in the birthing bed is the first step in the sequence of events that culminates in the birth of the baby (Fig. 15.6; see also Figs. 15.3–15.5). During the period around birth, the nurse reduces factors that contribute to injuries.

Positioning for Birth

Upright positions promote effective pushing and take advantage of gravity. Squatting is a good position for uncomplicated birth but limits accessibility to the client's perineum and may not be an option for clients with epidural analgesia. Positions with the upper body leaning forward promotes expulsive efforts, directs the fetus efficiently toward the pelvic outlet, and increases the diameter of the pelvic outlet.

Other upright positions for the birth include standing and kneeling positions. The semirecumbent position limits

POSITIONS FOR SECOND-STAGE LABOR

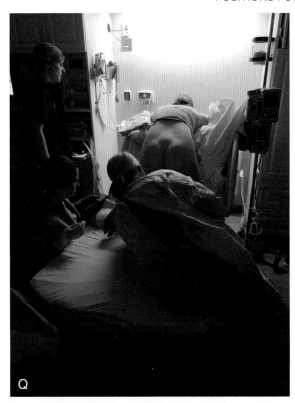

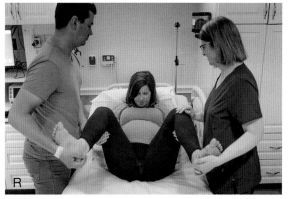

Open knees positioning allows more direct access to the client's pelvis for the provider and nursing staff. Clients with decreased mobility may find this position is more easily attainable for pushing. Closes off sacral movement by applying direct pressure from the bed. Placing hands on posterior aspect of the thigh increases the risk of lower extremity nerve injury (LENI).

Pressure should not be applied when sacral movement is noted as pictured here. The rhombus of Michaelis (sometimes called the quadrilateral of Michaelis) is a kite-shaped area, which includes the three lower lumbar vertebrae, the sacrum, and the long ligament, which reaches down from the base of the scull to the sacrum. This wedge-shaped area of bone moves backward during the second stage of labor and as it moves back, it pushes the wings of the ilea out, increasing the diameters of the pelvis. This happens as part of the physiologic second stage and is an integral part of an active normal birth. (Photo credit Melissa Espey-Mueller)

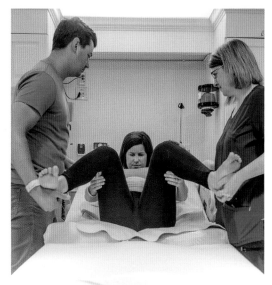

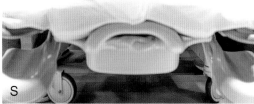

Closed knees opens the outlet (bottom of the pelvis). It may seem counterintuitive, but it provides an alternate method of pushing to facilitate fetal movement through the pelvis. It may be used with epiduralized or natural clients. May use handles or position hands on top of knees instead of on the posterior aspect of the thigh.

Fig. 15.5 cont'd

POSITIONS FOR SECOND-STAGE LABOR

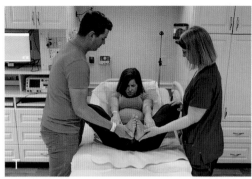

Diamond changes the relationship of the pelvis and provides an alternative for pushing. Not all clients can achieve this position. Assess whether this position/exercise has previously been achieved by the client before attempting during labor. Exercise care in the epiduralized client (who may not feel the discomfort of nerves pulling or stretching).

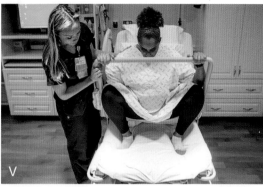

Squatting increases pelvic diameter, gives more power/biofeedback to clients, gravity assists, and might be attainable with epidural and support with squat bar in the bed. This position may be tiring, and access to the client's perineum is challenging. Leaving the bed intact allows for a soft surface should fetal descent and birth occur rapidly.

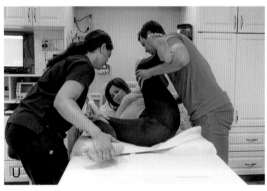

Side-lying is often associated with decreased tearing. It may be achieved with an epidural. This is a restful position for pushing. It assists with fetal rotation and navigation of the pelvis; it also allows sacral movement.

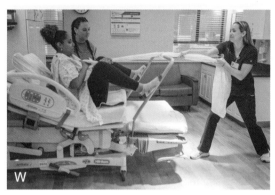

Tug of war provides muscle memory for epiduralized clients. The body uses muscles without thinking about how to do it. It also incorporates the C curve but can be tiring. It can cause injury to client or support person if not correctly positioned.

Fig. 15.5 cont'd

movement of the sacrum as the fetus descends during birth but maintains some advantages of gravity (Berta et al., 2019). Sitting on a birthing bed with a cutout for the perineal area maintains many advantages of squatting, may be less tiring, and may allow for sacrum movement, which enlarges the pelvic outlet. The hands-and-knees position may be helpful for the fetus in the occiput posterior position and to rotate wide fetal shoulders.

Many clients and providers are more comfortable using stirrups and foot rests to support the client's legs and feet and make the perineum more accessible. If the client has limited leg movement related to an anesthetic motor block, raise and lower the legs together and do not separate them too widely. Surfaces that contact the popliteal space behind the knee should be padded because pressure on veins and nerves near the surface could lead to thrombus formation or peroneal nerve injury. The client's upper body should be in the semi-Fowler's or sitting position rather than the supine position.

Observe the Perineum

Birth is near when the fetal head progresses anteriorly in the mechanism of extension and the occiput moves under the symphysis pubis. Observe the client's perineum, especially during late second-stage labor.

A classic sign of imminent birth is the client's urgent cry, "The baby's coming!" Look at the perineum, and if the baby delivers before the provider arrives, remain calm and support the infant's head and body with gloved hands as it emerges. Ask the support person to push the call button to summon help (See Box 15.1, Assisting with an Imminent Birth).

Evaluation

The goal or expected outcome for this client problem is evaluated throughout the postpartum period because injuries such as muscle strains, nerve injuries, or thrombus formation are not evident until later. The provider notes lacerations after the delivery of the infant and makes necessary repairs.

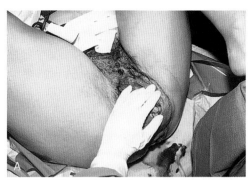

A, Crowning. The fetal head distends the labial and perineal tissues. The anus is stretched wide, and it is not unusual to see the client's anterior rectal wall at this time. Any feces expelled are wiped posteriorly to avoid contaminating the vulva. The provider is not holding the fetal head back but rather controlling its exit by using gentle pressure on the fetal occiput. Continue to observe the fetal heart rate during this time and alert the provider if there are changes that require interventions to speed up birth. If an episiotomy is needed, the provider will perform it when the head is well crowned to minimize blood loss.

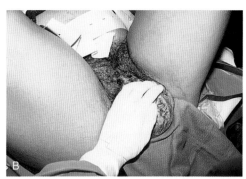

B, Ritgen Maneuver. Pressure is applied to the fetal chin through the perineum at the same time pressure is applied to the occiput of the fetal head. This action aids the mechanism of extension as the fetal head comes under the symphysis and allows the head to gradually deliver. This support minimizes perineal tissue trauma.

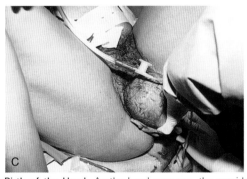

C, Birth of the Head. As the head emerges, the provider prepares to wipe the mouth and nose to avoid aspiration of secretions when the infant takes the first breath.

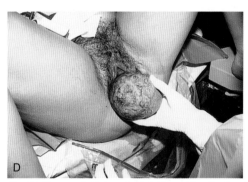

D, Restitution and External Rotation. After the head emerges, it realigns with the shoulders (restitution). External rotation occurs as the fetal shoulders internally rotate, aligning their transverse diameter with the anteroposterior diameter of the pelvic outlet. The provider feels for a cord around the fetal neck (nuchal cord). If it is loose, the cord is slipped over the head. If tight, it is clamped and cut between the two clamps before the rest of the baby is born.

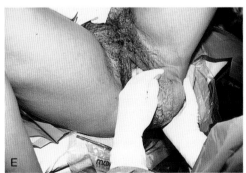

E, Birth of the Anterior Shoulder. The provider gently pushes the fetal head toward the client's perineum to allow the anterior shoulder to slip under the symphysis. The bluish skin color of the fetus is normal at this point; it becomes pink as the infant begins breathing air.

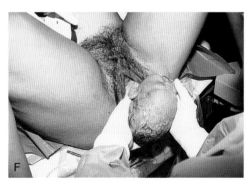

F, Birth of the Posterior Shoulder. The provider now pushes the fetal head upward toward the client's symphysis to allow the posterior shoulder to slip over the perineum.

FIG. 15.6 Vaginal birth.

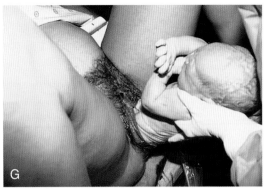

G, **Completion of the Birth.** The provider supports the fetus during expulsion. Note that the fetus has excellent muscle tone, as evidenced by facial grimacing and flexion of the arms and hands.

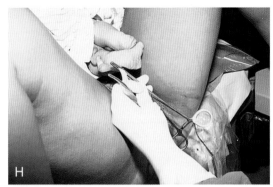

H, **Cord Clamping.** While the infant is skin-to-skin with the client, delayed cord clamping (DCC) for 30-60 seconds may be performed for the stable infant (ACOG, 2017). Once the preferred time for DCC has passed or if the infant needs resuscitation, the provider double clamps the umbilical cord. The cord is then cut between the two clamps. Samples of cord blood are collected after it is cut. If the client has chosen to bank cord blood, the health care team follows the instructions in the cord blood banking collection kit.

I, **Birth of the Placenta.** The provider applies gentle traction on the cord to aid expulsion of the placenta. Note the fetal membranes that surrounded the fetus and amniotic fluid during pregnancy. The chorionic vessels that branch from the umbilical cord are readily visible on the fetal surface of the placenta.

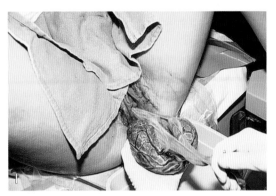

FIG. 15.6 cont'd

KNOWLEDGE CHECK

15. When stirrups are used to position the client for birth, what safety precautions should be used?
16. Why is it important to watch the perineum as the client pushes?

ALTERATIONS IN THE LABOR PROCESS

Although labor is a normal process, some clients may require interventions, such as versions, labor induction, or labor augmentation.

Version

When the fetal lie is oblique or transverse or the presentation is breech, the provider may attempt to turn the baby to a cephalic presentation. Either of two methods may be used: **external cephalic version (ECV)** or internal version. Each has different indications and technique. ECV is the more common method.

Indications

The goal of ECV is to change the fetal position from a breech, shoulder (transverse lie), or oblique presentation. Successful version may allow the client to avoid a cesarean birth by increasing the chance for vaginal birth. Version of a fetus with a transverse lie has a higher success rate than breech presentations (Cunningham et al., 2022). Research has shown that, in many cases, spontaneous version occurs by 37 weeks' gestation (ACOG, 2020a).

Internal version is an uncommon procedure, most often for the second twin after the first delivers in the cephalic presentation. The physician reaches into the uterus with one hand and, with the other hand on the client's abdomen, moves the fetus into a longitudinal lie (cephalic or breech) to allow vaginal birth (ACOG, 2021b).

Contraindications

ECV is not done if a client is unlikely to deliver vaginally, which is the goal of the procedure. Contraindications are similar for internal and external procedures. Conditions that may contraindicate ECV or reduce its success include the following (AAP & ACOG, 2017; Cunningham et al., 2022; Thorp & Grantz, 2019):

- Uterine malformations that limit the room available to perform the version and may be the reason for the abnormal fetal presentation.
- Previous cesarean birth or other significant uterine surgery is a relative contraindication. Manipulation of the fetus within the uterus may strain and rupture the old incision.
- Placenta abnormalities (abruption or previa). Manipulation of the fetus within the uterus may cause hemorrhage, endangering both client and fetus.
- Third-trimester bleeding.

- Disproportion between fetal size and pelvic size.
Fetal conditions that may contraindicate the use of version include the following:
- Multifetal gestation, which reduces the room available to turn the fetus or fetuses. Version may be attempted after the first twin is born vaginally in a cephalic presentation.
- Oligohydramnios, ruptured membranes, and a cord around the fetal body or neck **(nuchal cord).** These conditions limit the room to turn the fetus and may lead to cord compression and fetal hypoxia.
- Intrauterine growth restriction (IUGR).
- Uteroplacental insufficiency. Uterine contractions occurring during the version and labor may worsen the insufficiency and cause fetal compromise.
- Engagement of the fetal head into the pelvis.

Risks

Complications occur in 1% to 2% of attempted versions (ACOG, 2020a; Thorp & Grantz, 2019). Changes to FHR pattern are common, but the pattern usually returns to normal after the version. Serious risks involving the fetus include umbilical cord entanglement or cord prolapse, compressing its vessels and resulting in hypoxia, and placental abruption if fetal manipulation disrupts the placental site, leading to fetal compromise and even death (ACOG, 2020a; Cunningham et al., 2022; Thorp & Grantz, 2019). The client's blood and the fetal blood could become mixed within placental vessels, possibly resulting in client sensitization to the fetal blood type. Cesarean birth may be needed for fetal compromise at the time of the version or later if the fetus returns to an abnormal presentation.

Technique

ECV is performed at a location and time to allow emergency cesarean delivery if necessary (ACOG, 2020a; Cunningham et al., 2022). A nonstress test or biophysical profile is done before the procedure to evaluate fetal health and placental function. If fetal well-being is not present, the version is not performed. An ultrasound examination confirms fetal gestational age and presentation and identifies adequacy of amniotic fluid and placental location (Cunningham et al., 2022).

ECV usually is attempted at 37 weeks' gestation or later, but before the client is in labor, for the following reasons:
- The fetus may spontaneously turn to a cephalic presentation before 37 weeks.
- The fetus is more likely to return to an abnormal presentation if version is attempted before 37 weeks of gestation.
- If fetal compromise or onset of labor occur, a fetus born after 37 weeks of gestation is not likely to have problems associated with preterm birth, such as respiratory distress syndrome.

The client often is given a tocolytic to relax the uterus while the version is performed. Epidural or spinal block may be given to reduce the client's discomfort as the provider manipulates the fetus. Ultrasonography guides fetal manipulations during ECV and monitors the FHR. The provider gently pushes the breech out of the pelvis in a forward or backward roll (ACOG, 2020a; Thorp & Grantz, 2019) (Fig. 15.7).

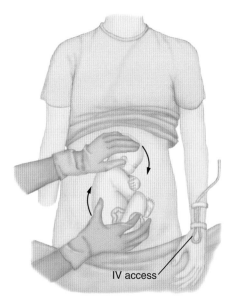

FIG. 15.7 External Cephalic Version. Intravenous access is established, if needed. If terbutaline is used as a tocolytic or uterine relaxant medication, it is given by subcutaneous injection.

Rh immunoglobulin is given to the Rh-negative client after external version to prevent Rh sensitization. Labor induction may be done immediately after a successful ECV, or the client may await spontaneous labor or a later induction. A nonstress test (NST) or EFM is performed after the version for evaluation of fetal condition (Thorp & Grantz, 2019).

Nursing Considerations

When providing care during an external version, the nurse provides information, assesses the client and fetus, and helps reduce the client's anxiety.

Provide information. The provider completes informed consent by explaining the indications and risks for ECV to clients before they sign the consent. Purposes and side effects of any planned tocolytic drug are reviewed. If epidural or other analgesia is planned, its purposes and side effects are explained by the person who will administer the treatment, and the client signs additional consents. The nurse verifies the client's understanding of the purposes, risks, and limitations of the procedure and related treatments. Cesarean birth may be required suddenly; therefore, surgical consents and initial newborn care consents are signed.

Promote client and fetal health. Admission information is collected as if the client were in labor or having a cesarean birth because the need for operative intervention may arise suddenly. The client should have nothing by mouth 6 hours before and during this short procedure in case a cesarean is needed quickly (ACOG, 2018a; Simpson & O'Brien-Abel, 2021). An IV line is placed for possible drug administration or fluid resuscitation.

Obtain vital signs and baseline FHR values to establish well-being. Indeterminate or abnormal (category II or III) FHR patterns should be reported to the provider. Administer the tocolytic medication as ordered. Real-time ultrasonography is used to guide the version and check the FHR periodically during the procedure.

The client and fetus are observed for at least 1 hour after the procedure. Fetal bradycardia may occur during the procedure, but the FHR usually returns to normal when manipulation ends (Thorp & Grantz, 2019). Reassuring fetal signs are a heart rate within the same range as on admission, resolution of any bradycardia, and the presence of moderate variability and FHR accelerations.

The client's vital signs are taken every 15 to 30 minutes until they return to baseline. The pulse rate should be no higher than 120 bpm. Discomfort should diminish quickly after the version, regardless of whether fetal position changes are successful. Persistent and continuous pain suggests a complication such as placental abruption.

If epidural or spinal analgesia was used and is now discontinued, observe for return of sensation before ambulation. Accompany the client while ambulating until gait remains steady and no additional assistance is required.

Regular contractions suggest onset of labor. SROM sometimes occurs, with leakage of fluid from the client's vagina. Rh immunoglobulin is given if indicated. The IV line is discontinued after the client and fetal conditions return to normal unless labor will be induced the same day.

Because the client having ECV is near term, the nurse should review the signs of labor with the client and explain guidelines for returning to the hospital after discharge.

Reduce anxiety. The client may be anxious before version because its success is not certain, and complications may require emergency cesarean delivery. Anxiety may continue after a successful version because the fetus can return to its previous position, and vaginal birth is not certain. The nurse should keep the client informed about what is occurring during the version to reduce the fear of the unknown.

The nurse can point out reassuring fetal monitor patterns such as a normal rate and accelerations to help reduce anxiety about the baby. If a problem such as bradycardia develops, the nurse should explain what has happened, what steps are being done to relieve it, and the result of these interventions.

KNOWLEDGE CHECK

17. Why is observing the FHR important before, during, and after ECV?
18. Why should the UA be monitored after ECV?

Induction and Augmentation of Labor

Induction and augmentation of labor use artificial methods to stimulate uterine contractions. Techniques and nursing care are similar for both induction and augmentation.

Induction of labor is an increasingly common procedure in intrapartum units. Induction rates more than doubled from 1990 to 2010. Although data from the National Vital Statistics System previously showed that the induction rate was declining as recently as 2015, the statistics showed an increase from 27.1% in 2018 to 29.3% in 2019 (Martin et al., 2021; Simpson, 2020).

Inductions have been associated with a higher cesarean birth rate. This increased risk for cesarean section can be mitigated if the cervix is dilated (at least 2 cm) and somewhat effaced before labor (Thorp & Grantz, 2019). Induction is more likely to be successful at term because prelabor cervical changes favor dilation. In 2019 the national cesarean rate was 31.7% for clients of all racial origins, which continued the downward trend noted since 2009 (Martin et al., 2021). This decline is partly attributed to the focus on reducing nonmedically indicated (elective) cesarean sections and induction of labor before 39 weeks.

Indications

Induction of labor may be medically necessary for an obstetric, fetal, or other medical indication, or it may be elective (i.e., performed at the convenience of the client and/or provider). Labor induction is not done if the fetus must be delivered more quickly than the process permits, in which case a cesarean birth is performed. Induction is indicated in the following conditions (ACOG, 2020c; Cunningham et al., 2022; Thorpe & Grantz, 2019):

- The intrauterine environment is hostile to fetal well-being (e.g., IUGR, isoimmunization [maternal-fetal blood incompatibility], oligohydramnios)
- SROM at or near term without onset of labor, also called **premature rupture of the membranes** (PROM). If pregnancy is preterm, less than 37 weeks, the term **preterm premature rupture of the membranes** (PPROM) is used (see Chapter 16)
- Postterm pregnancy
- Chorioamnionitis (infection and inflammation of the amniotic sac)
- Hypertension associated with pregnancy or chronic hypertension, both of which are associated with reduced placental blood flow
- Placental abruption (large abruptions require immediate delivery)
- Medical conditions that worsen with continuation of the pregnancy (e.g., diabetes, hypertension, renal disease, pulmonary disease, heart disease, antiphospholipid syndrome)
- Fetal demise

Induction solely for convenience is not recommended. Valid reasons to induce labor include having a history of rapid labor and living a long distance from the hospital because of the possibility of birth in uncontrolled circumstances (ACOG, 2020c; Simpson & O'Brien-Abel, 2021). Elective inductions have two major risks: twofold increase in cesarean section compared with spontaneous labor and increased risk for neonatal respiratory complications (Thorp & Grantz, 2019). Therefore confirmation of fetal gestational age is paramount before elective induction. Recent recommendations suggest waiting until 39 to 40 weeks before considering elective induction (ACOG, 2020c; AWHONN, 2021; Simpson

& O'Brien-Abel, 2021; Spong et al., 2012; Thorp & Grantz, 2019). This gestational age is associated with decreased risk for cesarean delivery and neonatal respiratory morbidity.

Prenatal testing sometimes identifies a fetal anomaly that will require specialized neonatal care at a facility providing a higher level of care. The client may be transported to such a facility for labor induction or cesarean birth.

Augmentation of labor with oxytocin is considered when labor has begun spontaneously but progress has slowed or stopped, even if contractions seem to be adequate. Nonpharmacologic augmentation may be possible with nipple stimulation (Thorp & Grantz, 2019).

Contraindications

Any contraindication to labor and vaginal birth is a contraindication to induction or augmentation of labor. Possible contraindications and cautions associated with induction may include the following (ACOG, 2020c; Simpson & O'Brien-Abel, 2021; Thorp & Grantz, 2019):

- **Placenta previa**, or placental implantation in the lower uterine segment, which could result in hemorrhage during labor
- **Vasa previa**, a velamentous insertion of the umbilical cord (umbilical cord vessels branch over the amniotic membrane rather than inserting into the placenta, therefore lacking protection of Wharton's jelly); these vessels cross the cervical os; fetal hemorrhage is a possibility if the membranes rupture
- Umbilical cord prolapse because immediate cesarean is indicated to stop cord compression
- Abnormal fetal presentation for which vaginal birth is often more hazardous (i.e., transverse fetal lie)
- Active genital herpes
- Previous uterine surgery, including a previous classical cesarean incision or myomectomy (removal of uterine fibroids) that entered the endometrial cavity

Other conditions that are not contraindications to induction but require individual evaluation include the following (ACOG, 2020c; Thorpe & Grantz, 2019):

- One or more previous low transverse cesarean deliveries
- Breech presentation
- Conditions in which the uterus is overdistended, such as a multifetal pregnancy and polyhydramnios, because the risk for uterine rupture is higher
- Client conditions such as heart disease and severe hypertension
- Fetal presenting part above the pelvic inlet, which may be associated with cephalopelvic disproportion or a preterm fetus
- Inability to adequately monitor the fetal status during labor or presence of indeterminate or abnormal (Category II or III) FHR

Risks

Induction and augmentation of labor, like spontaneous labor, are associated with the following risks (ACOG, 2020c; Cunningham et al., 2022; Simpson & O'Brien-Abel, 2021):

- Excessive UA (increased frequency, duration, or insufficient relaxation time or resting tone) can reduce placental perfusion and fetal oxygenation. Uterine tachysystole may or may not be accompanied by an indeterminate or abnormal (Category II or III) FHR pattern.
- Uterine rupture may occur, which is more likely with overdistention of the uterus with excess amniotic fluid or a multifetal pregnancy or in cases of excessive UA.
- Water intoxication can occur, which is more likely if a hypotonic IV solution is used to dilute the oxytocin and with rates greater than 20 milliunits/minute.
- Chorioamnionitis and cesarean birth
- Postpartum hemorrhage

Elective labor induction at term is associated with increased risk for cesarean birth and newborn respiratory problems. Studies have demonstrated that nulliparous clients who have their labor induced are two to three times more likely to have a surgical birth. A Bishop score (Table 15.2) of 6 or less is associated with an increased risk for cesarean birth compared with spontaneously laboring clients (Simpson, 2020; Simpson & O'Brien-Abel, 2021; Thorpe & Grantz, 2019). The risk for cesarean after failed induction was similar whether clients had medical or elective inductions. Risk for chorioamnionitis increases as the duration of ruptured membranes increases (Cunningham et al., 2022).

Technique

Pharmacologic and mechanical methods may be used for labor induction and augmentation. Cervical assessment estimates whether the cervix is favorable for induction. The Bishop scoring system (see Table 15.2) is used to estimate cervical readiness for labor with five factors: cervical dilation, effacement, consistency, position, and fetal station. Vaginal birth is more likely to result if a Bishop score is higher than 8 (ACOG, 2020c; Simpson & O'Brien-Abel, 2021).

Cervical ripening. Cervical ripening is a process used to ripen (soften) the cervix and make it more likely to dilate with the forces of labor. Typically, this procedure is performed before the scheduled induction. Cervical ripening is recommended for a Bishop score of 6 or less (ACOG, 2020c; Cunningham et al., 2022).

Pharmacologic methods. Prostaglandin is a drug that may be used to cause cervical ripening. Prostaglandin E_2 (PGE_2) preparations may be given as an intravaginal gel, an intracervical gel, or a timed-release vaginal insert (Table 15.3). PGE_2 preparations are administered in a setting where fetal monitoring and emergency care, including immediate cesarean birth, are readily available.

Misoprostol (Cytotec) is a prostaglandin E_1 (PGE_1) analog usually given for gastric ulcers. Misoprostol can be used for both cervical ripening and induction of labor. Misoprostol for cervical ripening is currently an off-label use, and its manufacturer does not plan to seek United States (US) Food and Drug Administration (FDA) approval for these purposes. In addition to its effectiveness, misoprostol is attractive for its lower cost and stability at room temperature (ACOG, 2020c; Cunningham et al., 2022; FDA, 2015). It should not be given, however, to a client who has had a previous cesarean birth or major uterine surgery (ACOG, 2020c; Simpson & O'Brien-Abel, 2021).

TABLE 15.2 Bishop Scoring System to Evaluate the Cervix[a]

Factor	SCORE			
	0	**1**	**2**	**3**
Dilation	0 cm	1–2 cm	3–4 cm	5–6 cm
Effacement	0%–30%	40%–50%	60%–70%	≥80%
Fetal station	−3	−2	−1 or 0	+1 or +2
Cervical consistency	Firm	Medium	Soft	
Cervical position	Posterior	Midposition	Anterior	

[a]This system is used to estimate how easily a client's labor can be induced. Higher scores are associated with a greater likelihood of successful induction because the cervix has undergone prelabor changes, often called *ripening*. Vaginal delivery is most likely after induction if the Bishop score is 8 or higher.
(Modified from Bishop, E. H. [1964]. Pelvic scoring for elective induction. *Obstetrics & Gynecology, 24*[2], 266–268.)

Misoprostol is available in 100- and 200-mcg tablets. The usual dose is 25 or 50 mcg vaginally, orally, or sublingually, one-quarter or one-half of an unscored 100-mcg tablet (ACOG, 2020c). A pharmacist should prepare the tablet to ensure dose accuracy when using an unscored tablet. The 25-mcg preparation of misoprostol is placed high in the vagina. An oral dose of misoprostol 25-mcg has been associated with fewer episodes of tachysystole and indeterminate or abnormal (Category II or III) FHR changes (ACOG, 2020c; Simpson & O'Brien-Abel, 2021).

The major adverse effect of prostaglandins is tachysystole; therefore, the medication is administered in a setting in which fetal monitoring and emergency care, including cesarean birth, are immediately available.

After vaginal insertion of prostaglandins, the client should remain recumbent for at least 30 minutes. The FHR and UA should be monitored continuously for a period of 30 minutes to 4 hours (ACOG, 2020c; Simpson, 2020).

Mechanical methods. Mechanical methods for cervical ripening are efficacious and have decreased risk for excessive UA. These methods include placement of a transcervical balloon catheter, membrane stripping, or placement of hygroscopic inserts (i.e., *Laminaria*—sterile cone-shaped preparations of dried seaweed).

Transcervical catheters are placed through the internal cervical os, and downward tension is created by either taping the catheter to the thigh or attaching the catheter to a dependent IV bag. The double balloon device (Fig. 15.8) is designed to compress the cervix with simultaneous placement of fluid in an intrauterine and intravaginal balloon. Once 4 to 6 centimeters of cervical dilation is achieved, the balloon typically falls out (Simpson & O'Brien-Abel, 2021).

Membrane stripping is the digital separation of the amniotic membrane from the wall of the cervix and the lower uterine segment. Spontaneous labor may occur within 48 hours and reduces the need for other induction methods (ACOG, 2020c; Simpson & O'Brien-Abel, 2021).

Hygroscopic inserts (*Laminaria*) are placed into the cervical canal, where they absorb water and swell, gradually dilating the cervix. Placement requires a speculum and can be cumbersome and uncomfortable (ACOG, 2020c; Cunningham et al., 2022; Simpson & O'Brien-Abel, 2021).

Oxytocin administration. Oxytocin is the most common drug given for induction and augmentation of labor (see Drug Guide). Oxytocin is a powerful drug, and predicting a client's response to it is impossible. Several precautions reduce the chance of adverse reactions in the client and fetus.

- Oxytocin should be diluted in an isotonic solution and given as a secondary (piggyback) infusion so it can be stopped quickly if complications develop.
- The oxytocin line should be inserted into the primary (nonadditive or maintenance) IV line as close as possible to the venipuncture site (the proximal port) to limit the amount of drug infused if discontinued.
- Oxytocin should be started slowly, increased gradually, and regulated with an infusion pump. The primary line is also regulated with an infusion pump.
- UA and fetal heart patterns should be monitored before induction for a baseline, when oxytocin is started, and throughout labor.

Oxytocin receptor sites become desensitized from prolonged exposure. Continual rate increases can result in abnormal UA (tachysystole), coupling or tripling of contractions, or low-intensity contractions (Simpson & O'Brien-Abel, 2021). The rate of oxytocin infusion may be gradually reduced once the active phase of labor is reached (6 cm of cervical dilation) to decrease the receptor site saturation (Simpson & O'Brien-Abel, 2021). It may be stopped or the rate reduced after the client's membranes rupture. When labor is augmented with oxytocin, a lower total dose usually is needed to achieve adequate contractions compared with the dose needed for labor induction.

Nursing considerations

When providing care during cervical ripening and labor induction or augmentation, the nurse observes the client and fetus for complications and takes corrective actions if abnormalities are noted. The nurse has a responsibility to closely monitor the client and fetus when administering uterine stimulants. The nurse initiates, titrates, and discontinues the oxytocin infusion using the facility's protocols and medical orders. Facility policies related to oxytocin must clearly

TABLE 15.3 Prostaglandin Preparations for Cervical Ripening at Term

Prostaglandin Gel (Dinoprostone [Prepidil])(PGE2)	Vaginal Insert (Dinoprostone [Cervidil]) (PGE2)	Misoprostol (Cytotec)(PGE1)
Dosage[a]		
0.5 mg applied in the cervix; may be repeated 6–12 hr later. Maximum recommended dose is 1.5 mg applied in the cervix in a 24-hr period. 2.5 mg applied in the vagina.	10 mg in a time-release vaginal insert left in place for up to 12 hr. Remove with onset of active labor, membrane rupture, or uterine tachysystole.	One-quarter to one-half of 100-mcg tablet vaginally (~25–50 mcg[a]; see following precautions) or up to 100 mcg orally. Dosing for labor induction includes repeating 25-mcg dose every 3–6 hr. A 50-mcg dose, every 6 hr, has been associated with excessive uterine activity. Oral dosing may be administered every 2 hrs.
Actions for Excessive Uterine Activity, With or Without Indeterminate or Abnormal Fetal Heart Rate Patterns		
Place client in side-lying position. Provide oxygen by nonrebreather face mask at 10 L/min. Administer tocolytic drug such as terbutaline. Typically begins 1 hr after gel application. Higher incidence with vaginal application.	Same as for dinoprostone gel. Remove insert. Hypertonic uterine activity may occur up to 9.5 hr after insert placement. Greater incidence than with lower dose intracervical dinoprostone gel.	Same as for dinoprostone gel. Higher dose or more frequent administration is more likely to cause excessive contractions, which may or may not be accompanied by indeterminate or abnormal fetal heart rate pattern.
When Oxytocin Induction May Begin		
Safe interval has not been established. Delaying oxytocin administration for 6–12 hr after total intracervical dose of 1.5-mg or 2.5-mg vaginal dose recommended.	30–60 min after removal of insert.	At least 4 hr after last dose.
Precautions and Comments		
Limit dinoprostone gel to maximum of 1.5 mg in the cervix in 24 hr. Client should remain recumbent with lateral uterine displacement for 15–30 min after application. Has increased effect if combined with other oxytocics such as oxytocin (Pitocin). Use caution in clients with asthma, glaucoma, epilepsy, cardiovascular disease, severe renal or hepatic dysfunction.	Remove after 12 hr or when active labor begins. Adverse effects can be reduced within 15 min of removal. Most expensive of prostaglandin options.	Misoprostol is currently FDA-approved only for treatment of peptic ulcers but is widely used for cervical ripening and induction of labor. Manufacturer does not intend to seek approval, but the ACOG supports its use for these purposes. 100-mcg tablet is not scored. The hospital pharmacy should prepare the 25- or 50-mcg dose for greater accuracy. Cost is approximately 1%–2% that of other prostaglandin preparations. Contraindicated in clients with a previous cesarean or other uterine surgery in the third trimester. Increase in meconium-stained amniotic fluid has been reported. Buccal and sublingual routes have limited data and therefore are not recommended for cervical ripening or induction until further studies are completed.

ACOG, American College of Obstetricians and Gynecologists; *FDA*, U.S. Food and Drug Administration.
[a]Doses may be higher in cases of fetal death.

(From American Academy of Pediatrics & American College of Obstetricians and Gynecologists [AAP & ACOG, 2017]. *Guidelines for perinatal care* [8th ed.]; American College of Obstetricians and Gynecologists [ACOG]. [2020c]. Induction of Labor. *ACOG Practice Bulletin 107*. Published 2009, reaffirmed 2020; Dinoprostone: Drug information [2021]. *UpToDate*. https://www.uptodate.com/contents/dinoprostone-drug-information?search=dinoprostone&source=panel_search_result&selectedTitle=1~96&usage_type=panel&kp_tab=drug_general&display_rank=1; Levine, L.D., L., & Srinivas, S.K. [2021]. Induction of labor. In M. Landon, H. Galan, E. Jauniaux, D. Driscoll, V. Berghella, W. Grobman, S. Kilpatrick, & A. Cahill [Eds.]. *Gabbe's obstetrics: Normal and problem pregnancies.* [8th ed., pp. 226–239]. Elsevier; Misoprostol: Drug information. [2021]. *UpToDate*. https://www.uptodate.com/contents/misoprostol-drug-information?search=misoprostol &source=panel_search_result&selectedTitle=1~122&usage_type=panel&kp_tab=drug_general&display_rank=1; Oxytocin: Drug information. [2021]. *UpToDate*. https://www.uptodate.com/contents/oxytocin-drug-information?search=oxytocin&source=panel_search_result&selectedTitle=1~132&usage_type=panel&kp_tab=drug_general&display_rank=1; U.S. Food and Drug Administration [FDA]. [2015]. Misoprostol [marketed as Cytotec] information [2015]. www.fda.gov/Drugs/DrugSafety/PostmarketDrugSafetyInformationforPatientsandProviders/ucm111315.htm.)

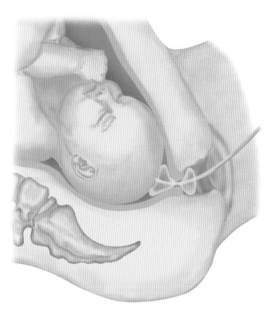

FIG. 15.8 Double balloon catheter.

support nursing and medical actions, which promote client safety.

Observe the fetal response. Oxytocin stimulates uterine contractions, and they may become too frequent (tachysystole). Tachysystole may reduce placental blood flow (uteroplacental insufficiency), which decreases exchange of fetal oxygen and waste products. Before induction and augmentation of labor, the nurse assesses the FHR and contraction pattern to ensure fetal well-being is present. ACOG and AWHONN set forth standards for FHR assessment based on risk stratification of the client (Miller et al., 2022; Simpson, 2020; Simpson & O'Brien-Abel, 2021; Wisner & Ivory, 2021). Individual facilities set documentation guidelines incorporating those recommendations.

The nurse remains alert for FHR patterns, which suggest reduced placental exchange secondary to excessive UA. Examples are fetal bradycardia, tachycardia, pathologic decelerations, and decreased FHR variability. The nurse should assess the client and fetus carefully to identify the most likely cause of the problem and institute corrective actions. See Chapter 14 for more detailed information on fetal monitoring.

DRUG GUIDE

Oxytocin (Pitocin)

Classification
Oxytocic.

Action
Synthetic compound identical to the natural hormone released from the posterior pituitary. Stimulates uterine smooth muscle, resulting in increased strength, duration, and frequency of uterine contractions. Uterine sensitivity to oxytocin increases gradually until 34 weeks' gestation, and then a rapid increase in sensitivity is noted during labor. Oxytocin has vasoactive and antidiuretic properties.

Indications
Induction or augmentation of labor at or near term. Maintenance of firm uterine contractions after birth to control postpartum bleeding. Management of inevitable or incomplete abortion.

Dosage and Route
Induction or Augmentation of Labor
1. Intravenous (IV) infusion via a secondary (piggyback) line. Oxytocin infusion is controlled with a pump. Various dilutions of oxytocin and balanced electrolyte solution may be used. Common mixtures of oxytocin include (1) 15 units of oxytocin (1.5 mL) plus 250 mL of solution; (2) 30 units (3 mL) of oxytocin plus 500 mL of solution; and (3) 60 units (6 mL) of oxytocin plus 1000 mL of solution. Concentrations that result in a 1:1 solution decrease calculation errors. The Institute for Safe Medication Practices (2018) noted that oxytocin was a high-alert medication in the acute care setting, requiring safety checks to be completed with administration. Therefore oxytocin solutions should be standardized in a 1:1 solution and premixed in the pharmacy to reduce risk for error.

2. Guidelines for oxytocin administration from ACOG (2020c) provide examples of low-dose and high-dose oxytocin labor induction protocols. Protocols may recommend: (1) starting doses of 0.5 to 2 milliunits/min for the low-dose protocol and 6 milliunits/min for the high-dose protocol, and (2) increasing the dose in 1 to 2 milliunits/min increments every 15 to 40 minutes for low dose; high-dose protocols may increase the dose in increments of 3 to 6 milliunits/min. The actual oxytocin dose is based on uterine response and absence of adverse effects. Higher starting doses, higher dose increases, and shorter intervals between dose increases are most likely to result in uterine tachysystole. A lower starting dose and lower rate increase increments are usually required to augment labor.

3. Once active labor is achieved and an adequate contraction pattern exists, oxytocin may be reduced or discontinued.

Control of Postpartum Bleeding
IV infusion: Dilute 10 to 40 units in 1000 mL of IV solution. The rate of infusion must control uterine atony. Begin at a rate of 20 to 40 milliunits/min, increasing or decreasing the rate according to uterine response and the rate of postpartum bleeding. Any identifiable cause of the hemorrhage should also be corrected.

Inevitable or Incomplete Abortion
Dilute 10 units in 500 mL of IV solution and infuse at a rate of 10 to 20 milliunits/min. Other dilutions are acceptable.

Intramuscular Injection
Inject 10 units after placenta delivery if there is no IV access.

Onset of Action
IV, within 1 minute; intramuscular (IM), 3 to 5 minutes.

DRUG GUIDE—CONT'D

Excretion
Renal (urine).

Contraindications and Precautions
Include, but are not limited to, placenta previa, vasa previa, indeterminate or abnormal (Category II or III) fetal heart rate (FHR) patterns, abnormal fetal presentation, prolapsed umbilical cord, previous classic or other fundal uterine incision, active genital herpes infection, and invasive cervical carcinoma.

Adverse Reactions
Most result from hypersensitivity to drug or excessive dosage. Adverse reactions include excessive UA (e.g., tachysystole, hypertonus, inadequate relaxation time), impaired uterine blood flow, uterine rupture, and placental abruption. Uterine hypertonicity may result in fetal bradycardia, fetal tachycardia, reduced FHR variability, and late or prolonged decelerations. Fetal arrhythmias (including premature ventricular contractions) may also occur. Fetal asphyxia may occur with diminished uterine blood flow. Fetal or client trauma, or both, may occur from rapid birth. Prolonged administration may cause client fluid retention, leading to water intoxication. Hypotension (seen with rapid IV injection), tachycardia, cardiac arrhythmias, and subarachnoid hemorrhage are rare adverse reactions.

Drug interactions include vasopressors and the herb ephedra, which cause hypertension; carboprost tromethamine, which may cause enhanced oxytocic effects; and haloperidol or QT prolonging agents, which may enhance QT prolonging effect.

Nursing Considerations
Intrapartum
Assess the FHR for at least 20 minutes before induction to identify fetal well-being. Confirm cephalic fetal presentation via Leopold's or vaginal examination. If indeterminate or abnormal FHR patterns are identified or if fetal presentation is other than cephalic, notify the provider and do not begin induction until fetal presentation and fetal well-being are confirmed.

Observe UA for establishment of effective labor pattern: contraction frequency every 2 to 3 minutes, duration of 40 to 90 seconds. Observe for excessive UA: more than five contractions in a 10-minute window, averaged over 30 minutes, contractions with a rest interval shorter than 60 seconds in first-stage labor and 45 to 50 seconds in second-stage labor, duration longer than 120 seconds, or an elevated resting tone firm by palpation or greater than 20 to 25 mm Hg (if measured with an intrauterine pressure catheter), and Montevideo units (MVUs) greater than 250 in first-stage and 400 in second-stage labor.

Observe FHR for patterns such as tachycardia, bradycardia, minimal to absent variability, and pathologic (late, variable, or prolonged) decelerations. If uterine tachysystole or FHR patterns, as indicated previously, occur, intervene to reduce UA and increase fetal oxygenation: stop the oxytocin infusion, increase the rate of nonadditive solution, position the client in a side-lying position, and consider oxygen administration by nonrebreather face mask at 10 L/min. Notify the provider of adverse reactions, nursing interventions, and client response. Record the blood pressure, pulse rate, and respirations every 30 to 60 minutes or with each dose increase. Record intake and output.

Postpartum
Observe the uterus for firmness, height, and deviation. Massage until firm if uterus is soft ("boggy"). Observe lochia for color, quantity, and presence of clots. Notify the provider if the uterus fails to remain contracted or if lochia amount is large or contains large clots. Assess for cramping. Assess vital signs every 15 minutes or according to protocol for the recovery period. Monitor intake and output and breath sounds to identify fluid retention or bladder distention.

Inevitable or Incomplete Abortion
Observe for cramping, vaginal bleeding, clots, and passage of products of conception. Observe vital signs and intake and output as noted under postpartum nursing implications.

(From American College of Obstetricians and Gynecologists [ACOG]. [2020c]. *Induction of labor*. ACOG Practice Bulletin 107. Published 2009, reaffirmed 2020; Miller, L.A., Miller, D.A., & Cypher, R.L. [2022]. *Mosby's pocket guide to fetal monitoring: A multidisciplinary approach* [9th ed.]. Mosby; Oxytocin: Drug information. [2021]. UpToDate. https://www.uptodate.com/contents/oxytocin-drug-information?search=oxytocin&source=panel_search_result&selectedTitle=1~132&usage_type=panel&kp_tab=drug_general&display_rank=1; and Simpson, K.R., & O'Brien-Abel, N. [2021]. Labor and birth. In K. Simpson, P. Creehan, N. O'Brien-Abel, C. Roth & A. Rohan [Eds.], *AWHONN's perinatal nursing*. [5th ed., pp. 326–412]. Wolters Kluwer.)

⚡ SAFETY CHECK

Signs of Excessive Uterine Activity

- Contraction duration longer than 120 seconds
- Less than 60 seconds relaxation time between contractions in first-stage labor and 45 to 50 seconds in second-stage labor
- Uterine resting tone firm by palpation or higher than 20 to 25 mm Hg (with intrauterine pressure catheter)
- **Montevideo units** (MVUs; unit of measure for uterine contraction intensity) exceeding 250 in first-stage labor to 400 in second-stage labor (Miller et al., 2022)
- More than five contractions in a 10-minute window, averaged over 30 minutes

(From American College of Obstetricians and Gynecologists [ACOG]. [2021a]. Management of intrapartum fetal heart rate tracing. *ACOG Practice Bulletin 116*. Published 2010, reaffirmed 2021; and Simpson, K.R., & O'Brien-Abel, N. (2021). Labor and birth. In K. Simpson, P. Creehan, N. O'Brien-Abel, C. Roth & A. Rohan (Eds.), *AWHONN's perinatal nursing*. [5th ed., pp. 326–412]. Wolters Kluwer.)

BOX 15.2   Suggested Protocol for Nursing Actions in the Presence of Excessive Uterine Activity

The following are the suggested protocols for nursing actions in the presence of excessive uterine activity with normal FHR patterns and abnormal FHR patterns (ACOG, 2021a; Simpson & O'Brien-Abel, 2021).

With Normal Fetal Heart Rate Patterns
• Position the client laterally.
• Administer an IV fluid bolus of at least 500 mL.
• If the tachysystole does not resolve in 10 to 15 minutes, the oxytocin infusion rate should be decreased by half.
• If tachysystole persists after another 10 to 15 minutes, the oxytocin infusion should be stopped until the uterine activity is normal.

With Abnormal Fetal Heart Rate Patterns
• Stop the oxytocin infusion and administer an IV fluid bolus of at least 500 mL.
• Keep the client in a side-lying position to prevent aortocaval compression and increase placental blood flow.
• Consider oxygen administration at 10 L/min via nonrebreather face mask until FHR pattern improves.
• Notify the provider; anticipate order for terbutaline (Brethine 0.25 mg subcutaneously) if no improvement occurs with other interventions.
   In both cases, if the provider orders oxytocin to be restarted, oxytocin administration can occur when the tachysystole resolves and the FHR pattern returns to normal. The oxytocin should be restarted at no more than half the previous rate if it has been turned off for less than 20 to 30 minutes. If more than 30 to 40 minutes has elapsed, it should be restarted at the initial dose.

Observe the client's response. The uterus must be assessed for excessive UA, which may reduce fetal oxygenation and contribute to uterine rupture. Contractions are assessed for frequency, duration and intensity, uterine resting tone, and relaxation time of at least 60 seconds between contractions in first-stage labor and 45 to 50 seconds in second-stage labor (Bakker et al., 2007; Miller et al., 2022). UA observations are charted at the same intervals as the FHR. Corrective actions for excessive UA should be treated per hospital guidelines (see Safety Check: Signs of Excessive Uterine Activity and Box 15.2).

If the oxytocin must be discontinued, the medical decision about resuming is individualized. The oxytocin infusion may be restarted at the same or a lower dose if the contractions are no longer too frequent and the FHR is reassuring. If the oxytocin has been discontinued for 40 minutes or longer, the drug that was in the client's system has been metabolized. Therefore it should be restarted at the beginning dose ordered and advanced more slowly to prevent a recurrence of uterine tachysystole and indeterminate or abnormal FHR patterns.

The client's blood pressure and pulse rate are taken hourly or with each oxytocin dose increase to identify changes from baseline. Temperature is assessed every 2 hours, if amniotic membranes are intact; if the membranes are ruptured, it is assessed hourly to identify infection (Simpson & O'Brien-Abel, 2021).

The client may need to use pharmacologic and nonpharmacologic pain management techniques sooner than in a spontaneous labor. Although the goal of induced and augmented labor is to mimic natural labor, stimulated contractions often increase in intensity more quickly. Cervical ripening may increase the discomfort felt by the client.

Recording intake and output identifies fluid retention, which may precede water intoxication. Signs and symptoms of water intoxication include headache, blurred vision, behavioral changes, increased blood pressure and respirations, decreased pulse rate, auscultatory crackles and wheezing, and coughing.

After birth, the client is observed for postpartum hemorrhage caused by uterine relaxation. Postpartum uterine atony is more likely with prolonged use of oxytocin. The uterine muscle becomes fatigued and does not contract effectively to compress vessels at the placental site, and the oxytocin receptor sites may be saturated and less responsive. Atony is manifested by a soft uterine fundus and excess amounts of lochia, usually with large clots. Hypovolemic shock may occur with hemorrhage (see Chapter 19).

? KNOWLEDGE CHECK

19. What precautions are taken to enhance the safety of oxytocin administration for the client and fetus?
20. How may oxytocin administration differ if labor is being augmented rather than induced?
21. What signs may indicate an unfavorable fetal response to oxytocin stimulation?
22. What are the signs of excessive uterine activity?
23. How can induction of labor with oxytocin contribute to postpartum hemorrhage?

NURSING CARE: PREPARATION AND BIRTH

Responsibilities During Birth

The nurse's responsibilities during birth may include the following:
• Preparation of a delivery table with sterile gowns, gloves, drapes, solutions, and instruments (Fig. 15.9)
• Prewarming all equipment and linens that will be used on the newborn
• Perineal cleansing preparation
• Ongoing assessments of client and fetus
• Supporting the client and partner with final pushing efforts
• Initial care and assessment of the newborn
• Administration of medications (usually oxytocin) to contract the uterus and control blood loss

At least one person, usually an additional nurse, certified to provide neonatal resuscitation should be present at all births. This person's role is dedicated to the assessment and resuscitation of the newborn infant (AAP & ACOG, 2017; AAP & AHA, 2021). If the newborn is at risk for complications, this is likely to be a nurse or resuscitation team from the nursery. The client's nurse continues to assist the provider as needed and supports the client and partner.

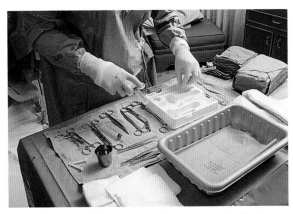

FIG. 15.9 The provider arranges instruments in final preparation for birth. Although the vagina is not sterile, a sterile table is prepared to limit introduction of outside organisms into the birth canal. Included on the sterile table are infant care materials (e.g., cord clamp, cord blood tube), instruments for repair of lacerations or episiotomy, and anesthesia materials (if needed).

Personal protective equipment, including eye shields, should be worn as protection from fluid and blood exposure. The newborn is covered with blood, amniotic fluid, vernix, and other body substances. The first bath usually occurs several hours after birth, so team members involved in infant care should wear gloves and other needed protective equipment to avoid contact with potentially infectious secretions.

ALTERATIONS IN THE BIRTH PROCESS

Operative Vaginal Birth

Operative vaginal birth, also called *forceps* or *vacuum extraction,* may be used by the provider to apply traction to or assist descent or rotation of the fetal head during birth, aiding the client's expulsive efforts. As the rate of cesarean birth has increased, vaginal births assisted by either forceps or vacuum extractor have declined. Among vaginal births in 2019, 3.0% were delivered with instrumentation, with 0.5% delivered with forceps and 2.5% with vacuum extraction. Use of either method is down from 9.01% in 1990 (Martin et al., 2021; Simpson & O'Brien-Abel, 2021).

A vacuum extractor uses suction to grasp the fetal head while traction is applied (Fig. 15.10). Its use is similar to that of forceps and carries the following contraindications to use: breech, face, or brow presentation; cephalopelvic disproportion; unengaged fetal head; incompletely dilated cervix; suspected bone demineralization condition (i.e., osteogenesis imperfecta); bleeding disorder (i.e., hemophilia, von Willebrand's disease); or premature infant. The fetus of 34 weeks or less of gestation is more likely to injure the head, scalp, and intracranial vessels from vacuum suction (ACOG, 2020d; Thorp & Grantz, 2019). Typically, facility policies

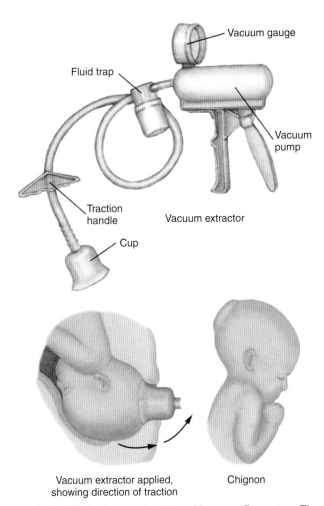

FIG. 15.10 Birth Assisted with a Vacuum Extractor. The chignon is scalp edema, which often forms under the suction cup when the vacuum extractor is used.

do not support more than three "pop-offs" of the vacuum extractor or proceeding to forceps after failed attempts to deliver with vacuum because a higher incidence of injury to the client and neonate can occur (ACOG, 2020d; Simpson & O'Brien-Abel, 2021; Thorp & Grantz, 2019).

Forceps are curved, metal instruments with two curved blades that can be locked in the center. Many styles are available for different needs. The blades may be closed or open and are shaped to grasp the fetal head (Fig. 15.11). Piper forceps are a special type used to assist birth of the head in a vaginal breech birth. Forceps and a vacuum extractor also may be used during cesarean birth if assistance is needed in delivering the head.

Indications

Forceps or vacuum extraction is considered if the second stage should be shortened for the well-being of the client, fetus, or both and if vaginal birth can be accomplished quickly. Client indications may include exhaustion, inability to push effectively, infection, and cardiac or pulmonary disease (AAP & ACOG, 2017; Cunningham et al., 2022).

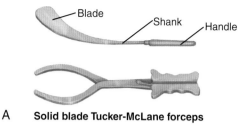

A   **Solid blade Tucker-McLane forceps**

Application of forceps with an open (fenestrated) blade

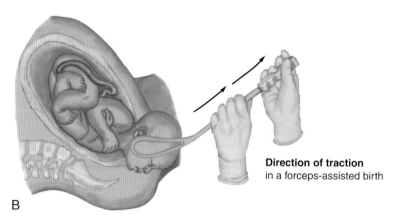

Direction of traction
in a forceps-assisted birth

B

FIG. 15.11 **Obstetric Forceps and Their Application.** (A) Solid-blade Tucker-McLane forceps. (B) Direction of traction in a forceps-assisted birth.

Fetal indications may include failure of the fetal presenting part to fully rotate and descend in the pelvis, partial separation of the placenta, or abnormal FHR patterns near the time of birth.

Contraindications

Cesarean birth is preferable if the client and fetal conditions mandate a more rapid birth than can be accomplished with forceps or vacuum extraction or if the procedure would be too traumatic. Examples of these conditions are severe fetal compromise, acute client conditions such as congestive heart failure and pulmonary edema, a high fetal station, and disproportion between the size of the fetus and client pelvis.

Risks

The main risk in forceps and vacuum extraction is trauma to the pregnant client and fetus. Because of the relative safety of cesarean birth, the attempt at an instrumental birth usually is abandoned if the fetal head does not descend easily.

Client risks include laceration and hematoma of the vagina, pelvic floor disorders, anal sphincter disruption, and infection. The infant may have ecchymoses, facial and scalp lacerations and abrasions, facial nerve injury, cephalohematoma, subgaleal hemorrhage, intracranial hemorrhage, and jaundice. A vacuum extractor may create scalp edema called a *chignon* at the application area (see Fig. 15.10) (AAP & ACOG, 2017; Simpson & O'Brien-Abel, 2021).

Technique

Preparation for vacuum extraction or forceps is similar to that for any vaginal birth. The presentation, position, and station of the fetal presenting part are verified. Membranes must be ruptured and the cervix completely dilated for forceps or vacuum extraction birth. The client needs adequate anesthesia, usually a regional block such as an epidural.

Forceps and vacuum extractor–assisted births are classified according to the extent of descent of the fetal head into the pelvis during the procedure and necessary degree of rotation for the fetal head to be born. Describing descent in centimeters below the ischial spines is preferred (AAP & ACOG, 2017; ACOG, 2020d; Simpson & O'Brien-Abel, 2021; Thorp & Grantz, 2019).

- Outlet operative vaginal delivery—The fetal head is at or on the perineum, with the scalp visible at the vaginal opening without separating the labia, rotation does not exceed 45 degrees. The position is either right or left occiput anterior (ROA, LOA) or right or left occiput posterior (ROP, LOP).
- Low operative vaginal delivery—The leading edge of the fetal skull is at station +2 cm or lower and not on the pelvic floor. Low operative vaginal birth is subdivided according to the amount of rotation of the fetal head needed. Births requiring 45 degrees or less of fetal head rotation are simpler.
- Midpelvis or midforceps operative vaginal delivery—The leading edge of the fetal skull is between 0 (at the level of the ischial spines or engaged) and +2 cm station.

The provider determines the presentation, position, and station of the fetal head and amount of cervical dilation. When the blades are correctly applied, the long axis of the blades lies over the fetal cheeks and parietal bones. After checking for proper application, the provider articulates or locks the two blades in the center and pulls gently as the client pushes, following the curve of the pelvis. An **episiotomy** (surgical incision of the perineum) may be performed as the fetal head distends the perineum. The provider may keep the forceps on until the head is born or may remove the blades just before expulsion.

For vacuum extraction, a hand pump is used to create suction to hold the vacuum cup on the fetal head in the midline of the occiput. The provider applies traction intermittently, as in a forceps-assisted birth. A vacuum release allows easy removal of the cup.

Nursing Considerations

When a forceps or vacuum extraction birth is anticipated, a catheter is often added to the instrument table for the birth to empty the bladder before the procedure. The provider specifies the type of vacuum cup or forceps needed. If the nurse must apply the suction to the cup, suction should not go outside the green zone on the suction indicator. Fetal tolerance of the procedure should be monitored through FHR assessment.

After birth, the client and infant are observed for trauma. The client may have vaginal wall lacerations or a hematoma (see Chapter 18). Cold applications for the first 24 hours reduce pain by numbing the area and limit bruising and edema of the tissues. Heat applications may then be applied to aid resolution of the edema and bruising.

The infant often has reddening and mild bruising of the skin where the forceps were applied. These areas do not need treatment. Cold treatment is not done for an infant because of hypothermia. Skin breaks that allow entry of microorganisms should be noted and kept clean. Facial asymmetry, which is most obvious when the infant cries, suggests facial nerve injury. Temporary caput or scalp edema (**chignon**) is common at the location of the vacuum extractor cup.

After an operative vaginal birth, a parent may ask questions about the infant's condition (e.g., bruising, redness, edema). A good response is to explain the pressure of the forceps on the baby's delicate skin may cause minor bruising, which usually resolves without treatment. Point out improvement in the area during the postpartum stay. Parents may need an explanation for the scalp edema, or chignon, after a vaginal birth assisted with a vacuum extractor.

Episiotomy

Episiotomy, or incision of the perineum just before birth, was once routine for vaginal births. The presumed benefits, which included reducing pain, perineal tearing, and later pelvic floor dysfunction or pelvic organ prolapse, have not proved true (ACOG, 2018b; Cunningham et al., 2022). However, the provider must decide if one is needed based on the clinical picture.

Indications

Examples of situations in which the provider may perform an episiotomy are as follows (Cunningham et al., 2022):

- Rapid resolution of fetal shoulder dystocia, in which the shoulder of a fetus becomes lodged under the client's symphysis during birth
- Vacuum extractor–assisted or forceps-assisted births
- Birth with the fetus in an occiput posterior (face-up) position
- Breech delivery
- Macrosomic fetus
- Markedly short perineal length

Risks

Infection is the main risk in episiotomy. Perineal pain occurs with both episiotomy and spontaneous tears. However, perineal pain may last longer with episiotomy because of the tendency to extend into deeper lacerations. Prolonged perineal pain impairs resumption of sexual intercourse and makes it uncomfortable for the client.

Data since the 1980s have confirmed midline episiotomies, more frequently done than mediolateral episiotomies, increase a client's risk for the more extensive third-degree (into the anal sphincter) or fourth-degree (through the rectal sphincter) tear. Fecal incontinence was increased, blood loss was greater, and more infection and pain were experienced compared with clients who delivered with an intact perineum (ACOG, 2018b; Cunningham et al., 2022; Simpson & O'Brien-Abel, 2021). Spontaneous lacerations are more likely to occur if a client had an episiotomy with a previous pregnancy. However, despite data confirming benefits of avoiding episiotomies, approximately 12% of vaginal deliveries have routine episiotomies performed (ACOG, 2018b; Cunningham et al., 2022).

Technique

An episiotomy is done when the fetal presenting part has crowned to a diameter of approximately 3 to 4 cm. The two types of episiotomies, median (midline) and mediolateral, have different advantages and disadvantages (Fig. 15.12).

Nursing Considerations

An episiotomy sometimes can be avoided or limited in length with nursing measures. An upright position while pushing promotes gradual stretching of the client's perineum. Delaying pushing until the urge is felt also gradually distends the soft tissue of the pelvic floor. Pushing with an open-glottis technique rather than prolonged breath-holding when pushing also promotes gradual perineal stretching.

Daily perineal massage and stretching by the client from 34 weeks until birth has been shown to reduce the risk for perineal trauma during birth. During second stage, the use of perineal massage decreased the incidence of third- or fourth-degree lacerations (ACOG, 2018b).

Nursing interventions during the recovery and postpartum periods are similar for episiotomy and perineal laceration. The perineum should be observed for hematoma and edema. Use of the acronym REEDA (redness, edema, ecchymosis, discharge, and approximation of episiotomy edges) guides the assessment aspects (James & Suplee, 2021). As with use of forceps, perineal cold applications are done for at least the first 24 hours, followed by perineal heat applications.

Median or Midline

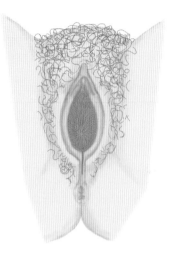

Mediolateral

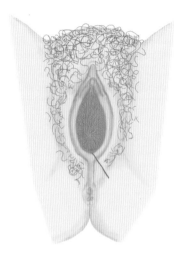

Advantages
Minimal blood loss
Neat healing with little
　scarring
Less postpartum pain
　than the mediolateral
　episiotomy

Disadvantages
An added laceration may
　extend the median
　episiotomy into the
　anal sphincter
Limited enlargement of the
　vaginal opening because
　perineal length is limited
　by the anal sphincter

Advantages
More enlargement of
　the vaginal opening
Little risk that the
　episiotomy will extend
　into the anus
Protective from fecal
　incontinence
Less time and suture
　needed for repair

Disadvantages
More blood loss
Increased postpartum
　pain
More scarring and
　irregularity in the
　healed scar
Prolonged dyspareunia
　(painful intercourse)

FIG. 15.12 Types of Episiotomies.

KNOWLEDGE CHECK

24. Why should an additional nurse or other qualified professional be present at birth?
25. What are the similarities in the uses of vacuum extractors and forceps? What are the differences? Do limits exist for the number of attempts with these instruments?
26. Why should the nurse add a urinary catheter to the instrument table if a forceps-assisted or vacuum extractor–assisted birth is expected?
27. What newborn injury is suggested by an asymmetric facial appearance when the infant cries?

Cesarean Birth

In 1965 the cesarean birth rate in the United States was approximately 5% of all births, rising to almost 21% in 1996. From 1996 to 2009, the number of cesareans steadily increased among all age groups, with a peak in 2009 at 32.9%. Data for 2019 show cesarean deliveries have continued the steady downward trend started in 2010, with the current rate being 31.7% of all births (Martin et al., 2021). Despite this recent decline, the increase in cesarean birth rate in the U.S. remains significant.

Many factors contribute to the rise in the national cesarean birth rate, including the following (Martin et al., 2021; Simpson & O'Brien-Abel, 2021; Thorp & Grantz, 2019):

- Clients having their first baby are more likely to deliver by cesarean than clients who have had one or more previous births vaginally.
- Clients having labor induction with their first baby have a greater risk for a cesarean.
- The 25.6% primary (first) cesarean rate adds to the overall rate because more clients will have repeat cesareans rather than attempting vaginal birth for subsequent children.
- Clients are having children later, and cesareans are more common in the older pregnant population.
- Increasing body mass index.
- Cesarean birth may be chosen if the baby remains in a breech presentation.
- A high threat of litigation if birth outcomes are not good causes physicians to opt for surgery quickly if the client or fetal condition or both seem to be at risk.
- Cesarean upon request rather than medical need.
- Operative vaginal delivery incidence is decreasing.

Evidence linking labor induction to increased risk for cesarean birth continues to accumulate. Studies have demonstrated that clients who have their labor induced are two to three times more likely to have a surgical birth. Clients having a Bishop score of less than 6 at the time of induction, indicating a cervix which is not favorable, had a greater risk for cesarean than clients who had a score of 8 or more. The likelihood of a cesarean increases as the duration of induced labor increases. The risk for cesarean after failed induction was similar whether clients had medical or elective inductions (Simpson & O'Brien-Abel, 2021; Thorp & Grantz, 2019).

A national goal for the *Healthy People 2030* initiative is to reduce the rate of first-time cesarean births in low-risk clients to no more than 23.6% using a baseline of 25.9% of births in 2018 (U.S. Department of Health and Human Services,

2020). Promotion of vaginal birth after cesarean (VBAC) in clients for whom it is appropriate is one way to decrease overall cesarean births. Data suggests **labor dystocia** (difficult or prolonged labor) is the primary reason for cesarean section in the United States (AAP & ACOG, 2017; Simpson & O'Brien-Abel, 2021). Attempts to decrease the primary cesarean rate include a more careful evaluation of labor dystocia and careful selection of clients who are appropriate candidates for vaginal breech birth. ECV may be an option to attempt to change the presentation of a near-term fetus in the breech presentation to a cephalic presentation.

Vaginal Birth after Cesarean

With the high cesarean rate and the desire to lower the incidence, many clients are faced with the decision about whether to have a trial of labor after a cesarean (TOLAC), hopefully resulting in a vaginal birth after cesarean (VBAC). At one time, the saying "Once a cesarean, always a cesarean" was accepted without question (ACOG, 2019; Cunningham et al., 2022). For many years, the only clients who had VBACs were those who entered the hospital in such advanced labor that there was no time for a repeat cesarean. Current literature states VBAC is associated with decreased morbidity and decreased risk for complications in future pregnancies, but a failed TOLAC is associated with more complications for the client and infant than a repeat cesarean section (American Academy of Family Physicians [AAFP], 2019; AAP & ACOG, 2017; ACOG, 2019).

A higher incidence in uterine rupture is noted with vertical uterine incisions (AAFP, 2019; ACOG 2019). As low transverse uterine incisions became the norm for almost all clients having cesarean births, the safety of a TOLAC became established. VBAC gradually became an accepted way to lower the rise in cesarean births.

The AAP and ACOG (2017) have affirmed their support for VBAC (Box 15.3) but have urged caution when considering a TOLAC because VBAC is associated with a small but significant risk for uterine rupture. The risks and benefits of VBAC must be considered by the client and physician. Evidence suggests up to two prior low-transverse uterine incisions are candidates for TOLAC without increased risk of uterine rupture (AAFP, 2019; ACOG, 2019; Thorp & Grantz, 2019). Uterine rupture increases the risk that the client and infant are more likely to have complications, such as bleeding or infection, which further complicate recovery and add to costs. The hospital also incurs greater costs for personnel and supplies.

When making the decision about whether to attempt VBAC, clients need to know that surgical birth has risks just as all surgeries have risks. Besides risks common to any surgery, multiple cesarean births have risks including greater risk for placental abnormalities such as placenta previa (low-lying placenta) or placenta accreta (abnormal adherence of the placenta to the uterine wall, often along the previous incision area) (AAFP, 2019; ACOG, 2019). Therefore the client and physician must consider the risks and benefits of both.

Clients may be anxious about attempting vaginal birth in a later pregnancy. Although they may be a good candidate for

---

BOX 15.3 Vaginal Birth after Cesarean

1. Approximately 60% to 80% of clients who attempt a trial of labor after cesarean (TOLAC) have successful vaginal births.
2. Clients who had their previous cesarean for a nonrecurring reason, such as breech presentation, are more likely to have a successful vaginal birth after cesarean birth (VBAC) than clients who had their previous cesarean because of dystocia ("failure to progress").
3. Clients who have had a vaginal birth, before or since the prior cesarean birth, are more likely to have successful VBAC.
4. There is a higher probability of success in the client who has spontaneous labor.

Possible Candidates and Requirements for Vaginal Birth After Cesarean

1. A client who has one to two previous low transverse uterine incision.
2. A client with two prior cesarean deliveries may have a low risk of uterine rupture with VBAC.
3. Absence of other uterine scars (e.g., removal of fibroid tumors) or a previous uterine rupture.
4. A pelvis that is clinically adequate for the estimated fetal size.
5. Immediate availability of a physician during active labor if an emergency cesarean is needed.
6. Availability of anesthesia and personnel to perform an emergency cesarean.

Management of Clients Who Plan Vaginal Birth After Cesarean

1. External cephalic version is not contraindicated for the client with a previous cesarean.
2. Epidural analgesia may be used.
3. Induction and augmentation of labor with oxytocin may be done.
4. Mechanical methods of cervical ripening with transcervical catheters may be an option for TOLAC candidates with an unfavorable cervix. Misoprostol (Cytotec) should not be used.
5. Most authorities recommend continuous electronic fetal monitoring.

(Data from American College of Obstetricians and Gynecologists [ACOG, 2019]. Vaginal birth after cesarean delivery. *Practice Bulletin 205*; American Academy of Pediatrics & American College of Obstetricians and Gynecologists [AAP & ACOG]. [2017]. *Guidelines for perinatal care* [8th ed.]; Dalton, J., & Strehlow, S. [2019]. Maternal obesity. In N. Troiano, C. Harvey, & B. Chez [Eds.], *AWHONN high-risk & critical care obstetrics* [4th ed., pp. 232–243]. Wolters Kluwer.)

VBAC, it can be hard to disregard risks. Scheduling a repeat cesarean may seem safer and simpler. The prospect of laboring and perhaps still needing a cesarean birth can also be worrisome.

The physician discusses VBAC during prenatal care if it is a reasonable option. The nurse reinforces these explanations and identifies misunderstandings. If the client chooses VBAC, the nurse should reinforce the appropriateness of attempting VBAC and advantages of a vaginal birth, such as fewer overall complications individually. VBAC should be presented in a positive way if it is a real option, yet the possibility of cesarean delivery should be acknowledged (see Box 15.3).

BOX 15.4   Enhanced Recovery After Cesarean Birth

This guideline covers care of the client from 30–60 minutes before surgery starts until hospital discharge. Enhanced recovery guidelines have been shown to decrease length of stay, surgical complications, pain and need for analgesia postoperatively, costs, and readmissions. In the event of an emergent cesarean section, some aspects can be completed postoperatively.

Phase 1 (Preoperative Care)
- Begins 30–60 minutes before surgery start time.
- No solid food for at least 6 hours before surgery.
- Clear fluids encouraged until 2 hours before surgery; encourage oral carbohydrate drinks for nondiabetic clients 2 hours before surgery if possible.
- Administer antacid and histamine H2 receptor antagonists to decrease aspiration risk.
- Administer acetaminophen 1000 mg to decrease postoperative pain.

Phase 2 (Intraoperative Care)
Client Pathway
- Begins upon entrance to the operating room (OR) and ends upon exit from OR.
- Administer intravenous (IV) antibiotics (cephalosporins are recommended) within 60 minutes of skin incision to decrease infection risk.
- Prep abdomen with chlorhexidine-alcohol solution to prevent surgical site infection.
- Prep vagina with povidone-iodine solution to reduce endometritis after surgery.
- Regional anesthesia is preferred.
- Avoid hypothermia by using forced air warming, IV fluid warming, and increased OR temperature

- Recommendations for the type of uterine incision and repair are included to decrease blood loss and intraoperative time
- Maintain **euvolemia** (normal blood volume status) pre- and intraoperatively.

Neonate Pathway
- Delayed cord clamping for 30 seconds (preterm infant) to 1 minute (term infant) after delivery decreases anemia and improves neurodevelopmental outcomes.
- Maintain body temperature between 36.5° and 37.5°C.
- Have necessary personnel present to initiate immediate neonatal resuscitation.

Phase 3 (Postoperative Care)
- Begins at surgery completion and transfer to recovery room and ends at facility discharge.
- Encourage chewing gum to increase recovery of gastrointestinal function (may be redundant if early oral intake is used).
- Combine administration of fluid bolus, phenylephrine or ephedrine, and antiemetics intraoperatively with lower limb compression to decrease postoperative nausea and vomiting.
- Use multimodal postoperative analgesia with nonsteroidal antiinflammatories (NSAIDs) and acetaminophen to provide pain control.
- Client should be consuming a regular diet within 2 hours of delivery.
- Strict control of blood sugars after delivery.
- Early ambulation and immediate removal of urinary catheter placed during surgery.

(From American College of Obstetricians and Gynecologists [ACOG]. [2018a]. Perioperative pathways: Enhanced recovery after surgery. *ACOG Committee Opinion 750;* Caughey, A. B., Wood, S. L., Macones, G. A., Wrench, I. J., Huang, J., Norman, M., Pettersson, K., Fawcett, W. J., Shalabi, M. M., Metcalfe, A., Gramlich, L., Nelson, G., & Wilson, R. D. [2018]. Guidelines for antenatal and preoperative care in cesarean delivery: Enhanced recovery after surgery society recommendations [part 2]. *American Journal of Obstetrics & Gynecology, 219*[6], 533–544; Killion, M. M. (2019). Enhanced recovery after cesarean birth. *MCN: The American Journal of Maternal Child Nursing, 44*[6], 296; Macones, G. A., Caughey, A. B., Wood, S. L., Wrench, I. J., Huang, J., Norman, M., Pettersson, K., Fawcett, W. J., Shalabi, M. M., Metcalfe, A., Gramlich, L., Nelson, G., & Wilson, R. D. [2019]. Guidelines for antenatal and preoperative care in cesarean delivery: Enhanced recovery after surgery society recommendations [part 3]. *American Journal of Obstetrics & Gynecology, 221*[3], 247.e1–247.e9; and Wilson, R. D., Caughey, A. B., Wood, S. L., Macones, G. A., Wrench, I. J., Huang, J., Norman, M., Pettersson, K., Fawcett, W. J., Shalabi, M. M., Metcalfe, A., Gramlich, L., & Nelson, G. [2018]. Guidelines for antenatal and preoperative care in cesarean delivery: Enhanced recovery after surgery society recommendations [part 1]. *American Journal of Obstetrics & Gynecology, 219*[6], 523.E1–513.E15.)

Cesarean Section Indications

Cesarean birth is typically performed when vaginal birth would compromise the client, the fetus, or both. Possible indications for cesarean birth include, but are not limited to, the following (AAP & ACOG, 2017; Cunningham et al., 2022; Simpson & O'Brien-Abel, 2021; Thorp & Grantz, 2019):
- Labor dystocia
- Cephalopelvic disproportion
- Hypertension, if prompt delivery is necessary
- Diseases such as diabetes, heart disease, or cervical cancer if labor is not advisable
- Active genital herpes
- Some previous uterine surgical procedures, such as a classic cesarean incision or myomectomy (removal of fibroid tumors)

- Persistent indeterminate or abnormal (Category II or III) FHR patterns
- Prolapsed umbilical cord
- Fetal malpresentations, such as breech or transverse lie
- Multiple gestation
- Hemorrhagic conditions, such as placental abruption or placenta previa
- Client request

Contraindications

Few absolute contraindications exist, but cesarean birth in some conditions is not desirable because the risks are too great compared with the potential benefits to the client and fetus. These conditions include a fetus too immature to survive, a current fetal demise, or coagulation defects, which could cause harm to the client in surgery.

Risks

Cesarean birth is one of the safest major surgical procedures. However, it poses greater risk for the client than vaginal birth. Risks include the following (Cunningham et al., 2022; Thorp & Grantz, 2019):

- Infection
- Hemorrhage
- Urinary tract trauma or infection
- Thrombophlebitis, thromboembolism
- Bowel dysfunction, such as paralytic ileus, obstruction, sigmoid volvulus
- Atelectasis
- Endomyometritis
- Anesthesia complications
- Wound complications, such as hematoma, dehiscence, infection, necrotizing fasciitis

Cesarean delivery poses added risks to the infant, which may include the following (Cunningham et al., 2022; Thorp & Grantz, 2019):

- Iatrogenic prematurity
- Transient tachypnea of the newborn caused by delayed absorption of lung fluid
- Injury, such as laceration, bruising, fractures, or other trauma

Lung immaturity is the greatest risk if the fetus is delivered preterm. Therefore tests for fetal lung maturity may be done if elective cesarean birth is planned. Other criteria for assuring fetal lung maturity at the time of cesarean birth include the following (AAP & ACOG, 2017):

- Documentation of fetal heart tones for 30 weeks by Doppler
- Passage of 36 weeks since positive results from a pregnancy test performed by a laboratory
- Ultrasound measurement at less than 20 weeks, which supports a gestation of 39 weeks or more

Technique

Enhanced Recovery After Cesarean Delivery is a guideline with evidence-based recommendations for preoperative, intraoperative and postoperative client care (Box 15.4). Many facilities have used these guidelines to implement protocols or client care pathways for cesarean births.

Preparation. Routine admission assessments including allergies, last oral intake (time of intake and what was consumed), any medications or herbal preparations and the time of the last dose, and laboratory studies are completed. The client's condition, risk factors, and type of anesthesia may affect the laboratory studies ordered. The provider may order one or more units of blood to be typed and crossmatched to have available for transfusion if the client's hemoglobin and hematocrit values are low or if the client has a high risk for hemorrhage, such as grand multiparity (five or more births). The provider may also request the client to begin skin preparation the night before scheduled surgery by washing the skin with an antimicrobial soap (Caughey et al., 2018). The client signs informed consents for care, including surgery and anesthesia.

Consent for blood transfusion is also included at most facilities as a precautionary measure. IV access is started with a large-bore (18-gauge or larger) catheter.

Epidural or combined spinal–epidural block is common for cesarean birth. General anesthesia may be required for either known or unexpected reasons. For emergency cesarean with no epidural in place, a general anesthetic may be chosen because it can be established the most quickly. A drug such as famotidine (Pepcid) or sodium citrate with citric acid (Bicitra) may be given to reduce gastric acidity before surgery.

Additional preoperative care includes a "time out," in which all members of the team validate the client's identity, surgical site, and consents. Staff members identify themselves and their roles during this process (Cunningham et al., 2022; Simpson & O'Brien-Abel, 2021).

Fetal surveillance should be individualized, and fetal heart tones should be documented before surgery. For unscheduled surgeries, surveillance should continue until just before the sterile abdominal skin preparation (intermittent auscultation or external monitor) or just after the preparation (internal monitor) (AAP & ACOG, 2017). A wedge placed under one hip prevents aortocaval compression and promotes placental blood flow (Cunningham et al., 2022; Simpson & O'Brien-Abel, 2021).

A single IV dose of a prophylactic antibiotic, such as ampicillin or a cephalosporin, is given to the client within 60 minutes of surgery (AAP & ACOG, 2017; Caughey et al., 2018; Simpson & O'Brien-Abel, 2021; Thorp & Grantz, 2019). Additional antibiotic doses for 24 hours are common to prevent postoperative infections in clients with an increased infection risk (i.e., prolonged rupture of membranes or a lengthy labor).

If a Pfannenstiel (transverse or "bikini") skin incision is planned, the client's lower abdominal hair is clipped from about 3 inches above the pubic hairline to the mons pubis, where the legs come together. The fronts of the upper thighs are also clipped. For a vertical skin incision, the upper border of the abdominal hair clipping is near the umbilicus. Cordless electric clippers with disposable heads reduce skin nicks, which provide an entry point for microorganisms.

Before surgery, an indwelling catheter should be inserted after the regional block is established to allow comfortable insertion and to keep the bladder away from the operative area, reducing the risk for injury (Cunningham et al., 2022). The catheter also may be placed before the block. The catheter allows for accurate observation of urine output during and after surgery, which helps evaluate circulatory status.

Risk for thromboembolism almost doubles for the client undergoing cesarean delivery. Therefore sequential pneumatic compression devices are applied before surgery initiation (Caughey et al., 2018; Cunningham et al., 2022; Simpson & O'Brien-Abel, 2021; Witcher & Hamner, 2019). A grounding pad for the electrocautery is applied to an area with no bony prominences, usually the thigh. After application of the pad, the client's legs are secured to the operating table with a wide, padded strap.

Sterile abdominal skin preparation is completed and allowed to dry before sterile drapes are applied. Surgical skin preparations vary in methods of application (friction vs. paint).

Application begins at the center of the operative site upward and from the pubic area downward on each upper thigh. It may be necessary to secure excess abdominal fat (the panniculus, or "apron") away from the skin incision area. Methods include using tape or a commercially prepared retraction device for this process. Vaginal preparation should be considered for clients with ruptured membranes or those who have been laboring before surgery (ACOG, 2018a; Cunningham et al., 2022; Simpson & O'Brien-Abel, 2021).

If a general anesthetic is required, preoperative preparations are completed before anesthesia is begun to reduce newborn exposure to anesthesia. The team scrubs, dons gowns and gloves, and drapes the client before general anesthesia is induced.

Incisions. Two incisions are made, one in the abdominal wall (skin incision) and the other in the uterine wall. Either of two skin incisions are used: a midline vertical incision between the umbilicus and the symphysis or a low transverse (Pfannenstiel) incision just above the symphysis (Cunningham et al., 2022) (Fig. 15.13).

Three types of uterine incisions are possible, each with different indications and limitations: (1) low transverse, (2) low vertical, and (3) classic, a vertical incision into the upper uterus (Cunningham et al., 2022) (Fig. 15.14). The low transverse uterine incision is preferred because of its low risk for rupture in subsequent pregnancies. The uterine incision does not always match the skin incision. For example, a client may have a vertical skin incision and a low transverse uterine incision, particularly if the client is obese or has a preexisting vertical scar.

The low transverse uterine incision may not be suitable if the fetus is very large. The length of this incision is limited because the uterine artery and vein enter the uterus at its lower right and left sides. The low transverse incision may not be large enough to deliver a large fetus without tearing these large vessels. Sometimes, a vertical uterine incision must be added to a transverse one (making an inverted T or a J) to deliver a very large baby. If an additional vertical incision is needed bilaterally, a U incision is formed (Cunningham et al., 2022).

A classic uterine incision occasionally must be used when the other two incisions are not possible, such as when a placenta previa is located in the lower anterior uterus. The vertical uterine incision, especially the classic one, is more likely to rupture during later pregnancies.

Sequence of events in a cesarean birth. The sequence of events in a cesarean birth is similar to that of a vaginal birth. When the client is anesthetized and draped, the physician makes the skin incision. The uterus is incised, usually in a low transverse incision. If the membranes are intact, they are ruptured with a sharp instrument and amniotic fluid is suctioned from the operative field. As in vaginal births, the color and odor of the amniotic fluid are noted and the time of rupture is recorded.

The physician lifts the fetal presenting part through the uterine incision. The infant's face is wiped, and the mouth and nose may be suctioned to remove secretions that would impair breathing. The cord is clamped and cut. Evidence suggests that a 30- to 60-second delay in cord clamping increases total body iron stores, expands blood volume, decreases anemia, and decreases rate of intraventricular hemorrhage in the preterm infant (AAP & ACOG, 2017; ACOG, 2017; Cunningham et al., 2022). The physician collects cord blood for analysis.

After the infant's birth, the physician removes the placenta. IV oxytocin is given to contract the uterus. The physician then closes the uterine and abdominal incisions, approximating each layer separately.

Vertical

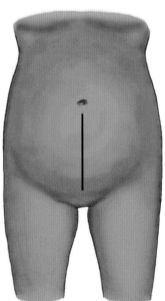

Advantages
Quicker to perform
Better visualization of the uterus
Can quickly extend upward for greater visualization if needed
Often more appropriate for obese clients

Disadvantages
Easily visible when healed
Greater chance of dehiscence and hernia formation
More postoperative pain

Pfannenstiel

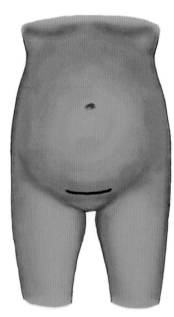

Advantages
Less visibility when healed and the pubic hair grows back
Less chance of dehiscence or formation of a hernia

Disadvantages
Less visualization of the uterus
Cannot be done as quickly, which may be important in an emergency cesarean birth
Cannot easily be extended to give greater operative exposure
Reentry at a subsequent cesarean birth may require more time

FIG. 15.13 Skin (abdominal wall) incisions for cesarean birth.

Low Transverse **Low Vertical** **Classic**

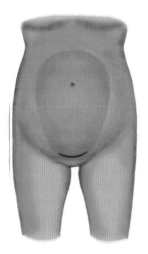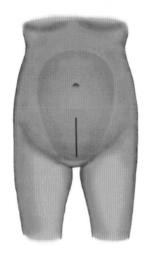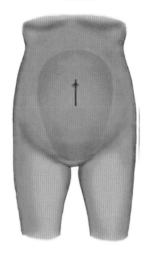

Advantages
Unlikely to rupture during a subsequent
birth
Makes VBAC possible for subsequent
pregnancy
Less blood loss
Easier to repair
Less adhesion formation

Disadvantage
Limited ability to extend laterally to enlarge the incision

Advantage
Can be extended upward to make a larger
incision if needed

Disadvantages
Slightly more likely to rupture during a
subsequent birth
A tear may extend the incision downward
into the cervix

Advantage
May be the only choice in these situations:
Implantation of a placenta previa on the
lower anterior uterine wall
Presence of dense adhesions from
previous surgery
Transverse lie of a large fetus with the
shoulder impacted in the mother's pelvis

Disadvantages
Most likely of the uterine incisions to rupture during a subsequent birth
Eliminates VBAC as an option for birth of
a subsequent infant

FIG. 15.14 Uterine Incisions for Cesarean Birth. The abdominal and uterine incisions do not always match. *VBAC,* Vaginal birth after cesarean.

Nursing care for the infant is similar to the care after vaginal birth. Resuscitation equipment should be readied for use before delivery. Professional personnel who care for the infant born by cesarean vary with the baby's anticipated condition and facility policy. A pediatrician, neonatal or pediatric nurse practitioner, or neonatal team usually attends the at-risk infant at the time of cesarean birth (AAP & ACOG, 2017; AAP & AHA, 2021). Newborn care personnel must be prepared for unexpected resuscitation measures as in any birth. Implementation of skin-to-skin contact has shown stabilization of infant heart and respiratory rate, temperature, and blood sugars; therefore, this contact should be promoted when possible (Simpson & O'Brien-Abel, 2021).

Nursing Considerations

Nursing care for a client who has a cesarean birth varies according to the situation. The client may be planning a cesarean birth, or a surgical birth may be unexpected. Even in these two situations, clients differ. For example, is the planned cesarean the first or has the client had a cesarean birth before? Was the previous cesarean planned? An unplanned cesarean birth may occur after hours of unsuccessful labor or may be needed quickly in an emergency.

Nursing care for clients having cesarean childbirth is similar to vaginal birth, but the approach in each situation is different. For example, although preoperative teaching is important, it must be abbreviated or even omitted in a true emergency.

Emotional support. Emotional support may begin before and extend after the birth. A client with a history of a previous cesarean birth may harbor unresolved feelings of grief, guilt, or inadequacy because of the perception that the client somehow failed in the expected birth experience. The client may feel anxious about choosing repeat cesarean when given the choice of a TOLAC. Therapeutic communication techniques help identify stressors and misunderstandings to promote a positive childbirth experience.

Anxiety is an expected and normal reaction to surgery. The staff's behavior can either reduce or increase the client's anxiety. A calm and confident manner helps the client feel cared for by competent professionals. A quiet, low voice is calming. The nurse and the client's significant others are important sources of emotional support. The nurse should remain with the client to establish rapport so the client can express fears. Therapeutic communication helps clarify concerns, so explanations to reduce fear of the unknown can be most effective.

The support person should be encouraged to remain during surgery if regional anesthesia is used. In some hospitals, the support person may come into the operating room after the client is intubated for general anesthesia to foster attachment with the infant and help the client integrate the birth experience afterward.

Nurses also support a client's partner and significant others during the cesarean birth. The partner may be as anxious as the client but afraid to express it because the client needs so much support. The partner may be physically exhausted after hours of labor coaching. The staff should not expect more support from partners than can be reasonably provided.

Although cesarean births are routine in the intrapartum unit, they are not routine to clients who undergo them and to their families. Avoid belittling their fears by telling clients and their families not to worry and that everything will be all right, especially if an emergency occurs.

After birth, in the postanesthesia care unit (PACU), the nurse begins to answer questions about the surgery and fill in any gaps in the client and family's understanding. This helps promote a positive perception of the birth.

Teaching. Knowledge may reduce fear of the unknown and increase a client's sense of control over the birth. The nurse cannot assume a client who had a previous cesarean birth already knows what will happen and why. If the previous surgery was done after a long labor or in an emergency, clients may recall only parts and not understand those parts they remember. Teaching should be given in simple language and include the support person.

The nurse explains preoperative procedures such as hair clipping in the incisional area, indwelling catheter, IV lines, and dressings and their purposes. The catheter and IV lines usually remain in place less than 24 hours after birth. Sequential compression devices (SCDs) may be used throughout surgery and until ambulating well to reduce the risk for deep vein thrombosis.

Clients who have regional anesthesia such as an epidural or a subarachnoid block often fear they will feel pain during surgery. They do feel pressure and pulling, but these sensations do not mean the anesthesia is wearing off. The nurse reassures the client that pain management is regularly assessed by the anesthesia provider.

If a client is having general anesthesia, the nurse explains why operative preparations are completed before anesthesia is started. Clients should be reassured that surgery will not begin until anesthesia has been administered and they will not wake up during the procedure.

The nurse describes the operating room (OR) and who will be present to make it less intimidating to the client. Staff in the OR should introduce themselves, if possible. The client's labor nurse often is the circulating nurse during surgery and reassures the client with a familiar face and voice. The OR is very cool in most cases, and the surgery table is narrow.

The support person should be told when to expect to come into the OR. If it is not already in place, an epidural block often is established after the client goes to the OR. Preparations may take 30 to 45 minutes if no rush exists. Support persons should be told they will not be forgotten and apparent delays do not indicate problems. Surgery preparation time, which moves quickly and efficiently for staff, often moves very slowly for family and the main support person.

The PACU and any equipment that will be used, such as, a pulse oximeter, electrocardiogram monitor, and automatic blood pressure cuff, are explained to the client. The nurse reviews routine assessments and interventions such as fundus and lochia checks, coughing, and deep breathing. The nurse reassures the client that every effort will be made to promote comfort with medication, positioning, and other interventions.

Promoting safety. See Table 15.3. The client's food intake is assessed for type and time on admission because general anesthesia occasionally is necessary. Oral intake and emesis during labor are recorded and reported to the anesthesia clinician. Oral intake other than ordered medications and possibly ice chips is discontinued if a cesarean birth becomes likely. Medications to control gastric and respiratory secretions are administered, as ordered.

The client is transferred and positioned carefully to prevent injury, especially when regional anesthesia is being administered. Regional anesthesia reduces motor control and sensation. Bariatric operating tables are used for clients with increased body mass index. Bony prominences are cushioned. A safety strap, used to secure the client to the OR table, is placed across the thighs. A wedge under one hip or a tilted operating table avoids aortocaval compression and reduced placental blood flow. During positioning the drain tube of the indwelling catheter should be routed under the leg to promote drainage and keep the tubing away from the operative area. The catheter bag is made visible so the urine output may be monitored during surgery, an important measure of fluid balance. The nurse applies sequential compression devices to the client's lower limbs.

The nurse verifies proper function of equipment such as suction devices, monitors, and electrocautery. Leads for the cardiac monitor, temperature, and pulse oximeter are placed to observe vital functions. A grounding pad permits safe use of electrocautery.

After the surgery, the incision area is cleansed with sterile water and a sterile dressing is applied. Blood and amniotic fluid are cleaned from the client's abdomen, buttocks, and back before transferring to a bed. Lateral transfer devices are available to assist with transition off the operating table safely. Smooth transfers reduce pain and hypotension.

NURSING CARE AFTER BIRTH

Intrapartum nursing care extends through the fourth stage of labor and includes care of the infant, the client, and the family unit.

Care of the Infant

Nursing care of the newborn includes recording the time of birth, supporting cardiopulmonary and thermoregulatory function, and identifying the infant. In addition, the nurse assesses the infant for approximate gestational age and examines them for obvious anomalies and birth injuries. A full neonatal assessment may be delayed to allow time for uninterrupted skin-to-skin contact with the parents after birth.

The initial assessment can usually be done with the infant skin-to-skin with the parent.

Maintain Cardiopulmonary Function

Assess the infant's Apgar score (Table 15.4) at 1 and 5 minutes and every 5 minutes thereafter until the Apgar score is greater than 7 (AAP & ACOG, 2017; Fraser, 2021). This scoring system after birth allows for rapid evaluation of early cardiopulmonary adaptation. If the Apgar score is 7 or higher, no intervention is needed other than supporting thermoregulation and promoting normal respiratory efforts by positioning and wiping secretions from the mouth and nose. If the infant is in obvious distress (no or low heart rate and respirations, limp muscle tone, lack of response to stimulation, blue or pale color), interventions to correct the problem are instituted immediately rather than waiting for the 1-minute Apgar score (AAP & AHA, 2021).

A newborn with a vigorous cry and minimal secretions is usually sufficiently warmed by skin-to-skin contact with the client or support person, but a prewarmed warmer should be available. Avoid an extended time with the infant in a head-dependent position because upward pressure from the intestines limits diaphragmatic movement. An infant in a warmer should be placed in the flat position or turned to one side with the head flat or slightly elevated. Temperature probes should be used when the infant remains under the radiant warmer to prevent overheating. Wipe secretions from the infant's face and mouth. Suction the infant's mouth and nose with a bulb syringe, if needed. Suctioning with a catheter may be necessary for more copious secretions.

Support Thermoregulation

Hypothermia raises the infant's metabolic rate and oxygen consumption, worsening any respiratory problems. Place the infant skin to skin with the client or, if necessary, on a prewarmed warmer. Quickly dry with warm towels to reduce evaporative heat loss. The head should be dried well because substantial heat loss can occur from the head, which is about one-fourth of the neonate's body surface area. The stimulus of drying the skin promotes vigorous crying and lung expansion in most healthy infants.

Delaying the first bath for several hours allows the temperature to stabilize. Avoid positioning yourself between the infant and the radiant heat source in the warmer. The infant should be wrapped in dry, warm blankets when not in the warmer or making skin-to-skin contact. Remove wet linens, replacing them with warm, dry ones. A stockinette cap further reduces heat loss if it is placed on the baby's *dry* head. A cap is not worn while the infant is in the radiant warmer because the cap slows transfer of heat to the baby.

Identify the Infant

Bands with matching imprinted numbers and identifying information are the primary means to ensure the right baby goes to the right client after any separation. Verify the imprinted band number and client's name are identical on each set of bands and have the client or support person verify this information at the time of banding. Apply identification band(s) on the infant, preferably on the ankle to prevent facial scratching. Infant bands are applied more snugly than those worn by an adult because of

TABLE 15.4 Apgar Score[a]

	POINTS		
Assessment	**0**	**1**	**2**
Heart rate	Absent	Below 100 beats per minute (bpm)	100 bpm or higher
Respiratory effort	No spontaneous respirations	Slow respirations or weak cry	Spontaneous respirations with strong, lusty cry
Muscle tone	Limp	Minimal flexion of extremities; sluggish movement	Flexed body posture; spontaneous and vigorous movement
Reflex response	No response to suction or gentle slap on soles	Minimal response (grimace) to suction or gentle slap on soles	Responds promptly to suction or gentle slap to sole with cry or active movement
Color	Pallor or cyanosis	Bluish hands and feet only (acrocyanosis)	Pink (light-skinned) or absence of cyanosis (dark-skinned); pink mucous membranes

0	1	2	3	4	5	6	7	8	9	10
Infant needs resuscitation.[b]			Gently stimulate by rubbing infant's back while administering oxygen. Determine whether client received narcotics, which may have depressed infant's respirations.				Provide no action other than support of infant's spontaneous efforts and continued observation.			

[a]The Apgar score is a method for rapid evaluation of the infant's cardiorespiratory adaptation after birth. The nurse scores the infant at 1 minute and 5 minutes in each of five areas. The infant is assigned a score of 0 to 2 in each of the five areas, and the scores are totaled. Resuscitation should not be delayed until the 1-minute score is obtained. However, general guidelines for the infant's care are based on three ranges of 1-minute scores: 0 to 2, 3 to 6, 7 to 10.

[b]Neonatal resuscitation measures, if needed, do not await 1-minute Apgar scoring but are instituted at once.

anticipated infant weight loss, with about one adult finger width of slack in the bands. Trim the excess band ends and apply the longer band to the client's wrist. The client's primary support person usually wears a fourth band. The infant will not be released to any adult who is not wearing a band with a matching name and number. A set of bands is needed for each baby in a multiple birth. Some facilities take an early photo of the infant, when the infant is alert, which serves two purposes: as a keepsake for the parents and identification in the event of abduction. Other facilities use footprints for the same purposes.

Care of the Client

Nursing care of the client during the fourth stage of labor focuses on observing for hemorrhage and promoting comfort and safety (Table 15.5).

Observe for Hemorrhage

Important assessments related to hemorrhage are the client's vital signs, uterine fundal location and tone, bladder, lochia, and perineal and labial areas.

Vital signs. Assess the client's temperature when fourth-stage care begins. Blood pressure, pulse, and respirations should be assessed every 15 minutes during the first 2 hours or as indicated (James, 2021). A rising pulse rate is an early sign of excessive blood loss because the heart pumps faster to compensate for reduced blood volume. The blood pressure falls as the blood volume diminishes, but this is a late sign of hypovolemia. A rising pulse rate also may reflect medications administered.

Fundus. The most common reason for excessive postpartum bleeding is failure of the uterus to firmly contract and compress open vessels at the placental site. Assess the firmness, height, and positioning of the uterine fundus while supporting the lower uterine segment during uterine massage to prevent inversion or prolapse (James & Suplee, 2021). Uterine assessment is typically performed with each vital sign assessment. The fundus should be firm, in the midline, and below the umbilicus (about the size of a large grapefruit). If the fundus is firm, no massage is needed, but if it is soft (boggy), it should be massaged until it is firm. Nipple stimulation from the infant's suckling releases oxytocin from the client's posterior pituitary gland to maintain firm uterine contraction. IV or intramuscular (IM) oxytocin has the same effect.

Bladder. A full bladder interferes with contraction of the uterus and may lead to hemorrhage. A full bladder is suspected if the fundus is above the umbilicus or displaced to one side, usually the right. The first two to three voidings are often measured until it is evident that the client voids without difficulty and empties the bladder completely. If no contraindication, such as altered sensation, is present, the client can walk to the bathroom (with assistance the first few times; see the "Promote Comfort and Safety" section).

Lochia. Assess for lochia with each vital sign and fundal assessment. The amount of lochia seems large to the inexperienced nurse. Perineal pads vary in their absorbency, but saturation of one standard pad (one that does not contain a cold pack) within the first hour is a guideline for excessive lochia flow. Turn the client to check for lochia pooling under the buttocks and back. Small clots may be present, but the presence of large clots is not normal, and the provider should be notified.

Perineal and labial areas. Observe perineal and labial areas for bruising and hematoma formation. Small hematomas

TABLE 15.5 Maternal Problems During the Fourth Stage of Labor

Sign	Potential Problem	Immediate Nursing Action
Rising pulse rate and/or falling blood pressure; possibly accompanied by low or no urine output	An early sign of hypovolemia caused by excessive blood loss (visible or concealed) is increased pulse. Hypotension is a late sign of blood loss.	Identify probable cause of blood loss, usually a poorly contracted uterus. Take steps to correct it. Indwelling catheter may be inserted to observe urine output.
Soft (boggy) uterus	A poorly contracted uterus does not adequately compress large open vessels at placental site, resulting in hemorrhage	With one hand securing uterus just above symphysis and other hand on fundus, massage uterus until firm. Push downward on *firm* uterus to expel any clots. Empty client's bladder (by voiding or catheterization) if that is contributing to uterine atony.
High uterine fundus, often displaced to one side	Suggests a full bladder, which can interfere with uterine contraction and result in hemorrhage	Massage uterus if it is not firm. Help client urinate in bathroom or on bedpan. If the client cannot void, catheterize the client (usually a routine postpartum order).
Lochia exceeding one saturated perineal pad per hour during fourth stage	Suggests hemorrhage; however, perineal pads vary in their absorbency, and this must be considered	Identify cause of hemorrhage, usually uterine atony, which is manifested by a soft uterus. Correct cause. If lacerations are suspected cause (excess bleeding with a firm fundus), notify provider. Keep client on NPO status until birth attendant completes their evaluation.
Intense perineal or vaginal pain, poorly relieved with analgesics	Hematoma, usually of vaginal wall or perineum; signs of hypovolemia may occur with substantial blood loss into tissues	If hematoma is visible, apply cold packs to area to slow bleeding into tissues. Notify provider and anticipate possible surgical drainage. Keep client on NPO status.

NPO, Nothing by mouth.

usually are easily limited by ice packs, which are also applied for comfort. Large and rapidly expanding hematomas may cause significant enlargement of the tissues involved, a bluish color, and pain. Observe the episiotomy using the acronym REEDA (redness, edema, ecchymosis, discharge, approximation of edges of episiotomy) for assessment guidelines (James, 2021).

Promote Comfort and Safety

Uterine contractions (afterpains) and perineal trauma are common causes of pain after birth. A postpartum chill often adds to discomfort. Pain usually is mild and readily relieved by simple measures. Notify the provider if pain is intense or does not respond to common relief measures.

Ice packs. Apply an ice pack to the perineum promptly after vaginal birth to reduce edema and limit hematoma formation. Some perineal pads include chemical cold packs. These pads absorb less lochia than ordinary pads, so this should be considered when estimating pad saturation. Evidence shows ice applied for the first 24 to 48 hours in 10- to 20-minute intervals, rather than continuously, is most beneficial (James, 2021).

Analgesics. Afterpains and perineal pain respond well to mild oral analgesics. Regular urination reduces the severity of afterpains because the uterus contracts most effectively when the bladder is empty. The nurse should encourage the client to take analgesics as needed for both perineal and afterpain discomfort.

Warmth. A warm blanket shortens the chill common after birth. A portable radiant warmer provides warmth to both the client and infant. The client may enjoy warm drinks initially.

Safety. Before any ambulation, such as for urination after birth, test the client's ability to raise and move legs. Have the client push their legs against your hands to determine the leg strength, demonstrate the ability to move legs back and forth, and raise the knees. The client should sit on the side of the bed to make sure no dizziness or lightheadedness is present because of postural (orthostatic) hypotension, which may occur in any postpartum client regardless of the pain management methods during labor. Accompany the client when ambulating and monitor the client's ability to move.

Postoperative Care

Postoperative care for the client who has had a cesarean birth is similar to care after a vaginal birth, with additional assessments and interventions related to the incision and anesthesia. Temperature is assessed on admission to the PACU and according to protocol thereafter. If the client's condition is stable, other assessments are done every 15 minutes during the first 2 hours and progress to every 1 hour until transferred to the postpartum room. In addition to temperature, routine postoperative assessments include the following:

- Vital signs, electrocardiogram pattern, respiratory character, and oxygen saturation
- Return of motion and sensation if a regional block was given

- Level of consciousness, particularly if general anesthesia and sedating drugs were given
- Abdominal dressing
- Uterine firmness and position (height; midline or deviated to one side)
- Lochia (color, quantity, presence and size of any clots)
- Urine output (quantity, color, other characteristics; patency of catheter and tubing)
- IV infusion (fluid, rate, condition of IV site)
- Pain relief needs
- Function of the SCD

The nurse observes for return of motion and sensation if the client had epidural or subarachnoid block anesthesia. The level of consciousness and respiratory status (skin and mucous membrane color, rate and quality of respirations, pulse oximeter readings) are important observations if the client had general anesthesia. Respiratory observations also are important if the client received epidural opioid narcotics, which can cause delayed respiratory depression. Naloxone (Narcan) should be available to reverse opioid-induced respiratory depression.

The pulse rate, respirations, blood pressure, and oxygen saturation level provide important clues to the client's circulatory and respiratory status. If oxygen saturation falls below 92%, it usually can be raised with several deep breaths. A persistent respiratory rate of less than 12 breaths per minute suggests respiratory depression. Deep breathing and coughing move secretions out of the lungs. A small pillow to support the incision reduces pain when the client coughs. Hourly position changes with deep breathing and coughing improve ventilation, reduce pooling of lung secretions, and decrease discomfort from constant pressure.

As with vaginal birth, the fundus is assessed for height, firmness, and position. This examination is painful after regional anesthesia wears off, but the postcesarean client also can have uterine atony. To relax the abdominal muscles and thus reduce pain from fundus checks, have the client flex their knees and take slow, deep breaths. The nurse can gently "walk" the fingers toward the fundus to determine uterine firmness. The client who has a Pfannenstiel skin incision usually has less pain with fundus checks than the client with a vertical skin incision. A firm fundus does not need massage. The dressing is checked for drainage with each fundus check.

The nurse assesses the lochia and urine output with other assessments. Lochia may pool under the client's buttocks and lower back. Urine may be bloody temporarily if the cesarean delivery was done after a long labor or an attempted forceps delivery. The urine drain tubing should be observed for gradual clearing of the blood. Urine should drain freely to prevent bladder distention, which worsens pain and increases the risk for postpartum hemorrhage. The nurse should remember that falling urine output is an early sign of hypovolemia.

The client's needs for pain relief should be regularly assessed. The client who received an epidural opioid may not need other analgesia during the early postpartum period. If additional pain relief is needed while the epidural opioid is still in effect, the dose ordered often is lower than if the client had not had that form of analgesia. Oral analgesics usually replace parenteral ones the day after surgery. A nonsteroidal anti-inflammatory drug, such as ibuprofen, provides long-acting analgesia to supplement the epidural opioid. If the client did not receive an epidural opioid, analgesia usually is given by client-controlled analgesia pump.

🔘 KNOWLEDGE CHECK

28. Why is the low transverse uterine incision preferred for cesarean birth?
29. What should a client who expects a cesarean birth be taught about the OR? The recovery room or the PACU?
30. How should the nurse modify recovery room care of the client who had a cesarean birth from the care of the client who had a vaginal delivery?
31. What does the acronym REEDA mean?

Promote Early Family Attachment

The first hour after birth is ideal for parent-infant attachment because the healthy neonate is alert and responsive. Provide privacy while unobtrusively observing the client, support person, and infant. The infant can remain in the client or support person's arms or skin-to-skin while the nurse takes vital signs, administers intramuscular (IM) medications as ordered, and suctions small amounts of secretions. Many newborn admission assessments can be performed while the parent holds the baby.

If breastfeeding is the preferred feeding method, assist the client with this process during the recovery period. The infant is usually attentive and nurses briefly. Early nipple stimulation helps initiate milk production and contract the uterus.

When the parents are ready, siblings, other family members, and friends should be allowed to visit. Help siblings see and touch their new brother or sister by putting a stool at the bedside or letting them sit on the bed.

Observe for signs of early parent-infant attachment. Parent behaviors are tentative at first, progressing from fingertip touch to palm touch to enfolding of the infant. Parents usually make eye contact with the infant and talk to the baby in higher-pitched, affectionate tones.

Cultural variations should be considered when assessing early attachment. The nurse should be knowledgeable about the typical practices of the populations commonly served. In some cultures, great attention to the newborn is considered unlucky ("evil eye").

SUMMARY CONCEPTS

- Some clients do not have symptoms typical of true labor. They should enter the birth center for evaluation if they are uncertain and have concerns other than those listed in the guidelines.
- The childbearing family's first impression on admission to the intrapartum unit is important to promote a therapeutic relationship with caregivers and a positive birth experience.
- Initial intrapartum assessments quickly evaluate the client's and fetal health and labor status.
- The fetus is the more vulnerable of the maternal-fetal pair because of complete dependence on the client's physiologic systems.
- A supine position can reduce placental blood flow because the uterus compresses the aorta and inferior vena cava (aortocaval compression).
- Regular changes in position during labor promote comfort and help the fetus adapt to the pelvis, promoting the progress of labor.
- The nurse must be alert for signs of impending birth: The client may state, "The baby's coming," make grunting sounds, and bear down.
- Prolapse and compression of the umbilical cord are the primary risks of amniotomy. As the fluid gushes out, the cord can become compressed between the fetal presenting part and the client's pelvis.
- Infection is more likely to occur when membranes have been ruptured for a long time (e.g., 24 hours or longer).
- Induction of labor may be done if continuing the pregnancy is more hazardous to the client and fetal health than the induction. It is not done if a client or fetal contraindication to labor and vaginal birth exists.

- Oxytocin-stimulated uterine contractions may be excessive, decreasing placental perfusion.
- External cephalic version is done to promote vaginal birth by changing the fetal presentation from a breech or transverse lie to a cephalic presentation. Internal version may be used to change presentation of a second twin after the birth of the first twin.
- Trauma to the client and neonatal tissue is the primary risk associated with use of forceps and vacuum extraction. Possible trauma to the client includes vaginal wall laceration and hematoma. Trauma to the infant may include ecchymoses, lacerations, abrasions, facial nerve injury, and intracranial hemorrhage.
- The midline episiotomy is less painful but more likely to extend into the rectum than the mediolateral episiotomy.
- The preferred uterine incision for cesarean birth is the low transverse incision because it is least likely to rupture in a subsequent pregnancy. The skin incision does not always match the uterine incision and is unrelated to the risk for later uterine rupture.
- Some clients have feelings of guilt and inadequacy if they have a cesarean birth or if they choose not to try trial of labor after cesarean (TOLAC) when given the choice. Therapeutic communication and sensitive, family-centered care are essential to help them achieve a positive perception of their birth experience.
- Enhanced recovery guidelines have been shown to decrease length of stay, surgical complications, pain, need for analgesia postoperatively, and costs and readmissions.

- The priority nursing care of the newborn immediately after birth is to promote normal respirations, maintain normal body temperature, and promote attachment.

- The priority nursing care of the client after birth is to assess for hemorrhage and promote firm uterine contraction, comfort, and parent-infant attachment.

Clinical Judgment and Next-Generation NCLEX® Examination-Style Questions

A 27-year-old G1 P0 at 39+0 weeks' gestation presents to the birth center at 0130 complaining of contractions occurring 2 to 10 minutes apart over the last several hours accompanied by a small amount of thick pink vaginal discharge mixed with mucus.

1. **Which of the following are the priorities for the nurse to assess at this time? Select all that apply.**
   A. Status of amniotic membranes (intact or ruptured)
   B. Preparation for labor and birth
   C. Last oral intake
   D. Medical and obstetric histories
   E. Client perception of recent fetal movement
   F. Spiritual beliefs
   G. Client vital signs
   H. Fetal heart rate
   I. Presence of advance directives

The client was examined and found to be 1 cm dilated, 20% effaced, and −3 station with intact membranes. The pain scale is rated as 3/10 and is acceptable to the client. The fetal heart rate baseline is 130 beats per minute (bpm) with moderate variability and accelerations present. Vital signs: temperature = 98.0°F (36.6°C), pulse = 86 beats per minute, respirations = 18 breaths per minute, and blood pressure = 126/68. The client is observed for 2 hours. The cervical exam remains unchanged, and the client reports the contractions have become farther apart. At 0400, orders are received from the provider to discharge the client with labor warnings.

2. **What discharge teaching is appropriate to instruct the client regarding when to return to labor and delivery (L&D)? Select all that apply.**
   A. Loss of mucous plug
   B. Contractions continuing current pattern after 24 hours
   C. Trickle or gush of fluid from the vagina
   D. Presence of bloody show (spotting)
   E. Bright red vaginal bleeding (requires a pad)
   F. Decreased fetal movement

At 1600, the client returns to the birth center reporting a gush of vaginal fluid 3 hours before. The fluid is clear with no odor. The fetal heart rate tracing is a Category 1. The contractions remain irregular, and the cervix remains unchanged at 1 cm. The provider orders oxytocin to induce labor.

3. **Choose the best options for the information missing from the statement below by selecting from the lists of options provided.**
   The client is at highest risk for ___1___ because of ___2___, ___3___, and ___4___.

Options for 1	Options for 2	Options for 3 and 4
Precipitous delivery	Postdates	Primipara
Infection	Ruptured membranes	Gestational age
Shoulder dystocia	Fetal distress	Not in active labor
Cesarean birth	Oxytocin administration	Amniotic fluid characteristics

At 2200, the client is 4 cm dilated and 100% effaced, and the fetal head is at 0 station. You note that the fetal heart rate baseline is 165 bpm with moderate variability and late decelerations. Contractions are firm to palpation, occurring every 2 minutes, lasting 100 to 120 seconds. With palpation, you note that the client's uterus does not fully relax before another contraction begins.

4. **Use an "X" to identify nursing actions that are indicated (necessary), contraindicated (could be harmful), or nonessential (not necessary) for the client's care at this time. Only one selection can be made for each nursing action.**

Nursing Action	Indicated	Contra-indicated	Nonessential
Position client supine for better electronic fetal monitoring (EFM) tracing quality.			
Position client in a lateral position.			
Stop the oxytocin infusion.			
Decrease oxytocin to half of the current rate.			
Notify the provider.			
Consider oxygen administration.			
Prepare for emergency cesarean birth.			
Adjust the EFM to improve the tracing quality.			

REFERENCES

Academy of American Family Physician (AAFP). (2019). *Planning for labor and vaginal birth after cesarean delivery: Guidelines from the AAFP.* https://www.aafp.org/afp/2015/0201/p197.html.

American Academy of Pediatrics & American College of Obstetricians and Gynecologists (AAP & ACOG). (2017). *Guidelines for perinatal care* (8th ed.).

American Academy of Pediatrics & American Heart Association (AAP & AHA). (2021). *Neonatal resuscitation textbook* (8th ed.).

American College of Obstetricians and Gynecologists (ACOG). (2017). *Delayed umbilical cord clamping after birth.* ACOG Committee Opinion 814.

American College of Obstetricians and Gynecologists (ACOG). (2018a). *Perioperative pathways: Enhanced recovery after surgery.* ACOG Committee Opinion 750.

American College of Obstetricians and Gynecologists (ACOG). (2018b). *Prevention and management of obstetric lacerations at vaginal delivery.* ACOG Practice Bulletin 198.

American College of Obstetricians and Gynecologists (ACOG). (2019). *Vaginal birth after previous cesarean delivery.* ACOG Practice Bulletin 205.

American College of Obstetricians and Gynecologists (ACOG). (2020a). *External cephalic version.* ACOG Practice Bulletin 221.

American College of Obstetricians and Gynecologists (ACOG). (2020b). *Gestational hypertension and preeclampsia.* ACOG Practice Bulletin 222.

American College of Obstetricians and Gynecologists (ACOG). (2020c). *Induction of labor.* ACOG Practice Bulletin 107. Published 2009, reaffirmed 2020.

American College of Obstetricians and Gynecologists (ACOG). (2020d). *Operative vaginal birth.* ACOG Practice Bulletin 219.

American College of Obstetricians and Gynecologists (ACOG). (2020e). *Ultrasound in pregnancy.* ACOG Practice Bulletin 175. Published 2016, reaffirmed 2020.

American College of Obstetricians and Gynecologists (ACOG). (2021a). *Management of intrapartum fetal heart rate tracing.* ACOG Practice Bulletin 116. Published 2010, reaffirmed 2021.

American College of Obstetricians and Gynecologists (ACOG). (2021b). *Multifetal gestations: Twin, triplet, and high-order multifetal pregnancies.* ACOG Practice Bulletin 231. Published 2016, reaffirmed 2021.

Association of Women's Health, Obstetric and Neonatal Nurses (AWHONN). (2018). Continuous labor support for every woman: AWHONN position statement. *Journal of Obstetric Gynecologic and Neonatal Nursing, 47*(1), 73–74. https://doi.org/10.1016/j.jogn.2017.11.010.

Association of Women's Health, Obstetric and Neonatal Nurses (AWHONN). (2019). *Nursing care and management of the second stage of labor: Evidence-based clinical practice guidelines* (3rd ed.).

Association of Women's Health, Obstetric and Neonatal Nurses (AWHONN). (2020). Lower extremity nerve injury in childbirth: AWHONN practice brief number 11. *Journal of Obstetric Gynecologic and Neonatal Nursing, 49*(6), 622–624. https://doi.org/10.1016/j.jogn.2020.08.004.

Association of Women's Health, Obstetric and Neonatal Nurses (AWHONN). (2021). 40 reasons to go the full 40. www.health4mom.org/go-the-full-40.

Bakker, P. C., Kurver, P. H., Kuik, D. J., & Van Geijin, H. P. (2007). Elevated uterine activity increases the risk of fetal acidosis at birth. *American Journal of Obstetrics and Gynecology, 196*(4), 313.e1–313.e6. https://doi.org/10.1515/jpm.2007.116.

Berta, M., Lindgren, H., Christensson, K., Mekonnen, S., & Adefris, M. (2019). Effect of maternal birth positions on duration of second stage of labor: Systematic review and meta-analysis. *BMC Pregnancy and Childbirth, 19,* 466. https://doi.org/10.1186/s12884-019-2620-0.

Bishop, E. H. (1964). Pelvic scoring for elective induction. *Obstetrics & Gynecology, 24*(2), 266–268.

Bohren, M. A., Hofmeyr, G. J., Sakala, C., Fukuzawa, R. K., & Cuthbert, A. (2017). Continuous support for women during childbirth. *Cochrane Database of Systematic Reviews, 2017* (7), CD003766. https://doi.org/10.1002/14651858.CD003766.pub6.

California Maternal Quality Care Collaborative. (2017). *Toolkit to support vaginal birth and reduce primary cesareans.* https://www.cmqcc.org/VBirthToolkitResource.

Callister, L. C. (2021). Integrating cultural beliefs and practices when caring for childbearing women and families. In K. Simpson, P. Creehan, N. O'Brien-Abel, C. Roth, & A. Rohan (Eds.), *AWHONN's perinatal nursing* (5th ed., pp. 18–47). Wolters Kluwer.

Caughey, A. B., Wood, S. L., Macones, G. A., Wrench, I. J., Huang, J., Norman, M., Pettersson, K., Fawcett, W. J., Shalabi, M. M., Metcalfe, A., Gramlich, L., Nelson, G., & Wilson, R. D. (2018). Guidelines for antenatal and preoperative care in cesarean delivery: Enhanced recovery after surgery society recommendations (part 2). *American Journal of Obstetrics and Gynecology, 219*(6), 533–544. https://doi.org/10.1016/j.ajog.2018.08.006.

Cunningham, F. G., Leveno, K. J., Bloom, S. L., Dashe, J. S., Hoffman, B. L., Casey, B. M., & Spong, C. Y. (2022). *Williams obstetrics* (26th ed.). McGraw-Hill Companies.

Dalton, J., & Strehlow, S. (2019). Maternal obesity. In N. Troiano, C. Harvey, & B. Chez (Eds.), *AWHONN high-risk & critical care obstetrics* (4th ed., pp. 232–243). Wolters Kluwer.

Dinoprostone: Drug information. (2021). *Up to date.* https://www.uptodate.com/contents/dinoprostone-drug-information?search=dinoprostone&source=panel_search_result&selectedTitle=1~96&usage_type=panel&kp_tab=drug_general&display_rank=1.

Fairchild, E., Roberts, L., Zelman, K., Michelli, S., & Hastings-Tolsma, M. (2017). Implementation of Robert's coping with labor algorithm in a large tertiary care facility. *Midwifery, 50,* 208–218. https://doi.org/10.1016/j.midw.2017.03.008.

Fenwick, L., & Simkin, P. (1987). Maternal positioning to prevent or alleviate dystocia in labor. *Clinical Obstetrics and Gynecology, 30*(1), 83–89.

Fraser, D. (2021). Newborn adaptation to extrauterine life. In K. Simpson, P. Creehan, N. O'Brien-Abel, C. Roth, & A. Rohan (Eds.), *AWHONN's perinatal nursing* (5th ed., pp. 564–578). Wolters Kluwer.

Gupta, J. K., Sood, A., Hofmeyr, G. J., & Vogel, J. P. (2017). Position in the second stage of labour for women without epidural anaesthesia. *Cochrane Database of Systematic Reviews, 2017,* CD002006. pub4. https://doi.org/10.1002/14651858.CD002006.pub4.

Hickey, L., & Savage, J. (2019). Effect of peanut ball and position changes in women laboring with an epidural. *Nursing for Women's Health, 23*(3), 245–252. https://doi.org/10.1016/j.nwh.2019.04.004.

Institute for Safe Medication Practices. (2018). *ISMP list of high alert medications in the acute care setting.* https://www.ismp.org/sites/default/files/attachments/2018-08/highAlert2018-Acute-Final.pdf.

James, D. C., & Suplee, P. D. (2021). Postpartum care. In K. Simpson, P. Creehan, N. O'Brien-Abel, C. Roth, & A. Rohan (Eds.), *AWHONN's perinatal nursing* (5th ed., pp. 509–563). Wolters Kluwer.

Killion, M. M. (2019). Enhanced recovery after cesarean birth. *MCN: The American Journal of Maternal Child Nursing, 44*(6), 296. https://doi.org/10.1097/NMC.0000000000000572.

Kilpatrick, S. J., Garrison, E., & Fairbrother, E. (2021). Normal labor and delivery. In M. Landon, H. Galan, E. Jauniaux, D. Driscoll, V. Berghella, W. Grobman, et al. (Eds.), *Gabbe's obstetrics: Normal and problem pregnancies* (8th ed., pp. 204–225). Elsevier.

Levine, L. D. ,L., & Srinivas, S. K. (2021). Induction of labor. In M. Landon, H. Galan, E. Jauniaux, D. Driscoll, V. Berghella, W. Grobman, et al. (Eds.), *Gabbe's obstetrics: Normal and problem pregnancies* (8th ed., pp. 226–239). Elsevier.

Macones, G. A., Caughey, A. B., Wood, S. L., Wrench, I. J., Huang, J., Norman, M., Pettersson, K., Fawcett, W. J., Shalabi, M. M., Metcalfe, A., Gramlich, L., Nelson, G., & Wilson, R. D. (2019). Guidelines for antenatal and preoperative care in cesarean delivery: Enhanced recovery after surgery society recommendations (part 3). *American Journal of Obstetrics and Gynecology, 221*(3), 247. e1–247.e9. https://doi.org/10.1016/j.ajog.2019.04.012.

Macones, G. A., Hankins, G. D., Spong, C. Y., Hauth, J., & Moore, T. (2008). The 2008 National Institute of Child Health and Human Development workshop report on electronic fetal monitoring: Update on definitions, interpretation, and research guidelines. *Journal of Obstetric Gynecologic and Neonatal Nursing, 37*(5), 510–515. https://doi.org/10.1111/j.1552-6909.2008.00284.x.

Martin, J. A., Hamilton, B. E., Osterman, M. J. K., & Driscoll, A. K. (2021). Births: Final data for 2019. *National Vital Statistics Reports, 68*(13). www.cdc.gov/nchs/products/index.htm.

Mercer, B. M., & Chien, E. K. S. (2019). Premature rupture of the membranes. In R. Resnik, C. Lockwood, T. Moore, M. Greene, J. Copel, & R. Silver (Eds.), *Creasy & Resnik's maternal-fetal medicine: Principles and practice* (8th ed., pp. 663–672). Elsevier.

Miller, L. A., Miller, D. A., & Cypher, R. L. (2022). In *Mosby's pocket guide to fetal monitoring: A multidisciplinary approach* (9th ed.). Elsevier.

Misoprostol: Drug information. (2021). *UpToDate.* https://www.uptodate.com/contents/misoprostol-drug-information?search=misoprostol &source=panel_search_result&selectedTitle=1~122&usage_type=panel&kp_tab=drug_general&display_rank=1.

O'Brien-Abel, N., & Simpson, K. R. (2021). Fetal assessment during labor. In K. Simpson, P. Creehan, N. O'Brien-Abel, C. Roth, & A. Rohan (Eds.), *AWHONN's perinatal nursing* (5th ed., pp. 413–465). Wolters Kluwer.

Oxytocin: Drug information. (2021). *UpToDate.* https://www.uptodate.com/contents/oxytocin-drug-information?search=oxytocin &source=panel_search_result&selectedTitle=1~132&usage_type=panel&kp_tab=drug_general&display_rank=1.

Roberts, L., Gulliver, B., Fisher, J., & Cloyes, K. G. (2010). The coping with labor algorithm: An alternative pain assessment tool for the laboring woman. *Journal of Midwifery & Women's Health, 55*(2), 107–116. https://doi.org/10.1016/j.jmwh.2009.11.002.

Rohan, A. J. (2021). Common neonatal complications. In K. Simpson, P. Creehan, N. O'Brien-Abel, C. Roth, & A. Rohan (Eds.), *AWHONN's perinatal nursing* (5th ed., pp. 651–688). Wolters Kluwer.

Roth, C., Dent, S. A., Parfitt, S. E., Hering, S. L., & Bay, R. C. (2016). Randomized control trial of use of the peanut ball during labor. *MCN: The American Journal of Maternal Child Nursing, 41*(3), 140–146. https://doi.org/10.1097/nmc.0000000000000232.

Simpson, K. R. (2020). In *Cervical ripening and induction and augmentation of labor* (5th ed.). Association of Women's Health, Obstetric and Neonatal Nurses.

Simpson, K. R., & O'Brien-Abel, N. (2021). Labor and birth. In K. Simpson, P. Creehan, N. O'Brien-Abel, C. Roth, & A. Rohan (Eds.), *AWHONN's perinatal nursing* (5th ed., pp. 326–412). Wolters Kluwer.

Spinning Babies. (2021a). *Flying cowgirl.* https://www.spinningbabies.com/pregnancy-birth/techniques/other-techniques/flying-cowgirl/.

Spinning Babies. (2021b). *Side-lying-release.* https://www.spinning-babies.com/pregnancy-birth/techniques/side-lying-release/.

Spong, C. Y., Berghella, V., Wenstrom, K. D., Mercer, B. M., & Saade, G. R. (2012). Preventing the first cesarean delivery: Summary of a joint Eunice Kennedy Shriver National Institute of Child Health and Human Development, Society for Maternal-Fetal Medicine, and American College of Obstetricians and Gynecologists Workshop. *Obstetrics & Gynecology, 120*(5), 1181–1193. https://doi.org/10.1097/aog.0b013e3182704880.

The Joint Commission. (2019). *Language access: Improve health outcomes for limited English proficient patients.* Retrieved from https://www.jointcommission.org/resources/news-and-multimedia/blogs/ambulatory-buzz/2019/01/language-access-improve-health-outcomes-for-limited-english-proficient-patients/.

Thorp, J. M., & Grantz, K. L. (2019). Clinical aspects of normal and abnormal labor. In R. Resnik, C. Lockwood, T. Moore, M. Greene, J. Copel, & R. Silver (Eds.), *Creasy & Resnik's maternal-fetal medicine: Principles and practice* (8th ed., pp. 723–757). Elsevier.

Tussey, C. M., Botsios, E., Gerkin, R. D., Kelly, L. A., Gamez, J., & Mensik, J. (2015). Reducing length of labor and cesarean surgery rate using a peanut ball for women laboring with an epidural. *The Journal of Perinatal Education, 1*(24), 16–24. https://doi.org/10.1891/1058-1243.24.1.16.

U.S. Department of Health and Human Services. (2020). *Healthy People 2030. Reduce cesarean births among low-risk women with no prior births – MICH-06.* www.health.gov/healthypeople/objectives-and-data/browse-objectives/pregnancy-and-childbirth/reduce-cesarean-births-among-low-risk-women-no-prior-births-mich-06.

U.S. Food and Drug Administration (FDA). (2015). *Misoprostol (marketed as Cytotec) information (2015).* www.fda.gov/Drugs/DrugSafety/PostmarketDrugSafetyInformationforPatientsandProviders/ucm111315.htm.

Wilson, R. D., Caughey, A. B., Wood, S. L., Metcalfe, A., Gramlich, L., & Nelson, G. (2018). Guidelines for antenatal and preoperative care in cesarean delivery: Enhanced recovery after surgery society recommendations (part 1). *American Journal of Obstetrics and Gynecology, 219*(6), 523.e1–523.e15. https://doi.org/10.1016/j.ajog.2018.09.015.

Wisner, K., & Ivory, C. (2021). Documentation of fetal heart monitoring information. In A. Lyndon, & K. Wisner (Eds.), *Fetal heart monitoring principles and practices* (6th ed., pp. 245–276). Kendall Hunt.

Wisner, K., & Larry-Osman, C. (2021). Maternal-fetal assessment. In A. Lyndon, & K. Wisner (Eds.), *Fetal heart monitoring principles and practices* (6th ed., pp. 51–82). Kendall Hunt.

Witcher, P. M., & Hamner, L. (2019). Venous thromboembolism in pregnancy. In N. Troiano, C. Harvey, & B. Chez (Eds.), *AWHONN High-risk & critical care obstetrics* (4th ed., pp. 176–193). Wolters Kluwer.

Intrapartum Complications

Cheryl K. Roth

For most clients, birth is a normal process that is free of major complications. However, complications sometimes make childbearing hazardous for the client or the baby. The nurse's challenge is to identify complications promptly and provide effective care for the client while nurturing the entire family at this significant time of life.

The complications addressed in this chapter are often interrelated. For example, dysfunctional labor is likely to be prolonged, and the client is more vulnerable to infection, psychological distress, and fetal compromise. Also, clients who have complications are more likely to need interventions such as lengthy hospitalization before vaginal or cesarean birth. The nurse provides care that relates to all problems experienced by the client.

DYSFUNCTIONAL LABOR

Normal labor is characterized by progression of cervical effacement, dilation, and fetal descent. Dysfunctional labor is one that does not result in normal progress. A dysfunctional labor may result from problems with the powers of labor, the passenger, the passage, the psyche, or a combination of these. This type of labor can be associated with shortened or prolonged time frames.

An operative birth (assisted with a vacuum extractor or forceps, or cesarean birth) may be needed if dysfunctional labor does not resolve or compromise occurs with the fetus or client. Signs of possible compromise include persistent abnormal fetal heart rate (FHR) patterns (see Chapter 14), fetal acidosis, and meconium passage. Maternal infection or exhaustion can also occur with a long labor. Nursing measures enhance labor progress and maternal comfort and promote fetal well-being.

Problems of the Powers

The powers of labor may not be adequate to expel the fetus because of ineffective contractions or maternal pushing efforts.

Ineffective Contractions

Effective uterine activity is characterized by coordinated contractions that are strong and numerous enough to propel the fetus past the resistance of the client's bony pelvis and soft tissues. It is not possible to say how frequent, long, or strong labor contractions must be to achieve a vaginal delivery. One client's labor may progress with contractions that would be inadequate for another client. Possible causes of ineffective contractions include the following:

- Maternal fatigue
- Maternal inactivity
- Fluid and electrolyte imbalance
- Hypoglycemia
- Excessive analgesia or anesthesia
- Maternal catecholamines secreted in response to stress or pain
- Disproportion between the maternal pelvis and fetal presenting part
- Uterine overdistention such as with multiple gestation or **polyhydramnios** (or hydramnios—excess volume of amniotic fluid)
- Poor application of the presenting part to the cervix

Two patterns of ineffective uterine contractions are labor dystocia and tachysystole. The characteristics and management of each are different, but both result in poor labor progress if they persist.

Labor Dystocia. **Labor dystocia** means difficult labor and may be used to describe any form of dysfunctional labor. However, it is most often used to describe labor that does not progress as expected. When labor dystocia, or "failure to progress," occurs, contractions may be coordinated but too weak to be effective. They may be infrequent and brief and, when palpated, can be indented easily with fingertip pressure at the peak.

Labor dystocia, or secondary arrest, occurs during the active phase of labor when progress normally quickens. The active phase usually begins by 6 cm of cervical dilation.

The client may be fairly comfortable due to weaker contractions. However, they often are frustrated because labor slows at a time when they expect to be making faster progress. Labor dystocia is tiring as a result of the duration of labor.

Management depends on the cause. Many clients respond to simple measures. Administration of adequate intravenous (IV) or oral fluids corrects maternal fluid and electrolyte imbalances or hypoglycemia. Position changes, particularly different upright positions, favor fetal descent and promote effective contractions. The client who actively changes positions typically has better labor progress and is more comfortable than the client who remains in one position. Standing or sitting in a shower provides the comfort of warm water and an upright position. Pain management techniques may have outcomes that reduce the effectiveness of contractions, requiring interventions specific to that factor. Effective pain management may, however, improve the progress of labor.

The nurse uses therapeutic communication to help the client identify anxieties or beliefs about labor and its progress. Identifying anxieties is important because the stress response could slow labor.

The maternal pelvis, fetal presentation, and position should be evaluated by the provider to identify abnormalities. Measures such as amniotomy and oxytocin infusion may be needed to promote labor progress. Reducing undesired maternal effects of a prolonged latent phase such as exhaustion or infection is a goal of the provider. However, the provider considers the possibility a client is in false labor rather than in a prolonged latent phase when choosing interventions to correct the labor progress.

Amniotomy or augmentation, usually with oxytocin, may be used to stimulate an established, yet ineffective labor pattern. The risks of amniotomy include umbilical cord prolapse, infection, and placental abruption (premature separation of placenta). Reduced placental perfusion caused by excessive uterine contractions is the most common risk for labor augmentation using oxytocin (Hobson et al., 2019; Simpson, 2020).

Tachysystole. Tachysystole can be either spontaneous or induced and is defined as excessive uterine activity. Tachysystole is more than five contractions in 10 minutes, averaged over 30 minutes (Macones et al., 2008a, 2008b). In addition to tachysystole, contractions lasting 2 minutes or longer, contractions with less than 1 minute resting time between, or failure of the uterus to return to resting tone between contractions via palpation or intrauterine pressure above 25 mm Hg measured by an intrauterine pressure catheter may also be of concern. Contractions may be uncoordinated and erratic in their frequency, duration, and intensity (Simpson, 2020).

Although each contraction varies in its intensity, the **uterine resting tone** (uterine muscle tone when not having contraction) between contractions may be higher than normal, reducing uterine blood flow. The reduction of blood flow to the uterus decreases fetal oxygen supply and causes the client to have almost constant cramping pain. With a high uterine resting tone and complaints of continuous pain, the nurse is alert to a possibility of placental abruption as the symptoms can be the same.

The client becomes very tired because of nearly constant discomfort, creating doubt in their ability to give birth and cope with labor. Frustration and anxiety further reduce the client's pain tolerance and interfere with the normal processes of labor. Cervical dilation should not be equated with the amount of pain a client "should" experience.

First, management of uterine tachysystole depends on the cause. If oxytocin is being administered, the dose is decreased or stopped. Oxytocin can intensify the already high uterine resting tone. Second, pain relief is an important intervention to promote a normal labor pattern. In the latent phase of labor, warm showers and baths promote relaxation and rest, often allowing a normal labor pattern to ensue. Systemic analgesics or, occasionally, low-dose epidural analgesia may be required to achieve this purpose.

Tocolytic medications (inhibit uterine contractions) may be ordered to reduce uterine resting tone and improve placental blood flow. The decision to order uterine stimulant or relaxant drugs is very individualized, based on each client's labor pattern.

Ineffective Pushing

A reflexive urge to push with contractions usually occurs as the fetal presenting part reaches the pelvic floor during second-stage labor. However, ineffective pushing may result from the following:

- Use of nonphysiologic pushing techniques and positions
- Fear of injury because of pain and tearing sensations felt by the client when pushing
- Decreased or absent urge to push
- Maternal exhaustion
- Analgesia or anesthesia that suppresses the client's urge to push
- Psychological unreadiness to "let go" of the baby

Management focuses on correcting causes contributing to ineffective pushing. There is no limit for the duration of the second stage of labor if the client and fetus are stable with normal vital signs and FHR patterns. Each client is evaluated individually by the provider to determine whether labor may be appropriately ended with an operative delivery or can continue safely.

Nursing care to promote effective pushing helps the client make each effort more productive. Most clients, including those with epidural analgesia, can detect the urge to push.

Upright positions, such as squatting, add gravity to the client's pushing efforts. Semisitting, side-lying, and pushing while sitting on the toilet are other options. If the client prefers side-lying, the upper leg is moved toward the chest with each push. Leaning forward while in the sitting or squatting position maintains the best alignment of the fetal head with the pelvis.

The client who fears injury because of the sensations felt when pushing may respond to accurate information about the process of fetal descent. If they understand the sensations of tearing often accompany fetal descent and the tissues can expand to accommodate the baby, they may be more willing to push with contractions.

Epidural analgesia for labor uses a mixture of a local anesthetic agent and an epidural opioid analgesic to provide pain control without the major loss of sensation that is likely if local anesthetic is used alone. However, if a client cannot feel the urge to push after the fetus has descended, the nurse can direct them how to push with each contraction.

The client who is exhausted may push more effectively when encouraged to rest and push only when the urge is felt or pushing with every other contraction. Oral and IV fluids can provide energy for the strenuous work of second-stage labor. Reassuring the client about fetal well-being and working with the body's efforts seems most effective. This reassurance also helps the client who may be emotionally readying to "let go" of the fetus in exchange for a newborn as labor progresses.

Problems with the Passenger

Fetal problems associated with dysfunctional labor are related to the following:

- Fetal size
- Fetal presentation or position
- Multifetal pregnancy
- Fetal anomalies

These variations may cause mechanical problems and contribute to ineffective labor.

Fetal Size

Macrosomia. The **macrosomic** infant weighs more than 8 lb 8 oz (4000 g) at birth, although some authorities define it as a weight of 9 lb 9 oz (4500 g) or greater (American College of Obstetricians and Gynecologists [ACOG], 2020b). The head or shoulders may not be able to adapt to the pelvis if they are too large (**cephalopelvic disproportion**). In addition, distention of the uterus by the large fetus reduces the strength of contractions both during and after birth.

Size, however, is relative. The client with a small or abnormally shaped pelvis may not be able to deliver an average-size or small infant. The client with a large pelvis may easily give birth to an infant heavier than 8 lb 8 oz (4000 g). Fetal position as the baby descends through the pelvis is another important factor in terms of fetal size and maternal pelvic size.

Use of different maternal positions open the pelvis, promoting vaginal delivery. Positions promoting the C-curve of the spine, in which the client leans the shoulders forward and causes the spine to curve forward, directing the fetus toward the back of the pelvis rather than the front, narrower part of the pelvis. Use of labor balls, large inflated physiotherapy balls, to sit on can cause the pelvic diameter to increase and the perineal muscles to relax. Use of side-lying positions with the peanut ball (a peanut-shaped labor ball) between the knees can allow the sacrum and coccyx to fall farther back, increasing the pelvic diameter.

Shoulder Dystocia. Delayed or difficult birth of the shoulders may occur as they become impacted against the maternal symphysis pubis. Shoulder dystocia is more likely to occur when the fetus is large but many cases occur in pregnancies with no identifiable risk factors. Labor may be long, but shoulder dystocia also may occur after a normal labor (ACOG, 2020g).

Shoulder dystocia is an emergency that can result in maternal and fetal injury and is both unpredictable and unpreventable (ACOG, 2020g). One of the initial signs of shoulder dystocia is known as the "turtle sign." After the head is born, it retracts against the perineum, much like a turtle's head drawing into its shell. When the turtle sign is identified, the delivery team calls for additional help and prepares for delivery. Although the infant's head is out of the vaginal canal, the chest is inside, preventing respirations. Any of several methods may be used to quickly release the impacted fetal shoulders (Fig. 16.1). McRobert's maneuver is a nursing action that is taken immediately, pulling the client's knees up as far toward the shoulders as possible. Fundal pressure should be avoided so the fetal shoulders are not pushed even harder against the symphysis. Suprapubic pressure may assist in moving the impacted shoulder past the symphysis. The provider may take additional measures to affect delivery. After delivery of the infant, the clavicles are checked for crepitus, deformity, and bruising, each of which suggests fracture (see Chapter 21). Documentation of all care is essential, including a clear description of the maneuvers used to assist with delivery. One person is usually designated the "timekeeper" for accuracy of records (Barth, 2021; Simpson, 2020).

Abnormal Fetal Presentation or Position

An unfavorable fetal presentation or position may interfere with cervical dilation or fetal descent.

Rotation Abnormalities. Persistence of the fetus in the occiput posterior (OP) or occiput transverse (OT) position can contribute to dysfunctional labor. These positions prevent the mechanisms of labor (cardinal movements) from occurring normally. Most fetuses beginning in the OP position rotate spontaneously to the occiput anterior (OA) position, promoting normal extension and expulsion of the head. The fetus may not rotate or may partly rotate and remain in the OT position. Although clients may experience difficulty in delivering a fetus in the OP position, the client with a pelvis larger than the fetal size or the client who is positioned correctly to open the pelvic inlet and outlet at different stages of labor may be able to deliver the OP fetus without difficulty.

Labor usually is longer and more uncomfortable when the fetus remains in the OP or OT position. Intense back or leg pain, which may be poorly relieved with analgesia, makes coping with labor difficult for the client. "Back labor" aptly describes the sensations a client may feel when the fetus is in the OP position. Some clients who have a fetus in the OP position during labor continue to feel more pain in the back or coccyx during the postpartum period. Maternal position changes promote fetal head rotation to the OA position and descent (see other examples in Chapter 15).

Upright maternal positions promote descent, which usually is accompanied by fetal head rotation. The hands-and-knees and side-lying positions promote rotation

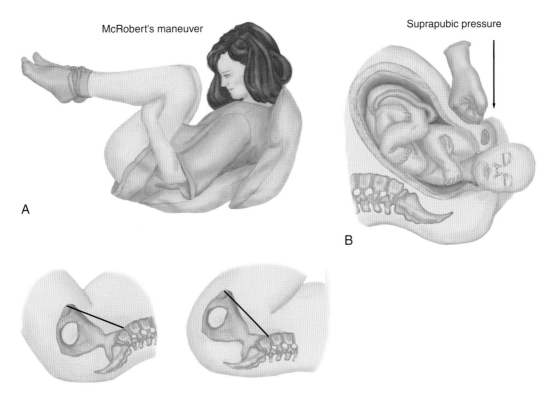

FIG. 16.1 Methods that may be used to relieve shoulder dystocia. (A) McRobert's maneuver. The client flexes their thighs sharply against the abdomen, which straightens the pelvic curve somewhat. (B) Suprapubic pressure by an assistant pushes the fetal anterior shoulder downward to displace it from above the client's symphysis pubis. Fundal pressure is not used because it will push the anterior shoulder even more firmly against the client's symphysis.

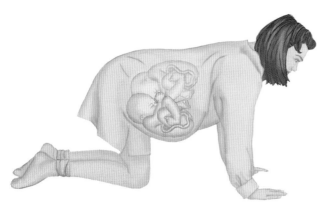

FIG. 16.2 A hands-and-knees position helps this fetus rotate from a left occiput posterior (LOP) position to an occiput anterior position.

because the client's abdomen is dependent in relation to the spine. In the hands-and-knees position, the convex surface of the fetal back tends to rotate toward the convex anterior uterus, similar to nesting of two spoons (Fig. 16.2). The side-lying position has a similar effect, although not quite as pronounced. These positions decrease the client's discomfort by reducing the pressure of the fetal head on the sacrum. All variations of the squatting position aid rotation and fetal descent by straightening the pelvic curve and enlarging the pelvic outlet. They add gravity to the force of maternal pushing.

If spontaneous rotation does not occur, the physician may assist with the rotation and descent of the head by manual rotation or using forceps. The vacuum extractor cannot always be applied to the fetal head when it remains in the OP position. However, some styles of vacuum extractors may be used to correct minor degrees of malrotation because the fetal head tends to rotate as it descends with downward traction. Cesarean birth may be needed if these methods are unsuccessful or cannot be used.

Deflexion Abnormalities. The poorly flexed fetal head presents a larger diameter to the pelvis than if flexed with the chin on the chest (see Fig. 12.8). In vertex presentation, the head diameter is smallest. In military and brow presentations, the head diameter is larger. In face presentation, the head diameter is similar to a vertex presentation, but the maternal pelvis can be traversed only if the fetal chin (mentum) is anterior.

Breech Presentation. Cervical dilation and effacement often are slower when the fetus is in breech presentation because the buttocks or feet do not form a smooth, round dilating wedge like the head. The greatest risk is the head—the largest fetal part—is the last to be born. By the time the lower body is born, the umbilical cord is well into the pelvis and may be compressed. The shoulders, arms, and head are delivered quickly so the infant can breathe.

A breech presentation is common well before term, but only 3% to 5% of term fetuses remain in this presentation. Reasons for breech presentation may include the following:

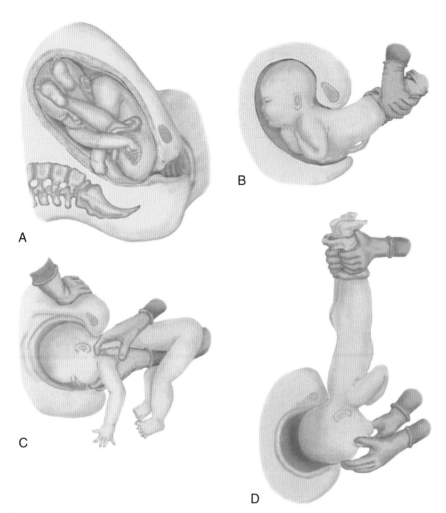

FIG. 16.3 Sequence for vaginal birth in a frank breech presentation. (A) Descent and internal rotation of the fetal body. (B) Internal rotation complete; extension of the fetal back and neck as the trunk slips under the symphysis pubis. The provider uses a towel for traction when grasping the fetal legs. (C) After the birth of the shoulders, the provider maintains flexion of the fetal head by using the fingers of the left hand to apply pressure to the lower face. The fetal body straddles the provider's left arm. An assistant provides suprapubic pressure to help keep the fetal head well-flexed. (D) After the fetal head is brought under the symphysis pubis, an assistant grasps the fetal legs with a towel for traction while the provider delivers the face and head over the client's perineum.

- Low birth weight as a result of preterm gestation, multifetal pregnancy, or intrauterine growth restriction
- Fetal anomalies contributing to breech presentation, such as hydrocephalus
- Complications secondary to placenta previa or previous cesarean birth

External cephalic version may be attempted to manually move the fetus in breech presentation or transverse lie to cephalic presentation (see Chapter 15). If the fetus remains in the abnormal presentation, cesarean section usually is performed to avoid complications. Birth for the nulliparous client with a fetus that remains in breech presentation is almost always by cesarean section. The fetus remaining in a transverse lie is delivered by cesarean section as well.

Some clients are admitted in advanced labor with the fetus in breech presentation, so providers and intrapartum nurses should prepare to care for the client having either a planned or an unexpected vaginal breech birth. (Fig. 16.3 illustrates the mechanisms of vaginal birth for an infant in breech presentation.)

Multifetal Pregnancy

Multifetal pregnancy may result in dysfunctional labor because of uterine overdistention, which contributes to labor dystocia, and abnormal presentation of one or both fetuses (Fig. 16.4). Similar to a large overstretched rubber band, the overdistended uterine muscle does not contract evenly or with great force. In addition, the potential for fetal hypoxia during labor is greater because the client must supply oxygen and nutrients to more than one fetus. There is greater risk for postpartum hemorrhage resulting from uterine atony because of uterine overdistention.

Many clients with multifetal pregnancy deliver preterm or late preterm. Placentation and fetal indications make timing of delivery complex and must be carefully planned. Twins generally are delivered by 37 to 38^{6/7} weeks, whereas triplets and higher order multiples may be delivered at 32 to 35 weeks

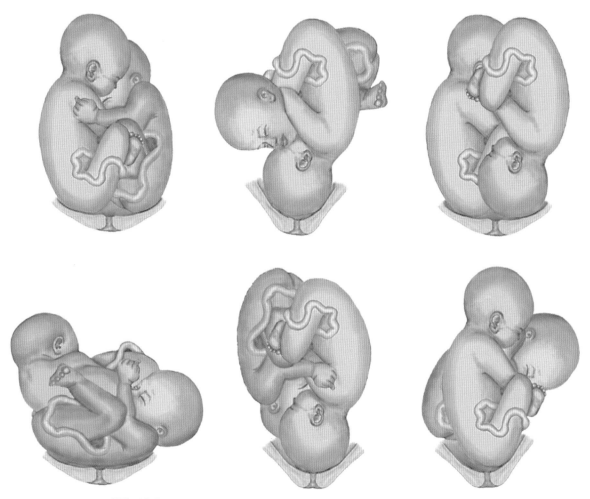

FIG. 16.4 Twins can present in any combination of presentations and positions.

as the prospective risk of fetal mortality increases after those dates (ACOG, 2021b; Bowers, 2021; Malone & D'Alton, 2019).

Some clients with twin A in the vertex position may have a vaginal delivery, especially when Twin B is also vertex. Due to the risk for cord prolapse, placental shearing, and potential bleeding problems, many clients with multifetal pregnancies opt for cesarean birth. If three or more fetuses are involved, the birth is almost always cesarean. The physician considers fetal viability, fetal presentations, maternal pelvic size, and presence of other complications such as preeclampsia or chronic hypertension when determining the best plan of care for the client and fetuses.

Each twin's FHR is monitored during labor. When in bed, the client remains in the lateral position to promote adequate placental blood flow. After vaginal birth of the first twin, assessment of the second twin's FHR continues with ultrasound and fetal monitoring until birth (Bowers, 2021).

The delivery staff is prepared for the care and possible resuscitation of multiple infants. Radiant warmers, resuscitation equipment, medications, and identification materials are prepared for each infant. One or more neonatal nurses, a neonatal or pediatric nurse practitioner, and a pediatrician or a neonatologist may be available to care for each infant. One nurse is dedicated to caring for the client.

? KNOWLEDGE CHECK

1. How does labor dystocia differ from tachysystole?
2. How can maternal position changes facilitate rotation of the fetus from the OT or OP position to the OA position?
3. Why is cesarean birth usually the delivery method of choice for infants in breech presentation?
4. How does preparation for the birth of multiple infants (vaginal or cesarean) differ from preparation for a single infant's birth?

Fetal Anomalies

Fetal anomalies such as hydrocephalus or a large fetal tumor may prevent normal descent of the fetus. Abnormal presentations such as breech or transverse lie also are associated with fetal anomalies. These abnormalities often are discovered by ultrasound examination before labor. Cesarean birth is scheduled if vaginal birth is not possible or is inadvisable.

Problems with the Passage

Dysfunctional labor may occur because of variations in the maternal bony pelvis or soft tissue problems that inhibit fetal descent.

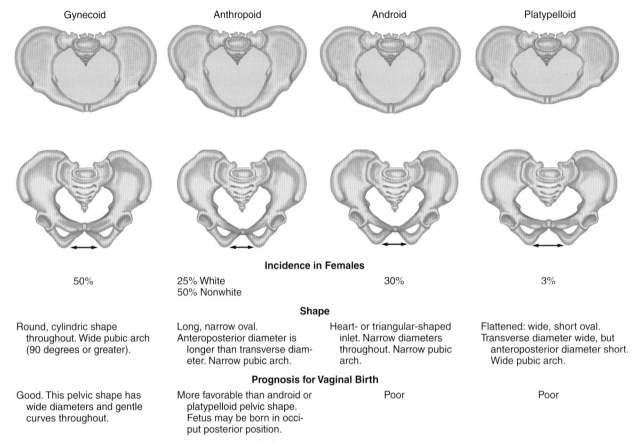

Gynecoid	Anthropoid	Android	Platypelloid

Incidence in Females

50%	25% White 50% Nonwhite	30%	3%

Shape

Round, cylindric shape throughout. Wide pubic arch (90 degrees or greater).	Long, narrow oval. Anteroposterior diameter is longer than transverse diameter. Narrow pubic arch.	Heart- or triangular-shaped inlet. Narrow diameters throughout. Narrow pubic arch.	Flattened: wide, short oval. Transverse diameter wide, but anteroposterior diameter short. Wide pubic arch.

Prognosis for Vaginal Birth

Good. This pelvic shape has wide diameters and gentle curves throughout.	More favorable than android or platypelloid pelvic shape. Fetus may be born in occiput posterior position.	Poor	Poor

FIG. 16.5 Pelvic shapes.

Pelvis

A small (contracted) or abnormally shaped pelvis may slow labor and obstruct fetal passage. The client may experience poor contractions, slow dilation, slow fetal descent, and a long labor.

Four basic pelvic shapes exist, each with different implications for labor and birth (Fig. 16.5). Most clients do not have a pure pelvic shape but instead have mixed characteristics from two or more types.

Soft Tissue Obstructions

During labor, a full bladder is a common soft tissue obstruction. Bladder distention reduces available space in the pelvis and intensifies maternal discomfort. The client is assessed for bladder distention regularly and encouraged to void every 1 to 2 hours. Catheterization may be needed if the client is unable to urinate or if epidural analgesia depresses the urge to void. There are mixed opinions in the literature as to whether intermittent catheterization or Foley placement is more appropriate.

Problems of the Psyche

Labor may be a stressful event for clients. A perceived threat caused by pain, fear, lack of support, or personal situations can result in impaired coping ability and interfere with normal labor progress. Responses to excessive or prolonged stress interfere with labor in the several ways:

- Increased glucose consumption reduces the energy supply available to the contracting uterus.
- Secretion of catecholamines (epinephrine and norepinephrine) by the adrenal glands stimulates uterine beta receptors, which inhibit uterine contractions (an action similar to tocolytic drugs such as terbutaline).
- Adrenal secretion of catecholamines diverts blood supply from the uterus and placenta to the client's skeletal muscles.
- Labor contractions and maternal pushing efforts are less effective because these powers are working against the resistance of tense abdominal and pelvic muscles.
- Pain perception is increased, and pain tolerance is decreased, further increasing maternal anxiety and stress.

Assisting the client to relax allows the body to work more effectively with the forces of labor. Nursing measures may involve the following:

- Establishing a trusting relationship with the client and significant other
- Making the environment comfortable by adjusting temperature and light
- Identifying coping measures the client finds useful
- Promoting physical comfort such as cleanliness
- Providing accurate information
- Implementing nonpharmacologic and pharmacologic pain management

Abnormal Labor Duration

An unusually long or abnormally short, or precipitous, labor may result in maternal, fetal, or neonatal complications.

Prolonged Labor

Reasons for prolonged labor are multifaceted. Traditional thought based on the Friedman curves developed in the 1970s indicated after the client reached the active phase of labor, cervical dilation should proceed at a minimum rate of 1.2 cm/hr in the nullipara and 1.5 cm/hr in the parous client. The fetal presenting part was expected to descend at a minimal rate of 1 cm/hr in the nullipara and 2 cm/hr in the parous client.

Zhang et al. (2010), with the Consortium for Safe Labor, studied normal labor duration in a 2010 trial funded by the National Institute of Child Health and Human Development. This multicenter retrospective study abstracted detailed labor and delivery information from electronic medical records in 19 hospitals across the United States. A total of 62,415 clients were selected who had a singleton term gestation, spontaneous onset of labor, vertex presentation, vaginal delivery, and an optimal perinatal outcome. They found labor may take over 6 hours to progress from 4 to 5 cm and over 3 hours to progress from 5 to 6 cm of dilation. Nulliparas and multiparas appeared to progress at a similar pace before 6 cm. However, after 6 cm, multiparas accelerated much faster than nulliparas. The 95th percentile of the second stage of labor in nulliparas with epidural analgesia was 3.6 hours, and without epidural analgesia was 2.8 hours. They concluded allowing labor to continue for a longer period before 6 cm of cervical dilation may reduce the rate of primary and subsequent repeat cesarean births in the United States.

Possible maternal and fetal problems in prolonged labor include the following:

- Maternal infection, intrapartum, or postpartum
- Neonatal infection, which may be severe or fatal
- Maternal exhaustion
- High levels of anxiety and fear
- Malposition of the fetus

Maternal and neonatal infections are more likely if the membranes have been ruptured for a prolonged time because organisms ascend from the vagina.

Nursing measures for the client who has prolonged labor include promotion of comfort, conservation of energy, emotional support, position changes that favor normal progress, and assessments for infection. Nursing care for the fetus includes observation for signs of intrauterine infection and compromised fetal oxygenation.

Precipitous Labor

Precipitous labor is one in which birth occurs within 3 hours of its onset. Intense contractions often begin abruptly rather than gradually increasing in frequency, duration, and intensity, as is typical of most labors.

Precipitous labor is not the same as a precipitous birth. A **precipitous birth** occurs after a labor of any length, in or out of the hospital or birth center, when a provider is not present to assist. A client in precipitous labor may have both a precipitous labor and a precipitous birth. If the obstetrics (OB) provider will not arrive in time for the baby's birth, the nurse wears gloves and supports the infant's body as it emerges. If the maternal pelvis is adequate and the soft tissues yield easily to fetal descent, little maternal injury is likely. However, if the soft tissues are firm and resist stretching, trauma of the vagina or vulva (vaginal wall lacerations, cervical lacerations, sulcus or vulvar tears, and hematoma) may occur.

Several conditions that can be associated with precipitous labor include placental abruption, fetal meconium, maternal cocaine use, postpartum hemorrhage, and low Apgar scores for the infant (Cunningham et al., 2022). Trauma from rapid labor may result in genital tract lacerations in the client and neonatal birth injuries (Francois & Foley, 2021; Rozance & Wright, 2021). The fetus may become hypoxic because intense contractions with a short relaxation period reduce the time available for gas exchange in the placenta. Abnormal electronic fetal monitoring (EFM) patterns may include bradycardia and late decelerations. The fetus may suffer direct trauma such as intracranial hemorrhage or nerve damage during a precipitous birth from the sudden release of pressure on the fetal head.

Priority nursing care of the client in precipitous labor includes promotion of fetal oxygenation and maternal comfort. The side-lying position enhances placental blood flow and reduces the effects of aortocaval compression. An added benefit of the side-lying position is to slow the rapid fetal descent and minimize perineal tears. Additional measures to enhance fetal oxygenation include administering oxygen to the client and maintaining adequate blood volume with nonadditive IV fluids. If oxytocin is being used, it is stopped. A tocolytic medication may be ordered.

Promoting comfort is difficult in a precipitous labor because intense contractions give the client little time to prepare and use coping skills such as breathing techniques. Pharmacologic measures, such as analgesics or epidural block, may not be useful if rapid labor progress does not allow time for them to become effective. Possible newborn respiratory depression is considered if opioid analgesia is given near birth. The nurse assists the client to focus on techniques to cope with pain, one contraction at a time. The nurse remains at bedside to provide support and assist with an emergency birth if it occurs.

APPLICATION OF THE NURSING PROCESS: DURING DYSFUNCTIONAL LABOR

Several client problems may be appropriate when caring for an individual having dysfunctional labor. The potential complication of fetal compromise is a part of all intrapartum management (see Chapter 14). Pain management is especially important to clients in labor because they may find their coping skills are inadequate or difficult to use because of fatigue, possibly to the point of exhaustion. Anxiety or fear often is higher with abnormal labor, which limits the client's ability to cope with labor. Anxiety or fear may reduce the effectiveness of pain medications or regional block analgesia.

In addition to these problems, nursing care is directed toward two other client problems: possible intrauterine infection and maternal exhaustion.

POSSIBLE INTRAUTERINE INFECTION

Infection can occur with both normal and dysfunctional labors. The interdisciplinary team works within the criteria for **Triple I** (intraamniotic inflammation and infection) (ACOG, 2017b; Sloane et al., 2019) and the protocols or order sets that are in place in their institution. Triple I is also known as *chorioamnionitis*, *intraamniotic infection*, or *intrauterine infection*. Triple I is the preferred term as it is more general and descriptive.

The following parameters are suggestive of a possible infection (ACOG, 2017b, Sloane et al., 2019):
- Maternal fever—defined as an oral temperature of 39.0° C or greater (102.2° F) on one reading or 38.0° C (100.4° F) or greater but less than 39.0° C (102.2° F) on two readings 30 minutes apart

with one or more of the following:
- Fetal tachycardia—baseline greater than 160 bpm × at least 10 minutes
- Maternal white blood cell (WBC) count greater than 15,000 in the absence of corticosteroids
- Purulent fluid emanating from the cervical os
  - Cloudy, yellowish, thick discharge confirmed visually on sterile speculum examination

A confirmed infection is based on the following:
- Biochemical or microbiologic amniotic fluid results consistent with microbial invasion of the amniotic cavity (confirmed testing), includes the following:
  - Positive Gram stain for bacteria
  - Low amniotic fluid glucose.
- Placenta pathology demonstrating evidence of infection or inflammation

NOTE: If *only* maternal temperature is elevated, with no other markers, it is not Triple I.

> Fever plus one indicator = Suspected Triple I
> Fever plus confirmed testing = Confirmed Triple I

Assessment

Assess maternal temperature every 2 hours during labor and every 1 hour after the membranes have ruptured. Assess maternal pulse, respirations, and blood pressure hourly if elevated temperature.

Assess amniotic fluid for clear color and mild odor. Small flecks of white vernix are normal in amniotic fluid. Yellow or cloudy fluid or fluid with a foul or strong odor suggests infection. The strong odor may be noted before birth or afterward on the infant's skin.

Identification of Client Problems

For the client without signs of infection but with risk factors, the problem identified is potential for infection because of the presence of favorable conditions for development. The nurse may specify the client-specific conditions that may cause infection when choosing this client problem.

Planning: Expected Outcomes

Expected outcomes relate to detecting the onset of infection:
- Maternal temperature will remain below 38°C (100.4°F).
- The FHR will remain near the baseline with an average baseline rate no higher than 160 bpm.
- The amniotic fluid will remain clear and without a foul or strong odor.

Interventions
Reducing the Risk for Infection

Nurses should wash their hands before and after each contact with all clients to reduce transmission of organisms. Limit vaginal examinations to reduce transmission of vaginal organisms into the uterine cavity and maintain aseptic technique during essential vaginal examinations. The intrapartum nurse learns to estimate a client's progress with few vaginal examinations. For example, increased bloody show and heightened anxiety may occur when the cervix is approximately 6 cm dilated. The client may become irritable and lose control at about 8 cm dilation if unmedicated.

Keep under pads as dry as possible to reduce the moist, warm environment that favors bacterial growth. Periodically clean excess secretions from the vaginal area in a front-to-back direction to limit fecal contamination and promote the client's comfort. Use personal protective equipment to avoid contact with body secretions.

Identifying Infection

Assess the client and fetus for signs of infection. Increase the frequency of assessments if labor is prolonged, if other risk factors are present, or if any signs of infection are found. If signs of infection are noted, report them to the provider for further evaluation and treatment. Note the time at which the membranes ruptured to identify prolonged rupture, which adds to the risk for infection.

After birth, the provider may collect specimens from the uterine cavity or placenta for culture to identify infectious organisms and determine antibiotic sensitivity. Aerobic and anaerobic culture specimens may be collected in containers specifically made for these two types of organisms. Follow directions on the container for proper handling and prevention of contamination with extraneous organisms, which would result in inaccurate results. Transport specimens to the laboratory promptly because living organisms are required for culture and sensitivity study. Antibiotic therapy is started without delay after collecting specimens.

Inform the newborn nursery staff if signs of infection are noted or if increased maternal risk factors exist. Specimens of infant secretions also may be obtained for testing before administration of antibiotics. The infant may receive prophylactic antibiotics to prevent neonatal sepsis. If results of maternal or infant cultures indicate no infection is present, the antibiotic is discontinued. Culture and sensitivity testing may reveal an infection and indicate a different antibiotic would be more effective, in which case the antibiotic is changed.

Evaluation

The goals and expected outcomes are achieved if the following occur:
- The client's temperature remains below 38°C (100.4°F).
- The FHR remains within the expected range, not showing tachycardia, whether sudden or gradual in onset.
- The amniotic fluid has no abnormal characteristics that are typical of infection (abnormal or yellow color, foul or strong odor).

The goals are continually reevaluated throughout labor with hourly temperature assessments and more frequent FHR evaluations. Periodically the nurse will provide pericare and evaluate the amniotic fluid. Even if they have no signs of infection, the client remains at higher risk for postpartum infection and observation for signs and symptoms of infection occurs throughout the hospital stay.

EXHAUSTION

Assessment

Many clients begin labor with a sleep deficit because of fetal movement and frequent urination associated with advanced pregnancy. As labor drags on, their reserves are further depleted. Some clients do not choose to or cannot have epidurals. Even with epidural analgesia, a long labor drains the client's energy. The labor nurse is skilled in helping the client deal with exhaustion.

Assess for the following signs of exhaustion:
- Verbal expression of tiredness, fatigue, or exhaustion
- Verbal expression of frustration with a prolonged, unproductive labor ("I can't go on any longer. Why doesn't the doctor just take the baby?")
- Ineffectiveness of or inability to use coping techniques (e.g., patterned breathing) previously used effectively
- Changes in the client's pulse rate, respiration, and blood pressure (increased or decreased)

Identification of Client Problems

The intense energy demands of a dysfunctional labor may exceed a client's physical and psychological ability to meet them. For this reason, exhaustion due to depletion of maternal energy reserves is an appropriate problem.

Planning: Expected Outcomes

Contractions must continue for labor to progress; therefore two realistic outcomes include:

- Rest between contractions with muscles relaxed
- Effective use of coping skills such as breathing and relaxation techniques

Interventions
Conserving Energy

Reduce the factors that interfere with the client's ability to relax.
- Lower the light level—turn off overhead lights.
- Reduce noise—close the door, play music, water sounds, or other comforting sounds.
- Maintain a comfortable temperature with blankets or a fan.
- If not contraindicated, a warm shower or bath is soothing.

Position the client to encourage comfort, promote fetal descent, and enhance fetal oxygenation. Support the client with pillows or birth balls to reduce muscle strain and added fatigue. Assist with position changes regularly (about every 20–30 minutes) to reduce muscle tension from constant pressure.

A soothing back rub reduces muscle tension and thus decreases fatigue. Firm sacral pressure and use of some positions discussed in the section on fetal OP positions may reduce back pain. Using the birthing ball can relax and provide support in some positions. Warmth to the lower back can reduce back pain. (See Chapters 13 and 15 for added comfort measures.)

Maintain IV fluids at the rate ordered to provide fluid, electrolytes, and possibly glucose. Assess intake and output to identify dehydration, which may accompany prolonged labor. Dehydration also may cause maternal fever. If not contraindicated, provide juice, lollipops, frozen juice bars, or other clear liquids, as ordered by the OB provider to moisten the client's mouth and replenish energy.

Promoting Coping Skills

When position changes or medical therapies are used to enhance labor, explain their purpose and expected benefits. Generous praise and encouragement of the client's use of skills such as breathing and visualization techniques provide motivation to continue even when they are discouraged. As with any laboring client, communicate their labor progress, fetal status, and uterine activity patterns. Knowing this information provides the client courage to continue.

Evaluation

Goals are met if the client
- Rests and relaxes between contractions. If unable to relax and verbalizes a desire for help, discuss alternative coping methods, including analgesia options.
- Continues to demonstrate adequate use of learned skills to cope with labor.

PREMATURE RUPTURE OF THE MEMBRANES

Rupture of the amniotic membranes before onset of true labor is called *premature rupture of the membranes* (PROM), regardless of gestational age. A precise term, *preterm premature rupture of the membranes* (PPROM, sometimes abbreviated as pPROM), refers to the rupture of membranes earlier than 37 weeks, with or without contractions. PPROM is associated with preterm labor and birth. (ACOG, 2020f; Parfitt, 2021).

Etiology

Several conditions are associated with PROM and PPROM, but the exact cause often remains unclear. Conditions associated with preterm ruptured membranes include the following:

- Triple I may be associated with group B *Streptococcus* (GBS), *Neisseria gonorrhoeae*, *Listeria monocytogenes*, or species from the genera *Mycoplasma*, *Bacteroides*, and *Ureaplasma* in the amniotic fluid
- Infections, possibly asymptomatic, of the vagina or cervix, such as *N. gonorrhoeae*, *Chlamydia trachomatis*, *Trichomonas vaginalis*, GBS, or *Gardnerella vaginalis* (bacterial vaginosis)
- Amniotic sac with a weak structure
- Previous preterm birth, especially if preceded by PPROM
- Fetal abnormalities or malpresentation
- Incompetent cervix or a short cervical length (25 mm or less)
- Overdistention of the uterus, such as multiple gestation or polyhydramnios
- Maternal hormonal changes
- Maternal stress or low socioeconomic status
- Maternal nutritional deficiencies and diabetes

Complications

Both client and newborn are at risk for infection during the intrapartum and postpartum periods. Infection can be both a cause and a result of PROM. Organisms that cause Triple I weaken the amniotic membrane, leading to the rupture. The client is at higher risk for postpartum infection, and the newborn is vulnerable to neonatal sepsis.

Triple I, characterized by maternal fever and uterine tenderness, is most likely to precede preterm birth in the infant born before 34 weeks of gestation. Preterm infants with the lowest maturity, such as 23 weeks of gestation, have higher risk for the infection than preterm infants who are even a few weeks more mature. The exact time at which infection occurs cannot be predicted for either term or preterm infants. Frequent performance of digital examination of the cervix increases the risk for all gestations. If Triple I does not precede PROM, it is more likely to occur if a long time elapses between membrane rupture and birth because vaginal organisms can readily enter the uterus. The risk for Triple I is known to increase when the membranes are ruptured for 24 hours or longer.

Membranes that rupture before term may form a seal, stopping the fluid leak and allowing the amniotic fluid to become reestablished. However, membranes may continue to leak, resulting in low levels of amniotic fluid (**oligohydramnios**) and prolonging the loss of the amniotic fluid cushion

for the fetus. Umbilical cord compression, reduced lung volume, and deformities resulting from compression may occur. The earlier in gestation the rupture occurs, the greater the risks associated with prolonged oligohydramnios.

If preterm birth occurs, the infant is more likely to have respiratory distress syndrome (RDS) and complications related to prematurity. The hazards of prematurity are greatest before 34 weeks of gestation, especially if the client did not receive steroids to accelerate fetal lung maturation before birth.

Therapeutic Management

Management of PROM depends on the gestation and whether evidence of infection or other fetal or maternal compromise exists. If the fetus is less than 36 weeks, therapeutic management is more complex and may involve short-term tocolytic medications to delay delivery until steroids can be administered to enhance fetal lung maturity and antibiotics can be started to reduce transmission of bacteria, including GBS. Risks for infection or preterm birth complications are weighed against risks of labor induction or cesarean birth. For a client at or near term (37 weeks or more of gestation), PROM may herald the imminent onset of true labor.

Determining True Membrane Rupture

The first step is to verify ruptured membranes. Urinary incontinence, increased vaginal discharge, or loss of the mucous plug can be mistaken for ruptured membranes. A digital vaginal examination is avoided, particularly if the gestation is preterm and no evidence of labor exists. Instead, a sterile speculum exam is performed to look for a pool of fluid near the cervix and estimate cervical dilation and effacement. A pH test or fern test may be done on the fluid to verify the liquid is amniotic fluid. Tests are available that check for the presence of placental alpha microglobulin-1 (PAMG-1), found only in amniotic fluid. Tests to assess fetal lung maturity and identify infection are often performed. A transvaginal ultrasound examination may be performed to measure cervical length. A short (25 mm or less) cervix is more likely to continue effacement and dilation even if the gestation is far from term. Serial abdominal ultrasounds will follow fluid levels and fetal growth status.

Gestation Near Term. If labor does not begin spontaneously, the client's pregnancy is at or near term, the cervix is favorable, and fetal lungs are mature, labor is usually induced (see Chapter 15). If the cervix is not favorable and no infection is evident, induction may be delayed 24 hours or longer to allow cervical softening and administration of antibiotics. Steroids to accelerate fetal lung maturity are not indicated if the fetus is 37 or more weeks of gestation (ACOG, 2020a). If induction is unsuccessful or if infection or other complications develop, a cesarean birth is most common. Cesarean birth also increases the risk for maternal infection after birth.

Preterm Gestation. If the gestation is preterm, the physician weighs the risks for maternal-fetal infection against the newborn's risk for complications of prematurity. Many variables are considered by the provider and client to determine the best course of management. Medical management changes as fetal maturation and conditions of the client and fetus change with the continuation of pregnancy.

The cervix usually is not favorable for induction far from term. Factors such as gestational age, amount of amniotic fluid remaining, fetal lung maturity, and any signs of fetal compromise are considered. A **cerclage** (suture encircling the cervix) may have been placed earlier in the pregnancy to prevent premature cervical dilation. If infection is not already present, the physician considers whether leaving the cerclage in place or removing the cerclage is the best course of action for each individual client (ACOG, 2020a).

If no evidence of infection exists and the fetal lungs are immature, the client usually is observed for infection or onset of labor in the hospital (**expectant management**). Daily nonstress tests or continuous fetal monitoring are performed to watch for FHR nonreactivity, which may occur with intraamniotic infection. Biophysical profiles, in which sonographic evaluation is added to the nonstress test, may be done one or more times per week. Fetal lung maturity testing may be done as term approaches to identify the best time for delivery unless other complications require delivery before fetal lung maturity. Antibiotics are given during labor.

Maternal Antibiotics

A 7-day course of parental and oral maternal antibiotics are usually prescribed for PPROM because of the increased infection risk or further complications caused by PPROM for both client and fetus. Antibiotics may prevent an infection from developing or stop the infection that caused the rupture initially, thereby delaying the onset of labor and allowing the fetus to mature. Common antibiotics may include ampicillin, amoxicillin, and erythromycin (ACOG, 2020f; Parfitt, 2021). Guidelines for specific medications to correct infection associated with early membrane rupture may vary with culture and sensitivity test results, other maternal laboratory results, or changes in the current guidelines.

Nursing Considerations

If the fetus is previable, the client may be managed with at home care. Once viability is reached, ACOG (2020f) recommends inpatient management related to the increased risk for umbilical cord compression and potential rapid onset of infection. When hospitalized, the nurse observes for signs of infection that may include temperature elevation, white count elevation, uterine tenderness, contractions, body aches, chills, or a generalized feeling of illness.

Preparation for home management includes teaching the client the following:

- Avoid sexual intercourse, orgasm, or insertion of anything into the vagina, which increases the risk for infection caused by ascending organisms and can stimulate contractions.
- Avoid breast stimulation if the gestation is preterm because it may cause release of oxytocin from the posterior pituitary and thus stimulate contractions.
- Take their temperature at least four times a day, reporting any temperature of more than 37.8°C (100°F).
- Maintain any activity restrictions.
- Note and report uterine contractions or a foul odor to vaginal drainage.

❓ KNOWLEDGE CHECK

10. How does PROM differ from PPROM?
11. What is the relationship of infection to PROM?
12. What is the usual therapeutic management of PROM if the client is at or near term? What if the gestation is preterm?
13. What are the nursing considerations for a client with PPROM?

PRETERM LABOR

In 2019, the preterm birth rate in the United States was 10.2% (March of Dimes, 2021). The March of Dimes (2021) reports in 2019, the rate of preterm birth in the United States was highest for Black infants (14.0%), followed by American Indian/Alaska Natives (11.7%), Hispanics (9.8%), Whites (9.2%), and Asian/Pacific Islanders (8.8%). Understanding the disparities of these populations is critical to moving forward in the hope of limiting preterm birth.

Preterm labor begins after the 20th week but before the start of the 37th week of pregnancy. The physical risk to the client is no greater than labor at term unless complications such as infection, hemorrhage, or the need for a cesarean delivery also exist. Preterm labor, however, may result in the birth of an infant who is ill equipped for extrauterine life, particularly if earlier than 32 weeks of gestation. Adverse effects of prematurity may include cerebral palsy, developmental delay, and vision and hearing impairment. Families may suffer heavy emotional and economic burdens.

Many possible risk factors exist that might trigger preterm labor (Box 16.1). A client who has previously delivered a preterm infant is more likely to have preterm labor. Having a multifetal pregnancy or use of assisted reproductive technology carries higher risks for both clients and their infants, such as cesarean birth, prematurity, and infant disability or death. Smoking cigarettes when combined with smoking marijuana increases risk for delivering preterm (Nawa et al., 2020).

Infants born at "early term," $37^{0/7}$ to $38^{6/7}$ weeks of gestation, have an increased risk for poor outcomes than those born after 39 weeks (Rohan, 2021; Simhan & Romero, 2021).

Associated Factors

Just as all causes of onset of labor at term are not known, the causes of preterm labor are not fully known. Over half of the clients who have preterm labor and birth do not have known risk factors. Other clients who have many risk factors deliver at term.

Preterm labor is thought to be initiated by multiple factors, including infection or inflammation, uteroplacental

BOX 16.1 Risk Factors for Preterm Labor

Medical History
Low weight for height
Obesity
Uterine or cervical anomalies, uterine fibroids
History of cone biopsy
Diethylstilbestrol (DES) exposure as a fetus
Chronic illness (e.g., cardiac, renal, diabetes, clotting disorders, anemia, hypertension)
Periodontal disease

Obstetric History
Previous preterm labor
Previous preterm birth
Previous first-trimester spontaneous abortion (more than 2)
Previous second-trimester spontaneous abortion
History of previous pregnancy losses (2 or more)
Incompetent cervix
Cervical length 25 mm (2.5 cm [1 inch]) or less at midtrimester of pregnancy
Number of embryos implanted (assisted reproductive techniques)

Present Pregnancy
Uterine overdistension (e.g., multifetal pregnancy, hydramnios)
Abdominal surgery during pregnancy
Uterine irritability
Uterine bleeding
Dehydration
Infection
Anemia
Incompetent cervix
Preeclampsia
Preterm premature rupture of membranes
Fetal or placental abnormalities

Lifestyle and Demographics
Little or no prenatal care
Poor nutrition
Age younger than 18 years or older than 40 years
Low educational level
Low socioeconomic status
Smoking more than 10 cigarettes daily
Nonwhite
Employment with long hours and/or long time standing
Chronic physical or psychological stress
Domestic violence
Substance abuse

ischemia or hemorrhage (abruption or previa), uterine overdistension as with multiple gestations, stress, and other immunologically mediated processes. Some of the possible causes of preterm labor are the following (Simhan & Romero, 2021):

- Maternal medical conditions, including infections of the urinary tract, reproductive organs, or systemic organs; dental disorders (periodontal disease); preexisting or gestational diabetes; connective tissue disorders; chronic hypertension; and drug abuse

- Conceptions enhanced by assisted reproductive technology, including conceptions resulting in a single fetal gestation rather than a multifetal gestation
- Present and past obstetric conditions such as short cervical length (25 mm or less), multifetal gestation, preterm membrane rupture, preeclampsia, and bleeding disorders that involve the client, fetus, or placental implantation area
- Fetal conditions such as growth restriction, inadequate amniotic fluid volume, chromosome abnormalities, and other birth defects
- Social and environmental factors such as inadequate or absent prenatal or dental care, maternal domestic violence episodes, maternal smoking, and housing deficiency such as homelessness
- Demographic factors such as race and ages of the parents, financial stability, and the number and birth intervals of the client's other children

As we learn more about COVID-19 and the effects on pregnancy, emerging science would indicate an increased risk of preterm birth for clients infected with the COVID-19 virus related to the increased risk of severe morbidity. Current recommendations include administration of the COVID-19 vaccine to pregnant clients (see the Maternal Immunization Task Force Joint Statement, 2021).

Signs and Symptoms

Signs and symptoms of early preterm labor are more subtle than those of labor at term and often occur in normal pregnancies as well. Prenatal visits and routine ultrasounds may reveal evidence of cervical changes that have been occurring over several weeks during the second and third trimesters. The client may be only vaguely aware that something seems different, or they may not detect anything is amiss. Only when preterm labor reaches the active phase is it likely to have characteristics typical of term labor. Symptoms vary among clients, but common ones are as follows:

- Uterine contractions may or may not be painful (the client may not feel contractions at all)
- A sensation of the baby frequently "balling up"
- Cramps similar to menstrual cramps
- Constant low backache; irregular or intermittent low back pain
- Sensation of pelvic pressure or feeling like the baby is pushing down
- Pain, discomfort, or pressure in the vagina or thighs
- Change or increase in vaginal discharge (increased, watery, "spotting," bleeding)
- Abdominal cramps with or without diarrhea
- A sense of "just feeling bad" or "coming down with something"

Preventing Preterm Birth
Community Education

Preterm birth can impose substantial physical, emotional, and financial burdens on the child, family, and society. Ideally, nursing strategies to prevent preterm birth begin before conception, with community education. Topics may include the following:

- Role of early and regular prenatal care, including dental care, in preventing preterm birth
- Duration of normal pregnancy
- Consequences of preterm birth
- Conditions that increase the risk for preterm birth
- Signs and symptoms of preterm labor
- Consequences of preterm birth for client, baby, and family members

Clients who are aware of the consequences of preterm birth may be more likely to take action to prevent it. If they recognize they have risk factors, they may seek prenatal care earlier in pregnancy. Recognizing the onset of labor in early gestation has subtle signs and symptoms compared with labor near term may prompt the client to seek care promptly rather than waiting for more definite signs of labor.

During Pregnancy

During pregnancy, measures to prevent preterm birth include the following:

- Reducing barriers and improving access to early prenatal care
- Assessing for risk factors to permit changes, if possible
- Promoting adequate nutrition
- Promoting cessation of the use of tobacco and recreational drugs
- Teaching clients and their partners about the subtle signs and symptoms of preterm labor and ways in which they differ from normal pregnancy changes
- Empowering clients and their partners to take an active approach in seeking care if they have signs and symptoms of preterm labor

Improving Access to Care. Community needs assessment determines how resources can be made available for each setting. What works in one area may be inappropriate for another. Accessibility of care at public clinics may be a serious problem. Long waits, fragmented care, language barriers, and insensitivity of caregivers discourage clients from obtaining care. Expanding the number of caregivers by using advanced practice nurses such as certified nurse–midwives and nurse practitioners can significantly increase access to care. Nurses can help coordinate appointments clients need to obtain complete care. As work toward equity of care continues, models of care that fit the needs of the community such as Group Prenatal Care or Centering Pregnancy (ACOG, 2019a; Adams, 2021) and moving clinics to be community-based must be explored.

Identifying Risk Factors. Identification of risk factors may allow reduction or elimination of these factors. Clients should be rescreened regularly to identify new risks that emerge as pregnancy progresses. High-risk clients benefit from interventions such as more frequent prenatal care appointments, reinforcement of the symptoms of preterm labor, telephone contacts, and added assessments of fetal growth and health.

Some risk factors can be reduced or eliminated if the client makes lifestyle changes. Many pregnant clients stop smoking or using nontherapeutic drugs to benefit their babies. A client may need to rest more or stop working, which may be difficult or impossible for many. Nurses and social workers can help the client reduce risks by helping identify sources of support.

Infections of the urinary and reproductive tracts are associated with PPROM and preterm labor. Screening at the appropriate times for pathogenic organisms in the urine, vagina, and cervix identifies clients who may benefit from antibiotic therapy.

Promoting Adequate Nutrition. An adequate maternal diet contributes positively to the length of gestation and the infant's birth weight. The client's height is measured at the first prenatal visit, and the weight is taken at each visit to evaluate adequacy of weight gain. Every pregnant client should be offered culturally sensitive dietary counseling. Some conditions require additional supplements, like iron to treat anemia, or increased calorie intake to support multifetal pregnancies. The Special Supplemental Nutrition Program for Women, Infants, and Children (WIC) is available to supplement the diet of clients from low-income groups.

Educating Clients and Their Partners about Preterm Labor. All pregnant clients and their partners should be taught about symptoms of preterm labor, because half of preterm births occur in clients with no identified risk factors. Information about the vague signs and symptoms of early preterm labor are reinforced regularly as part of prenatal care. Clients who often have uterine irritability may be given guidelines to observe at home before they go to the hospital. Preterm labor often has vague sensations to the client, so any home care guidelines are individualized according to the client's risk for a preterm birth, the gestation and prenatal status, and the likelihood that specific interventions are beneficial to client and baby. In addition, clients are taught to enter the hospital for evaluation if they are not sure about the seriousness of their symptoms. Examples of home care guidelines include the following:

- Drink an adequate amount of water to improve hydration or reduce bladder irritation that may accompany a urinary tract infection (UTI).
- Empty the bladder frequently because a full bladder may be associated with uterine irritability and contractions.
- Rest in the side-lying position to promote uterine blood flow. Limiting physical activity may increase diuresis. Prolonged limitation of physical activity is not usually beneficial or safe for prevention of premature labor, although it may be required for serious maternal disorders such as cardiac disease.
- Palpate contractions for 1 hour or as instructed. However, notify the provider or go directly to the labor unit for assessment if contractions increase in frequency, duration, or sensitivity.

The nurse performs teach-back instruction and verifies the client's understanding of the education given by having the client restate signs and symptoms of preterm labor. Interpreters who are culturally acceptable to the client and printed materials in the client's primary language should be used. Diagrams should supplement the words of any language for clients with limited reading skills. Respecting cultural norms of the client and their family is an essential part of prenatal care that encourages compliance with care and the possibility of identifying problems early.

Empowering Clients and Their Partners. Delaying birth depends on early identification of preterm labor. Clients are encouraged to seek treatment promptly if they suspect preterm labor. The client must communicate concerns clearly upon arrival at the clinic or hospital. The client should indicate to the triage nurse what symptoms they are experiencing regardless of the subtlety of the symptoms. Nurses should listen to the client without judgment. Otherwise, the client may not seek care for recurrent episodes of labor, and the opportunity to delay preterm birth may be lost.

Therapeutic Management

Management focuses on identifying those at risk for preterm birth, identifying preterm labor early, and delaying birth if possible. If preterm birth is likely, the emphasis is accelerating fetal lung maturity and providing neonatal neuroprotection.

Predicting Preterm Birth

Onset of changes that lead to preterm labor and birth may be subtle. The client may not perceive any changes in the pregnancy. Research has focused on predicting which clients will deliver early. Better identification of these clients would allow more intensive treatment, ideally before preterm labor or rupture of membranes occurs. Many signs and symptoms of preterm labor occur in clients who deliver at term, possibly exposing them to unneeded treatment. The key is to identify which clients are really at risk for preterm birth and treat them intensively while continuing regular prenatal care for clients who are not truly at risk. A good screening test would provide quick results and would be inexpensive, usable for all pregnant clients, noninvasive, and highly specific for predicting preterm birth. No screening test meeting these criteria is currently available. For this reason, many evaluations may be used in an attempt to determine the best medical management for the client.

Cervical Length. A short cervix (25 mm or less) measured by transvaginal ultrasound at 22 to 24 weeks gestation is associated with an increase in preterm birth. Although the pathologic process is not clearly understood, current evidence suggests it is not a weakness in cervical resistance to uterine contractions (Simhan & Romero, 2021). An updated meta-analysis and systematic review following and including the OPPTIMUM study (Norman et al., 2016) showed evidence of vaginal progesterone reducing the risk for both preterm birth and neonatal morbidity and mortality, when studying clients with a singleton gestation and a midtrimester cervical length of 25mm or less, without negative effects on neurodevelopmental outcome (Norman et al., 2016). The study recommends universal transvaginal cervical length screening be done at 18 to 24 weeks of gestation in clients with a singleton gestation and vaginal progesterone offered to those with a cervical length 25mm or less (Norman et al., 2016). However, ACOG (2020e) cautions the predictive value of a short

cervix as the only indicator of preterm labor is limited and recommends against its exclusive use to direct management of clients with symptoms of preterm labor.

Preterm Premature Rupture of Membranes in a Previous Birth. Some clients may have a predisposition to weak amniotic membrane structure which predates the actual leaking of fluid. This predisposition seems to repeat in subsequent pregnancies (Mercer & Chien, 2021).

Fetal Fibronectin. Fetal fibronectin (fFN) and PAMG-1 are present in the layers of the amniotic membrane. They are normally found in cervical and vaginal secretions until 16 to 20 weeks of gestation and again at or near term. If it appears too early, it suggests labor may begin early. Maternal or fetal infections may be present if the fFN or PAMG-1 are positive during midpregnancy. Cervical examination, recent sexual intercourse, and vaginal bleeding can result in a false-positive test when preterm labor is not truly present. To reduce false-positive results, the test specimen should be collected at least 24 hours after significant vaginal manipulation. Both the fFn test and PartoSure test, which tests PAMG-1, are available in the United States (Hologic, 2009). Predictability data on each were published by Varley-Campbell et al. (2019). ACOG (2020f) does not support the exclusive use of either PAMG-1 or fFN to solely direct the medical management of a client with preterm contractions.

Infections. Infections often increase the risk for preterm membrane rupture or birth, even if the client does not initially have clinical signs or symptoms with the preterm labor. A UTI is common with preterm labor, so catheterized or midstream urine is often obtained for urinalysis and for culture and sensitivity testing.

A client with an infection not related to pregnancy may seek care. Relevant testing may relate to acute gastrointestinal or respiratory tract infections that affect pregnant clients, as well as other people of both genders. More serious maternal infections may require cultures of maternal blood or respiratory tract or other secretions to determine the ideal treatment. Maternal pneumonia increases the risk for fetal or maternal death, as well as increasing the preterm birth risk. Other poor health conditions during pregnancy (such as crowded living conditions) or a chronic medical condition (such as asthma) may increase a client's risk for pneumonia as well (Roth, 2021).

Stopping Preterm Labor

Once the diagnosis of preterm labor is made, management focuses on stopping uterine activity. Preterm delivery may be inevitable, but steroid therapy promotes earlier fetal lung maturation. Particularly for very early gestations, such as 23 weeks, treatment may add enough time for the steroids to be effective. Even one more day of fetal maturation may make a great difference in the outcome for the very premature infant.

Initial Measures. The provider initially determines whether any maternal or fetal problems exist that contraindicate continuing the pregnancy. Some examples are maternal complications such as hypertension or hypotension, hypovolemia, hypoxemia, cardiac disease, and sepsis. Fetal problems needing prompt delivery may be demonstrated by persistent abnormal FHR patterns.

Initial measures to stop preterm labor include identifying and treating infections, identifying other causes of preterm labor that may be treatable, and reducing activity.

Identifying and Treating Infections. Infection, both systemic and local, has a strong association with preterm birth and PROM. However, it may be unclear whether various microorganisms found at diagnosis of preterm labor are significant if the membranes remain intact. Hematologic studies identify signs of infection and also conditions such as anemia that are associated with preterm labor or affect its management. Common studies include a complete blood cell count with differential white blood cell analysis and cultures for GBS, chlamydia, gonorrhea, or other suspected infections. **Amniocentesis** (transabdominal puncture of amniotic sac) may be done to obtain amniotic fluid for culture if Triple I is suspected, because this infection would contraindicate stopping preterm labor. Fetal lung maturity testing will likely be done on an amniotic fluid specimen as well (Simhan & Romero, 2021). Urinalysis with culture and sensitivity testing may be performed to determine whether treatment for a UTI is indicated.

Culture results require a minimum of 24 to 48 hours to complete; therefore, antibiotics that are effective against probable organisms are started as soon as the specimen is obtained. The medication can be changed if culture results indicate a different antibiotic would be more effective.

Prompt treatment of acute infections such as pyelonephritis improves maternal and fetal outcomes. Broad-spectrum antibiotics (e.g., ampicillin, penicillin) and an aminoglycoside (e.g., gentamicin), which are effective against many organisms, may be ordered. Medications such as clindamycin or metronidazole may be prescribed for a client who requires a cesarean birth and is at risk for infection from anaerobic organisms (Sloan et al., 2019).

Identifying Other Causes for Preterm Contractions. The client with polyhydramnios, identified by ultrasonography, may have preterm contractions because the uterine musculature is stretched more than normal. Therapeutic amniocentesis options include removal of some amniotic fluid to reduce uterine irritability and relieve maternal dyspnea. Multifetal gestations also can be identified by ultrasonography if not previously diagnosed. These clients may benefit from improved nutrition, stress reduction, assistance with household care, and other interventions.

Limiting Activity. Activity limits, usually by relaxing in the side-lying or semisitting position, increase placental blood flow and reduce fetal pressure on the cervix. However, lengthy and substantial activity restriction (e.g., complete bed rest) has not been shown to significantly prolong pregnancy (ACOG, 2020e). As in other individuals, activity restriction is associated with serious maternal side effects, some of which develop within as little as 24 hours. Adverse effects of substantial activity restriction during pregnancy may include the following:

- Muscle weakness, including aching, muscle atrophy, and bone loss

- Diuresis as the body tries to reduce the normally higher fluid level of pregnancy
- Poor nutrition as a result of appetite loss, lower food intake, and increased indigestion; weight loss or inadequate weight gain
- Orthostatic hypotension caused by the change in blood pressure regulation by baroreceptors
- Psychological effects such as increased stress about separation from family, anxiety about the pregnancy's outcome, depression, frustration from a decreased activity level and reduced contact with other people, and concerns about finances if the client's income is essential to the family
- Sleep changes as depression increases or usual activities that direct the sleep–wake cycles are not present

Because of the adverse effects and lack of benefits for most clients, bed rest is no longer routine. If necessary, individualized activity reductions may be prescribed. Changes may be relatively simple, such as a change in work hours or duties or finding ways to help the client meet the needs for their other children, for example, transportation to school or other activities. Several rest periods during the day may be prescribed. Positions for rest may include the semisitting position with the feet and legs elevated. If lying down for rest, a client's frequent change of the side-lying position reduces discomfort from the pressure of remaining on one side for a prolonged time.

Clients hospitalized for preterm labor may have greater activity restrictions. Ambulating to the bathroom may be limited because of maternal sedative effects from medications. If preterm labor stops, the client may walk to the restroom for showers, voiding, and bowel movements. If remaining hospitalized for longer term care, the client may have activity orders that include sitting in a chair periodically or taking occasional short trips to another area in a wheelchair with family or friends.

Whether the client is expected to be hospitalized briefly or for a longer time, the following services may improve client outcomes:

- Physical therapy to help maintain muscle strength and coordination and to reduce muscle aching, fatigue, and bone loss
- Recreational therapy to identify appropriate activities
- Occupational therapy to help the client cope physically with lifestyle changes, particularly if discharge home is anticipated
- Complementary therapy to reduce stressors and enhance physical care measures
- Social work to identify how needs such as financial and childcare can be met
- Consultation with a psychologist to help the client and family cope with the added stressors

Hydrating the Client. Hydration to stop preterm contractions has not been shown to be beneficial for all clients. High-volume IV infusions may cause maternal respiratory distress if tocolytic medications are also administered, especially if given in combination with steroids.

However, dehydration may contribute to uterine irritability for some clients. This is often the case in those who have had an infection such as an acute gastrointestinal infection, in which loss of fluid through diarrhea may exceed the nauseated client's ability to drink water or other fluids. Infections with maternal fever (temperature of 38°C [100.4°F] or greater) increase the client's metabolic rate and may result in dehydration. IV fluids are ordered according to their expected benefit. Oral fluids are usually encouraged because hydration may reduce uterine irritability and the risk for UTIs.

Tocolytics. Tocolytic medications have not demonstrated a decrease in the rate of preterm birth. However, they may successfully delay the birth of a preterm infant. Delay of preterm birth with tocolysis may provide time for the following (ACOG, 2020e; Simhan & Romero, 2021):

- Administration of maternal corticosteroids to reduce respiratory distress in the newborn
- Administration of antibiotics to prevent neonatal infection with GBS
- Transferring the client to a facility with a higher level neonatal intensive care unit (NICU)
- Administration of magnesium sulfate for neuroprotection of a fetus less than 32 weeks gestation

Tocolysis is considered appropriate for clients, 23 to 34 weeks gestation with regular uterine contractions and cervical change.

Because tocolytic drugs have significant side effects, the decision about whether to treat for preterm labor is individualized, based on risk factors, cervical dilation, and other signs and symptoms. EFM helps identify uterine contractions or irritability and establish fetal status. A PAMG-1 or fFN test may be done to determine whether the client is likely to deliver in the next 7 days. Ultrasound imaging provides information that may be useful to determine fetal age, adequacy of placental supply, and status of the cervix. Tests for infection are done if indicated.

Current tocolytic medications are used primarily for conditions other than preterm labor and therefore have effects on body systems other than the reproductive system. Risks and possible benefits of the medication chosen should be considered and communicated clearly to the client. The lowest possible dose that inhibits contractions is used. Four types of medications are used for tocolysis: (1) magnesium sulfate, (2) calcium antagonists, (3) prostaglandin synthesis inhibitors, and (4) beta-adrenergics. Table 16.1 summarizes doses and routes of administration for each of these drugs.

Magnesium sulfate. Magnesium sulfate is used in management of preeclampsia to prevent seizures and in the treatment of preterm labor. It causes smooth muscle relaxation, including quieting uterine activity, which may inhibit preterm labor. Magnesium sulfate therapy has a well-established record of safety during pregnancy. When given to suppress preterm labor, magnesium sulfate has side effects (such as lethargy and sedation) similar to those seen in its use to prevent seizures related to hypertension. ACOG Practice Bulletin 171: Management of Preterm Labor supports use of magnesium sulfate as a short-term tocolytic to provide for steroid therapy and for neonatal neuroprotection; long-term therapy is not supported (ACOG, 2020e).

Common assessment criteria for magnesium sulfate therapy include the following:

- Urine output of at least 30 milliliters per hour (mL/hr)
- Presence of deep tendon reflexes
- At least 12 breaths per minute

In addition, the nurse assesses heart and lung sounds frequently because fluid overload and electrolyte imbalances can lead to pulmonary edema or cardiac dysrhythmias. Oxygen saturations are often included with vital signs and other assessments. Bowel sounds are checked when therapy begins and every 4 to 8 hours because the smooth muscle in the intestinal tract may be relaxed just as the uterus is relaxed. Serum magnesium level measurements guide maintenance of therapeutic levels (4.8 to 8.4 milligrams per deciliter [mg/dL]). EFM identifies fetal effects such as reduced variability or a slight decrease in the baseline rate.

Calcium gluconate (10%) must be available to reverse magnesium toxicity and prevent respiratory arrest, which can occur if serum levels rise above 12 mg/dL. Excess serum levels of magnesium are less likely when the medication is given for preterm labor, compared with when it is given for preeclampsia, because the renal function of the client in preterm labor is usually normal. However, the nurse remains alert for this complication of magnesium sulfate therapy.

Calcium Antagonists. Nifedipine (Adalat, Procardia) is a calcium channel blocker usually given for hypertension. Calcium is essential for muscle contraction in smooth muscles such as the uterus, so blocking calcium reduces the muscular contraction. Flushing of the skin, headache, and a transient increase in the maternal and FHR are common side effects. Headache generally resolves in 48 hours. Nifedipine is a potent vasodilator that may cause postural hypotension.

The nurse observes for side effects of nifedipine and reports a maternal pulse rate greater than 120 bpm. The client is given information about possible dizziness or faintness with nifedipine's hypotensive effects. Encourage the client to sit or stand slowly and call for assistance, if needed.

Prostaglandin Synthesis Inhibitors. Because prostaglandins stimulate uterine contractions, medications can be used to inhibit their synthesis. Indomethacin (Indocin) and ibuprofen are the prostaglandin synthesis inhibitors most often used for tocolysis.

Maternal side effects are minimal because of the brief duration of therapy. Gastrointestinal side effects are usually limited to nausea, vomiting, and heartburn. The nurse observes the client for gastrointestinal side effects. Because indomethacin and ibuprofen can prolong bleeding time, the nurse observes for abnormal bleeding such as prolonged bleeding after injections and bruising with no apparent cause. The antiinflammatory effect of these medications can mask infection.

Fetal adverse effects are more serious and may include constriction of the ductus arteriosus, pulmonary hypertension, and oligohydramnios. The ductus arteriosus remains open before birth and will close 12 to 48 hours after birth. Fetal adverse effects of prostaglandin synthesis inhibitors are unlikely if treatment is no longer than 48 to 72 hours and

TABLE 16.1 Drugs Used in Preterm Labor

Drug and Purpose	Common Dose Regimens*	Side or Adverse Effects
Magnesium sulfate (use as tocolytic) Therapeutic range: 4.8–8.4 mEq/L. ~10 mEq/L = Depression of DTRs ~12 mEq/L = Respiratory depression ~18 mEq/L = Cardiac depression	IV: Loading dose: 4–6 g over 20–30 min Maintenance dose for tocolysis: 1–3 g/hr When contraction frequency is no higher than 1 per 10 min (≤6 per hr), maintain infusion rate for 12–48 hr, then discontinue drug.	Side- and adverse effects are dose-related, occurring at higher maternal serum levels. Depression of DTRs, may be present Respiratory or cardiac depression if serum levels are high; greatest risk is in client with poor urinary elimination of drug Less serious side effects: Lethargy, weakness, visual blurring, headache, hot flashes, nausea, vomiting, constipation Fetal–neonatal effects: Reduced FHR variability in the first 24 hr, labor dystocia
Nifedipine (Procardia), nicardipine (Cardene) (calcium channel blockers for tocolysis)	Oral loading dose: 10–20 mg Continued oral therapy (if needed): 10–20 mg every 3–6 hr for a maximum of 72 hours	Maternal flushing, dizziness, headache, nausea Transient maternal tachycardia Mild hypotension Modest increases in blood glucose levels
Indomethacin (Indocin), sulindac (Clinoril) and ibuprofen (prostaglandin synthesis inhibitors - NSAIDS)	Limit use to preterm labor before 32 wk of gestation. Use indomethacin for no longer than 48–72 consecutive hr. Indocin: Loading dose: 50 mg (oral) Maintenance dose: 25 mg orally every 6 hr for 48 hr Ibuprofen: 600 mg (oral) every 6 hr (used ≤32 wk gestation) Ultrasound examinations and fetal echocardiography help determine whether maternal indomethacin has adverse effects on the fetus.	Epigastric pain, nausea, gastrointestinal bleeding Asthma in aspirin-sensitive client Increased BP in hypertensive client Fetus: Adverse fetal effects may include constriction of ductus arteriosus, particularly if client receives indomethacin for more than 48–72 hr and gestation is later than 32 wk; impairs fetal renal function, which may reduce volume of amniotic fluid and result in cord compression.
Terbutaline (beta-adrenergic for tocolysis); should not be used beyond 48–72 hr for preterm labor	Subcutaneous (most common parenteral route): Intermittent injections, 0.25 mg, initially every 20–30 min × 3, followed by rescue doses only.	Terbutaline is not approved by the FDA for inhibiting uterine activity and now carries a *boxed warning and contraindications* ("black box") against use as a tocolytic rather than its intended use as a bronchodilator. Dose may be held if maternal pulse rate exceeds 120 bpm or systolic BP falls below 80–90 mm Hg or FHR <180. Adverse reactions: 1. Cardiovascular: Maternal and fetal tachycardia, palpitations, cardiac dysrhythmias, chest pain, wide pulse pressure 2. Respiratory: Dyspnea, chest discomfort 3. Central nervous system: Tremors, restlessness, weakness, dizziness, headache 4. Metabolic: Hypokalemia, hyperglycemia 5. Gastrointestinal: Nausea, vomiting, reduced bowel motility 6. Skin: Flushing, diaphoresis
Betamethasone and dexamethasone (corticosteroids)	See Drug Guide: Betamethasone, Dexamethasone (p. 456)	
Makena (17-P alpha-hydroxyprogesterone caproate)	IM: 250 mg (1 mL) every 7 days Begin treatment between $16^{0/7}$ wks and $20^{6/7}$ wks Continue until 37 wks or delivery	Drug is a progestin indicated to reduce the risk for preterm birth in a client who had a previous preterm birth; not intended for clients with multiple gestation or other risk factors for preterm birth.

BP, blood pressure; *bpm*, beats per minute; *DTRs*, deep tendon reflexes; *FDA*, U.S. Food and Drug Administration; *FHR*, fetal heart rate; *IM*, intramuscularly; *IV*, intravenously; *NSAIDs*, nonsteroidal antiinflammatory drugs.
*Doses and frequency of administration are examples; actual protocols may vary.
Source: Data from American Academy of Pediatrics & American College of Obstetricians and Gynecologists (AAP & ACOG). (2017). *Guidelines for perinatal care* (8th ed.). Authors; Simhan, H.N. & Romero, R. (2021). Preterm labor and birth. In M. Landon, H. Galan, E. Jauniaux, D. Driscoll, V. Berghella, W. Grobman, S. Kilpatrick, & A. Cahill (Eds.). *Gabbe's obstetrics: Normal and problem pregnancies* (8th ed., pp. 663-693). Elsevier; and U.S. Food and Drug Administration (FDA). (2011). FDA drug safety communication: new warnings against use of terbutaline to treat preterm labor. http://www.fda.gov.

the gestation is less than 32 weeks. Amniotic fluid levels are monitored and the medication stopped if volume is trending downward. The amniotic fluid volume usually returns to its previous level when treatment is discontinued. Regular ultrasound examinations and fetal echocardiography help determine whether the medication is having adverse effects on the fetus. Decreased fetal movements and absent FHR accelerations with fetal movement may occur if the fetal condition deteriorates. After birth, assessment of the infant may be performed for other complications such as pulmonary hypertension or intracranial hemorrhage, depending on the duration of treatment and the infant's gestation.

Beta-adrenergic Drugs. Terbutaline (Brethine), a bronchodilator, is the most frequently used beta-adrenergic for treatment of preterm labor. It is used to delay preterm birth to allow administration of corticosteroids and antibiotics (approximately 48 hours).

The main side effects for beta-adrenergic drugs, including terbutaline, involve the cardiorespiratory system. Maternal and fetal tachycardia are common (see Table 16.1). Propranolol (Inderal), an agent that blocks beta-adrenergic drugs, is used to reverse severe adverse effects.

Because of reported cardiovascular events, terbutaline now carries a *boxed warning and contraindications* ("black box") against prolonged parenteral use for more than 48 to 72 hours and for use of oral terbutaline for treatment of preterm labor. (See www.fda.gov for the FDA drug safety report.)

The nurse assesses a client's apical heart rate and lung sounds before administering each intermittent dose of terbutaline. A maternal heart rate over 120 bpm or respiratory findings such as "wet" lung sounds or tachypnea, possibly accompanied by shortness of breath, suggest drug toxicity and may be a reason to discontinue terbutaline. Abnormal maternal and fetal assessments are promptly reported to the physician.

Accelerating Fetal Lung Maturity

ACOG (2020a) recommends administration of a single course of corticosteroids to pregnant clients, 24 to 34 weeks gestation who are at risk of preterm birth within 7 days. It may be administered as early as 22–23 weeks gestation, based on the family's decisions regarding resuscitation of an extremely preterm newborn. Administration of a single course may also be considered for a client at risk of preterm birth within 7 days who is between 34 and 37 weeks gestation. Steroid therapy may reduce the incidence and severity of RDS and intraventricular hemorrhage in the preterm infant (ACOG, 2020a). Betamethasone (Celestone) or dexamethasone (Decadron) may be used for this purpose (ACOG, 2020a).

Corticosteroids are indicated if the gestation period is between 24 and 34 weeks due to the high incidence of problems such as RDS that affect an infant born at this gestation. Delay of preterm birth for at least 24 hours after initiation of corticosteroid therapy provides the greatest benefit in reducing the incidence and severity of RDS associated with prematurity. One indication for tocolytic therapy is to delay preterm birth to allow the fetus to receive the benefits of the

DRUG GUIDE
Betamethasone and Dexamethasone

Classification
Corticosteroids.

Indications
Acceleration of fetal lung maturity to reduce the incidence and severity of respiratory distress syndrome. Studies suggest antenatal steroids can reduce the incidence of intraventricular hemorrhage and neonatal death in the preterm infant. Greatest benefits accrue if at least 24 hours elapses between the initial dose and birth of the preterm infant, but the medication is indicated if birth is not imminent.

Dosage and Route
Betamethasone: 12 mg intramuscularly (IM) for two doses, 24 hours apart.
  Dexamethasone: 6 mg IM every 12 hours for four doses.

Absorption
Rapid and complete after IM administration.

Excretion
Metabolized in the liver. Excreted in urine.

Contraindications
Active infection such as Triple I is a relative contraindication. ACOG (2020a) recommends use of corticosteroids for the client who has preterm rupture of the membranes (24 to 34 weeks of gestation).

Precautions
Possible infection. Pregnancies complicated by diabetes.

Adverse Reactions
Few, owing to the short-term use of the medication. Pulmonary edema is possible secondary to sodium and fluid retention.

Nursing Considerations
Explain to the client the potential benefits of corticosteroid administration for the preterm neonate. Explain the medication cannot prevent or lessen the severity of all complications of prematurity. If the client has diabetes, explain more frequent blood glucose assessments are common because these levels are often elevated for up to 7 to 10 days after taking either of the corticosteroids. A temporary rise in platelet and WBC levels may last 72 hours. WBC levels greater than 20,000/mm^3 may indicate infection. Assess lung sounds. Report chest pain or heaviness or dyspnea.

corticosteroid. Evidence shows an infant born sooner than 24 hours after administration of corticosteroid may have some fetal lung maturation benefits. Concerns regarding the probability of delaying the birth should not prevent administration of corticosteroids.

Vital signs are assessed to identify fever and elevated pulse rate that may indicate infection. Lung sounds are assessed with vital signs because corticosteroids can cause sodium retention with accompanying fluid retention and pulmonary edema. The nurse observes for symptoms of pulmonary edema. The client is taught to report any chest pain, heaviness, or any difficulty breathing because these symptoms could indicate pulmonary edema.

Neuroprotection

Neonatal complications of preterm birth include neurologic problems such as cerebral palsy (CP). Current evidence supports the administration of magnesium sulfate to the client before birth to decrease this risk. The ACOG and the Society for Maternal Fetal Medicine (SMFM) recommend its use for pregnant clients less than 32 weeks gestation and with anticipated preterm birth (ACOG, 2020c). Protocols for the administration of magnesium sulfate for fetal neuroprotection are similar to protocols for its use in preeclampsia or as a tocolytic agent (Parfitt, 2021; Sinham & Romero, 2021).

Periviable Birth

The ACOG and SMFM Obstetric Care Consensus No. 4 (2019b) addresses "periviable birth," which is defined as birth at $20^{0/7}$ weeks to $25^{6/7}$ weeks gestation. Prenatal and postnatal counseling regarding the anticipated neonatal outcome based on the specific circumstances of each client should be provided. If the family desires resuscitative efforts of a periviable neonate, management strategies may include "short-term tocolytic therapy to allow time for administration of antenatal steroids, antibiotics to prolong latency after preterm premature rupture of membranes or for intrapartum group B streptococci (GBS) prophylaxis, and delivery, including cesarean delivery, for concern regarding fetal well-being or fetal malpresentation" (ACOG, 2019b, p. 1). If birth of a periviable neonate is anticipated, administration of magnesium sulfate for fetal neuroprotection is supported. It is recommended periviable births occur in hospitals with expertise and support services for high-risk maternal and neonatal care (ACOG, 2019b).

> **❓ KNOWLEDGE CHECK**
>
> 14. What symptoms of preterm labor should be taught to clients at risk?
> 15. Why is it important to identify preterm labor early?
> 16. What four classifications of drugs may be used to stop preterm labor contractions?
> 17. What is the purpose of giving corticosteroids to a client who is in preterm labor at 27 weeks of gestation? Why is it important for birth to be delayed at least 24 hours?

APPLICATION OF THE NURSING PROCESS: PRETERM LABOR

Nursing care for the client experiencing preterm labor often includes interventions related to tocolytic, corticosteroid, or antibiotic drug therapy. If labor cannot be halted, care is similar to other laboring clients, with additional care to prepare for a preterm infant's needs at birth. Support for anticipatory grieving may be needed if the infant has lethal fetal anomalies or is very immature and not expected to live.

Care for the family when an extremely preterm infant (~20–24 weeks of gestation) is expected to be born can be heavily laden with ethical and legal issues. For example, what is the true accuracy of the gestational age? Has a corticosteroid to accelerate fetal lung maturity been administered? Has magnesium sulfate been administered for neuroprotection? Abnormal fetal monitoring patterns in the very immature fetus can distress parents and caregivers alike. However, knowledge of the fetal response to labor helps the neonatologist make better decisions about how to treat the infant. In addition, ultrasound estimates of gestational age at this time have shown considerable variations. A fetus presumed to be 23 weeks of gestation before birth may be assessed to be 25 weeks or older after birth and suited to more intense treatment than planned, especially if the client had no prenatal care before entering the hospital.

Much of the general nursing care for a client having preterm labor also applies to clients experiencing other types of high-risk pregnancies. Clients may need multiple hospitalizations which occur unexpectedly, disrupting family routines. Other clients may have attended a routine prenatal visit and be shocked to discover they may be in preterm labor. These clients often have some activity modifications and may have to stop working if the best outcome for their pregnancy is to be achieved. This section focuses on the family's psychosocial concerns, management of home care, and the client's activity limitations.

PSYCHOSOCIAL CONCERNS

Assessment

The entire family is affected by stressors associated with a high-risk pregnancy. Assess how the client and their family usually cope with crisis situations and how they are coping with this one. Identify their greatest concerns to prioritize care. For example, the nurse might say, "This development in your pregnancy must have been a shock." The following are other questions the nurse might ask: "How are you handling things?" "In what ways do you usually handle crisis situations in your family?" "What concerns you the most right now?" Rather than asking questions in a rapid-fire manner, the nurse gives the client time to answer assessment questions because stress may have narrowed their focus.

The client or their family may have physical, emotional, and cognitive impairments because of the unexpected problems. Physical signs of emotional distress such as tremulousness, palpitations, and restlessness also are side effects of beta-adrenergic drugs and corticosteroids. The client may express fear, helplessness, or disbelief. They may be irritable and tearful. Their ability to concentrate may be impaired at a time when new information needs to be absorbed.

The partner may feel like they are losing control. They struggle to keep the household running if the client decreases their activity level. Young children recognize their parents' anxiety and may misbehave or regress. They may feel abandoned if they must be temporarily placed with relatives or friends.

The client may need to stop working, straining family finances. If they do not have sick time or other benefits, the family sustains an abrupt drop in income at a time when medical expenses are mounting. The client may be transferred to a tertiary care referral center with a higher level NICU and maternity care. The increased distance from home can make it more challenging to receive support from friends, family, or support groups.

In addition to the sudden change in lifestyle is the family's concern for their baby's well-being. A client may feel pulled in many directions by the needs of all the children—those already born and those of the current pregnancy. Clients may be concerned about the effects of medication therapy on the fetus and their own body.

Identification of Client Problems

Unexpected development of complications during pregnancy can prevent a client and family from using their normal coping mechanisms. The problem selected for the client and family is apprehension due to the uncertain outcome of the pregnancy, disruption of relationships with family and friends, and financial concerns.

Planning: Expected Outcomes

The outcome of any pregnancy is never certain, especially when the pregnancy is a high-risk one. Goals and expected outcomes focus on the family's ability to cope with the crisis of preterm labor. The appropriate goal is:

- The client and family will identify one or more constructive method to cope with this temporary disruption in their lives.

Interventions
Providing Information

Knowledge decreases anxiety and fear related to the unknown. Include appropriate family members so they are more likely to be supportive. Appropriate family members may include the client's partner or in-laws, adult siblings, and others, but this may vary according to culture. Determine the extent of the client's knowledge about preterm birth and the specific therapy recommended. Determine what information the parents need about problems a preterm infant may face. Use this opportunity to correct misinformation and reinforce accurate information.

Initially, the client for whom activity modification is prescribed may be highly motivated. Contractions often diminish, even if for only a short time, making the client restless. They may question the need for any activity restriction. Explain what is currently known about the benefits of activity modification for the pregnancy complication and assure the client recommendations to restrict activity often lessen as the pregnancy progresses. Initiate consultations from caregivers such as physical, occupational, and recreational therapists; social workers; and other professionals whose services might benefit the client.

The Sidelines National Support Network (www.sidelines. org) is an online network of local groups across the country for clients experiencing high-risk pregnancy, including the risk for preterm birth. The site has information for clients "sidelined" by pregnancy complications, including articles, information about reimbursement from insurance, and contact via e-mail with others who have been "sidelined."

Promoting Expression of Concerns

Encourage the client and family to express their concerns. Begin by exploring common concerns of clients with problem pregnancies. For example, "Most clients are worried when they must adjust their work schedules. How has this affected your family?" An open-ended question gives the client and family a chance to express their feelings so they can take the next step—identifying constructive methods to cope with the situation. Collaboration with a social worker may identify financial or other community resources available. Offer chaplain services for support.

Teaching What May Occur During a Preterm Birth

Because preterm birth often occurs despite all interventions, a pregnant client and partner should be prepared for this possibility. If the hospital has a NICU, a nurse often visits the parents to explain what might occur if their baby is born early. One or both parents may tour the unit to see the equipment and care given to preterm infants.

In hospitals with NICUs, one or more neonatal nurses, a neonatal or pediatric nurse practitioner, a neonatologist, or a combination of these are present at birth to care for the infant. The client who has planned to give birth in a hospital without a NICU may be transferred to a facility with this type of unit before the birth to allow immediate care and stabilization of the newborn. The infant also may be transferred after birth if there is no time to transfer the client before birth or if the infant has more problems than were anticipated. Hospitalization of the client, infant, or both at a distant location adds to the stress on the family and can impair the attachment process.

Evaluation

The expected outcome for this client problem is achieved if the client and family can identify one or more constructive methods to deal with their anxiety. This outcome is assessed throughout pregnancy. If the goal is not met, the nurse provides additional support and reviews other coping strategies as appropriate.

MANAGEMENT OF HOME CARE
Assessment

Care of clients with high-risk pregnancies may be managed in the hospital or in their homes if the gestation is sufficiently advanced and the signs and symptoms of preterm labor and birth have diminished significantly. Many daily household activities are managed by the client, even if only by giving directions to others. However, when labor complications become greater, family roles are again disrupted because of the changed relationships among family members. Multiple professionals are likely to be involved in home care, including home care nurses and assistants, social workers, therapists (physical, occupational), and others.

Clarify the level of activity prescribed by the provider and identify the role of each member of the household. A good way to do this is to have the client describe a usual day before any limitations were recommended. Determine the number and ages of children in the home.

Evaluate the home itself, either by visual inspection or by questioning the family. Does the home or apartment have more than one level? Determine whether a telephone is available for emergency contact. If the client works, is working online a possibility?

Evaluate the family's resources and their willingness to use them. Ask whether family members and friends in the area are available to help. Explore local support groups such as churches or parent networks the family might contact for assistance. Determine financial reimbursement which may be available through insurance coverage.

Identification of Client Problems

Activity limitations for the client may require adjustment in roles and responsibilities of all members of the family resulting in possible changes in the home environment because of altered roles and responsibilities.

Planning: Expected Outcomes

Two goals and expected outcomes are appropriate for this client problem. The short-term goal may change over time if the client remains pregnant.
- Short-term goal—The family will identify methods for management of daily household routines.
- Long-term goal—The client will be able to maintain the prescribed levels of activity and drug therapy.

Interventions

The pregnancy threatened by preterm labor or other complications that require activity modification is a self-limiting situation, making temporary adjustments somewhat easier. Needed changes in home routines may be brief but sometimes extend over several weeks. Even if the restriction consists only of added rest periods during the day, the client still is unable to fulfill all the usual roles. For the client who is prescribed more restricted activity, the disruptions are greater.

Caring for Children

The client with children has different concerns from the client without children. Toddlers and preschoolers rarely understand why their parent does not play with them as usual. If they already are in daycare, this can continue if the family can afford it. They may temporarily live with a relative or friend. Toddlers may feel their parents have abandoned them if they are sent away, although this may be the only realistic solution if no one except the client is available to supervise them.

School-age children can understand the situation better and often are quite helpful. They may assist with care of other children, but they should not be put into the role of an adult. They may resent responsibility that is excessive for their age.

School-age children often enjoy learning new facts about their client's pregnancy and tests the baby may need.

Adolescents may welcome their parents' trust but also resent the intrusion on independent activities with their peers. Teenagers who drive can be very helpful in taking younger siblings to school and other activities. They may be enlisted for grocery shopping and meal preparation. If resentment flares, remind them the situation is temporary, and they are valuable contributors to the health of the new baby.

Maintaining the Household

The first step to household maintenance during this time may be for the client to lower the housekeeping standards. The partner may take over some household tasks, but these may compete with responsibilities outside the home. Talk to the client about prioritizing the health of the fetus and letting household chores go unfinished if necessary.

Advise the client to have a list of tasks ready when friends and family ask, "Can I do anything to help?" If they offer to bring a meal or do laundry, encourage acceptance of this help. Remind the client, people who offer to help mean it and the opportunity to return the favor may occur later. Homemaker services may be an option to help the family deal with the client's temporary disability.

Transportation of school-aged children may be a concern. If no family or friends are available, the school nurse or the Parent–Teacher Association may help find someone willing to take the children to school each day.

Evaluation

Identification of short-term goals and expected outcomes helps the nurse, client, and the family identify resolution of immediate needs like managing household care. Longer term outcomes may be evaluated over a series of days or weeks as the prescribed therapy for the complicated pregnancy changes.

POSTTERM PREGNANCY

The normal length of a pregnancy is 40 to $41^{0/7}$ weeks, with full term being regarded as delivery between weeks $39^{0/7}$ to $40^{6/7}$ weeks (ACOG, 2017a; Cunningham et al., 2022). The late-term pregnancy is defined as the period between $41^{0/7}$ weeks and $41^{6/7}$ weeks (ACOG, 2017a; Cunningham et al., 2022). A postterm pregnancy is one that lasts longer than $42^{0/7}$ weeks (ACOG, 2017a, 2020c; Cunningham et al, 2022). Most clients in the United States who receive prenatal care and have reliable dates are induced before 42 weeks gestation. Average gestational age at term birth is now 39 weeks rather than 40 weeks. Some apparent cases of prolonged pregnancy are actually miscalculations of the estimated due date (EDD) because the client has irregular menstrual periods or forgot the date of the last normal period. Late or no prenatal care limits the accuracy of clinical methods such as ultrasound for determining EDD and avoiding potential problems associated with prolonged gestation. Although clients are encouraged to allow their babies to develop as much as possible, there are risks to the baby that can occur if a pregnancy goes past 42 weeks.

Complications

The greatest physical risk in prolonged pregnancy is to the fetus or newborn. Insufficiency of the placental function secondary to aging and infarction reduces transfer of oxygen and nutrients to the fetus and removal of waste. The fetus with placental insufficiency has less reserve to tolerate uterine contractions, and signs of fetal compromise such as late decelerations and minimal to absent variability may develop during labor. In addition, reduced amniotic fluid volume (oligohydramnios) that often accompanies placental insufficiency can result in umbilical cord compression. The infant may have late growth restriction and appear to have lost weight, with a normal-size head and thin body. **Meconium aspiration syndrome** caused by the aspiration of meconium in the amniotic fluid before or during birth may result in respiratory distress in the newborn.

Many postterm fetuses do not suffer from placental insufficiency and may continue growing. If the fetus becomes large, the client and fetus then may have complications related to dysfunctional labor, increased shoulder dystocia risk, increased risk of operative vaginal delivery, inadequate postpartum uterine contraction to control bleeding, and lacerations or infections (ACOG, 2020d). Although the absolute risk for stillbirth and neonatal mortality in postterm pregnancy is low, late-term and postterm pregnancies have an increase in fetal mortality after 41 weeks of gestation compared with 40 weeks of gestation (ACOG, 2020d).

Psychologically, the client often feels as though the pregnancy will never end. The added fatigue imposed by a pregnancy that extends significantly beyond the due date diminishes the client's resources for tolerating the added stress and anxiety about labor and birth.

Therapeutic Management

If the client has no prenatal care or receives care late in pregnancy, therapeutic management begins by determining the gestation as accurately as possible. Several markers used to determine gestation, such as ultrasound examination, fundal height measurements, dates of quickening, and first identification of fetal heart tones, may be less accurate or lost if a client begins prenatal care very late. Also, the client may have forgotten the date of the last menstrual period or may have irregular menstrual cycles.

Another factor in management decisions is whether the fetus is thriving in the uterus. If antepartum tests such as a biophysical profile indicate the fetus is doing well and placental function is not diminished, the provider can take a more conservative approach and allow labor to begin naturally. According to the Cochrane review, data are insufficient to define the optimal type or frequency of antepartum testing (ACOG, 2021a).

Clients are at risk for oligohydramnios with late-term and postterm pregnancies. Oligohydramnios is defined as an amniotic fluid index of 5 cm or less or a single deep pocket of amniotic fluid of 2 cm or less on ultrasound. With decreased amniotic fluid, the risk for stillbirth is increased. Additionally, there is an increased rate of meconium-stained fluid and FHR abnormalities such as decelerations and bradycardia associated with oligohydramnios (ACOG, 2020d)

If the gestation appears to be truly postterm, induction is usually indicated as a result of an increased risk for perinatal morbidity and mortality (ACOG, 2020d). Many providers may choose to perform membrane sweeping to begin the process of labor. Membrane sweeping or "stripping of membranes" involves the provider digitally separating the membranes from the lower uterine segment when the cervix is dilated. According to the Cochrane review, stripping of membranes was associated with significant reductions in the number of pregnancies that progressed beyond 41 weeks of gestation (ACOG, 2020d; Finucane et al., 2020).

Nursing Considerations

Nursing care for the client with a prolonged pregnancy is tied to the medical management. The nurse's role may include the following:

- Teaching the client about antepartum testing to include fetal movement counting
- Supporting the client's psychological and physical fatigue
- Providing nursing care related to specific procedures such as induction of labor

> ### ❓ KNOWLEDGE CHECK
>
> 18. What are three risks to the fetus or neonate when pregnancy lasts longer than 42 weeks?

INTRAPARTUM EMERGENCIES

Placental Abnormalities

Clients with placental abnormalities may experience hemorrhage during the antepartum or intrapartum period. Placental abnormalities include placenta accreta, placenta increta, or placenta percreta. It is unknown as to why the placenta embeds into the uterine tissue as deep as it does, but the theory is a defective decidua basalis. The strongest risk for abnormal placentation is prior uterine surgery, usually one or more cesarean births. Additional risk factors include smoking, advanced maternal age, artificial reproductive technology, dilation and curettage or other minor surgical procedures, and a short interconceptional period (ACOG, 2021c; Salera-Vieira, 2021). Abnormal placentation may cause intrapartum hemorrhage, or hemorrhage may occur after birth because the placenta does not separate cleanly, often leaving small fragments that prevent full uterine contraction. Placenta accreta occurs when the placenta is implanted into the uterine wall (ACOG, 2021c). All or part of the placenta may be involved. Placenta increta occurs when the chorionic villi invade the myometrium (ACOG, 2021c). Placenta percreta is described as complete perforation through the uterine musculature and onto the adjacent organs such as the bladder (ACOG, 2021c).

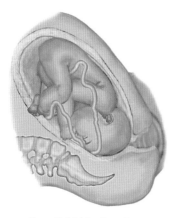

Occult (hidden) prolapse

The cord is compressed between the fetal presenting part and pelvis but cannot be seen or felt during vaginal examination.

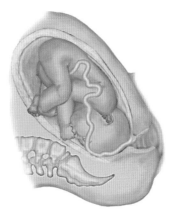

Cord prolapsed in front of the fetal head

The cord cannot be seen but can probably be felt as a pulsating mass during vaginal examination.

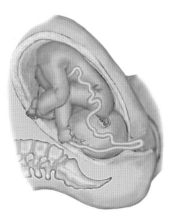

Complete cord prolapse

The cord can be seen protruding from the vagina.

FIG. 16.6 Variations of prolapsed umbilical cord.

A hysterectomy may be required if a large portion of the placenta is abnormally adherent (Foley et al., 2018; Jauniaux et al., 2021). An ultrasound evaluation to determine placental location and rule out an implantation abnormality is useful for a pregnant client with a history of a previous cesarean birth. If placental adherence is suspected, magnetic resonance imaging is recommended to further determine the extent of placental abnormality. Multidisciplinary planning for delivery is crucial and involves the obstetrician, perinatologist, interventional radiologist, urologist, and neonatologist. In addition, gynecologic oncologists or a general surgeon may need to be available at delivery. The average blood loss at delivery can be significant, ranging from 3000 to 5000 mL. It is important to have blood products and clotting factors on hold in the blood bank for use in the operating room. An additional IV line is usually started for emergency use. Clients who are diagnosed with placental abnormalities are at an increased risk for maternal mortality, reported as high as 7% (ACOG, 2021c).

Prolapsed Umbilical Cord

A **prolapsed umbilical cord (prolapsed cord)** slips downward after the membranes rupture, subjecting it to compression between the fetus and pelvis (Fig. 16.6). It may slip down immediately with the fluid gush or long after the membranes rupture. Interruption in blood flow through the cord interferes with fetal oxygenation and is potentially fatal for the fetus.

Causes

Prolapse of the umbilical cord is more likely when the fit is poor between the fetal presenting part and the maternal pelvis. When the fit is good, the fetus fills the pelvis, leaving little room for the cord to slip down. Although prolapse of the cord is possible during any labor, it is more likely if the following conditions are present:
- High fetal station

- Very small or preterm fetus
- Breech presentations (the footling breech is more likely to be complicated by a prolapsed cord because the feet and legs are small and do not fill the pelvis well)
- Transverse lie
- Polyhydramnios (often associated with abnormal presentations; also, the unusually large amount of fluid exerts more pressure to push the cord out)

Signs of Prolapse

Prolapse may be complete, with the cord visible at the vaginal opening, or it may not be visible but may be palpated on vaginal examination as it pulsates synchronously with the fetal heart. An **occult prolapse** of the cord is one in which the cord slips alongside the fetal head or shoulders. The prolapse cannot be seen and may not be palpated but is suspected because of changes in the FHR, such as sustained bradycardia, variable decelerations or prolonged decelerations.

Therapeutic Management

Medical and nursing management often overlap, as they do in many emergency situations. Either the nurse or the provider may be the first to discover umbilical cord prolapse. Birth is almost always cesarean unless vaginal delivery can be accomplished more quickly and less traumatically. If fetal death has occurred, usually before client arrival, management will focus on the best care for the client based on other complications.

When cord prolapse occurs, the priority is to relieve pressure on the cord to improve umbilical blood flow until delivery. Interventions should not delay the prompt delivery of a living fetus. Have someone push the call light to summon help. Other nurses can call the physician and prepare for birth while the nurse caring for the client relieves pressure on the cord vaginally if the provider is not doing so. Neonatal nurses and a pediatrician or neonatologist are notified, and the staff prepares for neonatal resuscitation.

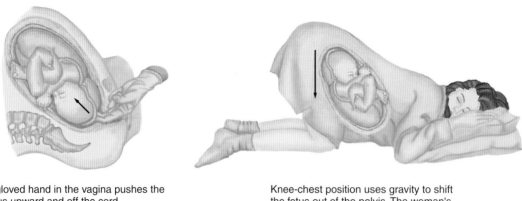

A gloved hand in the vagina pushes the fetus upward and off the cord.

Knee-chest position uses gravity to shift the fetus out of the pelvis. The woman's thighs should be at right angles to the bed and her chest flat on the bed.

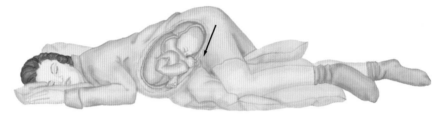

The woman's hips are elevated with two pillows; this is often combined with the Trendelenburg (head down) position.

FIG. 16.7 Measures that may be used to relieve pressure on a prolapsed umbilical cord until delivery can take place.

Prompt actions reduce cord compression and increase fetal oxygenation:
- Position the client's hips higher than their head to shift the fetal presenting part toward the diaphragm. Any of these methods (Fig. 16.7) may be used:
  - Knee–chest position
  - Trendelenburg position
  - Hips elevated with pillows, with side-lying position maintained
- Maintain vaginal elevation of the presenting part using a gloved hand while the client is transferred to the operating room (OR) until the physician orders cessation of vaginal elevation. Minimize cord compression from the hand that is elevating the presenting part as much as possible during the client's transport to the OR.
- Avoid or minimize manual palpation or handling of the cord as much as possible to minimize cord vessel vasospasm.
- Ultrasound examination may be used to confirm presence of fetal heart activity before cesarean delivery.

While preparing for surgery, consider giving the client oxygen at 10 liters per minute (L/min) by face mask to increase maternal blood oxygen saturation, making more available for the fetus.

Other actions may be used to enhance fetal oxygenation, but prompt delivery is the priority. A tocolytic drug such as terbutaline inhibits contractions, increasing placental blood flow and reducing intermittent pressure of the fetus against the pelvis and cord.

Prognosis for the client is good because the only additional risks are those associated with cesarean birth. Prognosis for the infant depends on how long and how severely blood flow through the cord has been impaired. With prompt recognition and corrective actions, the infant usually does well.

Nursing Considerations

In addition to taking prompt corrective actions, the nurse considers the client's anxiety. The nurse remains calm while working quickly during this time and acknowledges the client's anxiety. Explanations are simple because anxiety interferes with the client's ability to comprehend them. The partner and family are included as much as possible.

Uterine Rupture

Sometimes a tear in the wall of the uterus occurs because the uterus cannot withstand the pressure against it (Fig. 16.8). Uterine rupture may occur at home rather than in the hospital. Uterine rupture may precede labor's onset. Three variations of uterine rupture exist:
- *Complete rupture* is a direct communication between the uterine and peritoneal cavities.
- *Incomplete rupture* is a rupture into the peritoneum lining of the uterus or into the broad ligament but not the peritoneal cavity.
- *Dehiscence* is a partial separation of an old uterine scar. Little or no bleeding may occur. No signs or symptoms may exist, and the rupture ("window") may be found

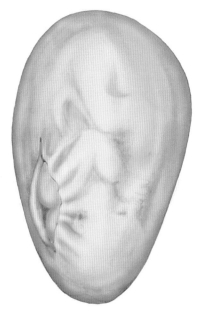

FIG. 16.8 Uterine rupture in the lower uterine segment.

incidentally during a subsequent cesarean birth or other abdominal surgery.

Causes

Uterine rupture is rare and is usually associated with previous uterine surgery such as cesarean birth or surgery to remove fibroids. However, there have been incidences of uterine rupture on an unscarred uterus. The risk for rupture in a client who has had a prior cesarean birth depends on the type of uterine incision. The risk for rupture is greater in clients with a classic uterine incision (vertical into the upper uterine segment) than in clients with a low transverse incision. For this reason, vaginal birth after cesarean (VBAC) is not recommended for clients who have had a previous birth through a classic cesarean incision (see Fig. 15.14 [types of uterine incisions]). The decision to attempt a trial of labor after cesarean (TOLAC) is made by the client and provider after discussion of the benefits, as well as potential problems associated with VBAC (Foley et al., 2018; Landon & Grobman, 2021).

Rupture of the unscarred uterus is more likely for clients of high parity with a thin uterine wall, clients sustaining blunt abdominal trauma, and those having intense contractions, especially if fetopelvic disproportion is present. Excessively strong contractions may cause the intrauterine pressure to exceed the tensile strength of the uterine wall. If the fetus cannot be expelled downward through the pelvis, contractions may push it through the lower uterine segment. Intense contractions are more likely to occur when uterine stimulants such as oxytocin and misoprostol are administered for induction or augmentation of labor, but they also may occur spontaneously.

Signs and Symptoms

Dehiscence does not have symptoms initially and may not interfere with labor or vaginal birth if the area is small. However, labor progress may stop because the open area prevents efficient expulsion of the fetus. Intrauterine pressures may have little change during contractions. A larger area of dehiscence may cause abdominal pain that persists despite analgesia.

Manifestations of uterine rupture vary with the degree of rupture and may mimic other complications. Possible signs and symptoms of uterine rupture are as follows:

- Abdominal pain and tenderness—The pain may not be severe; it may occur suddenly at the peak of a contraction. The client may say they felt something "gave way" or "ripped." This may be blunted if the client has epidural analgesia.
- Chest or shoulder pain, pain between the scapulae, or pain on inspiration—Pain occurs because of the irritation of blood below the client's diaphragm.
- Hypovolemic shock caused by hemorrhage—Tachycardia, tachypnea, falling blood pressure, pallor, cool and clammy skin, and anxiety. Signs of shock may not occur until after birth. The fall in blood pressure is often a late sign of hemorrhage.
- Signs associated with impaired fetal oxygenation, such as late decelerations, minimal to absent variability, tachycardia, and bradycardia.
- Absent fetal heart sounds with a large disruption of the placenta; absent fetal heart activity by ultrasound examination.
- Cessation of uterine contractions.
- Palpation of the fetus outside the uterus (usually occurs only with a large, complete rupture).
- Loss of station (fetus previously at a lower station and is now no longer engaged in the pelvis).

If the rupture is incomplete, blood loss is slower, and signs of shock, chest pain, or interscapular pain may be delayed. Complete rupture results in massive blood loss. Signs of shock and pain develop quickly. External bleeding may not be impressive, however, because most blood is lost into the peritoneal cavity. The fetus often dies in complete rupture because the placental blood supply is disrupted.

Therapeutic Management

Initial management is to stabilize the client and the fetus for a cesarean birth. If the rupture is small and the client wants other children, it may be repaired. A client with a large uterine rupture may require hysterectomy. Blood and blood products are replaced as needed.

Nursing Considerations

The nurse has increased awareness of clients who are at increased risk for uterine rupture and stays alert for the signs and symptoms. Administer uterine stimulant drugs cautiously to reduce the likelihood of excessive contractions. However, tachysystole also can occur spontaneously. Notify the provider if tachysystole occurs. A tocolytic drug may be needed to reduce excessive contractions.

Uterine rupture may not be detected before birth. If postpartum bleeding is excessive and the fundus is firm, injury to the birth canal, including uterine rupture, is possible. Bleeding may be concealed if the ruptured area bleeds into the broad ligament. In this case, signs of hypovolemic shock are likely to develop quickly.

Uterine Inversion

An inversion occurs when the uterus completely or partly turns inside out, usually during the third stage of labor. Such an event is uncommon but potentially fatal.

Causes

Often, no single cause is identified. Predisposing factors are as follows:

- Excessive traction on the umbilical cord before the placenta detaches from the uterine wall spontaneously
- Fundal pressure during birth
- Fundal pressure on an incompletely contracted uterus after birth
- Increased intraabdominal pressure
- An abnormally adherent placenta
- Congenital weakness of the uterine wall
- Fundal placenta implantation

Signs and Symptoms

The provider notes either the uterus is absent from the abdomen or a depression in the fundal area is present. The interior of the uterus may be seen through the cervix or protruding into the vagina, appearing as a red, beefy mass. Massive hemorrhage, shock, and pain quickly become evident. The client has severe pelvic pain.

Management

Quick action by nursing and medical personnel is essential to reduce maternal morbidity and mortality. The provider tries to replace the uterus through the vagina into a normal position. Anesthesia may be required to produce enough relaxation to allow the uterus to be replaced. If replacement is not possible, a laparotomy may be necessary. Several units of blood are usually ordered immediately (Francois & Foley, 2021; Thorp & Grantz, 2019).

Nursing Considerations

Nursing care during the emergency supplements care provided by other staff members. Postpartum nursing care is directed toward observing and maintaining maternal blood volume and correcting shock. The client may be transferred to the intensive care unit after birth.

Assess the uterine fundus (if a hysterectomy was not required) for firmness, height, and deviation from the midline. Assess vital signs every 15 minutes or more frequently until stable and then according to recovery room routine. Observe for tachycardia and falling blood pressure, which

are associated with shock. Remember when the blood pressure decreases it is often a late sign of hemorrhagic shock. A cardiac monitor identifies dysrhythmias, which may occur with shock; a pulse oximeter displays the client's pulse rate and oxygen saturation. Invasive hemodynamic monitoring with central venous pressure and arterial lines is common to directly evaluate functions such as heart rate, venous and arterial pressures, blood gases, circulation to the lungs, venous functions, and other tests that may be needed.

An indwelling catheter usually is inserted to observe fluid balance and keep the bladder empty so the uterus can contract well. Assess the catheter for patency, and record intake and output. Urine output should be at least 30 mL/hr. A fall in urine output may indicate hypovolemia or an obstructed catheter.

The client is allowed nothing by mouth until their condition is stable. They usually can receive fluids and progress to solid foods quickly because **uterine inversion** does not usually recur in the current postpartum period. It may recur in a future pregnancy if conditions favor its development.

APPLICATION OF THE NURSING PROCESS: INTRAPARTUM EMERGENCIES

Nursing care of the client with an intrapartum emergency overlaps with care in other situations discussed elsewhere. Much of the nursing care is collaborative and supports medical management. Parents may suffer loss if the fetus dies or the client loses the ability to bear other children, as may occur with uterine rupture. One problem expected in any emergency situation is the emotional distress of the client and their family.

Assessment

When an emergency occurs, the client and family have little time to absorb what has happened, simply because of its suddenness. In umbilical cord prolapse, for example, labor often has been uneventful. Suddenly, nurses place the client in a strange position, administer oxygen, and transfer to the operating room. The staff is clearly excited as well.

Under such circumstances, the client and family have a very narrow focus. They are obviously apprehensive and feel out of control. The client or their partner may be immobilized by fear.

Identification of Client Problem

The problem is "apprehension because of the sudden development of complications." This problem is expected to differ from the anxiety associated with preterm labor because the onset is acute. The apprehension also may lessen more quickly because the emergency is sometimes resolved quickly. Grief may occur because of ill effects of the emergency on the client and baby.

Planning: Expected Outcomes

The focus of a goal is very narrow in an emergency situation. Two appropriate outcomes, during and after the emergency, are the client and their family will do the following:

- Indicate an understanding of emergency procedures.
- Express their feelings about the complication.

Interventions

Although little time for discussion exists, explain honestly and simply what is occurring. To reduce fear and anxiety of the unknown, tell the client what is happening and why. Include the partner and family, if appropriate. Provide continued reassurance and support to the client because the partner often must be excluded from the emergency or operating room when an emergency occurs.

The infant born in an emergency situation may need resuscitation or other supportive measures. Nurses and a neonatal or pediatric nurse practitioner or pediatrician from the NICU usually are present at the birth to attend the infant. A neonatologist also may be present. Explain to the family who the other professionals are and their roles. If possible, explain what is being done to care for the baby.

After the emergency, give the client and family a chance to ask questions. The ability to absorb new knowledge during periods of severe anxiety is very limited. Adequate explanations afterward help them understand and assimilate the experience.

Although the nurse is usually anxious in an emergency situation, keeping a calm attitude is important. The client and family quickly pick up on the staff's anxiety, and consequently their anxiety escalates. Remain with the client to reduce fears of abandonment. If possible, hold the client's hand; speak in a low, calm voice; and debrief after the occurrence to help assimilate the event.

Evaluation

Evaluation of the goals is probably impossible until the emergency is over and the client's physical condition stabilizes. Expected outcomes for this client problem are achieved if the client and family do the following:

- Indicate they understand the problem and the rationale for emergency procedures.
- Express, possibly over several days, their feelings about what has occurred.

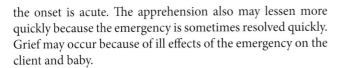

SUMMARY CONCEPTS

- Dysfunctional labor may occur because of abnormalities in the powers, the passenger, the passage, or the psyche. Combinations of abnormalities are common.
- Nursing care in labor focuses on prevention or prompt identification and action to correct additional complications such as fetal hypoxia, infection, injury to the client or fetus, and postpartum hemorrhage.
- Premature rupture of the membranes is associated with infection as both a cause and a complication.
- Early indications of preterm labor are often vague. Prompt identification of preterm labor enables the most effective therapy to delay preterm birth.
- Nursing care for the client at risk for a preterm birth before 37 weeks of gestation focuses on helping delay birth long enough to provide time for fetal lung maturation with corticosteroids, administration of antibiotics to decrease the risk of neonatal GBS infection, allow transfer to a facility with a neonatal intensive care, or reach a gestation at which the infant's problems with immaturity are less.

- The main risk in prolonged pregnancy is reduced placental function. This may compromise the fetus during labor and result in meconium aspiration in the neonate. Dysfunctional labor may occur if a fetus continues growing during the prolonged pregnancy.
- The key intervention for umbilical cord prolapse is to relieve pressure on the umbilical cord and to expedite delivery.
- Be aware of clients at risk for uterine rupture, and observe for signs and symptoms such as signs of shock, abdominal pain, a sense of tearing, chest pain, shoulder pain, pain between the scapulae, abnormal FHR patterns, cessation of contractions, palpation of the fetus outside the uterus, and loss of fetal station. However, lesser degrees of uterine rupture or dehiscence may have minimal symptoms.
- Uterine inversion can be accompanied by massive blood loss and shock. Recovery care promotes uterine contraction and maintenance of adequate circulating volume.

Clinical Judgment And Next-Generation NCLEX® Examination-Style Questions

1. **Highlight the findings that would require follow-up.**
   An American Indian 19-year-old, who identifies as female, walks into your OB emergency department stating she is cramping and bleeding for the past 2 hours. She is 5 ft 2 in and 255 lbs. She appears mildly uncomfortable. She had two prenatal visits but cannot tell you the name of the provider she saw, only the clinic where she was seen. She states she had an ultrasound once, and they said her due date was a couple months from now. She did have labs drawn on her first visit but does not know the results. Her boyfriend dropped her off, and she can call him if needed.

Initial Assessment: BP 130/80, P 100, R 16, T 97.2, O2 Sats 99% FHR Category I. Contractions palpate mild, q 7 minutes × 60 seconds, resting tone soft. She has a small amount of watery bloody fluid on her underwear.

Upon full assessment, the client reveals this is her first pregnancy, she has no allergies, and she does not have high blood pressure or diabetes, but both her parents have diabetes and high blood pressure. She last ate and drank 2 hours ago and has not had intercourse in the past week. She denies taking any medications or recreational drugs, but she does take a vitamin sometimes. The fetal monitor continues to show a baseline of 150 with moderate variability and accelerations that are 15 bpm × 15 seconds.

2. **Which of the following provider orders would the nurse anticipate initially? Select all that apply.**
   A. Routine admission labs for a client with no prenatal care (CBC with diff, type and screen, CMP, RPR, chlamydia and gonorrhea culture, HIV, Hep B, Hep C, urine drug screen)
   B. IV of LR 500 cc bolus and then 125 cc/hr
   C. OB ultrasound, complete, with BPP
   D. Amnisure test for rupture of membranes
   E. Continuous fetal monitoring
   F. Bed rest with bathroom privileges
   G. NPO
   H. Administration of corticosteroids
   I. Administration of tocolytic
   J. Administration of magnesium sulfate

Vital signs continue to be similar to her baseline with a Category 1 FHR. Contractions decrease to irregular after an IV bolus of 500 cc. All labs are normal except her glucose, which is 182, and she is O positive. Amnisure is positive. The physician does a speculum exam and sees clear fluid coming from the cervical os, which appears closed. Ultrasound reveals a 28-week gestation fetus in the breech position, AFI is 4, cervical length (abdominal view) is 3.5 cm. Placenta is posterior, and no abruption is noted. BPP is 8/8. The physician orders admission to the antepartum unit for PPROM.

3. **Place an X to indicate if the findings are expected or require follow-up.**

Assessment finding	Expected	Requires follow-up
Contractions decrease to irregular		
Normal labs		
Blood sugar 182		
Positive amnisure		
Cervical exam—appears to not be dilated (closed)		

4. **Use an X to indicate which potential problems listed in the left column are a priority for prevention.**

Potential problem	Priority for prevention
Preterm birth	
Immobility	
Infection	
Umbilical cord prolapse	
Pain	
Anxiety	
Venous thromboembolism	

The physician orders betamethasone 12 mg IM now and the second dose in 24 hours. The antibiotic protocol for PPROM is begun. A 3-hour glucose tolerance test (GTT) is done that meets the criteria for gestational diabetes, and the diabetes protocol orders are instituted with metformin po and a diabetic diet. The client remains stable with minimal contractions, leaking clear fluid, and with a Category 1 FHR pattern for 4 days. On day 5, she appears to have increased contractions and complains of some cramping. The physician orders magnesium sulfate for neuroprotection, starting a 6-g bolus and then 2 g per hour for 24 hours. Contractions decrease to irregular after the magnesium bolus.

5. **Highlight the findings that would require follow-up.**
   The magnesium bolus is discontinued after 24 hours, and the client once again appears stable on day 6. On day 8, she complains of not feeling well and aching. Her vital signs are BP 139/82, P 110, R 20, T 100.6, O2 Sats 96%. A CBC is drawn, and her white blood cell count is 21,000. Contractions are increasing, and she is becoming more restless.

REFERENCES & READINGS

Adams, E. (2021). Antenatal care. In K. Simpson, P. Creehan, N. O'Brien-Abel, C. Roth, & A. Rohan (Eds.), *Perinatal nursing* (5th ed., pp. 66–98). Wolters Kluwer.

American Academy of Pediatrics and American College of Obstetricians and Gynecologists (AAP & ACOG). (2017). *Guidelines for perinatal care* (8th ed.).

American College of Obstetricians and Gynecologists (ACOG). (2017a). *Definition of term pregnancy.* ACOG Committee Opinion, 579. Originally published 2013, reaffirmed 2017.

American College of Obstetricians and Gynecologists (ACOG). (2017b). *Intrapartum management of intraamniotic infection.* ACOG Committee Opinion, 712.

American College of Obstetricians and Gynecologists (ACOG). (2019a). *Group prenatal care.* ACOG Committee Opinion, 731. Originally published 2018, reaffirmed 2019.

American College of Obstetricians and Gynecologists (ACOG). (2019b). *Periviable birth.* Obstetric Care Consensus No. 4. Originally published 2017, reaffirmed 2019.

American College of Obstetricians and Gynecologists (ACOG). (2020a). *Antenatal corticosteroid therapy for fetal maturation.* ACOG Committee Opinion No. 713. Originally published 2017, reaffirmed 2020.

American College of Obstetricians and Gynecologists (ACOG). (2020b). *Macrosomia.* Practice bulletin No. 216. Originally published 2016, reaffirmed 2020.

American College of Obstetricians and Gynecologists (ACOG). (2020c). *Magnesium sulfate before anticipated preterm birth for neuroprotection.* ACOG Committee Opinion, 455. Originally published 2010, reaffirmed 2020.

American College of Obstetricians and Gynecologists (ACOG). (2020d). *Management of late-term and postterm pregnancies.* Practice Bulletin No. 146. Originally published 2014, reaffirmed 2020.

American College of Obstetricians and Gynecologists (ACOG). (2020e). *Management of preterm labor.* Practice Bulletin No. 171. Originally published 2016, reaffirmed 2020.

American College of Obstetricians and Gynecologists (ACOG). (2020f). *Prelabor rupture of membranes.* Practice Bulletin No. 217. Originally published 2018, reaffirmed 2020.

American College of Obstetricians and Gynecologists (ACOG). (2020g). *Shoulder dystocia.* Practice Bulletin No. 178. Originally published 2017, reaffirmed 2020.

American College of Obstetricians and Gynecologists (ACOG). (2021a). *Antepartum fetal surveillance.* Practice Bulletin No. 229. Originally published 2014, reaffirmed 2021.

American College of Obstetricians and Gynecologists (ACOG). (2021b). *Multifetal gestations: Twin, triplet, and higher-order multifetal pregnancies.* Practice Bulletin No. 231.

American College of Obstetricians and Gynecologists (ACOG). (2021c). *Placenta accreta spectrum.* Obstetric Care Consensus No. 7. Originally published 2018, reaffirmed 2021.

Barth, W. H. (2021). Malpresentations and malposition. In M. Landon, H. Galan, E. Jauniaux, D. Driscoll, V. Berghella, W. Grobman, S. Kilpatrick, & A. Cahill (Eds.), *Gabbe's obstetrics: Normal and problem pregnancies* (8th ed., pp. 319–342). Elsevier.

Bowers, N. (2021). Multiple gestation. In K. Simpson, P. Creehan, N. O'Brien-Abel, C. Roth, & A. Rohan (Eds.), *Perinatal nursing* (5th ed., pp. 249–295). Wolters Kluwer.

Cunningham, F. G., Leveno, K. J., Bloom, S. L., Dashe, J. S., Hoffman, B. L., Casey, B. M., & Spong, C. Y. (2022). *Williams obstetrics* (26th ed.). McGraw-Hill Companies.

Finucane, E. M., Murphy, D. J., Biesty, L. M., Gyte, G. M. L., Cotter, A. M., Ryan, E. M., Boulvain, M., & Devane, D., (2020). Membrane sweeping for induction of labour. *Cochrane Database of Systematic Reviews, 2020*(2), CD000451. https://doi.org/10.1002/14651858.CD000451.pub3.

Foley, M., Strong, T., Jr., & Garite, T. (2018). *Obstetric intensive care manual* (5th ed.). McGraw-Hill Medical Education.

Francois, K. E., & Foley, M. R. (2021). Antepartum and postpartum hemorrhage. In M. Landon, H. Galan, E. Jauniaux, D. Driscoll, V. Berghella, W. Grobman, S. Kilpatrick, & A. Cahill (Eds.), *Gabbe's obstetrics: Normal and problem pregnancies* (8th ed., pp. 343–374). Elsevier.

Hobson, S. R., Abdelmalek, M. Z., & Farine, D. (2019). Update on uterine tachysystole. *Journal of Perinatal Medicine, 47*(2), 152–160. https://doi.org/10.1515/jpm-2018-0175.

Hologic. (2009). *Enzyme immunoassay and rapid fFN™ for the TLiIQ® System.* http://www.fFNtest.com/pdfs/rapid_fFN_product_insert_lettersize.pdf.

Jauniaux, E. R. H., Silver, R. M., & Wright, J. D. (2021). Placenta accreta. In M. Landon, H. Galan, E. Jauniaux, D. Driscoll, V. Berghella, W. Grobman, S. Kilpatrick, & A. Cahill (Eds.), *Gabbe's obstetrics: Normal and problem pregnancies* (8th ed., pp. 408–420). Elsevier.

Landon, M. B., & Grobman, W. A. (2021). Vaginal birth after cesarean delivery. In M. Landon, H. Galan, E. Jauniaux, D. Driscoll, V. Berghella, W. Grobman, S. Kilpatrick, & A. Cahill (Eds.), *Gabbe's obstetrics: Normal and problem pregnancies* (8th ed., pp. 395–407). Elsevier.

Macones, G. A., Hankins, G. D., Spong, C. Y., Hauth, J., & Moore, T. (2008a). The 2008 National Institute of Child Health and Human Development workshop report on electronic fetal monitoring: Update on definitions, interpretation, and research guidelines. *Journal of Obstetric, Gynecologic, and Neonatal Nursing, 37*(5), 510–515.

Macones, G. A., Hankins, G. D., Spong, C. Y., Hauth, J., & Moore, T. (2008b). The 2008 National Institute of Child Health and Human Development workshop report on electronic fetal monitoring: Update on definitions, interpretation, and research guidelines. *Obstetrics & Gynecology, 112*, 661–666.

Malone, F. D., & D'Alton, M. E. (2019). Multiple gestation: Clinical characteristics and management. In R. Resnik, C. Lockwood, T. Moore, M. Greene, J. Copel, & R. Silver (Eds.), *Creasy & Resnik's maternal–fetal medicine: Principles and practice* (8th ed., pp. 654–675). Elsevier.

March of Dimes. (2021). *2019 Premature birth report card.* http://www.marchofdimes.org.

Maternal Immunization Task Force. (2021). *Maternal immunization task force and partners urge that covid-19 vaccine be available to pregnant individuals.* https://www.acog.org/-/media/project/acog/acogorg/files/pdfs/news/joint-statement_covid-vaccine-for-pregnant-ppl-final.pdf?la=en&hash=4B504FA716FB9845C8297B84414ED58A.

Mercer, B. M., & Chien, E. K. S. (2021). Premature rupture of the membranes. In M. Landon, H. Galan, E. Jauniaux, D. Driscoll, V. Berghella, W. Grobman, S. Kilpatrick, & A. Cahill (Eds.), *Gabbe's obstetrics: Normal and problem pregnancies* (8th ed., pp. 694–707). Elsevier.

Nawa, N., Garrison–Desany, H. M., Kim, Y., Ji, Y., Hong, X., Wang, G., Pearson, C., Zuckerman, B. S., Wang, X., & Surkan, P. J.

(2020). Maternal persistent marijuana use and cigarette smoking are independently associated with shorter gestational age. *Paediatric & Perinatal Epidemiology, 34*(6), 696–705. https://doi.org/10.1111/ppe.12686.

Norman, J. E., Marlow, N., Messow, C., Shennan, A., Bennett, P. R., Thornton, S., Robson, S., McConnachie, A., Petrou, S., Sebire, N.J., Lavender, T., Whyte, S., & Norrie, J. (2016). Vaginal progesterone prophylaxis for preterm birth (the OPPTIMUM study): A multicentre, randomised, double-blind trial. *Lancet, 387*(10033), 2106–2116.

Parfitt, S. (2021). Preterm labor and birth. In K. Simpson, P. Creehan, N. O'Brien-Abel, C. Roth, & A. Rohan (Eds.), *Perinatal nursing* (5th ed.). Wolters Kluwer.

Rohan, A. J. (2021). Common neonatal complications. In K. Simpson, P. Creehan, N. O'Brien-Abel, C. Roth, & A. Rohan (Eds.), *Perinatal nursing* (5th ed.). Wolters Kluwer.

Roth, C. K. (2021). Pulmonary complications in pregnancy. In K. Simpson, P. Creehan, N. O'Brien-Abel, C. Roth, & A. Rohan (Eds.), *Perinatal nursing* (5th ed., pp. 221–248). Wolters Kluwer.

Rozance, P. J., & Wright, C. J. (2021). The neonate. In M. Landon, H. Galan, E. Jauniaux, D. Driscoll, V. Berghella, W. Grobman, S. Kilpatrick, & A. Cahill (Eds.), *Gabbe's obstetrics: Normal and problem pregnancies* (8th ed., pp. 430–458). Elsevier.

Salera-Vieira, J. (2021). Bleeding in pregnancy. In K. Simpson, P. Creehan, N. O'Brien-Abel, C. Roth, & A. Rohan (Eds.), *Perinatal nursing* (5th ed., pp. 124–141). Wolters Kluwer.

Simhan, H. N., & Romero, R. (2021). Preterm labor and birth. In M. Landon, H. Galan, E. Jauniaux, D. Driscoll, V. Berghella, W. Grobman, S. Kilpatrick, & A. Cahill (Eds.), *Gabbe's obstetrics: Normal and problem pregnancies* (8th ed., pp. 663–693). Elsevier.

Simpson, K. R. (2020). *Cervical ripening and labor induction and augmentation* (5th ed.). AWHONN.

Sloane, A. J., Aghai, Z., Roman, A., Cruz, Y., Carola, D., McElwee, D., & Solarin, K. (2019). Impact of new "Triple I" classification on the incidence of clinical chorioamnionitis and antibiotic use in neonates. *Pediatrics, 144*(2 MeetingAbstract), 648. https://doi.org/10.1542/peds.144.2_MeetingAbstract.648.

Thorp, J. M., & Grantz, K. L. (2019). Clinical aspects of normal and abnormal labor. In R. Resnik, C. Lockwood, T. Moore, M. Greene, J. Copel, & R. Silver (Eds.), *Creasy & Resnik's maternal–fetal medicine: Principles and practice* (8th ed., pp. 723–757). Elsevier.

U.S. Food and Drug Administration. (2011). *FDA drug safety communication: New warnings against use of terbutaline to treat preterm labor*. http://www.fda.gov.

Varley-Campbell, J., Mujica-Mota, R., Coelho, H., Ocean, N., Barnish, M., Packman, D., Dodman, S., Cooper, C., Snowsill, T., Kay, T., Liversedge, N., Parr, M., Knight, L., Hyde, C., Shennan, A., & Hoyle, M. (2019). Three biomarker tests to help diagnose preterm labour: A systematic review and economic evaluation. *National Institute for Health Research, 23*(13), 1–226. https://doi.org/10.3310/hta23130.

Zhang, J., Landy, H. J., Branch, D. W., Burkman, R., Haberman, S., Gregory, K. D., Hatjis, C. G., Ramirez, M. M., Bailit, J. L., Gonzalez-Quintero, V. H., Hibbard, J. U., Hoffman, M. K., Kominiarek, M., Learman, L. A., Velduisen, P. V., Troendle, J., & Reddy, U. M. (2010). Contemporary patterns of spontaneous labor with normal neonatal outcomes. *Obstetrics & Gynecology, 116*(6), 1281–1287.

17

Postpartum Adaptations and Nursing Care

Emily Drake

OBJECTIVES

After studying this chapter, you should be able to:

1. Explain the physiologic changes occurring during the postpartum period.
2. Explain maternal psychosocial adaptation to childbirth, including the process of bonding and attachment and the stages of maternal role attainment.
3. Discuss the cause, manifestations, and interventions for postpartum blues.
4. Describe the processes of family adaptation to the birth of a baby and factors impacting the process.
5. Discuss cultural influences on family adaptation.
6. Apply the nursing process to the care of the postpartum family.
7. Discuss expected outcomes and interventions for common postpartum problems.
8. Explain the role of the nurse in health education of the postpartum family and identify important areas of teaching.
9. Compare postpartum nursing assessments and care for clients who have undergone cesarean birth and vaginal birth.
10. Describe criteria for postpartum discharge and available follow-up health care services.

The first 6 weeks after the birth of an infant are known as the *postpartum period,* or **puerperium**. During this time, clients experience physiologic and psychosocial changes. Family members also experience psychosocial changes as they adapt to the new infant.

PHYSIOLOGIC CHANGES

Many of the physiologic changes are retrogressive: Changes that occurred in body systems during pregnancy are reversed as the body returns to the nonpregnant state. Progressive changes such as the initiation of lactation also occur.

Reproductive System

Involution of the Uterus

Involution refers to the changes the reproductive organs, particularly the uterus, undergo after childbirth to return to their nonpregnant size and condition. Uterine involution involves three processes: (1) contraction of muscle fibers, (2) **catabolism** (the process of converting cells into simpler compounds), and (3) regeneration of the uterine epithelium. Involution begins immediately after delivery of the placenta, when uterine muscle fibers contract firmly around blood vessels at the area where the placenta was attached. This contraction controls bleeding from the area left denuded when the placenta separated. The uterus decreases in size as muscle fibers contract and gradually regain their former contour and size.

Regeneration of the uterine epithelial lining begins soon after childbirth. The outer portion of the endometrial layer is expelled with the placenta. Within 2 to 3 days, the remaining **decidua** (the endometrium during pregnancy) separates into two layers. The first layer is superficial and is shed in the lochia. The basal layer containing the residual endometrial glands and blood vessels remains to provide the source of new endometrium. Regeneration of the endometrium, except at the site of placental attachment, occurs by 2 to 3 weeks after birth (Blackburn, 2018).

Healing at the placental site occurs more slowly and requires approximately 6 weeks (Blackburn, 2018). This site, which is approximately 3.5 inches (9 cm) in diameter immediately postpartum, heals by a process of *exfoliation* (scaling off of dead tissue). New endometrium is generated at the site from glands and tissue remaining in the lower layer of the decidua after separation of the placenta (Cunningham et al., 2022; Isley, 2021). This process leaves the endometrial layer smooth and spongy, as it was before pregnancy, and the uterine lining is free of scar tissue unless the birth was cesarean. Scarring of the uterine lining may interfere with implantation of future pregnancies.

Descent of the Uterine Fundus. The location of the uterine fundus helps determine whether involution is progressing normally. Immediately after birth, the uterus is about the size of a large grapefruit or softball and weighs approximately 2.2 lb (1000 g). The fundus can be palpated midway between the symphysis pubis and umbilicus and in the midline of the abdomen. Within 12 hours the fundus rises to approximately the level of the umbilicus (Blackburn, 2018).

The fundus descends by approximately 1 cm, or one fingerbreadth, per day. By the 14th day, it has descended into the pelvic cavity and cannot be palpated abdominally (Fig. 17.1) (Blackburn, 2018). When the process of involution does not occur properly, **subinvolution** occurs. Subinvolution can cause postpartum hemorrhage (see Chapter 18).

Descent of the fundus is documented in relation to the umbilicus. For example, *U-1* or ↓1 indicates the fundus is palpable about 1 cm (one fingerbreadth) below the umbilicus. Within 1 week, the weight of the uterus decreases to approximately 1 lb (500 g); at 4 weeks, the uterus weighs 2 to 3 oz (100 g) or less (Cunningham, et al., 2022).

Afterpains

Etiology. Intermittent uterine contractions, known as **afterpains**, are a source of discomfort for many clients. The discomfort is more acute for multiparas because repeated stretching of muscle fibers leads to loss of muscle tone, which causes repeated contraction and relaxation of the uterus.

The uterus of a primipara tends to remain contracted; however primiparas may experience severe afterpains if the uterus has been overdistended or if retained blood clots are present. Afterpains are particularly severe during breastfeeding. Oxytocin, released from the posterior pituitary to stimulate the **milk-ejection reflex** (release of milk from the ducts of the breasts), causes strong contractions of uterine muscles.

Nursing Considerations. Analgesics are frequently used to lessen the discomfort of afterpains. Many breastfeeding clients are reluctant to take medication for fear it will pass into the breast milk and harm the infant. However, health care experts generally agree the most common analgesics may be used for short-term pain relief without harm to the infant. The benefits of pain relief such as comfort and relaxation facilitate the milk-ejection reflex and usually outweigh the small effect of the medication on the infant. The client should check with the health care provider before taking any medication. The nurse can reassure the client that afterpains are self-limiting and decrease in frequency and intensity by the third day (Cunningham et al., 2022).

Lochia. Changes in the color and amount of lochia (the vaginal drainage after childbirth) also provide information about whether involution is progressing normally. Table 17.1 summarizes the characteristics of normal and abnormal lochia.

Changes in Color. On days 1 to 3 after childbirth, lochia consists almost entirely of blood, with small particles of decidua and mucus. It is called **lochia rubra** because of its dark red or red–brown color. The amount of blood decreases when leukocytes begin to invade the area, as they do in any healing surface. The color of lochia then changes from red to pink or brown-tinged (**lochia serosa**). It lasts from days 3 to 10. Lochia serosa is composed of serous exudate, erythrocytes, leukocytes, and cervical mucus. By about the 10th day, the erythrocyte component decreases. The discharge becomes white, cream, or light yellow in color (**lochia alba**). Lochia alba contains leukocytes, decidual cells, epithelial cells, fat, cervical mucus, and bacteria. It may end by day 14 or persist until the end of the third to the sixth week (Blackburn, 2018; Cunningham et al., 2022).

Amount. Because estimating the amount of lochia on a peripad (perineal pad) is difficult, nurses frequently document lochia in terms that are difficult to quantify, such as *scant, moderate,* and *heavy.* Agreement on the meanings of terms in an agency is important to make charting accurate. One method for recording the amount of lochia in 1 hour uses the following labels (Whitmer, 2016):

- Scant—Less than a 1-inch (2.5-cm) stain on the peripad
- Light—Less than a 4-inch (10-cm) stain on the peripad
- Moderate—Less than a 6-inch (15-cm) stain on the peripad
- Heavy—Saturated peripad in 1 hour
- Excessive—Saturated peripad in 15 minutes

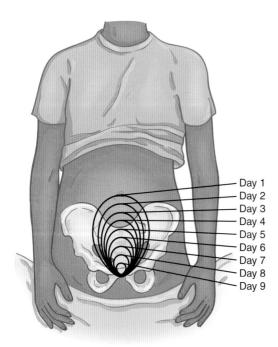

Day 1
Day 2
Day 3
Day 4
Day 5
Day 6
Day 7
Day 8
Day 9

FIG. 17.1 Involution of the Uterus. Height of the uterine fundus decreases by approximately 1 cm per day. The fundus is no longer palpable by 14 days.

TABLE 17.1	**Characteristics of Lochia**	
Time and Type	**Normal Discharge**	**Abnormal Discharge**
Days 1–3: Lochia rubra	Bloody; small clots; fleshy, earthy odor; dark red or red–brown	Large clots; saturated perineal pads; foul odor
Days 3–10: Lochia serosa	Decreased amount; serosanguineous; pink or brown-tinged	Excessive amount; foul smell; continued or recurrent reddish color
Days 10–14 (or up to 3rd–6th week): Lochia alba	White, cream, or light yellow color; decreasing amounts	Persistent lochia serosa; return to lochia rubra; foul odor; discharge continuing

Determining the time a peripad has been in place is important when assessing lochia. What appears to be a light amount of lochia may be a moderate flow if the peripad has been in use for less than an hour (Fig. 17.2).

The time between delivery and assessment of lochia also is important. Lochia flow will be greater immediately after birth but will gradually decrease. It is less after cesarean birth because some of the endometrial lining is removed during surgery. Post-cesarean birth lochia will go through the same phases as lochia from a vaginal birth, but the amount will be reduced.

Lochia flow is often heavier when the client first gets out of bed after birth or after sleeping because gravity allows blood to pool in the vagina during the hours of rest and flow freely when standing.

Some clients have a sudden, short episode of bleeding 7 to 14 days after birth. This bleeding occurs when the eschar over the placental site sloughs. Increased bleeding lasting longer than 1 to 2 hours should be evaluated by the health care provider (Isley, 2021).

Cervix

Immediately after childbirth the cervix is dilated, edematous, and bruised. Small tears or lacerations may be present. Rapid healing takes place, and by the end of the first week the external cervical os narrows, and the cervix thickens (Cunningham et al., 2022). There may be some edema for as long as 3 to 4 months (Blackburn, 2018). The internal os closes as before pregnancy, but the shape of the external os is permanently changed. It remains slightly open and appears slit-like rather than round, as in the nulliparous client.

Vagina

The vagina and vaginal introitus are greatly stretched during birth to allow passage of the fetus. Soon after childbirth, the vaginal walls appear edematous, and multiple small lacerations may be present. Very few vaginal rugae are present.

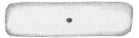

Scant: <2.5-cm (1-inch) stain

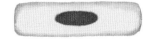

Light: 2.5- to 10-cm (1- to 4-inch) stain

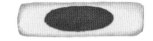

Moderate: 10- to 15-cm (4- to 6-inch) stain

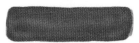

Heavy: Saturated in 1 hour

FIG. 17.2 Guidelines for Assessing the Amount of Lochia on the Perineal Pad.

Although rugae begin to reappear by 3 to 4 weeks, 6 to 10 weeks are needed for the vaginal epithelium to be restored. The vagina regains tone and decreases in size, although it does not completely return to the prepregnancy state (Blackburn, 2018).

During the postpartum period, vaginal mucosa becomes atrophic, and vaginal walls do not regain their thickness until estrogen production by the ovaries is reestablished. Ovarian function and estrogen production are not well-established during lactation; therefore, breastfeeding clients are likely to experience vaginal dryness and may experience **dyspareunia** (discomfort during intercourse).

Perineum

The muscles of the pelvic floor stretch and thin greatly during the second stage of labor, a result of pressure from the fetal head. After childbirth, the perineum may be edematous and bruised. If the client had an **episiotomy**, a surgical incision of the perineal area, it will begin to heal in 2 to 3 weeks. Complete healing of the episiotomy site may take 4 to 6 months (Blackburn, 2018).

Lacerations of the perineum also may occur during the birth. Lacerations and episiotomies are classified according to tissue involved (Box 17.1). See Chapter 15 for further discussion of episiotomies and lacerations.

Discomfort. Although the episiotomy is relatively small, the muscles of the perineum are involved in many activities (walking, sitting, stooping, squatting, bending, urinating, and defecating). An incision or laceration in this area can cause a great deal of discomfort. In addition, many postpartum clients are affected by hemorrhoids (distended rectal veins),

---

BOX 17.1 Lacerations of the Birth Canal

Perineum

Perineal lacerations are classified in degrees to describe the amount of tissue involved. Some physicians or nurse–midwives also use degrees to describe the extent of midline episiotomies.

First-degree—involves the superficial vaginal mucosa or perineal skin.

Second-degree—involves the vaginal mucosa, perineal skin, fascia, and muscles of the perineum.

Third-degree—same as second-degree lacerations but extends into or through the external anal sphincter.

Fourth-degree—extends through the anal sphincter and into the rectal mucosa.

Periurethral Area

A laceration in the area of the urethra may cause a client to have difficulty urinating after birth.

An indwelling catheter may be necessary for a day or two.

Vaginal Wall

A laceration involves the mucosa of the vaginal wall.

Cervix

Tears in the cervix may be a source of significant bleeding after birth.

which are pushed out of the rectum during the second stage of labor. Hemorrhoids, as well as perineal trauma, can make physical activity or bowel elimination difficult during the postpartum period. Relief of perineal discomfort is a nursing priority. It includes teaching self-care measures such as applying ice, taking sitz baths, performing perineal care, using topical anesthetics and cooling astringent pads, and taking prescribed analgesics (Cunningham et al., 2022; Isley, 2021).

Resumption of Ovulation and Menstruation

Although the first few menstrual cycles for both lactating and nonlactating clients are often anovulatory, ovulation may occur before the first menses (Cunningham et al., 2022). For some clients, ovulation may resume before their postpartum follow-up appointment. Therefore, contraceptive measures are important considerations when sexual relations are resumed for both lactating and nonlactating clients. Nonlactating clients will usually resume menstruation in 6 to 10 weeks (Blackburn, 2018; Isley, 2021).

Breastfeeding delays the return of both ovulation and menstruation. Menses usually resumes between 10 weeks and 6 months for these clients (Cunningham et al., 2022). Generally, clients who breastfeed more frequently and use fewer nutritional supplements with infant feeding are likely to ovulate and menstruate later than clients who breastfeed less often, use more supplements, and wean earlier (Kennedy & Trussell, 2018). For the client who is breastfeeding frequently and without supplements, contraception should be used by the time the infant is 6 months old or earlier because ovulation and menses are increasingly likely by that time (Isley, 2021).

Lactation

During pregnancy, estrogen and progesterone prepare the breasts for lactation. Although prolactin also rises during pregnancy, lactation is inhibited at this time by the high level of estrogen and progesterone. After expulsion of the placenta, estrogen and progesterone levels decline rapidly, and prolactin initiates milk production within 2 to 3 days after childbirth. Once milk production is established, it continues because of frequent suckling by the infant and removal of milk from the breast. Therefore, the more the infant nurses, the more milk the client produces.

? KNOWLEDGE CHECK

1. Which three processes are involved in involution of the uterus?
2. How is the fundus expected to descend after childbirth?
3. Which clients are most likely to experience afterpains? How are they treated?
4. What are the differences among lochia rubra, lochia serosa, and lochia alba in appearance and expected duration?
5. When should a formula-feeding client expect menses to resume? When should a breastfeeding client expect menses to resume?
6. How does breastfeeding affect the resumption of ovulation and menstruation?

Oxytocin is necessary for milk ejection or "let-down." This hormone causes milk to be expressed from the alveoli into the lactiferous ducts during suckling (see Chapter 23).

Cardiovascular System

Hypervolemia, which produces an average 40% to 50% increase in blood volume at term, allows the client to tolerate a substantial blood loss during childbirth without ill effect. Up to 500 milliliters (mL) of blood is lost in vaginal deliveries, and up to 1000 mL is lost in cesarean births (Blackburn, 2018).

Cardiac Output

Despite the blood loss, a transient increase in maternal cardiac output occurs after childbirth. This increase is caused by (1) an increased flow of blood back to the heart when blood from the uteroplacental unit returns to the central circulation, (2) decreased pressure from the pregnant uterus on the vessels which increases blood return to the heart, and (3) the mobilization of excess extracellular fluid into the vascular compartment.

The rise in cardiac output returns to prelabor values within an hour after delivery. Gradually, cardiac output returns to prepregnancy levels in most clients by 6 to 12 weeks after childbirth (Blackburn, 2018).

Plasma Volume

The body rids itself of the excess plasma volume needed during pregnancy by diuresis and diaphoresis.

- Diuresis (increased excretion of urine) is facilitated by a decline in the adrenal hormone aldosterone and a decrease in oxytocin. A urinary output of up to 3000 mL/day may occur, especially on postpartum days 2 through 5 (Blackburn, 2018).
- Diaphoresis (profuse perspiration) also rids the body of excess fluid. It can be uncomfortable and unsettling for the client who is not prepared for it. Explanations of the cause and provision of comfort measures such as showers and dry clothing are generally sufficient.

Hematologic System

Several components of the blood change during the postpartum period. Marked leukocytosis may occur, with the white blood cell (WBC) count increasing to as high as 30,000/mm³ during labor and the immediate postpartum period (Blackburn, 2018; Cunningham et al., 2022). The WBC count falls to normal values within 1 to 2 weeks after birth (Antony et al., 2021; Blackburn, 2018).

Maternal hemoglobin (Hgb) and hematocrit (Hct) values are difficult to interpret during the first few days after birth because of the remobilization and rapid excretion of excess body fluid. The Hct is low when plasma increases and dilutes the concentration of blood cells and other substances carried by the plasma. As excess fluid is excreted, the dilution is gradually reduced. The Hct should return to normal limits within 4 to 6 weeks unless excessive blood loss has occurred (Blackburn, 2018).

Coagulation

During pregnancy, plasma fibrinogen and other factors necessary for coagulation increase. As a result, the client's body has a greater ability to form clots and thus prevent excessive bleeding. Fibrinolytic activity is decreased during pregnancy. Elevations in clotting factors continue for several days or longer, causing a continued risk for thrombus formation. It takes 4 to 6 weeks before the hemostasis returns to normal nonpregnant levels (Blackburn, 2018). Although the incidence of thrombophlebitis has declined greatly as a result of early postpartum ambulation, clients are still at increased risk for thrombus formation (see Chapter 18). If needed, thromboprophylaxis can be pharmacologic with the use of anticoagulation agents or mechanical agents such as intermittent pneumatic compression devices (Pacheco et al., 2020).

Gastrointestinal System

Soon after childbirth, digestion begins to be active. The client is usually hungry because of the energy expended in labor and thirsty because of decreased oral intake during labor and fluid loss from exertion, mouth breathing, and early diaphoresis.

Constipation is a common problem during the postpartum period for a variety of reasons. Bowel tone and motility, which were diminished during pregnancy as a result of progesterone, remain sluggish for several days. In addition, relaxation of the abdominal muscles increases constipation and distention with gas. Decreased food and fluid intake during labor often results in small, hard stools. Perineal trauma, episiotomy, and hemorrhoids cause discomfort and interfere with effective bowel elimination. Many clients anticipate pain when they attempt to defecate and are unwilling to exert pressure on the perineum. Clients who are taking iron have an added cause of constipation.

Temporary constipation is not harmful, although it can cause a feeling of abdominal fullness and flatulence. Stool softeners and laxatives frequently are prescribed to prevent or treat constipation. The first stool usually occurs within 2 to 3 days postpartum. Normal patterns of bowel elimination generally resume by 8 to 14 days after birth (Blackburn, 2018).

Urinary System

The kidneys return to normal function by 2 weeks after delivery. The dilation of the renal pelvis and the ureters, which occurs during pregnancy, ends within 2 to 8 weeks (Cunningham et al., 2022). Both protein and acetone may be present in the urine for the first few postpartum days secondary to the catabolic processes involved in uterine involution and dehydration, which often occurs during the exertion of labor.

Changes during pregnancy cause the bladder of postpartum clients to have increased capacity and decreased muscle tone. During childbirth, the urethra, bladder, and tissue around the urinary meatus may become edematous and traumatized. The result is often diminished sensitivity to fluid pressure, and many clients have little or no sensation of needing to void even when the bladder is distended.

The bladder fills rapidly because of diuresis following childbirth. It is not unusual for a postpartum client to void

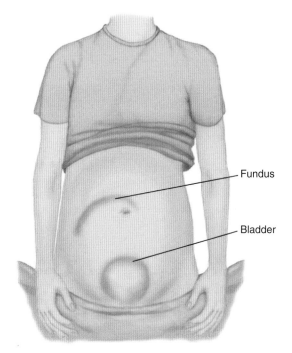

FIG. 17.3 A full bladder displaces and prevents contraction of the uterus.

500 to 1000 mL at a time (Blackburn, 2018). The client is at risk for overdistention of the bladder, incomplete emptying of the bladder, and retention of residual urine. Urinary retention is more common after the first vaginal birth, regional anesthesia, and catheterization during labor. Retention occurs in 1.7% to 17.9% of postpartum clients (Blackburn, 2018).

Urinary retention and overdistention of the bladder may cause urinary tract infection (UTI) and increased postpartum bleeding. UTI occurs when urinary stasis allows time for bacteria to multiply. Risk for bleeding increases because uterine ligaments, which were stretched during pregnancy, allow the uterus to be displaced upward and laterally by the full bladder (Fig. 17.3). The displacement results in decreased contraction of the uterine muscles (uterine **atony**), a primary cause of excessive bleeding.

Stress incontinence may occur during pregnancy or after giving birth. Approximately one-third of clients have urinary incontinence at 8 weeks postpartum, but only approximately 15% of postpartum clients still have a problem at 12 weeks (Isley, 2021). For some clients, the problem resolves with pelvic floor exercises and time for healing, while others may have continued problems.

Musculoskeletal System
Muscles and Joints

In the first 1 to 2 days after childbirth, many clients experience muscle fatigue and aches, particularly of the shoulders, neck, and arms, because of exertion during labor. Warmth and gentle massage increase circulation to the area and provide comfort and relaxation.

During the first few days, levels of the hormone relaxin gradually subside, and ligaments and cartilage of the pelvis

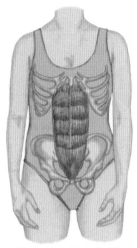

Normal location of rectus
muscles of the abdomen

Diastasis recti: separation
of the rectus muscles

FIG. 17.4 Diastasis recti occurs when the longitudinal muscles of the abdomen separate during pregnancy.

begin to return to their prepregnancy positions. These changes can cause hip and joint pain, which interferes with ambulation and exercise. The client should be told the discomfort is temporary and does not indicate a medical problem. Good body mechanics and correct posture are important during this time to help prevent low back pain and injury to the joints.

Abdominal Wall

During pregnancy, the abdominal walls stretch to accommodate the growing fetus, and muscle tone is diminished. Many clients, expecting the abdomen to return to the prepregnancy condition immediately after childbirth, are dismayed to find the abdominal muscles weak, soft, and flabby.

In addition, the longitudinal muscles of the abdomen may separate (**diastasis recti**) during pregnancy (Fig. 17.4). The separation may be minimal or extensive but is usually 1 to 2.5 inches (2 to 4 cm). The client may benefit from gentle exercises to strengthen the abdominal wall, which usually returns to normal position by 6 weeks after birth.

Integumentary System

Many skin changes of pregnancy are caused by an increase in hormones. When estrogen, progesterone, and melanocyte-stimulating hormones decline after childbirth, the skin gradually reverts to the nonpregnant state. This change is particularly noticeable when melasma, the "mask of pregnancy," and linea nigra fade and disappear for many clients. In addition, spider nevi and palmar erythema, which may develop during pregnancy as a result of increased estrogen level, gradually disappear.

Striae gravidarum (stretch marks), which develop during pregnancy when connective tissues in the abdomen and breasts are stretched, gradually fade to silvery lines but do not disappear. Loss of hair may especially concern the client. This is a normal response to the hormonal changes causing decreased hair loss during pregnancy. Hair loss begins at 4 to 20 weeks after delivery and is regrown in 4 to 6 months for

two-thirds of clients and by 15 months for the remainder of clients (Blackburn, 2018).

Neurologic System

Discomfort and fatigue after childbirth are common. Afterpains, an episiotomy, laceration or incision, muscle aches, and breast engorgement may increase a client's discomfort and inability to sleep.

Analgesia or anesthesia may cause temporary neurologic changes such as lack of feeling in the legs and dizziness. During this time, prevention of injury from falling is a priority.

Complaints of headache require careful assessment. Frontal and bilateral headaches are common in the first postpartum week and may be a result of changes in fluid and electrolyte balance (Blackburn, 2018). Severe headaches are not common but may be postdural puncture headaches resulting from regional anesthesia (see Chapter 13). They may be most severe when the client is in an upright position and are relieved by assuming the supine position. They should be reported to the appropriate health care provider, usually an anesthesiologist. Headache, along with blurred vision, photophobia, proteinuria, and abdominal pain, may indicate development or worsening of preeclampsia (see Chapter 10).

Endocrine System

After expulsion of the placenta, placental hormones such as estrogen, progesterone, and human placental lactogen decline fairly rapidly. High prolactin levels trigger the body to make milk for breastfeeding. In clients who are not breastfeeding, prolactin levels return to normal and help regulate the menstrual cycle.

Weight Loss

Approximately 10 to 13 lb (4.5 to 5.8 kg) are lost during childbirth. This includes the weight of the fetus, placenta, and amniotic fluid and blood lost during the birth. An additional 5 to 8 lb (2.3 to 3.6 kg) are lost as a result of diuresis and 2 to 3 lb (0.9 kg to 1.4 kg) from involution and lochia by the end of the first week (Blackburn, 2018).

Weight loss continues with the greatest loss during the first 3 months. If the client's weight gain during pregnancy has not been excessive, it is likely all but about 2.2 lb (1 kg) will be lost within a year if following a well-balanced diet. Younger clients with lower prepregnant weight lose more weight and lose it sooner than other clients (Blackburn, 2018).

Many clients are frustrated because they want an immediate return to prepregnancy weight. Nurses can provide information about diet and exercise that will produce an acceptable weight loss without depleting the client's energy or impairing their health (see Chapter 8).

NURSING CARE OF THE POSTPARTUM FAMILY

Postpartum Assessments

Providing essential, cost-effective postpartum care to new families is a challenge for maternity nurses. Most clients stay in the birth facility for up to 48 hours after an uncomplicated vaginal birth and up to 96 hours after a cesarean birth. Some clients choose to go home at an earlier time. Although the length of stay is short, the family's need for care and information is extensive.

Initial Assessments

Postpartum assessments begin during the fourth stage of labor (the first 1 to 2 hours after childbirth). The client is examined for physical stability. Initial assessments include the following:

- Vital signs
- Skin color
- Location and firmness of the fundus
- Amount and color of lochia
- Perineum (edema, episiotomy, lacerations, hematoma, hemorrhoids)
- Presence, degree, and location of pain
- Intravenous (IV) infusions—type of fluid, rate of administration, type and amount of added medications, patency of the IV line, and redness, pain, or edema of the site
- Urinary output—time and amount of last void or catheterization, presence of a catheter, color and character of urine, presence or absence of bladder distention
- Status of abdominal incision and dressing, if present
- Level of feeling and ability to move if regional anesthesia was administered

Chart Review

When the initial assessments confirm the client's physical condition is stable, nurses should review the chart to obtain pertinent information and determine whether there are factors that increase the risk for complications during the postpartum period. Relevant information includes the following:

- Gravida, para
- Time and type of birth (use of vacuum extractor, forceps, cesarean)
- Presence and degree of episiotomy or lacerations
- Anesthesia or medications administered
- Significant medical and surgical history, such as diabetes, hypertension, heart disease
- Medications given during labor or birth or routinely taken and the reasons for their use

- Food and drug allergies
- Chosen method of infant feeding
- Condition of the baby

Laboratory data also are examined. Of particular interest are the prenatal Hgb and Hct values, blood type and Rh factor, hepatitis B surface antigen, rubella immune status, syphilis screen, and group B *Streptococcus* status.

Risk Factors for Hemorrhage and Infection. Nurses should be aware of conditions that increase the risk for hemorrhage or infection, the two most common complications of puerperium. These risk factors should be identified upon admission, in hand-off reports, and in chart reviews.

CRITICAL TO REMEMBER

Postpartum Risk Factors

Hemorrhage
- Multiparity
- History of postpartum hemorrhage
- Overdistention of the uterus (large baby, twins, polyhydramnios, large fibroids)
- Precipitous labor (less than 3 hours)
- Prolonged labor
- Retained placenta
- Placenta previa or accreta or placental abruption
- Coagulopathy, low platelets (<100,000/mm^3)
- Trauma—lacerations, hematoma
- Infection—chorioamnionitis, sepsis
- Medications (tocolytics, magnesium sulfate, general anesthesia, prolonged use of oxytocin)
- Operative procedures (cesarean birth, vacuum extraction, forceps)

Infection
- Operative procedures (cesarean birth, vacuum extraction, forceps)
- Multiple cervical examinations
- Prolonged labor
- Prolonged rupture of membranes
- Manual extraction of placenta or retained fragments
- Diabetes
- Catheterization
- Bacterial colonization of lower genital tract

Need for Rho(D) Immune Globulin. Prenatal and neonatal records are checked to determine whether Rho(D) immune globulin should be administered. The Rh-negative client with a Rh-positive newborn is an indication for administration. Rho(D) immune globulin should be administered within 72 hours after childbirth to prevent the development of maternal antibodies which could affect subsequent pregnancies.

Immunizations

Rubella Vaccine. A prenatal rubella antibody screen is performed on each pregnant client to determine immunity. If the client is rubella nonimmune, the vaccine is recommended after childbirth to prevent acquiring rubella during subsequent pregnancies, when it can cause serious fetal anomalies.

There is a theoretic risk for fetal defects if the rubella vaccine is administered during pregnancy because the vaccine is a live virus. Therefore, clients are advised not to become pregnant for at least 30 days after receiving the vaccine (Centers for Disease Control and Prevention [CDC], 2021). The nurse should document in the chart that the risk has been explained and the parents have verbalized their understanding.

DRUG GUIDE

Rubella Vaccine

Classification
Attenuated live virus vaccine.

Action
Produces a modified rubella (German measles) infection that is not communicable, causing the formation of antibodies against rubella virus.

Indications for Childbearing Clients
Administered at least 30 days before pregnancy or after childbirth or abortion to clients whose antibody screen shows they are not immune to rubella. This vaccine prevents rubella infection and possible severe congenital defects in the fetus during a subsequent pregnancy.

Dosage and Route
0.5 mL subcutaneously.

Absorption
Well absorbed.

Contraindications and Precautions
The vaccine is contraindicated in clients who are immunosuppressed, pregnant, or sensitive to vaccine component or have a moderate or severe illness. The attenuated virus may appear in breast milk, and some infants may develop a rash, but this is not a contraindication to vaccination of lactating clients. It can be given near the time of Rho(D) immune globulin administration. Clients receiving the vaccine should be tested for immune status at 6 to 8 weeks to verify immunity.

Adverse Reactions
Transient stinging at site, fever, lymphadenopathy, arthralgia, and transient arthritis are most common.

Nursing Implications
Vials should be refrigerated. Reconstitute only with diluent supplied with the vial. Use immediately after reconstitution and discard if not used within 8 hours. Protect from light. Birth of infants with congenital rubella syndrome has not been documented when the vaccine has been given inadvertently during pregnancy.

From Centers for Disease Control and Prevention (CDC). (2021). *Measles, mumps, and rubella (MMR) vaccination: What everyone should know.* https://www.cdc.gov/vaccines/vpd/mmr/public/index.html.

Pertussis Vaccine. Recent outbreaks of pertussis have had serious effects in infants and young children. Although most adults were vaccinated as children, the effectiveness fades with time. Full protection of vaccinated infants does not occur until the entire series is completed. The CDC (2019) recommends all adults in contact with infants and young children get a booster dose of pertussis vaccine. It is usually administered along with diphtheria and tetanus vaccines (Tdap). (See the CDC website at https://www.cdc.gov/vaccines for current information.)

Varicella Vaccine. Varicella (chicken pox) in pregnant clients can cause infection and serious complications in the fetus and newborn. Therefore, the American Academy of Pediatrics (AAP) and American College of Obstetricians and Gynecologists (ACOG) (AAP & ACOG, 2017) recommend clients who are not immune to varicella should receive the first dose of varicella vaccine after delivery and before discharge from the birth facility. They should be advised not to become pregnant for 1 month after receiving the vaccine.

Focused Assessments after Vaginal Birth

Nurses perform postpartum assessments according to facility protocol. For example, a protocol might require assessment as follows:

- Every 15 minutes for the first 2 hours
- Every 4 hours for the next 12 to 24 hours
- Every 8 to 12 hours thereafter until discharge

Assessments are made more frequently if findings are abnormal or the client has additional risk factors. Although assessments vary depending on the particular problems presented, a focused assessment for a vaginal birth generally includes the vital signs, fundal height and tone, lochia, perineum, bowel and bladder elimination, breasts, and lower extremities.

Vital Signs

Blood Pressure. Blood pressure (BP) varies with position and the arm used. To obtain accurate results, BP should be measured on the same arm with the client in the same position each time. Postpartum BP should be compared with the prenatal period so deviations from what is normal for the client can be quickly identified. An increase from the baseline may be caused by pain or anxiety. If the BP is 140/90 mm Hg or higher, preeclampsia may be present. A decrease may indicate dehydration or hypovolemia resulting from excessive bleeding.

Orthostatic Hypotension. After birth a rapid decrease in intraabdominal pressure results in dilation of blood vessels supplying the viscera. The resulting engorgement of abdominal blood vessels contributes to a rapid fall in BP of 15 to 20 mm Hg systolic when the client is repositioned from the recumbent position to the sitting position. This change may cause the client to feel dizzy or lightheaded or to faint when they stand.

Hypotension also may indicate hypovolemia. Careful assessments for hemorrhage (location and firmness of the fundus, amount of lochia, pulse rate) should be made if the postpartum BP is significantly less than the prenatal baseline.

Pulse. Bradycardia, defined as a pulse rate of 60 beats per minute (bpm), may occur during the early postpartum period. The lower pulse rate may reflect the large amount of blood returning to central circulation after delivery of the placenta. The increase in central circulation results in increased stroke volume and allows a slower heart rate to provide adequate maternal circulation.

Tachycardia may indicate pain, excitement, anxiety, fatigue, dehydration, hypovolemia, anemia, or infection. If tachycardia is noted, additional assessments should include degree of pain, BP, temperature, location and firmness of the uterus, amount of lochia, blood loss at birth, and Hgb and Hct values. The objective of the additional assessments is to rule out excessive bleeding and to intervene at once if hemorrhage is suspected.

Respirations. A normal respiratory rate of 12 to 20 breaths per minute should be maintained. Assessing breath sounds is especially important for clients who have a cesarean birth, are smokers, have frequent or recent upper respiratory tract infections, have a history of asthma, or are receiving magnesium sulfate.

Temperature. A temperature of up to 100.4°F (38°C) is common during the first 24 hours after childbirth and may be caused by dehydration or normal postpartum leukocytosis. If the elevated temperature persists for longer than 24 hours, exceeds 100.4°F (38°C), or if the client shows other signs of infection, the nurse should notify the obstetric provider.

Pain. Pain should be assessed along with other vital signs to determine the type, location, and severity on a pain scale. Some clients are too excited by the birth of their child to complain of discomfort. Others do not want to "bother the nurse" or may be from cultures in which complaining is not acceptable. Nurses should remain alert to signs of pain or discomfort. Nonspecific signs of discomfort include an inability to relax or sleep, a change in vital signs, restlessness, irritability, facial grimaces, or guarding. The nurse should encourage clients to take prescribed medications as needed and should also assess the effectiveness of pain-relief measures.

Fundus. The fundus should be assessed for consistency and location. It should be firmly contracted and at or near the level of the umbilicus. If the uterus is above the expected level or shifted from the middle of the abdomen or midline position, the bladder may be distended. The location of the fundus should be rechecked after the client voids.

If the fundus is difficult to locate or is soft or "boggy," the nurse stimulates the uterine muscle to contract by gently massaging the uterus. The nondominant hand should support and anchor the lower uterine segment during palpation and massage. Uterine massage is not necessary if the uterus is firmly contracted.

The uterus can continue to contract only if it is free of intrauterine clots. To expel clots, the nurse should support the lower uterine segment and massage the fundus until firm, as illustrated in Procedure 17.1. This lower segment support helps prevent inversion of the uterus (turning inside out) when the nurse applies firm pressure downward toward the vagina to express clots that have collected in the uterus. Nurses should observe the perineum for the number and size of clots expelled. If lochia is excessive or large clots are expelled, they should be weighed to quantify the amount of blood loss (see Chapter 18). Table 17.2 describes normal and abnormal findings of the uterine fundus and includes follow-up nursing actions for abnormal findings.

Medications are sometimes needed to maintain contraction of the uterus and thus prevent postpartum hemorrhage. The most commonly used medication is oxytocin (Pitocin).

Other medications for excessive postpartum bleeding are discussed in Chapter 18.

Lochia. Important assessments include the amount, color, and odor of lochia. Nurses observe the lochia on peripads while assessing the perineum. They also assess vaginal discharge while palpating or massaging the fundus to determine the amount of lochia and the number and size of any clots expressed during these procedures. Important guidelines include the following:

- A constant trickle, dribble, or oozing of lochia indicates excessive bleeding and requires immediate attention.
- Excessive lochia in the presence of a contracted uterus suggests lacerations of the birth canal. The health care provider should be notified so lacerations can be located and repaired.

The odor of lochia is usually described as fleshy, earthy, or musty. A foul odor suggests endometrial infection, and assessments should be made for additional signs of infection. These signs include maternal fever, tachycardia, uterine tenderness, and pain.

Absence of lochia, like the presence of a foul odor, may indicate infection. If the birth was cesarean, lochia may be scant because the uterine cavity was wiped by sponges, removing some of the endometrial lining. Lochia should not be entirely absent, however.

Perineum. The acronym REEDA is used as a reminder about five signs of an episiotomy or a perineal laceration assessment: redness (R), edema (E), ecchymosis (E), discharge (D), and approximation (A). Redness of the wound may indicate the usual inflammatory response to injury. If accompanied by excessive pain or tenderness, however, it may indicate the beginning of localized infection. Ecchymosis or edema indicates soft tissue damage may delay healing; no discharge should come from the wound. Rapid healing requires the edges of the wound be closely approximated. (Procedure 17.2 describes the perineal examination.)

Bladder Elimination. Because the client may not experience the urge to void even if the bladder is full, nurses should rely on physical assessment to determine whether the bladder is distended. Bladder distention often produces an obvious or palpable bulge that feels like a soft, movable mass above the symphysis pubis. Other signs include an upward and lateral displacement of the uterine fundus and increased lochia. Frequent voids of less than 150 mL suggest urinary retention. Signs of an empty bladder include a firm fundus in the midline and a nonpalpable bladder.

Two to three voids should be measured after birth or the removal of a catheter to determine whether normal bladder function has returned. When the client can void at least 300 to 400 mL, the bladder is usually empty. Regardless of the amount voided, if the fundus was displaced when assessed, it should be assessed again after the client voids to confirm the bladder is empty. Subjective symptoms of urgency, frequency, or dysuria suggest UTI and should be reported to the health care provider.

Breasts. For the first day or two after birth, the breasts should be soft and nontender. Breast changes depend largely on whether the client is breastfeeding. The breasts should be

NURSING PROCEDURE 17.1   Assessing the Uterine Fundus

Purpose

To determine the location and firmness of the uterus.

1. Explain the procedure and rationale before beginning the procedure. *Explanations reduce anxiety and elicit cooperation.*
2. Ask the client to empty her bladder if she has not voided recently. *A distended bladder lifts and displaces the uterus.*
3. Place the client in the supine position with her knees flexed. *This relaxes the abdominal muscles and permits accurate location of the fundus.*
4. Put on clean gloves and lower the perineal pad to observe lochia as the fundus is palpated. *Gloves are necessary whenever contact with body fluids may occur.*
5. Place your nondominant hand above the client's symphysis pubis. *This supports and anchors the lower uterine segment.*

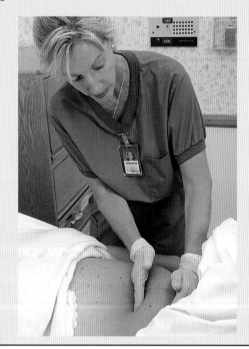

6. Use the flat part of your fingers (not the fingertips) for palpation. Palpation may be painful, particularly for the client who had a cesarean birth. *The larger surface of the fingers provides more comfort.*
7. Begin palpation at the umbilicus and palpate gently until the fundus is located. It should be firm, in the midline, and approximately at the level of the umbilicus. Locating the fundus is more difficult if the client is obese or if the abdomen is distended. *Palpation helps determine the firmness and location of the fundus.*
8. If the fundus is difficult to locate or is "boggy," (soft) keep the nondominant hand above the client's symphysis pubis and massage the fundus with the dominant hand until the fundus is firm. *The nondominant hand anchors the lower segment of the uterus and prevents inversion while the uterus is massaged. The uterus contracts in response to tactile stimulation, and this helps control excessive bleeding.*
9. After massaging a boggy fundus until it is firm, press firmly to expel clots. Do not attempt to expel clots before the fundus is firm. Keep one hand pressed just above the symphysis (over the lower uterine segment) throughout. *Removing clots allows the uterus to contract properly. Attempting to expel clots in a boggy uterus might result in uterine inversion. A firm fundus and pressure over the lower uterine segment help prevent uterine inversion.*
10. If the fundus is above or below the umbilicus, use your fingers to determine the number of fingerbreadths between the fundus and the umbilicus. *Using the fingers to measure allows an approximation of the number of centimeters.*
11. Document the consistency and location of the fundus. Record consistency as "fundus firm," "firm with massage," or "boggy." Record fundal height in fingerbreadths or centimeters above or below the umbilicus. For example, "fundus firm, midline, ↓1" (one fingerbreadth or 1 cm below the umbilicus); "fundus firm with light massage, U +2 (two fingerbreadths or 2 cm above the umbilicus), displaced to right." *This promotes accurate communication and identifies deviations from expected so potential problems can be identified early.*

TABLE 17.2   Assessments of the Uterine Fundus and Nursing Actions

Normal Findings	Abnormal Findings	Nursing Actions
Fundus is firmly contracted.	Fundus is soft, "boggy," uncontracted, or difficult to locate.	Support lower uterine segment. Massage until firm.
Fundus remains contracted when massage is discontinued.	Fundus becomes soft and uncontracted when massage is stopped.	Continue to support lower uterine segment. Massage fundus until firm; then apply pressure to express clots. Notify health care provider, and begin oxytocin or other drug administration, as prescribed, to maintain a firm fundus.
Fundus is located at or below the level of umbilicus and midline.	Fundus is above umbilicus and/or displaced from midline.	Assess bladder elimination. Assist the client to urinate, or catheterize, if necessary, to empty bladder. Recheck the position and consistency of fundus after bladder is empty.

examined even if the client chooses formula feeding because engorgement may occur despite preventive measures. The size, symmetry, and shape of the breasts should be observed. The skin should be inspected for dimpling or thickening, which, although rare, can indicate a breast tumor.

The areola and nipple should be carefully examined for potential problems such as flat or retracted nipples, which may make breastfeeding more difficult. Signs of nipple trauma (redness, blisters, or fissures) may be noted during the first days of breastfeeding, especially if the client needs assistance in positioning the infant correctly (see Chapter 23).

NURSING PROCEDURE 17.2
Assessing the Perineum

Purpose
To assess perineal trauma and the state of healing.
1. Provide privacy and explain the purpose of the procedure. *This elicits cooperation and reduces anxiety.*
2. Put on clean gloves. *Implements standard precautions to provide protection from possible contact with body fluids.*
3. Ask the client to assume a side-lying position and flex her upper leg. Lower the perineal pads, and lift her superior buttock. If necessary, use a flashlight to inspect the perineal area. *Position provides an unobstructed view of the perineum and allows assessment of lochia that may be under the client; light allows better visualization.*
4. Note the extent and location of edema or bruising. *Extensive bruising or asymmetric edema may indicate formation of a hematoma.*
5. Examine the episiotomy or laceration for redness, ecchymosis, edema, discharge, and approximation (REEDA). *Redness, edema, or discharge may indicate infection of the wound; extensive bruising may delay healing; wound edges should be in direct contact for uncomplicated healing to occur.*
6. Note the number and size of hemorrhoids. *Swollen, painful hemorrhoids interfere with activity and bowel elimination.*

The breasts should be palpated for firmness and tenderness, which indicate increased vascular and lymphatic circulation and may precede milk production. The breasts may feel "lumpy" as various lobes begin to produce milk.

The breast assessment is an excellent opportunity to provide information or reassurance about breast care and breastfeeding techniques. It is also an opportunity to teach the client how to perform this assessment while in the hospital and after discharge.

Lower Extremities. The legs are examined for varicosities and signs or symptoms of thrombophlebitis. Indications of thrombophlebitis include localized areas of redness, heat, edema, and tenderness. Pedal pulses may be obstructed by a thrombus and should be palpated with each assessment.

Edema and Deep Tendon Reflexes. Pedal or pretibial edema may be present for the first few days, until excess interstitial fluid is remobilized and excreted. (Fig. 17.5 shows how to assess for pitting edema.) Diuresis is highest between days 2 and 5 after birth. Fluid and electrolyte balance should return to nonpregnant status by 21 days (Blackburn, 2018).

Deep tendon reflexes should be 1+ to 2+. Report brisker-than-average or hyperactive reflexes (3+ to 4+), which suggest preeclampsia, to the provider (see Procedure 10.1 for a description of assessing deep tendon reflexes).

KNOWLEDGE CHECK

11. What causes orthostatic hypotension? What are the typical signs and symptoms of orthostatic hypotension?
12. What additional assessments are necessary when tachycardia is noted? Why?
13. When is uterine massage necessary? How is the uterus supported during massage?
14. What does excessive bleeding suggest when the uterus is firmly contracted?

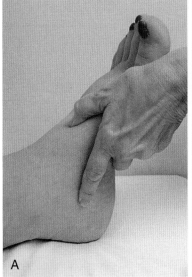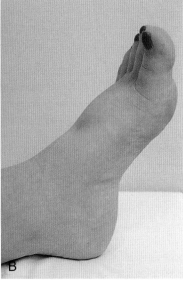

FIG. 17.5 Pedal edema. (A) Apply pressure to foot. (B) "Pit" appears when fluid moves into adjacent tissue and away from point of pressure.

Interventions in the Immediate Postpartum Period

Care of the client during the immediate postpartum period focuses on physiologic safety, comfort measures, bladder elimination, and health education.

Providing Comfort Measures

Both cold and warmth are used to alleviate perineal pain after childbirth.

Ice Packs. Ice causes vasoconstriction and is most effective if applied soon after the birth to prevent edema and numb the area. Chemical ice packs and plastic bags or nonlatex gloves filled with ice may be used after a vaginal birth. The ice pack is wrapped in a washcloth or paper before it is applied to the perineum. It should be left in place until the ice melts. It is removed for 10 minutes before a fresh pack is applied. Some peripads have cold packs incorporated in them. Condensation from ice may dilute lochia and make it appear heavier than it actually is.

Although some clients may prefer to use cool gel pads or ice, there is limited evidence of the overall effectiveness of these to relieve pain (East et al., 2020), and clients may need to combine the use of topical applications with analgesia. Care should be taken for clients who are still numb from an epidural as they cannot feel how cold the area becomes.

Sitz Baths. In some facilities, sitz baths may be offered two to four times a day to clients with episiotomies, painful hemorrhoids, or perineal lacerations or edema. Sitz baths provide continuous circulation of water, cleansing, and comfort to the traumatized perineum. Cool water reduces pain caused by edema and may be most effective within the first 24 hours. Ice can be added to cool the water to a comfortable level as the client sits in it. Warm water increases circulation, promotes healing, and may be most effective after 24 hours. Nurses should be sure the emergency call light is within easy reach in case the client feels faint during the sitz bath. Clients often take the disposable sitz bath container home. They should be instructed to clean it well between uses (Isley, 2021).

Analgesics. Clients should be encouraged to take prescribed medications for afterpains and perineal discomfort. Many analgesics are combinations that include acetaminophen. The nurse should be careful the client receives no more than 4 g of acetaminophen in a 24-hour period. Nonsteroidal antiinflammatory medications, such as ibuprofen, are often prescribed to decrease swelling and pain.

Perineal Care

Perineal care consists of squirting warm water over the perineum after each voiding or bowel movement. This is important for all postpartum clients whether the birth was vaginal or cesarean. The bottle should not touch the perineum. Perineal care cleanses, provides comfort, and prevents infection, which can accompany an episiotomy or lacerations. The perineum is gently patted dry rather than wiped dry.

Topical Medications. Local anesthetic decreases surface discomfort. It is available as a spray or foam. The client is instructed to hold the nozzle of the spray 6 to 12 inches from the body and direct it toward the perineum. The spray should be used after perineal care and before clean pads are applied. Foam is placed directly on the clean perineal pad. Astringent compresses should be placed directly over the hemorrhoids to relieve pain. Hydrocortisone ointments may also be applied over hemorrhoids to increase comfort.

Sitting Measures. Clients should be advised to squeeze their buttocks together before sitting and to slowly lower their weight onto their buttocks. This measure prevents stretching of the perineal tissue and avoids sharp impact to the traumatized area. Sitting slightly to the side is also helpful to prevent the full weight from resting on the episiotomy site.

Promoting Bladder Elimination

Many clients have difficulty voiding because of edema and trauma of the perineum and diminished sensitivity to fluid pressure in the bladder. As soon as they are able to ambulate safely, clients should be assisted to the bathroom. Providing privacy and allowing adequate time for the first voiding are important. Common measures to promote relaxation of the perineal muscles and stimulate the sensation of needing to void include the following:

- Providing pain medication to assist with relaxation
- Running water in the sink or shower, placing the client's hands in warm water, and pouring water over the vulva
- Providing hot tea or fluids of choice
- Asking the client to blow bubbles through a straw
- Using the shower or sitz bath and encouraging voiding when the urge is felt

A nonpalpable bladder and firm fundus at or below the umbilicus and in the midline confirm the bladder is empty and rule out urinary retention.

A distended bladder lifts and displaces the uterus, making it difficult for it to remain contracted. The resulting uterine atony permits excessive bleeding. In addition, stasis of urine in the bladder increases the risk of UTI. Therefore, the client should be catheterized in the following situations:

- Unable to void.
- The amount voided is less than 150 mL, and the bladder can be palpated.
- The fundus is elevated or displaced from the midline.

Repeated catheterizations increase the chance of UTI. An indwelling catheter may be ordered for 24 hours if edema is excessive or catheterization is necessary more than once or twice.

CRITICAL TO REMEMBER

Signs of a Distended Bladder

Location of the fundus above the baseline level (determined when the bladder is empty)
Fundus displaced to the side from midline
Excessive lochia
Bladder discomfort
Bulge of bladder above symphysis
Frequent voidings of less than 150 mL of urine, which may indicate urinary retention

Providing Fluids and Food

Adequate fluids help restore the balance altered by fluid loss during labor and the birth process. Encourage clients to drink approximately 2500 mL of fluids each day. Offering ice water or cold drinks may be culturally inappropriate for some clients; others may prefer hot or room-temperature water instead. If the client is unable to tolerate oral fluids, IV administration may be necessary. Ice chips may be offered soon after cesarean birth, and, although protocols vary, most are able to progress to a regular diet in a short time.

Postpartum clients generally have a hearty appetite, and nurses should encourage healthy food choices with respect for ethnic background. Meals and snacks should be available at all times.

Preventing Thrombophlebitis. The client should be assisted to ambulate early after childbirth to prevent the development of thrombi. Frequent trips to the bathroom will help accomplish this.

Nursing Care after Cesarean Birth

In 2019, 31.7% of births in the United States were by cesarean delivery (Martin et al., 2021). These clients must recover from childbirth along with a major surgery and need special care. The usual length of stay after a cesarean birth is 72 to 96 hours after surgery.

Pain Relief

Assessment of pain and the effectiveness of pain relief is an important aspect of nursing care after cesarean birth. These clients differ from typical postoperative clients in four important ways. First, they often are eager to be alert so they can interact with their newborn infants. Second, they are concerned the analgesics they receive may pass into their breast milk and harm their infants. Third, compared with other postoperative clients, after cesarean births, clients want to have more input and control of their care. Fourth, they are often healthier than clients who had surgery to correct a problem.

Pain relief is provided in various ways. Patient-controlled analgesia (PCA) is administered by continuous IV infusion of a low-concentration narcotic solution using a pump specifically designed for that purpose. If analgesia is insufficient, the client can self-administer intermittent small doses of narcotic from the infusion pump. The machine limits the amount of narcotic available within a specified time interval to prevent an overdose. This allows the client to have pain relief immediately when needed without waiting for a nurse to administer it. Side effects include respiratory depression, itching (pruritus), nausea and vomiting, and urinary retention.

Neuraxial administration of a single dose of opioid (such as preservative-free morphine or fentanyl) injected into the epidural or subarachnoid space is another method of pain management which may provide 18 to 24 hours of postcesarean analgesia (see Chapter 13). Itching and nausea are the major side effects. Other side effects are the same as for PCA. Oral analgesics usually are effective if additional pain-relief measures are needed. Occasionally, IV or intramuscular analgesics are needed for one or two doses of breakthrough pain.

Assessment

In addition to the usual postpartum evaluation, after cesarean birth the assessment should be the same as any other postoperative client.

Respirations. When clients receive epidural narcotics for postoperative pain relief, respirations should be assessed frequently because narcotics depress the respiratory center. A pulse oximeter or apnea monitor is used for 18 to 24 hours to detect low oxygen saturation from a decreased respiratory rate or depth. Oxygen saturation and respiratory rate are documented hourly or according to facility policy. If a client receiving epidural narcotics has a respiratory rate of 12 breaths per minute or less or the pulse oximeter shows a persistent oxygen saturation less than 95%, the nurse should do the following:

- Notify the anesthesia provider.
- Elevate the head of the bed to facilitate lung expansion, and instruct the client to breathe deeply.
- Administer oxygen, and apply a pulse oximeter (if not already in place).
- Follow facility protocol to administer narcotic antagonists, such as naloxone hydrochloride (Narcan).
- Observe for recurrence of respiratory depression because the duration of naloxone is only approximately 30 minutes.
- Recognize naloxone may reduce the level of pain relief.

In addition to observing the respiratory rate and depth, the nurse should auscultate the client's breath sounds because depressed respirations and a longer period of immobility allow secretions to pool in the bronchioles.

Abdomen. Nurses assess gastrointestinal function by auscultating for bowel sounds until normal peristalsis is noted in all abdominal quadrants. Although paralytic ileus (lack of movement in the intestines) is rare after cesarean birth, nurses should be aware of the signs. They include abdominal distention, absent or decreased bowel sounds, and failure to pass flatus or stool.

If a surgical dressing is present, it should be assessed for intactness and drainage. When the dressing is removed, nurses observe the incision, and use the acronym REEDA to assess for approximation and signs of infection such as redness and edema (Fig. 17.6). A topical skin adhesive may be used instead of staples. Assessment of the wound is the same.

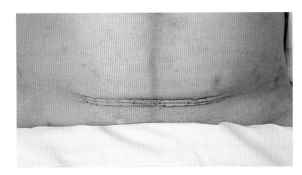

FIG. 17.6 This cesarean incision is closed with staples. Note the absence of all signs of infection, such as redness, edema, bruising (ecchymosis), discharge, and loss of approximation.

It is just as important to assess the fundus after cesarean birth as it is with vaginal birth. However, palpation should be gentle because of increased discomfort caused by the abdominal incision.

Intake and Output. The IV line should be monitored for patency, the rate of flow, and the condition of the site. Any signs of infiltration (edema, coolness at the site, pain) or signs of infection (edema, redness, warmth, pain) should be reported. Ice chips and clear fluids are allowed soon after birth. The amount, color, and clarity of urine should be monitored.

Interventions

Assisting the Client with Infant Feeding. Pain after cesarean may interfere with the client's ability to breastfeed and to provide infant care. Ensuring adequate pain relief is important so the client can focus on the infant.

It is important to help the client find a comfortable position for holding and feeding the infant. Some clients prefer sitting with a pillow on the lap to protect the incisional area. A side-lying position or football hold may be more comfortable because the infant is not putting pressure against the incision (see Chapter 23). A support person or the nurse should provide assistance with infant care until the client is able to do it independently.

The First 24 Hours. Nursing care for the client who gave birth by cesarean is similar to other postoperative clients.

Providing Pain Relief and Comfort Measures. The nurse should determine the need for pain relief on a regular basis. If a client has a PCA, the nurse should check how often it is being used. The effectiveness of analgesics should be evaluated. Pain relief enhances the client's ability to increase activity, helps prevent thrombophlebitis, promotes healing and facilitates attachment with the baby. For clients with epidural or spinal opioids, the nurse should continue to assess the respiratory status and ability to stand and ambulate safely. Assisting with first ambulation can help reduce fall risk. Placing a pillow behind the back and one between the client's knees while in bed prevents strain and discomfort when in the side-lying position. Excellent physical care (oral hygiene, perineal care, a sponge bath, clean linen) comforts and refreshes the client.

Overcoming Effects of Immobility. Client who delivered by cesarean are usually on bed rest for the first 6 to 12 hours. To prevent pooling of secretions in the airways, they should be assisted to turn, cough, and expand the lungs by breathing deeply at least every 2 hours while awake. Splinting the abdomen with a small pillow reduces incisional discomfort when they cough. Incentive spirometers help expand the lungs to prevent hypostatic pneumonia, which can result from immobility and shallow, slow respirations.

Clients should be encouraged to flex their knees and move their legs and feet frequently while in bed to improve peripheral circulation and to prevent thrombi. Compression stockings and pneumatic compression devices may be used to prevent the pooling of blood in the lower extremities (Cunningham et al., 2022).

Activity will be gradually increased. Encourage and assist the client to sit and dangle their feet the first few times before getting out of bed. They should be helped to get out of bed and walk short distances within 12 hours to decrease risk for thrombi. They will need support ambulating when the IV line and catheter are still in place.

After 24 Hours

Resuming Normal Activities. Twenty-four hours after a cesarean birth, several normal functions return, and clients are able to participate more actively in their own care:

- Both the indwelling catheter and the IV line are discontinued.
- The dressing, if present, is removed. If staples are present, they are removed before discharge. Steri-Strips (small strips of adhesive) may be placed over the incision when staples are removed. A small nonstick dressing may be placed over the incision to protect it from friction from clothing or adipose tissue, or the incision may be left open to air.
- The client is helped to ambulate the first postpartum day and is comfortable sitting in a chair for brief periods.
- The diet is advanced as tolerated. In some agencies, solid foods are provided immediately postoperatively, while other institutions do not offer solid food until bowel sounds are audible and the client is passing flatus.

Nurses should encourage the client to increase activity and ambulation each postpartum day. By the second day, they are usually allowed to shower.

Preventing Abdominal Distention. Abdominal distention is a major source of discomfort. Measures to prevent or minimize it include the following:

- Early, frequent ambulation.
- Tightening and relaxing the abdominal muscles.
- Avoidance of carbonated beverages and the use of straws, which increase the accumulation of intestinal gas.
- Pelvic lifts—Lying supine with knees bent, the client lifts the pelvis from the bed and repeats the exercise up to 10 times, several times each day.
- Simethicone, as ordered, to help disperse upper gastrointestinal flatulence.
- Rectal suppositories, as ordered, to help stimulate peristalsis and passage of flatus.

Teaching for Discharge. After cesarean births, clients receive the same overall teaching as those who had vaginal births. Information about care of the incision and signs to report to the health care provider are added. In addition, clients should have support at home because they are recovering from major surgery as well as childbirth.

KNOWLEDGE CHECK

15. What additional assessments are necessary for the client after a cesarean birth?
16. How can hypostatic pneumonia be prevented?
17. Which nursing measures are used to prevent or minimize abdominal distention?

APPLICATION OF THE NURSING PROCESS: KNOWLEDGE OF SELF-CARE

Assessment

Regardless of the method of birth, nurses are responsible for providing health education before the family is discharged from the birth facility. Much should be taught during this short time, which can be challenging when clients are not fully recovered from the birth process.

Before beginning teaching, determine the learning needs and major concerns of the family. Multiparas remember some aspects of self-care but may benefit from a review. Primiparas may be anxious about self-care measures and all aspects of infant care. They may need more thorough teaching and more time for practice. Identify the most common barriers to learning: age and developmental level, cultural factors, or difficulty understanding the language.

Identification of Client Problems

In general, clients adapt well to the physiologic changes after childbirth, and most nursing care is wellness-oriented. A common client problem is a lack of knowledge of personal care, signs of complications, and preventive measures.

Planning: Expected Outcomes

Expected outcomes for this problem are the client will do the following:
- Verbalize or demonstrate understanding of self-care instructions by discharge.
- Verbalize understanding of health promotion practices by discharge.
- Describe plans for follow-up care and signs and symptoms that should be reported to the health care provider by discharge.

Interventions

Preparing for Teaching

Before beginning teaching sessions, be sure the client is comfortable. Give pain medication, if needed. Provide teaching at times that do not interfere with meals, infant care needs, or visitors. Make a teaching plan with the client to include topics most important to them. Identify the client's educational needs, which helps with engagement and making best use of the short time available. Topics of less interest may require just a brief review. This review may elicit questions from the client and interest in more in-depth information.

Teaching about the Process of Involution

Provide the client with basic information about involution, including how to assess lochia and locate and palpate the fundus. This information allows the client to recognize abnormal signs such as prolonged lochia, reappearance of bright-red lochia after lochia rubra has ended, and uterine tenderness, which should be reported to the health care provider. If the client is a young adolescent, another family member also may need the information.

Teaching Self-Care

Handwashing. Emphasize the importance of thoroughly washing their hands before they touch their breasts, after diaper changes, after bladder and bowel elimination, before and after handling peripads, and always before handling the infant. Observing nurses helps model this behavior and reinforces this parent teaching.

Breast Care for Lactating Clients. Instruct breastfeeding clients to avoid using soap on their nipples because it will remove the natural lubrication secreted by the Montgomery's glands. Keeping the nipples dry between feedings helps prevent tissue damage, and wearing a good bra provides necessary support as breast size increases.

Measures to Suppress Lactation. If the client chooses not to breastfeed, initiate measures to minimize lactation and increase the client's comfort. Techniques such as binding the breasts, applying an infrared lamp, fluid and diet restrictions, external application of jasmine flower and ice packs have all been used to suppress lactation without convincing evidence. Current recommendations include instructing the client to wear a firm fitted bra 24 hours a day until breasts are soft and nontender. Avoid breast stimulation, but if experiencing severe discomfort, express only a small amount of milk or take a warm shower, which may stimulate milk leakage if absolutely necessary for pain relief. The client may use cold compresses or gel packs inside the bra for comfort. Cold cabbage leaves also promote comfort. They should be washed and dried. The client should place the cabbage leaves in the bra and change them out every 2 hours or as they become limp. If cold is not acceptable due to cultural reasons, then warmth may also provide comfort. Explain warmth can stimulate further milk let-down and should not be used routinely. Analgesic medications may be recommended by the provider (Australian Breastfeeding Association, 2020; Janke, 2021).

Care of the Cesarean Incision. If the birth was by cesarean, the client may have concerns about care of the incision. Staples, if used, are usually removed before the client is discharged. The obese client may go home with staples and have them removed by the health care provider after discharge. If adhesive strips have been applied over the incision, teach the client that it is possible to shower with them in place, and the strips will gradually detach.

If a topical skin adhesive was applied in surgery instead of staples or adhesive strips, there is no dressing, and the client is generally allowed to shower. For each method, explain the incision is closed and is unlikely to come apart. There should be little or no drainage from the incision. Instruct the client to call the provider if the incision separates or drainage increases or has a foul odor.

Perineal Care. Teach clients how to clean their perineum. The most common method is to fill a squeeze bottle with warm water and spray the perineal area from the front toward the back. Remind the client not to separate the labia during this procedure to avoid allowing water to enter the vagina. The tip of the bottle should not touch the perineum.

Toilet paper or moist antiseptic towelettes are used in a patting motion to dry the perineum. Teach the client to dry from front to back to prevent fecal contamination of the vaginal introitus from the anal area. Perineal cleansing and changing peripads should occur after each voiding or defecation.

Some clients do not use peripads for menstrual protection and should be taught how to use them correctly. Mesh panties and adhering pads are used in most facilities. Careful handling to avoid contamination of the pads is important to prevent perineal infection.

- Thorough handwashing is a must before and after changing pads.
- Unused pads should be stored inside their packages.
- Pads should be applied without touching the side that comes into contact with the perineum.
- The pads should be applied and removed in a front-to-back direction to prevent contamination of the vagina and the perineum.
- Used pads should be wrapped and disposed of in a covered container.

Kegel Exercises. All clients should become familiar with Kegel exercises. These movements strengthen the muscles surrounding the vagina and urinary meatus. The exercise helps prevent the loss of muscle tone, which can occur after childbirth and may decrease urinary incontinence.

Promoting Rest and Sleep

Many clients experience fatigue after childbirth, which continues for weeks or months. Clients are often tired when they begin the postpartum period because they slept poorly during the third trimester and are further exhausted by the exertion of labor. Feelings of excitement and euphoria after childbirth interfere with rest. Numerous visitors and phone calls, hospital routines, noise, frequent interruptions, and an unfamiliar environment also interfere with rest. Afterpains, discomfort from an episiotomy or incision, muscle aches, and breast **engorgement** (swelling from increased blood flow, edema, and presence of milk) further contribute to a client's discomfort and inability to sleep.

Most clients are discharged from the facility within 24 to 48 hours after vaginal birth or 72 to 96 hours after cesarean birth, and they go home with a tremendous deficit in sleep and energy. Yet new parents may be unprepared for the conflict between their need for sleep and the infant's need for care and attention.

A telephone call to screen for prolonged postpartum fatigue may be helpful in the days after discharge. Anemia, infection, and thyroid dysfunction also may cause postpartum fatigue. Clients at risk for these conditions or suffering postpartum fatigue after the first 2 weeks should be evaluated and treated, if necessary.

Rest at the Birth Facility. Hospital routines continue around the clock, making undisturbed rest difficult to obtain during the birth facility stay. Make every effort to avoid interruptions and allow clients adequate time for uninterrupted rest periods and relaxed time with their infants.

Cluster assessments and care and try to correlate them with times when the client will be awake, such as just before or after meals, infant feeding times, and visiting hours.

Make plans with the client for napping. Suggest they restrict phone calls and visitors during planned nap times. A quiet, softly lit environment also promotes sleep.

Rest at Home. Help clients understand how their energy will be negatively impacted by physical discomfort and the demands of the newborn and other family members during the first few weeks. If they understand fatigue is normal and will continue for some time, they can plan ways to obtain extra help and conserve their energy. Suggest energy-saving measures such as the following:

- Maintain a relaxed, flexible routine focusing on self and infant care.
- Nap or rest when the infant sleeps.
- Plan simple meals and flexible meal times.
- Limit visitors.
- Accept assistance with food shopping, meal preparation, laundry, and housework.
- Ask family or friends to care for the infant to provide nap times for the client.
- Put off housework that is not absolutely necessary.
- Postpone major household projects.
- Involve friends and family to provide care for other children.
- Avoid heavy meals or vigorous exercise near bedtime.

Advise the client to restrict intake of caffeine or to use caffeine-free versions for the first few weeks. Suggest relaxation exercises (lying quietly, alternately tightening and relaxing the muscles of the neck, shoulders, arms, legs, and feet) when a nap is not possible.

Emphasize to the client the importance of asking for help when beginning to feel exhausted or overwhelmed. Encourage sharing these feelings with partners, other family members, friends, and other new parents.

Infant Sleep and Feeding Schedules. Many families require information about infant sleep cycles, frequency of feeding, and probable crying episodes during the first weeks. Although newborns sleep much of the time, they may awaken every 2 to 3 hours for feeding. If possible, having the partner or another helper assist with nighttime care of the infant allows the client longer sleep periods. For the breastfeeding client, this would mean the helper gets up, changes the baby's diaper, and brings the baby to the client to nurse and returns the baby to the crib or bassinet after nursing.

Providing Nutrition Counseling

Food Supply. Low-income families might benefit from referral to government-sponsored programs such as Temporary Assistance for Needy Families (TANF) or the Special Supplemental Nutrition Program for Women, Infants, and Children (WIC). Determining the facilities available for cooking and storing food also may be necessary. The new family may need referral to a social worker to identify the best solutions for their unique problems.

Diet. Although many clients are unsatisfied with slow weight loss, they should avoid severe restriction of caloric intake. A balanced, low-fat diet with adequate protein, complex carbohydrates, fruits, and vegetables provides the energy and nutrients needed.

Promoting Regular Bowel Elimination

Explain the role of progressive exercise, adequate fluid, and dietary fiber in preventing constipation. Walking is an excellent exercise, and the distance can be increased as strength and endurance increase. Drinking at least eight glasses of water daily helps maintain normal bowel elimination. Unpeeled fruits and vegetables are high in fiber, and prunes are natural laxatives. Additional fiber is found in whole-grain cereals, bread, and pasta.

A regular schedule of bowel elimination is important in overcoming constipation. For example, bowel elimination after breakfast allows the client to take advantage of the gastrocolic reflex (stimulation of peristalsis induced in the colon when food is consumed on an empty stomach). Comfort measures for reducing perineal and hemorrhoid pain include witch hazel astringent compresses and hydrocortisone ointments, which also facilitate bowel elimination.

Promoting Good Body Mechanics

Exercise. Exercise has beneficial physical and psychological effects during the postpartum period. Teach exercises in the early postpartum period to strengthen the abdominal muscles and firm the waist (Fig. 17.7). These mild exercises can be started soon after childbirth with five repetitions, twice a day. The number of exercises is increased gradually as the client gains strength.

Exercise routines may be resumed gradually after pregnancy as soon as medically safe, depending on the mode of delivery, vaginal or cesarean, and the presence or absence of medical or surgical complications. Some clients are capable of resuming physical activities within days of birth. In the absence of medical or surgical complications, rapid resumption of these activities has not been found to result in adverse effects. Pelvic floor exercises could be initiated in the immediate postpartum period (ACOG, 2020a). Walking is a common exercise, and clients can take the infant with them on walks. Clients who exercise with a friend are more likely to fit it into their schedules.

Counseling about Sexual Activity

The couple may have concerns about resuming sexual intercourse and contraceptive choices. Some couples will ask questions; for others, the nurses should be sensitive to unasked questions and provide anticipatory guidance. Many new parents are reluctant to ask about when to resume sexual activity and potential changes in sexuality resulting from pregnancy and childbirth. Fatigue, pain, fear of pregnancy, concerns about the baby, and a feeling of unattractiveness may interfere with a client's sexual desire. Some clients who breastfeed have nipple tenderness and should be advised this should subside after the first week, and ongoing nipple pain is not normal.

Couples can begin intercourse as early as 2 weeks after giving birth, if desire and comfort allow (Cunningham et al., 2022). Low estrogen levels during the early postpartum period and during lactation cause vaginal dryness. Application of a water-soluble vaginal lubricant may increase comfort during intercourse. Clients with third- or fourth-degree lacerations or episiotomies may need more time to allow for healing.

Cultural or religious convictions may restrict the choice of contraceptive method for some couples. The availability of health care or limited finances may dictate the choice for others. Discuss previous experience with contraceptives and the satisfaction with those methods.

Instructing about Follow-Up Appointments

Remind the client to make an appointment with the provider for a postpartum examination at the time suggested. This is often 3 to 6 weeks after vaginal birth and 2 weeks after cesarean birth. It is recommended all postpartum clients contact a health care provider at least once within the first 3 weeks postpartum followed by a comprehensive visit within 4 to 12 weeks (ACOG, 2018; Paladine et al., 2019).

Emphasize the importance of the postpartum examination. It allows early assessment of postpartum healing and identification and treatment of problems that may develop. It also provides an opportunity for contraceptive counseling and planning for future pregnancies. Clients who have had complications during the pregnancy or postpartum period may need to see their health care provider sooner or have more extensive follow-up than those without complications.

Teaching about Signs and Symptoms to Report

Teach the client and at least one family member which physical signs and symptoms should be reported to the health care provider immediately. These include the following:

- Fever (greater than 100.4°F)
- Localized area of redness, swelling, or pain in either breast
- Persistent abdominal tenderness
- Feelings of pelvic fullness or pelvic pressure
- Persistent perineal pain
- Frequency, urgency, or burning on urination
- Abnormal change in character of lochia (increased amount, resumption of bright red color, passage of clots, foul odor)
- Localized tenderness, redness, edema, or warmth of the legs
- Redness, separation or edema of, or foul drainage from an abdominal incision
- Headache (severe) or vision changes

The following symptoms should prompt a call to emergency services immediately:

- Pain in the chest
- Difficulty breathing or shortness of breath
- Seizures
- Thoughts about hurting themselves or someone else

Ensuring All Elements Have Been Taught

Organize information so it can be presented and absorbed in the time available. Many facilities have a television channel for client teaching. If this format is used, the nurse should follow up, clarifying any misunderstandings and answering any

ABDOMINAL BREATHING

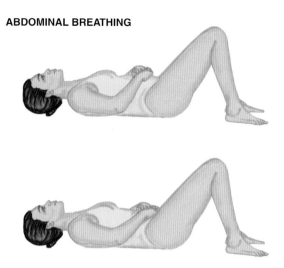

This is one of the simplest exercises and can be started on the first postpartum day. The client assumes a supine position with knees bent. Inhaling through the nose, keeping the rib cage as stationary as possible, and allowing the abdomen to expand. Then the client contracts the abdominal muscles while exhaling slowly through the mouth.

HEAD LIFT

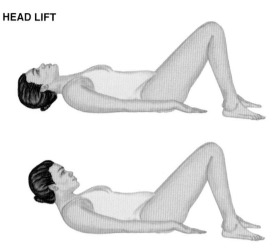

This exercise can be started within a few days after childbirth. The client assumes a supine position with knees bent. Inhaling deeply to begin, then exhaling while lifting the head slowly. Hold this position for a few seconds and relax.

KNEE AND LEG ROLLS

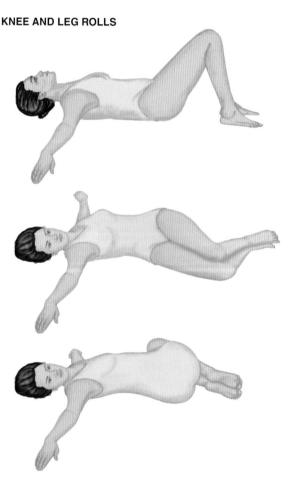

MODIFIED SIT-UPS

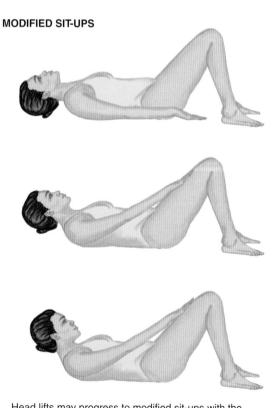

Head lifts may progress to modified sit-ups with the approval of the healthcare provider; the client should follow the advice of the healthcare provider about the number of repetitions.

The exercise begins with the client supine with arms outstretched and knees bent. Raising the head and shoulders while reaching for the knees. The client raises the shoulders only as far as the back will bend; the waist remains on the floor.

This is an excellent exercise to begin firming the waist. The client lies supine with knees bent and feet flat on the floor or bed; keeping the shoulders and feet stationary and rolling the knees to touch first one side of the bed, then the other. Maintaining a smooth motion as the exercise is repeated five times. Later, as flexibility increases, the exercise can be varied by rolling of one knee only. The client rolls the left knee to touch the right side of the bed, returns to center, and rolls the right knee to touch the left side of the bed.

FIG. 17.7 Postpartum exercises. Exercises should be approved by the client's provider before beginning them.

CHEST EXERCISES

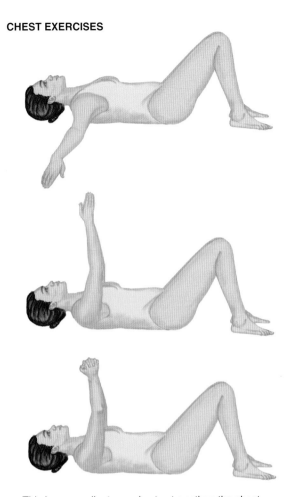

This is an excellent exercise to strengthen the chest muscles. The client lies supine with arms extended straight out to the side; bringing the hands together about the chest while keeping the arms straight; holding for a few seconds and returning to the starting position. Repeat the exercise five times initially and follows the advice of the healthcare provider for increasing the number of repetitions.

Isometric exercises also increase strength and tone; the client bends their elbows, clasps hands together above chest, and presses hands together for a few seconds. This is repeated at least five times.

FIG. 17.7, cont'd

questions. In some cases, clients are given information pertaining to postpartum self-care during the prenatal period. During the hospital stay, the nurse reviews and checks the parents' understanding of previous teaching.

Although there are many topics to discuss in parent teaching, avoid covering too much information at a time. Interspersing small segments of teaching into normal care throughout the day will keep the client from being overwhelmed and help them remember information better. Written instructions, including a phone number for questions, should also be provided at discharge for the family's reference. Organizations such as the Council on Patient Safety in Women's Healthcare and the Association of Women's Health Obstetric and Neonatal Nurses (AWHONN) provide handouts outlining urgent maternal and post-birth warning signs (AWHONN, 2017; Council on Patient Safety in Women's Health Care, 2020; Suplee & Janke, 2020).

Documenting Teaching

Documentation is an important aspect of teaching, just as it is for other aspects of nursing care. Documentation of discharge teaching and the client's comprehension of teaching is required by accrediting agencies. To prevent omissions, many hospitals use teaching checklists for topics to be included (Box 17.2) (see Chapter 22 for teaching about infant care).

Evaluation

The demonstration of correct breast and perineal hygiene provides evidence of the client's ability to perform self-care measures. The ability to discuss practices that promote health in the areas of diet, exercise, rest, and sleep confirms understanding of these measures. The plan for future appointments with the health care provider for examinations or follow-up of complications increases the likelihood the client will experience an uncomplicated recovery.

KNOWLEDGE CHECK

18. How is lactation suppressed when the client elects not to breastfeed?
19. What are challenges nurses have in preparing new parents for discharge?

POSTPARTUM DISCHARGE AND COMMUNITY-BASED CARE

Criteria for Discharge

Most clients leave the hospital when they are just beginning to recover from giving birth and starting to learn how to care for themselves and their infants. Criteria for discharge have been developed by the AAP and ACOG (2017) and includes the following:

- The client has no complications, and assessments (including vital signs, pain level, lochia, fundus, urinary output, incisions, ambulation, ability to eat and drink, and emotional status) are normal.
- Pertinent laboratory data, including blood type and Hgb or Hct have been reviewed, and Rho(D) immune globulin has been administered, if necessary.
- The client has received instructions on self-care, deviations from normal, and proper response to danger signs and symptoms.
- The client demonstrates knowledge, ability, and confidence to care for themselves and their baby.
- The client has received instructions on postpartum activity, exercises, and relief measures for common postpartum discomforts.
- Arrangements have been made for postpartum follow-up care.
- Family members or other support persons are available to the client for the first few days after discharge.

Community-Based Care

Many assessments and interventions of postpartum clients occur in the clinic or outpatient setting. Clients leave the birth facility when they are not fully recovered from the childbirth experience. New parents should be made aware of local community care services. Information lines, websites, telephone calls from birth facility staff, nurse-managed postpartum outpatient clinics, and, in some areas, home visits provide information and guidance for postpartum families. Breastfeeding and parenting classes, "baby and me" walks or exercise sessions, and postpartum support groups also may be available.

> **? KNOWLEDGE CHECK**
>
> 20. What are the criteria for discharge of the postpartum client?

PSYCHOSOCIAL ADAPTATIONS

Perhaps no other event requires such rapid change in family structure and function as the birth of a baby. The addition of a new baby requires all family members adjust their roles. The postpartum client progresses through restorative phases to replenish the energy lost during labor and childbirth and to gain confidence in the role as parent. Both parents continue the process of attachment with the newborn that began during pregnancy. Siblings must adapt to a new standing in the family structure. Numerous factors such as previous experience, available support system, and culture influence the family's adaptation.

The role of maternity nurses includes not only the care of the client-infant dyad but also the well-being of the entire family. Nurses are concerned with the family's adjustment to childbearing during the hospital stay and during the early weeks at home. The first 12 weeks, as the family makes the transition to parenthood and adapts to changes in the family structure, are often called the **fourth trimester**.

The Process of Becoming Acquainted

Nursing literature has described how parents and newborns become acquainted and progress to develop feelings of love, concern, and deep devotion, which last throughout life. The terms *bonding* and *attachment* are commonly used to describe the initial steps. Although the terms are sometimes used interchangeably, their meanings differ.

Bonding

Bonding refers to the rapid initial attraction felt by parents for their infant. It is unidirectional, from parent to child, and is enhanced when parents and infants are permitted to touch and interact during the first 30 to 60 minutes after birth. During this time the infant is in a quiet, alert state and seems to gaze directly at the parents (Fig. 17.8).

Infants should be placed skin-to-skin on the client's chest or abdomen for bonding time immediately after the birth, if possible. Nurses frequently delay procedures, such as measurements and medication administration that would interfere with this time so that parents can focus on their newborn baby.

Early and sustained contact between the parents and infant can enhance bonding and attachment. However, if early contact between parent and infant is limited because of an obstetric emergency or neonatal condition, bonding and attachment can still occur at a later time.

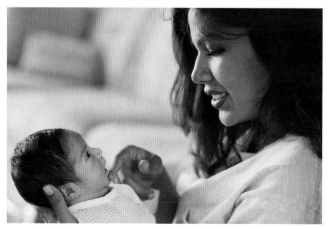

FIG. 17.8 The infant is quiet and alert during the initial sensitive period. The newborn gazes at the client and responds to their voice and touch.

Attachment

Attachment is the process by which an enduring bond between a parent and child is developed through pleasurable, satisfying interaction. The process begins in pregnancy and extends for many months after childbirth. The infant receives warmth, food, and security from the parent. The parent accepts responsibility for the infant's care and places the child's needs above his or her own for years to come. In return, the parent receives enjoyment and establishes his or her identity as a father, mother or parent. Both infant and parent benefit from the formation of irreplaceable links that continue long after the child ceases to be dependent.

Attachment follows a progressive or developmental course that changes over time. It is rarely instantaneous. Attachment behaviors of inexperienced or first-time parents do not differ significantly from those of experienced parents (Mercer & Ferketich, 1994). Attachment occurs through mutually satisfying experiences. Therefore, if the client is in pain or physically exhausted, pain relief and assistance are needed to facilitate enjoyable, early experiences with the baby.

Attachment is reciprocal—it occurs in both directions between parent and infant. It is facilitated by positive feedback, either real or perceived, from the infant. For example, an infant's grasp reflex around a parent's finger means "I love you" to the parent. Alert infants have a repertoire of responses called **reciprocal attachment behaviors**. These behaviors are the infant's part in the process of early attachment that progresses to lifelong, mutual devotion.

CRITICAL TO REMEMBER

Reciprocal Attachment Behaviors

Newborn infants have the ability to do the following:
Make eye contact and engage in prolonged, intense, mutual gazing.
Move their eyes and attempt to "track" the parent's face.
Grasp and hold the parent's finger.
Move synchronously in response to rhythms and patterns of the parent's voice (called **entrainment**).
Root, latch onto the breast, and suckle.
Be comforted by the parent's voice or touch.

Maternal Touch

Classic research by Rubin (1963) and Klaus, Kennell et. al (1970) described the progression of touch used by postpartum clients, identified as mothers, during the initial and early interactions as they move through a discovery phase with the infant. Initially mothers may not reach for the infant, but if the infant is placed in their arms, they hold the baby in an **en face** position with the infant's face in the same vertical plane as their own so they can have eye contact. When the infant is awake, the two engage in prolonged, mutual gazing.

Mothers need time to get acquainted with the tiny stranger. At first, they may gently explore the infant's face, fingers, and toes with their fingertips only.

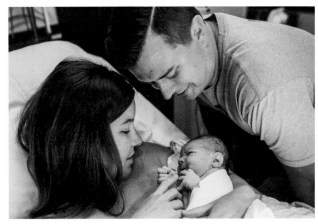

FIG. 17.9 During the binding-in or claiming process the client identifies the baby's specific features and relates them to other family members. This client states, "Her fingers are long, just like mine."

After using fingertips to explore the new infant, the mother begins to stroke the baby's chest and legs with their palm. Next, they use their entire hand and arms to enfold the infant and to bring the baby close to their body. They hold the newborn closer, stroke the baby's hair, press their cheek against the infant's cheek, and finally feel comfortable enough to engage in a full range of consoling behaviors.

The mother next begins to identify specific features of the newborn: "Look how bright his eyes are." Then they begin to relate features to family members: "He has his father's chin and nose" (Fig. 17.9). This identification process has been called **claiming** or binding-in (Rubin, 1977).

Verbal Behaviors

Verbal behaviors are also important indicators of attachment. Most clients speak to the infant in a high-pitched voice. Although many have been calling the baby by name since seeing it on an ultrasound scan during pregnancy, others wait until after the birth to progress from calling the baby "it" to "he" or "she," and then to using the given name. "I can't believe it's here" rapidly becomes "Michele is such a good baby." Verbal behaviors may provide clues to a client's early psychological relationship with their infant. Nurses observe the interactions of clients and their infants and, if necessary, teach and model interactions that foster early attachment between them. Referrals can be made to a social worker or home visit if needed to further assess bonding behaviors.

KNOWLEDGE CHECK

21. How do bonding and attachment differ?
22. How does maternal touch change over time?
23. How does verbal behavior of the parents change over time?

The Process of Maternal Adaptation
Puerperal Phases

Rubin (1961) identified restorative phases postpartum clients (mothers) go through to replenish the energy lost during labor and attain comfort in their new role. The puerperal phases are called *taking-in, taking-hold,* and *letting-go* and provide one method to observe progressive change in maternal behavior. Although they should not be used as strict guidelines for assessment, the phases can help the nurse anticipate needs and intervene to meet those needs.

Taking-In Phase. During the **taking-in** phase, mothers are focused primarily on their own need for fluid, food, and sleep. Inexperienced nurses may be puzzled by the passive, dependent behavior as they take in or receive attention and physical care. They also take in every detail of the neonate but may seem content to allow others to make decisions.

A major task for mothers during this time is to integrate the birth experience into reality. To do this, they discuss their labor and delivery many times on the telephone or with visitors. They attempt to piece together all the details from those who were involved in the birth. This process helps the new mother realize the pregnancy is over and the newborn is now a separate individual.

Although Rubin believed the taking-in phase lasted for approximately 2 days, it probably lasts a day or less today. The phase may be prolonged when a cesarean birth, especially in an emergency, has been necessary. These mothers may have difficulty assimilating the unfamiliar and intrusive procedures that occurred in rapid succession and may have negative perceptions of the birth experience. Clients who have had cesarean births need continued attention and sensitive care taking into account their physical and psychological needs.

Taking-Hold Phase. Mothers become more independent during the **taking-hold** phase. They exhibit concern about managing their own body functions and assume responsibility for their own care. When they feel more comfortable and in control of their body, they shift their attention to the behaviors of the infant. They compare the infant with other infants to validate wellness and wholeness. They welcome information about the wide variety of behaviors exhibited by newborns.

During the taking-hold phase, mothers may verbalize anxiety about their competence as a parent. They may compare their caretaking skills unfavorably with those of the nurse.

Nurses should be careful not to assume the primary role in caring for the infant. Instead, they should encourage new mothers to perform as much of the caretaking as possible. Both parents should be encouraged to participate in caretaking as they take on a new role. Nurses should praise each attempt, even if the parents' early care is awkward.

The taking-hold phase, which extends over several days, has been called the *teachable, reachable, referable moment.* Nurses who provide home or clinic care can take advantage of this ideal time to review previously taught material and provide additional instructions and demonstrations.

Letting-Go Phase. The **letting-go** phase is a time of relinquishment for the parents. If this is their first child, the couple must give up their previous role as a childless couple and acknowledge the loss of their more carefree lifestyle. Many must also give up idealized expectations of the birth experience. For example, they may have planned to have a vaginal birth with minimal or no anesthesia but instead required a cesarean birth.

In addition, some parents are disappointed in the size, sex, or characteristics of the infant who does not "match up" with the fantasy baby of pregnancy. They must relinquish the infant of their fantasies and accept the real infant.

These losses often provoke feelings of grief, which are so subtle they may be unexamined or unacknowledged. Both parents may benefit, however, if given the opportunity to discuss unexpected feelings and realize these feelings are common. If the client is very young or the pregnancy was unplanned, the feelings of loss and grief may be acute.

During this phase, clients refocus on the relationship with their partner. They may also return to work at this time. This requires relinquishing a portion of infant care to other adults.

Maternal Role Attainment and Role Conflict

Role attainment is a process by which clients achieve confidence in their ability to care for their infant and becomes comfortable with their identity as a parent. The process begins during pregnancy and continues for several months after childbirth.

The transition to the maternal role includes the following four stages (Mercer, 1995b):

1. The anticipatory stage begins during the pregnancy when the pregnant client chooses a provider and a location for the infant's birth. They may attend childbirth classes to be prepared and feel they have some control over the birth experience. They seek out role models to help them learn the new role.
2. The formal stage begins with the birth of the infant and continues for approximately 4 to 6 weeks (Mercer, 1995a). During this stage, behaviors are largely guided by others, such as health professionals, close friends, and parents. A major task during this stage is for the new parents to become acquainted with their infants so they can mesh their caregiving with infant cues.
3. The informal stage, which may overlap the formal stage, begins when mothers have learned appropriate responses to their infants' cues and signals. The mothers begin to respond according to the unique needs of their infants and develop their own version of the maternal role rather than following textbooks or health professionals' directives.
4. The personal stage is attained when the mother feels a sense of harmony in the role, enjoys the infant, sees the infant as a central person in their life, and has internalized the parental role. They accept the role of parent and feel comfortable in this role. The range of time for achieving the maternal role is highly variable, with some reaching that point in the first month and others taking much longer.

Maternal role attainment implies an end point when the client adjusts to motherhood. However, this motherhood role grows and evolves as the client responds to the challenges of their child's growth and development. This process is sometimes called *becoming a mother* (Mercer, 2004). Most mothers do not feel competent and self-confident in this new role until about 4 months after childbirth (Mercer & Walker, 2006).

Role conflict occurs when a person's perception of role responsibilities differs significantly from reality. For example, conflict may occur if the parent perceives their responsibility is providing most of the care and comfort for the infant, but reality dictates they must place the infant with a caregiver and return to full-time employment. In the United States 66% of mothers with children under 6 years of age were employed in 2019 (U.S. Department of Labor, 2020). The amount of maternity leave, now often called parental or family leave, may vary. In the United States the Family and Medical Leave Act (FMLA) entitles most workers to up to 12 weeks of unpaid leave for birth or adoption. Most other countries offer paid maternity leave from 14 weeks up to a year or more to care for the new child. Many parents feel guilty and experience intense "separation grief" when they first leave the infant with a caregiver. Some report feeling jealous of the caregiver, whom they fear will supplant them in the infant's affection.

The nurse can help by acknowledging these feelings and reassuring the parent these emotions are normal. Anticipatory guidance from the nurse is important. Parents need to plan for time to reestablish feelings of closeness when they come home from work. They need to develop a schedule which allows maximum time with the infant when they are at home. They may have to negotiate with another family member to take over some of the household tasks until they feel more comfortable with the situation (see Nursing Care Plan).

NURSING CARE PLAN

Adaptation of the Working Parent

Assessment

Claire, a 30-year-old single mother who identifies as female, gave birth to a baby boy, Drew, by cesarean delivery 6 days ago. She has made a good recovery, and breastfeeding is going well. During her visit to a nurse-managed postpartum clinic, Claire discusses her need to return to work as a sales executive in 6 weeks. She states that she hates the thought of leaving the baby with someone else while she works. "I've always planned to stay home for at least 6 months when I had a baby, but it's impossible. How can I be a mother and work full-time?"

Identification of Client Problems

Emotional distress as a result of inability to perform the parental role as she wishes because of the need to return to full-time employment.

Critical Thinking

Emotional distress or grief may be related to loss. What has Claire lost, or what must she give up?

Answer

Claire must give up her idealized picture of motherhood. She also must give up mothering tasks and time with the infant to a caregiver. She will have to modify her self-concept based on the perception of these losses.

Expected Outcomes

Claire will do the following:
1. Describe concerns and feelings about leaving Drew with a caregiver.
2. Verbalize plans to achieve maximal satisfaction in the parental role by the time she returns to work.

Interventions and Rationales

1. Allow Claire to describe her perception of her role as a mother and express concerns about how employment will interfere with her ability to fulfill this role. *Venting can help Claire cope with the role of conflict, stress, and grief, which can result when a mother who envisions her role as the primary caregiver must leave her infant with another caregiver and return to her job.*
2. Suggest Claire openly express her feelings of anxiety, guilt, and jealousy to significant others and to her baby's care provider. *Candid expression of feelings helps resolve them and allows for a discussion of measures that will help overcome the intense feelings that cause conflict.*
3. Acknowledge Claire's feelings are difficult and reassure her they are common. *Knowledge that the feelings are not trivial and are experienced by others reinforces their validity and importance.*
4. Recommend Claire investigate several daycare providers before choosing one. She should check references, make unannounced visits, see required licenses and certification, discuss the number and ages of children cared for and the daily schedule, ask about the provider's philosophy of infant care and training in emergency measures, and know what emergency plans are in place. *A great deal of stress is eliminated if parents feel confident that a competent and nurturing daycare provider has been found. Mothers are more content with their return to work if they are satisfied with their child care arrangements.*
5. Suggest she leave the infant with the chosen daycare provider for 2 to 3 days before resuming full-time employment. *Allowing both mother and infant to "practice separating" while their schedules are still somewhat flexible helps ease the transition and makes it less traumatic.*
6. Recommend Claire pump her breasts and feed Drew by bottle at least once per day in the week or two before returning to work. *Becoming proficient at pumping the breasts and introducing the infant to bottle feeding prepares both the mother and the infant for all-day separation.*
7. Help Claire develop a schedule allowing her maximum time with Drew. *Feelings of frustration and stress can be alleviated if the mother has a plan that allows her long periods of uninterrupted time with the infant.*
   a. Make a list of errands and supplies needed to avoid frequent stops that delay getting home from work.
   b. Double the recipe when cooking and freeze half for future use.
   c. Pick up nutritious takeout meals to avoid cooking every evening.
   d. Purchase nutritious prepackaged frozen meals to have available when needed.
   e. Schedule appointments on the same day when possible.
   f. Include Drew in daily walks, exercise, and social visits.

Continued

◎ NURSING CARE PLAN—cont'd

Adaptation of the Working Parent

8. Recommend Claire allow 30 to 45 minutes to hold Drew when she first gets home. Delay all other activities until this need is met for both mother and infant. *Time is needed to make the transition between work and home. It helps to reestablish feelings of closeness, comfort, and attachment.* 9. Advise Claire to try to get more rest in the early weeks after returning to work. *The return to work may increase fatigue. Extra rest will help Claire avoid undue fatigue or illness.*	**Evaluation** Claire freely expressed her feelings of guilt, anxiety, and concern about leaving Drew. She made a plan to investigate daycares in her area and discussed plans to reorganize her work and social schedule so she can spend as much time as possible with her son.

Major Maternal Concerns

As the postpartum client gains confidence in their ability to care for the infant and physical discomfort decreases, emotional concerns related to self become more important. Body image and the experience of postpartum blues are particularly important.

Body Image. Postpartum clients are very concerned about regaining their normal figures. Some have unrealistic expectations about weight loss and the time it takes for the body to regain its nonpregnant shape. Nurses should emphasize that weight loss should be gradual. Rigid restriction of calories can lead to depleted energy and decreased immunity.

In addition, nurses should teach the importance of safe activities such as walking and graduated exercises to regain muscle tone. Some birth facilities offer classes for postpartum clients that include exercise and nutrition as well as the opportunity to share concerns with other parents.

THERAPEUTIC COMMUNICATIONS

Body Image

Mary Kay delivered 48 hours ago. Aubrey, the client's nurse, is reviewing self-care measures before Mary Kay's discharge from the birth facility.

Mary Kay: Look at me! I still look pregnant, and my husband calls me Tubby.

Aubrey: You were looking forward to your abdomen being flat after the baby was born. *(This clarifies the concern by reflecting content.)*

Mary Kay: Well, I never had a big belly before. I thought it would all go away after I had the baby. I can't believe I look this fat.

Aubrey: Remember, it took 9 months for those muscles to stretch. You can't expect them to snap back in a few days. *This blocks communication by ignoring the feeling expressed. A more helpful response would be to acknowledge Mary Kay's distress and to delay giving information until feelings have been expressed. For example: "How disappointing for you! If you like, we can discuss some exercises that will help."*

Smoking. Many clients give up smoking during pregnancy to protect the health of the fetus. However, many resume smoking at some point during the first 6 months to 1 year postpartum. Factors that increase the likelihood of relapse include weight concerns, failure to breastfeed, depression, living with a smoker, stress, and planning to quit only during the pregnancy (ACOG, 2020b).

Nurses should discuss smoking with postpartum clients to offer resources for those who stopped smoking prenatally and are at risk for relapse in the postpartum period. Explanations of the hazards to the infant from smoking also may be helpful because some parents may think the harmful effects occur only during pregnancy.

Exposure to secondhand smoke increases the risk for sudden infant death syndrome (SIDS) and has been associated with cognitive impairments, behavior problems, ear infections, asthma, and other respiratory problems in children. Cigarettes themselves present a poisoning risk for small children; the amount of nicotine in just one cigarette butt is enough to poison a child. In addition, children of smokers are more likely to grow up to become smokers themselves.

There are many reasons to quit smoking after the baby is born. Nurses can provide support for smoking cessation, reducing smoking, and avoiding environmental tobacco smoke and nicotine exposure around the baby. Provide encouragement and information. Refer clients to support groups and their primary health care provider for further assistance.

Postpartum Blues. **Postpartum blues,** *baby blues,* or *maternity blues* is a frequent concern for new parents. This mild, transient condition affects 50% to 80% of clients who have given birth. The condition begins in the first week, peaks around day 5, and ends within 2 weeks. If it lasts beyond 2 weeks, it may be a more serious condition (Isley, 2021; Wisner et al., 2021).

Postpartum blues is characterized by irritability, fatigue, tearfulness, mood swings, headaches, confusion, forgetfulness, and anxiety. The symptoms are usually unrelated to events, and the condition does not seriously affect the client's ability to care for the infant (James & Suplee, 2021). Nurses should prepare clients and family members for the occurrence of postpartum blues symptoms, let them know it is normal, and offer emotional support and encouragement. Explain the difference between the transient postpartum blues and more serious postpartum depression and anxiety, which may require treatment.

Although the direct cause is unknown, postpartum blues may be a result of the emotional letdown that occurs after birth, postpartum discomforts, sleep deprivation, anxiety about the ability to care for the infant, and body image concern (Cunningham et al., 2022). Hormonal fluctuations have not been proved to be a cause, but associations with thyroid dysfunction, serotonin, and progesterone levels have been suggested.

Although postpartum blues is self-limiting, clients benefit greatly when empathy and support are freely given by the family and the health care team. Because the condition is so common in postpartum clients, caregivers or family members may not be as empathetic as they would be for a condition deemed more serious (James & Suplee, 2021). Yet clients need adequate attention to move through this period. Encourage rest, taking time for themselves, and discussing their feelings. In addition, provide reassurance that such feelings are normal and generally last less than 2 weeks.

Postpartum blues should be distinguished from postpartum depression and postpartum psychosis, which are disabling conditions and require therapeutic management for full recovery. Screening for risk factors (e.g., previous history of depression or mental illness or limited social support) along with initial screening and education about early warning signs and symptoms is important during the birth facility stay (see Chapter 11). Many hospitals conduct a baseline Edinburgh Postnatal Depression Screen (EPDS) before discharge. Nurses should teach the client and the family to call the health care provider if depression becomes severe or lasts longer than 2 weeks, or if the client is unable to cope with daily life. Early detection and early intervention improve treatment success. Nurse home visits, parenting support groups, therapy, or medication can be options for treating postpartum depression.

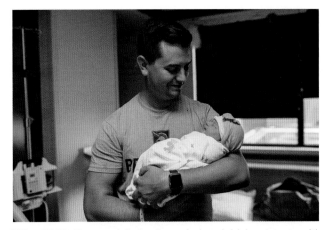

FIG. 17.10 Partners' behaviors during initial contact with their infants often correspond to behaviors of the postpartum client. The intense fascination that partners exhibit is called *engrossment.*

KNOWLEDGE CHECK

24. How do maternal behaviors in the taking-in phase differ from those in the taking-hold phase?
25. What does the mother relinquish in the letting-go phase?
26. How do mothers progress through the stages of role attainment?
27. How is postpartum blues different from postpartum depression? How can nurses intervene for this common emotional response?

The Process of Family Adaptation

The birth of an infant requires the reorganization of roles and relationships within the family. The previously childless couple now must integrate a new member into the family unit. Fathers or partners must learn new skills and often adjust to new roles. Siblings must adapt to a new standing in the family structure. Expectations and involvement of grandparents vary widely. Each family member is affected.

Partners

The partner's developing bond with the newborn is facilitated by engrossment. **Engrossment** is an intense fascination and face-to-face observation between the parent and newborn. It is characterized by the parent's intense interest in how the infant looks and responds and a desire to touch and hold the baby. Many parents comment on the baby's distinctive features and view the baby as perfect. They experience strong attraction to the infant and elation after the birth. The partner's attachment behaviors increase when the infant is awake, makes eye contact, and responds to their voice (Fig. 17.10).

Many partners eagerly look forward to coparenting with their mate. However, they may lack confidence in providing infant care and are sensitive to being left out of instructions and demonstrations of infant care. They may feel others expect them only to provide support to the client. Nurses can assist partners by involving them in child care activities soon after birth to help them feel more confident and competent.

Although first-time partners may attend prenatal classes about parenting, they often do not know what to expect from infants and need more information about normal growth and development during infancy. A review of information about child care presented in the prenatal period is helpful after the baby is born, when the information seems more relevant and the partner is ready to learn.

The additional work involved in care of a newborn may be a source of concern for both parents. Partners should be encouraged to negotiate the division of household chores during pregnancy or shortly after delivery.

Siblings

Siblings' response to the birth of a new brother or sister depends on their age and developmental level. Toddlers usually are not completely aware of the impending birth. When the baby arrives, they may view the infant as competition and fear they will be replaced in the parents' affection. They may have feelings of jealousy and resentment when they must share time and attention with a baby. Some toddlers exhibit hostile behaviors toward the mother, particularly when holding or feeding the newborn. Sleep problems, an increase in attention-seeking efforts, and regression to more infantile behaviors such as renewed bed wetting and thumb sucking are common. These behaviors show the jealousy and frustration young children feel as they observe the mother's attention being given to another.

The parents can be taught to accept without judgment the strong feelings expressed by the toddler and to continue to reinforce the child's feelings of being loved. Plans for changes in routine, such as beginning toilet training, should

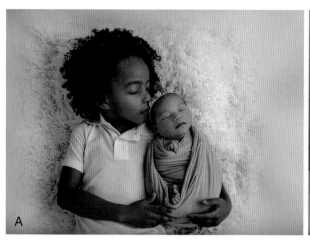

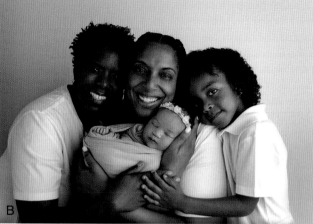

FIG. 17.11 (A) Although they may be hesitant to touch the infant, children often want to be close. (B) This boy's joy is obvious as he snuggles in with his parents.

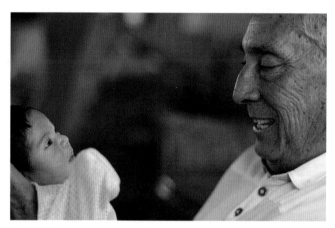

FIG. 17.12 Grandparents may develop strong bonds with grandchildren.

be postponed until family adjustments have been made. Expecting 2-year-old children to welcome a "stranger" is not realistic until they feel secure in the affection of their parents.

Preschool siblings may engage in looking more than touching. Most spend at least some time in proximity to the infant and talk to the parents about the infant (Fig. 17.11). Older children may adapt more easily. All siblings need extra attention from the parents and reassurance they are loved and important. Sibling classes, available in many agencies, may help ease the transition. Siblings are often allowed to visit the client on the postpartum unit, where they can interact with the new baby.

At home, a relaxed approach without time constraints may facilitate interactions between young children and infants. Special care should be taken by the parents, visitors, and nurses to pay as much attention to the sibling as to the new baby. Parents can emphasize the advantages of being an older sibling and allow siblings to participate in age-appropriate aspects of infant care.

Grandparents

The involvement of grandparents with grandchildren depends on many factors. One of the most important is proximity. Grandparents who live near the child frequently develop a strong attachment. This evolves into unconditional love and a special relationship bringing joy to the grandparents and an added sense of security to the grandchildren (Fig. 17.12).

When grandparents live many miles from grandchildren and have sporadic contact, forming a close attachment is more difficult. Grandparents must try to devise ways to foster a relationship with grandchildren they seldom see.

Expectations of the role of grandparents are also a factor in their adaptation to the birth of a grandchild. Many grandparents strive to be fully involved in the care and upbringing of the child, but others desire less involvement. The degree of grandparent involvement may cause some conflict with parents, or it may be a comfortable arrangement for both families.

Grandparents are often a major part of the support system for new parents. They may provide assistance with household tasks and infant care, which helps the client recover from childbirth and make the transition to parenthood. Grandparents who were very busy providing for their own children may enjoy the opportunity to nurture their grandchildren.

Factors Affecting Family Adaptation

Numerous factors influence the family's adjustment. Some, such as discomfort and fatigue, can be anticipated because they are so common. Additional factors include knowledge of infant needs, expectations about the infant, previous experience, age of the parents, and temperaments of the parents and infant. Other events such as cesarean birth, birth of a preterm or ill infant, and birth of more than one infant also affect the ease and speed with which the family adjusts.

Discomfort and Fatigue

Normally, discomforts associated with childbirth resolve within the first days after birth but may make it difficult to focus on the newborn's needs. Fatigue often remains a problem during the first few weeks and months, when the infant's schedule is erratic and the chance for uninterrupted sleep is minimal. When the infant begins to sleep through the night (usually by 3 to 4 months), the parents can reestablish familiar patterns, and fatigue often becomes less of a factor.

Knowledge of Infant Needs

Parents experience powerful feelings of protectiveness when they discover they can console their infant and the infant responds to their care. First-time parents, who are often unsure about how to care for a newborn, become very anxious if they are unable to console a crying infant. In addition, many are concerned about feeding and specific procedures such as care of the umbilical cord or circumcision. Breastfeeding benefits both the client and the infant but may add to the stress initially experienced by parents who lack sufficient knowledge and support.

Some parents have concerns about spoiling the infant. They may think responding each time the infant cries causes the baby to cry to get attention. It may be necessary to teach parents that infants cry to indicate hunger, cold, wetness, and a need for cuddling or gentle stimulation and responding to crying does not spoil the child. Suggest a variety of methods to cope with crying. Prompt, gentle response to crying helps the infant develop trust in the world as a safe, secure place. Trust is a basic developmental task of infancy and depends on the child learning that caregivers respond consistently and gently in meeting his or her needs.

Previous Experience

Previous experience with newborns also may affect family adjustment. Multiparas are more comfortable with infants and exhibit attachment behaviors earlier than primiparas, who may spend many more hours in the early discovery phase of attachment. Typically, multiparas are more relaxed in caring for the new baby but have to establish new routines that fit the expanded family. The multiparous client may find it more difficult to have time alone with their partner. They may need more help from family and friends than the primipara because of the lack of sleep and the time and energy involved in meeting the needs of all family members. Clients with other children may need encouragement to take time for themselves and time alone with their partner. Support groups for multiparas may be helpful.

Parents who have had a long interval between pregnancies may have forgotten much of the teaching received with the last birth and may need more instruction. Those who previously gave birth to infants with anomalies or infants who did not survive may need more time to feel comfortable with this infant.

Expectations about the Newborn

Unrealistic expectations of the infant may influence adjustment. Parents who have little experience with newborns may be surprised and disappointed at the newborn's appearance. They may be unprepared for normal newborn characteristics such as cranial molding, blotchy skin, and newborn rash.

Nurses should teach normal newborn characteristics and early growth and development. They should assist parents in working through misconceptions about newborn behavior. For example, the capacity of an infant's stomach is small, and the infant should be fed frequently. Also, infants are neurologically unable to sleep through the night during the early weeks. Increasing the time the client spends with the infant during the postpartum stay provides extra opportunities to gain comfort with the physical characteristics, as well as to learn infant care while a nurse is available to help.

Some clients may be very disappointed in the sex of their infants or sense their partners are disappointed. These feelings should be acknowledged and resolved before attachment can take place. For example, a client may be tearful when the fifth child is another male. This disappointment might delay attachment and result in situations like refusing to pick out a name at first. Later, when holding the baby and observing differences between this infant and the other sons, the client can begin the discovery period with this unique child.

Maternal Age

Adjustment to parenthood is a challenge for the teenager who has not achieved a strong sense of their own identity. In general, the adolescent may talk less, respond less, and appear more passive or less affectionate with the infant than older parents. They need special assistance to develop necessary parenting skills that promote optimal development of the infant (see Chapter 11).

Parental Temperament

Parental personality traits greatly influence attachment. Clients who are calm, secure in their ability to learn, and free from unnecessary anxiety adjust more easily to the demands of parenthood. Conversely, clients who are excitable, insecure, and anxious have more difficulty.

Temperament of the Infant

The infant's temperament also affects parental adjustment. Infants who are calm, easily consoled, and enjoy cuddling increase parental confidence and feelings of competence. In contrast, irritable infants who are difficult to console and do not respond to cuddling increase parental frustration and interfere with attachment.

Availability of a Strong Support System

A strong, consistent support system is a major factor in the adjustment of the new family. Friends and relatives who are parents can provide role modeling to first-time parents. They also can provide encouragement, praise, and reassurance to the new parents. Support may be needed for an extended period after childbirth. In addition, the client needs practical assistance with household tasks such as meal preparation, laundry, and shopping.

Postpartum support groups are often available and can help the client with early concerns during this period. These groups provide an opportunity to share thoughts and feelings with others who are having similar experiences. Some groups are focused on breastfeeding or exercise, but others simply provide an opportunity for interacting with other new parents. Partners may be included occasionally or at all meetings. There are also support groups just for new fathers or partners.

Other Factors

Cesarean Birth. A cesarean birth, especially an unexpected one, can make parental adjustment more difficult. Cesarean childbirth includes a longer recovery time and additional discomfort for the client, increased stress for the family, and possible financial strain. The client's needs for recovery and attachment with the newborn should be considered in planning nursing care.

Preterm or Ill Infant. Birth of a preterm or ill infant results in additional concerns. Prolonged separation of parents and child may be necessary. Although attachment can occur in these situations, the separation may delay the process and create stress on the normally functioning family.

Birth of Multiple Infants. The birth of twins or triplets often follows a high-risk pregnancy in which the client was confined to limited activity. There may have been one or more hospitalizations for preterm labor or other complications. The infants may be preterm and have health problems. Financial strain may occur because the client had to stop work earlier than expected and expenses associated with the birth and future health care are higher. In addition, birth of more than one infant makes family relationships more complex, especially if there are other children.

Problems of attachment may occur when there is more than one newborn. Rooming-in helps the parents gain confidence in caretaking and facilitates the attachment process. If infants are in a neonatal intensive care unit, early, frequent contacts should be arranged.

Parents attach to the infants separately as they get to know each infant's unique characteristics. They need help relate to each infant as an individual rather than part of a unit by pointing out the individual responses and characteristics of each infant. Arranging time for the parents to interact with each child alone, especially in the early, getting-acquainted period, is important.

Clients may be overwhelmed at the prospect of breastfeeding more than one infant. They need reassurance they will produce an ample supply of milk for each infant because supply increases with demand.

❓ KNOWLEDGE CHECK

28. What does a partner mean when saying they feel "out of place"?
29. What feelings may siblings experience when a new baby is born into the family?

Cultural Influences on Adaptation

A major goal of nursing practice in the postpartum period is to provide culture-specific nursing care incorporating the health beliefs, values, and practices of each client. This can be difficult because of the wide ethnic diversity in countries such as the United States and Canada. A major challenge for nurses is to be aware of cultural beliefs and acknowledge their importance in family adaptation. The postpartum period often is thought to be a time of vulnerability for the client and infant. Many cultural factors relevant to this time can be grouped into communication, health beliefs, and dietary practices.

Communication

Verbal communication may be difficult because of the numerous dialects and languages spoken. An interpreter should be fluent in the language, possibly of the same religion and of the same country of origin.

Care of the non-English speaking client will be challenging for the English-speaking nurse and health care team. Clients who are not able to speak or understand the primary language spoken at the hospital require extra vigilance and support. Extra time and patience may be needed to provide the best possible care. Making an effort by speaking a few words in their language, demonstrating a caring attitude, and using nonverbal communication is a first step. Using an interpreter improves understanding and subsequent adherence to discharge instructions, satisfaction with care, and outcomes.

Hospitals are required to provide professionally trained health care interpreter services and translated printed materials for limited English-proficient clients. Culturally and linguistically appropriate services may include telephone or video interpreters, trained volunteer interpreters, or computer-assisted translation. Using the client's family and friends, children under 18, other clients or visitors, or untrained volunteers is not best practice. Try to meet briefly with the interpreter in advance to make a plan. Speak slowly and in short segments; speak directly to the client, not to the interpreter; and ask the client or family member to repeat back what he or she understands.

When the nurse and family speak different primary languages, verifying the family's understanding is important. Nodding or saying "Yes" may be a sign of courtesy rather than understanding or agreement. To be certain the message has been received, the nurse should ask family members to repeat in their own words what they have been told.

A client may not indicate disagreement with what the nurse is saying or instructing as to not show disrespect. The client may simply not follow the nurse's instructions or might follow cultural requirements that differ from nursing expectations. Even if clients do not really believe the cultural requirements are necessary, they may follow them to avoid offending close relatives.

Respect for privacy and modesty of all people is important, but modesty is especially important in Hispanic, Middle-Eastern, and Asian cultures. Laws of modesty require that Muslim clients cover their hair, body, arms, and legs except when at home with family or in all-female company (Giger, 2017).

Health Beliefs

Cultural beliefs and practices provide a sense of security for new parents. Provision of care for the client and baby by female relatives is a common thread among cultures.

For many Southeast Asians, the postpartum period is important to ensure health in later years. New parents are expected to rest for 1 to 3 months while the grandmother or other female relatives assume the client's usual responsibilities of cooking or housework and care for the client, the baby, and other children. Care for the Korean client and baby is traditionally performed by the mother-in-law (Callister, 2021).

Client's activities are often restricted for a period after birth to allow rest and recuperation. The time involved varies. Laotian clients stay home for 1 month near a fire or heater to help "dry up the womb." Native Americans and their infants stay indoors and rest for 20 days or until the umbilical cord falls off (Callister, 2021).

"Doing the month" is very important for Chinese clients. Postpartum clients and their babies are cared for by a grandmother. They do not go outside and must keep warm to avoid "wind chill." They wear long sleeves and long pants and restrict bathing and washing their hair (Liu et al., 2015).

Many Southeast Asian and Hispanic persons believe the postpartum client should be kept warm to avoid upsetting the balance of hot and cold (Callister, 2021). Use of ice for perineal edema or breast engorgement may not be acceptable to these clients.

Many Mexican clients follow the customs of *la cuarentena*. This 40-day period is a time when the client is considered at risk because the entire body is open and subject to entrance of air, which would cause illness and various body aches. The client may bind the abdomen and wear more clothes than usual to avoid becoming cold, even when the weather is hot. Sexual intercourse is avoided to prevent serious illness to both parents and the infant (Waugh, 2011).

When clients are unwilling to take baths or showers in the postpartum period, nurses may be concerned about hygiene. Perineal cleansing is generally acceptable. Although an opportunity to wash or shower should be offered, it is up to the client. Tact and sensitivity are necessary to determine what care is appropriate for each client and to find a compromise, if necessary. In some cultures, baths are an important part of postpartum recovery. Navajo clients take a ritual bath on the fourth postpartum day (Mattson, 2015).

Specific religious practices should be accepted and supported. For instance, Muslim clients are exempted from their obligation to pray while they are bleeding. However, the partner and other family members kneel, place their heads on the floor, and pray five times per day. If possible, a clean, quiet room should be provided so this obligation can be fulfilled without having to leave the birthing center.

Dietary Practices

Some cultural dietary practices to consider center on the hot–cold theory of health and diet. This theory refers to the intrinsic properties of certain foods instead of the temperature or spiciness of foods. Although ice water is commonly given to hospital patients, it is not acceptable to many Asians. For example, Southeast Asian clients may refuse cold or ice water and prefer hot water or other warm beverages to keep warm. See Chapter 8 for more information about cultural practices and nutrition.

Food brought from home is a welcome sign of caring in many cultures. This is especially true if traditional foods are eaten after a client gives birth. Nurses should encourage this practice and discuss any dietary restrictions with the family.

Home and Community-Based Care

Because many clients and infants are discharged from the birth facility soon after childbirth, some assessments and interventions described in this chapter occur in the home or clinic setting. Clients may leave the birth facility when they still have discomfort and are just beginning to recover from the childbirth experience. Consequently, most psychosocial concerns, such as family adaptation and postpartum blues, surface later, when support from health care professionals is not as readily available.

Methods currently used to provide care for clients and infants after discharge include telephone calls, nurse-managed postpartum clinics, home visits, and "baby lines" staffed by nurses who provide information and guidance for callers. Comprehensive psychosocial support including telephone calls, home and clinic visits, and breastfeeding and parenting education may decrease the incidence of hospital readmission of normal newborns. Some programs use postpartum doulas or paraprofessionals to help extend the work of nurses in providing support to postpartum clients. All methods have advantages and disadvantages.

The overlap between nursing care in the birth facility and home makes communication among nurses extremely important. Nurses in the birth facility, who perform the initial assessments, should make information available to nurses who provide follow-up care.

APPLICATION OF THE NURSING PROCESS: MATERNAL ADAPTATION

Assessment

Several factors such as the client's progress through the puerperal phases, mood, interaction with the infant, and unanticipated events affect adaptation to the birth (Table 17.3).

Identification of Client Problems

Adjustment to parenting may be altered when one or more caregivers experience difficulty creating or continuing a nurturing environment. Multiple factors such as fatigue, discomfort, and lack of knowledge of infant care may interfere with parent and family adaptation.

Planning: Expected Outcomes

Expected outcomes are that the client will do the following:
* Verbalize feelings of comfort and support through the phases of recovery.
* Demonstrate progressive attachment behaviors (enfolding the infant, calling the infant by name, and responding gently when the infant cries) by discharge.
* Participate in care of the newborn (diapering, feeding, and care of the umbilical cord and circumcision) by discharge.

Interventions

Assisting the Client through Recovery Phases

Supporting the Client. The early, taking-in phase is a time to support the client to help the transition to more complex tasks of adjustment. During the first few hours after childbirth, the client has a great need for physical care and comfort. Provide ample fluids and favorite foods. Keep linens dry, tuck warm blankets around the client until chilling has stopped, and use warm water for perineal care.

Monitor and Protect. Nurses monitor and protect the client throughout the hospital or birth center stay. Remind the client to void, assist with ambulation, assess the level of comfort frequently, and offer analgesia before discomfort is severe and analgesia is less effective. Instruct the client not to delay requesting analgesia because it is more effective and the postpartum course is smoother if pain stays well controlled. Encourage rest.

Listen to the Birth Experience. Be prepared to listen to details of the birth experience and offer sincere praise for the effort during labor. Use open-ended questions to determine

TABLE 17.3   Assessing Adaptation

Assessments	Nursing Considerations
Progression through Puerperal Phases	
Taking-in (passive, dependent)	Consider client's need to rest, need to tell the details of the labor and childbirth, and the readiness to learn infant care and assume control of self-care.
Taking-hold (autonomous, seeks information)	Avoid taking over the primary role in care of the infant. Praise and encourage client's efforts. Ideal time to teach.
Letting-go (relinquishes fantasy baby, begins to see self as mother)	
Mood	
Mood and energy level, eye contact, posture, and comfort	Tense body posture, crying, or anxiety (may indicate fatigue, discomfort, or beginning of postpartum blues).
Factors Affecting Adaptation	
Age of client	May need additional support if under 18 years of age.
Previous experience	Primiparas progress through puerperal phases more slowly and may need more assistance than multiparas. Previous birth of an infant with anomalies or death of an infant may delay adaptation.
Parental and infant temperaments	Clients who are calm, secure, and free from anxiety need less assistance. More teaching is necessary for parents of infants who are difficult to console.
Other factors	Cesarean birth causes increased discomfort and longer recovery. Attachment challenges may occur with birth of a preterm or ill infant or more than one infant.
Interaction with Infant	
Touch	Progresses from fingertipping to enfolding and other comforting behaviors.
Verbal interaction	Parent may call infant "it" initially but progresses quickly to using given name and identifying specific characteristics.
Response to infant cues or signals	Prompt, gentle, consistent response indicates progressive adaptation to parenting role.
Preparation for Parenting	
Classes in breastfeeding, parenting, and infant care	Many parents feel more prepared after completing classes and participate in care sooner.

the client's perception of the birth. The opportunity to discuss feelings about the experience helps integrate it and clarify concerns. Many clients spend so much time on the telephone that completing nursing care is difficult. The client's need to relate the experience to family and friends is important, and nurses may be reluctant to interrupt. When assessments and care are necessary for the client's physical safety, a compromise can be effective. Offering a choice is often helpful: "Excuse me for a moment. I need to check you soon. I can do it now or come back in 10 minutes."

Foster Independence

As clients become more independent, allow them to schedule their care as much as possible. Collaborate with them to plan when such care as ambulation or a shower will be performed. Encourage them to assume responsibility for self-care, and emphasize the nurse's role at this point is to assist and teach.

Promote Bonding and Attachment

Early, unlimited contact between parents and infants is of primary importance to facilitate the attachment process. In most hospitals and birth centers, infants remain in the room with the parents unless complications occur. This arrangement may be called *rooming-in, mother-baby care, couplet care,* or *dyad care.* One nurse is responsible for both the client and the baby and provides teaching and help with bonding as part of ongoing nursing care. The client participates as they are able. The nurse assists as the client learns to care for their baby and gradually takes overall care. This provides continuity of care and helps prepare the parents for discharge.

Prolonged contact between parents and infants leads to parents caring for their infants as they learn the infants' characteristics and needs. Nursing measures to promote bonding and attachment include the following:

- Assist the parents in unwrapping the baby to inspect the toes, fingers, and body. Inspection fosters identification and allows the parents to become acquainted with the "real" baby, which must replace the fantasy baby many parents imagined during the pregnancy.
- Position the infant in an en face position and discuss the infant's ability to see the parent's face. Face-to-face and eye-to-eye contact is a first step in establishing mutual interaction between the infant and parent.
- Point out the reciprocal bonding activities of the infant: "Look how she holds your finger." "He hasn't taken his eyes off you."
- Encourage the parents to take as much time as they wish with the infant. This allows them to progress at their own speed through the discovery or getting-acquainted phase.
- Encourage and assist with putting the infant to the breast. Provide positive reinforcement. Answer questions about feeding.
- Model behaviors by holding the infant close, making eye contact with the infant, and speaking in high-pitched, soothing tones.
- Point out the characteristics of the infant in a positive way: "She has such pretty little hands and beautiful eyes."

- Provide comfort and ample time for rest because the client must replenish their energy and be relatively free of discomfort before they can progress to initiating infant care. A client who seems uninterested may just need a period of rest or pain intervention to be comfortable enough to focus on the infant.

Involve Parents in Infant Care

Providing infant care fosters feelings of responsibility and nurturing and is an important component of attachment. In addition, it allows parents to develop confidence in their ability to care for their infant before they go home. Begin with demonstrations, as necessary, and provide assistance while the parents gradually assume all infant care as their confidence in their abilities grows.

Although teaching begins during pregnancy, review information and repeat demonstrations. Demonstrate the simpler tasks, such as care of the cord, before progressing to more complicated procedures such as bathing.

Agreement among the entire staff about how to teach basic care is important. Parents seek confirmation of information, and they become confused and lose faith in the credibility of the staff if information varies. Allow time for practice and repeated encouragement. Parents become easily discouraged if they feel unsuccessful with early attempts to care for their infants.

Suggestions for care should be tactfully phrased to avoid the implication the parents are inept. "You burped the baby like a professional. There are a couple of little hints I can share about diapering."

Evaluation

The expected outcomes are met when the client independently performs self-care and verbalizes feelings of comfort and support during the progression through the phases of recovery. They should show progressive attachment behaviors, including enfolding the infant, calling the infant by name, and responding gently when the infant cries. Their participation in infant care should include diapering, feeding, and care of the umbilical cord and circumcision.

APPLICATION OF THE NURSING PROCESS: FAMILY ADAPTATION

Assessment

Partners

The partner's emotional status and interaction with the infant are particularly important because they usually serve as the client's primary support person. Is the partner involved with the client and infant? How do they interact with the infant? How much information do they have about infant characteristics and care? What are their expectations about their partner's recovery? Unrealistic expectations of the infant (will sleep through the night, smile, be easily consoled) may lead to problems. In addition, if the partner expects the client to recover energy and libido rapidly, they may become resentful if the recovery takes longer than anticipated.

Siblings

Note the ages of siblings and their reactions to the newborn. Are they interested and helpful? Are they hostile and aggressive? How do the parents respond to sibling behaviors?

Support System

Family members often provide a powerful support system, and their involvement is important to the adaptation of the family. Are grandparents available and involved? Do sisters and brothers live nearby? Are they available to help the new parents? If the family is unavailable, who provides support? What arrangements have been made for assistance?

Nonverbal Behavior

Nonverbal behavior is equally important. Are the parents' words congruent with their actions? Validate impressions and conclusions during a psychosocial assessment. One of the best ways to do this is to ask questions such as, "How much experience have you had with newborns?" "How are newborns fed in Vietnam until the breast milk comes in?" "What are your plans when you go home?" "How long can your mother stay?"

Intersperse questions over time during normal caregiving. The client should not be made to feel they are being interrogated because the nurse asks so many questions at once. Table 17.4 summarizes family assessment.

Identification of Client Problems

Family assessment identifies strengths and areas in which nursing interventions could promote family adaptation or prevent disruptions in family functioning. Sometimes a family that usually functions effectively is unable to cope because of a specific event, such as the birth of a baby. Lack of knowledge of an infant's needs and behaviors, stress during the early weeks at home, and sibling rivalry can interfere with the usual family functioning.

Planning: Expected Outcomes

Goals and expected outcomes may overlap with care after discharge because they often cannot be evaluated before the family leaves the birth facility. By (specific date) the family will do the following:

- Verbalize understanding of the infant's needs and behaviors
- Identify methods for reducing stress during the early weeks at home
- Describe measures to reduce sibling rivalry
- Identify external resources and the family's support system

TABLE 17.4 **Assessing Family Adaptation**	
Assessment	**Nursing Considerations**
Characteristics of Infant That May Affect Family Adaptation	
Sex and size of infant	Disappointment about sex or concern about small size may interfere with bonding.
Unexpected characteristics (cephalhematoma, jaundice, cranial molding, newborn rash)	Explain unexpected appearance or behavior in language parents can comprehend. Reassure normalcy and temporary nature, if accurate.
Congenital anomaly or illness	Explain the condition to parents; assist them during visits and in learning care.
Infant behavior (irritable, easily consoled, cuddles)	Infants who are easy to manage increase bonding and attachment.
Partner Adaptation	
Response to the client and the infant	The partner often provides the most important support for the client. Their involvement with the infant indicates acceptance of parenting role.
Knowledge of infant care	The partner's knowledge determines the teaching they will need.
Response to infant cues or signals (crying, fussing)	Many partners feel awkward handling infant but want to become proficient in infant care.
Ages and Developmental Levels of Siblings	
Reaction of siblings	Young children often fear the newborn will replace them in the affection of the parents. Parents may need anticipatory guidance about sibling rivalry.
Support System	
Interest and availability of family or friends to assist during early weeks	Families may need assistance in identifying available support.
Plans for first few days at home	Suggest parents plan for support and rest. Provide resources such as telephone "baby lines," postpartum clinics, or support groups.
Follow-up plans	Appointments for the client and infant are generally scheduled at 2–6 weeks with clinic or health care provider.
Cultural Factors	
Cultural beliefs and practices which may affect nursing care	Culture-specific care can be planned for hygiene, dietary preferences, usual care and feeding of infants, and role of the partner and family in child care.
Expectations of health care team	Expectations may vary in different cultures.

Interventions

Teaching the Family about the Newborn

Many families access the internet for information about infant care. A free service from the National Healthy Mothers, Healthy Babies Coalition provides texts with information about pregnancy and infants through 1 year. The service can be accessed by going to the website at https://www.text4baby.org or texting BABY to 511411 on a mobile phone.

Infant Needs. Some new parents have unrealistic expectations of the newborn. Provide them with information about the infant's capabilities, emotional needs, and physical needs.

Infant Signals. Discuss the importance of responding promptly and gently to cues such as crying and fussing indicating the infant needs attention. Reassure parents that responding to cues does not "spoil" their baby but helps the infant learn they are in a safe, secure place.

Help parents recognize signals indicating when their infant has had enough interaction and wants to avoid further stimulation. These avoidance cues, such as looking away, splaying the fingers, arching the back, and fussiness indicate the infant needs quiet time.

Helping the Family Adapt

Providing Anticipatory Guidance about Stress Reduction. Help the family plan for the demands of the first weeks at home by providing anticipatory guidance. This is a time when the need for rest is great but the opportunity for uninterrupted sleep is minimal. As a result, fatigue is a common problem for both parents. The nurse should do the following:

- Emphasize the priority during the first 4 to 6 weeks should be caring for the client and the baby.
- Recommend parents establish a relaxed home atmosphere and flexible meal schedule because attempts to maintain a rigid schedule or meticulous environment increase tension within the family.
- Recommend the client sleep when the infant sleeps and conserve energy for care of the baby.
- Encourage parents to let friends and relatives know sleep and nap times and request they telephone and visit at other times.
- Advise parents to place a "Do Not Disturb" sign on the door and to silence the ring on their phones during rest times.
- Suggest the parents limit coffee, tea, colas, and chocolate because they contain caffeine and will interfere with rest.
- Teach breathing exercises and progressive relaxation to reduce stress and energize, especially when a nap is not possible.
- Encourage both parents to delay tiring projects until the infant is older. Remind them although schedules are chaotic for a while, the infant's behavior is generally more predictable by 12 to 16 weeks of age.
- Encourage open expression of feelings between parents as a first step in coping with stress.
- Remind parents of the need for healthy nutrition and recreation. Fatigue and tension easily can overwhelm the anticipated joys of parenting if no respite is available from constant care.
- Suggest new parents enlist grandparents, other relatives, and friends to help with cooking, cleaning, shopping, and care of other children.

Helping the Partner Coparent. Help the partner become involved with the infant by including them in teaching. Provide opportunities to participate in diapering, comforting activities, and feeding or helping the client breastfeed. Offer frequent encouragement and praise. If classes or chat rooms for new parents are available, refer fathers and partners to them.

Providing Ways to Reduce Sibling Rivalry. Suggest parents plan time alone with older children. Frequent praise and expressions of love and affection help reassure older children of their places in the family. Suggest visitors and relatives do not focus exclusively on the infant but include older children in their gift giving and attention.

Emphasize the importance of responding calmly and with understanding when a sibling regresses to more infantile behaviors or expresses hostility toward the infant. Acknowledging the child's feelings and offering prompt reassurance of continued love are the most valuable actions.

Some children, particularly those older than 3 years of age, enjoy being a big brother or sister and respond well when they are included in infant care. This participation may not be possible with younger children, and setting aside separate time with them to participate in a favorite activity may be more worthwhile for the parents.

Identifying Resources. In many homes, the postpartum client assumes the major responsibilities of day-to-day homemaking. With the birth of an infant, this task becomes more difficult. A division of labor should be negotiated to prevent undue stress and fatigue. This division of labor is particularly important when other children in the home also need time, attention, and comfort.

Although the client's primary support often is the partner, extended family members and friends also provide valuable support. Community resources such as daycare centers, parenting classes, and breastfeeding support groups are available in many areas. In addition, close friends and neighbors often share solutions to specific problems. Remind the client resources are available when they begin to feel isolated and exhausted.

Evaluation

A prompt, gentle response to infant crying and fussing and verbalizations of acceptance of normal newborn behaviors indicate parental understanding of the infant's need. Devising a plan for obtaining rest and lessening anxiety in siblings is a first step in reducing stress and sibling rivalry. Identifying resources in the family, neighborhood, and community may help the family function to meet its needs during the early weeks at home.

SUMMARY CONCEPTS

- After childbirth the uterus returns to its nonpregnant size and condition by involution.
- The site of placental attachment heals by a process of exfoliation, which leaves the endometrium smooth and without scars.
- Involution can be evaluated by measuring the descent of the fundus (~1 cm/day). By about the 14th day after childbirth the fundus should no longer be palpable abdominally.
- Afterpains, or intermittent uterine contractions, cause discomfort for many clients, particularly multiparas who breastfeed.
- Vaginal discharge (lochia) progresses from lochia rubra (dark red or red–brown) to lochia serosa (pink or brown-tinged) to lochia alba (white, cream, or light yellow) in a predictable timeframe. Lochia should be assessed for amount, type, and odor. Foul odor suggests endometrial infection.
- Orthostatic hypotension occurs when the client moves from the supine to standing position quickly.
- Tachycardia may be caused by pain, excitement, anxiety, fatigue, dehydration, hypovolemia, anemia, or dehydration. Additional assessments (e.g., lochia, fundus) are required to determine whether excessive bleeding is the cause.
- The postpartum client should be afebrile, but the temperature may be higher during the first 24 hours after delivery because of dehydration and leukocytosis.
- Hemorrhoids and perineal trauma can cause a great deal of discomfort and interfere with activity and bladder and bowel elimination.
- Cardiac output increases after birth when blood from the uterus and placenta returns to the central circulation, uterine pressure on the vessels decreases, and extracellular fluid moves into the vascular compartment. Excess fluid is excreted by diuresis and diaphoresis.
- Increased clotting factors predispose the postpartum client to thrombus formation. Early, frequent ambulation helps prevent thrombophlebitis.
- Constipation may occur from decreased food and fluid intake during labor, reduced activity, decreased muscle and bowel tone, and fear of pain during defecation.
- Increased bladder capacity and decreased sensitivity to fluid pressure may result in urinary retention. Stasis of urine allows time for bacteria to grow and can lead to urinary tract infection. A distended bladder displaces

the uterus and can interfere with uterine contraction and cause excessive bleeding.
- Exercises to strengthen the abdominal muscles, good posture, and body mechanics may reduce musculoskeletal discomfort.
- Breastfeeding may delay the return of ovulation and menstruation, but ovulation may occur before the first menses. All postpartum clients need information about family planning.
- After cesarean birth, the client requires postoperative and postpartum assessments and care. There may be problems with immobility and discomfort.
- Attachment is a gradual process which begins before childbirth and progresses to feelings of love and deep devotion lasting throughout life.
- Nurses foster bonding and attachment by providing early, unlimited contact between the parents and infant and modeling attachment behaviors.
- Maternal touch changes over time as many parents progress from exploratory "fingertipping" to enfolding and finally demonstrating a full range of comforting behaviors.
- Verbal behaviors are important indicators of maternal attachment. Nurses often model how to speak to the infant and point out the infant's response to the verbal stimulation.
- Maternal adjustment to parenthood is a gradual process involving restorative phases of taking-in, taking-hold, and letting-go. Nurses play a valuable role in the process by first supporting and then fostering independence as the client becomes ready.
- Mothers usually progress through four stages of role attainment—anticipatory, formal, informal, and personal—before they attain a sense of comfort and can structure their parenting behaviors to mesh with the infant's unique needs.
- Postpartum blues is a temporary, self-limiting period of tearfulness and mood instability. It should not last longer than 2 weeks.
- The birth of a baby requires reorganization of family structure and renegotiation of family responsibilities. Nurses can assist the partner in coparenting the infant and help the new parents identify family resources.
- Siblings may be jealous and fearful they will be replaced by the newborn in the affection of the parents. Nurses can lessen the negative feelings by providing information about ways to reduce sibling rivalry.
- Attention to cultural concerns of postpartum clients is important in helping them meet cultural, physical, and psychosocial needs.

Clinical Judgment and Next-Generation NCLEX® Examination-Style Questions

Taylor, 34-year-old gravida 3 para 3, delivered a term infant vaginally approximately 12 hours ago. No obstetric or significant medical history was noted upon admission. The client has no known drug allergies, O positive blood type, Hgb 12.3, and Hct 34. Taylor had a successful natural childbirth with no medications required. Quantified blood loss at delivery was

375 mL. The recovery period was uneventful, and Taylor was transferred to the postpartum unit.

Client identity and provider orders verified upon transfer to postpartum. 18 gauge IV in right arm with 30 units of Pitocin in 1000 mL of LR infusing at 125 mL/hour. Vital signs stable: Blood pressure (BP) 123/74, heart rate (HR) 82, respiratory rate (RR) 16, temperature (temp) 98.4°F. Fundus firm 1 cm above the umbilicus. Light amount of lochia rubra (about 4-inch stain) noted on the peripad. No vaginal lacerations were noted at delivery. Perineum slightly swollen. Client states no pain at this time. Oriented to room and call light. Infant in crib at bedside.

One hour later, client up to the bathroom. 200 mL voided. Moderate lochia rubra noted. Pericare completed. Client denies pain except when breastfeeding and states, "It feels crampy when I feed him."

Assessment the following morning, almost 24 hours after delivery reveals the following:

Vital signs: BP 129/72, HR 102, RR 21, temp 100.4°F

Fundus: firm at umbilicus and midline, moderate lochia rubra noted

Pain: cramping associated with breastfeeding, headache that started around 1 a.m. when client was breastfeeding

Head to toe assessment: within normal limits (WNL) except 1+ pedal edema bilaterally, client complains of "night sweats"

Laboratory work from 5 a.m. today: Hgb 11.1, Hct 30, WBC 20,000

1. **Use an X to indicate whether the nursing assessment findings listed below are important (require nursing follow up) or expected findings for the client's care at this time.**

Assessment Finding	Important	Expected Findings
BP 129/72		
HR 102		
RR 19		
Temp 100.5°F		
Fundus firm, midline at umbilicus		
Moderate lochia rubra		
Cramping while breastfeeding		
Headache		
1+ pedal edema bilaterally		
Night sweats		
Hgb 11.1		
Hct 30		
WBC 20,000		

2. **Determine the sequence in which the nurse should perform each action to assess Taylor's fundus.**

Nursing Action	Sequence of Actions
Place Taylor in a supine position with knees flexed	
Place nondominant hand above symphysis pubis	
Have Taylor empty bladder	
Palpate using flat fingers of dominant hand starting at umbilicus	
Explain procedure and rationale	
Put on clean gloves and lower perineal pad	

3. **Choose the most likely options for the information missing from the statement below by selecting from the lists of options provided.**

The nurse is providing postpartum discharge teaching for Taylor Pedersen.

The nurse needs to include _____ 1 _____ in the discharge teaching. Should _____ 2 _____ occur after discharge, Taylor should notify the health care provider. The nurse knows the client understands the discharge follow-up instructions when Taylor states _____ 3 _____ during teach-back.

Option 1	Option 2	Option 3
Immediately resume prepregnancy exercise regimen	Intermittent perineal pain	"I should contact my provider within the first 3 weeks"
Use soap on nipples in shower	Foul odor of lochia	"I need to keep my nipples moist between feedings"
Dry the perineum front to back	Feeling of fullness in breasts	"I can expect to be at my prepregnant weight in 1 month"
Increase caffeine to help with fatigue	Vaginal dryness during intercourse	"I should try to get my work done while the baby naps"

REFERENCES & READINGS

American Academy of Pediatrics & American College of Obstetricians and Gynecologists (AAP & ACOG). (2017). In *Guidelines for perinatal care* (8th ed.).

American College of Obstetricians and Gynecologists (ACOG). (2018). *Optimizing postpartum care.* ACOG Committee Opinion (No. 736). Published 2016, reaffirmed 2018.

American College of Obstetricians and Gynecologists (ACOG). (2020a). *Physical activity and exercise during pregnancy and the postpartum period.* ACOG Committee Opinion (No. 804).

American College of Obstetricians and Gynecologists (ACOG). (2020b). *Tobacco and nicotine cessation during pregnancy.* ACOG Committee Opinion (No. 807). Published 2017, reaffirmed 2020.

Antony, K. M., Racusin, D. A., Aagaard, K., & Dildy, G. A. (2021). Maternal physiology. In M. Landon, H. Galan, E. Jauniaux, D. Driscoll, V. Berghella, W. Grobman, et al. (Eds.), *Gabbe's obstetrics: Normal and problem pregnancies* (8th ed., pp. 43–67). Elsevier.

Association of Women's Health, Obstetric and Neonatal Nurses. (2017). *Post birth warning signs.* https://www.awhonn.org/education/hospital-products/post-birth-warning-signs-education-program/.

Australian Breastfeeding Association. (2020). *Lactation suppression.* https://www.breastfeeding.asn.au/bfinfo/lactation-suppression.

Blackburn, S. T. (2018). In *Maternal, fetal, and neonatal physiology: A clinical perspective* (5th ed.). Elsevier.

Callister, L. C. (2021). Integrating cultural beliefs and practices when caring for childbearing women and families. In K. Simpson, & P. Creehan (Eds.), *AWHONN's perinatal nursing* (5th ed.). Wolters Kluwer.

Centers for Disease Control and Prevention (CDC). (2019). *Pertussis.* https://www.cdc.gov/pertussis/.

Centers for Disease Control and Prevention (CDC). (2021). *Measles, mumps, and rubella (MMR) vaccination: What everyone should know.* https://www.cdc.gov/vaccines/vpd/mmr/public/index.html.

Council on Patient Safety in Women's Health Care. (2020). *Urgent maternal warning signs.* https://safehealthcareforeverywoman.org/council/patient-safety-tools/urgent-maternal-signs/.

Cunningham, F. G., Leveno, K. J., Bloom, S. L., Dashe, J. S., Hoffman, B. L., Casey, B. M., et al. (2022). In *Williams' obstetrics* (26th ed.). McGraw-Hill Companies.

East, C., Dorward, E., Whale, R., & Liu, J. (2020). Local cooling for relieving pain from perineal trauma sustained during childbirth. *Cochrane Database of Systematic Reviews, 10.* https://doi.org/10.1002/14651858.CD006304.pub4.

Giger, J. N. (2017). In *Transcultural nursing: Assessment and intervention* (7th ed.). Elsevier.

Isley, M. M. (2021). Postpartum care and long-term health considerations. In M. Landon, H. Galan, E. Jauniaux, D. Driscoll, V. Berghella, W. Grobman, et al. (Eds.), *Gabbe's obstetrics: Normal and problem pregnancies* (8th ed., pp. 459–474). Elsevier.

James, D. C., & Suplee, P. D. (2021). Postpartum care. In K. Simpson, P. Creehan, N. O'Brien-Abel, C. Roth, & A. Rohan (Eds.), *AWHONN's perinatal nursing* (5th ed., pp. 509–563). Wolters Kluwer.

Janke, J. (2021). Newborn nutrition. In K. Simpson, P. Creehan, N. O'Brien-Abel, C. Roth, & A. Rohan (Eds.), *AWHONN's perinatal nursing* (5th ed., pp. 609–650). Wolters Kluwer.

Kennedy, K. I., & Trussell, J. (2018). Postpartum contraception and lactation. In D. Kowal, R. A. Hatcher, A. L. Nelson, J. Trussell, C. Cwiak, P. Cason, et al. (Eds.), *Contraceptive technology* (21st ed.). Managing Contraception LLC.

Klaus, M. H., Kennell, J. H., Plumb, N., & Zuehlke, S. (1970). Human maternal behavior at the first contact with her young. *Pediatrics, 46*(2), 187–192.

Liu, Y. Q., Petrini, M., & Maloni, J. A. (2015). 'Doing the month': Postpartum practices in Chinese women. *Nursing and Health Sciences, 17*(1), 5–14.

Martin, J. A., Hamilton, B. E., Osterman, M. J. K., & Driscoll, A. K. (2021). Births: Final data for 2019. *National Vital Statistics Reports, 68*(13).

Mattson, S. (2015). Ethnocultural considerations in the childbearing period. In S. Mattson, & J. E. Smith (Eds.), *AWHONN Core curriculum for maternal-newborn nursing* (5th ed., pp. 61–79). Elsevier.

Mercer, R. T. (1995a). *Becoming a mother: Research on maternal identity from Rubin to the present.* Springer.

Mercer, R. T. (1995b). Predictors of maternal role attainment. *Nursing Research, 34*(4), 198–204.

Mercer, R. T. (2004). Becoming a mother versus maternal role attainment. *Journal of Nursing Scholarship, 36*(3), 226–232.

Mercer, R. T., & Ferketich, S. L. (1994). Maternal-infant attachment of experienced and inexperienced mothers during infancy. *Nursing Research, 43*(6), 344–351.

Mercer, R. T., & Walker, L. O. (2006). A review of interventions to foster becoming a mother. *Journal of Obstetric, Gynecologic, and Neonatal Nursing, 35*(5), 568–582.

Pacheco, L. D., Saade, G., & Metz, T. D. (2020). Society for maternal-fetal medicine Consult series #51: Thromboembolism prophylaxis for cesarean delivery. *American Journal of Obstetrics and Gynecology, 223*(2), B11–B17. https://doi.org/10.1016/j.ajog.2020.04.032.

Paladine, H. L., Blenning, C. E., & Strangas, Y. (2019). Postpartum care: An approach to the fourth trimester. *American Family Physician, 100*(8), 485–491.

Rubin, R. (1961). Puerperal change. *Nursing Outlook, 9*(12), 743–755.

Rubin R. (1963). Maternal Touch. *Nursing Outlook, 11,* 828–829.

Rubin, R. (1977). Binding-in in the postpartum period. *MCN: The American Journal of Maternal/Child Nursing, 6*(1), 65–75.

Suplee, P. D., & Janke, J. (2020). AWHONN Compendium of postpartum care. In *Association of Women's Health, Obstetric and Neonatal Nurses* (3rd ed.).

U.S. Department of Labor, Bureau of Labor Statistics. (2020). *Employment characteristics of families—2019.* https://www.bls.gov/news.release/archives/famee_04212020.pdf.

Waugh, L. J. (2011). Beliefs associated with Mexican immigrant families' practice of La Cuarentena during postpartum recovery. *Journal of Obstetric, Gynecologic, and Neonatal Nursing, 40*(6), 732–741.

Whitmer, T. (2016). Physical and psychological changes. In S. Mattson, & J. E. Smith (Eds.), *AWHONN core curriculum for maternal-newborn nursing* (5th ed., pp. 301–314). Elsevier.

Wisner, K. L., Sit, D. K. Y., & Miller, E. S. (2021). Mental health and behavioral disorders in pregnancy. In M. Landon, H. Galan, E. Jauniaux, D. Driscoll, V. Berghella, W. Grobman, et al. (Eds.), *Gabbe's obstetrics: Normal and problem pregnancies* (8th ed., pp. 1147–1168). Elsevier.

Postpartum Complications

Kristin L. Scheffer, Karen S. Holub

OBJECTIVES

After studying this chapter, you should be able to:

1. Describe postpartum hemorrhage: predisposing factors, causes, signs, and management.
2. Explain major causes, signs, and management of subinvolution.
3. Describe three major thromboembolic disorders (superficial venous thrombosis, deep vein thrombosis, pulmonary embolism) and their predisposing factors, causes, signs, and management.
4. Discuss puerperal infection in terms of location, predisposing factors, causes, signs and symptoms, and management.
5. Describe the role of the nurse in the management of clients who have a postpartum complication.

Pregnancy and childbirth are natural events from which most clients recover without complication. However, nurses should be aware of potential problems and their effect on the family. The most common physiologic complications during the postpartum period are hemorrhage, thromboembolic disorders, and infection. Peripartum mood and anxiety disorders, the major psychological disorders during childbearing, are discussed in Chapter 11.

POSTPARTUM HEMORRHAGE

Postpartum hemorrhage (PPH) is a leading cause of maternal mortality and morbidity worldwide (California Maternal Quality Care Collaborative [CMQCC], 2015; James & Suplee, 2021; Texas Department of Health and Human Services [DHHS], 2021). Anticipated blood loss for a vaginal birth is up to 500 mL and up to 1000 mL for a cesarean birth (Cunningham et al., 2022; James & Suplee, 2021). The American College of Obstetricians and Gynecologists (ACOG) revised the definition of PPH as "cumulative blood loss of greater than or equal to 1000 mL or blood loss accompanied by sign or symptoms of hypovolemia within 24 hours after the birth process" (ACOG, 2017, p. e168). Estimated blood loss is frequently inaccurate. With excessive blood loss, literature notes underestimation occurs, and with lower volumes, overestimation is noted (ACOG, 2019; Cunningham et al., 2022). Underestimation is usually only about half the actual loss, and therefore blood loss should be quantified by weighing or measuring and documentation of cumulative loss maintained (ACOG, 2019; Association of Women's Health, Obstetric and Neonatal Nurses [AWHONN], 2021b). Underestimation has been associated with a delayed response in PPH management. Of note, 54% to 93% of obstetric hemorrhage–related maternal deaths may have been preventable (ACOG, 2019). Hemorrhage is further defined in regard to timing. *Early PPH,* or primary PPH, occurs in the first 24 hours after childbirth. Hemorrhage after 24 hours or up to 12 weeks after birth is called *late PPH,* or secondary PPH (ACOG, 2017; James & Suplee, 2021).

Early Postpartum Hemorrhage

Early PPH occurs during the first 24 hours after birth and is most often caused by uterine atony (ACOG, 2017; Cunningham et al., 2022; James & Suplee, 2021). **Atony** refers to lack of muscle tone resulting in failure of the uterine muscle fibers to contract firmly around blood vessels when the placenta separates. Trauma to the birth canal during labor and birth, **hematomas** (localized collections of blood in a space or tissue), retention of placental fragments, and abnormalities of coagulation are other causes. When determining the cause of PPH, many providers refer to the "Four Ts"—tone (atony), trauma, tissue, or thrombin (coagulation deficiencies) (ACOG, 2017). Hemorrhage from disseminated intravascular coagulation is discussed in Chapter 19. Other causes of hemorrhage include placenta previa (see Chapter 10), **placenta accreta** (abnormal adherence of the placenta to the uterine wall), and inversion of the uterus (see Chapter 16).

Uterine Atony

With uterine atony, the relaxed muscles allow rapid bleeding from the endometrial arteries at the placental site. Bleeding continues until the uterine muscle fibers contract to stop the flow of blood. Fig. 18.1 illustrates the effect of uterine contraction on the size of the placental site and the subsequent bleeding.

Predisposing factors. Knowledge of risk factors for uterine atony helps the nurse anticipate and therefore reduce excessive bleeding. Overdistention of the uterus from any cause such as multiple gestation, a large infant, uterine fibroids, or **polyhydramnios** (excessive volume of amniotic fluid) makes

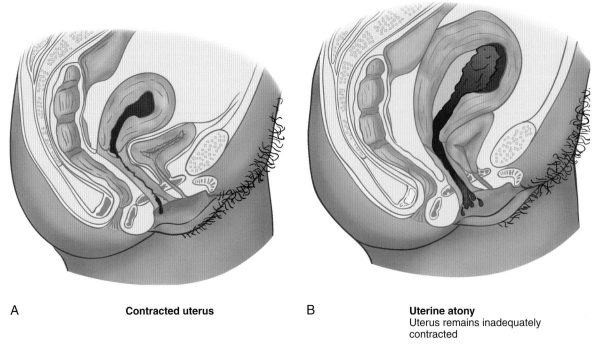

A   **Contracted uterus**   B   **Uterine atony**
Uterus remains inadequately
contracted

FIG. 18.1 (A) When the uterus remains contracted, the placental site is smaller, so bleeding is minimal. (B) If uterine muscles fail to contract around the endometrial arteries at the placental site, hemorrhage occurs.

it more difficult for the uterus to contract with enough firmness to prevent excessive bleeding. Multiparity results in repeatedly stretched muscle fibers, and these flaccid muscle fibers may not remain contracted after birth. (ACOG, 2017; Cunningham et al., 2022). Intrapartum factors include minimally effective contractions, resulting in prolonged labor; excessively vigorous contractions, resulting in precipitous labor; and labor that was induced or augmented with oxytocin. Retention of a large segment of the placenta does not allow the uterus to contract firmly and therefore can result in uterine atony. Additional related causes of uterine atony include **chorioamnionitis** (inflammation of the amniotic sac, usually caused by bacterial and viral infections), general anesthesia, and uterine inversion (ACOG, 2017). Box 18.1 summarizes predisposing risk factors for PPH.

Clinical manifestations. Major signs of uterine atony include the following:

- A uterine fundus that is difficult to locate
- A soft or "boggy" feel when the fundus is located
- A uterus that becomes firm as it is massaged but loses its tone when massage is stopped
- A fundus located above the expected level
- Excessive lochia, especially if it is bright red
- Excessive clots expelled, either with or without uterine massage

For the first 24 hours after childbirth, the uterus should feel like a firmly contracted ball roughly the size of a large grapefruit. It should be located at about the level of the umbilicus. Lochia should be dark red and scant to moderate in amount. Saturation of one peripad in 1 hour represents excessive blood loss. The nurse should realize profuse and dramatic

> **BOX 18.1**   **Common Predisposing Factors for Postpartum Hemorrhage**
>
> Overdistention of the uterus (multiple gestation, large infant, polyhydramnios)
> Multiparity (five or more)
> Precipitous labor or birth
> Prolonged labor
> Use of forceps or vacuum extractor (operative vaginal delivery)
> Cesarean birth
> Difficult third stage (manual removal of the placenta, aggressive fundal manipulation or cord traction)
> Uterine inversion or rupture
> Abnormal placentation (placenta previa, accreta, increta, or percreta)
> Medications: Oxytocin, prostaglandins, tocolytics, or magnesium sulfate
> General anesthesia
> Chorioamnionitis, sepsis
> Coagulopathies, low platelets, disseminated intravascular coagulation
> Previous postpartum hemorrhage or family history of postpartum hemorrhage in first-degree relative
> Uterine leiomyomas (fibroids)
> Trauma, lacerations, or hematomas

bleeding may be as dangerous as a constant steady trickle, dribble, or slow seeping.

Therapeutic management. Medical management of third-stage labor (from birth of the baby to birth of the placenta) may be expectant or active. Expectant management allows the placenta to deliver spontaneously or with the aid

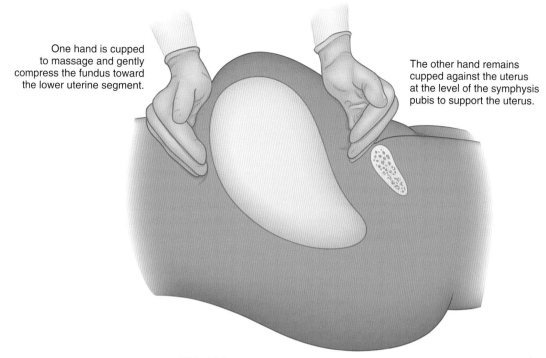

FIG. 18.2 Technique for fundal massage.

One hand is cupped to massage and gently compress the fundus toward the lower uterine segment.

The other hand remains cupped against the uterus at the level of the symphysis pubis to support the uterus.

of nipple stimulation or gravity. Active management of the third stage of labor is recommended as an effective intervention to prevent PPH (ACOG, 2017; AWHONN, 2021a). Active management includes three steps: early prophylactic uterotonic administration (preferably Pitocin), fundal massage, and controlled placenta cord traction. Of the three components, administration of uterotonics has the most impact on decreasing the rates of early PPH (Cunningham et. al. 2022; Gallos et. al., 2018; Salati et. al, 2019). Intravenous (IV) infusion of dilute oxytocin (not IV push) should be given during the third stage of labor. Oxytocin also may be administered intramuscularly (ACOG, 2017; AWHONN, 2021a) (see Drug Guide: Oxytocin in Chapter 15). Nurses remain with the client during the hours after childbirth and are responsible for assessments and initial management of uterine atony. If the uterus is not firmly contracted, the first intervention is to massage the fundus until it is firm and to express clots that may have accumulated in the uterus. One hand is placed just above the symphysis pubis to support the lower uterine segment while the other hand gently but firmly massages the fundus in a circular motion (Fig. 18.2). The evidence supporting the last component of active management of the third stage of labor, controlled cord traction, is mixed. Cord traction is thought to decrease the PPH risk by shortening the third stage through assisted placental removal. More studies are needed to demonstrate the benefits of controlled cord traction (AWHONN, 2021a).

Clots in the uterine cavity may interfere with effective uterine contractility. Clots are expressed by applying firm but gentle pressure on the fundus in the direction of the vagina. It is critical that the uterus is contracted firmly before attempting to express clots. *Pushing on a uterus that is not contracted could invert the uterus and cause massive hemorrhage and rapid shock.*

If the uterus does not remain contracted as a result of uterine massage or if the fundus is displaced, the bladder may be distended. A full bladder lifts the uterus, typically moving it up and laterally, away from midline, preventing effective contraction of the uterine muscles. Emptying the bladder takes priority in this situation. If the client is unable to void, then catheterization may be required.

If atony persists despite prophylactic oxytocin and uterine massage, further pharmacologic measures may be necessary. Initially, additional oxytocin may be ordered. Methylergonovine (Methergine) is a common medication used when oxytocin is not effective. Methergine elevates blood pressure and should not be given to a hypertensive client. The usual route of administration is intramuscularly (see Drug Guide: Methylergonovine). Misoprostol (Cytotec), a synthetic prostaglandin E1 (PGE$_1$) given orally or sublingually also may be used to control bleeding (ACOG, 2017; CMQCC, 2022). Analogs of prostaglandin F2-alpha (PGF2α; carboprost tromethamine [Hemabate; Prostin/15M]) are also effective when given intramuscularly (CMQCC, 2022) (see Drug Guide: Carboprost Tromethamine).

In 2010 the World Maternal Antifibrinolytic Trial (WOMAN) compared the efficacy of tranexamic acid (TXA), an antifibrinolytic medication, with a placebo for PPH treatment. A significant decrease in mortality from PPH was noted (Shakur et al., 2010). Although initial use of TXA in obstetrics focused on treatment of PPH, a small body of work emerged regarding routine prophylactic use. The primary benefit noted was in the cesarean section client. Studies reported decreased blood loss, reduction in blood product administration, and decreased use of additional uterotonics (ACOG, 2017; Alam & Choi, 2015; Cleveland Clinic, 2021; Naeiji et al., 2021; Stortreon et al., 2020). The limitations of the majority of these studies are sample size; therefore further research is needed for both vaginal and cesarean births.

If uterine massage and pharmacologic measures are ineffective in stopping uterine bleeding, the health care provider may use bimanual compression of the uterus. In this procedure, one hand is inserted into the vagina and the other compresses the uterus through the abdominal wall (Fig. 18.3). A balloon may be inserted into the uterus to apply pressure against the uterine surface to stop bleeding (ACOG, 2017; CMQCC, 2022; Cunningham et al., 2022) (Fig. 18.4). Uterine packing also may be used. It may be necessary to explore the uterine cavity and remove placental fragments, which may interfere with uterine contraction.

A laparotomy may be necessary to identify the source of the bleeding. Uterine compression sutures (B-lynch) may be placed to stop severe bleeding. Ligation of the uterine or hypogastric artery or embolization (occlusion) of pelvic arteries may be required if other measures are not effective. Hysterectomy is a last resort with uncontrollable PPH.

Hemorrhage requires prompt replacement of intravascular fluid volume. Lactated Ringer's solution, whole blood, packed red blood cells, normal saline, or other plasma expanders are used. Enough fluid should be given to maintain a urine flow of at least 30 milliliters per hour (mL/hr) (Cunningham et al., 2022). Typically, the nurse is responsible for obtaining properly typed and cross-matched blood and inserting large-bore IV lines capable of carrying whole blood.

Trauma

Trauma to the birth canal is the second most common cause of early PPH. Trauma includes vaginal, cervical, or perineal lacerations and hematomas.

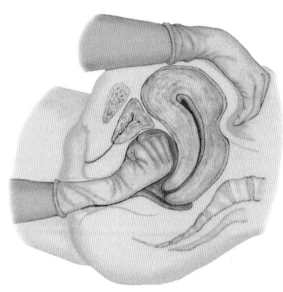

FIG. 18.3 Bimanual compression. One hand is inserted in the vagina, and the other compresses the uterus through the abdominal wall.

💊 DRUG GUIDE

Methylergonovine (Methergine)

Classification
Ergot alkaloid, uterine stimulant.

Action
Stimulates sustained contraction of the uterus and causes arterial vasoconstriction.

Indications
Used for the prevention and treatment of postpartum or postabortion hemorrhage caused by uterine atony or subinvolution.

Dosage and Route
Usual dosage is 0.2 mg intramuscularly every 2 to 4 hours for a maximum of five doses. If continued dosing is ordered, providers will change to the oral route 0.2 mg every 6 to 8 hours for a maximum of 7 days. Intravenous use is not recommended; use in life-threatening emergency only and give over at least 60 seconds with close monitoring of blood pressure (BP) and pulse; may cause severe hypertension and possible cerebrovascular accident.

Absorption
Well absorbed after oral or intramuscular route.

Excretion
Metabolized by the liver; excreted in the feces and urine.

Contraindications and Precautions
Methylergonovine should not be used during pregnancy or to induce labor. Do not use if the client is hypersensitive to ergot. Contraindicated for clients with hypertension, severe hepatic or renal disease, or cardiovascular disease.

Adverse Reactions
Nausea, vomiting, severe hypertension, dizziness, headache, dyspnea, chest pain, palpitations, peripheral ischemia, seizure, and uterine and gastrointestinal cramping.

Nursing Considerations
Before administering the medication, assess the BP. Follow facility protocol to determine at what BP level medication should be withheld. Monitor BP and pulse every 15 minutes until stable. Assess extremities for signs of decreased perfusion. Caution the client to avoid smoking because nicotine constricts blood vessels. Teach the client to report any adverse reactions.

(American College of Obstetricians and Gynecologists [ACOG]. [2017]. Postpartum hemorrhage. *ACOG Practice Bulletin No. 183*, Replaces *Practice Bulletin 76*; and Methylergonovine (methylergometrine): Drug Information. [2021]. *UpToDate.com*. https://www.uptodate.com/contents/search?search=methylergonovine-methylergometrine-drug-informaion&sp=0&searchType=PLAIN_TEXT&source=USER_INPUT&searchControl=TOP_PULLDOWN&searchOffset=1&autoComplete=false&language=&max=0&index=&autoCompleteTerm=&rawSentence=.

DRUG GUIDE

Carboprost Tromethamine (Hemabate, Prostin/15M)

Classification
Prostaglandin, oxytocic.

Action
Stimulates contraction of the uterus.

Indications
Used for the treatment of postpartum hemorrhage caused by uterine atony. Also used for pregnancy termination.

Dosage and Route
Postpartum hemorrhage: 250 mcg intramuscularly. May repeat at 15- to 90-minute intervals. Maximum total dose 2 mg.

Absorption
Metabolized by the liver and by enzymes in the lungs.

Excretion
Primarily excreted in urine.

Contraindications and Precautions
Contraindicated for clients with hypersensitivity to carboprost or other prostaglandins or asthma. Relative contraindication for acute pelvic inflammatory disease or cardiac, pulmonary, renal, or hepatic disease. Use caution if the client has a history of hypotension or hypertension.

Adverse Reactions and Side Effects
Excessive dose may cause tetanic contraction and laceration or uterine rupture. It may cause uterine hypertonus if used with oxytocin. Nausea, vomiting, diarrhea, fever, chills, facial flushing, headache, hypertension or hypotension, tachycardia, pulmonary edema, or bronchospasm.

Nursing Considerations
Should be refrigerated. Give via intramuscular injection. Rotate sites if repeated. Monitor vital signs. Administer antiemetics and antidiarrheals as ordered.

(American College of Obstetricians and Gynecologists [ACOG]. [2017]. Postpartum hemorrhage. *ACOG Practice Bulletin No. 183*, Replaces *Practice Bulletin 76*; and Carboprost tromethamine: Drug information. [2021]. *UpToDate.com*. https://www.uptodate.com/contents/search?search=hemabate&sp=0&searchType=PLAIN_TEXT&source=USER_INPUT&searchControl=TOP_PULLDOWN&searchOffset=1&autoComplete=false&language=en&max=10&index=&autoCompleteTerm=.

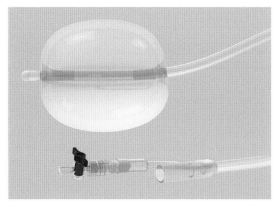

FIG. 18.4 Bakri Tamponade Balloon. (Courtesy of Cook Medical.)

Predisposing factors. Many of the same risk factors for uterine atony increase the risk for soft tissue trauma during childbirth. For example, trauma to the birth canal is more likely to occur if the infant is large or if labor and birth occur rapidly. Induction and augmentation of labor and use of assistive devices, such as a vacuum extractor or forceps, increase the risk for tissue trauma.

Lacerations. The perineum, vagina, cervix, and area around the urethral meatus are the most common sites for lacerations. Small cervical lacerations occur frequently and generally do not require repairs. Lacerations of the vagina, perineum, and periurethral area usually occur during the second stage of labor, when the fetal head descends rapidly or when assistive devices such as a vacuum extractor or forceps are used during birth.

Lacerations of the birth canal should be suspected if excessive uterine bleeding continues when the fundus is contracted firmly and remains midline. Bleeding from lacerations of the genital tract often is bright red, in contrast to the darker red color of lochia. Bleeding may be heavy or may appear to be minor with a steady trickle of blood.

Hematomas. Hematomas result from bleeding into loose connective tissue while overlying tissue remains intact. Hematomas develop because of blood vessel injury in spontaneous deliveries or with lacerations or episiotomies and in operative vaginal deliveries, in which vacuum extractors or forceps are used. Hematomas may be found in vulvar, vaginal, and retroperitoneal areas (Cunningham et al., 2022).

The rapid bleeding into soft tissue may cause a visible vulvar hematoma, a discolored bulging mass that is sensitive to touch (Fig. 18.5). Hematomas in the vagina or retroperitoneal areas cannot be seen. Hematomas produce deep, severe pain and feelings of pressure that are not relieved by usual pain-relief measures. Hematoma formation should be suspected if the client demonstrates systemic signs of concealed blood loss, such as tachycardia or decreasing BP, when the fundus is firm and lochia is within normal limits.

Therapeutic management. When PPH is caused by trauma of the birth canal, surgical repair is often necessary. Visualizing lacerations of the vagina or cervix is difficult, and it is necessary to move the client to an area where surgical lights are available. The client is placed in a lithotomy position and carefully draped. Surgical asepsis is required while the laceration is being visualized and repaired.

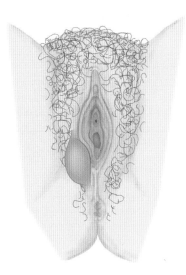

FIG. 18.5 A vulvar hematoma is caused by rapid bleeding into soft tissue, and it causes severe pain and feelings of pressure.

Small hematomas usually reabsorb naturally. Large hematomas may require incision, evacuation of the clots, and ligation of the bleeding vessel.

Late Postpartum Hemorrhage

Late PPH, also called *secondary PPH,* is defined as hemorrhage occurring between 24 hours and 12 weeks after birth (ACOG, 2017; Cunningham et al., 2022). The most common causes of late PPH are **subinvolution** (delayed return of the uterus to its nonpregnant size and consistency), retained placental fragments, and infection. Other causes of late PPH include uterine artery pseudoaneurysm and inherited coagulopathies (Cunningham et al., 2022; Francois & Foley, 2021). Normally the uterus descends at the rate of approximately 1 cm (one fingerbreadth) per day. By 14 days, it is no longer palpable above the symphysis pubis. The endometrial lining has sloughed off as part of the lochia, and the site of placental attachment is well healed by 6 weeks after childbirth. When placental fragments are retained, clots form around the retained fragments, and excessive bleeding can occur when the clots slough away several days after birth.

Clinical Manifestations

Signs of subinvolution include prolonged discharge of lochia, irregular or excessive uterine bleeding, and sometimes profuse hemorrhage. Pelvic pain or feelings of pelvic heaviness, backache, fatigue, and persistent malaise are reported by many clients. On bimanual examination, the uterus feels larger and softer than normal.

Predisposing Factors

Attempts to deliver the placenta before it separates from the uterine wall, manual removal of the placenta, placenta accreta, previous cesarean birth, and uterine leiomyomas are primary predisposing factors for retention of placental fragments.

Another factor associated with subinvolution is incompletely remodeled maternal spiral arteries that perfuse the placenta during pregnancy (Cunningham et al., 2022).

Therapeutic Management

Late PPH caused by retained placental fragments is generally preventable. When the placenta is delivered, the health care provider carefully inspects it to determine whether it is intact. If a portion of the placenta is missing, the provider manually explores the uterus, locates the missing fragments, and removes them.

Initial treatment for late PPH is directed toward control of the excessive bleeding. Oxytocin, methylergonovine, and prostaglandins are the most commonly used pharmacologic measures. Placental fragments may be dislodged and swept out of the uterus by the bleeding, and if the bleeding subsides when oxytocin is administered, no other treatment is necessary. Sonography may identify placental fragments that remain in the uterus. If bleeding continues or recurs, **dilation and curettage** (stretching of the cervical os to permit suctioning or scraping of the walls of the uterus) may be necessary to remove fragments. Broad-spectrum antibiotics may be given if postpartum infection is suspected because of uterine tenderness, foul-smelling lochia, or fever.

Nursing Considerations

In most cases, subinvolution is not obvious until the client has returned home after childbirth. Nurses should teach the client and family how to recognize its occurrence. Demonstrate how to locate and palpate the fundus and how to estimate fundal height in relation to the umbilicus. The uterus should become smaller each day (by approximately one fingerbreadth). Explain the progressive changes from lochia rubra to lochia serosa and then to lochia alba (see Chapter 17).

Instruct the client to report any deviation from the expected pattern or duration of lochia. A foul odor often indicates uterine infection for which treatment is necessary. Additional signs include pelvic or fundal pain, backache, and feelings of pelvic pressure or fullness. The client should be able to verbalize the warning signs before leaving the facility.

KNOWLEDGE CHECK

1. Why does the postpartum nurse examine the client's prenatal record and the labor and delivery record?
2. Why is a client who has given birth to twins at increased risk for PPH?
3. Can the nurse be positive that bleeding is controlled when the fundus is firm and the lochia is moderate? Why or why not?
4. How is uterine atony treated?
5. How are hematomas treated?
6. What are the major signs of subinvolution?
7. What is the nurse's primary responsibility in the management of subinvolution?

Hypovolemic Shock

During and after giving birth, the client can tolerate blood loss that approaches the volume of blood added during pregnancy (~1500 to 2000 mL). An anemic client or a preeclamptic client have less reserve than clients with uncomplicated pregnancies and normal blood values.

When blood loss is excessive, **hypovolemic shock** (acute peripheral circulatory failure resulting from loss of circulating blood volume) can ensue. **Hypovolemia** (abnormally decreased volume of circulating fluid in the body) endangers vital organs by depriving them of oxygen. The brain, heart, and kidneys are especially vulnerable to hypoxia and may suffer damage in a brief period.

Recognition of hypovolemic shock may be delayed because the body activates compensatory mechanisms that mask the severity of the problem. As shock worsens, the compensatory mechanisms fail and physiologic insults spiral and, if intervention is not performed, can result in maternal death.

The goals of therapy are to control bleeding and prevent hypovolemic shock from becoming irreversible. The health care team makes every effort to locate the source of bleeding and to stop the loss of blood. Many hospitals have massive transfusion protocols (MTP) to treat clients with severe hemorrhage. These protocols suggest transfusion of plasma, platelets, and packed red blood cells (PRBCs) in a 1:1:1 ratio. See Chapter 19 for more information about hypovolemic shock.

> ⚡ **SAFETY CHECK**
>
> Signs of postpartum hemorrhage include the following:
> A uterus that does not contract or does not remain contracted
> A large gush; slow, steady trickle; ooze; or dribble of blood from the vagina
> Saturation of one peripad per hour
> Severe, unrelieved perineal or rectal pain
> Tachycardia

APPLICATION OF THE NURSING PROCESS: THE CLIENT WITH EXCESSIVE BLEEDING

Assessment

The initial postpartum assessment includes a chart review to determine whether risk factors for hemorrhage are present. This alerts the nurse to an increased risk for hemorrhage.

Uterine Atony

Priority assessments for uterine atony include the fundus, bladder, lochia, vital signs, skin temperature, and color. Assess the consistency and the location of the uterine fundus. The fundus should be firmly contracted at or near the level of the umbilicus and midline. If the fundus feels soft (boggy), the uterus is not firmly contracted and bleeding from the placental site may be rapid and continuous. If the fundus is above the level of the umbilicus and displaced, a full bladder may be the cause of excessive bleeding. Assist the client to urinate or obtain an order for catheterization. Note urine output and then reassess the uterus (see Procedure 17.1 for assessing the fundus).

Assessment of the fundus may be difficult in the obese population. Monitor frequently for signs of uterine atony and attempt to assess the uterine fundus while watching for increased lochia flow or clots to be expelled.

Remember to check under the client's legs, buttocks, and back for lochia drainage by asking the client to turn to the side. Although bleeding may be profuse and dramatic, a continuing small but steady trickle may also lead to significant blood loss.

It is difficult to estimate the volume of lochia by visual examination of peripads. More accurate information is obtained by weighing peripads, linen savers, and, if necessary, bed linens. Weighing dry supplies, then weighing blood-saturated supplies and subtracting the difference provides a more accurate blood loss volume. One gram (weight) equals approximately 1 mL (volume).

Measure vital signs at least every 15 minutes or more often if necessary. Apply a pulse oximeter to determine oxygen saturation levels. Because the body initially compensates for excessive bleeding by constricting the peripheral blood vessels and shunting blood to vital organs, the vital signs may remain normal at first, even though the client is becoming hypovolemic. The preeclamptic client typically has low intravascular volume because of vasospasm and increased capillary permeability, leading to accumulation of fluid interstitially, and will be less tolerant of blood loss (Cunningham et al., 2022). The skin should be warm and dry, mucous membranes of the lips and mouth should be pink, and capillary return should occur within 3 seconds when the nails are blanched. These signs confirm adequate circulating volume to perfuse the peripheral tissue.

> ⚡ **SAFETY CHECK**
>
> The following are used to determine the amount of blood loss:
> Weigh all blood-soaked items (e.g., peripads, linens).
> Weigh similar clean, dry items.
> Subtract the weight of the dry items from the weight of the wet items.
> 1 g weight = 1 mL of blood.

Trauma

If the fundus is firm but bleeding is excessive, the cause may be lacerations of the cervix or birth canal. Inspect the perineum to determine whether a laceration is visible. Lacerations of the cervix or vagina are not visible, but bleeding in the presence of a firmly contracted uterus suggests a laceration. This warrants examination of the vaginal walls and the cervix by the health care provider.

Assess comfort level. If the client complains of deep, severe pelvic or rectal pain or if vital signs or skin changes suggest hemorrhage but excessive bleeding is not obvious, the cause may be concealed bleeding and the formation of a hematoma. Examine the vulva for bulging masses or discoloration. However, a hematoma developing in the vagina or in the retroperitoneal area will not be obvious when the vulva

TABLE 18.1   Nursing Assessments for Postpartum Hemorrhage

Assessments	Abnormal Signs and Symptoms	Nursing Implications
Chart review	Presence of predisposing factors	Perform more frequent evaluations.
Fundus	Soft, boggy, displaced	Massage, express clots, and assist to void or catheterize; notify primary health care provider if measures are ineffective.
Lochia	Bleeding (steady trickle, dribble, oozing, seeping, or profuse flow); heavy: saturation of 1 pad/hr; excessive: 1 pad/15 min	Assess for trauma; save and weigh pads, linen savers, and bed linens so estimation of blood loss will be more accurate. Notify health care provider.
Vital signs	Tachycardia, decreasing pulse pressure, falling blood pressure, decreasing oxygen saturation level	Report signs of excessive blood loss.
Urine output	Decreased urine output (should be at least 30 mL/hr)	Report decrease in output.
Comfort level	Severe pelvic or rectal pain	Assess for signs of hematoma, usually perineal or vaginal; examine vulva for masses or discoloration; report findings.
Skin	Cool, damp, pale	Look for signs of hypovolemia; vigilant assessment and management by entire health care team is necessary.

is examined. Table 18.1 summarizes assessments, abnormal signs and symptoms, and nursing implications for PPH.

Identification of Client Problems

Inadequate fluid volume and reduced tissue perfusion are examples of problems faced by a client with PPH. These problems require a team approach to prevent further complications such as hypovolemic shock.

Planning: Expected Outcomes

Hemorrhage requires an interprofessional approach; therefore the nursing plan of care will reflect both dependent and independent nursing care. Planning should reflect the nurse's responsibility to do the following:
- Monitor for signs of PPH.
- Perform actions that minimize PPH and prevent hypovolemic shock.
- Notify the provider if signs of excessive blood loss are observed or if the client does not respond as desired.

Interventions

Preventing Hemorrhage

The key to successful management of early PPH is early recognition and response. All postpartum clients are at risk for hemorrhage. However, awareness of risk factors and vigilance in monitoring these clients prepares the nurse to recognize excessive bleeding and intervene promptly.

When predisposing factors are present, initiate frequent assessments. Many hospitals and birth centers complete fundal and vital sign assessments every 15 minutes during the first 2 hours after birth. Assessment transitions to individual client needs, such as hourly or every 4, 8, or 12 hours depending on facility protocol, length of time since birth, and risk status. This plan may not be adequate for the client at known risk for PPH. A delay in assessment could result in excessive blood loss.

Collaborating with the Health Care Provider

When excessive bleeding is suspected and the fundus is boggy, begin uterine massage. Check the client's bladder for distention and empty it if necessary. If unable to void and the bladder is distended, obtain an order and catheterize the client. Weigh blood-soaked pads, linen savers, and linens to accurately determine the amount of blood lost. If massage is not effective in controlling bleeding, promptly notify the provider. Save any tissue or clots passed.

Follow facility protocols to initiate specific laboratory studies, such as hemoglobin (Hgb) and hematocrit (Hct) levels and type and crossmatch of blood, so blood may be available should transfusions become necessary. Coagulation studies may include fibrinogen, prothrombin time, partial thromboplastin time, fibrin split products, fibrin degradation products, platelets, D-dimer, and blood chemistry. Many protocols also allow the nurse to increase the flow rate of an existing IV line or insert a large-bore catheter to start IV fluids while the health care provider is being informed of the client's condition. These actions do not substitute for notifying the provider and obtaining additional orders, but they do allow nurses to make initial interventions quickly.

Keep the client on bed rest to increase venous return and maintain cardiac output. The full Trendelenburg position may interfere with cardiac and pulmonary function and is not advised. A modified Trendelenburg position may be used with the legs elevated 10 to 30 degrees to increase blood return from the legs, the trunk horizontal, and the head slightly elevated. Continue assessments, call for assistance, and save all blood-soaked materials so accurate blood loss can be determined. Assistance is necessary; one nurse should continue to massage the uterus and perform and record assessments while another notifies the health care provider of the client's condition and gathers medications and supplies needed.

Administer medications, fluids, and treatments as ordered by the health care provider or as stated in the facility's protocol. Evaluate the effects and relay the information to the provider. Because of oxytocin's antidiuretic effect, listen to breath sounds to identify signs of pulmonary edema from fluid overload if large amounts of oxytocin are given. If measures fail to control bleeding, notify the health care provider so additional procedures can be initiated. These may include preparation for operative intervention.

Providing Support for the Family

The unusual activity of the hospital staff may make the client and family anxious. Be alert to their nonverbal cues, and acknowledge their feelings when they appear frightened. Keeping the family informed is one of the most effective ways of reducing anxiety.

Acknowledge the anxiety and provide simple appropriate explanations of the activity. "I know all this activity must be frightening. The bleeding is a little more than we would like and we are doing several things at once."

Posthemorrhage Care

After the hemorrhage is controlled, continue to assess the client frequently for a resumption of bleeding. The client may be anemic and fatigued. Allow rest periods and cluster care to help conserve energy. The client may experience orthostatic hypotension; therefore assist with getting out of bed after dangling legs at bedside and assessing for dizziness and low BP. Encourage intake of fluids and foods high in iron. The client may need assistance with providing newborn care.

Home Care

Nurses who work in home care or nurse-managed postpartum clinics should be aware that clients who have had PPH are subject to a variety of complications. In general, they are exhausted; it may take weeks for them to feel well again. Anemia often results, and a course of iron therapy may be prescribed to restore Hgb levels. Activity may be restricted until strength returns. Some clients need extra assistance with housework and care of the new infant. Fatigue may interfere with attachment. Extensive blood loss increases the risk for postpartum infection; therefore the nurse should teach the client to observe for specific signs and symptoms.

Evaluation

The nurse collects and evaluates data with established norms and judges whether the data are within normal limits. If problems arise, the nurse acts to minimize hemorrhage and notifies the health care provider.

THROMBOEMBOLIC DISORDERS

A **thrombus** is a collection of blood factors, primarily platelets and fibrin, on a vessel wall. **Thrombophlebitis** occurs when the vessel wall develops an inflammatory response to the thrombus. This further occludes the vessel. An **embolus** is a mass, composed of a thrombus or amniotic fluid, released into the bloodstream that may cause obstruction of capillary beds in another part of the body, frequently the lungs. A **pulmonary embolus** is a potentially fatal complication that occurs when the pulmonary artery is obstructed by a blood clot that was swept into circulation from a vein or by amniotic fluid. The two most common thromboembolisms encountered during pregnancy and the postpartum period are deep vein thrombosis (DVT) and pulmonary embolism (PE). These two conditions are referred to as venous thromboembolism (VTE) (ACOG, 2018b). Superficial venous thrombophlebitis typically is not associated with morbidity but may develop into or be associated with a DVT or PE (Merriam & Pettker, 2021). DVT can involve veins from the foot to the iliofemoral region and is a major concern because it predisposes to developing a PE.

Incidence and Etiology

ACOG (2018b) notes the incidence of thromboembolic events is 0.5 to 2 per 1000 pregnancies. Thrombi can form whenever the flow of blood is impeded. Once started, the thrombus can enlarge with successive layering of platelets, fibrin, and blood cells as the blood flows past the clot. Thrombus formation is often associated with thrombophlebitis.

The three contributing factors to thrombus development are venous stasis, hypercoagulability, and injury to the endothelial surface (the innermost layer) of the blood vessel, often referred to as the **Virchow triad** (Merriam & Pettker, 2021). Two of these conditions—venous stasis and hypercoagulable blood—are present in all pregnancies; the third, blood vessel injury, is likely to occur during birth.

Venous Stasis

During pregnancy, compression of the large vessels of the legs and pelvis by the enlarging uterus causes venous stasis. Stasis is most pronounced when the pregnant client stands for prolonged periods. It results in dilated vessels that increase the potential for continued postpartum pooling of blood. Relative inactivity and activity restriction because of complications during pregnancy lead to venous pooling and stasis of blood in the lower extremities. Prolonged time in stirrups for birth and perineal repair may also promote venous stasis and increase the risk for thrombus formation.

Hypercoagulation

Pregnancy is characterized by changes in the coagulation and fibrinolytic systems that persist into the postpartum period. During pregnancy the levels of many coagulation factors are elevated. In addition, the fibrinolytic system, which causes clots to disintegrate (lyse), is suppressed. Clot formation factors are increased and factors that prevent clot formation are decreased to prevent maternal hemorrhage, resulting in a higher risk for thrombus formation during pregnancy and the postpartum period.

Blood Vessel Injury

Endothelial damage may occur during pregnancy, especially at birth. Lower extremity trauma, operative birth, and prolonged labor can cause vascular damage. Cesarean birth significantly increases the risk for thromboembolic disease

BOX 18.2 Factors That Increase the Risk for Thrombosis

History of previous thrombosis
Inherited thrombophilia—Factor V Leiden, Prothrombin G20210A
Acquired thrombophilia—antiphospholipid antibody syndrome (APS)
Prolonged bed rest (1 week or longer)
Obesity
Medical conditions—heart disease, diabetes, hypertension, autoimmune disorders, sickle cell
Surgical procedures—cesarean birth, dilation & curettage, postpartum sterilization
Forceps-assisted vaginal delivery
Infections—endometritis, wound infection, sepsis, pneumonia
Smoking
Varicose veins
Multiple gestation
Prolonged labor
Preeclampsia
Maternal age older than 35 years
Parity of 3 or higher
First-degree relative with thrombosis
Air travel

(ACOG, 2018b; Cunningham et al., 2022; Witcher & Hamner, 2019). Clients with varicose veins, obesity, a history of thrombophlebitis, and a history of smoking are at additional risk for thromboembolic disease (Box 18.2). Age older than 35 years doubles the risk (Leung et al., 2019).

Superficial Venous Thrombosis
Clinical Manifestations
Superficial thrombophlebitis is most often associated with varicose veins and occur in the calf area. It also can occur in the arms as a result of IV therapy or perineal area during pregnancy. Signs and symptoms include swelling of the involved extremity and redness, tenderness, and warmth. It may be possible to palpate an enlarged, hardened, cordlike vein. The client may experience pain, but some clients have no signs at all.

Therapeutic Management
Treatment includes analgesics, rest, and elastic support. Elevation of the lower extremity improves venous return. Anticoagulants are not usually needed, but antiinflammatory medications may be used. After a period of bed rest with the leg elevated, the client may ambulate gradually if symptoms have disappeared. Encourage the client to avoid standing for long periods and continue to wear support hose to help prevent venous stasis and a subsequent episode of superficial thrombosis. Little chance of pulmonary embolism exists if the thrombosis remains in the superficial veins of the lower leg.

Deep Vein Thrombosis
Depending on the size of the thrombus, signs and symptoms of DVT or PE may be absent in affected clients (Leung

et al., 2019; Roth, 2021). Signs and symptoms are caused by an inflammatory process and obstruction of venous return. The client may report pain in the leg, groin, lower back, or abdomen (Witcher & Hamner, 2019). Swelling of the leg, erythema, heat, and tenderness over the affected area are the most common signs. Reflex arterial spasms may cause the leg to become pale and cool to the touch with decreased peripheral pulses. Additional symptoms may include pain on ambulation, chills, general malaise, and stiffness of the affected leg. The most common extremity affected is the left leg. This is attributed to compression of the left iliac vein and compression of the vena cava by the gravid uterus.

Diagnosis
Venous ultrasonography with vein compression and Doppler flow analysis of the deep veins of the upper legs is most commonly used to detect alterations in blood flow that are diagnostic of DVT. Noncontrast magnetic resonance imaging (MRI) is considered very sensitive and accurate in diagnosing pelvic and leg thrombosis (Leung et al., 2019). d-Dimer tests may be performed, but the results are normally higher during pregnancy and postpartum, and the test may not be as accurate as at other times (Cunningham et al., 2022; Leung et al., 2019; Merriam & Pettker, 2021).

Risk Assessment
Risk assessment for development of VTE is recommended by ACOG and supported by the Joint Commission and Alliance for Innovation on Maternal Health (AIM) initiatives (ACOG, 2018b; AIM, 2020; Council on Patient Safety in Women's Health, 2015; The Joint Commission, 2021). Because of the hypercoagulability of pregnancy and increased risk of thrombosis formation for all pregnant clients, risk assessment helps determine appropriate interventions for each individual. Risk assessment is recommended to be completed during outpatient visits, antepartum and intrapartum hospitalization, and during the postpartum phase of care (AIM, 2020; Council on Patient Safety in Women's Health, 2015). The most significant individual risk factors for VTE development are a history of thrombosis and the presence of a thrombophilia. The highest risk for development of VTE is during the postpartum period, with more incidents noted in the first week postpartum (ACOG, 2018b).

Therapeutic Management
Preventing thrombus formation. Clients who have had a previous DVT or PE are at risk for another. High-risk clients may receive prophylactic heparin, which does not cross the placenta. Either standard unfractionated heparin (UH) or a low-molecular-weight heparin (LMWH) such as enoxaparin (Lovenox) may be used. LMWH is longer acting and can be given less frequently; is associated with fewer laboratory tests and side effects; and is less likely to cause bleeding. However, LMWH is more expensive than UH and must be given subcutaneously. UH is given via IV or subcutaneously.

Clients receiving LMWH during pregnancy may be changed to UH based on provider and institution preference.

Another management choice is to discontinue anticoagulation 12 to 24 hours before induction or scheduled surgery. The change is necessary because epidural anesthesia, which may be needed in labor, is contraindicated within 24 hours of the last dose of LMWH. Heparin is discontinued during labor and birth and resumed approximately 6 to 12 hours after uncomplicated birth and 12 hours after the epidural catheter is removed (ACOG, 2018b). For clients with a recent pulmonary embolus, iliofemoral thrombosis, or mechanical heart valves, anticoagulation may continue during labor and birth (Roth, 2021).

If stirrups must be used during the birth, they should be padded to prevent prolonged pressure against the popliteal angle during the second stage of labor. If possible, the time in stirrups should be no more than 1 hour.

Frequent and early ambulation is encouraged after birth. Ambulation prevents stasis of blood in the legs and decreases the likelihood of thrombus formation. If the client is unable to ambulate, range-of-motion and gentle leg exercises, such as flexing and straightening the knee and raising one leg at a time, should begin within 8 hours after childbirth. Extreme flexion at the groin should be avoided because this leads to pooling of blood in the lower extremities.

Sequential compression devices are used for clients with varicose veins, a history of thrombosis, or a cesarean birth. Sequential compression devices should be applied preoperatively for cesarean birth and should be continued until ambulation begins postpartum (ACOG, 2018b).

Initial treatment. Anticoagulant therapy is started to prevent extension of the thrombus. Clotting studies should be monitored to ensure a safe but therapeutic level. The client is placed on bed rest, with the affected leg slightly elevated to decrease interstitial swelling and to promote venous return from the leg. Analgesics may be prescribed to control pain, and antibiotics will be used as necessary to prevent or control infection. Moist heat provides relief of pain and increases circulation. Gradual ambulation is allowed when symptoms have disappeared.

Subsequent treatment. The long-term management of DVT depends on whether the client is pregnant or in the postpartum period. The pregnant client with a DVT receives anticoagulation therapy until labor begins. It is resumed 6 to 12 hours after birth and continued for 6 weeks to 6 months after birth (Witcher & Hamner, 2019). Warfarin (Coumadin) is contraindicated during pregnancy because of teratogenic effects and the risk for fetal hemorrhage. Therefore pregnant clients are given UH or LMWH, which do not cross the placenta.

During the postpartum period, warfarin is started before heparin is stopped to provide continuous anticoagulation. Heparin is discontinued when the international normalized ratio (INR) has been at therapeutic levels for 2 days. Warfarin is safe for use during lactation. The INR is used to monitor coagulation time when warfarin is used.

Before discharge from the birth facility, the client should be taught about lifestyle changes that can improve peripheral circulation. This includes avoiding both clothing that is constricting around the legs and prolonged sitting. If sitting for long periods is necessary, walking for a short time hourly or moving feet and legs frequently will help prevent circulatory stasis.

KNOWLEDGE CHECK

8. Why is the risk for thrombus formation increased in pregnancy and in the postpartum period?
9. How does the long-term treatment for DVT in the pregnant client differ from that in the client who is in the postpartum period?
10. Why is bed rest prescribed for the client with DVT?

CLIENT TEACHING

How to Prevent Thrombosis (Blood Clots)

The following methods to improve peripheral circulation will help prevent the occurrence of thrombophlebitis:

Improve your circulation with a regular schedule of activity, preferably walking.

Avoid prolonged standing or sitting in one position.

When sitting, elevate your legs and avoid crossing them. This will increase the return of venous blood from the legs.

Maintain a daily fluid intake of 12 or more 8-oz glasses to prevent dehydration and consequent sluggish circulation.

Stop smoking. Smoking is a risk factor for thrombosis and can cause respiratory problems in you and your newborn.

Pulmonary Embolism

Pathophysiology

Pulmonary embolism (PE) is a serious complication of DVT that can lead to maternal mortality. PE occurs when fragments of a blood clot dislodge and are carried to the lungs. An embolus can also consist of amniotic fluid and its debris, a condition called *anaphylactoid syndrome* of pregnancy (see Chapter 19). The embolus lodges in a vessel and partially or completely obstructs the flow of blood into the lungs. If pulmonary circulation is severely compromised, death may occur within a few minutes. If the embolus is small, adequate pulmonary circulation may be maintained until treatment can be initiated.

Clinical Manifestations

Clinical signs and symptoms depend on how much blood flow is obstructed. Dyspnea and chest pain are the most common signs (Leung et al., 2019; Witcher & Hamner, 2019). Clients typically have a sense of "impending doom" before the onset of other symptoms (Roth, 2021). Other signs and symptoms include hypoxemia, tachycardia, tachypnea, and hemoptysis. Hypotension and syncope are uncommon and may indicate massive emboli (Leung et al., 2019). Pulmonary crackles, cough, abdominal pain, and low-grade fever also may occur. Pulse oximetry shows decreased oxygen saturation. Arterial blood gas determinations show decreased partial pressure of oxygen, and chest radiography reveals areas of atelectasis, pulmonary edema, and pleural effusion.

Other diagnostic tests may include computed tomographic pulmonary angiography (CPTA) or ventilation-perfusion (V/Q) scan. A venous ultrasound is also performed to identify a DVT (Leung et al., 2019).

Therapeutic Management

Treatment of PE is aimed at dissolving the clot and maintaining pulmonary circulation. Oxygen is used to decrease hypoxia, and narcotic analgesics are given to reduce pain and apprehension. Bed rest with the head of the bed elevated is used to help reduce dyspnea. The level of care, including support of ventilation, depends on the client's pulmonary status. Pulse oximetry and arterial blood gases are evaluated. Heparin therapy is initiated and continued throughout pregnancy if the embolism occurs before birth. Therapy may be continued with warfarin for months after birth to prevent further emboli.

Nursing Considerations

Monitoring for signs. When caring for a client with DVT, nurses should be aware of the danger of PE and focus the assessment for early signs and symptoms. This includes frequent assessment of respiratory rate and thorough and frequent auscultation of breath sounds. Abnormalities such as diminished or unequal breath sounds or coughing should be reported immediately to the health care provider. Additional signs that require immediate attention include air hunger, dyspnea, tachycardia, pallor, and cyanosis.

Facilitating oxygenation. Oxygen should be administered at 8 to 10 L/min by face mask. The nurse should remain with the client to allay fear and apprehension. The head of the bed should be raised to facilitate breathing. Narcotic analgesics, such as morphine, may be used to relieve pain. Sedatives may be given to help control anxiety.

Seeking assistance. The client's condition is precarious until the clot is lysed or until it adheres to the pulmonary artery wall and is reabsorbed. The primary nurse should call for assistance to initiate interventions. These include continuous assessment of vital signs and administration of IV heparin and emergency drugs that may be needed. The client requires critical care nursing skills and is usually transferred to an intensive care unit.

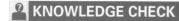

KNOWLEDGE CHECK

11. What additional nursing assessments are necessary when the client is receiving anticoagulants?

APPLICATION OF THE NURSING PROCESS: THE CLIENT WITH DEEP VENOUS THROMBOSIS

Assessment

Assessment focuses on determining the status of the venous thrombosis. Inspect both legs at the same time comparing the affected leg with the unaffected leg. DVT is most often unilateral, usually affecting the client's left side (Leung et al., 2019). Warmth or redness indicates inflammation; coolness or cyanosis indicates venous obstruction. Palpate the pedal pulses, comparing the strength of the right and left. Measure the affected and unaffected legs, comparing the circumferences to obtain an estimation of the swelling present in the affected leg. Record the measurements for ongoing assessment. A circumference 2 cm greater in the affected leg may be noted (Witcher & Hamner, 2019). It may be helpful to mark the client's legs at the location of the measurement for consistency in assessments. Assess for pain. Pain is caused by tissue hypoxia, and increasing pain indicates progressive obstruction.

Evaluate the clotting studies laboratory reports. Thrombocytopenia is a concern when heparin is administered for a prolonged time.

Identification of Client Problems

The treatment of DVT includes the administration of anticoagulants for a prolonged time. For many clients, a lack of knowledge of anticoagulant precautions places them at an increased risk.

Planning: Expected Outcomes

Expected outcomes for the client include:
- Remain free of bleeding from anticoagulant therapy.
- Verbalize precautions necessary when taking anticoagulants.
- Verbalize plan for changes necessary as a result of anticoagulant therapy.

Interventions

Monitoring for Signs of Bleeding

At least twice a day, inspect the client for the appearance of bruising or petechiae. Instruct the client to report any signs of bleeding: bruises, bloody nose, blood in urine or stools, bleeding gums, or increased vaginal bleeding. Be alert for signs of hemorrhage, such as tachycardia, falling BP, or other signs indicating internal bleeding.

Observe for excessive or bright red lochia. If the uterus is boggy, the cause is uterine atony. Massage the uterus and express clots. If the fundus is firm, bleeding may be from trauma or anticoagulant therapy. In either case, the provider should be notified.

Unless frank hemorrhage is present, the usual treatment for excessive anticoagulation is temporary discontinuation of the anticoagulant. Protamine sulfate, which is the antidote for UH and is partially effective against LMWH, should be available. The antidote for warfarin is vitamin K.

Explaining Continued Therapy

Teach the client how to prevent excessive anticoagulation. Carefully explain the treatment regimen, including the schedule of medication. Help develop a method for remembering to take the medication as directed. Caution the client not to "double up" if a dose is missed. If necessary, teach the client and another family member how to inject heparin or enoxaparin. Explain the need for repeated laboratory testing to regulate the anticoagulant dose. Emphasize the importance of careful attention to dosage changes to keep the medication at the appropriate blood levels.

Oral anticoagulants are associated with many clinically significant drug interactions; emphasize the importance of keeping the health care provider informed about any medications taken. Caution the client that common over-the-counter medications, such as aspirin and other nonsteroidal antiinflammatory medications, increase the risk for bleeding. Explain that some herbs and dietary supplements may affect the potency of anticoagulants, and the client should check with the health care provider before using them.

Instruct the client taking warfarin that eating large amounts of vitamin K–containing foods may interfere with anticoagulation. These foods include broccoli, cabbage, lettuce, spinach, and lentils. Caution against drinking alcohol, which inhibits the metabolism of oral anticoagulants. The client should use effective contraception while taking warfarin because of the risk of fetal developmental defects.

Suggest the client use a soft toothbrush and floss teeth gently to prevent bleeding from the gums. An electric toothbrush may be too vigorous and may cause bleeding. Using a depilatory or waxing product or shaving with an electric razor to remove unwanted hair is safer than using a blade razor during anticoagulant therapy. Remind the client not to go barefoot and to avoid activities that could cause injury. Emphasize the importance of reporting unusual bleeding.

Helping the Family Adapt to Home Care

Assess the family structure and function to determine how prepared the family is to cope with the client's illness. Determine the ages of any children and availability of support to help while the client is confined to bed or on limited activity. Help the family develop a plan of care that includes the temporary assistance needed.

Note interactions between the parents and the newborn. Although the health of the client is of primary importance, it is also important for the attachment process between the parents and infant to progress.

Evaluation

The expected outcomes are met when:
- The client demonstrates no signs of unusual bleeding or other side effects of the medication.
- The client discusses precautions taken to prevent hemorrhage.
- Necessary changes have been made in the home.

PUERPERAL INFECTION

Puerperal infection is a term used to describe bacterial infections after childbirth. Until the advent of antibiotics, puerperal infection often resulted in death. It remains a cause of maternal death, especially in developing nations. Common postpartum infections are **endometritis** (an infection of the inner lining of the uterus), wound infections, urinary tract infections (UTIs), **mastitis** (infection of the breast), and septic pelvic thrombophlebitis. **Endomyometritis** is an infection of the muscle and inner lining of the uterus. If the surrounding tissues are also involved, **endoparametritis** is present. **Metritis** is the infection of the decidua, myometrium, and parametrial tissues of the uterus.

Definition

The definition of **puerperal infection** is a temperature of 38°C (100.4°F) or higher after the first 24 hours and occurring on at least 2 of the first 10 days after childbirth (Cunningham et al., 2022). Although a slight elevation of temperature may occur during the first 24 hours because of dehydration or the exertion of labor, any client with fever should be assessed for other signs of infection.

Effect of Normal Anatomy and Physiology on Infection

Every part of the reproductive tract is connected, and organisms can move from the vagina, through the cervix, into the uterus, and through the fallopian tubes to infect the ovaries and peritoneal cavity. The entire reproductive tract is particularly well supplied with blood vessels during pregnancy and after childbirth. Bacteria that invade or are picked up by the blood vessels or lymphatics can carry the infection to the rest of the body, which can result in life-threatening septicemia.

The normal physiologic changes of childbirth increase the risk for infection. During labor and birth, the acidity of the vagina is reduced by the amniotic fluid, blood, and lochia, which are alkaline. An alkaline environment encourages growth of bacteria.

Necrosis of the endometrial lining and the presence of lochia provide a favorable environment for the growth of anaerobic bacteria. Many small lacerations, some microscopic in size, occur in the endometrium, cervix, and vagina during birth and allow bacteria to enter the tissue. Although the uterine interior is not sterile until 3 to 4 weeks after childbirth, infection does not develop in most clients, partly because granulocytes in the lochia and endometrium help prevent infection. Scrupulous aseptic technique during labor and birth and careful handwashing during the postpartum period are also major preventive factors.

Other Risk Factors

Other factors may predispose a client to infection (Table 18.2). Cesarean birth is a major predisposing factor because of the tissue trauma that occurs in surgery; the incision provides an entrance for bacteria, there is the possibility of contamination during surgery, and foreign bodies such as sutures can promote infection (Duff, 2019; Mackeen et al., 2015). In addition, clients who must have a surgical birth because of a problem during labor may have other risk factors, such as prolonged labor, that raise the chances of infection. Colonization of the vagina with organisms such as group B *Streptococcus, Chlamydia trachomatis, Mycoplasma hominis,* and *Gardnerella vaginalis* also predisposes the client to the development of infection after childbirth.

Any trauma to maternal tissues increases the hazard of infection. Trauma during vaginal birth may occur with rapid birth, birth of a large infant, use of a vacuum extractor or forceps, manual delivery of the placenta, or lacerations and episiotomies. Catheterization during labor increases the chance of introduction of organisms into the bladder and adds to the trauma to the urinary tract that occurs during normal childbirth.

TABLE 18.2   Risk Factors for Puerperal Infection

Risk Factor	Reason
History of previous infections (urinary tract infection, mastitis, thrombophlebitis)	May be more vulnerable to infectious process.
Colonization of lower genital tract by pathogenic organisms	Infections usually caused by several microbes that have ascended to the uterus from the lower genital tract.
Cesarean birth	Provides increased portals of entry for bacteria.
Trauma	Provides entrance for bacteria and makes tissues more susceptible.
Prolonged rupture of membranes	Removes barrier of amniotic membranes and allows access by organisms to interior of uterus.
Prolonged labor	Increases number of vaginal examinations; allows time for bacteria to multiply.
Catheterization	Could introduce organisms into bladder.
Excessive number of vaginal examinations	Increases chance that organisms from the vagina or outside source are carried into the uterus.
Retained placental fragments	Provide growth medium for bacteria and may interfere with flow of lochia.
Hemorrhage	Results in loss of infection-fighting components of blood.
Poor general health (excessive fatigue, anemia, frequent minor illnesses)	Increases vulnerability to infections and complications of labor.
Poor nutrition (decreased protein, vitamin C)	Less able to repair tissue and defend against infection.
Poor hygiene	Increases exposure to pathogens.
Medical conditions such as diabetes mellitus	Decreases ability to defend against infections of any kind; diabetes increases glucose level in urine.
Low socioeconomic status	More likely to have poor nutrition and inadequate prenatal care.

When prolonged rupture of membranes occurs during labor, organisms from the vagina are more likely to ascend into the uterine cavity. A long labor or many vaginal examinations during labor increases the danger of infection. Each vaginal examination increases the possibility of contamination from organisms in the vagina that are carried through the open cervix. Use of a fetal scalp electrode or intrauterine pressure catheter has the same effect. If part of the placenta remains inside the uterus after birth, the tissue becomes necrotic and provides a good place for bacteria to grow.

Additional factors include PPH, which causes loss of infection-fighting components of the blood, such as leukocytes, and leaves the client in a weakened condition. Prenatal conditions (poor nutrition, anemia) interfere with the client's ability to resist infection. Lack of knowledge of hygiene or lack of access to facilities that permit adequate hygiene increases the risk for postpartum infection.

KNOWLEDGE CHECK

12. In addition to assessment, physical care, and teaching, what should the nurse consider for the client with a DVT being treated at home?
13. Why is the client who had an assisted birth or cesarean birth at increased risk for postpartum infection?
14. Why do the normal physiologic changes of childbearing make a client especially susceptible to infection of the reproductive system?
15. Why is infection more likely to develop in a client who had prolonged labor?

Specific Infections
Endometritis

Incidence and etiology. Endometritis occurs in 1% to 3% of clients after vaginal birth and increases to 5% to 6% with risk factors such as ruptured membranes, prolonged labor, and multiple vaginal exams (Cunningham et al., 2022; Duff, 2021). An incidence of 5% to 15% is noted in clients after scheduled cesarean birth. If extended labor and rupture of membranes precede cesarean birth, infection occurs in 30% to 35% of clients who have no prophylactic antibiotics and 10% or less of those who receive prophylactic antibiotics (Duff, 2021).

Endometritis is usually caused by organisms that are normal inhabitants of the vagina and cervix. Most infections are polymicrobial with both aerobic and anaerobic organisms involved. Organisms most often found include aerobic and anaerobic streptococci, *Escherichia coli*, *Klebsiella pneumoniae*, *Proteus*, *Bacteroides*, and group B *Streptococcus* (Duff, 2019).

Clinical manifestations. The client with severe endometritis looks sick. The major signs and symptoms are temperature of 38°C (100.4°F) or higher, chills, malaise, abdominal pain and cramping, uterine tenderness, and purulent, foul-smelling lochia. Additional signs include tachycardia and subinvolution. In most cases, the signs and symptoms occur within 36 hours after birth (Duff, 2019).

Laboratory data may confirm the diagnosis. The results of a complete blood count (CBC) may show an elevation in the number of leukocytes ($15,000/mm^3$ to $25,000/mm^3$).

Leukocyte levels are normally elevated to as high as 25,000/mm³ during early postpartum (Cunningham et al., 2022); however, leukocytosis that is not decreasing should prompt further evaluation. A blood culture and catheterized urine specimen may be obtained. Cultures of the vagina or endometrium are not usually helpful.

Therapeutic management. Administration of IV antibiotics is the initial treatment for endometritis. The goal is to confine the infectious process to the uterus and prevent spread of the infection throughout the body. Broad-spectrum antibiotics, such as the cephalosporins, clindamycin plus gentamicin, or ampicillin plus aminoglycosides, are often used. Metronidazole with penicillin also may be given. Antibiotics are continued until the client has been afebrile and asymptomatic for 24 hours (Duff, 2019).

To decrease the incidence of endometritis and wound infections, a single prophylactic IV dose of an antibiotic should be given before skin incision for any client who is having a cesarean birth (ACOG, 2018a). Other medications include antipyretics for fever and oxytocics such as methylergonovine to increase drainage of lochia and promote involution.

Complications. If the infection spreads outside the uterine cavity, it may affect the fallopian tubes (salpingitis) or the ovaries (oophoritis), which could result in sterility. Peritonitis (inflammation of the membrane lining the walls of the abdominal and pelvic cavities) may occur and lead to formation of a pelvic abscess. In addition, the risk for pelvic thrombophlebitis is increased when pathogenic bacteria enter the bloodstream during episodes of endometritis. Fig. 18.6 illustrates complications of metritis.

Signs and symptoms of spreading infection may be similar to those of endometritis but more severe. Fever and abdominal pain will be particularly pronounced. Peritonitis may result in paralytic ileus and abdominal distention with absent bowel sounds.

Nursing considerations. The client with endometritis should be medicated as needed for abdominal pain or cramping, which may be severe. Monitor the client's response to treatment, and note signs of improvement or continued infection (nausea and vomiting, abdominal distention, absent bowel sounds, and severe abdominal pain). Assess vital signs every 2 hours while fever is present and every 4 hours afterward. Comfort measures include warm blankets, cool compresses, cold or warm drinks, or use of a heating pad. Foods high in vitamin C and protein to aid healing are encouraged along with oral fluids to maintain hydration.

Teaching should include signs and symptoms of worsening condition, side effects of therapy, and the importance of adhering to the treatment plan and follow-up care. If the client is separated from the infant, there is a risk for alteration in attachment. If the client is breastfeeding, initiate breast pumping to establish and maintain lactation.

Wound Infection

Wound infections are common types of puerperal infection because any break in the skin or mucous membrane

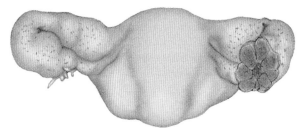
Salpingitis: Infection in fallopian tubes causes them to become enlarged, hyperemic, and tender.

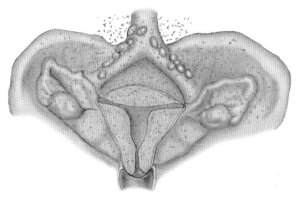
Peritonitis: Infection spreads through the lymphatics to the peritoneum; a pelvic abscess may form.

FIG. 18.6 Areas of spread of uterine infection.

provides a portal of entry for organisms. The most common sites are cesarean surgical incisions, episiotomies, and lacerations. Incisional infection occurs in 3% to 5% of clients after cesarean (Duff, 2021). Risk factors include obesity, diabetes, hemorrhage, chorioamnionitis, corticosteroid therapy, and multiple vaginal examinations.

Clinical manifestations. Signs of wound infection are edema, warmth, redness, tenderness, and pain. The edges of the wound may pull apart, and seropurulent drainage may be present. If the wound remains untreated, generalized signs of infection, such as fever and malaise, also may develop. As with other puerperal infections, cultures may reveal mixed aerobic and anaerobic bacteria. Necrotizing fasciitis is a rare infection that may occur at any incision site. The necrosis may spread and the condition may be fatal.

Therapeutic management. An incision and drainage of the affected area may be necessary. The wound exudate is cultured, and broad-spectrum antibiotics are ordered until a report of the organism is returned. Analgesics are often necessary, and warm compresses or sitz baths may be used to provide comfort and promote healing by increasing circulation to the area. Surgical debridement is performed for necrotizing fasciitis.

Nursing considerations. Despite their size, wound infections are painful. Perineal infections cause discomfort during many activities, such as walking, sitting, or defecating, and are particularly troublesome because they are not expected by the client.

Wound infections may require readmission to the hospital or home health care visits. The client requires reassurance and supportive care. Comfort measures include sitz baths, warm compresses, and frequent perineal care. Education should include to wipe from front to back and to change perineal pads frequently. Good handwashing techniques are emphasized. Adequate fluid intake and a healthy diet are important. Activity may be modified depending on the site, severity, and treatment of the wound infection.

The infant is not routinely isolated from the client with a wound infection; however, provide education regarding how to protect the infant from contact with contaminated articles such as dressings. Anticipatory guidance should include teaching side effects of medications, signs of worsening condition, self-care measures, and the importance of handwashing.

> ### ❓ KNOWLEDGE CHECK
> 16. What are the signs and symptoms of endometritis? How is it usually treated?
> 17. What are the most common sites for wound infections?
> 18. How does the nurse assess for wound infection?

Urinary Tract Infections

Etiology. During childbirth, the bladder and urethra are traumatized by pressure from the descending fetus. Insertion of a catheter, with its risk for infection, also may occur during labor. After childbirth, the bladder and urethra are hypotonic, with urinary stasis and retention common problems. Residual urine and reflux of urine may occur during voiding. Other risk factors for developing a UTI include the fact that females have a shorter urethra, contamination from vagina and rectum, incomplete bladder emptying, and frequent vaginal exams during labor (James & Suplee, 2021).

Clients who had bacteria in the urine during pregnancy, often without symptoms, are at increased risk for cystitis and pyelonephritis, which may result in preterm labor. Asymptomatic bacteriuria may be discovered during urine screens in 2% to 10% of pregnant clients. UTIs are most often caused by coliform bacteria, such as *E. coli*. Other organisms include *K. pneumoniae* and *Proteus* species (Burwick, 2021).

Clinical manifestations. Symptoms typically begin on the first or second postpartum day. They include dysuria, urgency, frequency, and suprapubic pain. Hematuria also may occur. A low-grade fever is sometimes the only sign. On the third or fourth day, some clients may develop an upper UTI, such as pyelonephritis, with chills, spiking fever, costovertebral angle tenderness, flank pain, and nausea and vomiting. This infection of the renal pelvis may result in permanent damage to the kidney if not promptly treated.

Therapeutic management. Most UTIs can be treated with antibiotics on an outpatient basis. Asymptomatic bacteriuria during pregnancy increases the risk for pyelonephritis. Treatment reduces the incidence of pyelonephritis significantly (Duff, 2019). Pyelonephritis during pregnancy may require hydration and IV administration of broad-spectrum antibiotics. In addition, the client should be observed for signs of preterm labor. Outpatient management is possible with postpartum pyelonephritis. Urinary analgesics such as phenazopyridine (Pyridium) also may be ordered. Antibiotics that are safe for use during lactation are given if the client is breastfeeding.

Nursing considerations. The client with a UTI should be instructed to take the medication for the entire time it is prescribed and not stop when symptoms abate. In addition, encourage oral fluid intake of at least 2500 to 3000 mL each day to help dilute the bacterial count and flush the infection from the bladder. Acidification of the urine inhibits multiplication of bacteria, and drinks that acidify urine, such as apricot, plum, prune, and cranberry juices, are frequently recommended. Grapefruit and carbonated drinks should be avoided because they increase urine alkalinity. Teaching also should include measures to prevent UTI, such as using proper perineal care, increasing fluid intake, and urinating frequently.

Mastitis

Incidence and etiology. Mastitis, an infection of the breast, occurs most often 2 to 4 weeks after childbirth, although it may develop at any time during breastfeeding. Approximately 5% of lactating clients are affected (Duff, 2019; James & Suplee, 2021). It usually affects only one breast. Mastitis is often caused by *Staphylococcus aureus,* methicillin-resistant *S. aureus* (MRSA), and streptococci (Duff, 2019). The bacteria are most often carried on the skin of the client or in the mouth or the nose of newborn. The organism may enter through an injured area of the nipple, such as a crack or blister, although no obvious signs of injury may be apparent. Soreness and pain of a nipple may result in insufficient emptying of the breast during breastfeeding.

Engorgement and stasis of milk may precede mastitis. This may occur when a feeding is skipped, when the infant begins to sleep through the night, when latch is inefficient to remove milk, or when breastfeeding is suddenly stopped. Constriction of or constant pressure on the breasts by a bra that is too tight may interfere with emptying of all the ducts and may lead to infection (Academy of Breastfeeding Medicine, 2014). The client who is fatigued or stressed or who has other health problems might have a lower immune system response and is at increased risk for mastitis.

Clinical manifestations. Initial symptoms may be flu-like with fatigue and aching muscles. Symptoms progress to include a temperature of 39°C (102.2°F) or higher, chills, malaise, and headache. Mastitis is characterized by a localized lump or wedge-shaped area of pain, redness, heat, inflammation, and enlarged axillary lymph nodes. A hard, tender area may be palpated (Fig. 18.7). Untreated mastitis may progress to breast abscess.

Therapeutic management. Antibiotic therapy and continued emptying of the breast by breastfeeding or breast pump constitute the first line of treatment. With early antibiotic treatment, mastitis usually resolves within 24 to 48 hours.

Early mastitis

Acute mastitis

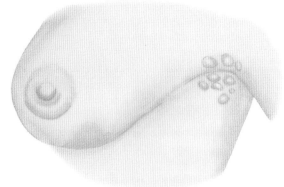
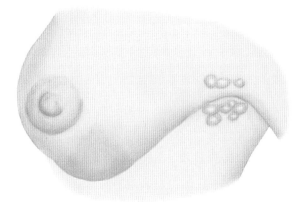

Enlarged, tender axillary lymph nodes
Tender "flush" without swelling

Enlarged, tender axillary lymph nodes
Area of inflammation is red, swollen,
hot, and tender

FIG. 18.7 Mastitis typically occurs after 2 to 4 weeks after birth in the breast of a client who breastfeeds.

Antibiotics should be continued for 7 to 10 days (Cunningham et al., 2022). Clients who develop a breast abscess are treated with surgical drainage and antibiotics.

Supportive measures include application of moist heat or ice packs, breast support, bed rest, fluids, and analgesics. The client should continue to breastfeed from both breasts. Regular and thorough emptying of the breast is important in preventing abscess formation. If an abscess forms and is surgically drained, breastfeeding can be continued as long as the incision is not near the areola and the client is comfortable.

Nursing considerations. Because mastitis rarely occurs before discharge from the birth facility, the nurse should provide adequate information for prevention. Measures to prevent mastitis include positioning the infant correctly and avoiding nipple trauma and milk stasis. The infant should breastfeed every 2 to 3 hours and avoid formula supplements. Nursing pads should not have a plastic layer and should be changed as soon as they are wet. Advise the client to avoid continuous pressure on the breasts from tight bras or infant carriers.

Once mastitis occurs, nursing measures are aimed at increasing comfort and helping the client maintain lactation. Moist heat promotes comfort and increases circulation. A disposable diaper, wet with warm water and placed over the breast, is an easy way to apply heat. The thickness helps maintain the temperature, and the plastic cover prevents dripping. A shower or hot packs should be used before feeding or pumping the breasts. The client should complete the entire course of antibiotics to prevent recurrence or a breast abscess.

The breast should be completely emptied at each feeding to prevent stasis of milk. If the client is too sore to breastfeed on the affected side, demonstrate how to express milk or use a pump to empty the breasts.

Breastfeeding or pumping every 1.5 to 2 hours makes the client more comfortable and prevents stasis. Starting the feeding on the unaffected side causes the milk-ejection reflex to occur in both breasts, making milk available in the painful breast as soon as the infant begins to nurse on that side. Massaging over the affected area before and during the feeding helps ensure complete emptying. The client should stay in bed during the acute phase of the illness. Fluid intake should be 2500 to 3000 mL per day. Analgesics may be required to relieve discomfort.

The client with mastitis is likely to be very discouraged. Some people decide to stop breastfeeding because of the discomfort involved. Weaning during an episode of mastitis may increase engorgement and stasis, leading to abscess formation or recurrent infection. The client may need much encouragement and help in arranging care for other children or with other responsibilities to allow adequate rest time.

Septic Pelvic Thrombophlebitis

Incidence and etiology. Septic pelvic thrombophlebitis is the least common of the puerperal infections, occurring in 1 in 2000 pregnancies (Duff, 2019). It usually is not seen until 2 to 4 days after childbirth. It occurs when infection spreads along the pelvic venous system and thrombophlebitis develops.

Clinical manifestations. The primary symptom is pain in the groin, abdomen, or flank. Fever, tachycardia, gastrointestinal distress, abdominal bloating, and decreased bowel sounds may be present. The only sign may be fever that does not respond to antibiotic therapy (Duff, 2019).

Laboratory data may be used to exclude other diagnoses and usually include CBC with differential, blood chemistries, coagulation studies, and cultures. Computed tomography (CT) or MRI may be performed to confirm the diagnosis (Duff, 2019).

Therapeutic management. Readmission to the hospital is usually necessary. Primary treatment includes anticoagulation therapy with IV heparin and IV antibiotics. Warfarin may be given when heparin is discontinued. Supportive care is similar to that for DVT and includes monitoring for safe levels of anticoagulation therapy and for signs and symptoms of PE.

APPLICATION OF THE NURSING PROCESS: INFECTION

Assessment

Although all clients are observed for indications of infection as part of routine nursing assessments, the nurse should practice increased vigilance for clients who are at increased risk for infection.

Pay particular attention to expected signs of infection, such as fever, tachycardia, pain, or unusual amount, color, or odor of lochia. Generalized symptoms of malaise and muscle aching may be significant. Examine all wounds each shift for signs of localized infection, such as redness, edema, tenderness, discharge, or pulling apart of incisions or sutured lacerations. Ask clients if they are experiencing difficulty emptying their bladder or discomfort related to urination.

Assess the client's knowledge of hygiene practices that prevent infections, such as proper handwashing, perineal care, and handling of perineal pads. Evaluate breastfeeding knowledge and any problems that might result in breast engorgement and stasis of milk in the ducts. Examine the nipples for signs of injury that might provide a portal of entry for organisms.

Identification of Client Problems

All clients have a potential for infection after childbirth; therefore most facilities have developed protocols and procedures to assess for and attempt to prevent infection. When predisposing factors increase the likelihood of infection, however, routine assessments and care should be modified and preventive measures intensified.

Planning: Expected Outcomes

Expected outcomes for the client include:
- Remain free of signs of infection during the postpartum period.
- Describe methods to prevent infection.
- List signs of infection that should be reported immediately.

⚡ SAFETY CHECK

Signs and symptoms of postpartum infection include the following:
Fever, chills
Pain or redness of wounds
Purulent wound drainage or wound edges not approximated
Tachycardia
Uterine subinvolution
Abnormal duration of lochia, foul odor
Elevated white blood cell count
Frequency or urgency of urination, dysuria, or hematuria
Suprapubic pain
Localized area of warmth, redness, or tenderness in the breasts
Body aches, general malaise

Interventions
Preventing Infection

Promoting hygiene. Nursing responsibilities for the client at risk for puerperal infection focus on prevention of initial infection. Preventive measures include using aseptic technique for all invasive procedures and paying attention to meticulous handwashing. Handwashing is important for the nursing staff and the client. Encourage handwashing before and after changing pads or touching the perineum. Instruct the client on care of the perineum and episiotomy site (see Chapter 17). Ensure client performs return demonstration of proper cleansing methods before discharge.

Preventing urinary stasis. An adequate intake of fluids (at least 2500 to 3000 mL/day) is important for preventing stasis of urine. Encourage the client to empty the bladder at least every 2 to 3 hours during the day. Some facility protocols include measuring the first two voids after childbirth or removal of a urinary catheter, followed by assessment of the bladder and fundus to be certain the bladder is empty. Instruct the client to report any signs of UTI immediately so that early treatment can be initiated.

Use appropriate measures to promote bladder emptying if the client has difficulty. Drinking hot fluids, such as tea, helps some clients void. Running water or having the client blow bubbles in a glass of water uses the sound of water to stimulate the urge to urinate. Pouring warm water over the perineum or having the client void in a sitz bath or shower may help relax the urinary sphincter. Administration of analgesics may help the client relax enough to urinate.

Teaching breastfeeding techniques. Clients often need assistance in establishing an effective pattern of breastfeeding that results in complete emptying of the breasts at each feeding and reduces the risk for nipple trauma (see Chapter 23).

Providing Information

Advise clients to obtain adequate rest and sufficient food of high nutritive value to replenish their energy and prevent infection. Identify foods high in protein and vitamin C, necessary for repair of damaged tissue. Red meat, poultry, fish, cheese, eggs, whole-grain breads, cereals, and pasta are some of the best sources of protein. This is particularly important if the client is breastfeeding.

Obtaining adequate rest is a problem for many clients. Nursing interventions focus on helping them plan a schedule allowing for rest while the infant sleeps and to identify family members or friends who are available to provide support and assistance.

Teaching Signs and Symptoms That Should Be Reported

Before discharge, teach the client signs and symptoms of infection to report to the health care provider. These include fever, chills, dysuria, and redness and tenderness of a wound. Malodorous lochia, discharge from a wound, and prolonged lochial discharge also should be reported.

Evaluation

The interventions can be judged to be successful if the client does the following:

- Shows no signs of infection
- Explains methods to prevent infection
- Lists signs and symptoms that should be reported to the health care provider

If infection occurs, the problem is no longer amenable to independent nursing actions but becomes a collaborative problem requiring medical and nursing interventions.

KNOWLEDGE CHECK

19. What measures can the client take to decrease the risk for UTI? How does the treatment for cystitis differ from that for pyelonephritis?
20. How can mastitis be prevented?

SUMMARY CONCEPTS

- PPH can sometimes be prevented by careful examination of factors that predispose to excessive bleeding.
- Overstretching of the muscle fibers during pregnancy and repeated stretching during past pregnancies predispose to uterine atony and excessive uterine bleeding.
- Initial management of uterine atony focuses on measures to contract the uterus and provide fluid replacement.
- Soft tissue trauma (lacerations, hematomas) can cause rapid loss of blood even when the uterus is firmly contracted. Management involves repairing the trauma before excessive blood loss occurs.
- Compensatory mechanisms maintain the blood pressure so that vital organs receive adequate oxygen. When these mechanisms fail, hypovolemic shock follows.
- The process of uterine involution may be delayed (subinvolution) when placental fragments are retained or when the uterus is infected.
- Subinvolution of the uterus develops after the client goes home. The nurse teaches the family the process of normal involution and the signs and symptoms that should be reported to the health care provider.
- Venous stasis that occurs during pregnancy, increased levels of coagulation factors, and decreased levels of thrombolytic factors that persist into the postpartum period increase the risk for thrombus formation during the puerperium.
- Treatment for deep venous thrombosis includes anticoagulants, analgesics, and bed rest with the affected leg elevated.

- Nurses who administer anticoagulant therapy assess the client to determine whether the laboratory results are within the recommended therapeutic range to prevent overmedication with anticoagulants that may result in unexpected bleeding.
- Pulmonary embolism occurs when a clot is dislodged from the vein, or amniotic fluid debris is carried by the blood to a pulmonary vessel, which may be completely or partially occluded.
- The risk for infection is increased with childbearing because there is open access to bacteria from the vagina through the fallopian tubes and into the peritoneal cavity. Increased blood supply to the pelvis and the alkalinization of the vagina by the amniotic fluid further increase the risk for infection.
- Any break in the skin or mucous membranes during childbirth provides a portal of entry for pathogenic organisms and increases the risk for puerperal infection. Nurses should assess clients with an incision or laceration for signs of localized wound infections.
- Urinary stasis and trauma to the urinary tract increase the risk for urinary tract infection. Nurses should initiate measures to prevent urinary stasis.
- Nurses should provide information about the importance of completely emptying the breasts at each feeding and about measures to avoid nipple trauma to prevent mastitis.

Clinical Judgment and Next-Generation NCLEX® Examination-Style Questions

A 28-year-old G_5P_{5005} client is admitted to the mother-baby unit 2 hours after vacuum-assisted vaginal birth of an 8 lb. 6 oz. live infant. The client's 10-hour labor was augmented with Pitocin because of arrest of labor at 6 cm dilation; epidural anesthesia was used for the labor and birth. A third-degree perineal laceration was repaired. Quantified blood loss at birth was 400 mL.

Current pain level is 2/10. The client is able to raise both legs and lift the buttocks off the bed. The nurse reviews the client's recovery medical record.

Birth time: 1155. Placenta: 1200
Quantified blood loss in Recovery: 150 mL

Time	T	PR	BP	Fundus	Lochia	Incision/perineum	Pain	Mobility
1215	98.1	98;25	130/75	Firm, at umbilicus, midline (F/U/ML)	Rubra Heavy	repair intact; edematous	1/10	None
1230		96;20	127/73	F/U/ML	Rubra Moderate	Intact/ edema; ice applied	1/10	none
1245		84;18	126/72	Massaged to firm/U/ML	Rubra Heavy; small clots	Intact/ice	2/10	Moves legs
1300	98.0	78; 16	123/70	F/U/ML	Rubra Light; no clots	Intact/ice	2/10	Moves legs
1330		78;16	124/70	F/U/ML	Rubra Light; no clots	Intact/ice	3/10 Ibuprofen 800 mg PO	Raises legs
1400	98.0	74;16	121/73	F/U/ML	Rubra Light; no clots	Intact/ice	2/10	Lifts buttocks

BP, Blood pressure; *PO*, by mouth; *PR*, pulse and respiratory rate; *T*, temperature.

The nurse assesses the client and finds

VS	T98.2, P110, R20
BP	100/66
Fundus	Boggy, midline, 2 cm above the umbilicus, nonresponsive to uterine massage
Lochia	Perineal pad and under buttocks drape are saturated with dark red blood with 4–5 quarter-sized clots
LOC	Alert

BP, Blood pressure; *LOC*, level of consciousness; *P*, pulse; *R*, respiratory rate *T*, temperature; *VS*, vital signs.

1. **Use an X to indicate whether the nursing actions below are Indicated (appropriate or necessary), Contraindicated (could be harmful), or Nonessential (not necessary at this time).**

Nursing Action	Indicated	Contraindicated	Nonessential
Assist the client to the bathroom to empty bladder			
Continue to massage the fundus			
Raise head of bed 90 degrees			
Call for help; notify provider			
Increase IV fluids per protocol			

Nursing Action	Indicated	Contraindicated	Nonessential
Dispose of linens as they become saturated with blood			

Two days ago, a thin, pale, 16-year-old primipara was admitted to the postpartum unit after a cesarean birth because of fetal distress. The client was in labor for 16 hours, and the fetal membranes were ruptured for 14 hours before the birth. The client was catheterized twice during labor, with insertion of an indwelling catheter shortly before surgery. The client is breastfeeding the infant.

2. **Place an "X" to indicate which assessment findings are normal/expected or abnormal/require follow-up.**

Assessment	Expected/Normal	Unexpected/Follow-up required
Breasts lumps palpated		
Temperature 101.3°F		
Strong, foul odor to lochia		
Abdominal pain, not relieved with prescribed medications.		
Uterine fundus at the umbilicus, midline, boggy but responds to uterine massage.		
Lochia rubra scant		

REFERENCES

Academy of Breastfeeding Medicine. (2014). *ABM clinical protocol #4: Mastitis, revised March 2014.* https://www.bfmed.org/protocols.

Alam, A., & Choi, S. (2015). Prophylactic use of tranexamic acid for postpartum bleeding outcomes: A systematic review and meta-analysis of randomized controlled trials. *Transfusion Medicine Reviews, 29*(4), 231–241. https://doi.org/10.1016/j.tmrv.2015.07.002.

Alliance for Innovation on Maternal Health (AIM). (2020). Maternal venous thromboembolism. https://safehealthcareforeverywoman.org/aim/patient-safety-bundles/maternal-safety-bundles/maternal-venous-thromboembolism-aim/.

American College of Obstetricians and Gynecologists (ACOG). (2017). Postpartum hemorrhage. ACOG Practice Bulletin No. 183. *Replaces Practice Bulletin, 76.*

American College of Obstetricians and Gynecologists (ACOG). (2018a). *Prevention of infection after gynecologic procedures.* ACOG Practice Bulletin No. 195, Replaces Practice Bulletin 104 and Committee Opinion 571.

American College of Obstetricians and Gynecologists (ACOG). (2018b). Thromboembolism in pregnancy. ACOG Practice Bulletin No. 196. *Replaces Practice Bulletin, 123.*

American College of Obstetricians and Gynecologists (ACOG). (2019). *Quantitative blood loss in obstetric hemorrhage.* ACOG Committee Opinion No. 794.

Association of Women's Health, Obstetric and Neonatal Nurses (AWHONN). (2021a). Active management of the third stage of labor using oxytocin: AWHONN Practice Brief No. 12. *JOGNN: Journal of Obstetric, Gynecologic & Neonatal Nursing, 50*(4), 499–502. https://doi.org/10.1016/j.jogn.2021.04.006.

Association of Women's Health, Obstetric and Neonatal Nurses (AWHONN). (2021b). Quantification of blood loss: AWHONN Practice Brief No. 13. *JOGNN: Journal of Obstetric, Gynecologic & Neonatal Nursing, 50*(4), 503–505. https://doi.org/10.1016/j.jogn.2021.04.007.

Burwick, R. M. (2021). Renal disease in pregnancy. In M. Landon, H. Galan, E. Jauniaux, D. Driscoll, V. Berghella, W. Grobman, S. Kilpatrick, & A. Cahill (Eds.). *Gabbe's Obstetrics: Normal and problem pregnancies.* (8th ed., pp. 857–870). Elsevier.

California Maternal Quality Care Collaborative (CMQCC). (2022). *Improving health care response to obstetric hemorrhage, version 3.0.* Stanford: California Department of Public Health. https://www.cmqcc.org/resource/improving-health-care-response-obstetric-hemorrhage-toolkit-version-30.

Carboprost tromethamine. (2021). *Drug information.* UpToDate.com. https://www.uptodate.com/contents/search?search=hemabate&sp=0&searchType=PLAIN_TEXT&source=USER_INPUT&searchControl=TOP_PULLDOWN&searchOffset=1&autoComplete=false&language=en&max=10&index=&autoCompleteTerm=.

Cleveland Clinic. (2021). *Prophylactic tranexamic acid may prevent hemorrhage following cesarean delivery.* https://consultqd.clevelandclinic.org/prophylactic-tranexamic-acid-may-prevent-hemorrhage-following-cesarean-delivery/.

Council on Patient Safety in Women's Health. (2015). *Maternal venous thromboembolism.* https://safehealthcareforeverywoman.org/council/patient-safety-bundles/maternal-safety-bundles/maternal-venous-thromboembolism-aim/.

Cunningham, F. G., Leveno, K. J., Bloom, S. L., Dashe, J. S., Hoffman, B. L., Casey, B. M., & Spong, C. Y. (2022). *Williams obstetrics* (26th ed.). McGraw-Hill Companies.

Duff, P. (2019). Maternal and fetal infections. In R. Resnik, C. Lockwood, T. Moore, M. Greene, J. Copel, & R. Silver (Eds.), *Creasy & Resnik's maternal-fetal medicine: Principles and practice* (8th ed., pp. 862–919). Elsevier.

Duff, P. (2021). Maternal and perinatal infection in pregnancy: Bacterial. In M. Landon, H. Galan, E. Jauniaux, D. Driscoll, V. Berghella, W. Grobman, S. Kilpatrick, & A. Cahill (Eds.). *Gabbe's Obstetrics: Normal and problem pregnancies.* (8th ed., pp. 1124–1146). Elsevier.

Francois, K. E., & Foley, M. R. (2021). Antepartum and postpartum hemorrhage. In M. Landon, H. Galan, E. Jauniaux, D. Driscoll, V. Berghella, W. Grobman, S. Kilpatrick, & A. Cahill (Eds.). *Gabbe's Obstetrics: Normal and problem pregnancies.* (8th ed., pp. 343–374). Elsevier.

Gallos, I. D., Papadopoulou, A., Man, R., Athanasopoulos, N., Tobias, A., Price, M. J., Williams, M. J., Diaz, V., Pasquale, J., Chamillard, M., Widmer, M., Tuncalp, O., Hofmeyr, G. J., Althabe, F., Gulmezoglu, A. M., Vogel, J. P., Olodapo, O. T., & Coomarasamy, A. (2018). *Uterotonic agents for preventing postpartum haemorrhage: A network meta-analysis.* Cochrane Database of Systematic Reviews. https://doi.org/10.1002/14651858.CD011689.pub3.

James, D. C., & Suplee, P. D. (2021). Postpartum care. In K. Simpson, P. Creehan, N. O'Brien-Abel, C. Roth, & A. Rohan (Eds.), *AWHONN's perinatal nursing* (5th ed., pp. 509–563). Wolters Kluwer.

Leung, A. N., Sottile, P., & Lockwood, C. J. (2019). Thromboembolic disease in pregnancy. In R. Resnik, C. Lockwood, T. Moore, M. Greene, J. Copel, & R. Silver (Eds.), *Creasy & Resnik's maternal-fetal medicine: Principles and practice* (8th ed., pp. 977–990). Elsevier.

Mackeen, A. D., Packard, R. E., Ota, E., & Speer, L. (2015). Antibiotic regimens for postpartum endometritis. *The Cochrane Database of Systemic Reviews 2*, CD001067.

Merriam, A. A., & Pettker, C. M. (2021). Thromboembolic disorders. In M. Landon, H. Galan, E. Jauniaux, D. Driscoll, V. Berghella, W. Grobman, S. Kilpatrick, & A. Cahill (Eds.), *Gabbe's obstetrics: Normal and problem pregnancies* (8th ed., pp. 972–986). Elsevier.

Methylergonovine (methlergometrine). (2021). *Drug Information.* UpToDate.com. https://www.uptodate.com/contents/search?search=methylergonovine-methylergometrine-drug-informaion&sp=0&searchType=PLAIN_TEXT&source=USER_INPUT&searchControl=TOP_PULLDOWN&searchOffset=1&autoComplete=false&language=&max=0&index=&autoCompleteTerm=&rawSentence=.

Naeiji, Z., Delshadiyan, N., Saleh, S., Moridi, A., Rahmati, N., & Fathi, M. (2021). Prophylactic use of tranexamic acid for decreasing the blood loss in elective cesarean section: A placebo-controlled randomized clinical trial. *Reproduction, 50*(1), 1–5. https://doi.org/10.1016/j.jogoh.2020.101973.

Roth, C. (2021). Pulmonary complications in pregnancy. In K. Simpson, P. Creehan, N. O'Brien-Abel, C. Roth, & A. Rohan (Eds.), *AWHONN's perinatal nursing* (5th ed., pp. 221–248). Wolters Kluwer.

Salati, J. A., Leathersich, S. J., Williams, J. J., Cuthbert, A., & Tolosa, J. E. (2019). Prophylactic oxytocin for the third stage of labour to prevent postpartum haemorrhage. *Cochrane Database of Systematic Reviews.* https://doi.org/10.1002/14651858.cd001808.pub3.

Shakur, H., Elbourne, D., Gulmezoglu, M., Alfirevic, Z., Ronsmans, C., Allen, E., & Roberts, I. (2010). The WOMAN trial (world maternal antifibrinolytic trial): Tranexamic acid for the treatment of postpartum haemorrhage: An international randomized, double blind placebo controlled trial. *Trial, 11*(40). https://doi.org/10.1186/1745-6215-11-40.

Stortroen, N. E., Tubog, T. D., & Shaffer, S. K. (2020). Prophylactic tranexamic acid in high-risk patients undergoing cesarean delivery: A systematic review and meta-analysis of randomized controlled trials. *American Association of Nurse Anesthesiology, 88*(4), 273–281.

Texas Department of Health and Human Services (DHHS). (2021). *Obstetric hemorrhage bundle.* https://dshs.texas.gov/mch/Obstetric-Hemorrhage-Bundle.aspx.

The Joint Commission. (2021). *Venous thromboembolism.* https://www.jointcommission.org/measurement/measures/venous-thromboembolism/.

Witcher, P. M., & Hamner, L. (2019). Venous thromboembolism in pregnancy. In N. Troiano, C. Harvey, & B. Chez (Eds.), *AWHONN high-risk & critical care obstetrics* (4th ed., pp. 176–193). Wolters Kluwer.

Critical Care Obstetrics

Emily Roberts, Suzanne McMurtry Baird

INTRODUCTION

Critical care is a subspecialty in obstetric (OB) nursing requiring advanced knowledge of physiology, pathophysiology, and a specialized skill set based on unit scope of service (Baird & Martin, 2019; Troiano & Baird, 2018). With the continued rise in maternal morbidity and mortality in the United States, there is increased need for this area of practice to meet client care needs and improve outcomes. Defined levels of care for hospitals that provide OB care and regionalization/transport systems promote client care in risk-appropriate facilities with clinicians who are prepared to provide high-risk, subspecialty consultation, and/or acute critical care. However, all facilities need to have the capability to provide initial interventions and stabilizing measures for any client who becomes critically ill while facilitating transfer or transport to a higher level of care.

Traditional training in nursing does not prepare a new graduate for expertise in care of the compromised and critically ill OB client. Likewise, nurses in other specialty areas, such as critical care, have training and skills associated with nonpregnant clients but may not understand the impact of anatomic, physiologic, and hemodynamic changes in the pregnant client. Therefore, it is essential for a nurse caring for a critically ill OB client to have additional education and skills. Training may be accomplished in several ways including didactic courses, simulation, and bedside clinical care. Example critical care OB (CCOB) nursing requirements include the following (Baird & Martin, 2019):

- Basic Life Support and Advanced Cardiac Life Support certifications
- Minimum of 1 year experience as a nurse on Labor and Delivery in an OB tertiary care setting
- Demonstrated interest in care for CCOB client population
- Favorable clinical skills as evidenced by performance evaluations
- Completion of an CCOB orientation course
- Completion of an CCOB skills competency checklist
- Annual validation of competency

Being proactive versus reactive is essential when preparing and training for clinical emergencies in OB. Literature mentions several ways to help manage clinical emergencies including development of a rapid response team, development of protocols that include clinical triggers, use of a standardized communication tool for huddles and briefs, and implementation of emergency drills and simulation. Allowing teams to practice high-risk, low-volume events assists in developing efficient systems and processes for emergency response, determines team member roles, instructs on management principles, maintains competencies, and promotes teamwork.

MATERNAL MORTALITY

There are several definitions related to the death of a client during pregnancy or the postpartum period (Table 19.1). All current identification systems lack sufficient details on contributors to death and prevention strategies and are limited by methods of data collection.

With constraints of current U.S. data surveillance systems to accurately measure maternal mortality and understand causation, maternal mortality review committees (MMRCs) have been developed through state health departments to better ascertain trends and disparities and identify opportunities for prevention. MMRCs review each death and determine answers for six key questions. The last four questions are unique to MMRCs and provide additional data.

1. Was the death pregnancy-related?
2. What was the underlying cause of death?
3. Was the death preventable?
4. What were the factors that contributed to the death?
5. What are the recommendations and actions that address those contributing factors?
6. What was the anticipated impact of those actions if implemented?

Additional information for committees is also gained through medical records and autopsy report review.

The Centers for Disease Control and Prevention (CDC) estimates 700 pregnancy-related deaths in the United States each year, with three out of five deaths noted to be preventable (CDC, 2019, CDC, 2020). To track data and better understand risk factors and causes, the CDC Division of Reproductive Health launched the Pregnancy Mortality Surveillance System (PMSS) in 1986 to calculate the estimated pregnancy-related deaths per 100,000 live births by linking the maternal death certificate to a live birth or fetal death certificate. From an estimated number of 7.2 deaths per 100,000 live births in 1987, the rate has more than doubled to the most recent data of 17.3 deaths per 100,000 live births in 2017 and 2018 (CDC, 2022c). During this time, data collection from the National Center for Health Statistics improved the detection of maternal deaths by implementing a standard pregnancy checkbox on the revised

TABLE 19.1   Maternal Mortality Terminology

Term	Definition
Pregnancy-related death (CDC)	During pregnancy or within 1 year of the termination of pregnancy that was caused by a pregnancy complication, a chain of events initiated by the pregnancy, or a condition or event unrelated to pregnancy that was aggravated by the physiologic effects of pregnancy.
Pregnancy-associated death (CDC)	During the pregnancy or within 1 year of the pregnancy and the course of the condition or event was unlikely to be impacted by the pregnancy.
Maternal death (NVS)	While pregnant or within 42 days of termination of the pregnancy, irrespective of the duration and site of the pregnancy, from any cause related to or aggravated by the pregnancy or its management, but not from accidental or incidental causes.

CDC, Centers for Disease Control and Prevention; *NVS,* National Vital Statistics.
Adapted from Witcher, P.M. & Lindsay, M.K. (2019). Maternal morbidity and mortality. In N.H. Troiano, P.M. Witcher, S.M. Baird, High Risk & Critical Care Obstetrics, 4th ed. Wolters Kluwer.

2003 death certificate (Hoyert et al., 2020). Before all states adopted the revision, maternal death was underreported. This enhanced data collection has provided improved data on this national public health crisis.

Timing of pregnancy-related death is important to consider when determining quality improvement initiatives and public health policy. According to CDC data, approximately one-third of deaths occur during pregnancy (31%), one-third occur during birth hospitalization (36%), and one-third occur 1 week to 1 year postpartum (33%) (CDC, 2019). This timing distribution is similar to aggregate data review from nine MMRCs indicating that 38% of deaths occurred during pregnancy, 45% within 42 days, and 18% between 43 days and 1 year postpartum (Building U.S. Capacity to Review and Prevent Maternal Deaths, 2018).

SEVERE MATERNAL MORBIDITY

In addition to maternal death, it is estimated that 50,000 clients suffer severe maternal morbidity (SMM) and life-threatening injuries each year (Callaghan et al., 2012; Kilpatrick et al., 2014). SMM includes unexpected physical or psychological conditions associated with or aggravated by pregnancy and/or birth. In 2012, the CDC identified an index of International Classification of Diseases Clinical Modification (ICD-CM) diagnosis and procedure codes associated with SMM (CDC, 2021). This index has been used in state and facility quality improvement and maternal health research to impact outcomes. The CDC SMM index has also led to the development of comorbidity scoring tools for prediction of SMM. Most SMM is

related to hemorrhage with blood transfusions, increasing 54% between 2006 and 2015 (Fingar et al., 2018). The three most common SMM index indicators most closely linked to maternal mortality are cardiac arrest/ventricular fibrillation, conversion of cardiac rhythm, and mechanical ventilation (Building U.S. Capacity to Review and Prevent Maternal Deaths, 2018).

Racial Ethnic Disparities

Considerable racial and ethnic disparities exist in SMM and mortality. Social determinants, implicit racial bias, racism, and inequities shape the health of each individual and affect pregnancy outcomes (Petersen et al., 2019; Scott et al., 2019; Havranek et al., 2015). Higher rates of SMM and mortality occur in clients who are non-Hispanic Black, American Indian, and Alaska Native race; those of Hispanic ethnicity; those who lack private insurance; and those with lower education levels (Wang et al., 2020). Initiatives to support and improve health care in vulnerable populations requires sustained, comprehensive public health programs to address disparities, especially for clients with chronic health conditions.

Causes of Severe Maternal Morbidity and Mortality

Due to earlier diagnosis, advances in care, and improvements in health outcomes, pregnancy is now considered for many clients with chronic medical disorders. However, preexisting conditions, such as obesity, heart disease, thrombophilia, diabetes, and chronic hypertension, place the pregnant client at increased risk for morbidity and mortality. Physiologic changes associated with pregnancy and childbirth (e.g., increased stroke volume and cardiac output, changes in pulmonary function, hypercoagulable state of pregnancy) may exacerbate such conditions and increase risk. Other conditions such as preeclampsia, infection, hemorrhage, embolism, and trauma may affect a previously healthy OB client and are often associated with serious sequelae.

Causes of maternal death vary by age, race, ethnicity, regions within the United States, and timing during pregnancy and the postpartum period. Overall, the most common causes in the United States are cardiovascular conditions (congenital or acquired), infection leading to sepsis, cardiomyopathy, hemorrhage, thrombotic pulmonary or other embolism, cerebrovascular accidents, hypertensive disorders of pregnancy, amniotic fluid embolism, anesthesia complications, and other noncardiovascular medical conditions (e.g., diabetic ketoacidosis) (CDC, 2022c).

Factors contributing to maternal death are also studied, including community, systems of care, facility, provider, and client/family factors. When linked to cause of death, improved understanding helps in prevention and policy adaptation or development. The most common contributing factors from MMRC review are listed below (Building U.S. Capacity to Review and Prevent Maternal Deaths, 2018).

- Client/family factors: lack of knowledge regarding warning signs and need to seek care
- Provider factors: misdiagnosis, ineffective treatments
- System factors: lack of coordination between providers

TABLE 19.2	Early Warning Criteria in the Pregnant or Postpartum Client	
	EARLY WARNING CRITERIA SYSTEMS	
	Early Warning Criteria	**REACT**
Temperature		<96°F or >100.4°F
Systolic blood pressure	>160 or <90 mm Hg	Sustained >160 or <90 mm Hg
Diastolic blood pressure	>100 mm Hg	Sustained >110 or <60 mm Hg
Heart rate	>120 or <50 beats/minute	Sustained >120 or <60 beats/minute
Respiratory rate	>30 or <10 breaths/minute	Sustained >24 or <12 breaths/minute
Oxygen saturation (SpO$_2$)	<95% on room air	<95% or change in oxygenation
Shortness of breath	With preeclampsia	Labored breathing
Neurologic status	Agitation, confusion, or unresponsiveness	Agitated, delirious, somnolent, difficult to arouse, confused or obtunded. Any other changes in mental status, such as sudden blown pupil, onset of slurred speech or unilateral limb or facial weakness
Urine output	Oliguria <35 mL/hour for >2 consecutive hours	<30 mL/hour for 2 consecutive hours
Headache	Nonrelenting headache	
Nurse concern		Worried or concerned, "gut" instinct, client "doesn't look good or act right"

Adapted from Mhyre, J. M., Tsen, L. C., Einav, S., Kuklina, E. V., Leffert, L. R., & Bateman, B. T. (2014). Cardiac arrest during hospitalization for delivery in the United States, 1998–2011. *Anesthesiology, 120*(4), 810–818; Baird, S. M., & Graves, C. R. (2015). REACT: An interprofessional education and safety program to recognize and manage the compromised obstetric client. *Journal of Perinatal & Neonatal Nursing, 29*(2), 138–148.

EARLY WARNING SIGNS

Severe morbidity and mortality events are usually preceded by early signs of compromise (Mhyre et al., 2014; Baird & Graves, 2015; Shields et al., 2016). If abnormal assessment parameters are ignored, communication and presence of the provider at the bedside for diagnosis and treatment may be delayed, potentially increasing the risk of morbidity and mortality. There are several early warning sign parameters in the literature that differ in defined abnormal assessment categories and parameters (Table 19.2). In addition, some early warning systems provide algorithms for initial management.

It is important to understand that early warning signs are more than provider orders on when to communicate abnormal assessment parameters. It is recommended that when one of the criteria is met, the provider is notified and comes to the bedside in a timely manner. Once at the bedside, the provider performs an assessment, discusses the history and evolution of the issue with the nurse, and develops a list of differential diagnoses and/or diagnoses the cause of the abnormal assessment (Mhyre et al., 2014; Baird & Graves, 2015). This process is documented in the medical record (Fig. 19.1).

MATERNAL LEVELS OF CARE

In 1976, the March of Dimes and its partners conceptualized an integrated system for regionalized perinatal care in a report titled Toward Improving the Outcome of Pregnancy (March of Dimes). This report outlined criteria for levels of neonatal and maternal care based on the complexity of care and recommended referral to the appropriate higher level of care based on resources and personnel to care for these clients. In many states, one of the outcomes of this report was

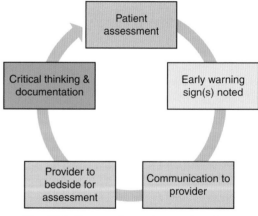

Fig. 19.1 Process for early warning signs.

a coordinated regionalization of perinatal care with "regional or tertiary care centers" identified. However, the concept for levels of care focused almost entirely on neonatal needs. It has taken 40 years for a coordinated effort to establish maternal levels of care that are distinct from, but complementary to, neonatal levels. In the interim, making sure that a client receives the appropriate care has been disorganized and left to individual discretion. This has meant that whether, when, where, and how a pregnant client is transported to another facility for care was not a structured process (ACOG & SMFM, 2019).

With U.S. data reflecting a substantial rise in SMM and mortality, there are renewed efforts to focus on maternal health conditions warranting designation as high risk and to define specific clinical care systems criteria to manage such conditions. In 2015 the American College of Obstetricians and Gynecologists (ACOG) and the Society for Maternal-Fetal

TABLE 19.3   Maternal Levels of Care

Level of Maternal Care	Description	Capabilities
Birthing center	• Peripartum care of low-risk clients • Uncomplicated singleton pregnancies • Vertex • Uncomplicated birth expected	• Capability and equipment for low-risk maternal care • Emergency procedures in place • Agreement with receiving hospital and procedures in place for timely maternal transport • Data collection, storage, and retrieval • Quality improvement programs • 24/7 medical consultation available
Level I basic care	• Uncomplicated pregnancies • Ability to detect, stabilize, and initiate management of unanticipated maternal-fetal complications until client transfer	Birth center plus: • Ability to do emergency cesarean birth • Access to obstetric ultrasound, laboratory testing, and blood bank supplies • Protocol for massive transfusion • Ability to establish formal transfer plans with higher level facility
Level II specialty care	Level I plus: • Care of appropriate high-risk antepartum, intrapartum, or postpartum conditions	Level I plus: • CT and MRI with interpretation • Maternal and fetal ultrasound services • Ability to accommodate care of obese clients
Level III subspecialty care	Level II plus: • Care of more complex maternal medical conditions, OB complications, and fetal conditions	Level II plus: • Advanced imaging services 24/7 • Ability to assist level I and II facilities with quality improvement and safety programs • Provide perinatal system leadership • Medical and surgical ICUs that accept pregnant women • Onsite critical care providers to collaborate with MFMs • Ability to ventilate and monitor clients in L&D until ICU transfer
Level IV regional tertiary care center	Level III plus: • Onsite medical and surgical care of the most complex maternal conditions, and critically ill pregnant women and fetuses	Level III plus: • Onsite ICU care for OB clients • Onsite medical and surgical care of complex maternal conditions • Perinatal system leadership • Facilitation of maternal referral and transport • Outreach education • Analysis of regional data and quality improvement

CT, Computerized tomography; *ICU*, intensive care unit; *L&D*, labor and delivery; *MFM*, maternal fetal medicine; *MRI*, magnetic resonance imaging; *OB*, obstetrics.

Adapted from American College of Obstetricians and Gynecologists, Society for Maternal-Fetal Medicine. (2019). Obstetric care consensus: Levels of maternal care. *Obstet Gynecol, 134*(2), e41-e55; Baird, S. M., & Martin, S. M. (2019). Critical care obstetric capabilities: Development strategies. In N. H. Troiano, P. Witcher, & S. M. Baird (Eds.), *AWHONN's high risk and critical care obstetrics* (4th ed., pp. 21–29). Wolters Kluwer/Lippincott.

Medicine (SMFM) outlined risk appropriate maternal care in their Obstetric Care Consensus statement (ACOG & SMFM, 2015). There were four objectives of this document:

1. To introduce uniform designations for levels of maternal care that are complementary but distinct from levels of neonatal care—addressing maternal health needs.
2. To develop standardized definitions and nomenclature for facilities.
3. To provide consistent guidelines according to level of maternal care for use in quality improvement and health promotion.
4. To foster the development and equitable geographic distribution of full-service maternal care facilities and systems

that promote proactive integration of risk appropriate antepartum, intrapartum, and postpartum services.

The levels outlined in the 2015 document are birthing centers, level 1, 2, 3, and 4 facilities, with incremental increases in capabilities at each level and as the client's care needs become more complex (Table 19.3). For each level of care there is an outlined definition of care, capabilities of the facility, types of health care providers, and examples of appropriate clients. In addition, nursing services, availability of primary delivery providers, OB surgeons, maternal-fetal medicine (MFM) providers, director of OB services, anesthesiology, intensive care, and subspecialty services are outlined. The CDC supports the outlined recommendations through the Levels of Care

Assessment Tool (LoCATE). Some states have also initiated independent, yet similar, description of services and capabilities. States coordinate these efforts through state health departments (CDC, 2022b).

COLLABORATION

If an OB client becomes compromised and critically ill, the decision is usually made to transfer the client to an intensive care unit (ICU) environment. Placing a pregnant client in off-service ICU settings prior to birth presents several clinical care challenges for the OB, ICU, anesthesiology, and neonatal teams. These challenges include, but are not limited to the following: (Troiano & Baird, 2018)

- Client assessment and monitoring by both the OB and ICU teams
- Determination of physician team leader for collaboration, communication, and management
- Treatment and medication effect on uterine perfusion and fetal/neonatal outcomes
- Potential for compromise in the status of the pregnant/postpartum client or the fetus despite initiation of appropriate interventions requiring delivery of the fetus(es)
- Availability of delivery and neonatal resuscitation supplies and equipment
- Cost of care
- Lack of research and data regarding care of the CCOB client

Irrespective of where care is provided, all health team members require enhanced knowledge and skills regarding reasons pregnant clients become compromised and principles of management to optimize outcomes.

Once a client has been transferred from OB services to an ICU, increased collaboration between physician and nursing teams is key to optimize client and neonatal outcomes. Healthy work environments require teamwork and collaboration for optimal outcomes. Over the last few decades, research has demonstrated that collaboration and communication are central to positive client outcomes in ICU environments (Ulrich et al., 2019). In addition to physiologic concepts which provide a framework for CCOB, significant psychosocial principles are incorporated into the plan of care. The most common causes for an OB client to be admitted to an ICU are listed in Table 19.4.

FETAL/NEWBORN IMPLICATIONS

As OB complexities increase, managing and balancing the care needs of the pregnant or postpartum client and the fetus can be challenging. Often in ICU, OB nurses are utilized at the bedside to assess pregnancy-related issues and interpret fetal heart rate (FHR) monitoring as ICU nurses do not typically have this skillset or knowledge (Cypher, 2018). Fetal surveillance will most likely depend on several factors such as the stability of the pregnant client (e.g., altered cardiac output, hypovolemia), gestational age, resources available, and neonatal services (Cypher, 2018). A fundamental physiologic understanding is needed regarding the maternal-fetal oxygen pathway and how interruptions can affect oxygen content and delivery to the fetus. Critical illness in pregnancy can negatively impact

TABLE 19.4	Causes for Admission to an Obstetric Intensive Care
Issue	**Examples**
Respiratory	• Pulmonary edema
	• Pulmonary embolus
	• Asthma
	• Pneumonia
	• Acute respiratory distress syndrome
Hypertensive disease	• Preeclampsia
	• Chronic hypertension
	• Hypertensive crisis
	• HELLP syndrome
	• Eclampsia
Cardiac	• Valve lesions
	• Rhythm disturbances
	• Cardiomyopathy
	• Myocardial infarction
Hemorrhage and hemorrhagic shock	• Postpartum
	• Placenta accreta spectrum disorder
	• Previa
	• Abruption
	• Disseminated intravascular coagulopathy (DIC)
Gastrointestinal	• Acute fatty liver disease of pregnancy
	• Pancreatitis
	• Inflammatory bowel disease
Sepsis and septic shock	• Infection
Endocrine	• Diabetic ketoacidosis (DKA)
	• Thyroid storm
Postoperative fetal surgery	• Pulmonary edema
Acute kidney injury	• Sepsis
	• Hemorrhage
	• DIC
	• Preeclampsia
Other	• Trauma
	• Amniotic fluid embolus
	• Pheochromocytoma

From Baird, S. M., & Martin, S. M. (2019). Critical care obstetric capabilities: Development strategies. In N. H. Troiano, P. Witcher, & S. M. Baird (Eds.), *AWHONN's high risk and critical care obstetrics* (4th ed., pp. 21–29). Wolters Kluwer/Lippincott; Guntupalli, K. K., Karnad, R. D., Bandi, V., Hall, N., & Belfort, M. (2015). Critical illness in pregnancy part II: Common medical conditions complicating pregnancy and puerperium. *Chest, 148*(5), 1333–1345; Shamshirsaz, A. A., & Dildy, G.A. (2018). Reducing maternal mortality and severe maternal morbidity: The role of critical care. *Clin Obstet Gynecol, 61*(2), 1–13.

oxygen transfer and lead to fetal compromise. Appreciation of small changes interpreted from fetal monitoring and careful attention toward the evolution of FHR patterns over time can help reveal a further compromise in the hemodynamic state of the pregnant client (Cypher, 2018). In a client with a viable pregnancy, assessment of fetal well-being and for signs of preterm labor is recommended (Chau & Tsen, 2014). As with any diagnosis, electronic fetal monitoring (EFM) is only indicated if fetal interventions, including cesarean birth, would be considered (Martin & Baird, 2018).

Betamethasone for fetal lung maturity is recommended between 23 and 36 6/7 weeks' gestation (Gyamfi-Bannerman et al., 2016). Magnesium sulfate for fetal neuroprotection is an option for clients at high risk for delivery between 23 and 32 6/7 weeks' gestation if a contraindication does not exist (Gentle et al., 2020).

NURSING ROLE

The high-risk and critically ill OB client requires care by nurses in the outpatient and inpatient clinical settings. Preconception care provides opportunities for risk assessment, including economic vulnerability and stress, medication adjustment when indicated, lifestyle modifications, and client education to assist in meeting individualized health goals. Group prenatal care, a collaborative team-based model of care that integrates nurses as facilitators, has demonstrated evidence of improved pregnancy outcomes, including prolonged gestational age, decreased rates of low birth weight in the newborn, and readiness for labor and birth (Robinson et al., 2018; Gareua et al., 2016; Rowley et al., 2016). Likewise, inpatient nurses have the responsibility to assess for risk factors upon admission and throughout the birth hospitalization, communicate abnormal assessment findings that are not improved by nursing interventions, and initiate protocols and care guidelines.

Another nursing role is the planning of care. Interprofessional, nurse-led bedside rounds allow for development and communication of the plan of care and involves client and family input. Bedside rounds can occur each shift or daily depending on client acuity and needs. This process has been well developed in adult ICUs and in some studies resulted in lower mortality rates, decreased length of stay, improved collaboration, and staff autonomy and satisfaction (Kim et al., 2010; Aparanji et al., 2018; Flannery et al., 2019). In addition, bringing the care team together to discuss client care needs decreases complications such as skin breakdown, infection, deep vein thrombosis, stress ulcers, and readmissions (Louzon et al., 2017; Abraham, et al., 2016).

Despite the emphasis on physical assessment and interventions, another essential role of the nurse is to provide support and address the emotional response of the client and family. Because many of the causes of critical illness in pregnancy are unanticipated, the client and family will most likely be anxious, fearful, confused, and overwhelmed. They may have little knowledge of the etiology, management, and fetal implications of the illness or complication. Preterm birth or surgical intervention may be necessary. Getting additional team members to the bedside will assist the nurse in management and client/family emotional needs.

Nurses can:
- Assist clients in the management of health and chronic conditions
- Provide appropriate risk assessment according to client needs
- Educate clients and family members about early warning signs and when to communicate with a provider
- Actively listen to client complaint(s), signs, and symptoms

- Provide focused assessments to determine abnormal parameters
- Increase frequency of assessments when abnormal parameters are determined
- Use tools to flag early warning signs of compromise
- Communicate to provider regarding abnormal assessment parameters
- Request the provider to come to the bedside for timely diagnosis and treatment
- Critically think to consider the most likely the cause(s) of abnormal assessment parameter(s)
- Facilitate transfer or transport to a higher level of care as indicated
- Practice evidence-based care
- Commit to lifelong learning

Hospitals and health systems can:
- Expect and demand a culture of safety
- Standardize care and response to OB emergencies
- Simplify processes that may interfere with efficiency and accuracy of care
- Improve delivery of quality prenatal, intrapartum, and postpartum care through best practice and/or evidence-based care recommendations
- Determine unit scope and practice and when clients should be transferred or transported to a higher level of care
- Define protocols for OB emergencies
- Train nonobstetric providers in care of critical illness during pregnancy and to consider recent pregnancy history (e.g., Emergency Department personnel)
- Commit to team training for OB emergencies
- Determine role delegation for emergency response and management
- Practice emergencies through interprofessional simulation

States and communities can:
- Require mandatory reporting of all maternal deaths
- Support the review of every maternal death through a formalized statewide MMRC
- Collect, analyze, and communicate data
- Assess and coordinate delivery hospitals for risk-appropriate care, including regionalization of care
- Determine barriers for access to care
- Expand postpartum Medicaid coverage for 1 year postpartum

Clients and families can:
- Plan pregnancy with OB health care provider if chronic health conditions exist
- Enter pregnancy with a healthy lifestyle
- Initiate prenatal care early and attend all prenatal care appointments as outlined by provider
- Communicate accurate and complete health and pregnancy information when seeking care
- Ask questions to understand the plan of care
- Know and communicate early warning signs and symptoms
- Note pregnancy history any time medical care is received in the year after birth

Cardiac output	Oxygen transport
• Preload (volume) • Systemic vascular resistance (pressure) • Contractility • Heart rate	• Oxygen content • Oxygen affinity • Oxygen delivery • Oxygen consumption

Fig. 19.2 Components of cardiac output and oxygen transport.

CRITICAL ILLNESS IN PREGNANCY

Thorough, accurate, and timely client assessment is essential with any critical illness. The two core components of noninvasive assessment are (1) cardiac output (formula for cardiac output is stroke volume x heart rate) and (2) oxygen transport. Fig. 19.2 outlines components that determine cardiac output and oxygen transport.

In the critically ill OB client, knowledge regarding the physiologic changes in pregnancy and how physical assessment parameters may be affected is foundational. Most conditions associated with critical illness in obstetrics place the client at risk for intravascular hypovolemia and decreased tissue oxygenation. Utilizing noninvasive assessment only may limit differentiation between hypovolemic, normovolemic, and hypervolemic states, since some parameters of assessment may be the same. For example, hypo- and hypervolemia cause tachycardia requiring assessment of additional parameters to determine etiology. Instead of focusing on a single isolated abnormal parameter, trending of data is helpful to determine significance and events that may have preceded the assessment (e.g., medication administration, pain) and previous assessment (Troiano & Baird, 2018). If a client requires invasive hemodynamic monitoring (e.g., arterial line, central venous pressure, pulmonary artery catheter) to gain additional hemodynamic information for stabilization and treatment guidance, advancing the level of care and ICU admission is required. Table 19.5 outlines noninvasive assessment of hypo and hypervolemia.

NOTE: The following topics represent some of the common causes of critical illness in pregnancy and the postpartum period that are not addressed in other areas of this textbook.

HYPOVOLEMIC SHOCK

Pathophysiology

Hypovolemic shock is a medical emergency requiring immediate recognition and management to minimize insufficient oxygen delivery and tissue perfusion resulting from decreased intravascular volume. Protective physiologic mechanisms provide compensation to maintain cardiac output and tissue perfusion during hypovolemic states such as sepsis (Fig. 19.3). As stroke volume decreases, endogenous catecholamine release is signaled, increasing heart rate, vascular tone in selected vessels, and myocardial contractility. Circulating blood volume redistributes with preferential shunting of blood to the heart, brain, liver, and lungs and away from nonessential organ systems, including the kidneys and uterus (Brown & Abdel-Razeq, 2019). In the absence of circulating volume restoration, these compensatory mechanisms begin to fail, ultimately resulting in decreased cardiac output, inadequate tissue and organ perfusion, tissue hypoxia, lactic acid production, metabolic acidosis, and end organ dysfunction or death (Brown & Abdel-Razeq, 2019).

Etiology

Hypovolemic shock can result from hemorrhage or as a result of extracellular fluid loss. Extracellular fluid loss has numerous etiologies:
- Gastrointestinal (vomiting, diarrhea)
- Renal (osmotic diuresis from hyperglycemia)
- Skin (hot, dry climate)
- Third-spacing (sepsis, preeclampsia)

The most common causes of hypovolemic shock in pregnancy are listed in Table 19.6.

Clinical Presentation

Early recognition and diagnosis of shock in OB clients is often delayed due to normalization of abnormal assessment parameters (e.g., vital signs, anxiety, pain). Physiologic attempts to compensate for decreased blood volume and oxygenation of essential organs is by increasing the rate and effort of the heart and lungs by preferential shunting of arterial blood from less essential organs, such as the skin, extremities, and uterus, to more essential organs such as the heart, brain, and lungs. Compensation results in signs and symptoms of hypovolemia listed in Table 19.5.

Clinical Management
Goals

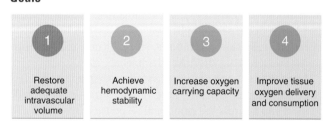

When hypovolemic shock is suspected, timely interventions are targeted to stabilize hemodynamics and tissue oxygenation. Increased client surveillance is critical to assess for worsening signs and symptoms and to evaluate effectiveness of interventions. Assessment of vital signs is increased to every 5 to 15 minutes including use of a continuous pulse oximeter and electrocardiogram (ECG) monitoring. Laboratory values such as complete blood count (CBC), coagulation studies (PT, PTT, and Fibrinogen), and electrolytes are evaluated at frequent intervals. Type and cross and notification of the blood bank for the possibility of the massive transfusion protocol (MTP) initiation facilitates quicker, type-specific blood product administration. Other interventions are listed below:

TABLE 19.5 Noninvasive Assessment Parameters

Parameter	Hypovolemia Assessment	Hypervolemia Assessment
Heart rate	Increased >110 beats per minute	Increased >110 beats per minute
Respiratory rate	Increased >24 breaths/minute	Increased >24 breaths/minute
Blood pressure	Initially increased, then decreased (late sign)	Increased
Pulse pressure (systolic BP - diastolic BP)	Decreased <30 mm Hg	Increased >65–70 mm Hg
SpO$_2$	Decreased <95%	Decreased <95%
Shortness of breath	None	Increased; use of accessory muscles
Capillary refill	Prolonged, sluggish >4 seconds	Normal
Peripheral pulse quality	Weak, thready, progressing to absent	Bounding 3+ to 4+
Urine output	Oliguria <30 mL/hour for 2 consecutive hours; concentrated	Increased; clear
Skin temperature of extremities	Cool to touch	Normal
Skin color and appearance	Pale and mottled	Normal
Mucous membranes	Dry, pale, increased thirst	Moist, production of sputum

Adapted from Brown, K. N., & Abdel-Razeq, S. S. (2019). Sepsis in pregnancy. In N. H. Troiano, P. Witcher, & S. M. Baird (Eds.), *AWHONN's high risk and critical care obstetrics* (4th ed., pp. 296–319). Wolters Kluwer/Lippincott; Abdel-Razeq, S. S., & Norwitz, E. R. (2019). Septic shock. In J.P. Phelan, et al., (Eds.), *Critical Care Obstetrics,* (6th ed., pp 599-629),; Kennedy, B. B., & Baird, S. M. (2017). Collaborative strategies for management of obstetric hemorrhage. In P. O'Malley, & J. Foster (Eds.), *Critical Care Nursing Clinics of North America, 29*(3), 315–330.

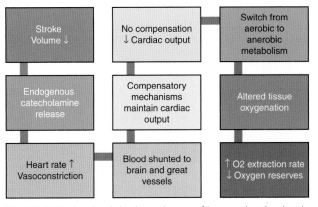

Fig. 19.3 Pathophysiologic pathway of hypovolemic shock.

Promote Tissue Oxygenation

- Lateral position to increase cardiac output and promote oxygenation to the placenta and vital organs
- Minimize activity to decrease oxygen consumption
- Provide oxygen per hospital protocol and provider order
- Keep the client warm as hypothermia can further impact tissue oxygenation and disseminated intravascular coagulation. Utilize fluid warmers, warm blankets, and/or warming devices.

Fluid/Volume Measurement and Replacement

- Ensure client has adequate peripheral IV access. Multiple peripheral lines are usually indicated. If possible, use large-bore IV catheters (16 to 18 gauge) to accommodate rapid IV fluid infusion and blood/volume replacement. Anticipate that a central line placement may be necessary.
- Administer IV fluids and blood products for replacement as directed by the provider or following the MTP.
- MTP is indicated if four or more units of blood products within the hour are anticipated and with continued

TABLE 19.6 Etiologies Leading to Hypovolemic Shock in Pregnancy

Etiology of Hypovolemic Shock in Pregnancy

- Hemorrhage
  - Postpartum hemorrhage
  - Previa
  - Placenta accreta spectrum disorder
  - Abruption
  - Uterine rupture
  - Postsurgical
  - Trauma
  - Ectopic pregnancy
  - Uterine inversion
- Disseminated intravascular coagulopathy (DIC)
- Amniotic fluid embolism
- Sepsis and septic shock
- Preeclampsia with severe features including hemolysis, elevated liver enzymes, low platelets (HELLP) and hepatic rupture
- Hyperemesis gravidarum
- Diabetic ketoacidosis (DKA)

From Baird, S. M., & Fox, K. (2019). Morbidly adherent placenta. In N. H. Troiano, P. Witcher, & S. M. Baird (Eds.), *AWHONN's high risk and critical care obstetrics* (4th ed., pp. 244–257). Wolters/Kluwer/Lippincott; Brown, K. N., & Abdel-Razeq, S. S. (2019). Sepsis in pregnancy. In N. H. Troiano, P. Witcher, & S. M. Baird (Eds.), *AWHONN's high risk and critical care obstetrics,* (4th ed., pp. 296–319). Wolters Kluwer/Lippincott.

bleeding (includes packed red blood cells, fresh frozen plasma, platelets, cryoprecipitate). An example MTP is in Fig. 19.4.
- If type-specific blood products are not available, emergent transfusion of O negative products may be necessary.
- Monitor intake and output by placing an indwelling urinary catheter.
- Measure and calculate cumulative, quantified blood loss (QBL).

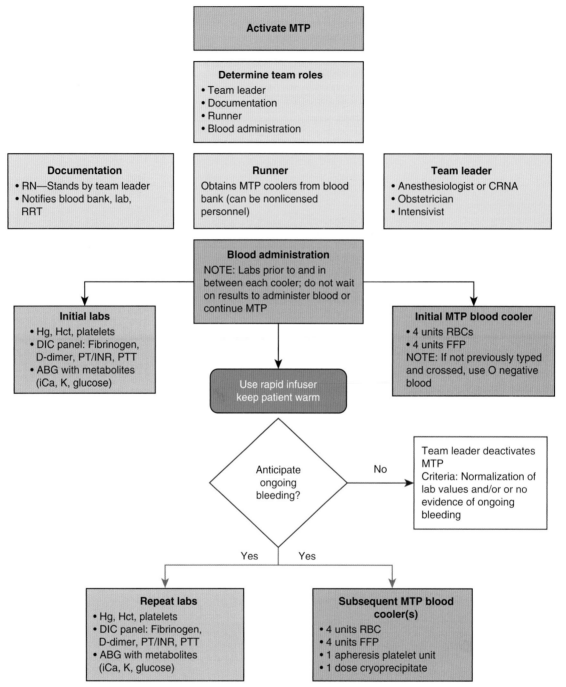

Fig. 19.4 Example massive transfusion protocol.

Other Interventions

- Depending on gestational age and client conditions, a combination of methods can be utilized to assess fetal well-being (Cypher, 2016). Evidence suggestive of fetal compromise in the presence of hypovolemia in the pregnant client may include fetal tachycardia, progressive decrease in baseline variability, late decelerations, and fetal bradycardia.
- Assess for signs and symptoms of pulmonary edema; anticipate mechanical ventilation with loss of consciousness, inability to oxygenate, or respiratory compromise.

⚡ SAFETY CHECK

Signs and symptoms of hypovolemic shock caused by blood loss include the following:
- Increased pulse rate, falling blood pressure, increased respiratory rate
- Weak, diminished, or "thready" peripheral pulses
- Cool skin; pallor; or cyanosis (late sign)
- Decreased (<30 mL/hour) or absent urinary output
- Decreased hemoglobin, hematocrit levels
- Change in mental status (restlessness, agitation, difficulty concentrating)

DISSEMINATED INTRAVASCULAR COAGULATION

Pathophysiology

Disseminated intravascular coagulation (DIC), also called consumptive coagulopathy, is a life-threatening condition involving systemic activation of coagulation, formation of fibrin clots, decreased tissue oxygenation, and consumption of coagulation factors. DIC is a secondary complication of an underlying condition. In each of the disease processes that cause DIC, tissue factors initiate massive release of clotting factors, resulting in systemic, rather than local, activation and circulation of thrombin, plasmin, and fibrin clot formation. This process is activated by one or more processes:

1. Trauma to tissues
2. Trauma to vascular endothelium
3. Trauma to red blood cells or platelets

When coagulation factors are consumed, there is an inability to form additional clots, and additional blood loss occurs. With the formation of microvascular clots, tissues become hypoxic, ischemic, and dysfunctional. To restore tissue perfusion, the breakdown of clots in the process of fibrinolysis occurs, and fibrin degradation/split products, or fibrin clot fragments, accumulate in the circulation. These fragments further interfere with normal hemostasis causing platelet dysfunction (bleeding), red blood cell hemolysis (decreased oxygen carrying capacity), damaging endothelial lining of pulmonary capillary bed (acute lung injury), and plugging the microcirculation (tissue hypoxia). These pathophysiologic processes lead to excessive bleeding and tissue ischemia resulting in catastrophic hemorrhage, profound hypovolemic shock, and multisystem organ failure (Fig. 19.5) (Sisson & Hamner, 2019).

Etiology

Normal physiologic changes in pregnancy result in a hypercoagulable state with decreased fibrinolytic capacity. OB conditions that predispose the client to DIC include:

- Placental abruption
- Preeclampsia with severe features/eclampsia
- HELLP syndrome
- Amniotic fluid embolism
- Sepsis
- Acute fatty liver disease of pregnancy
- Retained intrauterine fetal demise (IUFD)/demise of twin
- Massive hemorrhage

Clinical Presentation

The pathophysiologic process of DIC causes bleeding from any vulnerable area such as IV insertion site, incision, oral or nasal mucosa, or the site of placental attachment during the postpartum period. Other signs may include ecchymosis, petechiae, purpura, and hematuria. The process of DIC can occur rapidly and the client may exhibit signs and symptoms of profound circulatory shock including hypotension, respiratory distress, and altered level of consciousness.

Clinical Management

Clinical evaluation and serial coagulation studies determine the diagnosis of DIC and guide management. Coagulation studies and values are listed in Table 19.7. D-dimer, a common laboratory test used in the diagnosis of DIC, measures prior plasmin and thrombin formation. However, it is not a helpful test in pregnancy since levels are consistently elevated. The international normalized ratio (INR), used to dose oral anticoagulant therapy, is also not used to diagnose or monitor the DIC process. Thromboelastometry (ROTEM) and thromboelastography (TEG) tests allow for the assessment of the speed and quality of clot formation and are used in combination with clinical assessment to guide transfusion therapy (Baird et al., 2021).

NOTE: It is important to know normal and abnormal laboratory values for the OB client as normal and abnormal laboratory reference values provided on laboratory reports will reflect a nonpregnant population.

Anticipate aggressive volume resuscitation with IV fluids and blood products to replace decreased circulating blood volume and maintain perfusion to organs and tissues (McBride, 2018). Because DIC can progress rapidly and lead to profound blood loss and hypovolemic shock, MTP will most likely be initiated. Knowledge on how to set up and manage a rapid infusion/warming device is needed if responsible for this task. Additional peripheral IV access with a large bore catheter (16 or 18 gauge) are needed. Managing DIC requires an interprofessional team working together to

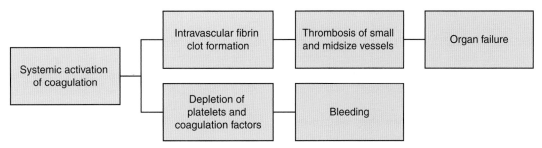

Fig. 19.5 Pathologic process of disseminated intravascular coagulation (DIC).

TABLE 19.7   Coagulation Values in DIC

Laboratory	Measures	Increased	Decreased
Fibrinogen	Function of common clotting pathway		√
Platelet count	Platelet number		√
Prothrombin time (PT)	Extrinsic and common clotting pathways	√ prolonged	
Activated partial thromboplastin (aPTT)	Intrinsic and common clotting pathways	√ prolonged	
Fibrin split or degradation products	Breakdown of fibrin clots	√	
Bleeding time	Platelet function	√	

DIC, Disseminated intravascular coagulopathy.
From Sisson, M., & Hamner, L. (2019). Disseminated intravascular coagulation in pregnancy. In N. H. Troiano, P. Witcher, & S. M. Baird (Eds.), *AWHONN's high risk and critical care obstetrics* (4th ed., pp 286–295). Wolters Kluwer/Lippincott; McBride, A.-M. (2018). Clinical presentation and treatment of amniotic fluid embolism. *AACN Advanced Critical Care, 29*(3), 336–342.

achieve the goals of correcting the underlying process, resolving signs and symptoms of shock, resuming normal oxygen delivery and consumption, and minimizing complications. Collaboration with other departments such as operative (OR) and ICU is beneficial to assist with care needs.

> **? KNOWLEDGE CHECK**
>
> 4. True or false: DIC is never the primary cause.
> 5. The process of DIC is caused by what three types of trauma?
> 6. What obstetric conditions predispose the client to DIC?
> 7. What laboratory values are needed to evaluate coagulopathy?

SEPSIS

Pathophysiology

Sepsis continues to be a leading cause of preventable pregnancy-related deaths. Sepsis is a physiologic, pathologic, and biochemical dysregulated host response to infection that results in organ dysfunction and/or failure and can progress to septic shock (Rhodes, 2017). In the United States, sepsis accounts for 12.5% of maternal deaths, is the second most common cause of pregnancy-related death, and has become the second most common cause of death in the first week postpartum (Plante, 2019; Petersen et al., 2019).

Because of normal physiologic compensatory mechanisms in pregnancy, early warning signs may be masked, and a diagnosis of sepsis may be delayed and progress to septic shock

very rapidly. Widespread activation and dysfunction of the immune system in sepsis leads to several hemodynamic and oxygen transport pathophysiologic processes:

1. Hypovolemia
2. Hypotension
3. Decreased tissue perfusion

In addition, the offending pathogen may trigger diffuse activation of the clotting cascade, resulting in the potential for DIC, and microvascular thrombosis (Parfitt et al., 2017; Brown & Abdel-Razeq, 2019).

Etiology

Obstetric and non-obstetric etiologies can lead to sepsis in the pregnant or postpartum client. Risk factors in the antepartum period include multiple gestation, ruptured membranes, urinary tract infection, and stillbirth. In the intrapartum and immediate postpartum period, additional risk factors include cesarean or operative vaginal birth, hemorrhage, manual placental extraction or curettage, and the potential for retained products of conception (Parfitt et al., 2017).

Assessment

As sepsis is considered a medical emergency, the intake history and physical assessment is crucial to ensure that early recognition and treatment are not delayed. The depth and detail of the history is driven by the presenting chief complaint following a brief assessment for immediate life-threatening signs and symptoms. A complete and thorough interview includes timing of onset, location, duration, and severity of symptoms. If pain is present, quality and numerical scale application is completed. Questions regarding medications and therapeutics used by the client to relieve symptoms, and reconciliation of previous medication history are necessary. If infection is suspected, an assessment of recent exposure to sick persons, previous or recurrent infection, and travel out of the country is crucial as this information may assist the provider with possible source identification (Albright, 2017).

Frequent assessment of the client and fetus is principle for early recognition, determination of pathophysiology, guidance of management, stabilization, and improved outcomes. Abnormal physical assessment findings provide clinical clues of sepsis pathology, which trigger increased frequency of assessments, communication to the provider, and bedside provider assessment of the client (Kennedy & Baird, 2017). Components of noninvasive assessment are outlined in Table 19.5.

Interventions

The Surviving Sepsis Campaign (SSC) is an international collaborative organization that provides guidelines for management of clients with known or suspected sepsis. It should be noted that obstetric considerations were not specifically identified when establishing these guidelines, and most scientific data utilized in the development of the SSC bundle excluded pregnant clients. Therefore, it is essential to consider physiologic and hemodynamic changes in pregnancy when adapting these guidelines (Singer et al., 2016).

When sepsis is suspected, timely implementation of bundle components while simultaneously determining etiology is crucial to optimize outcomes for the client and fetus. Fundamental sepsis management principles of fluid resuscitation, correction of hypotension to maintain tissue perfusion, and timely administration of antibiotics still apply to the OB population and are discussed in detail below.

Fluid Resuscitation

Fluid resuscitation in sepsis is a dynamic process and not an end point or specific value. Adequacy of resuscitation is judged in part by resolution of hypotension and normal lactate levels. Lateral positioning ensures that the uterus is not compressing the vena cava which aids fluid resuscitation by improving blood return to the heart. In addition to IV fluid resuscitation, blood component replacement may be necessary to replace clotting factors and increase oxygen carrying capacity (Baird & Belfort, 2019).

Management of Hypotension

Decreased systemic vascular resistance (SVR) is a normal physiologic change in pregnancy and can be exacerbated rapidly by sepsis. A drop in SVR contributes to decreased mean arterial pressure (MAP) and impairs blood return to the heart (decreased preload) and ultimately impairs cardiac output and organ perfusion (Baird & Belfort, 2019). Hypotension is usually progressive, requiring rapid assessment and initiation of interventions to maintain organ perfusion, including the pregnant uterus. If hypotension persists despite aggressive fluid resuscitation and client positioning, vasopressor therapy is recommended to achieve MAP >65 mm Hg and improve cardiac output (Plante et al., 2019).

Antibiotic Therapy

Whenever possible, necessary cultures should be obtained prior to antibiotic initiation. However, empiric antibiotic therapy should not be delayed beyond the first hour of bundle implementation as mortality rates increase appreciably with every hour delay (Mohamed-Ahmed et al., 2016). The initial antibiotic choice for a pregnant or postpartum client provides broad spectrum coverage for Gram-positive, Gram-negative, and possibly anaerobic bacteria, as these are the most likely causes of sepsis in these clients (Brown & Abdel-Razeq, 2019). As culture results become available, antibiotics are tailored to target specific organisms.

Bacterial Cultures

The timing of cultures should be aimed at 1 hour to determine the causative organism(s) for targeted antimicrobial therapy. Blood cultures are obtained from two different sites and include aerobic and anaerobic (Singer et al., 2016). Additionally, cultures may also be obtained from the presumptive infection source, if possible. If chorioamnionitis is suspected, amniocentesis may be indicated.

Lactate

A serum lactate level is recommended in the first hour of bundle implementation (Rhodes et al., 2017). Lactate levels increase in response to anaerobic metabolism from poor tissue perfusion in a septic client. Normal lactate levels are <2 mmol/L. Levels >4 mmol/L are associated with increased mortality rates in nonpregnant clients and nonlaboring pregnant clients; however, levels may exceed 4 mmol/L in a laboring client in the absence of sepsis, making diagnosis difficult (Bauer et al., 2019). Elevated lactate levels in pregnant clients have also been associated with positive blood cultures, longer hospital stays, increased risk of ICU admission, fetal tachycardia, and preterm birth (Albright et al., 2014).

Other Management Considerations

All pregnant or postpartum clients with sepsis should receive venous thrombosis embolism (VTE) prophylaxis measures due to the increased risk of deep vein thrombosis. In addition to sequential compression devices and in the absence of contraindications, pharmacologic prophylaxis with either low molecular weight heparin or unfractionated heparin is recommended.

> ### ❓ KNOWLEDGE CHECK
>
> 8. What are some OB and non-OB risk factors for sepsis in the pregnant or postpartum client?
> 9. What are some interventions used to improve hypotension associated with sepsis in obstetric clients?
> 10. When should antibiotics be initiated in a client with suspected sepsis?

AMNIOTIC FLUID EMBOLUS/ ANAPHYLACTOID SYNDROME OF PREGNANCY

Pathophysiology

Amniotic fluid embolism (AFE), also referred to as anaphylactoid syndrome of pregnancy, is an extremely rare and unpredictable event with high morbidity and mortality for the client and fetus/newborn. AFE is thought to occur when amniotic fluid enters the client's circulation, triggering a sequence of life-threatening proinflammatory immune reactions at or close to the time of birth. There are specific diagnostic criteria for AFE (Pacheco et al., 2016):

1. Sudden onset of cardiopulmonary arrest, or both hypotension and respiratory compromise
2. Documentation of overt DIC following initial signs and symptoms
3. Clinical onset during labor or within 30 minutes of placental delivery
4. No fever during labor

Although there is usually some exchange between fetal and client components around the time of birth, it is unclear why some clients experience an intense pathophysiologic response to fetal antigen exposure and why in most clients this exchange is benign (Drummond & Yeomans, 2018). Although AFE remains associated with a high mortality rate, data now shows rates closer to 15% to 20% (Benson, 2017). In 2016 to 2018, the CDC reported AFE contributed to 5.7% of all pregnancy-related deaths (CDC, 2022c). Of those that survive, it is

TABLE 19.8   Phases of Amniotic Fluid Embolism

	PHASES OF AMNIOTIC FLUID EMBOLISM		
Phase	Pathophysiology	Clinical Presentation	Immediate Supportive Treatment
Phase 1	Amniotic fluid enters the client's circulation and leads to right-sided ventricular failure	• Hypoxia, acidosis, profound respiratory distress	• Start immediate high-quality CPR • Consider immediate delivery • Avoid excessive fluid resuscitation
Phase 2	Release of inflammatory mediators and leads to pulmonary edema and left ventricular failure	• Hypotension, acute renal failure, cardiac failure, shock, lung injury, neurologic changes	• Maintain hemodynamic status with use of inotropes such as dobutamine or norepinephrine • Avoid excessive fluid administration
Phase 3	Overwhelming coagulopathy	• Profound bleeding, disseminated intravascular coagulation	• Activate massive blood transfusion protocol • Treat uterine atony

Adapted from Pacheco, L.D., Saade, G., Hankins, G.D.V., & Clark, S. (2016) Amniotic fluid embolism: diagnosis and management. *American Journal of Obstetrics and Gynecology, 215*(2):B16-24. Drummond, S., & Yeomans, E. (2018). Amniotic fluid embolism. In N. H. Troiano, P. Witcher, & S. M. Baird (Eds.), *AWHONN's high risk and critical care obstetrics* (4th ed., pp. 320–330). Wolters Kluwer/Lippincott.

estimated that 85% have severe neurologic morbidity resulting from hypoxia (Clark et al., 1995; Sultan et al., 2016).

Risk factors related to AFE are not well understood. The most frequent cited risk factors include advanced client age, multiple gestation, placental abnormalities, preeclampsia/eclampsia, and operative vaginal and cesarean birth (Barnhart & Rosenbaum, 2019). Many clients have a preceding aura, progressive change in mental status, or sense of impending doom prior to an AFE event. If still pregnant, fetal compromise due to shunting of oxygenated blood away from the uterus results in sudden bradycardia. There are three phases with corresponding signs and symptoms (Table 19.8). The first phase involves profound respiratory failure followed by cardiopulmonary arrest. If the client survives the initial insult and phase, the second phase complications such as acute renal failure, cardiac failure, and lung injury occur. The third phase involves overwhelming coagulopathy (Pacheco, et al, 2016).

Clinical Management
Goals

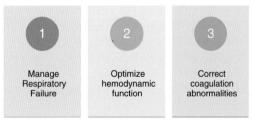

| Manage Respiratory Failure | Optimize hemodynamic function | Correct coagulation abnormalities |

Amniotic fluid embolus is a clinical emergency requiring rapid, coordinated emergent care. Nursing staff is most likely to the first to respond and prompt recognition and action is crucial. Initial interventions involve calling for the rapid response team and getting help to the bedside, administering cardiopulmonary support if needed, and placing the client in a left lateral uterine displacement position. If a code persists, anticipate a perimortem cesarean birth beginning at 4 minutes with the baby delivered by 5 minutes after the onset of cardiac arrest. The cesarean is performed in the same location where the event is taking place. Due to poor neonatal outcomes secondary to profound hypoxia, the neonatal team should be called to the bedside and ready for neonatal resuscitation. Be prepared to initiate large-bore IV access and carry out the massive blood transfusion protocol as DIC is likely to follow delivery. Many resources for families can be found at https://www.afesupport.org.

❓ KNOWLEDGE CHECK

11. What are some risk factors associated with AFE?
12. Recognition of what signs and symptoms should alert the nurse to be suspicious of an AFE?
13. What are the initial interventions for AFE that should be initiated by the nurse?

DIABETIC KETOACIDOSIS

Pathophysiology

Diabetic ketoacidosis (DKA) in pregnancy is a critical complication of diabetes and can be life-threatening to both the pregnant client and fetus. While maternal mortality rates from DKA have decreased in recent years, there is still significant fetal loss at 10% to 25% (Sibai & Viteri, 2014). DKA occurs mostly in clients with type 1 diabetes but has increased in poorly controlled type 2 diabetes (Sibai & Viteri, 2014). DKA is an acute form of decompensated diabetes caused by abnormal carbohydrate, protein, and fat metabolism due to an absolute (decreased amount) or relative (decreased utilization) insulin deficiency. The breakdown of noncarbohydrate sources (proteins, fats) is called gluconeogenesis. Gluconeogenesis leads to hyperglycemia and ketogenesis (ketonemia and acidosis).

Hormonal, metabolic, and respiratory changes lead to insulin resistance, an accelerated starvation state, and compensated respiratory alkalosis to predispose the pregnant client to DKA (Witcher & Graves, 2019). Blood glucose levels of a pregnant client with DKA may be lower (>180 mg/dL) than those of a nonpregnant client with DKA (Witcher & Graves, 2019). As a result of insulin resistance from placental

TABLE 19.9 Laboratory Values in Diabetic Ketoacidosis

Laboratory Assessment in DKA	Abnormal Values
Blood glucose	• Elevated: 180 mg/dL to >300 mg/dL
Ketones	• Positive ketones in blood (ketonemia) • Positive ketones in urine (ketonuria)
Arterial blood gas	• Arterial pH <7.30 • Bicarbonate <15 mEq/L • Base deficit >4 mEq/L
Serum electrolytes	• Anion gap >12 mEq/L (NA^+ - [Cl^- + $HCO3^-$]) • Potassium deficits

Adapted from Witcher, P., & Graves, C. (2019) Diabetic ketoacidosis. In N. H. Troiano, P. Witcher, & S. M. Baird (Eds.), *AWHONN's high risk and critical care obstetrics* (4th ed., pp. 203–211). Wolters Kluwer/Lippincott; Sibai, B. M., & Viteri, O. A. (2014). Diabetic ketoacidosis in pregnancy. *Obstetrics and gynecology, 123*(1), 167–178.

hormones, there is an elevation in fatty acids which convert to ketones in the liver and circulate in the client's system leading to metabolic acidosis (Witcher & Graves, 2019). Ketones along with lactic acid cross the placenta and may interrupt fetal oxygenation, resulting in cardiac arrhythmias and fetal demise (Witcher & Graves, 2019).

Etiology

DKA in pregnancy may be precipitated by several factors (Witcher & Graves, 2019).
- Nausea/vomiting resulting in decreased caloric intake
- Missed/miscalculation of insulin doses
- Pump failure
- Eating disorders
- Infection (e.g., pyelonephritis, intraamniotic infection, pulmonary, urinary)
- Hyperglycemia after medication (e.g., corticosteroids and beta-sympathomimetics)

Clinical Presentation

Prompt recognition and treatment is crucial to optimize outcomes for the client and fetus. The client may present with hallmark signs and symptoms such as elevated glucose levels, polyuria, polydipsia, nausea/vomiting, fruity ketonic breath, tachycardia, hypotension, dehydration/dry mucous membranes, weakness, altered mental status, and coma (Morrison & Everett, 2016). Initial laboratory evaluation is paramount in the diagnosis. Common laboratory findings in DKA are listed in Table 19.9. Anion gap metabolic acidosis, hyperglycemia, and positive ketones are seen in most cases of DKA.

Clinical Management

Clients with DKA are critically ill. Therefore, early referral to an ICU with collaboration between OB and ICU clinicians is essential to improve outcomes for the client and fetus. Management of DKA in a pregnant client is similar to that of the nonpregnant population. Initial treatment utilizing a DKA protocol involves four key principles.

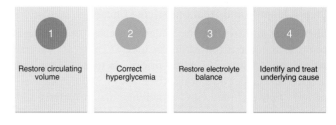

1. Restore circulating volume
2. Correct hyperglycemia
3. Restore electrolyte balance
4. Identify and treat underlying cause

Step 1: Restore Circulating Volume

Fluid resuscitation is prioritized as a primary intervention to promote perfusion to tissues and organs and help disseminate insulin into the cells (Sibai & Viteri, 2014). Most literature recommends 100 mL/kg over 1 to 2 hours of isotonic solution of normal saline (NS). This amount may be equal to 1 to 2 L of IV fluid initially, followed by a maintenance rate of 250 to 500 mL/hour over the next 2 hours depending on the degree of volume deficit and hypotension (Sibai & Viteri, 2014). After the initial fluid bolus, 0.45% NS is typically administered to prevent excessive chloride buildup (Witcher & Graves, 2019). When blood glucose levels reach 250 mg/dL or less, 5% dextrose is added to IV fluids (Witcher & Graves, 2019). Whenever aggressive fluid resuscitation is initiated, the client is monitored for signs and symptoms of pulmonary edema. Vital signs are obtained frequently to assess hemodynamic status.

Step 2: Correct Hyperglycemia

Short-acting regular insulin is administered intravenously as a primary treatment to reduce hyperglycemia. A bolus of regular insulin is administered at 0.1 units/kg, which usually correlates to a dose of 6 to 10 units. After the initial bolus, the maintenance rate is 0.1 units/kg/hour with a goal of resolving acidosis and closing the anion gap (Witcher & Graves, 2019). Insulin is not infused with other medications, therefore a second peripheral line is needed. Oral intake may be reestablished if the client is stabilized, has normal mentation, has no further gastrointestinal symptoms, and no further interventions are anticipated that would require an NPO status. Regular insulin may be given subcutaneously (SQ) when oral intake is tolerated. Because subcutaneous (SQ) absorption is altered and has a slower onset to action than the IV route, it is important to keep IV regular insulin infusing for at least 2 hours after the first SQ dose (Sibai & Viteri, 2014).

Step 3: Restore Electrolyte Balance

Severe volume depletion leads to abnormal serum electrolytes, which are evaluated every 2 hours until stable. Hypokalemia or hyperkalemia are anticipated due to the shifting of potassium from extracellular to intracellular space after volume replacement and insulin administration. The goal is a target serum potassium between 4 and 5 mEq/L (Sibai & Viteri, 2014). Based on laboratory values and the client's clinical situation, other electrolytes such as phosphate, magnesium, and calcium may need to be replaced as well. Because of the arrhythmogenic potential of hypokalemia, continuous ECG monitoring is recommended.

Step 4: Identify and Treat Underlying Cause

Identifying and treating the underlying cause of DKA is a priority to reverse the pathophysiology. There are several precipitating factors. A central priority is to assess for and determine whether infection is the etiology. Laboratory evaluation would include a CBC with differential, urinalysis, and cultures of any suspected site of infection. A thorough history including review of the client's glucose and insulin log, evaluation of mechanical insulin pump function, and assessment for increased levels of stress assists the provider in diagnosis.

KNOWLEDGE CHECK

14. What physiologic changes of pregnancy predispose the pregnant client to DKA?
15. What are the hallmark signs and symptoms in pregnant clients with DKA?
16. What are the four key principles in management of DKA in pregnant clients?

TRAUMA

Although the majority of trauma during pregnancy does not result in major injury, 1 in 12 pregnant clients experience significant trauma with a negative impact on client and/or fetal outcomes. (Ruth & Mighty, 2019). The leading causes of trauma-related injuries are motor vehicle crashes (MVCs), falls, and interpersonal violence (Ruth & Mighty, 2019). Trauma is one of the leading causes of non-OB maternal death and is associated with an increased risk of spontaneous abortion, preterm labor, preterm premature rupture of membranes, fetal injury, and stillbirth (Mendez-Figueroa et al., 2013) The mechanisms of injury in trauma are outlined in Table 19.10.

The anatomic and physiologic changes of pregnancy make trauma care challenging. During early pregnancy, the uterus is surrounded by the pelvis and is well-protected from direct damage. As the uterus enlarges and lifts out of the pelvis, exposure to injury increases. However, the uterus may shield other organs, such as the kidneys and bowel, often protecting them from direct trauma. Pregnancy increases blood volume up to 50%, which masks signs and symptoms of hypovolemia until 1200 mL or approximately 15% to 20% of circulating blood volume is lost (Owattanapanich et al., 2021). Decreased perfusion may result from damage to the uterus, placental abruption, and traumatic injury, and it may lead to hemodynamic instability in the client and fetal compromise.

Although the trauma injury may not be fatal, infant neurologic deficits may be identified after birth. Direct fetal trauma such as skull fracture or intracranial hemorrhage may occur with fracture of the client's pelvis, penetrating wounds, or blunt trauma. Indirect causes of fetal injury or death include placental

TABLE 19.10   Mechanisms of Traumatic Injury

Mechanism	Examples	Notes
Blunt	• Motor vehicle crash • Falls • Interpersonal violence	• Risk of placental abruption and fetal injury • Retroperitoneal injury and hematomas are more frequent due to increased vascularity • Uterine rupture is rare but risk increases with gestational age
Penetrating	• Gun shot • Stab wound	• Small bowel injury more frequent with upper abdominal injury • Consider fetal injury
Chest	• Airway obstruction • Pneumothorax • Cardiac tamponade • Contusion	• Control airway • Chest tube or needle thoracostomy for pneumothorax
Head	• Concussion • Intracranial injury	• Use of Glasgow Coma Scale helpful
Burns and Thermal		• Maternal and fetal mortality related to total body surface area involved • Hypovolemia concern

abruption and disruption of the placental blood flow secondary to hypovolemia of the pregnant client or uterine rupture. The most common cause of fetal death resulting from trauma is death of the pregnant client (Mendez-Figueroa et al., 2013).

Clinical Management

Management of a pregnant trauma client is similar to that of the nonpregnant population (Fig. 19.6). The advanced trauma life support course of the American College of Surgeons Committee on Trauma recommends focusing on two initial surveys when assessing trauma (Ruth & Mighty, 2019).

Primary Survey

The primary survey assesses Airway, Breathing, Circulation, Disability and Displacement, and Exposure to focus on identifying life-threatening injuries and implementing lifesaving interventions. The primary survey is completed within minutes and includes a visual physical assessment (Ruth & Mighty, 2019). Assessment and treatment priorities are listed in Table 19.11.

Secondary Survey

The secondary survey focuses on wounds, injuries, and pregnancy/fetal status after initial stabilization. The pregnancy/fetal assessment would include gestational age, uterine

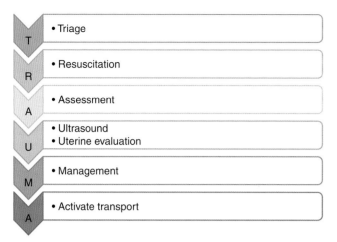

Fig. 19.6 Management of pregnant trauma clients.

TABLE 19.11 Advanced Trauma Life Support Primary Assessment	
Airway and cervical spine	• Assess and maintain airway • Any client with trauma who is unconscious or has a neck injury above the clavicle is regarded as having a cervical neck injury until proven otherwise
Breathing	• Oxygen administration • Brief neurologic examination prior to intubation and neuromuscular blockade • Continuous SpO$_2$ monitoring
Circulation	• Identify hypovolemia and signs of shock • Assess peripheral circulation • Frequent vital signs • Control obvious external hemorrhage • Volume resuscitation • If signs and symptoms of shock persist after 2–3 L of crystalloid, administer blood products • Vasopressors as indicated after initial volume resuscitation
Disability and displacement	• Assess level of consciousness and sensorimotor function • Displace uterus in pregnant women
Exposure	• Undress to allow fully assess injuries • Avoid hypothermia

Data from ATLS Advanced Trauma Life Support Student Course Manual, 10th ed.

tenderness, vaginal bleeding, leaking of amniotic fluid, presence or absence of uterine contractions, and fetal movement. In addition, assessment for signs and symptoms of placental abruption and labor are ongoing.

Nursing Considerations

Nursing care of the pregnant trauma victim initially focuses on the pregnant client and then shifts to fetal stabilization. To help improve placental perfusion and optimize cardiac output, the client is placed in a lateral tilt position. Placing a wedge under the client's hip displaces the uterus away from the major blood vessels such as the vena cava. If a cervical spine injury has not been ruled out and the client remains on a stabilizing board, the board may be tilted to displace the uterus. The frequency of vital signs are based on the client's condition.

There are various assessment tools utilized in trauma. The Focused Assessment with Sonography for Trauma (FAST) is utilized to assess for intraperitoneal hemorrhage, which may be difficult to assess in pregnancy (Mendez-Figueroa et al., 2013). An OB ultrasound is performed to determine gestational age, fetal heart rate, placental location, amniotic fluid amount, and fetal activity. If required for diagnosis, additional imaging studies should not be delayed or eliminated from the plan of care due to concerns of radiation exposure in pregnancy (Ruth & Mighty, 2019). Consultation with the radiology team allows for coordination of care and client teaching.

Laboratory trauma panels typically include type and screen, Rh status if not known, a Kleinhuaer–Betke test to detect maternal-fetal hemorrhage, and coagulation panel (PT, PTT, Fibrinogen) (Mendez-Figueroa et al., 2013). Pregnancy parameters must be considered when interpreting laboratory results as trauma victims may be present in the adult emergency room or adult ICU where the OB population is not common.

A focused fetal assessment occurs after initial stabilization of the pregnant client. A fetus with an estimated gestational age greater than 23 to 24 weeks and determined to be viable may have continuous electronic fetal monitoring depending on location of wound(s) and if the plan of care includes intervention with evidence of fetal compromise. If gestational age is less than 23 weeks, fetal heart rate can be intermittently auscultated.

KNOWLEDGE CHECK

17. What are some leading causes of trauma related injuries?
18. What physiologic alteration of pregnancy can lead to masked signs/symptoms of blood loss due to trauma?
19. What is the most common cause of fetal death during trauma?
20. What is assessed during the primary survey of a pregnant trauma victim?

CARDIAC ARREST

Although cardiac arrest in a pregnant or postpartum client is a rare event, it requires a highly skilled, coordinated, prepared, practiced, interprofessional team response. Determining etiology of the arrest, utilization of advanced cardiac life support algorithms, and early delivery are key components of resuscitation. The reversible etiologies of cardiac arrest are listed in Table 19.12. The most common causes during pregnancy or postpartum are hypovolemia (hemorrhage, sepsis, preeclampsia), hypoxia (respiratory compromise), acidosis (hypovolemia, DKA), and pulmonary embolus (Martin & Arafeh, 2018).

Clinical Management

Management of a cardiac arrest in a pregnant client is the same as nonpregnant resuscitation with a few modifications due to the physiologic and anatomic changes in pregnancy.

TABLE 19.12   Reversible Causes Leading to Cardiac Arrest

Hypovolemia	Tension pneumothorax
Hypoxia	Tamponade, cardiac
Hydrogen ion (acidosis)	Toxins
Hypo/Hyperkalemia	Thrombosis, pulmonary
Hypothermia	Thrombosis, coronary

From American Heart Association (2020). ACLS Advanced Cardiovascular Support Provider Manual, AHA.

TABLE 19.13   OB Cardiac Arrest Checklist

CALL FOR HELP		
☐ OB team		☐ Get code cart
☐ Code blue team		☐ Bed to CPR position
☐ NICU team		☐ Assign timer/documenter
C	Circulation	☐ Left uterine displacement
		☐ Backboard (or bed in CPR mode)
		☐ Hand placement: slightly above center of sternum
		☐ 100 compressions/minute
		☐ Push hard, push fast
		☐ Change compressors Q 2 minutes
A	Airway	☐ Chin lift/jaw thrust if not trauma victim
		☐ Oral airway
B	Breathing	☐ Intubated: 8–10 breaths/minute
		☐ Not intubated: 30 compressions: 2 breaths
		☐ 100% oxygen at 15 L/minute
D	Defibrillate, displace, deliver	☐ Apply pads front and side
		☐ Analyze, defibrillate via AED
		☐ Immediately resume CPR x 2 minutes
		☐ Prepare for cesarean/operative vaginal birth
		☐ Reanalyze Q 2 minutes with AED
		☐ Begin delivery within 4–5 minutes

From Jeejeeboy, F. M., Zelop, C. M., Lipman, S., Carvalho, B., Joglar, J., Mhyre, J. M., Lapinsky, S. E., Elnav, S., Warnes, C. A., Page, R. L., Griffin, R. E., Jain, A., Dainty, K. N., Arafeh, J., Windrim, R., Koren, G., & Callaway, C. W. (2015). Cardiac arrest in pregnancy: A scientific statement from the American Heart Association. *Circulation, 132*(18), 1747–1773; Martin, S., & Arafeh, J. (2018). Cardiac disease in pregnancy. *AACN Advanced Critical Care, 29*(3), 295–302.

Effective cardiac compressions, defibrillation, and medication administration are performed in the same order that is recommended in basic life support (BLS) and advanced cardiac life support (ACLS). A common acronym used to outline care during pregnancy: CABD. See Table 19.13.

An early key intervention is to provide continuous manual displacement of the uterus upward and laterally to optimize circulation and return of blood to the heart (Roth et al., 2014). Fetal assessment is not performed during resuscitation with monitors removed or detached to expose the abdomen (Jeejeeboy et al., 2015). Early intubation is performed by the most experienced provider available due to the physiologic changes of pregnancy and tissue edema making endotracheal intubation difficult (Martin & Arafeh, 2018). If return of spontaneous circulation (ROSC) has not been achieved and the code has persisted for 4 minutes, it is recommended to proceed with a perimortem cesarean birth if gestational age is greater than 20 weeks' gestation. Decrease in aortocaval compression is thought to improve outcomes for the client and newborn (Jeejeeboy et al., 2015; Martin & Arafeh, 2018). To help avoid delay in care when seconds matter, the client is not moved to the operating room for delivery as a perimortem cesarean birth can occur in any location (Martin & Arafeh, 2018).

Nursing Implications

Often the first person to recognize arrest is the bedside nurse. Bundled emergency call procedures that include all key stakeholders such as the adult code team, OB responders, and the neonatal team in one call facilitates quicker response and resuscitation interventions (Arafeh & Abir, 2019). Nurses have significant roles during a code, which include but are not limited to:

- Giving a brief report/history to teams presenting to bedside
- Calming and organizing the room
- Making sure there is an identified team leader
- Determining whether the right team members are present
- Determining that each person present has a specific role; if no role, asking that person to wait outside the room
- Documenting and timing events
- Initiating additional large-bore IV access
- Preparing and administering code medications
- Performing chest compressions
- Assisting with airway and breathing
- Administering blood (may include assisting with rapid infusion device)

Delineated roles outside of the room include a "runner" to the blood bank or laboratory, getting additional equipment to the bedside, or providing care for other clients on the unit.

? KNOWLEDGE CHECK

21. What are the most common causes of cardiac arrest in pregnancy and postpartum?
22. What early key intervention is performed that is unique to the pregnant cardiac arrest client?
23. After how many minutes into cardiac arrest should a perimortem cesarean birth occur?
24. What are some roles/interventions unique to nursing during a code of a pregnant client?

PULMONARY EDEMA

Pathophysiology

Pulmonary edema is the abnormal accumulation of fluid outside of the vascular space in the lungs and is a common cause of respiratory compromise in the OB population.

The fluid can accumulate in the interstitial space, alveoli, and cells. Excess fluid within the interstitial space and alveolar spaces results in decreased gas exchange between the alveoli and blood vessels. Decreased oxygen diffusion results in hypoxemia and potentially tissue hypoxia (Mason & Burke, 2019).

Respiratory conditions during pregnancy account for one-third of adult ICU admissions (Cypher, 2018). Normal physiologic and anatomic alterations in pregnancy lead to significant changes within the respiratory system and result in a compensated respiratory alkalosis (Mason & Burke, 2019).

Etiology

There are two types of pulmonary edema, cardiogenic and noncardiogenic, with specific etiology and treatment. However, similar presentation can make it difficult to diagnose type and etiology (Cypher, 2018). Cardiogenic pulmonary edema results from increased hydrostatic pressure in the pulmonary capillaries (hypervolemia). Noncardiogenic pulmonary edema results when there is increased permeability within the capillary system allowing passive fluid leak out of the vessel resulting in low intravascular pressure (hypovolemia). Noncardiogenic pulmonary edema is usually a complication of a disease process, such as preeclampsia and sepsis (Mason & Burke, 2019; Cypher, 2018). A variety of etiologies can lead to pulmonary edema and are covered in Table 19.14.

Clinical Presentation

Acute pulmonary edema can be mistaken for other respiratory complications with similar presentation of symptoms and client complaints. It is important to understand the pathophysiology, risk factors, and signs and symptoms of pulmonary edema to improve recognition and differentiation from other respiratory complications. Regardless of etiology and type, the clinical signs and symptoms of pulmonary edema are similar. Dyspnea is often the first sign that is recognized and may be associated with anxiety or agitation if hypoxemia is present (Cypher, 2018). The client may report or show signs of coughing, chest discomfort (tightness), tachypnea, tachycardia, and downward trending pulse oximetry values less than 95% (Mason & Burke, 2019; Cypher, 2018). Upon physical examination, the client may be diaphoretic, utilize abdominal accessory muscles, express the need to "sit up straight," or show air hunger. Auscultation of the lungs may or may not reveal crackles, especially in the early stages of pulmonary edema (Mason & Burke, 2019). A common sign associated with pulmonary edema is tachycardia, and although the client's heart rate is elevated slightly during pregnancy, a sustained heart rate over 120 beats per minute is an early warning sign of compromise and warrants further investigation by the provider (Cypher, 2018). Additionally, a respiratory rate greater than 24 breaths per minute is also evaluated by the provider to determine the underlying cause (Cypher, 2018).

Clinical Management
Diagnostic and Laboratory Tests

Laboratory assessment may assist in determining the etiology and type of pulmonary edema. A CBC with differential is needed to detect systemic infection or anemia as an underlying cause. A complete metabolic profile (CMP) is helpful to guide fluid management and can evaluate for adequate renal and liver function prior to diuresis. Other helpful laboratory tests include a B-type natriuretic peptide (BNP) to distinguish between hydrostatic and nonhydrostatic pulmonary edema. If the BNP is elevated (>100), this suggests overstretching of the myocardium in a hypervolemic state associated with cardiogenic pulmonary edema (Cypher, 2018). Arterial blood gases determine impending respiratory failure and guide treatment. See Table 19.15 for normal pregnancy arterial blood gas values (compensated respiratory alkalemia).

TABLE 19.14 Disorders and Risk Factors for Pulmonary Edema in Pregnancy

Cardiogenic	Noncardiogenic
Valvular disease	Preeclampsia
Cardiomyopathy	Sepsis
Medications (B-mimetic tocolytics)	Pneumonia/aspiration syndrome
Hypertension	Transfusion-related lung injury (TRALI)
Ischemic heart disease	Conditions requiring massive blood transfusion (Postpartum hemorrhage, DIC, AFE)
Multifetal pregnancy	Amniotic fluid embolism
Dysrhythmias	Anaphylaxis

Adapted from Mason, B., & Burke, C. (2019). Pulmonary disorders in pregnancy. In N. H. Troiano, P. Witcher, & S. M. Baird (Eds.), *AWHONN's high risk and critical care obstetrics*, (4th ed., pp. 155–175). Wolters Kluwer/Lippincott; Lapinsky, S. (2017). Management of acute respiratory failure in pregnancy. *Seminars in Respiratory and Critical Care Medicine, 38*(02), 201–207; Cypher, R. L. (2018). Pulmonary edema in obstetrics: Essential facts for critical care nurses. *AACN Advanced Critical Care, 29*(3), 327–335.

TABLE 19.15 Blood Gas Values During Pregnancy

Values	Normal Adult Arterial Blood Gas Values	Normal Pregnancy Arterial Blood Gas Values
pH	7.35–7.45	7.40–7.45
$Paco_2$	35–45	27–32
Pao_2	90–100	104–108
HCO_3	22–26	18–22
Sao_2	96%–99%	98%–100%

From Mason, B., & Burke, C. (2019). Pulmonary disorders in pregnancy. In N. H. Troiano, P. Witcher, & S. M. Baird (Eds.), *AWHONN's high risk and critical care obstetrics* (4th ed., pp. 155–175). Wolters Kluwer/Lippincott; Lapinsky, S. (2017). Management of acute respiratory failure in pregnancy. *Seminars in Respiratory and Critical Care Medicine, 38*(02), 201–207.

Radiographic tests, such as a chest x-ray, aids in diagnosis and should not be withheld due to concerns of radiation exposure (Mason & Burke, 2019).

Nursing Implications

The main goal in management of pulmonary edema is adequate oxygenation by maintaining $SpO_2 > 95\%$ and $PaO_2 > 70$ mm Hg (Mason & Burke, 2019). Key nursing interventions include providing supplemental oxygen therapy and client positioning. An upright position decreases return to the right side of the heart and is recommended with cardiogenic pulmonary edema. Lateral recumbent positioning optimizes cardiac output in a noncardiogenic pulmonary client with evidence of hypovolemia. However, the client may not tolerate and may feel air hunger. Another nursing goal is decreasing oxygen consumption by limiting client activity, controlling pain, and decreasing anxiety (Mason & Burke, 2019). To assess fluid balance and response to treatment, nursing assessment of hourly intake and output utilizing an indwelling catheter and placing all IV lines on an infusion pump are essential interventions. As rapid deterioration can occur (especially with noncardiogenic pulmonary edema), anticipation of potential changes in assessment and preparation for intubation is critical.

ⓘ KNOWLEDGE CHECK

25. What disease processes can cause noncardiogenic pulmonary edema?
26. What are the signs and symptoms of pulmonary edema?
27. What are important nursing considerations when caring for clients with pulmonary edema?

CARDIOVASCULAR DISEASE IN PREGNANCY

During pregnancy, significant physiologic cardiovascular changes occur to support oxygenation and metabolic demands of the pregnant client and the fetus. These changes can have substantial effects on the client with preexisting cardiovascular disease (CVD). Such changes include increased blood volume, decreased SVR, increased clot formation (hypercoagulable state), and increase in heart rate and cardiac output starting as early as 5 weeks' gestation (Martin & Arafeh, 2018).

CVD complicates 1% to 4% of pregnancies and is currently responsible for over one-third of pregnancy-related deaths in the United States (CDC, 2022c). CVD is classified as:
1. Congenital
2. Acquired
3. Ischemic
4. Other conditions

The diagnosis of congenital and acquired CVD has trended upward, with recent literature indicating an increase in maternal mortality from acquired heart disease (ACOG, 2019; Briller et al., 2017).

Congenital

Congenital heart disease (CHD) is the most common birth defect affecting 1% or approximately 40,000 births per year in the United States (CDC, 2022a). Advances in early diagnosis and surgical treatment has increased lifespan, with many lesions corrected in early childhood (ACOG, 2019). Examples of congenital lesions include septal defects (atrial and ventricular), pulmonary stenosis, aortic stenosis, patent ductus arteriosus, tetralogy of Fallot, coarctation of the aorta, mitral valve prolapse, and transposition of the great vessels.

Acquired

Acquired heart disease develops after birth and has many etiologies. One etiology is rheumatic heart disease caused by group A streptococci. Rheumatic fever (a complication of streptococcal pharyngitis) may cause scarring of the heart valves, resulting in stenosis (narrowing) of the openings between the chambers of the heart and affecting forward blood flow through the heart. Endocarditis from IV substance use or viral infection is another etiology.

Ischemic

Ischemic heart disease is defined as insufficient blood flow and oxygenation of the myocardium. Examples include acute myocardial infarction (MI) and acute coronary syndrome. Even though ischemic heart disease is uncommon during pregnancy and postpartum, the incidence has increased, affecting 2.8 and 8 per 100,000 pregnancy/postpartum hospitalizations (Smilowitz et al., 2018), and is associated with significant maternal morbidity and mortality (ACOG, 2019). Risk factors associated with MI include the following: (ACOG, 2019; Krening et al., 2019)

- Tobacco use
- Non-Hispanic Black race
- Hyperlipidemia—increased total cholesterol, increased low-density lipoprotein (LDL), decreased high-density lipoprotein (HDL)
- Family history of MI
- Previously existing CVD (hypertension, diabetes)
- High body mass index (BMI)
- Advanced age >30

Other

Cardiomyopathy is a disease of the myocardium resulting in enlargement, thickened, or rigid muscle. Cardiomyopathy can be preexisting, hypertrophic, or occur during pregnancy—peripartum. Peripartum cardiomyopathy has uncertain etiology with strict diagnostic criteria which includes:

- New onset of cardiomyopathy with systolic dysfunction (left ventricular ejection fraction <45%)
- No other identifiable cause and no previously diagnosed heart disease
- Onset of symptoms occurring near the end of pregnancy or in the first few months postpartum (AHA, 2020; ACOG, 2019).

Most clients recover and return to normal cardiac function; however, approximately 40% to 50% have partial recovery with

TABLE 19.16 **Common Signs and Symptoms of Normal Pregnancy versus Abnormal Signs Indicative of Underlying Cardiac Disease**

	ROUTINE CARE	CAUTION*	STOP**
	Reassurance	*Nonemergent Evaluation*	*Prompt Evaluation Pregnancy Heart Team*
History of cardiovascular disease	None	None	Yes
Self-reported symptoms	None or mild	Yes	Yes
• Shortness of breath	No interference with activities of daily living; with heavy exertion only	With moderate exertion, new-onset asthma, persistent cough, or moderate or severe OSA	At rest; paroxysmal nocturnal dyspnea or orthopnea; bilateral chest infiltrates on CXR or refractory pneumonia
• Chest pain	Reflux related that resolves with treatment	Atypical	At rest or with minimal exertion
• Palpations	Few seconds, self-limited	Brief, self-limited episodes; no lightheadedness or syncope	Associated with near syncope
• Syncope	Dizziness only with prolonged standing or dehydration	Vasovagal	Exertional or unprovoked
• Fatigue	Mild	Mild or moderate	Extreme
Vital signs	Normal		
• Heart rate (beats per minute)	<90	90–119	>120
• Systolic blood pressure (mm Hg)	120–139	140–159	>160 (or symptomatic low BP)
• Respiratory rate (per minute)	12–15	16–25	>25
• Oxygen saturation	>97%	95%–97%	<95% (unless chronic)
Physical examination	Normal		
• Jugular venous pressure	Not visible	Not visible	Visible >2 cm above clavicle
• Heart	S3, barely audible soft systolic murmur	S3, systolic murmur	Loud systolic murmur, diastolic murmur, S4
• Lungs	Clear	Clear	Wheezing, crackles, effusion
• Edema	Mild	Moderate	Marked

From Thorne S. (2016). Pregnancy and native heart valve disease. *Heart*, 102:1410-1417.

persistent congestive heart failure or other cardiac dysfunction (Krening et al., 2019). Peripartum cardiomyopathy often recurs with subsequent pregnancies, particularly in clients who did not have complete recovery of left ventricular function (Krening et al., 2019). Other conditions in this classification include heart rhythm disturbances and Marfan's syndrome.

Risk and Assessment

Preferably, care of a client with known CVD begins prior to conception for pregnancy risk assessment and counseling, testing/procedures to determine or enhance cardiac function, identification of modifiable risks, optimization of health, and adjustment of medications. There are several CVD risk assessment tools utilized for pregnancy, such as CARPREG, ZAHARA, and the mWHO (Modified World Health Organization Classification of Maternal Cardiovascular Risk). The risk of perinatal morbidity and/or mortality associated with CVD depends on:
- Specific cardiac lesion
- Functional ability to adapt to physiologic changes in pregnancy, labor, birth, and postpartum
- Development of pregnancy-related complications

During pregnancy, there may be difficulty differentiating signs and symptoms of heart disease from normal pregnancy related complaints. Table 19.16 is an evaluation tool that outlines signs and symptoms common to normal pregnancy and those concerning for CVD.

The New York Heart Association (NYHA) clinical classification system assesses the effect of activity on the heart and is listed in Table 19.17 (Dolgin et al., 1994). Although this system helps determine the care needed for the pregnant woman with cardiac disease, it lacks the ability to predict the risk for adverse outcomes in pregnancy.

Laboratory and Diagnostic Assessment

There are specific laboratory, imaging, and diagnostic studies that are unique to a client with known or suspected CVD. Routine laboratories such as hemoglobin and hematocrit are evaluated at regular intervals to determine anemia, which can be severe in clients with heart failure or MI (ACOG, 2019). An elevated BNP and N-terminal pro-BNP (NT-proBNP) are found in clients with heart failure and can be helpful when determining a diagnosis (Martin & Arafeh, 2018). In pregnant clients with suspected MI, monitoring cardiac enzymes such

TABLE 19.17 New York Heart Association (NYHA) Classification (2017)

Grade	Symptoms
Class I	No limitations of physical exercise, ordinary activity does not cause undue fatigue, palpitations, dyspnea (shortness of breath).
Class II	Slight limitations of physical exercise, ordinary activity results in fatigue, palpitations, dyspnea, or angina. Comfortable at rest.
Class III	Marked limitations of physical activity, less than ordinary activity causes symptoms. Still comfortable at rest.
Class IV	Inability to perform any physical activity, without symptoms. Symptoms of cardiac insufficiency with minimal activity or at rest.

Adapted from Krening, C., Troiano, N., & Shah, S. (2019). Maternal cardiac disorders. In N. H. Troiano, P. Witcher, & S. M. Baird (Eds.), *AWHONN's high risk and critical care obstetrics* (4th ed., pp. 134–154). Wolters Kluwer/Lippincott; Dolgin M., Association NYH, Fox A.C., Gorlin R., Levin R.I. (1994). New York Heart Association. Criteria Committee. Nomenclature and criteria for diagnosis of diseases of the heart and great vessels. 9th ed. Lippincott.

as troponin studies (troponin I and troponin T) are preferred since other cardiac enzymes such as total serum creatinine kinase and MB fractions (CK-MB$_{mass}$) can be elevated due to uterine contractions (Krening et al., 2019). Other testing and evaluation may include a 12-lead ECG, echocardiogram, chest x-ray, computed tomography, and magnetic resonance imaging.

Clinical Management

For clients with moderate to high-risk CVD, referral to a higher level of care (level 3 or level 4) with management by an interprofessional pregnancy heart team is recommended (ACOG, 2019). The pregnancy heart team includes MFM, obstetrics, cardiology, anesthesiology, neonatology, nursing, social work, pharmacy, case management, and other ancillary staff as needed based on conditions of the pregnant client and fetus (Davis & Walsh, 2019; ACOG, 2019). A plan of care outlining appropriate resources aimed to reduce complications is developed and reviewed at regular team meetings. This plan of care should be readily available in the medical record to all health care team members. An example CVD care plan is outlined in Table 19.18.

Although there are unique intrapartum management plans specific to different cardiac lesions, careful assessment and interventions should be targeted to avoid tachycardia (heart rate >100 bpm), hypotension, tachypnea, and decreased oxygen saturation (<95%) (Martin & Arafeh, 2018). Assessment for other warning signs of decreased cardiac output including decreased urine output; delayed capillary refill; cool, pale, mottled skin; and weakened peripheral pulses is ongoing. Additional understanding of cardiac output effects related to specific cardiac lesions is needed to implement appropriate interventions. The two most common intrapartum cardiac complications are:

1. Pulmonary edema (cardiogenic)
2. Arrhythmias

Avoid supine and lithotomy positioning during labor. Lateral positioning enhances cardiac output; if the client experiences fluid overload and/or develops pulmonary edema, the client may need to be placed into high Fowler's.

> **? KNOWLEDGE CHECK**
>
> 28. What are the classifications of CVD in pregnancy?
> 29. What does the risk of perinatal morbidity and/or mortality associated with CVD depend on?
> 30. What disciplines may make up a pregnancy heart team?
> 31. What are the two most common intrapartum cardiac complications?

SUMMARY CONCEPTS

- The CDC estimates 700 pregnancy-related deaths in the United States each year, with three out of five deaths noted to be preventable.
- In addition to maternal death, it is estimated that 50,000 clients suffer severe maternal morbidity (SMM) and life-threatening injuries each year. SMM includes unexpected physical or psychological conditions associated with or aggravated by pregnancy and/or birth.
- Higher rates of severe maternal morbidity and mortality occur in clients who are non-Hispanic Black, American Indian, and Alaska Native race; who are of Hispanic ethnicity; who lack private insurance; and who have lower education levels.
- Preexisting conditions, such as obesity, CVD, thrombophilia, diabetes, and chronic hypertension, place the pregnant client at increased risk for morbidity and mortality.

- The most common causes of pregnancy-related death in the United States are cardiovascular conditions (congenital or acquired), infection leading to sepsis, cardiomyopathy, hemorrhage, thrombotic pulmonary or other embolism, cerebrovascular accidents, hypertensive disorders of pregnancy, AFE, anesthesia complications, and other noncardiovascular medical conditions (e.g., DKA).
- Severe morbidity and mortality events are usually preceded by early warning signs of compromise in the pregnant or postpartum client.
- Levels of neonatal and maternal care are determined by the complexity of care, available resources, and subspecialty care. It is recommended that a client is referred and transported to risk-appropriate care.
- Nurses caring for high-risk and critically ill OB clients require enhanced knowledge and skills regarding principles of management.

TABLE 19.18 Example Cardiovascular Care Plan

Prenatal and Antepartum

Plan of care	Assemble pregnancy heart team and develop plan of care for labor, birth, and postpartum. Document in electronic medical record.
Assessment	Perform NYHA functional assessment at each prenatal visit. Tolerance to physiologic changes in pregnancy. Monitor weight gain and encourage client to avoid excessive weight gain, which may increase cardiac workload. Fetal echocardiogram screening at 18–22 weeks' gestation. Monitor fetal growth trends. Fetal surveillance testing at 32 weeks' gestation.
Medications	Avoid beta-agonist medications for preterm labor or tachysystole to prevent tachycardia. Administer cardiovascular medications as ordered; evaluate client response. If on anticoagulant therapy, monitor coagulation laboratory trends for therapeutic range. Plan for birth and anticoagulant management.
Client teaching	Need for increased surveillance, physical activity, fetal and newborn risks, signs of worsening CVD and when to contact provider, medications

Intrapartum

Plan of care	Review and implement pregnancy heart team plan of care Anticipate planned induction of labor and vaginal birth for most CVD clients. Review current medications and understand administration and monitoring requirements. Determine need for continuous ECG monitoring and interpretation. Determine need for invasive hemodynamic monitoring and increased level of care. Understand cardiac output influences related to structural defects, surgical repair, function, or arrhythmia potential. Continuous electronic fetal and uterine monitoring. Avoid Valsalva, breath holding pushing. Allow "laboring down" or gentle pushing. Anticipate operative vaginal birth.
Assessment	Frequent vital signs. Note and report sustained heart rate >100 or hypotension. Continuous pulse oximetry. Administer oxygen for any sustained valued <95%. Assess for signs and symptoms of cardiogenic pulmonary edema immediately postpartum with delivery of the placenta. Intake and output. All IV lines on a pump.
Pain management	Early consultation with anesthesiology provider. Provide effective pain control to decrease oxygen consumption. Anticipate regional anesthesia for most CVD clients.
Medications	Endocarditis prophylaxis according to American Heart Association recommendations in high-risk clients. Have diuretic medication readily available immediate postpartum for clients with left-sided lesions or cardiomyopathy. Avoid terbutaline for tachysystole. Regulate oxytocin administration to avoid tachysystole.
Client teaching	Labor and birth process, indicated monitoring, pain management

Postpartum

Plan of care	Measure cumulative, quantified blood loss. Be prepared to treat postpartum hemorrhage and implement protocol as indicated to prevent hypovolemia.
Assessment	Continue frequent noninvasive assessments of cardiac output and oxygenation. Extended monitoring in high acuity unit for 24 hours postpartum. Intake and output Assess for signs and symptoms of cardiogenic pulmonary edema.
Medications	Avoid methergine for postpartum hemorrhage. Provide effective pain control Administer stool softener to avoid constipation and Valsalva.
Client teaching	Contraception, pregnancy spacing, signs and symptoms of compromise and when to call provider/return to hospital, medications, future CVD risk, physical activity, early planned postpartum visit, follow-up with cardiology provider

NOTE: This example plan of care is not all-inclusive and should be tailored to each client's care needs.
CVD, Cardiovascular disease; *ECG,* electrocardiogram; *IV,* intravenous; *NYHA,* New York Heart Association.
From Cardiovascular Considerations in Caring for Pregnant Clients. (2020). A Scientific Statement From the American Heart Association. *Circulation,* 141(23), e884-e903; American College of Obstetricians and Gynecologists. (2019). Practice Bulletin No. 212: Pregnancy and Heart Disease. *Obstetrics & Gynecology, 133*(5), e320-356.

- Interprofessional, nurse-led bedside rounds allow for development and communication of the plan of care and include client and family input.
- Several ways to help prepare and manage clinical emergencies include development of a rapid response team, development of protocols that include clinical triggers, use of a standardized communication tool for huddles and briefs, and implementation of emergency drills and simulation.
- The two core components of noninvasive assessment are (1) cardiac output and (2) oxygen transport.
- Hypovolemic shock requires immediate recognition and management to minimize insufficient oxygen delivery and tissue perfusion resulting from decreased intravascular volume.
- Circulating blood volume redistributes with preferential shunting of blood to the heart, brain, liver, and lungs, and away from nonessential organ systems, including the kidneys and uterus.
- Two main goals for managing hypovolemic shock include promoting tissue oxygenation and replacement of adequate fluid/volume.
- Initiate massive blood transfusion if four or more units of blood products are needed due to hemorrhage.
- DIC is a secondary complication of an underlying condition.
- DIC is activated by trauma to tissues, trauma to vascular endothelium, or trauma to red blood cells or platelets.
- DIC pathophysiologic processes lead to excessive bleeding and tissue ischemia resulting in catastrophic hemorrhage, profound hypovolemic shock, and multisystem organ failure.
- During DIC, anticipate aggressive volume resuscitation with IV fluids and blood products to replace decreased circulating blood volume and maintain perfusion to organs and tissues.
- Sepsis is a physiologic, pathologic, and biochemical dysregulated host response to infection that results in organ dysfunction and/or failure and can progress to septic shock.
- Sepsis in the pregnant or postpartum client leads to hypovolemia, hypotension, and decreased tissue perfusion.
- Fundamental sepsis management principles include fluid resuscitation, correction of hypotension to maintain tissue perfusion, and timely administration of antibiotics.
- AFE is thought to occur when amniotic fluid contents such as fetal cells, tissue, and other debris enter the client's circulation signaling a sequence of life-threatening reactions at or close to the time of birth.
- Abrupt respiratory distress, depressed cardiac function with circulatory collapse, and massive hemorrhage occur with rapid onset in AFE clients.
- Many clients have a preceding aura, progressive change in mental status, or sense of impending doom prior to an AFE event.
- Initial interventions during an AFE involve calling for the rapid response team and getting help to the bedside;

administering cardiopulmonary support if needed; and placing the client in a left lateral uterine displacement position.
- DKA occurs mostly in clients with type 1 diabetes but is increasing in poorly controlled type 2 diabetes with uncontrolled hyperglycemia, metabolic acidosis, and ketosis.
- Blood glucose levels in a pregnant DKA client may be lower (>180 mg/dL) than those of a nonpregnant client with DKA.
- The DKA OB client may present with hallmark signs and symptoms such as elevated glucose levels, polyuria, polydipsia, nausea/vomiting, fruity ketonic breath, tachycardia, hypotension, dehydration/dry mucous membranes, weakness, altered mental status, and coma.
- Initial treatment utilizing a DKA protocol includes (1) restore circulating volume, (2) correct hyperglycemia, (3) restore electrolyte imbalance, (4) identify and treat underlying cause.
- Trauma may be blunt in nature, such as that sustained in an automobile accident; penetrating, such as gunshot or knife wounds; or others such as burns or electrical injuries.
- Management of the pregnant trauma client includes Trauma, Resuscitation, Assessment, Ultrasound/Uterine evaluation, Management, Activate transport.
- Nursing care of the pregnant trauma victim initially focuses on the pregnant client and then shifts to fetal stabilization.
- An early key intervention during cardiac arrest in a pregnant client is to continuously manually displace the uterus upward and laterally to optimize circulation and return of blood to the heart.
- Fetal assessment is not performed during resuscitation; monitors removed or detached to expose abdomen.
- If return of spontaneous circulation (ROSC) has not been achieved and the code has persisted for 4 minutes, it is recommended to proceed with a perimortem cesarean birth when gestational age is greater than 20 weeks.
- Due to decreased colloid osmotic pressure, pregnant clients are more susceptible to an accumulation of fluid in the pulmonary interstitial spaces known as pulmonary edema.
- Excess fluid within the interstitial space impedes oxygen diffusion, leading to decrease oxygen delivery, and tissue hypoxia.
- Cardiogenic pulmonary edema results from increased hydrostatic pressure in the pulmonary capillaries (hypervolemia). Noncardiogenic pulmonary edema results when there is increased permeability within the capillary system creating an environment where fluid is able to move in and out of the vessel leading to low intravascular pressure.
- Key nursing interventions for clients with pulmonary edema include supplemental oxygen therapy as needed, client positioning in an upright position with uterine displacement to help optimize cardiac output, and conserving oxygen consumption by limiting client activity and controlling pain and anxiety.

- Cardiovascular disease complicates 1% to 4% of pregnancies and is responsible for over one-third of pregnancy-related deaths in the United States.
- Although there are unique intrapartum management plans specific to different cardiac lesions, careful assessment and interventions should be targeted to avoid

tachycardia (heart rate >100 bpm), hypotension, tachypnea, and decreased oxygen saturation (<95%) in OB clients with cardiac disease.
- The two most common intrapartum cardiac complications are pulmonary edema and arrythmias.

Clinical Judgment And Next-Generation NCLEX® Examination-Style Questions

1. The nurse is assessing a 38-year-old, G3 P2 client at 34 weeks' gestation with complaints of shortness of breath during work. The nurse completes an assessment with the following data. **Highlight or place a check mark next to assessment findings that require follow-up by the nurse.**

Vital Signs:
    Temperature: 97.8°F
    Blood pressure: 146/94
    Pulse: 114 beats/minute
    Respirations: 26 breaths/minute
    Oxygen saturation: 91% (on room air)

Current OB History:
    Estimated weeks of gestation: 34 weeks
    Routine prenatal care
    Pregnant with twins
    Medications: prenatal vitamins, calcium, and Baby ASA

Past Medical History:
    Cardiac: mitral stenosis

Physical assessment:
    Skin cool and clammy
    Sitting upright in bed
    Alert and oriented
    Tearful
    Significant other at bedside
    Lungs: wheezes noted lower lungs bases bilaterally
    Cardiac: S1 S2 heard; midsystolic ejection murmur heard
    Uterus: occasional contractions every 7 to 10 minutes, palpate moderate with relaxation
    Fetus: twin A: baseline FHTs 145, moderate variability, no decelerations
    Twin B: baseline FHTs 155, minimal variability, late decelerations
    Cervix: closed, 0% effaced, −5 station, intact membranes

2. **Use an X to indicate whether the nursing actions listed below are emergent (appropriate or immediately necessary) or nonemergent (not appropriate or not immediately necessary) for the client's care at this time.**

Nursing Action	Emergent	Nonemergent
Place oxygen at 8–10 L per nonrebreather FM		
Insert a peripheral intravenous line		
Monitor vital signs every 30 minutes		
Administer morphine sulfate 1–2 mg SIVP		
Instruct the client of radiology coming to perform a bedside CXR		
Obtain admission laboratory work: CBC, CMP, type, and screen		
Insert Foley catheter		

3. Initial actions were performed to stabilize the client. **For each assessment finding, use an X to indicate whether the intervention was effective (met expected outcomes), ineffective (did not meet expected outcomes), or unrelated (not related to the expected outcomes).**

Assessment Finding	Effective	Ineffective	Unrelated
Oxygen saturation 95%			
Heart rate: 110 bpm			
Respirations: 20 breaths per minute			
Blood pressure: 136/78			
Temperature: 98.2ºF			
Uterus: irritability noted; mild to palpation			
Fetus: twin B: FHTs 150; moderate variability; no decelerations			
Lying semi-Fowler's wedged to the right side			
Intermittent wheezing in the lower lobes bilaterally			

REFERENCES

Abdel-Razeq, S. S., & Norwitz, E. R. (2019). Septic Shock. In J.P. Phelan, L.D. Pacheoco, M.R. Foley, G.R. Saade, G.A. Dildy, & M.A. Belfort (Eds.), *Critical Care Obstetrics* (6th ed., 599–629). Wiley Blackwell.

Abraham, J., Kannampallil, T. G., Patel, V. L., Patel, B., & Almoosa, K. F. (2016). Impact of structured rounding tools on time allocation during multidisciplinary rounds: An observational study. *JMIR Hum Factors, 3*(2), e29.

Advanced Trauma Life Support. American College of Surgeons. (n.d.). https://www.facs.org/quality-programs/trauma/atls.

Albright, C. (2017). Sepsis in Pregnancy. In *obstetric triage and emergency care protocols, second edition* (2nd ed., pp. 256–282). Springer Publishing Company.

Albright, C., Ali, T., Lopes, V., Rouse, D., & Anderson, B. (2014). 571: Lactic acid measurement to identify risk of morbidity in pregnancy. *American Journal of Obstetrics and Gynecology, 210*(1) p. S281. doi.org/10.1016/j.ajog.2013.10.604.

American College of Obstetricians and Gynecologists (ACOG). (2019). Practice Bulletin No. 212: Pregnancy and heart disease. *Obstetrics & Gynecology, 133*(5), e320–e356.

American College of Obstetricians and Gynecologists, Society for Maternal-Fetal Medicine ((ACOG & SMFM). (2015). Obstetric Care Consensus: Levels of Maternal Care. *Obstet Gynecol, 125*(2), 502–515.

American College of Surgeons Committee on Trauma. (2018). *ATLS Advanced Trauma Life Support Student Course Manual* (10th ed.).

American College of Obstetricians and Gynecologists, Society for Maternal-Fetal Medicine (ACOG & SMFM). (2019). Obstetric care consensus: Levels of maternal care. *Obstet Gynecol, 134*(2), e41–e55.

Aparanji, K., Kulkarni, S., Metzke, M., Schmudde, Y., White, P., & Jaeger, C. (2018). Quality improvement of delirium status communication and documentation for intensive care unit clients during daily multidisciplinary rounds. *BMJ Open Qual, 7*(2), e000239.

Arafeh, J. M. R., & Abir, G. (2019). Cardiopulmonary resuscitation in pregnancy. In N. H. Troiano, P. Witcher, & S. M. Baird (Eds.), *AWHONN's High Risk and Critical Care Obstetrics* (4th ed., pp. 359–368). Wolters Kluwer/Lippincott.

ATLS subcommittee; American College of Surgeons' Committee on Trauma; & International ATLS working group. (2013). Advance trauma life support (ATLS), 9th ed. *Journal of Trauma Acute Care Surgery, 74*(5), 1363–1366.

Baird, S. M., & Belfort, M. (2019). Critical pharmacologic agents. In N. H. Troiano, P. Witcher, & S. M. Baird (Eds.), *AWHONN's High Risk and Critical Care Obstetrics* (4th ed., pp. 81–97). Wolters/Kluwer/Lippincott.

Baird, S. M., & Fox, K. (2019). Morbidly adherent placenta. In N. H. Troiano, P. Witcher, & S. M. Baird (Eds.), *AWHONN's High Risk and Critical Care Obstetrics* (4th ed., pp. 244–257). Wolters Kluwer/Lippincott.

Baird, S. M., & Graves, C. R. (2015). REACT: An interprofessional education and safety program to recognize and manage the compromised obstetric client. *The Journal of Perinatal and Neonatal Nursing 29*(2), 138–148.

Baird, S. M., & Martin, S. M. (2019). Critical care obstetric capabilities: development strategies. In N. H. Troiano, P. Witcher, & S. M. Baird (Eds.), *AWHONN's High Risk and Critical Care Obstetrics* (4th ed., pp. 21–29). Wolters Kluwer/Lippincott.

Baird, S. M., Martin, S., & Kennedy, M. B. (2021). Goals for collaborative management of obstetric hemorrhage. *OBGYN Clinics of North America, 48*(1), 151–171.

Barnhart, M. L., & Rosenbaum, K. (2019). Anaphylactoid syndrome of pregnancy. *Nursing for Women's Health, 23*(1), 38–48.

Bauer, M. E., Housey, M., Bauer, S. T., Behrmann, S., Chau, A., Clancy, C., & Bateman, B. T. (2019). Risk factors, etiologies, and screening tools for sepsis in pregnant women. *Anesthesia & Analgesia, 129*(6), 1613–1620.

Benson, M. D. (2017). What is new in amniotic fluid embolism? Best articles from the past year. *Obstetrics and Gynecology, 129*(5), 941–942.

Briller, J., Koch, A. R., & Geller, S. E. (2017). Maternal cardiovascular mortality in Illinois, 2002–2011. *Obstetrics & Gynecology, 129*(5), 819–826.

Brown, K. N., & Abdel-Razeq, S. S. (2019). Sepsis in pregnancy. In N. H. Troiano, P. Witcher, & S. M. Baird (Eds.), *AWHONN's High Risk and Critical Care Obstetrics* (4th ed., pp. 296–319). Wolters Kluwer/Lippincott.

Building U.S. Capacity to Review and Prevent Maternal Deaths. (2018). *Report from nine maternal mortality review committees.* http://reviewtoaction.org/Report_from_Nine_MMRCs.

Callaghan, W. M., Creanga, A. A., & Kuklina, E. V. (2012). Severe maternal morbidity among delivery and postpartum hospitalizations in the United States. *Obstetrics & Gynecology, 120*(5), 1029–1036.

Cardiovascular Considerations in Caring for Pregnant Clients. (2020). A scientific statement from the American Heart Association. *Circulation, 141*(23) e884-e903.

Centers for Disease Control and Prevention. (2019). *Vital signs: Pregnancy related deaths.* https://www.cdc.gov/vitalsigns/maternal-deaths/index.html.

Centers for Disease Control and Prevention. (2020). *Maternal mortality.* https://www.cdc.gov/reproductivehealth/maternal-mortality/index.html.

Centers for Disease Control and Prevention. (2021). *Severe maternal morbidity in the United States.* https://www.cdc.gov/reproductivehealth/maternalinfanthealth/severematernalmorbidity.html.

Centers for Disease Control and Prevention. (2022a). *Data and statistics on congenital heart defects.* https://www.cdc.gov/ncbddd/heartdefects/data.html.

Centers for Disease Control and Prevention. (2022b). *CDC Levels of care assessment toolSM (CDC LOCATeSM).* https://www.cdc.gov/reproductivehealth/maternalinfanthealth/cdc-locate/index.html?CDC_AA_refVal=https%3A%2F%2Fwww.cdc.gov%2Freproductivehealth%2Fmaternalinfanthealth%2FLOCATe.html.

Centers for Disease Control and Prevention. (2022c). *Pregnancy mortality Surveillance system.* https://www.cdc.gov/reproductivehealth/maternal-mortality/pregnancy-mortality-surveillance-system.htm.

Chau, A., & Tsen, L. C. (2014). Fetal optimization during maternal sepsis. *Current Opinion in Anaesthesiology, 27*(3), 259–266.

Clark, S. L., Hankins, G. D. V., Dudley, D. A., Dildy, G. A., & Porter, T. F. (1995). Amniotic fluid embolism: Analysis of the national registry. *American Journal of Obstetrics and Gynecology, 172*(4), 1158–1169. Part 1 https://doi.org/10.1016/0002-9378(95)91474-9.

Cypher, B. (2016). A standardized approach to electronic fetal monitoring in critical care obstetrics. *Journal of Perinatal and Neonatal Nursing, 32*(3), 212–221.

Cypher, R. L. (2018). Pulmonary edema in obstetrics: Essential facts for critical care nurses. *AACN Advanced Critical Care, 29*(3), 327–335.

Davis, M. B., & Walsh, M. N. (2019). Cardio-obstetrics. *Circulation: Cardiovascular Quality and Outcomes, 12*(2).

Dolgin M., Association NYH, Fox A.C., Gorlin R., Levin R.I. (1994). New York Heart Association. Criteria Committee. Nomenclature and criteria for diagnosis of diseases of the heart and great vessels. 9th ed. Lippincott.

Drummond, S., & Yeomans, E. (2018). Amniotic fluid embolism. In N. H. Troiano, P. Witcher, & S. M. Baird (Eds.), *AWHONN's High Risk and Critical Care Obstetrics* (4th ed., pp. 320–330). Wolters Kluwer/Lippincott.

Fingar, K. R., Hambrick, M. M., Heslin, K. C., & Moore, J. E. (2018). *Trends and disparities in delivery hospitalizations involving severe maternal morbidity, 2006-2015. HCUP Statistical Brief #243. September 2018.* Rockville, MD: Agency for Healthcare Research and Quality. https://www.hcup-us.ahrq.gov/reports/statbriefs/sb243-Severe-Maternal-Morbidity-Delivery-Trends-Disparities.pdf.

Flannery, A. H., Thompson Bastin, M. L., Montgomery-Yates, A., Hook, C., Cassity, E., Eaton, P. M., & Morris, P. E. (2019). Multidisciplinary prerounding meeting as a continuous quality improvement tool: leveraging to reduce continuous benzodiazepine use at an academic medical center. *J Intensive Care Med, 34*(9), 707–713.

Gareua, S., Lopez-De Fede, A., Loudermilk, B. L., et al. (2016). Group prenatal care results in Medicaid savings with better outcomes: A propensity score analysis of centering pregnancy participation in South Carolina. *Maternal Child Health J, 20*(7), 1384–1393.

Gentle, S. J., Carlo, W. A., Tan, S., Gargano, M., Ambalavanan, N., Chawla, S., Bell, E. F., Bann, C. M., Hintz, S. R., Heyne, R. J., Tita, A., Higgins, R. D., & Eunice Kennedy Shriver National Institute of Child Health and Human Development (NICHD) Neonatal Research Network. (2020). Association of Antenatal Corticosteroids and Magnesium Sulfate Therapy With Neurodevelopmental Outcome in Extremely Preterm Children. *Obstetrics and Gynecology, 135*(6), 1377–1386.

Guntupalli, K. K., Karnad, R. D., Bandi, V., Hall, N., & Belfort, M. (2015). Critical illness in pregnancy part II: Common medical conditions complicating pregnancy and puerperium. *Chest, 148*(5), 1333–1345.

Gyamfi-Bannerman, C., Thom, E. A., Blackwell, S. C., Tita, A. T., Reddy, U. M., Saade, G. R., Rouse, D. J., McKenna, D. S., Clark, E. A., Thorp, J. M., Jr., Chien, E. K., Peaceman, A. M., Gibbs, R. S., Swamy, G. K., Norton, M. E., Casey, B. M., Caritis, S. N., Tolosa, J. E., Sorokin, Y., VanDorsten, J. P., & NICHD Maternal–Fetal Medicine Units Network. (2016). Antenatal betamethasone for women at risk for late preterm delivery. *The New England Journal of Medicine, 374*(14), 1311–1320.

Havranek, E. P., Mujahid, M. S., Barr, D. A., Blair, I. V., Cohen, M. S., Cruz-Flores, S., et al. (2015). Social determinants of risk and outcomes for cardiovascular disease: A scientific statement from the American Heart Association. *Circulation, 132*, 873–898.

Hoyert, D. L., Uddin, S. F. G., & Minino, A. M. (2020). Evaluation of the pregnancy status checkbox on the identification of maternal deaths. *Natl Vital Stat Rep, 69*, 1–25.

Jeejeeboy, F. M., Zelop, C. M., Lipman, S., Carvalho, B., Joglar, J., Mhyre, J. M., Lapinsky, S. E., Elnav, S., Warnes, C. A., Page, R. L., Griffin, R. E., Jain, A., Dainty, K. N., Arafeh, J., Windrim, R., Koren, G., & Callaway, C. W. (2015). Cardiac arrest in pregnancy: A scientific statement from the American Heart Association. *Circulation, 132*(18), 1747–1773.

Kennedy, B. B., & Baird, S. M. (2017). Collaborative strategies for management of obstetric hemorrhage. P. O'Malley, & J. Foster

(Eds.). (2017). *Critical Care Nursing Clinics of North America, 29*(3), 315–330.

Kilpatrick, S. J., Berg, C., Bernstein, P., Bingham, D., Delgado, A., Callaghan, W. M., et al. (2014). Standardized severe maternal morbidity review: Rationale and process. *Obstetrics & Gynecology, 124*, 361–366.

Kim, M. M., Barnato, A. E., Angus, D. C., Fleisher, L. A., & Kahn, J. M. (2010). The effect of multidisciplinary care teams on intensive care unit mortality. *Archives of Internal Medicine, 170*(4), 369–376.

Krening, C., Troiano, N., & Shah, S. (2019). Maternal cardiac disorders. In N. H. Troiano, P. Witcher, & S. M. Baird (Eds.), *AWHONN's High Risk and Critical Care Obstetrics* (4th ed., pp. 134–154). Wolters Kluwer/Lippincott.

Louzon, P., Jennings, H., Ali, M., & Kraisinger, M. (2017). Impact of pharmacist management of pain, agitation, and delirium in the intensive care unit through participation in multidisciplinary bundle rounds. *Am J Health Syst Pharm, 74*(4), 253–262.

March of Dimes. Toward improving the outcome of pregnancy III. (2010). *Enhancing perinatal health through quality, safety and performance initiatives. White Plains (NY): March of Dimes.* https://www.marchofdimes.org/toward-improving-the-outcome-of-pregnancy-iii.pdf.

Martin, S., & Arafeh, J. (2018). Cardiac disease in pregnancy. *AACN Advanced Critical Care, 29*(3), 295–302.

Martin, S., & Baird, S. M. (2018). *Sepsis and septic shock in pregnancy.* Contemporary OB/GYN. https://www.contemporaryobgyn.net/view/sepsis-and-septic-shock-pregnancy.

Mason, B., & Burke, C. (2019). Pulmonary disorders in pregnancy. In N. H. Troiano, P. Witcher, & S. M. Baird (Eds.), *AWHONN's High Risk and Critical Care Obstetrics* (4th ed., pp. 155–175). Wolters Kluwer/Lippincott.

McBride, A.-M. (2018). Clinical presentation and treatment of amniotic fluid embolism. *AACN Advanced Critical Care, 29*(3), 336–342.

Mendez-Figueroa, H., Dahlke, J. D., Vrees, R. A., & Rouse, D. J. (2013). Trauma in pregnancy: An updated systematic review. *American Journal of Obstetrics and Gynecology, 209*(1), 1–10.

Mhyre, J. M., Tsen, L. C., Einav, S., Kuklina, E. V., Leffert, L. R., & Bateman, B. T. (2014). Cardiac arrest during hospitalization for delivery in the United States, 1998–2011. *Anesthesiology, 120*(4), 810–818.

Mohamed-Ahmed, O., Nair, M., Acosta, C., Kurinczuk, J. J., & Knight, M. (2016). Progression from severe sepsis in pregnancy to death: A UK population-based case-control analysis. *Obstetric Anesthesia Digest, 36*(3), 154 154.

Morrison, J., & Everett, M. (2016). *Diabetic ketoacidosis during pregnancy.* http://www.kenkyugroup.org/images/articles/dd555956c4ac7ff86cbec84b8326b83d.pdf.

Lapinsky, S. (2017). Management of acute respiratory failure in pregnancy. *Seminars in Respiratory and Critical Care Medicine, 38*(02), 201–207.

Owattanapanich, N., Lewis, M. R., Benjamin, E. R., Wong, M. D., & Demetriades, D. (2021). Motor vehicle crashes in pregnancy: Maternal and fetal outcomes. *Journal of Trauma & Acute Care Surgery, 90*(5), 861–865. https://doi-org.ezproxy.baylor.edu/10.1097/TA.0000000000003093.

Pacheco, L. D., Saade, G., Hankins, G. D., & Clark, S. L. (2016). Amniotic fluid embolism: Diagnosis and management. *American Journal of Obstetrics and Gynecology, 215*(2), B16–B24.

Parfitt, S. E., Bogat, M. L., Hering, S. L., Ottley, C., & Roth, C. (2017). Sepsis in obstetrics. *MCN: The American Journal of Maternal/Child Nursing, 42*(4), 199–205.

Petersen, E. E., Davis, N. L., Goodman, D., Cox, S., Mayes, N., Johnston, E., Syverson, C., Seed, K., Shapiro-Mendoza, C. K., Callaghan, W. M., & Barfield, W. (2019). Vital signs: Pregnancy-related deaths, United States, 2011–2015, and strategies for prevention, 13 states, 2013–2017. *MMWR Morbidity and Mortality Weekly Report, 68*(18), 423–429.

Pijuan-Domènech, A., Galian, L., Goya, M., Casellas, M., Merced, C., Ferreira-Gonzalez, I., et al. (2015). Cardiac complications during pregnancy are better predicted with the modified WHO risk score. *International Journal of Cardiology, 195*, 149–154.

Plante, L. A., Pacheco, L. D., & Louis, J. M. (2019). SMFM consult series #47: Sepsis during pregnancy and the puerperium. *American Journal of Obstetrics and Gynecology, 220*(4), B2–B10.

Rhodes, A., Evans, L. E., Alhazzani, W., Levy, M. M., Antonelli, M., Ferrer, R., Kumar, A., Sevransky, J. E., Sprung, C. L., Nunnally, M. E., Rochwerg, B., Rubenfeld, G. D., Angus, D. C., Annane, D., Beale, R. J., Bellinghan, G. J., Bernard, G. R., Chiche, J. D., Coopersmith, C., De Backer, D. P., & Dellinger, R. P. (2017). Surviving sepsis campaign: international guidelines for management of sepsis and septic shock. *Intensive Care Medicine, 43*(3), 304–377.

Robinson, K., Garnier-Villarreal, M., & Hanson, L. (2018). Effectiveness of centering pregnancy on breastfeeding initiation among African Americans: A systematic review and meta-analysis. *J Perinat Neonatal Nurs, 32*(2), 116–126.

Roth, C. K., Parfitt, S. E., Hering, S. L., & Dent, S. A. (2014). Developing protocols for obstetric emergencies. *Nursing for Women's Health, 18*(5), 378–390.

Rowley, R., Phillips, L., O'Dell, L., Husseini, R., Carpino, S., & Hartman, S. (2016). Group prenatal care: A financial perspective. *Maternal Child Health Journal, 20*, 1–10.

Ruth, D., & Mighty, H. (2019). Trauma in pregnancy. In N. H. Troiano, P. Witcher, & S. M. Baird (Eds.), *AWHONN's High Risk and Critical Care Obstetrics* (4th ed., pp. 331–343). Wolters Kluwer/Lippincott.

Scott, K. A., Britton, L., & McLemore, M. R. (2019). The ethics of perinatal care for Black women. *J Perinat Neonatal Nurs, 33*(2), 108–115.

Shamshirsaz, A. A., & Dildy, G. A. (2018). Reducing maternal mortality and severe maternal morbidity: The role of critical care. *Clin Obstet Gynecol, 61*(2), 1–13.

Shields, L. E., Wiesner, S., Klein, C., Pelletreau, B., & Hedriana, H. L. (2016). Maternal trigger tool and severe maternal morbidity. *Am J Obstet Gynecol, 1*, 527.e1–527.e6.

Sibai, B. M., & Viteri, O. A. (2014). Diabetic ketoacidosis in pregnancy. *Obstetrics and Gynecology, 123*(1), 167–178.

Singer, M., Deutschman, C. S., Seymour, C. W., Shankar-Hari, M., Annane, D., Bauer, M., & Angus, D. C. (2016). The third international consensus definitions for sepsis and septic shock (Sepsis-3). *JAMA, 315*(8), 801–810.

Sisson, M., & Hamner, L. (2019). Disseminated intravascular coagulation in pregnancy. In N. H. Troiano, P. Witcher, & S. M. Baird (Eds.), *AWHONN's High Risk and Critical Care Obstetrics* (4th ed., pp. 286–295). Wolters Kluwer/Lippincott.

Smilowitz, N. R., Gupta, N., & Berger, J. S. (2018). Trends in cardiovascular risk factor and disease prevalence in clients undergoing non-cardiac surgery. *Heart, 104*(14), 1180–1186.

Sultan, P., Seligman, K., & Carvalho, B. (2016). Amniotic fluid embolism: Update and review. *Current Opinion in Anaesthesiology, 29*(3), 288–296.

Troiano, N. H., & Baird, S. M. (2018). Critical care obstetric nursing. In J. P. Phelan, L. D. Pacheco, M. R. Foley, G. R. Saade, G. A. Dildy, & M. A. Belfort (Eds.), *Critical Care Obstetrics* (6th ed., pp. 27–40). Boston, MA: Blackwell Publications.

Ulrich, B., Barden, C., Cassidy, L., & Varn-Davis, N. (2019). Critical care nurse work environments 2018: Findings and implications. *Critical Care Nurse, 39*(2), 67–84.

Wang, E., Glazer, K. B., Howell, E. A., & Janevic, T. M. (2020). Social determinants of pregnancy-related mortality and morbidity in the United States. *Obstetrics & Gynecology, 135*(4), 896–915.

Witcher, P., & Graves, C. (2019). Diabetic ketoacidosis. In N. H. Troiano, P. Witcher, & S. M. Baird (Eds.), *AWHONN's High Risk and Critical Care Obstetrics* (4th ed., pp. 203–211). Wolters Kluwer/Lippincott.

Witcher, P. M. & Lindsay, M. K. (2019). Maternal morbidity and mortality. In N.H. Troiano, P. M. Witcher, S. M. Baird (Eds.), *AWHONN's high risk and critical care obstetrics*, (4th ed.). Wolters Kluwer.

Newborn: Processes of Adaptation

Lisa Wallace

OBJECTIVES

After studying this chapter, you should be able to:

1. Explain the physiologic changes that occur in the respiratory and cardiovascular systems during the transition from fetal to neonatal life.
2. Describe thermoregulation in the newborn.
3. Compare gastrointestinal functioning in the newborn and adult.
4. Explain the causes and effects of hypoglycemia.
5. Describe the steps in bilirubin excretion and the development of physiologic, nonphysiologic, breastfeeding, and true breast milk jaundice.
6. Describe kidney functioning in the newborn.
7. Explain the functioning of the newborn's immune system.
8. Describe the periods of reactivity and the six behavioral states of the newborn.

At birth neonates must make profound physiologic changes to adapt to extrauterine life and meet their own respiratory, digestive, and regulatory needs. This chapter focuses on these changes and provides a foundation for discussion of nursing assessment and care detailed in Chapters 21 and 22.

INITIATION OF RESPIRATIONS

The first vital task the newborn must accomplish is the initiation of respirations. Forces occurring throughout pregnancy and during birth bring about this change.

Development of the Lungs

Beginning around 6 weeks of gestation, the epithelium of the alveoli produces **fetal lung fluid**, which expands the alveoli and is essential for development of the lungs (Jha et al., 2020). Some of the fluid empties from the lungs into the amniotic fluid. The lung fluid is continuously produced at a rate of 4 to 6 mL/kg/hour (Gleason & Juul, 2018). As the fetus nears term, the amount of fetal lung fluid may peak at 25 to 30 mL/kg. Near the end of gestation and during labor this functional reserve capacity (FRC) decreases as production decreases, and the fluid moves into the interstitial spaces, where it is absorbed in preparation for birth (Alhassen et al., 2021). Absorption of lung fluid begins during early labor, and by the time of birth only approximately 35% of the original amount remains (Subramanian et al., 2020). Absorption is accelerated by secretion of fetal epinephrine and corticosteroids but may be delayed by cesarean birth without labor. Approximately one-third of the remaining fetal lung fluid is forced out of the lungs into the upper air passages as the fetal chest is compressed during vaginal birth. The fluid passes out of the mouth or nose as the head emerges from the vagina. The

removal of fetal lung fluid helps reduce pulmonary resistance to blood flow, which is present before birth, and enhances the advent of air breathing.

Surfactant, a slippery, detergent-like combination of lipoproteins, is detectable by 24 to 25 weeks of gestation (Ohning, 2019). Surfactant lines the inside of the alveoli and reduces surface tension, allowing the alveoli to remain partially open when the infant begins to breathe at birth. Without surfactant the alveoli collapse as the infant exhales, resulting in the need to reexpand with each breath, greatly increasing the work of breathing and possibly resulting in atelectasis. By 34 to 36 weeks of gestation, sufficient surfactant is usually produced to prevent respiratory distress syndrome (Gardner et al., 2021). Surfactant secretion increases during labor and immediately after birth to enhance the transition from fetal to neonatal life.

Corticosteroids, such as betamethasone or dexamethasone, administered to a pregnant client at risk for preterm birth within seven (7) days increases surfactant production and speeds maturation of the fetal lungs (American College of Obstetrics and Gynecologists [ACOG], 2020a). The fetus with intrauterine growth restriction or stressed by conditions such as maternal hypertension, heroin addiction, preeclampsia, infection, placental insufficiency, or premature rupture of membranes greater than 48 hours also may have accelerated lung maturation. Infants of clients with diabetes have slower lung maturation (National Health Service, 2018).

Causes of Respirations

At birth, the infant's first breaths must force the remaining fetal lung fluid out of the alveoli and into the interstitial spaces to allow air to enter the lungs. This requires a much larger negative pressure (suction) than subsequent

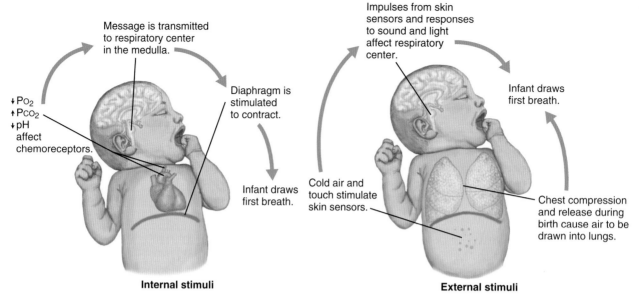

Fig. 20.1 Internal causes of the initiation of respirations are the chemical changes that take place at birth. External causes of respirations include thermal, sensory, and mechanical factors.

breathing. The initial breaths are short deep inspirations followed by long expiratory phases through a partially closed larynx.

Breathing is initiated by chemical, mechanical, thermal, and sensory factors that stimulate the respiratory center in the medulla and trigger respirations (Fig. 20.1).

Chemical Factors

Chemoreceptors in the carotid arteries and the aorta respond to changes in blood chemistry caused by the hypoxemia that occurs with birth. A decrease in the partial pressure of oxygen (Po_2) and pH and an increase in the partial pressure of carbon dioxide (Pco_2) in the blood cause impulses from these receptors to stimulate the respiratory center in the medulla. However, stimulation of the respiratory center and breathing do not occur if prolonged hypoxia causes central nervous system depression.

Mechanical Factors

During a vaginal birth the fetal chest is compressed by the narrow birth canal. When the pressure against the chest is released at birth, recoil of the chest draws a small amount of air into the lungs and helps remove some of the viscous fluid in the airways. This reduces the amount of negative pressure needed for the first breath after birth (Alhassen et al., 2021).

Thermal Factors

The temperature change that occurs with birth also stimulates the initiation of respirations. At birth, the infant moves from the warm, fluid-filled uterus into an environment where the temperature may be much cooler. Sensors in the skin respond to this sudden change in temperature by sending impulses to the medulla that stimulate the respiratory center and breathing.

Sensory Factors

Tactile, visual, auditory, and olfactory stimuli occur during and after birth to stimulate sensors. Nurses hold, dry, and place the infant skin-to-skin with the parent or wrap the infant in blankets, providing further stimulation to skin sensors. The stimulation of the light, sound, smell, and pain at birth also may aid in initiating respirations.

Continuation of Respirations

As the alveoli expand, surfactant allows them to remain partially open between respirations. Approximately 20 to 30 mL of air from the first few breaths remains in the lungs to become the functional residual capacity (FRC) (Ohning, 2019). Within the first hour after birth 80% to 90% of the FRC is established (Ohning, 2019). Because the alveoli remain partially expanded with this residual air, subsequent breaths require much less effort than the first one.

As the infant cries, pressure within the lungs increases, causing any remaining fetal lung fluid to move into the interstitial spaces where it is absorbed by the pulmonary circulatory and lymphatic systems. Complete absorption may take several hours. This explains why the lungs may sound moist when first auscultated but become clear a short time later.

Approximately 10% of newborns require interventions to establish adequate oxygenation at birth (Ohning, 2019). A minimum of one (1) skilled health care professional with the knowledge and skills to perform neonatal resuscitation should be present for every birth (Ohning, 2019).

KNOWLEDGE CHECK

1. How does hypoxemia, a cool room, and infant handling at birth stimulate the newborn to breathe?
2. Why is surfactant important to the newborn's ability to breathe easily?
3. How is fetal lung fluid removed before and after birth?

TABLE 20.1   Circulatory Changes at Birth

Structure	Purpose in Fetal Life	Change at Birth	Cause of Change at Birth	Results of Change at Birth	Time of Functional and Permanent Change
Umbilical vessels	Carry blood from placenta to fetus and back.	Obstruction of blood flow through vessels.	Clamping of cord.	Decreased pressure in RA and increased systemic resistance occur.	*Functional:* Immediately when clamped. *Permanent:* 1–2 week.
Ductus venosus	Shunts one-third of blood from umbilical vein to inferior vena cava and away from immature liver.	Blood flow occluded with end of umbilical circulation.	Occlusion of cord stops flow of blood from placenta through umbilical vein to ductus venosus.	Blood travels through liver to be filtered as in adult circulation.	*Functional:* When cord is clamped, becomes ligamentum venosum.
Foramen ovale	Provides flap valve between RA and LA so blood can bypass nonfunctioning lungs and go directly to LV and aorta; opens in R-to-L direction because of high RA pressure and low LA pressure.	Closes when pressure in LA becomes higher than pressure in RA.	Cord occlusion elevates systemic resistance; blood returns from PV to LA; both increase L heart pressure. Decreased pulmonary resistance allows free flow of blood into lungs and decreased pressure in RA.	Blood entering RA can no longer pass through to LA; instead it goes to RV and through PA to lungs.	Closes at birth because of pressure changes. *Functional:* 3 months but may be longer; becomes fossa ovale.
Pulmonary blood vessels	Narrowed vessels increase resistance to blood flow to lungs.	Dilation of all vessels in lungs.	Elevated blood oxygen and removal of fetal lung fluid.	Decreased pulmonary resistance allows blood to enter freely to be oxygenated.	Beginning with first breath.
Ductus arteriosus	Is widely dilated to carry blood from PA to aorta and avoid nonfunctioning lungs.	Constriction preventing entrance of blood from PA.	Increase of oxygen level in blood.	Blood in PA is directed to lungs for oxygenation.	*Functional:* Beginning within minutes after birth; complete constriction 1–8 days. *Permanent:* 1–4 months; becomes ligamentum arteriosum.

L, Left; *LA,* left atrium; *LV,* left ventricle; *PA,* pulmonary artery; *PV,* pulmonary veins; *R,* right; *RA,* right atrium; *RV,* right ventricle.

CARDIOVASCULAR ADAPTATION: TRANSITION FROM FETAL TO NEONATAL CIRCULATION

During fetal life, three shunts—the ductus venosus, foramen ovale, and ductus arteriosus—carry much of the blood away from the lungs and some blood away from the liver. High pressures within the collapsed, fluid-filled lungs permit only a small amount of blood flow into the narrow pulmonary vessels.

At birth, the shunts close and the pulmonary vessels dilate. These changes occur in response to increases in blood oxygen and shifts in pressure within the heart, pulmonary, and systemic circulations, as well as clamping of the umbilical cord. The functional alterations necessary for transition from fetal to neonatal circulation occur simultaneously within the first few minutes after birth. They are discussed separately here (Table 20.1; see also Fig. 5.9).

As the newborn takes the first breaths at birth, the rise in oxygen concentration causes the ductus arteriosus to constrict, preventing entry of blood from the pulmonary artery. The pulmonary blood vessels respond to the increased oxygenation by dilating. At the same time, fetal lung fluid shifts into the interstitial spaces and is removed by blood and lymph vessels. These changes decrease pulmonary vascular resistance by 80% and allow the vessels to expand to hold the suddenly increased blood flow from the pulmonary arteries.

At birth, pressures between the right and left sides of the heart are reversed. The sudden dilation of the vessels of the lungs allows blood to enter freely from the right ventricle and decreases pressure in the right side of the heart. Clamping of the umbilical cord closes the ductus venosus and further decreases pressure in the right side of the heart. Increased blood flow from the pulmonary veins into the left atrium causes pressure in the left side of the heart to build. Systemic resistance increases as blood flow to the placenta ends with clamping of the cord, and this also elevates pressure in the left heart.

The foramen ovale's flap valve closes when the pressure in the left atrium is higher than that in the right atrium. This change forces the blood from the right atrium into the right ventricle and pulmonary arteries. Because the ductus arteriosus is also closing, the blood continues into the lungs for oxygenation and returns to the left atrium through the pulmonary veins. Blood from the left atrium enters the left ventricle and leaves through the aorta to circulate to the rest of the body. Thus, blood flow through the heart and lungs changes from fetal to neonatal circulation and is similar to that in the adult (see Fig. 5.9).

Conditions such as **asphyxia** (insufficient oxygen and excess carbon dioxide in the blood and tissues) and persistent pulmonary hypertension (see Chapter 25) may reverse the pressures in the heart and cause the foramen ovale to reopen.

The ductus arteriosus closes gradually as oxygenation improves and prostaglandins, which helped keep it open, are metabolized. Complete closure may take 1 to 2 weeks, leaving a small amount of blood shunting through the ductus arteriosus (Ohning, 2019). A murmur may be heard as a result of blood flow through the partially open vessel.

Low levels of oxygen in the blood may lead to dilation of the ductus arteriosus and constriction of the pulmonary vessels, increasing resistance to blood flow to the lungs and pressure in the right side of the heart. The result may be a return to fetal circulation with a significant amount of blood being shunted away from the lungs. The increased pressure in the right side of the heart opens the foramen ovale and allows a right-to-left shunt of blood in the atria. The dilation of the ductus arteriosus allows blood to shunt from the pulmonary artery to the aorta. A patent ductus arteriosus may occur in the infant who experiences asphyxia at birth, becomes hypoxic, or is preterm.

🔍 KNOWLEDGE CHECK

4. What causes the closure of the ductus arteriosus, foramen ovale, and ductus venosus at birth?
5. What causes the pulmonary blood vessels to dilate and the ductus arteriosus to constrict?

NEUROLOGIC ADAPTATION: THERMOREGULATION

At birth the infant must assume **thermoregulation**, the maintenance of body temperature. Although the fetus produces heat in utero, the consistently warm temperature of the amniotic fluid and the mother's body makes thermoregulation unnecessary. The infant's temperature may drop as much as 2°C (1.8°F) within the first seconds up to 30 minutes after birth (Lubkowska et al., 2019). Neonates must produce and maintain enough heat to prevent cold stress, which can have serious and even fatal effects.

Newborn Characteristics that Lead to Heat Loss

Certain characteristics predispose newborns to lose heat. The skin is thin, and blood vessels are close to the surface. Little subcutaneous or white fat is present to provide a barrier to heat loss. Heat is readily transferred from the warmer internal areas of the body to the cooler skin surfaces and then to the surrounding air. Newborns have three times more surface area to body mass than adults, which provides more area for heat loss. Therefore newborns lose heat at a faster rate than adults.

The healthy full-term infant remains in a position of flexion, reducing the amount of skin surface exposed to the surrounding temperatures and decreasing heat loss. Sick or preterm infants have decreased muscle tone and are unable to maintain a flexed position. Preterm infants also have thinner skin and even less white subcutaneous fat than full-term infants. Therefore they are at increased risk for cold stress.

Methods of Heat Loss

Heat is lost in four ways: evaporation, conduction, convection, and radiation (Fig. 20.2). The nurse can prevent heat loss by each method and must be watchful for situations in which intervention is needed.

Evaporation

Evaporation is air-drying of the skin that results in cooling. Drying the infant, especially the head, as quickly as possible helps prevent loss of heat by evaporation. Insensible water loss from the skin and respiratory tract increases heat loss from evaporation.

Conduction

Movement of heat away from the body occurs when newborns have direct contact with objects that are cooler than their skin. Placing infants on cold surfaces or touching them with cool objects causes this type of heat loss. The reverse is also true: Contact with warm objects increases body heat by conduction. Warming objects that will touch the infant decreases heat loss by conduction. Placing the unclothed infant "skin to skin" against the parent (Fig. 20.3) uses conduction to keep the baby warm.

Convection

Transfer of heat from the infant to cooler surrounding air occurs in convection. When infants are in incubators, the circulating warm air helps keep them warm by convection. Providing a warm, draft-free environment avoids convective heat loss.

Radiation

Radiation is the transfer of heat to cooler objects that are not in direct contact with the infant. Infants in incubators transfer heat to the walls of the incubator. If the walls of the

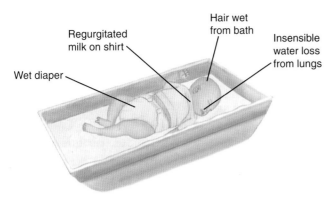

Evaporation can occur during birth or bathing from moisture on skin, as a result of wet linens or clothes, and from insensible water loss.

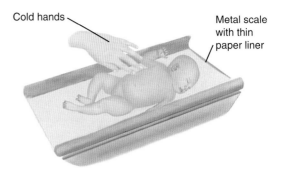

Conduction occurs when the infant comes in contact with cold objects or surfaces such as a scale, a circumcision restraint board, cold hands, or a stethoscope.

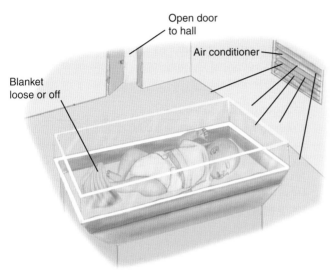

Convection occurs when drafts come from open doors, air conditioning, or even air currents created by people moving about.

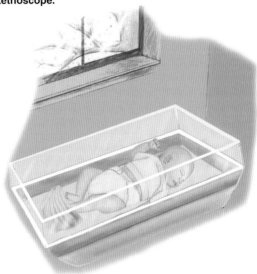

Heat is lost by radiation when the infant is near cold surfaces. Thus heat is lost from the infant's body to the sides of the crib or incubator and to the outside walls and windows.

Fig. 20.2 Methods of Heat Loss.

incubator are cold, the infant is cooled, even when the temperature of the air inside the incubator is warm. To combat this problem, incubators have double walls. Placing cribs and incubators away from windows and outside walls minimizes radiant heat loss. Newborns can gain heat by radiation, too. Using a radiant warmer transfers heat from the warmer to the cooler infant.

CRITICAL TO REMEMBER

Effects of Cold Stress:
Increased oxygen need/hypoxia
Decreased surfactant production
Respiratory distress
Hypoglycemia
Metabolic acidosis
Jaundice

Nonshivering Thermogenesis

Adults have the ability to shiver when cold, which increases muscle activity to produce heat and maintain warmth. Shivering is not an important method of **thermogenesis** (heat production) for newborns who rarely shiver except during prolonged exposure to low temperature (Blackburn, 2018). However, newborns may cry and become restless. This increased activity and their flexed position help generate some warmth and reduce the loss of heat from exposed surface areas. Exposure to cool temperatures also results in peripheral vasoconstriction, decreasing flow of warm blood to the skin. This helps prevent heat loss from the skin and causes the skin to feel cool to the touch.

The newborn's primary method of heat production is **non-shivering thermogenesis** (NST), which involves the metabolism of brown adipose tissue or fat (Ohning, 2019). **Brown fat** (also called *brown adipose tissue [BAT]*) contains a large number of blood vessels, which causes the brown color. Brown fat

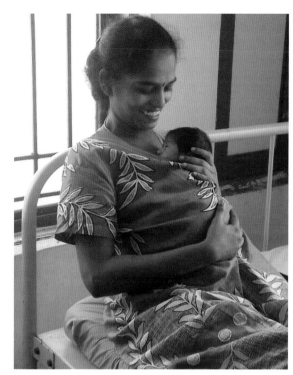

Fig. 20.3 Placing the newborn skin-to-skin with the parent promotes heat transfer by conduction. (From Dr. Arun Babu T: Pediatrics for medical graduates, New Delhi, 2018, Elsevier.)

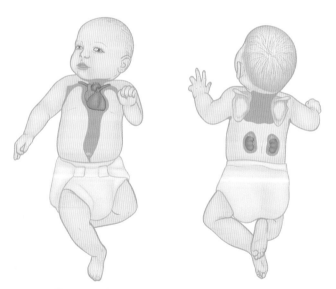

Fig. 20.4 Sites of Brown Fat in the Neonate.

is found primarily around the back of the neck; in the axillae; around the heart, kidneys, and adrenals; between the scapulae; and along the abdominal aorta (Fig. 20.4).

As brown fat is metabolized, it generates more heat than white subcutaneous fat. Blood passing through brown fat is warmed and carries heat to the rest of the body. NST increases the metabolic rate as much a 200% to 300% (Balest, 2021). The metabolism of brown fat uses significant amount of oxygen and glucose and produces acids as a byproduct, increasing the infant's risk for hypoxia, hypoglycemia, and acidosis (Brand & Shippey, 2021).

NST goes into effect when thermoreceptors in the skin detect a skin temperature of 35° to 36°C (95° to 96.8°F) (Blackburn, 2018), before a change occurs in core (interior) body temperature, as measured with a rectal thermometer. Activating thermogenesis before core temperature decreases allows the body to maintain internal heat at an even level. Therefore, NST may begin in an infant when skin temperature has been cooled, even though core measurements show normal readings. A decreased core temperature will not occur until NST is no longer effective.

Some infants have inadequate brown fat stores. Brown fat deposit begins around 26 weeks of gestation and continues throughout the third trimester of pregnancy (Blackburn, 2018; Lubkowska et al., 2019), so preterm infants may be born before adequate stores of brown fat have accumulated. Intrauterine growth restriction may deplete brown fat stores before birth. Hypoxia, hypoglycemia, and acidosis may interfere with the infant's ability to use brown fat to generate heat. These infants are not able to raise their body temperature if they are subjected to cold stress and may have serious complications.

Effects of Cold Stress

Cold stress causes many body changes (Fig. 20.5). The increased metabolic rate and metabolism of brown fat that result from cold stress can cause a significant rise in the need for oxygen. If an infant is having even mild respiratory distress, the problem may be exacerbated if added oxygen is used for heat production. Cold stress also causes a diminished production of surfactant, impeding lung expansion and leading to more respiratory distress.

Glucose is also necessary in larger amounts when the metabolic rate rises to produce heat. When glycogen stores are converted to glucose, they may be quickly depleted, causing hypoglycemia. Continued use of glucose for temperature maintenance leaves less available for growth.

Metabolism of glucose in the presence of insufficient oxygen causes increased production of acids. Metabolism of brown fat also releases fatty acids. The result can be metabolic acidosis, which can be a life-threatening condition. Elevated fatty acids in the blood can interfere with transport of **bilirubin** to the liver, increasing the risk for **jaundice** (yellow discoloration of the skin and sclera caused by excessive bilirubin in the blood).

As the infant's body attempts to conserve heat, vasoconstriction of the peripheral blood vessels occurs to reduce heat loss from the skin surface. Decreased oxygen concentration in the blood, however, also may cause vasoconstriction of the pulmonary vessels, leading to further respiratory distress.

Neutral Thermal Environment

A **neutral thermal environment** is one in which the infant can maintain a stable body temperature with minimal oxygen need and without an increase in metabolic rate. The range of environmental temperature that allows this stability is called the *thermoneutral zone.* In healthy, unclothed, full-term newborns, an environmental temperature of 32 to 33.5°C (89.6 to 92.3°F)

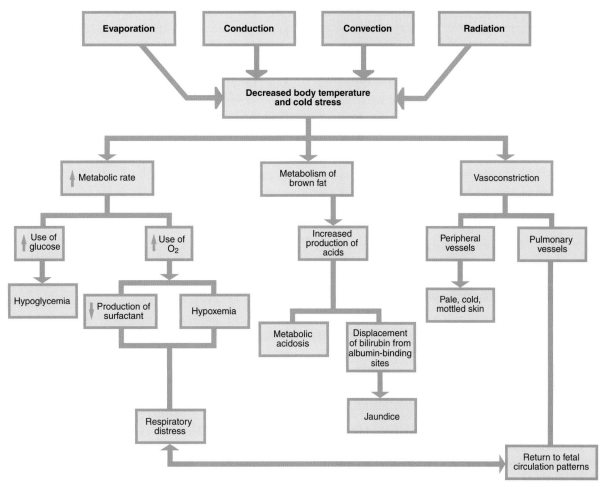

Fig. 20.5 Effects of Cold Stress.

provides a thermoneutral zone. When the infant is dressed, the thermoneutral range is 24° to 27°C (75.2 to 80.6°F) (Blackburn, 2018). The thermoneutral zone for each infant varies according to the infant's gestational age, size, and postnatal age.

Hyperthermia

Infants also respond poorly to hyperthermia. With an elevated temperature the metabolic rate rises, causing an increased need for oxygen and glucose and possible metabolic acidosis. In addition, peripheral vasodilation leads to increased insensible fluid losses. Sweating may occur but is often delayed because sweat glands are immature.

Newborns may be overheated by poorly regulated equipment designed to keep them warm. When radiant warmers, warming lights, or warmed incubators are used, the temperature mechanism must be set to vary the heat according to the infant's skin temperature and thus prevent heat that is too high or too low. Alarms to signal that the infant's temperature is too high or too low should be functioning properly.

⍰ KNOWLEDGE CHECK

6. Why are neonates more prone to heat loss than older children or adults?
7. What are the effects of low temperature in newborns?

HEMATOLOGIC ADAPTATION

Blood Volume

The blood volume of the term newborn is 80 to 100 mL/kg, but this varies according to the time of cord clamping and the gestational age of the infant (ACOG, 2020b). Preterm infants have a greater blood volume per kilogram than term infants. Blood samples drawn from the heel, where the circulation is sluggish, show higher hemoglobin (Hgb), hematocrit (Hct), and erythrocyte values than samples taken from central areas (Blackburn, 2018). Venous blood samples are more accurate and are taken when precise measurement is essential.

The benefits of delayed clamping of the umbilical cord following birth of term and preterm neonates include increased levels of Hgb and iron stores, decreased instances of anemia and blood transfusions, and lower rates of intraventricular hemorrhage (McDonald et al., 2013; Qian, 2019). Milking of the umbilical cord prior to clamping has also demonstrated benefits (Shirk et al., 2019); however, an increased risk of intraventricular hemorrhage among extremely preterm neonates resulted in the early termination of another study (Katheria et al., 2019). Therefore, the ACOG (2020b) recommends delayed cord clamping (30 to 60 seconds) for stable term and preterm newborns but advises against milking for extremely preterm infants (less than 28 weeks' gestation) and

TABLE 20.2 Laboratory Values in the Newborn

Test, Specimen, and Unit of Measurement	Age	Normal Ranges
Hemoglobin, whole blood	Newborn	15–24 g/dL
Hematocrit, whole blood (%)	Newborn	44–70
Leukocytes, whole blood	Birth	9.1–34 (thousand/mm^3)
Leukocyte differential count, whole blood		
Myelocytes (%)		0
Neutrophils ("bands") (%)		3–5
Neutrophils ("segs") (%)		54–62
Lymphocytes (%)		25–33
Monocytes (%)		3–7
Eosinophils (%)		1–3
Basophils (%)		0–0.75
Platelet count, whole blood	Newborn	150–450 (thousand/mm^3)
Glucose, serum (mg/dL)	Cord	45–96
	Newborn at 1 day	40–60
	Newborn >1 day	50–90
Calcium, total serum (mg/dL)	Cord	9–11.5
	3–24 hours	9–10.6
	24–48 hours	7–12
	4–7 days	9–10.9
Magnesium, plasma (mg/dL)	0–6 days	1.2–2.6
Bilirubin (mg/dL)	Cord	<2
Levels are interpreted based on gestational age, risk factors, and hours since birth. See Fig. 20.7.		

Modified from Lo, S. F. (2020). Reference intervals for laboratory tests and procedures. In R.M. Kliegman, J.W. St. Geme III, N.J. Blum, S.S. Shah, R.C. Tasker, K.M. Wilson, & R.E. Behrman (Eds.), *Nelson textbook of pediatrics* (21st ed., p. e5-e12). Elsevier; Pagana, K. D., & Pagana, T. J. (2019). *Mosby's diagnostic and laboratory test reference* (14th ed.). Elsevier Blackburn, S. T. (2018). *Maternal, fetal, and neonatal physiology: A clinical perspective* (5th ed.). Elsevier.

reports insufficient data to support or refute cord milking for neonates born at 32 weeks' gestation or greater (ACOG, 2020b).

Blood Components

Erythrocytes and Hemoglobin

At birth, especially with delayed cord clamping or milking, the infant has comparatively more erythrocytes (red blood cells [RBCs]) than the adult (Adler, 2019). This is necessary because in utero, fetal oxygen exchange is less efficient than the lungs, so the fetus needs additional RBCs (Alden, 2018). Adequate oxygenation of the cells is possible because fetal Hgb (Hgb F) carries a higher affinity to oxygen than adult Hgb (Kauffman et al., 2020). Newborn RBCs have a life span of 80 to 100 days, which is less than adults at 120 days. According to Ianni et al. (2020), newborn Hgb levels decrease approximately 5 g/dL the first 28 days of life. Fetal Hgb is replaced with adult Hgb within the first 6 to 12 months of life (Kauffman et al., 2020). (See Table 20.2 for specific newborn laboratory values.)

Hematocrit

The Hct level in the newborn is 44% to 64% for the first month (Pagana et al., 2019). An abnormal elevated level, defined as Hct >65% indicates **polycythemia** (an abnormally high erythrocyte count), which occurs in 1% to 5% of newborns (Garcia-Prats, 2021). Polycythemia increases the risk for jaundice and injury to the brain and other organs as a result of blood stasis. Respiratory distress and hypoglycemia are more common in these infants.

Leukocytes (White Blood Cells)

A newborn's immune system is immature. Neutrophils (a type of white blood cells [WBCs]) are responsible for killing or attacking bacteria. The WBC count at birth is 9000/mm^3 to 30,000/mm^3 (Pagana et al., 2019). Following birth, the WBCs fall, then increase. By 4 to 5 days after birth, the average WBC stabilizes at 6000/mm^3 to 15,000/mm^3 with a mean of 12,000/mm^3 (Blackburn, 2018). In newborns, an elevated WBC count does not necessarily indicate infection. In fact, the WBC count may decrease in infections. A differential count with a complete blood count will provide information on mature versus immature neutrophils. An increased number of immature leukocytes may be a sign of infection or sepsis in the neonate. The number of platelets (thrombocytes) also may decrease as a result of infections.

Platelets and Risk for Clotting Deficiency

Newborns are at risk for clotting deficiency during the first few days of life because they have low levels of vitamin K, which is necessary to activate several of the clotting factors (factors II [prothrombin], VII, IX, and X). Vitamin K is synthesized in the intestines, but food and normal intestinal flora are necessary for this process. At birth the intestines are sterile and therefore unable to produce vitamin K (Nimavat, 2019). To decrease the risk for hemorrhagic disease of the newborn, vitamin K is administered intramuscularly to most newborns in the United States during initial care. Drugs such as phenytoin (Dilantin), phenobarbital, and antituberculosis drugs taken by the mother during pregnancy interfere with clotting ability in the infant after birth (Blackburn, 2018).

The platelet (thrombocyte) count ranges from 150,000/mm^3 to 450,00/mm^3 (Blackburn, 2018). These platelet counts in term newborns are near adult levels, but their response to stimuli is decreased during the first few days of life.

GASTROINTESTINAL SYSTEM

Newborns must begin to take in, digest, and absorb food after birth because the placenta no longer performs these functions for them.

Stomach

The newborn's stomach capacity is about 6 mL/kg at birth. Gastric emptying may be delayed at first. The gastrocolic reflex is stimulated when the stomach fills, causing increased intestinal peristalsis. Infants frequently pass a stool during or after a feeding. Regurgitation and reflux are common in the newborn due in part to immaturity and relaxation of the lower esophageal sphincter (Blackburn, 2018).

Intestines

The intestines of the newborn are long in proportion to the infant's size and compared with those of the adult. The added length allows more surface area for absorption but makes infants more prone to water loss should diarrhea develop. Air enters the gastrointestinal tract soon after birth, and bowel sounds may be heard beginning within the first hour.

The digestive tract is sterile at birth. Once the infant is exposed to the external environment and begins to take in fluids, bacteria enter the gastrointestinal tract. Normal intestinal flora is established within the first few days of life. Breastfeeding supports the development of an intestinal microbiome (Blackburn, 2018).

Digestive Enzymes

Maturation of the ability to digest and absorb occurs at different rates for various nutrients. Pancreatic amylase, needed to digest complex carbohydrates, is deficient for the first 4 to 6 months after birth (Moore & Townsend, 2019). Amylase is also produced by the salivary glands, but in low amounts until about the third month of life. Amylase is present in breast milk.

The newborn is also deficient in pancreatic lipase, limiting fat absorption significantly. Lipase present in the mouth and stomach helps with some digestion of fat. Lipase is present in breast milk, which may make it more digestible for the newborn than formula. Protein and lactose, the major carbohydrate in the infant's milk diet, are both well digested.

Stools

Meconium is the first stool excreted by the newborn. It consists of particles from amniotic fluid such as vernix, skin cells, and hair, along with cells shed from the intestinal tract, bile, and other intestinal secretions. Meconium is greenish–black with a thick, sticky, tar-like consistency. Colostrum, the first milk produced by the breast, has a laxative effect and promotes the passage of meconium in breastfed infants. The first meconium stool is usually passed within 12 hours of life, and almost all neonates pass meconium within 48 hours (Alden, 2018). If meconium is not passed within that time, obstruction is suspected. Meconium stools are followed by transitional stools, a

---

BOX 20.1   Changes in Stooling Patterns of Newborns

Meconium
- The infant's first stool is composed of amniotic fluid and its constituents, intestinal secretions, shed mucosal cells, and possibly blood (ingested maternal blood or minor bleeding of alimentary tract vessels).
- Passage of meconium should occur within the first 24 to 48 hours, although it can be delayed up to 7 days in very-low-birth-weight infants. The passage of meconium can occur in utero and can be a sign of fetal distress.

Transitional Stools
- Usually appear by third day after initiation of feeding
- Greenish–brown to yellowish–brown; thin and less sticky than meconium; can contain some milk curds

Milk Stool
- Usually appears by the fourth day
- *Breastfed infants:* Stools yellow to golden, pasty in consistency; resemble a mixture of mustard and cottage cheese, with an odor similar to sour milk
- *Formula-fed infants:* Stools pale yellow to light brown, firmer consistency, with a more offensive odor

From Perry, S. E., Lowdermilk, D. L., Cashion, K., Alden, K. R., Olshansky, E. F., & Hockenberry, M. J. (2018). *Maternal child nursing care* (6th ed., p. 536). St. Louis, MO: Elsevier.

---

combination of meconium and milk stools. Transitional stools are greenish or yellowish–brown, of a looser consistency than meconium, and appear around day 3 of life. Milk stool characteristics vary based on the type of feeding given to the infant, and typically occur by about the fourth day of life. Milk stools of breastfed infants are yellow to golden in color, pasty, seedy, and smell like soured milk (Box 20.1). The breastfed infant generally has more frequent stools than the infant who is formula fed. A stool may be passed with each feeding. The breastfed newborn should have two to five stools daily, after the fourth day of life up to 6 weeks (La Leche League International, 2021).

Babies fed commercial formulas have milk stools that are pale yellow to light brown, firmer consistency, and malodorous, characteristic of feces. The infant may excrete several stools daily, or only one or two.

KNOWLEDGE CHECK

8. Why do newborns have higher levels of erythrocytes, hemoglobin, and hematocrit than adults?
9. How do the stools change over the first few days after birth?

HEPATIC SYSTEM

The liver assumes many different functions after birth. Some of the most important include maintenance of blood glucose levels, conjugation of bilirubin, production of factors necessary for blood coagulation, storage of iron, and metabolism of drugs.

Blood Glucose Maintenance

Throughout gestation, glucose is supplied to the fetus by the placenta. During the third trimester, glucose is stored as glycogen primarily in the fetal liver and skeletal muscles for use after birth. These stores are quickly depleted after birth due to stress from delivery and energy needed for respirations, heat production, activity, and transition into extrauterine life.

Until newborns begin regular feedings, and their intake is adequate to meet energy requirements, the glucose present in the body is used. As the blood glucose level falls over the first 1 to 2 hours of life, stored glycogen in the liver is converted to glucose for use. Although the brain can use alternative fuels such as ketones and fatty acids if necessary, glucose is the primary source of energy. Therefore, early initiation of breastfeeding in the first hour of life is recommended. Glucose concentration in the blood commonly falls to the lowest levels by 60 to 90 minutes after birth but rises and stabilizes in 2 to 3 hours after birth (Blackburn, 2018).

There is no consensus about the level of glucose defined as hypoglycemia. However, in the term infant, it is suggested that target glucose levels should be greater than 45 to 50 mg/dL prior to routine feedings (American Academy of Pediatrics [AAP] & ACOG, 2017; Abramowski et al., 2020; Sandberg, 2019). The need for intervention should be individualized based on the newborn's clinical situation and individual characteristics rather than a specific plasma glucose concentration (AAP & ACOG, 2017).

Many newborns are at increased risk for hypoglycemia. In the preterm, late preterm (born between 34 weeks and 36^{6/7} weeks of gestation), and small-for-gestational-age infant, adequate stores of glycogen or even fat for metabolism may not have accumulated. Stores may be used up before birth in the postterm infant because of poor intrauterine nourishment from a deteriorating placenta. Infants who are large for gestational age and those with diabetic mothers may produce excessive insulin that consumes available glucose quickly.

Infants exposed to stressors such as asphyxia or infection may exhaust their stores of glycogen. The cold-stressed infant may deplete glycogen to increase metabolism and raise body temperature.

Conjugation of Bilirubin

A major function of the liver in the newborn is conjugation of bilirubin (Fig. 20.6). The newborn's liver may not be mature enough to prevent jaundice during the first week of life. Jaundice results from **hyperbilirubinemia**, excessive

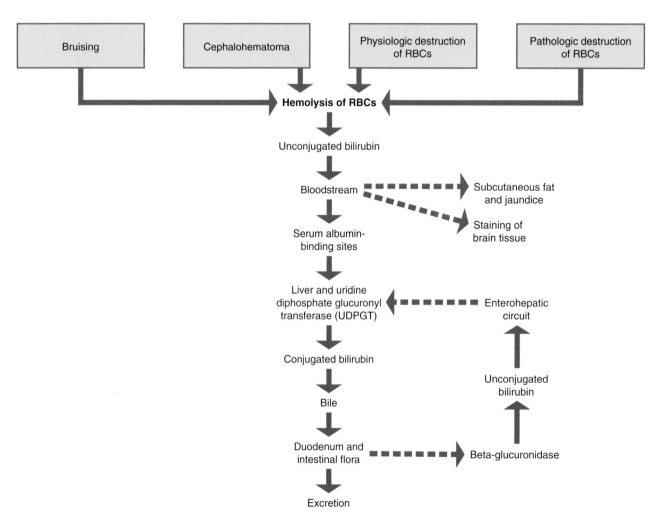

Fig. 20.6 Sources of Bilirubin and How It Is Removed from the Body. *RBCs,* Red blood cells.

bilirubin in the blood, and occurs in 60% of term newborns and 80% of preterm infants (Alden, 2018; Bratton et al., 2021).

Source and Effect of Bilirubin

The principal source of bilirubin is the hemolysis of erythrocytes (RBCs). This is a normal occurrence after birth when fewer erythrocytes are needed than during fetal life. The breakdown of RBCs releases their components into the bloodstream to be reused by the body. Bilirubin remains as an unusable residue in the blood. This substance is toxic to the body and must be excreted.

Bilirubin is released in an unconjugated form. Unconjugated bilirubin, also called *indirect bilirubin,* is soluble in fat but not in water. Before excretion can occur, the liver must change it to a water-soluble form by a process called *conjugation.* The bilirubin is then known as *conjugated* or *direct bilirubin.* Conjugated bilirubin is not toxic to the body and can be excreted.

Because unconjugated bilirubin is fat soluble, it may be absorbed by the subcutaneous fat, causing the yellowish discoloration of the skin called *jaundice.* If enough unconjugated bilirubin accumulates in the blood, staining of the tissues in the brain may occur. This may cause acute **bilirubin encephalopathy**, a neurologic condition resulting from bilirubin toxicity. If this condition becomes chronic, it causes permanent neurologic injury known as **kernicterus**. The level of bilirubin necessary to cause injury to the central nervous system is unknown and may be different for various infants.

Normal Conjugation

When unconjugated bilirubin is released into the bloodstream, it attaches to binding sites on albumin in the plasma and is carried to the liver. If an adequate number of albumin-binding sites are not available, bilirubin circulates as unbound or free unconjugated bilirubin. Bilirubin can be displaced from albumin by some medications. Free fatty acids, acidosis, and infection also decrease albumin binding of bilirubin (Alden, 2018). It is the free, unbound unconjugated bilirubin that can move into the tissues and cross the blood–brain barrier.

When the albumin-bound bilirubin reaches the liver, it is changed to the conjugated form of bilirubin by the enzyme uridine diphosphate glucuronyl transferase (UDPGT). Conjugated bilirubin is excreted into the bile and then into the duodenum. In the intestines the normal flora act to reduce bilirubin to urobilinogen and stercobilin, which are excreted in the stools. Some urobilinogen is excreted by the kidneys.

A small percentage of conjugated bilirubin may be deconjugated, or converted back to the unconjugated state, by the intestinal enzyme beta-glucuronidase. This enzyme is important in fetal life because only unconjugated bilirubin can be cleared by the placenta for conjugation by the mother's liver. In the newborn, deconjugated bilirubin in the intestines is reabsorbed into the portal circulation and carried back to the liver, where it again undergoes the conjugation process. This recirculation of bilirubin is called the *enterohepatic circuit,* and it creates additional work for the liver.

Blood tests for bilirubin measure total serum bilirubin (TSB) and direct (conjugated) bilirubin in the serum. TSB is a combination of indirect (unconjugated) and direct bilirubin.

Factors in Increased Bilirubin

A number of factors lead to the production of excessive amounts of bilirubin or interfere with the normal process of conjugation. These increase the incidence of jaundice during the first week of life (Table 20.3).

Physiologic and Nonphysiologic Hyperbilirubinemia

Physiologic Jaundice

Physiologic jaundice, also called *nonpathologic* or *developmental jaundice,* is a transient hyperbilirubinemia (excess bilirubin in the blood) and is considered normal, occurring in about 60% of term newborns. Physiologic jaundice is not present during the first 24 hours of life in the term infant but appears on the second or third day after birth. In term newborns, the TSB level gradually increases following birth, peaks between day 2 and 4 of age, then decreases to normal levels by day 5 to 7. Yellowish color of the skin and sclera (jaundice) becomes visible when the bilirubin level is greater than 6 to 7 mg/dL (Alden, 2018). The rate at which the bilirubin level in the blood rises and falls is important because it helps determine whether the rate for a particular infant is following the expected curve for age and birth weight. Since newborns excrete bilirubin through feces, early initiation of feedings is vital to decrease the risk of hyperbilirubinemia. Physiologic jaundice often resolves with adequate, frequent feedings and requires no additional interventions. Clinicians may use the BiliTool for infants >35 weeks of gestation developed by the AAP to determine risk based on the level and age in hours of the infant, guiding clinician interventions (Fig. 20.7).

Nonphysiologic Jaundice

Jaundice that is physiologic or normal must be differentiated from nonphysiologic or pathologic jaundice. One of the most important differences is the time at which jaundice appears. Pathologic jaundice may occur in the first 24 hours. When bilirubin rises higher or more rapidly than expected or stays elevated for longer than expected, earlier treatment is needed to prevent severe hyperbilirubinemia.

Nonphysiologic jaundice is a result of abnormalities causing excessive destruction of RBCs or problems in bilirubin conjugation. These include incompatibilities between the mother's and the infant's blood types, infection, and metabolic disorders. Nonphysiologic jaundice is often treated with phototherapy.

Charts such as the BiliTool (see Fig. 20.7) are available that show the rise and fall of bilirubin and the degree of risk at various levels of TSB according to the age of the infant in hours. For example, a full-term infant with no complications who is 24 hours old is considered at low risk if the TSB is 5 mg/dL or less and at high risk if the TSB is greater than 8 mg/dL. At 48 hours of age, that infant would be at low risk if the TSB was 8.5 mg/dL but high risk if the TSB was that high before 48

TABLE 20.3   Factors Contributing to Hyperbilirubinemia

Gestational age	• Preterm and late preterm infants have more immature conjugation abilities.
Excessive bilirubin production	• Newborns produce bilirubin at 8–10 mg/kg, which is twice the rate of an adult • Newborns have excessive production for 3–6 weeks after birth
Red blood cells	• More RBCs than adults per kg • Fetal RBCs break down faster than adult RBCs • Fetal RBCs lifespan is shorter than adults (term infants: 80–100 days; preterm infants 60–80 days) • Fetal RBCs more susceptible to injury
Albumin	• Lack of albumin-binding sites to bind bilirubin • Newborns have decreased affinity to bind to bilirubin than adults.
Liver immaturity	• Newborns may not produce adequate amounts of UDPGT and other substances the first few days of life, limiting the amount of bilirubin conjugated.
Blood incompatibility	• Rh, ABO, or other incompatible blood between the mother and the infant may increase RBC breakdown.
Gastrointestinal factors	• Breastfeeding • At birth the intestines of the newborn are sterile, and conjugated bilirubin cannot be reduced to urobilinogen or stercobilin for excretion without the action of intestinal flora • Newborn intestines have a large amount of the enzyme beta-glucuronidase, which changes bilirubin back to the unconjugated state • Intestinal motility is decreased, allowing more time for the enzyme to act, leading to higher levels of unconjugated bilirubin that may be reabsorbed into the circulating blood • Delayed or inadequate feeding interferes with the establishment of intestinal flora and prolongs the time until passage of meconium, which is high in bilirubin. Delayed passage of stool increases exposure time to beta-glucuronidase and the opportunity for conjugated bilirubin to convert back to the unconjugated state and reabsorb into the blood.
Birth trauma	• Cephalohematoma or bruising during birth can cause increased hemolysis of RBCs adding to a higher bilirubin level.
Fatty acids	• Cold stress, causing the metabolism of brown fat, and asphyxia with anaerobic metabolism produce free fatty acids. Fatty acids have a greater affinity than bilirubin for the binding sites on albumin and bind to albumin in place of bilirubin, increasing the level of unbound unconjugated bilirubin that cannot be excreted.
Maternal risk factors	• Asian, American Indian, or Native Alaskan ethnicity • Previous child who had jaundice • Diabetes • Preeclampsia • Sulfisoxazole taken during pregnancy
Other neonatal risk factors	• Male gender • Swallowing blood during birth process. • Hypoglycemia • Infection/sepsis • Hemolytic anemias

Alden, K. R. (2018). Physiologic and behavioral adaptations of the newborn. In Perry, S. E., Lowdermilk, D. L., Cashion, K., Alden, K. R., Olshansky, E. F., & Hockenberry, M. J. *Maternal child nursing care* (6th ed., pp. 462–479). St. Louis, MO: Elsevier; Blackburn, S. T. (2018). *Maternal, fetal, and neonatal physiology: A clinical perspective* (5th ed.). St. Louis, MO: Saunders.

hours. Infants who are preterm or late preterm or who have other risk factors may receive treatment for hyperbilirubinemia at lower TSB levels than full-term infants.

Jaundice Associated with Breastfeeding

Jaundice occurs more frequently in breastfeeding versus bottle fed infants (Bratton et al., 2020).

Breastfeeding or Early Onset Jaundice. The most common cause of jaundice in breastfed infants is insufficient intake. Jaundice begins within the first week of life, and serum bilirubin may reach dangerous levels if intake is not increased.

Infants who are sleepy, have a poor suck, or nurse infrequently may not receive enough colostrum—the substance that precedes true breast milk—to benefit from its laxative effect in eliminating bilirubin-rich meconium. When meconium is not eliminated, the bilirubin may be deconjugated by beta-glucuronidase in the intestine, absorbed and recirculated to the liver for conjugation again.

Lack of adequate suckling depresses production of breast milk and increases the problem further. Helping the client with breastfeeding to increase the infant's intake and stimulate milk production may be the most important treatment. Supplementing with formula interferes with the client's milk production. However, if breastfeeding is inadequate and the infant is dehydrated or losing excessive weight, supplements of expressed breast milk or formula may be necessary. Glucose-water will not reduce bilirubin levels and should be avoided.

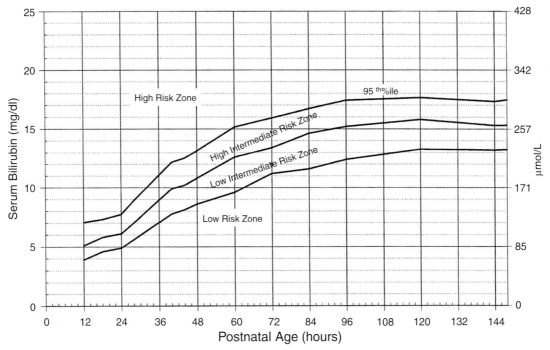

Fig. 20.7 BiliTool. (From American Academy of Pediatrics Subcommittee on Hyperbilirubinemia. (2004). Management of hyperbilirubinemia in the newborn infant 35 or more weeks of gestation. *Pediatrics, 114*(1), 297–316. doi: 10.1542/peds.114.1.297.)

True Breast Milk Jaundice. True breast milk jaundice, also called *late-onset breast milk jaundice,* occurs after the first 3 to 5 days of life. It lasts 3 weeks to as long as 3 months for some infants. The TSB usually peaks at 5 to 10 mg/dL and falls gradually over several months.

The exact cause of true breast milk jaundice is unknown. Substances in the breast milk may increase absorption of bilirubin from the intestine or interfere with conjugation. Infants have no signs of illness.

Treatment of breast milk jaundice includes close monitoring of TSB and at least 8 to 12 feedings each 24 hours. If bilirubin levels become too high, phototherapy is begun while the client continues frequent breastfeeding. Interruption of breastfeeding is generally not recommended. However, if the TSB levels are dangerously high, the health care provider may order formula feeding be given for 1 to 3 days while the client uses a breast pump to maintain milk supply. Temporarily switching to formula causes a rapid drop in bilirubin level. If the level rises while breastfeeding is interrupted, jaundice from another cause should be investigated. The level may rise again when breastfeeding is resumed but generally not high enough to interfere with further breastfeeding.

Blood Coagulation

Prothrombin and coagulation factors II, VII, IX, and X are produced by the liver and activated by vitamin K, which is deficient in the newborn.

Iron Storage

Iron is stored in the fetal liver and spleen during the last weeks of pregnancy. Full-term infants who are breastfeeding usually do not need added iron until 4 to 6 months of age. The AAP recommends 1 mg/kg iron supplementation starting at 4 months of age for breastfeeding infants; infants who are not breastfeeding should be given iron-fortified formula (AAP, 2016).

Metabolism of Drugs

The liver metabolizes drugs inefficiently in the newborn. This must be considered when drugs are given to the neonate. In addition, a breastfeeding client should alert the primary caregiver before taking medications because harmful amounts may be transferred to the infant via the breast milk.

> **? KNOWLEDGE CHECK**
>
> 10. Why is hypoglycemia a problem for the newborn?
> 11. Why are infants more likely than adults to become jaundiced?
> 12. What are the differences among physiologic, nonphysiologic, and breast milk jaundice?

URINARY SYSTEM

Kidney Development

By 34 to 35 weeks of gestation, the fetal kidneys have as many nephrons as adult kidneys (Hill, 2021). Blood flow to the kidneys increases after birth, and resistance in the renal vessels decreases. The improved perfusion results in a steady

BOX 20.2 Daily Intake and Output in the Newborn

First 3 to 5 Days of Life
Intake: 60 to 100 mL/kg (27 to 45 mL/lb)
Output: At least 1 or 2 voidings

After the First 3 to 5 Days
Intake: 150 to 175 mL/kg (68 to 80 mL/lb)
Output: At least 6 voidings by day 4

improvement in kidney function during the first few days of life.

Kidney Function

The placenta serves as the filtering system for the fetus while in utero. At birth, the newborn's kidney function is immature compared with that of the adult. The ability of the glomeruli to filter and the renal tubules to reabsorb is considerably less than in adults. The glomerular filtration rate increases rapidly. By 2 weeks of age, it has doubled but does not reach adult levels until 2 years of age (Blackburn, 2018). Therefore, infants have a decreased ability to remove waste products from the blood.

Small amounts of substances such as glucose and amino acids may escape into the urine of the neonate (Blackburn, 2018). They disappear within the first few days of life as kidney function improves. Uric acid crystals may give a reddish color to the urine that is sometimes mistaken for blood.

The average time for the first void is 7 to 9 hours after birth; most newborns will void within 24 hours and will void at least twice between 24 and 48 hours of life (Consolini, 2019). Failure to void within that time may be a result of hypovolemia from inadequate intake of fluids. Absence of kidneys or anomalies that interfere with excretion of urine are usually discovered before birth because they cause oligohydramnios (low amniotic fluid volume). This generally prompts investigation into the cause during pregnancy. Only one or two voids may occur during the first 2 days of life, although a higher number is common. In the term newborn, at least six voids per day by the fourth day indicates adequate fluid intake.

Fluid Balance

Newborns have a lower tolerance for changes in total volume of body fluid than do older infants. This is because of the location of water within the newborn's body and the inability of the kidneys to adapt to large changes in fluid volume. In addition, the fluid turnover rate is greater than that in adults. To maintain fluid balance, full-term infants need 60 to 100 mL/kg (27 to 45 mL/lb) daily during the first 3 to 5 days of life and then 150 to 175 mL/kg (68 to 80 mL/lb) (Bell, 2021) (Box 20.2).

Water Distribution

Seventy-eight percent of the newborn's body is composed of water. Intracellular water constitutes 34% of the body, and extracellular water makes up 44% of the body

(Blackburn, 2018). Because infants have more fluid for their size than adults, and because a larger proportion of it is located outside the cells, total body water is easily depleted. Conditions such as vomiting and diarrhea can quickly result in life-threatening dehydration.

Newborns diurese extracellular fluid the first week of life. This amount contributes to a weight loss in term infants up to 7% and up to 20% in preterm infants (Thulier, 2017). Term newborn weight loss greater than 10% needs investigation and intervention.

Insensible Water Loss

Water lost from the skin and respiratory tract contributes to insensible water loss. Insensible water losses are increased in the newborn because of the large surface area of the body and the rapid respiratory rate. Fluid losses increase greatly when infants are placed under radiant warmers or phototherapy lights, which accelerate evaporation from the skin. An elevated respiratory rate or low humidity in the air surrounding the infant raises insensible water losses even further.

Urine Dilution and Concentration

The ability of a newborn's kidneys to dilute urine is similar to that of adults, but they have less responsiveness to antidiuretic hormone (ADH), which influences their ability to concentrate urine (Bell, 2021). However, a newborn's kidneys cannot handle large increases in fluids, which result in fluid overload. This is most likely to happen if infants receive too much intravenous fluid. After the fourth day of age, expected urine output is 2 to 5 mL/kg/hour, and urine-specific gravity is 1.002 to 1.01 (Nyp et al., 2021). When abnormal conditions such as diarrhea cause excessive loss of fluid, the newborn's limited ability to conserve water may result in dehydration more quickly than in the older infant or child.

Acid–Base and Electrolyte Balance

The maintenance of acid–base and electrolyte balance is a primary function of the kidneys and may be precarious in neonates. Newborns tend to lose bicarbonate at lower levels than adults, increasing their risk for metabolic acidosis. The excretion of solutes also is less efficient in newborns. Although newborns conserve needed sodium well, they are limited in excretion of sodium (Blackburn, 2018). This is especially a problem if they receive excessive amounts.

IMMUNE SYSTEM

The neonate is less effective in fighting infection than the older infant or child. Leukocytes are delayed in moving to the site of invasion and are inefficient in destroying the invader. The infant's decreased ability to localize infection leads to a tendency toward generalized sepsis.

Fever and leukocytosis, which occur during infection of the older child, are often not present in the newborn with infection. This lack of response occurs because the hypothalamus and inflammatory responses are immature. Nonspecific signs such as changes in activity, color, tone, or feeding may be the only signs of sepsis.

Because of their immature immune system, infants are susceptible to some pathogens that do not usually affect older children. Full-term newborns receive antibodies across the placenta during the last trimester of pregnancy. The client continues to provide passive antibodies to the infant through milk if breastfeeding. Immunoglobulins (serum globulins with antibody activity) help protect the newborn from infection. The major immunoglobulins are IgG, IgM, and IgA, each of which performs a different function. The most abundant circulating antibodies in the newborn are IgG, which aid in providing adequate antimicrobial protection the first 3 months of life (Alden, 2018).

Immunoglobulin G

Only immunoglobulin G (IgG) crosses the placenta, with passage beginning in the first trimester. Preterm infants have less IgG because transfer is greatest during the third trimester. IgG provides the fetus with passive temporary immunity to bacteria, bacterial toxins, and viruses to which the mother has developed immunity. The full-term infant has IgG levels that are as high as or higher than those of the mother (Pierzynowska et al., 2020).

Although the fetus makes some IgG, significant production of IgG is delayed until after 6 months of age (Pierzynowska et al., 2020). The infant gradually produces larger quantities of the immunoglobulin to replace IgG from the mother, which is being catabolized. The passive immunity gradually disappears, reaching the lowest level at 2 to 4 months of age (Albrecht & Arck, 2020).

Immunoglobulin M

Immunoglobulin M (IgM) is the first immunoglobulin produced by the body when the newborn is challenged. This immunoglobulin helps protect against Gram-negative bacteria. Rapid production of IgM begins a few days after birth as a result of exposure to environmental antigens. IgM cannot cross the placenta because the molecules are too large. If IgM is found in cord blood, exposure to infection in utero has occurred. IgM level match adult levels by 2 years of age (Alden, 2018).

Immunoglobulin A

Immunoglobulin A (IgA) also does not cross the placenta and must be produced by the infant. IgA is important in protection of the gastrointestinal and respiratory systems, and newborns are particularly susceptible to infections of those systems. Secretory IgA is present in colostrum and breast milk (Crider, 2020). Therefore, breastfed infants may receive protection that formula-fed infants do not.

? KNOWLEDGE CHECK

13. How does the distribution of fluid in the newborn compare with that in the adult?
14. Why are IgG, IgM, and IgA important to the newborn?

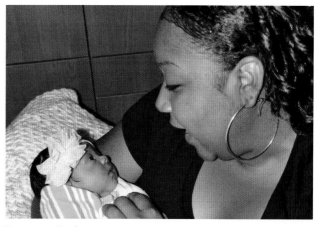

Fig. 20.8 En face position with the faces of the parent and infant about 20 cm apart and on the same plane encourages early eye contact. (From Lowdermilk, D.L., Cashion, M. C., Perry, S., et al. (2020). Maternity and women's health care (12th edition). St. Louis: Elsevier.)

PSYCHOSOCIAL ADAPTATION

Periods of Reactivity

In the early hours after birth, the infant goes through changes called *periods of reactivity* (Keehn & Lieben, 2020). The two periods of reactivity are separated by a period of sleep or decreased activity (Gardner & Niermeyer, 2021).

First Period of Reactivity

The **first period of reactivity** begins at birth and lasts for 30 minutes. Infants are active at this time and appear wide awake, alert, and interested in their surroundings (Keehn & Lieben, 2020). Parents enjoy watching the infant gaze directly at them when held in the en face (face-to-face) position (Fig. 20.8). Newborns move their arms and legs energetically, root, and appear hungry. A vigorous suck reflex is usually present; many newborns latch on to the nipple and suck well.

The temperature may be decreased during this period. Respirations may be as high as 80 breaths per minute. The heart rate may be elevated to 180 beats per minute (Gardner & Niermeyer, 2021). During this period, the lungs may sound wet; nasal flaring or retractions may be present, especially if the baby was born by cesarean section. The pulse and respiratory rates gradually slow, and the infant becomes sleepy.

Period of Sleep or Decreased Activity

After the first period of reactivity, infants become quieter or fall into a deep sleep. During this time the pulse and respirations drop into the normal range. Bowel sounds are audible, and meconium may be passed. This period usually lasts at 2 to 4 hours (Keehn & Lieben, 2020).

Second Period of Reactivity

The **second period of reactivity** lasts 2 to 5 hours as the infant awakes from the deep sleep (Keehn & Lieben, 2020). Infants have alert periods, and parents may enjoy the opportunity to get to know their infant at this time. Infants become interested in feeding and may pass meconium. There may be tachycardia and rapid respirations. Mucous secretions increase, and infants may gag or regurgitate.

Behavioral States

Six gradations in the behavioral state of the infant have been identified, ranging from quiet sleep to crying (Gardner & Goldson, 2021). The amount of time infants spend in the different sleep–wake states varies and is a key to their individuality.

Deep or Quiet Sleep State

During the quiet sleep state, the infant is in a deep sleep with closed eyes and no eye movements. Respirations are quiet, regular, and slower than in the other states. Although startles occur at intervals, the infant's body is quiet. The infant is very difficult to arouse and will not feed.

Light or Active Sleep State

The active sleep state is a lighter sleep in which the infant's eyes are closed. The infant moves its extremities, stretches, changes facial expressions, makes sucking movements, and may fuss briefly. During this period, respirations tend to be more rapid and irregular and rapid eye movements occur. The infant is more likely to startle from noise or disturbances and may return to sleep or move to an awake state.

Drowsy State

The drowsy state is a transitional period between sleep and waking similar to that experienced by adults as they awaken. The eyes may remain closed or, if open, appear glazed and unfocused. The infant startles and moves extremities slowly. The infant may go back to sleep or, with gentle stimulation, gradually awaken.

Quiet Alert State

The quiet alert state (also called *alert inactivity*) should be pointed out to parents because it is an excellent time to increase bonding. The infant focuses on objects or people, responds to the parents with intense gazing, and seems bright and interested in its surroundings. The infant responds to stimuli and interaction with others. Body movements are minimal as the infant seems to concentrate on the environment.

Active Alert State

In the active alert state, the infant seems restless, has increased motor movements, and may be fussy. The infant has faster and more irregular respirations, may hiccup or regurgitate, and seems more aware of feelings of discomfort from hunger or cold. Although the eyes may be open, the infant seems less focused on visual stimuli than during the quiet alert state.

Crying State

The crying state may quickly follow the active alert state if no intervention occurs to comfort the infant. The cries are continuous and lusty, active body movement occurs, and the infant does not respond positively to stimulation. Respirations are irregular and rapid. It may take a period of comforting to move the infant to a state in which feeding or other activities can be accomplished.

KNOWLEDGE CHECK

15. Describe the behaviors of newborns during the first and second periods of reactivity.
16. How do infant behavioral states vary?

SUMMARY CONCEPTS

- Chemical, mechanical, thermal, and sensory factors combine to stimulate the respiratory center in the brain and initiate respirations at birth.
- Surfactant lines the alveoli and reduces surface tension to keep the alveoli open. Fetal lung fluid moves into the interstitial spaces before, during, and after birth and is absorbed by the lymphatic and vascular systems.
- Increases in blood oxygen levels, shifts in pressure in the heart and lungs, and clamping of the umbilical vessels cause closure of the ductus arteriosus, foramen ovale, and ductus venosus at birth.
- Neonates must produce and maintain heat (thermogenesis) to prevent the effects of cold stress.
- Infants are predisposed to heat loss because they have thin skin with little subcutaneous (white) fat, blood vessels close to the surface, and a large skin surface area. They lose heat by evaporation, conduction, convection, and radiation.

- Heat is produced in newborns by increased activity, flexion, and metabolism; vasoconstriction; and nonshivering thermogenesis. These factors increase oxygen and glucose consumption and may cause respiratory distress, hypoglycemia, acidosis, and jaundice.
- Laboratory values for erythrocytes, hemoglobin, and hematocrit are higher for newborns than for adults because less oxygen is available in fetal life than after birth.
- The stools progress from thick, greenish–black meconium to loose, greenish–brown transitional stools to milk stools. Stools of breastfed infants are frequent, soft, seedy, and mustard-colored. Those of formula-fed infants are pale yellow to light brown, firmer, and less frequent.
- The neonate uses glucose rapidly and is at risk for hypoglycemia. Infants at an increased risk for hypoglycemia include those who are preterm, late preterm, small for gestational age, large for gestational age, born to diabetic mothers, or exposed to stressors.

- Physiologic jaundice occurs in newborns after the first 24 hours of life as a result of hemolysis of red blood cells and immaturity of the liver. Nonphysiologic (pathologic) jaundice begins within the first 24 hours and often requires treatment with phototherapy. Breastfeeding jaundice is often caused by insufficient intake. True breast milk jaundice begins later than physiologic jaundice and may be caused by substances in the milk.
- The newborn's kidneys filter, reabsorb, and maintain fluid and electrolyte balance less efficiently than the adult's kidneys. The newborn's body is composed of a greater percentage of water, with more located in the extracellular compartment, and fluid is more easily lost.
- Newborns receive passive immunity when immunoglobulin G crosses the placenta in utero. After birth, immunoglobulins M and A are produced to protect against infection.
- During the first and second periods of reactivity, newborns are active and alert and may be interested in feeding. They may have a low temperature, elevated pulse and respiratory rates, and excessive secretions.
- Newborns progress through six behavioral states: quiet sleep, active sleep, drowsy, quiet alert, active alert, and crying.

Clinical Judgment And Next-Generation NCLEX® Examination-Style Questions

1. The nurse is assessing a newborn. Vital signs: temperature 98.0°F, heart rate 130 bpm, and respirations 40. The skin has a slightly yellow color. **Choose the most likely options for the information missing from the statement below by selecting from the lists of options provided.** The nurse recognizes that _____1_____, _____2_____ and _____3_____ increase the risk of nonphysiologic (pathologic) jaundice.

Options for 1	Options for 2	Options for 3
Birth weight greater than 8 lb.	Maternal/newborn blood incompatibilities	Caucasian race
Preterm gestation	Effective breastfeeding	Vacuum-assisted birth
24 hours or more since birth	Formula feeding	Cesarean birth

2. A 6-lb 24-oz, 38-week estimated gestational age (EGA) female was born 1 hour ago following an uncomplicated pregnancy, labor, and birth.
   Place an "X" to indicate if the nursing action is indicated (appropriate or necessary), contraindicated (could be harmful), or nonessential (makes no difference or not necessary) to promoting neonatal thermoregulation.

	Indicated	Contraindicated	Nonessential
Place skin to skin with parents			
Keep infant, clothing, and linens dry			
Place bassinet next to window			
Prewarm objects before they touch the newborn			
Leave the door to the room open with the bassinet in sight so nursing staff can see the newborn as they pass by.			

REFERENCES & READINGS

Abramowski, A., Ward, R., & Hamdan, A. H. (2020). Neonatal hypoglycemia. In *StatPearls*. StatPearls Publishing. https://www.ncbi.nlm.nih.gov/books/NBK537105/.

Adler, L. C. (2019). *Polycythemia-newborn*. National Institution of Health U.S. National Library of Medicine (Medline Plus). https://medlineplus.gov/ency/article/000536.htm.

Albrecht, M., & Arck, P. C. (2020). Vertically transferred immunity in neonates: Mothers, mechanisms, and mediators. *Frontiers in Immunology*, 11, 555. https://doi.org/10.3389/fimmu.2020.00555.

Alden, K. R. (2018). Physiologic and behavioral adaptations of the newborn. In S. E. Perry, D. L. Lowdermilk, K. Cashion, K. R. Alden, E. F. Olshansky, & M. J. Hockenberry (Eds.), *Maternal child nursing care* (6th ed., pp. 462–479). Elsevier.

Alhassen, Z., Vali, P., Guglani, L., Lakshminrusimha, S., & Ryan, R. M. (2021). Recent advances in pathophysiology and management of transient tachypnea of newborn. *Journal of Perinatology*, 41, 6–16. https://doi.org/10.1038/s41372-020-0757-3.

American Academy of Pediatrics. (2016). *Vitamin D & iron supplements for babies: AAP recommendations. Healthychildren. org*. https://www.healthychildren.org/English/ages-stages/baby/feeding-nutrition/Pages/Vitamin-Iron-Supplements.aspx.

American Academy of Pediatrics & American College of Obstetricians and Gynecologists (AAP & ACOG). (2017). *Guidelines for perinatal care* (8th ed.).

American Academy of Pediatrics Subcommittee on Hyperbilirubinemia. (2004). Management of hyperbilirubinemia in the newborn infant 35 or more weeks of gestation. *Pediatrics, 114*(1), 297–316. https://doi.org/10.1542/peds.114.1.297.

American College of Obstetrics and Gynecologists. (2020a). *Delayed umbilical clamping after birth.* ACOG Committee Opinion 814.

American College of Obstetrics and Gynecologists. (2020b). *Antenatal corticosteroid therapy for fetal maturation.* ACOG Committee Opinion 713. Published 2017, reaffirmed 2020.

Balest, A. L. (2021). *Hypothermia in neonates.* Merck Manual Professional Version. https://www.merckmanuals.com/professional/pediatrics/perinatal-problems/hypothermia-in-neonates.

Brand, M. C., & Shippey, H. A. (2021). Thermoregulation. In M. T. Verklan, M. Walden, & S. Forest (Eds.), *Core curriculum for neonatal intensive care nursing* (6th ed., pp. 86–98). Elsevier.

Bell, S. G. (2021). Fluid and electrolyte management. In *Core curriculum for neonatal intensive care nursing* (6th ed., pp. 131–143). Elsevier.

Blackburn, S. T. (2018). *Maternal, fetal & neonatal physiology* (5th ed.). Elsevier.

Bratton, S., Cantu, R. M., & Stern, M. (2021). Breast milk jaundice. In *StatPearls*. StatPearls Publishing. https://pubmed.ncbi.nlm.nih.gov/30726019/.

Consolini, D. (2019). Evaluation and care of the normal neonate. *Merck Manual Professional Version.* https://www.merckmanuals.com/professional/pediatrics/care-of-newborns-and-infants/evaluation-and-care-of-the-normal-neonate.

Crider, C. (2020). *Breast milk antibodies and their magic benefits. Healthline Parenthood.* https://www.healthline.com/health/breastfeeding/breast-milk-antibodies.

Garcia-Prats, J. A. (2021). *Neonatal polycythemia. UpToDate.* https://www.uptodate.com/contents/neonatal-polycythemia.

Gardner, S. L., Enzman-Hines, M., & Nyp, M. (2021). Respiratory diseases. In S. L. Gardner, B. S. Carter, M. Enzman-Hineset, et al. (Eds.), *Merenstein & Gardner's handbook of neonatal intensive care* (9th ed., pp. 729–835). Elsevier.

Gardner, S. L., & Goldson, E. (2021). The neonate and the environment impact on development. In S. L. Gardner, B. S. Carter, M. Enzman-Hineset, et al. (Eds.), *Merenstein & Gardner's handbook of neonatal intensive care* (9th ed., pp. 334–405). Elsevier.

Gardner, S. L., & Niermeyer, S. (2021). Immediate newborn care after birth. In S. L. Gardner, B. S. Carter, M. Enzman-Hineset, et al. (Eds.), *Merenstein & Gardner's handbook of neonatal intensive care* (9th ed., pp. 93–136). Elsevier.

Gleason, C. A., & Juul, S. E. (2018). Lung development. In E. Plosa, & S. H. Guttentag (Eds.), *Avery's diseases of the newborn* (10th ed., pp. 586–599). Elsevier.

Hill, M. A. (2021). *Embryology Renal System Development.* https://embryology.med.unsw.edu.au/embryology/index.php/Renal_System_Development.

Ianni, B., McDaniel, H., Savilo, E., Wade, C., Micetic, B., Johnson, S., & Gerkin, R. (2020). Defining normal healthy term newborn automated hematologic reference intervals at 24 hours of life.

Archives of Pathology and Laboratory Medicine, 145(1), 66–74. https://doi.org/10.5858/arpa.2019-0444-OA.

Jha, K., Nassar, G. N., & Makker, K. (2020). Transient tachypnea of the newborn. In *StatPearls.* StatPearls Publishing. https://www.ncbi.nlm.nih.gov/books/NBK537354/.

Katheria, A., Reister, F., Essers, J., Mendler, M., Hummler, H., Subramaniam, A., et al. (2019). Association of umbilical cord milking vs delayed umbilical cord clamping with death or severe intraventricular hemorrhage among preterm infants. *JAMA, 322*(19), 1877–1886. https://doi.org/10.1001/jama.2019.16004.

Kauffman, D. P., Khattar, J., & Lappin, S. L. (2020). Physiology, fetal hemoglobin. In *StatPearls. StatPearls Publishing.* https://pubmed.ncbi.nlm.nih.gov/29763187/.

Keehn, N. F., & Lieben, K. (2020). *#32263: Newborn assessment. Netce [Internet].* https://www.netce.com/coursecontent.php?courseid=2068#chap.7.

La Leche League International. (2021). Constipation. https://www.llli.org/breastfeeding-info/constipation/.

Lo, S. F. (2020). Reference intervals for laboratory tests and procedures. In R.M. Kliegman, J.W. St. Geme III, N.J. Blum, et al. (Eds.), *Nelson textbook of pediatrics* (21st ed., pp. e5–e12). Elsevier.

Lubkowska, A., Szymański, S., & Chudecka, M. (2019). Surface body temperature of full-term healthy newborns immediately after birth-pilot study. *International journal of environmental research and public health, 16*(8), 1312. https://doi.org/10.3390/ijerph16081312.

McDonald, S. J., Middleton, P., Dowswell, T., & Morris, P. S. (2013). Effect of timing of umbilical cord clamping of term infants on maternal and neonatal outcomes. *Cochrane Database of Systematic Reviews.* https://doi: 10.1002/14651858.CD004074.pub3.

Moore, R. E., & Townsend, S. D. (2019). Temporal development of the infant gut microbiome. *Open Biology, 9.* pages 1-11. https://doi.org/10.1098/rsob.190128

National Health Service. (2018). *Newborn respiratory distress syndrome.* https://www.nhs.uk/conditions/neonatal-respiratory-distress-syndrome.

Nimavat, D. J. (2019). Vitamin K deficiency bleeding. Medscape. https://emedicine.medscape.com/article/974489-overview.

Nyp, M., Brunkhorst, J. L., Reavey, D., & Pallotto, E. K. (2021). Fluid and electrolyte management. In S. L. Gardner, B. S. Carter, M. Enzman-Hineset, et al. (Eds.), *Merenstein & Gardner's handbook of neonatal intensive care* (9th ed., pp. 407–430). Elsevier.

Ohning, B. L. (2019). In M. Aslam (Ed.), *Neonatal resuscitation* https://emedicine.medscape.com/article/977002-overview.

Pagana, K. D., Pagana, T. J., & Pagana, T. N. (2019). *Mosby's diagnostic and laboratory test reference* (14th ed.). Elsevier.

Pierzynowska, K., Wolinski, J., Westrom, B., & Pierzynowska, S. G. (2020). Maternal immunoglobulins in infants—Are they more than just a form of passive immunity? *Frontiers in Immunology, 11*, 855. https://doi.org/10.3389/fimmu.2020.00855.

Qian, Y., Ying, X., Wang, P., Lu, Z., & Hua, Y. (2019). Early versus delayed umbilical cord clamping on maternal and neonatal outcomes. *Archives of Gynecology and Obstetrics, 300*(3), 531–543. *https://doi: 10.1007/s00404-019-05215-8.*

Sandberg, E. S. (2019). Pediatric hypoglycemia. *Pediatric Endocrine Society.* https://pedsendo.org/clinical-resource/pediatric-hypoglycemia/.

Shirk, S. K., Manolis, S. A., Lambers, D. S., & Smith, K. L. (2019). Delayed clamping vs milking of umbilical cord in preterm infants: A randomized controlled trial. *American Journal of Obstetrics and Gynecology, 220*(5), 482. https://doi.org/10.1016/j.ajog.2019.01.234.

Subramanian, K. N. S., Gupta, A. O., Bahri, M., & Kicklighter, S. D. (2020). In T. Rosenkrantz, M. L. Windle, & B. S. Carter (Eds.), *Transient tachypnea of the newborn.* https://emedicine.medscape.com/article/976914-overview#a5.

Thulier, D. (2017). Challenging expected patterns of weight loss in full-term breastfeeding neonates born by cesarean section. *Journal of Obstetric, Gynecologic, and Neonatal Nurses, 46*(1), 18–28 https://www.jognn.org/article/S0884-2175(16)30433-6/pdf.

Assessment of the Newborn

Lisa Wallace

A very important role of the nurse is assessing the newborn to identify abnormalities and problems in adapting to life outside the uterus. The first complete assessment of the newborn is often called an *admission assessment.* Subsequent assessments are less detailed.

EARLY FOCUSED ASSESSMENTS

As soon as the infant is born, the nurse performs assessments that are most immediately crucial to determining the neonate's health status. These include the cardiorespiratory status, muscle tone, thermoregulation, estimation of the gestational age, and presence of anomalies. The nurse determines whether resuscitation or other immediate interventions are necessary. If no anomalies are present and the newborn is adapting to extrauterine life without difficulty, the nurse should facilitate parent-infant attachment and initiation of breastfeeding while continuing ongoing assessments of breathing, activity, and color. Completion of a more thorough admission assessment follows. If possible, this assessment should be performed in the parent's room to provide an opportunity for parent teaching and continued parent-infant attachment.

History

Information about the pregnancy, labor, and birth is important in assessing the likelihood of problems. The gestational age, maternal age, health problems, and any complications during the pregnancy or birth may affect the neonate's adaptation. For example, if narcotic analgesics were administered late in labor, depression of the fetal central nervous system (CNS) may interfere with initiation of respirations in the neonate. Preterm infants may not produce adequate amounts of surfactant, and atelectasis may occur because the alveoli do not remain open.

⚡ SAFETY CHECK

After newborns are dried at birth, it is easy to forget their skin is contaminated with blood and amniotic fluid. The nurse should wear gloves when handling newborns until they are bathed and all blood is removed from the skin and hair. Wearing gloves helps protect the nurse from blood-borne pathogens.

Assessment of Cardiorespiratory Status

Assessments of respiratory and cardiovascular status are performed together because transitional changes take place simultaneously in both systems. Problems of adaptation in one system are likely to result in problems in the other system.

Airway

During birth, some fetal lung fluid is forced into the upper airway and expelled. Excessive fluid and mucus in the infant's respiratory passages may cause respiratory difficulty for several hours after birth.

Respiratory rate. The nurse assesses respirations at least once every 30 minutes until the infant has been stable for 2 hours after birth (American Academy of Pediatrics & American College of Obstetricians and Gynecologists [AAP & ACOG], 2017). If abnormalities are noted, respirations are assessed more often.

The normal respiratory rate is 30 to 60 breaths per minute (Tappero, 2021). The average rate is 40 to 49 breaths per minute. The infant may breathe faster immediately after birth, during crying, and during the first and second periods of reactivity. Respirations should not be labored, and the chest movements should be symmetric. Because the pattern and depth of respirations are irregular, they should be counted for a full minute for accuracy (Procedure 21.1).

Counting the rapid, shallow, irregular respirations of a newborn can be a challenge at first. Differentiating between

PROCEDURE 21.1   Assessing Vital Signs in the Newborn

Respirations

1. Assess respirations when the infant is quiet or sleeping and before disturbing the infant for other assessments, if possible.
2. Observe, auscultate, and palpate the chest and abdomen, which should move synchronously.
3. Lift the infant's blanket and shirt to see the chest and abdomen. Observe the pattern of respirations before beginning to count.
4. If desired, place a hand lightly to the side of the infant's chest or abdomen to feel the movement. Avoid covering the chest completely so chest excursions can be watched and palpated.
5. To auscultate respirations, move a stethoscope over the chest until the respirations are easily heard. After counting, move the stethoscope to listen to breath sounds in all areas.
6. Count for a full minute.
7. If the infant is crying, allow the infant to suck on a pacifier or gloved finger. If crying continues, count the respirations and make a note on the chart. Recheck later when the infant is calm.
8. Expect the respiratory rate to be 30 to 60 breaths per minute, with an average rate of 40 to 49 breaths per minute when the infant is at rest. Report signs of respiratory distress, including tachypnea, retractions, flaring, cyanosis, grunting, seesawing, apneic periods, and asymmetry of chest movements. Continue to watch infants whose respiratory rate is near the extremes of the normal range.

Pulse

1. Listen to the apical pulse while the infant is quiet and before disturbing the infant for other assessments, if possible.
2. For maximum contact with the chest wall, use a stethoscope with a pediatric or neonatal head to listen to the apical pulse.
3. If the infant is crying, insert a pacifier or a gloved finger into the infant's mouth.
4. If the infant cannot be quieted, increase concentration and time spent listening.
5. Listen briefly before beginning to count. Tapping a finger in rhythm with the beat may be helpful. Count for a full minute. Expect the heart rate to be 120 to 160 bpm at rest.
6. Move the stethoscope to listen over the entire heart area. Assess for arrhythmias, murmurs, or other abnormal sounds. Refer any abnormalities.

Temperature
Axillary

1. Place the thermometer vertically along the chest wall with the tip of the thermometer against the skin in the center of the axillary space and the infant's arm held firmly against the body over the probe.
2. Read the thermometer at the proper time: electronic or digital, when indicator sounds; other types according to manufacturer's directions. Normal range: 36.5°C to 37.5°C (97.7°F to 99.5°F).

---

the respirations and other movements while observing the infant's chest may be difficult. Observation, auscultation, or palpation, alone or in combination, may be used to obtain an accurate respiratory rate.

The nurse observes for periodic breathing, pauses in breathing lasting 5 to 10 seconds without other changes followed by rapid respirations for 10 to 15 seconds. This occurs in some full-term infants during the first few days but is more common in preterm infants. Apnea is a pause in breathing lasting at least 20 seconds, or less if accompanied by cyanosis, pallor, bradycardia, or decreased muscle tone (Churchman, 2021). Apnea is abnormal and requires prompt intervention (Stewart & Rodgers, 2020).

Breath sounds. The anterior and posterior lung fields are auscultated for breath sounds, which should be present equally throughout. Breath sounds should be clear over most areas. Nevertheless, hearing crackles in the lungs during the first hour or two after birth is not unusual because fetal lung fluid has not been completely absorbed. Infants born by cesarean not preceded by labor do not experience the changes that occur in the lungs during labor and birth and are more likely to have coarse breath sounds for a short time. Wheezes, crackles, rhonchi, or stridor that persists should be reported.

Abnormal and diminished sounds should be reported to the primary care provider if they continue. They may indicate a pneumothorax. Bowel sounds in the chest may be a sign of diaphragmatic hernia.

Signs of respiratory distress. Throughout the assessment, the nurse should be alert for signs of respiratory distress, which may be present at birth or develop later. Whenever one sign of labored breathing is present, the assessment should be carefully expanded to identify others.

Tachypnea. Tachypnea, a respiratory rate of more than 60 breaths per minute, is the most common sign of respiratory distress. It is not unusual during the first hour after birth and during the periods of reactivity, but continued tachypnea is abnormal.

Retractions. Retractions occur when the soft tissue around the bones of the chest is drawn in with the effort of pulling air into the lungs. Xiphoid (substernal) retractions occur when the area under the sternum retracts each time the infant inhales. When the muscles between the ribs are drawn in so each rib is outlined, intercostal retractions are present. The muscles above the sternum and around the clavicles also may be used to aid in respirations (supraclavicular retractions). Retractions may be mild or severe, depending on the degree of respiratory difficulty. Occasional mild retractions are common immediately after birth but should not continue after the first hour.

Flaring of the nares. A reflex widening of the nostrils occurs when the infant is receiving insufficient oxygen. Nasal flaring helps decrease airway resistance and increase the amount of air entering the lungs. Intermittent flaring may occur in the first hour after birth. Continued flaring indicates a more serious respiratory problem.

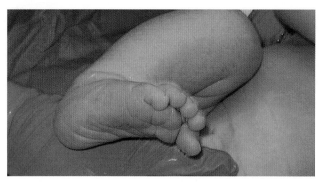

FIG. 21.1 Acrocyanosis. (Courtesy Todd Shires.)

Cyanosis. Cyanosis is a purplish–blue discoloration indicating the infant is not getting enough oxygen. It may be preceded by a dusky or gray hue to the skin. Central cyanosis involves the lips, tongue, mucous membranes, and trunk and indicates true hypoxia. This means not enough oxygen is reaching the vital organs and requires immediate attention.

Bruising of the face may occur from a tight nuchal cord or pressure during birth and may look like central cyanosis. To differentiate cyanosis from bruising, apply pressure to the area. A cyanotic area will blanch, but a bruised area remains blue. Central cyanosis in infants with dark skin tones can be checked by looking at the color of the mucous membranes. A pulse oximeter is used to determine oxygen saturation in infants with cyanosis.

Central cyanosis should be differentiated from acrocyanosis, which is peripheral cyanosis involving only the extremities. Acrocyanosis is normal during the first day after birth and if the infant becomes cold. It results from poor perfusion of blood to the periphery of the body (Fig. 21.1).

Cyanosis may be present at birth or may become apparent later. It is normal to see a cyanotic infant at birth whose color quickly turns pink as the infant begins to breathe. Cyanosis occurs whenever the infant's breathing is impaired. It may occur during feedings because of difficulty in coordinating sucking, swallowing, and breathing. Infants who become cyanotic on exertion or when crying may have a congenital heart defect.

Grunting. Grunting describes a noise made on expiration when air crosses partially closed vocal cords. This increases the pressure within the alveoli, which keeps the alveoli open and enhances the exchange of gases in the lungs. Grunting may be very mild and heard only with a stethoscope or loud enough to be heard unaided in an infant having severe respiratory difficulty. Persistent grunting is a common sign of respiratory distress syndrome and necessitates expanded assessment and referral for treatment.

Seesaw or paradoxical respirations. Normally the chest and abdomen rise and fall together during respiration. In the infant with severe respiratory difficulty, the chest falls when the abdomen rises and the chest rises when the abdomen falls, causing a seesaw effect.

Asymmetry. Chest expansion should be equal on both sides. Asymmetry or decreased movement on one side may indicate the collapse of a lung (pneumothorax).

Choanal atresia. The newborn airway is narrower and shorter than the adult, increasing the risk for obstruction or complications. Choanal atresia is blockage or narrowing of one or both nasal passages by bone or tissue. Although the concept is controversial, newborns may be obligate nose breathers for approximately 4 to 6 weeks after birth (Bush et al., 2019; Niermeyer & Clark, 2021; Tappero, 2021). This means they may breathe mostly through the nose except when crying. Therefore assessment for choanal atresia is important. Bilateral choanal atresia causes severe respiratory distress and requires surgery. Blockage of one side puts the infant at risk for respiratory distress if the other side becomes occluded by mucus or edema.

The nurse can assess for choanal atresia by closing the infant's mouth and occluding one nostril at a time. The infant is observed for breathing, and breath sounds are auscultated while each nostril is occluded. Another method of assessment is to pass a catheter through each nostril to check for patency. Infants with choanal atresia may become cyanotic when quiet but pink when crying because air is then drawn in through the mouth.

Color

In addition to cyanosis, the nurse assesses for pallor and ruddiness.

Pallor. Pallor can indicate the infant is slightly hypoxic or anemic. A laboratory examination of hemoglobin (Hgb) and hematocrit (Hct) or a complete blood count (CBC) may be ordered.

Ruddy color. A ruddy or reddish skin color (plethora) may indicate polycythemia, an excessive number of red blood cells (RBCs). Hct value above 65% confirms polycythemia. Infants with elevated Hct levels are at increased risk for jaundice from the normal destruction of excessive RBCs, which occurs after birth.

Heart Sounds

The heart is auscultated for rate, rhythm, and the presence of murmurs or abnormal sounds. The nurse should count the apical heart rate for a full minute for accuracy and listen for abnormalities. The rate should range between 120 and 160 beats per minute (bpm) with normal activity. It may elevate to 180 bpm when infants are crying or drop to as low as 100 bpm when they are in deep sleep.

If there are no problems present at birth, the heart rate should be recorded at least once every 30 minutes until the infant has been stable for 2 hours after birth (AAP & ACOG, 2017). Monitoring is more frequent if abnormalities are present. Once stable, the heart rate is checked once every 8 to 12 hours or according to hospital policy unless a reason for more frequent assessment develops.

Position. The apex of the heart is located at the point of maximum impulse, where the pulse is most easily felt and the sound is loudest. This is at the third or fourth intercostal space, left midclavicular line. Conditions that affect the position of the heart include pneumothorax and dextrocardia (a right-to-left reversal from the normal heart position).

Rhythm and murmurs. The rhythm of the heart should be regular, and the first and second sounds should be heard clearly. Abnormalities in rhythm and sounds such as murmurs should be noted. Murmurs are sounds of abnormal blood flow through the heart and may indicate openings in the septum of the heart or problems with blood flow through the valves. They occur in approximately 10% of newborns (Garner & Niermeyer, 2021). Most murmurs in the newborn are temporary and result from incomplete transition from fetal to neonatal circulation. A murmur is common until the ductus arteriosus is functionally closed. Although it may be a normal or functional murmur, any abnormal sounds of the heart are investigated because they may be signs of cardiac defects. Pulse oximetry screening for cardiac defects is performed before discharge (see Chapter 22).

Brachial and Femoral Pulses

The brachial and femoral pulses should be present and equal bilaterally. The brachial pulse is located over the antecubital space, and the femoral pulse is located at the groin. The brachial and femoral pulse rates should be the same. Femoral pulses that are weaker than the brachial pulses may result from impaired blood flow in coarctation of the aorta, a congenital heart defect. In this condition, a narrowed area of the aorta impedes blood flow to the lower part of the body and causes weaker pulses in the lower extremities.

Blood Pressure

Measurement of blood pressure (BP) is not a necessary part of a routine assessment of the newborn. Nevertheless, the BP is taken on all extremities if the infant has unequal pulses, murmurs, or other signs of cardiac complications. Doppler ultrasonography or other electronic measurement techniques are used. For accurate measurement, the infant should be quiet when the BP is taken because crying elevates it. The BP cuff width should be approximately 50% of the circumference of the limb (Dionne et al., 2020).

The average BP for full-term newborns soon after birth is 65 to 95 mm Hg systolic and 30 to 60 mm Hg diastolic (Gardner & Niermeyer, 2021). BP varies according to the infant's age, weight, and gestational age. Hypotension may occur in the sick infant.

The BP of the lower extremities should be the same or slightly higher than the upper extremities. A systolic BP in the upper extremities that is greater than 20 mm Hg higher than in the lower extremities may indicate coarctation of the aorta (Patnana & Selb, 2018).

Capillary Refill

Capillary refill is assessed to help determine whether perfusion is adequate. It is checked by depressing the skin over the forehead or sternum until the area blanches. Failure for color to return within 3 seconds or less may indicate hypoperfusion and needs additional investigation (Nyp et al., 2021).

Assessment of Thermoregulation

The neonate's temperature is taken soon after birth while the infant is being held by the parent or in a radiant warmer

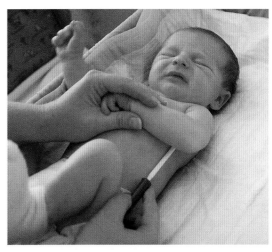

FIG. 21.2 The infant is held securely to prevent injury and obtain an accurate reading when taking the temperature.

BOX 21.1   Normal Vital Signs in the Newborn

Temperature: 36.5°C to 37.5°C (97.7°F to 99.5°F) axillary
Apical pulse: 120 to 160 bpm (100 sleeping, 180 crying)
Respirations: 30 to 60 breaths per minute

---

with a skin probe attached to the abdomen. The probe, which should not be attached over bony prominences or areas of brown fat, allows the warmer to measure and display the infant's skin temperature continuously. The temperature control is set to regulate the amount of heat produced according to the infant's skin temperature. The temperature should be assessed at least once every 30 minutes until the infant has been stable for 2 hours after birth (AAP & ACOG, 2017). It is often checked again at 4 hours and then once every 8 to 12 hours or according to facility policy as long as it remains stable (see Procedure 21.1).

The most common method of taking the neonate's temperature is axillary measurement (Fig. 21.2). The normal range for axillary temperature is 36.5°C to 37.5°C (97.7°F to 99.5°F; AAP & ACOG, 2017; Box 21.1). Taking axillary temperatures is safer than taking rectal temperatures because it avoids the possibility of irritation, perforation, or other injury to the rectum. The temperature method should always be charted along with the temperature measurement.

If a rectal temperature is necessary, the nurse should use great caution because inserting the thermometer too far could cause potentially fatal perforation of the intestinal wall. A thermometer should never be forced into the rectum because of the possible presence of an imperforate (closed) anus.

Temperatures are usually measured with an electronic digital thermometer. Inexpensive digital thermometers used while the infant is in the hospital are often given to the parents for home use. Tympanic thermometers are not recommend until infants are 6 months of age or older (Crumley, 2020). Some agencies use temporal artery thermometers.

General Assessment

If major abnormalities are present at birth, the nurse should maintain a calm, quiet demeanor to avoid frightening the parents. The provider should be alerted quietly and will explain the condition and possible plan of treatment to the parents.

Head

The newborn's head and neck constitute one-fourth of the body surface (Gardner & Niermeyer, 2021). It is much larger in proportion to the rest of the body than that of the adult. The head is palpated to assess the shape and identify abnormalities. The newborn who was delivered by cesarean not preceded by labor usually has a round head, whereas the infant born vaginally usually has some molding. The head of infants who were in a breech position may be flattened on the top. The degree of molding, size of the fontanels, and presence of the caput succedaneum or later development of a cephalohematoma are noted.

The hair should be fine, with a consistent pattern. Abnormal hair growth patterns may indicate genetic abnormalities. The nurse separates the hair, if necessary, to display bruises, rashes, or other marks on the scalp. A small, red mark is apparent if a fetal monitor electrode was inserted into the skin of the scalp. Later, a small scab forms. Occasionally this area becomes infected, and a topical antibiotic is applied.

Molding. Molding refers to changes in the shape of the head that allow it to pass through the birth canal. It is caused by overriding of the cranial bones at the sutures and is common, especially after a vaginal delivery. The parietal bones often override the occipital and frontal bones, and a ridge can be felt at those areas. The condition generally resolves within a few days to 1 week after birth. Often, dramatic improvement is seen by the end of the first day of life. Parents may need reassurance the infant's head is normal.

All sutures should be palpated. Separation may be the temporary result of molding or, if it persists or widens, may indicate increased intracranial pressure. If no space is found between suture lines, it may be the result of molding and overriding of the bones. Nevertheless, a hard, ridged area not resulting from molding may indicate premature closure of the sutures. This condition, called *craniosynostosis,* may impair brain growth and the shape of the head and requires surgery.

Fontanels. The fontanels are the areas of the head where sutures between the bones meet. In the newborn, the areas are not calcified but are covered by membrane to allow space for the brain to grow.

The nurse palpates the fontanels and notes the position in relation to the other bones of the skull (Fig. 21.3). The infant's

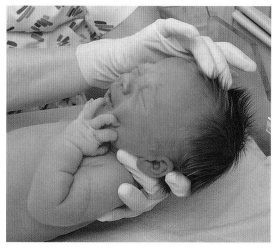

FIG. 21.3 Palpation of the anterior fontanel. Note elevation of the head.

head is elevated during palpation for accurate assessment. The infant may be placed in a semisitting position or held in an upright position. The fontanel should be palpated when the infant is quiet because vigorous crying may cause it to protrude.

The anterior fontanel is a diamond-shaped area where the frontal and parietal bones meet. It measures 4 to 6 cm from bone to bone, although this varies because of molding and individual differences. The fontanel closes by 18 months of age (National Institute of Health [NIH], 2021).

The anterior fontanel should be soft and flat (level with the surrounding bones) or only slightly sunken. After molding resolves, a depressed fontanel may be a sign of dehydration. Although the anterior fontanel may bulge slightly when the infant cries, bulging at rest may indicate increased intracranial pressure. A fontanel between flat and bulging is termed full. A larger-than-normal fontanel may be a sign of increased pressure within the skull. Abnormal signs are reported to the primary care provider.

The posterior fontanel is a triangular area where the occipital and parietal bones meet. It is much smaller than the anterior fontanel, measuring 0.5 to 1 cm, and feels like a dimple at the juncture of the occipital and parietal bones. This fontanel closes by the time the infant is 2 months of age (NIH, 2021).

Caput succedaneum. A caput succedaneum is an area of localized edema that appears over the vertex of the newborn's head as a result of pressure against the cervix during labor (Fig. 21.4). The pressure interferes with blood flow from the area, causing localized edema at birth. The edematous area crosses suture lines, is soft, and varies in size. It resolves quickly and generally disappears within 12 to 48 hours after birth (Gardner & Niermeyer, 2021). Caput also may occur when a vacuum extractor is used to assist birth. When a vacuum is used, the caput corresponds to the area where the extractor was placed on the skull. The amount of edema and presence of bruising are assessed.

Cephalohematoma. A cephalohematoma, bleeding between the periosteum and the skull, is the result of pressure

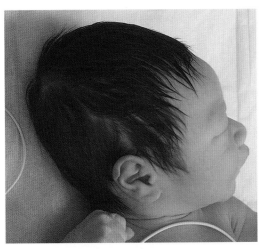

FIG. 21.4 Caput succedaneum is an edematous area on the head from pressure against the cervix. It may cross suture lines.

during birth (Fig. 21.5). It occurs on one or both sides of the head, usually over the parietal bones. The swelling may not be present at birth but may develop within the first 24 to 48 hours.

The area is carefully palpated to determine whether the swelling crosses suture lines. A cephalohematoma has clear edges that end at the suture lines. It does not cross the suture lines, unlike a caput succedaneum, because the bleeding is held between the bone and its covering, the periosteum. A cephalohematoma reabsorbs slowly and may take several months to completely resolve (Tappero, 2021). Because of the breakdown of the RBCs within the hematoma, affected infants are at greater risk for jaundice.

Both caput succedaneum and cephalohematoma may be frightening to parents. They need reassurance the conditions are not harmful to the infant. Even if parents do not ask, they need information about the causes and length of time required for the areas to resolve.

Face. The face is examined for symmetry, positioning of the facial features, movement, and expression. A transient asymmetry from intrauterine pressure may occur, lasting a few weeks or months. Drooping of the mouth appears as a one-sided cry and may be caused by facial nerve trauma. Irregularities of the facial features should be reported.

Neck and Clavicles

The nurse assesses the infant's neck visually and notes the ease and extent with which the head turns from side to side. The neck should have full range of motion. It is very short. Webbing or an unusually large fat pad between the occiput and the shoulders may indicate a chromosomal anomaly. No masses should be present. When lying in a prone position, the term newborn should be able to raise the head briefly and turn it to the other side.

Fractures of the clavicle are more likely to occur in large infants, especially when shoulder dystocia occurred. Sliding the fingers along each clavicle while moving the infant's arm helps identify a fractured clavicle. If a fracture is present, a lump, swelling, or tenderness over the bone may be observed. Crepitus (grating of the bone) and movement of the bone may be felt during palpation. Decreased movement of the affected arm also may occur. A difference in the movement of the arms is especially noticeable when the Moro reflex is elicited.

Injury to the brachial plexus may cause paralysis of the arm on the side of the fracture. Treatment of a fractured clavicle includes immobilization of the affected arm for a short time. The fracture heals quickly (Fig. 21.6).

Umbilical Cord

The umbilical cord should contain three vessels. The two arteries are small and may stand up at the cut end. The single vein is larger than the arteries and resembles a slit because its walls are more easily compressed. If only one artery is present, the infant is carefully assessed for other anomalies. A two-vessel cord may be an isolated abnormality or associated with chromosomal and renal defects. The amount of

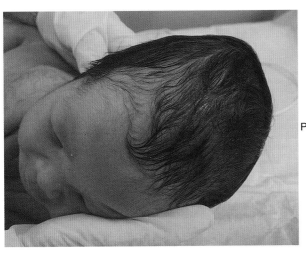

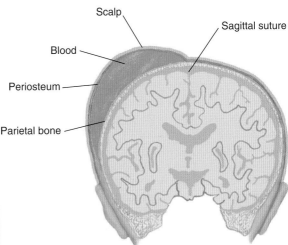

FIG. 21.5 A cephalohematoma is characterized by bleeding between the bone and its covering, the periosteum. It may occur on one or both sides and does not cross suture lines.

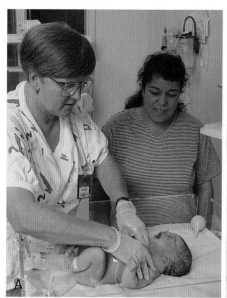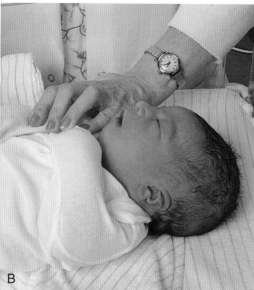

FIG. 21.6 A, The nurse palpates the clavicles to identify fractures. A fracture of the left clavicle is present. B, The arm on the side of the fractured clavicle is immobilized by pinning the sleeve to the shirt.

Wharton's jelly in the cord is noted. If the cord appears thin, the infant may have been poorly nourished in utero. A yellow–brown or green tinge to the cord indicates meconium was released at some time before birth, perhaps as a result of fetal compromise. No redness or discharge from the cord should be present.

Extremities

The infant should actively move the extremities equally in a random manner. The extremities of a term infant should remain sharply flexed and resist extension during examination. Poor muscle tone results in a limp or "floppy" infant, which may occur from inadequate oxygen during birth but should resolve within a few minutes as oxygen intake increases. Continued poor muscle tone may result from prematurity or neurologic injury. Infants with previously good muscle tone may show decreased flexion if they become hypoglycemic or experience respiratory difficulty.

All extremities are examined for signs of fractures such as crepitus, redness, lumps, or swelling. Lack of use of an extremity may indicate nerve injury with or without fractures.

Injury to the brachial nerve plexus may result in Erb's palsy (Erb–Duchenne paralysis), paralysis of the shoulder and arm muscles. Instead of the usual flexed position, the affected arm is extended at the infant's side with the forearm prone. Movement of this arm is diminished during the Moro reflex. The condition is treated by splinting, exercise, or both.

Hands and feet. The fingers and toes are examined for extra digits (polydactyly) and webbing between digits (syndactyly). Extra digits are often small and may not have bones. Tying the extra digits with sutures causes them to atrophy and fall off. The presence of a bone in the extra digit requires surgical removal. Webbed fingers or toes may be corrected by surgery. Nails in a term infant should extend to the end of the fingers or slightly beyond.

The creases in the hands also are examined. Normally, two long transverse creases extend most of the way across the palm. A single crease parallel with the base of the fingers that crosses the palm without a break is called a **single transverse palmar crease (STPC)**, previously known as a "simian" crease (Krause, 2019). It may be seen with incurving of the little finger in Down's syndrome (trisomy 21), but the crease alone is not diagnostic of trisomy 21 because it may also be a normal finding.

The feet are assessed for talipes equinovarus, or clubfoot, a common malformation of the feet. If a foot looks abnormal, it should be gently manipulated. If it moves to a normal position, the abnormality is probably temporary, resulting from the position of the infant in the uterus. In true clubfoot, the foot turns inward and cannot be moved to a midline position. Casting and manipulation are the usual treatment, but in some cases surgery is necessary.

Hips. The hips are examined for signs of developmental dysplasia. In this condition, instability of the hip joint occurs, and the head of the femur can be moved in and out of the acetabulum. Partial dislocation and inadequate development of the acetabulum may occur. Identifying a hip problem early is important to prevent permanent damage to the joint.

The infant's knees should be bent with the feet flat on the bed to compare the height of the knees. If the hip is dislocated, the knee on the affected side is lower. The legs are extended with the infant in the prone position to determine whether they are equal in length and if the thigh and gluteal creases are symmetric (Fig. 21.7). If the hip is dislocated, the leg on the affected side is shorter, and the creases are asymmetric. Because the hip may be unstable but not yet dislocated, these signs may not be present at birth.

Barlow and Ortolani tests are methods of assessing for hip instability in the newborn period (Fig. 21.8). These maneuvers are performed by the physician or advanced practice

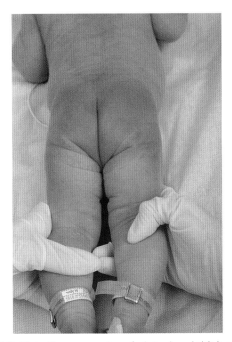

FIG. 21.7 Note the symmetry of gluteal and thigh creases.

nurse. Both legs should abduct equally in infants. Abducting the affected hip may be difficult. A hip click may be felt or heard but is usually normal and is different from the "clunk" of hip dysplasia when the femoral head moves in the hip socket (Tamai, 2020).

Treatment of developmental dysplasia of the hip involves immobilizing the leg in a flexed, abducted position, usually with a harness. Early identification and treatment are essential to provide the best results in correcting the problem. Treatment may involve casting or surgery if the condition is not discovered early.

Vertebral Column

The nurse palpates the entire length of the newborn's vertebral column to discover any defects in the vertebrae. An indentation is a sign of spina bifida occulta (failure of a vertebra to close). The defect is not obvious on visual inspection because it is covered with skin, but sometimes a tuft of hair grows over the area. Other more obvious neural tube defects include a meningocele (protrusion of spinal fluid and meninges) or a myelomeningocele (protrusion of spinal fluid, meninges, and the spinal cord) through the defect in the vertebrae. They appear as a sack on the back and may be covered by skin or only the meninges. The tissue should be covered with moist sterile saline dressings immediately after birth. A pilonidal dimple may be present at the base of the spine. It should be examined for a sinus and the depth noted.

Measurements

Measurements provide information about the infant's growth in utero. The weight, length, and head and chest circumferences are part of the initial assessment (Procedure 21.2). The measurements are compared with the norms for the infant's gestational age. When a difference is noted between the

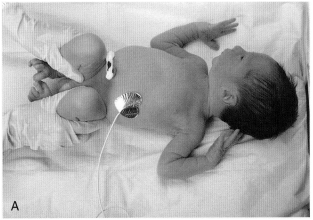
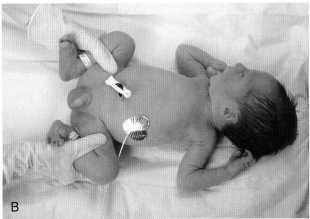

FIG. 21.8 Assessment of the hips. The physician or advanced practice nurse examining the infant places their fingers over the infant's greater trochanter and thumbs over the femur. The knees and hips are flexed. **A,** Barlow test. The provider adducts the hips and applies gentle pressure down and back with the thumbs. In hip dysplasia the examiner can feel the femoral head move out of the acetabulum. **B,** Ortolani test. The provider abducts the thighs and applies gentle pressure forward over the greater trochanter. A "clunking" sensation indicates a dislocated femoral head moving into the acetabulum. A hip click is from ligament movement and is not a problem.

expected and actual values, expanded assessments are necessary.

Weight

The weight of the term newborn ranges between 2500 and 4000 grams (g) (5 pounds [lb.], 8 ounces [oz] and 8 lb., 13 oz; Tappero, 2021). If the infant's weight is outside the normal range, possible causes are assessed. Factors affecting weight include gestational age; placental functioning; genetic factors such as race and parental size; and maternal diabetes, hypertension, and substance abuse.

Infants are weighed each day they are in the birth facility and at follow-up visits. They can be expected to lose 5% to 7% of their birth weight during the first week of life (Mersch, 2021). Weight loss of greater than 10% from birth weight needs further investigation. The weight loss results from excretion of meconium, normal loss of extracellular fluid, and inadequate intake of calories during the first few days. Infants normally regain or exceed their birth weight by 14 days of life. Newborns will double their weight by 4 to 6 months and triple the birth weight by 1 year of age (Mersch, 2021).

Length

The infant's length is measured from the top of the head to the heel of the outstretched leg. The average length of a full-term newborn is 48 to 53 cm (19 to 21 inches; Mersch, 2021). Some agencies also record the crown-to-rump measurement, which is approximately equal to the head circumference.

Head and Chest Circumference

The diameter of the head is measured around the occiput just above the eyebrows. The normal range of head circumference for the term newborn is 32 to 38 cm (13 to 14 inches; Gardner & Niermeyer, 2021). The measurement may be affected by molding of the skull during the birth process. If a large amount of molding occurred, the head is remeasured when it regains its normal shape. An abnormally small head may indicate poor brain growth and microcephaly. A very large head may be a sign of hydrocephalus.

The chest is measured at the level of the nipples. It usually is 1 to 2 cm smaller than the head. The normal circumference of

---

PROCEDURE 21.2   Weighing and Measuring the Newborn

Weight

1. Ensure the scale is properly cleaned.
2. Cover the scale with a warm blanket. Place a paper cover over the blanket if desired.
3. Balance or adjust the scale to 0 after the covering is placed.
4. Remove clothing and blankets from the infant and place the infant in the supine position on the scale. Keep one hand just above the infant and watch them constantly throughout the procedure.

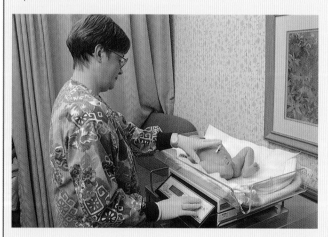

5. Wait until the infant is somewhat quiet. The electronic scale displays weight in pounds and ounces or in grams. Some electronic scales display an indicator when an accurate weight has been obtained. For a balance scale, move weights slowly until the arm is level.
6. Return the infant to the bassinet or skin to skin with the parent. Most electronic scales will retain the weight until it is cleared. As soon as the infant is safe and protected from cold stress, enter the weight in the electronic medical record (EMR). If necessary, the weight can be written on a scrap paper or report form until it can be charted in the EMR.
7. Compare weight with the normal range for term infants: 2500 to 4000 g (5 lb., 8 oz to 8 lb., 13 oz).
8. Clean and reset the scale according to policy.

Length
Ruler Printed on Scale or Crib

1. Place the infant in the supine position with their head at the upper edge of the ruler.

2. While holding the infant with one hand so the head does not move, use the other hand to fully extend the infant's leg along the ruler. Note the length at the bottom of the heel.

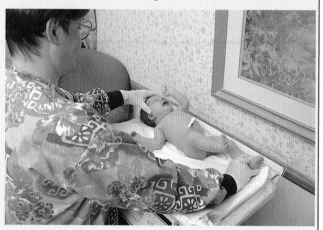

Tape Measure

1. Check for partial tears in a paper tape that could affect the accuracy of the measurement.
2. Place tape beside the infant, with the upper end at the top of the head. Tuck it beneath the shoulder and extend it down to the feet.
3. Hold the tape straight along the side of the infant's body while extending one of the infant's legs to its full length. Be sure the tape has not moved from the top of the head.

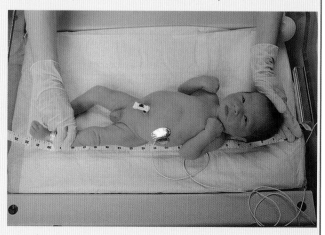

PROCEDURE 21.2 Weighing and Measuring the Newborn—cont'd

4. Another method is to mark the paper on which the infant is lying at the top of the head and the heel. Then measure the distance between the two marks.
5. Compare with the normal range of 48 to 53 cm (19 to 21 inches).
6. Enter the measurement in the EMR.

Head and Chest Circumference
1. Measure around the fullest part of the head, with the tape placed around the occiput and just above the eyebrows.

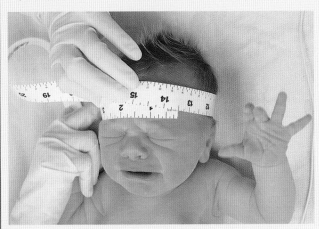

2. Move tape down to measure the chest at the level of the nipples. Keep the tape even and taut.

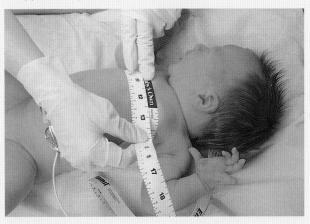

3. Remove the tape by lifting or rolling the infant instead of pulling the tape (which could cut the infant's skin).
4. Enter the measurements in the EMR. Compare measurements with normal range. Head: 32 to 38 cm (13 to 15 inches). Chest: 30 to 36 cm (12 to 14 inches).

---

the chest is 30 to 36 cm (12 to 14 inches; Azevedo et al., 2019; Gardner & Niermeyer, 2021). If molding of the head is present, the head and chest measurements may be equal at birth.

KNOWLEDGE CHECK

4. What are the differences among molding, caput succedaneum, and cephalohematoma?
5. Why are measurements of the neonate important?

ASSESSMENT OF BODY SYSTEMS

Neurologic System

Reflexes

Assessment of the reflexes is important to determine the health of the newborn's CNS. The nurse notes the presence and strength of the reflexes and whether both sides of the body respond symmetrically (Fig. 21.9). A diminished overall response occurs in preterm and ill infants. Absence of reflexes may indicate a serious neurologic problem. Asymmetric responses may indicate that trauma during birth caused nerve injury, paralysis, or fracture. Some newborn reflexes gradually weaken and disappear over a period of months (Table 21.1).

Sensory Assessment

Ears. The ears are assessed for placement, overall appearance, and maturity. An imaginary horizontal line drawn from the outer canthus of the eye should be even with the area where the upper ear (helix) joins the head (Fig. 21.10). Low-set ears may indicate chromosomal abnormalities. The ears should be almost vertical in placement on the head.

Abnormalities of the ear may indicate chromosomal abnormalities, hearing problems, or kidney defects. Skin tags, preauricular sinuses, and dimples, however, are most often isolated findings and do not require further evaluation (Rivers, 2019). The stiffness of the cartilage and degree of incurving of the pinna are checked as part of the gestational age assessment.

The fetus responds to sound by 28 weeks of gestation (Blackburn, 2018; Hibiya-Motegi et al., 2020). Infants can hear by the last trimester of pregnancy, and their hearing is very good after birth. Hearing is assessed by noting the infant's reaction to sudden loud noises, which should cause a startle response. Infants should respond to the sound of voices and prefer a high-pitched tone of voice and rhythmic sounds. They will turn toward the sound of the parent's voice or another interesting sound. A hearing screening is performed before discharge from most birth facilities.

Eyes. The eyes are examined for abnormalities and signs of inflammation. They should be symmetric and of the same size. The iris is dark gray, blue, or brown but may change color by 9 months of age (Rauch, 2021). Slanting epicanthal folds in a non-Asian infant may be a sign of trisomy 21 or other abnormal conditions.

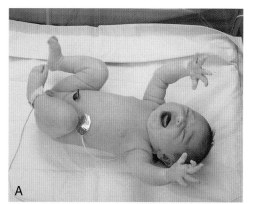

Moro reflex

The Moro reflex is the most dramatic reflex. It occurs when the infant's head and trunk are allowed to drop back 30 degrees when the infant is in a slightly raised position. The infant's arms and legs extend and abduct, with the fingers fanning open and thumbs and forefingers forming a C position. The arms then return to their normally flexed state with an embracing motion. The legs may also extend and then flex.

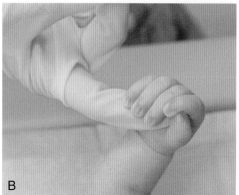

Palmar grasp reflex

The palmar grasp reflex occurs when the infant's palm is touched near the base of the fingers. The hand closes into a tight fist. The grasp reflex may be weak or absent if the infant has injury to the nerves of the arms.

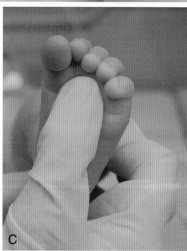

Plantar grasp reflex

The plantar grasp reflex is similar to the palmar grasp reflex. When the area below the toes is touched, the infant's toes curl over the nurse's finger.

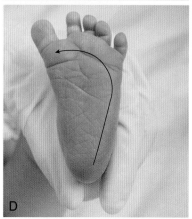

Babinski reflex

The Babinski reflex is elicited by stroking the lateral sole of the infant's foot from the heel forward and across the ball of the foot. This causes the toes to flare outward and the big toe to dorsiflex.

FIG. 21.9 Reflexes.

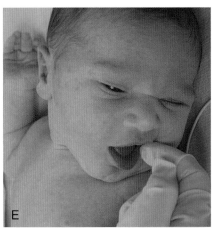

Rooting reflex
The rooting reflex is important in feeding and is most often demonstrated when the infant is hungry. When the infant's cheek is touched near the mouth, the head turns toward the side that has been stroked. This response helps the infant find the nipple for feeding. The reflex occurs when either side of the mouth is touched. Touching the cheeks on both sides at the same time confuses the infant.

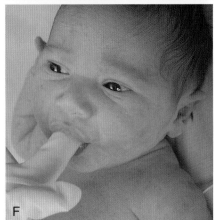

Sucking reflex
The sucking reflex is essential to life. When the mouth or palate is touched by the nipple or a finger, the infant begins to suck. The sucking reflex is assessed for its presence and strength. Feeding difficulties may be related to problems in the infant's ability to suck and to coordinate sucking with swallowing and breathing.

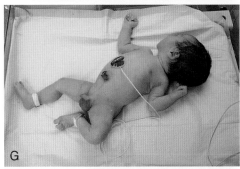

Tonic neck reflex
The tonic neck reflex refers to the posture assumed by newborns when in a supine position. The infant extends the arm and leg on the side to which the head is turned and flexes the extremities on the other side. This response is sometimes referred to as the "fencing reflex" because the infant's position is similar to that of a person engaged in a fencing match.

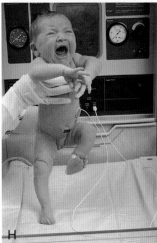

Stepping reflex
The stepping reflex occurs when infants are held upright with their feet touching a solid surface. They lift one foot and then the other, giving the appearance that they are trying to walk.

FIG. 21.9, cont'd

TABLE 21.1   Summary of Neonatal Reflexes

Reflex	Method of Testing	Expected Response	Abnormal Response/Possible Cause	Time Reflex Disappears
Babinski	Stroke lateral sole of foot from heel to across base of toes.	Toes flare with dorsiflexion of the big toe.	No response. Bilateral: CNS deficit. Unilateral: Local nerve injury.	1 yr.
Gallant (trunk incurvation)	With infant prone, lightly stroke along the side of the vertebral column.	Entire trunk flexes toward side stimulated.	No response: CNS deficit.	4 wk.
Grasp reflex (palmar and plantar)	Press finger against base of infant's fingers or toes.	Fingers curl tightly; toes curl forward.	Weak or absent: Neurologic deficit or muscle injury.	Palmar grasp: 5–6 mo. Plantar grasp: 9–12 mo.
Moro	Let infant's head drop back approximately 30 degrees.	Sharp extension and abduction of arms followed by flexion and adduction to "embrace" position.	Absent: CNS dysfunction. Asymmetry: Brachial plexus injury, paralysis, or fractured bone of extremity. Exaggerated: Maternal drug use.	5–7 mo.
Rooting	Touch or stroke from side of mouth toward cheek.	Infant turns head to side touched. Difficult to elicit if infant is sleeping or just fed.	Weak or absent: Prematurity, neurologic deficit, depression from maternal drug use.	3–4 mo.
Stepping	Hold infant so feet touch solid surface.	Infant lifts alternate feet as if walking.	Asymmetry: Fracture of extremity, neurologic deficit.	2 mo.
Sucking	Place nipple or gloved finger in mouth, rub against palate.	Infant begins to suck. May be weak if recently fed.	Weak or absent: Prematurity, neurologic deficit, maternal drug use.	1 yr.
Swallowing	Place fluid on the back of the tongue.	Infant swallows fluid. Should be coordinated with sucking.	Coughing, gagging, choking, cyanosis: Prematurity, tracheoesophageal fistula, esophageal atresia, neurologic deficit.	Present throughout life
Tonic neck reflex	Gently turn head to one side while infant is supine.	Infant extends extremities on side to which head is turned, with flexion on opposite side.	Prolonged period in position: Neurologic deficit.	May be weak at birth; disappears 5–7 mo.

CNS, Central nervous system.

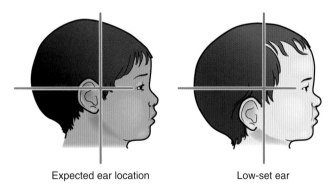

Expected ear location   Low-set ear

FIG. 21.10 An imaginary line is drawn from the outer canthus of the eye to the ear. The line should intersect with the area where the upper ear joins the head.

Edema of the eyelids and subconjunctival hemorrhages (reddened areas of the sclera) result from pressure on the head during birth, which causes capillary rupture in the sclera. The edema diminishes in a few days, and the hemorrhages resolve within a week (Rohan, 2021). The sclera should be white or bluish white. A yellow color indicates jaundice.

A blue color occurs in osteogenesis imperfecta, a congenital bone condition.

Conjunctivitis may result from infection or a chemical reaction to medications. *Staphylococcus, Chlamydia,* and *Neisseria gonorrhoeae* are common organisms that cause infection. Maternal infection can cause infection of the infant during birth. Ophthalmia neonatorum, which can cause blindness, results from infection of the newborn with gonorrhea or chlamydia. To decrease the risk of this condition, all newborns are treated prophylactically with antibiotics to the eyes. Any discharge from the eyes is reported for possible culture and treatment.

Transient strabismus (crossed eyes) is common because newborns have poor control of their eye muscles (Rohan, 2021). The doll's-eye sign is a normal finding in the newborn: When the head is turned quickly to one side, the eyes move toward the other side. The setting-sun sign (the iris appears low in the eye and part of the sclera can be seen above the iris) may be an indication of hydrocephalus.

The pupils should be equal in size and react equally to light. Cataracts (opacities of the lens) appear as white areas over the pupils. They may develop in infants who were exposed to rubella or other infections during the pregnancy. When a light is directed into the eyes, the normal red reflex may not be seen if large cataracts are present. Tears are scant or absent for the first several months after birth (Rohan, 2021). Excessive tearing may indicate a plugged lacrimal duct, which is treated with massage or surgery.

Visual acuity is approximately 20/600 (Horwood, 2019). The eyes cannot accommodate well, but newborns should show a visual response to the environment. They should make eye contact when held in a cradle position during a period of alertness. Although they focus best on objects which are 20 to 30 cm (8 to 12 inches) away, they can see objects to a distance of 76 cm (2.5 feet; Blackburn, 2018). They should respond well to human faces and geometric patterns of black and white or medium bright colors but show little interest in pastel colors.

Newborns should blink or close their eyes in response to bright lights. Any infant who does not respond to visual stimuli should be reported to the physician or nurse practitioner for further evaluation.

Sense of smell and taste. The sense of smell is demonstrated when infants recognize breast pads soaked with their mother's milk and differentiate them from pads soaked in water. Their ability to distinguish taste is shown by their preference for sweet liquids and aversion to sour or bitter tastes (Blackburn, 2018).

Other Neurologic Signs

The newborn is assessed for tremors or jitteriness. If tremors are present, the blood glucose should be checked because hypoglycemia is the most common cause. If blood glucose is within normal range, the cause may be low calcium or prenatal exposure to drugs. Tremors increase each time the infant is touched or moved but stop briefly if the extremity is flexed and held firmly.

Seizures indicate CNS or metabolic abnormality. To differentiate between tremors and seizures, the infant's extremities are held in a flexed position. This causes tremors to stop, but a seizure continues. Seizure activity also may include abnormal movements of the eyes and mouth and other subtle signs. Any infant thought to be having seizures is referred for further assessment and treatment.

⚡ SAFETY CHECK

Jitteriness or Tremors
Stop when the extremities are held firmly in a flexed position
Are commonly caused by low glucose or calcium levels

Seizures
Continue even if extremities are held
May include abnormal mouth or eye movements
Indicate central nervous system or metabolic abnormality

The pitch of the cry is important. Cries that are shrill, high-pitched, hoarse, and catlike (mewing) are abnormal. These cries may indicate a neurologic disorder or other problem.

Infants respond to holding and are quiet and appear content when their needs are met. Rocking motions are often effective in quieting an irritable infant. Most infants nestle or

---

BOX 21.2 Risk Factors for Neonatal Hypoglycemia

Prematurity
Postmaturity
Late preterm infant
Intrauterine growth restriction
Large or small for gestational age
Asphyxia
Problems at birth
Cold stress
Maternal diabetes
Maternal intake of terbutaline

---

mold their bodies to the body of the person holding them, making them easy to hold and cuddle. Neonates who stiffen the body, pull away from contact, or arch the back when held may be showing signs of CNS injury.

Infants should react to painful stimuli with crying and an increase in vital signs. Excessive irritability also may be a sign of injury to the CNS. All such abnormal signs are reported for further neurologic assessment.

Hepatic System

The major early assessments of the hepatic system are related to blood glucose and bilirubin conjugation.

Blood Glucose

The nurse should be alert for newborns at increased risk for hypoglycemia, which can cause brain damage. Factors that might have caused the infant to deplete available glucose are noted (Box 21.2). A quick estimate to determine whether the newborn appears to be near term and of appropriate size for gestational age is performed at birth.

Observing for signs of hypoglycemia is necessary throughout routine assessment and care. Early signs include jitteriness and other CNS signs and signs of respiratory difficulty, a decrease in temperature, and poor feeding. Some infants with hypoglycemia show no signs at all.

CRITICAL TO REMEMBER

Signs of Neonatal Hypoglycemia

Jitteriness, tremors
Poor muscle tone
Diaphoresis (sweating)
Poor suck
Tachypnea
Tachycardia
Dyspnea
Grunting
Cyanosis
Apnea
Low temperature
High-pitched cry
Irritability
Lethargy
Seizures, coma
No signs (some infants may be asymptomatic)

PROCEDURE 21.3   Obtaining Blood Samples from the Newborn by Heel Puncture

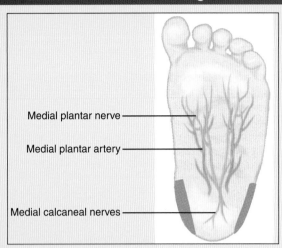

Medial plantar nerve

Medial plantar artery

Medial calcaneal nerves

Instructions are given here for measuring the infant's blood glucose level using a glucometer, but the same method applies to other testing.

1. Wash hands.
2. Gather supplies needed. Supplies vary with different glucose meters and for different tests. Common supplies include gloves, alcohol wipes, 2 × 2 inch gauze, glucometer, commercial lancing device, adhesive bandage, cotton balls, and blood-collecting devices (glucose screening reagent strips, blotting paper for metabolic screening tests, capillary tubes).
3. If the infant has not received a bath after birth, bathe the infant or thoroughly wash the puncture site before puncturing the skin.
4. Calibrate or program the glucose meter and use quality control measures according to the manufacturer's guidelines.

5. Warm the heel with a commercial heel warmer or a warm wet cloth according to agency policy. Take care not to burn the infant. Do not use a microwave to warm any item that will touch the infant.
6. Provide comforting measures (according to hospital policy) such as swaddling, providing a pacifier, allowing the parent to hold the infant or breastfeed, or giving the infant oral sucrose (unless testing blood glucose level). Rate the infant's pain level before, during, and after the procedure using an infant pain scale.
7. Apply gloves.
8. Hold the heel in one hand and locate the site. Palpate the bone of the heel and place the thumb or finger over the walking surface of the foot.
9. Avoiding the bone and the walking surface of the foot, choose a puncture site that has not been used previously (see diagram). The lateral heel is preferred, but the medial side may be used if necessary.
10. Clean the site with alcohol and wipe dry with sterile gauze or allow to air dry.
11. Puncture the side of the heel with a lancet or a spring-loaded heel incision device which punctures to the appropriate depth. Place the device in a sharps container.
12. Follow agency policy or manufacturer's directions regarding using or discarding the first drop of blood, collecting the sample, determining the amount of blood to collect, handling the specimen properly, and reading the results.
13. Avoid excessive squeezing of the foot.
14. Obtain blood sample. Apply adhesive bandage. Check site frequently and remove the bandage when the bleeding stops.
15. Document the procedure and the results. Send specimens to the laboratory as appropriate. Report abnormal readings and follow up according to agency policy.

Screening for blood glucose is not necessary for term infants who are low risk and asymptomatic (AAP & ACOG, 2017). Those at risk or showing early signs should be screened. The need for intervention should be individualized based on the newborn's clinical situation and individual characteristics rather than a specific plasma glucose concentration (AAP & ACOG, 2017). A suggested guideline includes a blood glucose target value of levels 45 mg/dL or greater before routine feedings and interventions for blood glucose levels less than 40 mg/dL in the first 4 hours of life (AAP & ACOG, 2017; Abramowski et al., 2020). Capillary blood is used in screening tests; these tests are less accurate than laboratory tests using venous blood. Therefore, a laboratory analysis (per agency policy) should be used to verify readings of 40 mg/dL or below (AAP & ACOG, 2017).

Early and frequent feedings of the healthy, term newborn decrease the risk for hypoglycemia. Corrective interventions, when indicated by the neonate's condition, facility protocol, and provider orders, include feeding the baby and rechecking the glucose in 1 hour. Intravenous (IV) glucose may be required for newborns with symptoms of hypoglycemia and those who do not respond to feedings (AAP & ACOG, 2017).

Infants who are at increased risk are usually monitored for 12 to 24 hours after birth (AAP & ACOG, 2017).

Avoiding injuries to the infant's foot is important when taking blood from the heel (Procedure 21.3). If the lancet goes into the calcaneus bone, osteomyelitis may result. Commercial devices for heel puncture are designed to puncture the heel to the proper depth. They are available for full-term and preterm infants. The site chosen should avoid injury to major nerves and arteries in the area. Other complications include cellulitis, abscess, scarring, bruising, and pain.

Bilirubin

The nurse assesses for jaundice at least every 8 to 12 hours and is particularly watchful when infants are at increased risk for hyperbilirubinemia. Jaundice is identified by pressing the infant's skin over a firm surface, such as the end of the nose or the sternum. The skin blanches as the blood is pressed out of the tissues, making it easier to see the yellow color which remains. Jaundice is more obvious when the nurse assesses in natural light. Jaundice begins at the head and moves down the body, and the areas of the body involved should be documented. Yellowish color of the skin and sclera (jaundice) becomes visible when the bilirubin level is greater than 6 to 7 mg/dL (Alden, 2018).

Jaundice appearing before the second day of life may indicate the bilirubin level is rising more quickly and to higher levels than normal and may not be physiologic. The physician or nurse practitioner may order laboratory determinations of the bilirubin level based on the nurse's assessment. In many facilities, protocols allow the nurse to obtain transcutaneous bilirubin (TcB) measurements using a bilirubinometer or laboratory measurement of total serum bilirubin (TSB) before notification of a nurse practitioner or physician. A bilirubinometer is a noninvasive device to measure bilirubin in the infant's skin, thus avoiding repeated skin punctures to obtain blood samples. Obtain TSB or TcB measurements on all infants jaundiced within the first 24 hours.

If serial bilirubin assays are ordered, the nurse notes change from one reading to the next and correlates the results with the infant's age. Abnormal results of TcB should be confirmed by measurement of TSB. Charts are available that show the degree of risk for infants at different ages (in hours) by the level of TSB (see Fig. 20.7).

The AAP and ACOG (2017) recommend obtaining TSB or TcB measurements on every infant before discharge. This helps determine whether discharge should be delayed or early follow-up arranged. All abnormal results should be documented and reported to the nurse practitioner or physician. Application of the nursing process in the care of infants at risk for hyperbilirubinemia is covered in Chapter 22, and a discussion of phototherapy is in Chapter 25.

? KNOWLEDGE CHECK

6. What are some signs of hypoglycemia in the newborn?
7. Why is it important to use the correct site for heel punctures when obtaining blood samples?

Gastrointestinal System

The initial assessment of the gastrointestinal tract occurs during the first hours after birth, when the nurse observes the parts that can be seen and the infant takes the initial feeding.

Mouth

The mouth is inspected visually and by palpation. Some infants are born with precocious teeth, usually lower incisors (Fig. 21.11). If the teeth are loose, the physician usually removes them to prevent aspiration. Epstein's pearls may be present on the hard palate or gums. These small, white, hard inclusion cysts are accumulations of epithelial cells and disappear without treatment within a few weeks. They are a form of milia.

The nurse examines the tongue for size and movement. A large, protruding tongue is present in hypothyroidism and some chromosomal disorders. Paralysis of the facial nerve affects the movement of the tongue and causes unilateral drooping of the mouth noticeable during crying or sucking. The tongue may appear to be tongue-tied because of the short

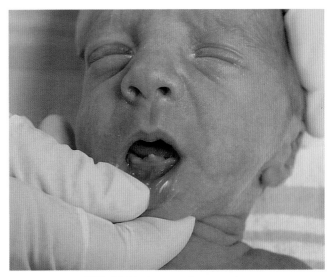

FIG. 21.11 A precocious tooth.

frenulum, but this is normal and usually has no effect on the infant's ability to feed. In a true tongue-tie, there is limited tongue movement. Clipping of the frenulum seldom is practiced because of the potential for infection.

Although candidiasis (thrush) is not apparent in the mouth immediately after birth, it may appear 1 or 2 days later. The lesions resemble milk curds on the tongue and cheeks, which bleed if attempts are made to wipe them away. Newborns may become infected with *Candida albicans* during passage through a candidal vaginal infection at birth. The infant is treated with antifungal medication such as nystatin suspension.

A cleft lip or palate results if the lip or palate fails to close. Cleft palate may involve the hard or soft palate or both and may appear alone or with a cleft lip. The palate is inspected when the infant cries. A gloved finger is inserted into the mouth to palpate the hard and soft palate. A very small cleft of the soft palate may be missed if only a visual examination is done.

Suck

The full-term infant should have a strong suck reflex, which is elicited when the lips or palate are stimulated. The reflex is weaker in the neonate who is preterm, is ill, or has just been fed. The newborn's cheeks have well-developed muscles and sucking pads, which enhance the ability to suck. These fatty sucking pads last until late in infancy, when sucking is no longer essential. Blisters may be present on the newborn's hands or arms from strong sucking before birth.

Initial Feeding

The initial feeding is an opportunity to further assess the newborn. Breastfeeding should begin in the first hour after the birth. The nurse can observe the infant's response unobtrusively while assisting the client to position the infant. If the newborn will be fed formula, the initial feeding should be no more than 1 oz to decrease regurgitation from overdistention of the stomach.

The nurse evaluates the infant's ability to suck, swallow, and breathe in a coordinated manner. Although the fetus sucks and swallows in utero, these acts may not have been performed together. The addition of breathing to sucking and swallowing is a new experience. Some newborns choke or gag during the first feeding. Others may become dusky or cyanotic because they become apneic while feeding. In either case the nurse should stop the feeding immediately, suction if necessary, and stimulate the infant to cry by rubbing the back. Most full-term infants learn to coordinate sucking, swallowing, and breathing very quickly.

Choking, coughing, cyanosis, or excessive oral secretions may indicate closure of the esophagus (esophageal atresia) or a connection between the trachea and esophagus (tracheoesophageal fistula). Neonates who continue to have difficulty with cyanosis during feedings may have a cardiac anomaly. Further assessment and referral are necessary.

Abdomen

The abdomen should be soft and rounded and should protrude slightly but should not be distended. The stomach may be distended by mucus, blood, and amniotic fluid swallowed during birth. An abdomen so distended that the skin is stretched and shiny may indicate obstruction. If the abdomen is distended, the nurse should measure the abdominal circumference periodically to note changes. The measurements should be recorded and reported to the health care provider. Loops of bowel should not be visible through the abdominal wall. Visible loops could indicate air and meconium are not passing through the intestines normally.

A sunken or scaphoid appearance of the abdomen occurs in diaphragmatic hernia, in which intestines are located in the chest cavity instead of the abdomen. This condition interferes with development of the lungs, resulting in respiratory difficulty at birth. The nurse listens over the abdomen for bowel sounds, which usually appear about 15 minutes after birth (Verklan, 2021). Bowel sounds heard in the chest may indicate diaphragmatic hernia.

An umbilical hernia occurs when the intestinal muscles fail to close around the umbilicus, allowing the intestines to protrude through the weak area. The condition is more common in low-birth-weight, male, and African American infants. By the time the infant is walking well, the muscles are usually stronger, and the hernia is no longer present. Some umbilical hernias require surgical repair.

Palpating the abdomen is easiest when the infant is relaxed and quiet. The abdomen should feel soft because the muscles are not yet well developed. Masses may indicate tumors of the kidneys. Palpation of the liver and kidneys usually is not part of routine nursing assessment of the abdomen but is performed by the primary care provider. The liver is normally 1 to 2 cm below the right costal margin. If the organ seems large, it should be reported to the physician or nurse practitioner because it may be a sign of congestive heart failure or congenital infection.

Stools

Stools should be assessed for type, color, and consistency. By the third to fourth day, stools reflect the type of feeding the infant receives. A "water ring" should never be present around the solid part of any stool. A water ring is a wet, stained area on the diaper where watery stool has been absorbed. There may be an area of more solid stool in addition, or all stool may have soaked into the diaper. A water ring indicates diarrhea and may be caused by formula intolerance or infection.

The first stool should be passed within 24 hours after birth (Verklan, 2021). The nurse should be aware of whether any stools have been passed since birth and, if so, when the infant's last stool occurred. If there is a question about whether the infant has had a stool, the nurse should investigate further. Feeding may cause the infant to pass a stool. Although rectal temperatures are not recommended, the provider may gently insert a thermometer into the rectum to determine patency and stimulate stool passage.

? KNOWLEDGE CHECK

8. Why is assessment of newborn reflexes important?
9. Why is it important for the nurse to observe the first feeding carefully?

Genitourinary System
Kidney Palpation

The health care provider palpates the kidneys just above the level of the umbilicus on each side of the abdomen during the first hours after birth. Abdominal masses may indicate enlargement or tumors of the kidneys.

The kidneys form early in fetal development when other systems are also developing. Therefore, kidney anomalies are often accompanied by other defects. For example, infants with only one umbilical artery or defects involving the ears may have renal anomalies. The nurse should observe carefully for urinary output in these infants to determine whether the kidneys are functioning adequately.

Urine

Most newborns void within 12 to 24 hours of birth and a few within 48 hours of birth. Because absence of urine output during this time may indicate anomalies, the first void should be carefully noted on the chart. The newborn's bladder empties as little as once or twice during the first 2 days, although more frequent voiding is common. Because of the small amount, the first void may be missed. Sometimes it occurs at birth but goes unnoticed because attention is focused on the infant's overall condition.

If there is a concern about whether the newborn has urinated, the delivery notes should be carefully read to see if the infant voided at birth. The nurse should ask the parents if they have changed a wet diaper. Increasing the infant's fluid intake often can initiate urination. If no void occurs in the expected time, the infant's fluid intake should be increased and the physician or nurse practitioner alerted.

By the fourth day of life, at least six wet diapers can be expected daily. Each void is recorded in the infant's chart, including the number of diapers changed by the parents. The total number is evaluated based on the age of the infant. Parent teaching should include the expectation for at least six wet diapers by the fourth day. This indicates the infant is taking adequate fluid.

If an infant is having feeding difficulties, noting the number of wet diapers is especially important. Disposable diapers are very absorbent, and the pale color of the newborn's urine may cause very little color change on the diaper. Wet diapers generally feel heavier than dry ones. If necessary, the nurse can put on gloves and take the diaper apart to examine it. The absorbent inner lining is damp if urine is present. Cotton balls or tissue placed in the diaper also may be used to increase visibility of small amounts of urine.

The newborn's urine may contain uric acid crystals, which cause a reddish or pink stain on the diaper. This is known as *brick dust staining* and may be frightening to parents, who may think the infant is bleeding. It does not continue beyond the first few days as the kidneys mature.

Genitalia

The nurse examines the newborn's genitalia for size, maturation, and presence of any abnormalities.

Female. In the full-term female infant, the labia majora should be large and completely cover the clitoris and labia minora. The labia may be darker than the surrounding skin, a normal response to exposure to pregnancy hormones before birth. Edema of the labia and white mucous vaginal discharge are normal. A small amount of vaginal bleeding, known as *pseudomenstruation,* may occur from the sudden withdrawal of these hormones. Hymenal (vaginal) tags are small pieces of tissue at the vaginal orifice. These are normal and disappear in a few weeks. The urinary meatus and vagina should be present.

Male. The scrotum should be pendulous at term and may be dark brown from pregnancy hormones. Pressure during a breech delivery may cause it to be edematous. Rugae (creases in the scrotum) are deep and cover the entire scrotum in the full-term infant.

Enlargement of one or both sides of the scrotum may result from a hydrocele. This collection of fluid around the testes may make palpating the testes difficult. Placing a flashlight against the sac may outline the testes. Parents should be told hydroceles are not painful and often reabsorb within 1 year. Some require later surgery.

Palpation of the scrotum determines whether the testes have descended (Fig. 21.12). Testes feel like small, round, movable objects that "slip" between the fingers. If the testes are not present in the scrotal sac, they may be felt in the inguinal canal. An empty scrotal sac appears smaller than one with testes.

Undescended testes (cryptorchidism) may occur on one or both sides. Approximately 50% of undescended testes in full-term infants will descend within 3 months. If the testes do not descend after 6 months, surgery may be performed to preserve fertility (Urology Care Foundation, 2021).

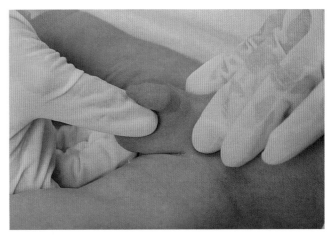

FIG. 21.12 The testes are palpated from front to back with the thumb and forefinger. Placing a finger over the inguinal canal holds the testes in place for palpation.

The meatus should be at the tip of the glans penis. It may be abnormally located on the underside of the penis (hypospadias), on the upper side (epispadias), or on the perineum. The prepuce or foreskin of the penis covers the glans and is adherent to it. Attempts to retract it in the newborn are unnecessary and can cause injury. Abnormal placement of the meatus may not be visible because it is covered by the prepuce, but often the prepuce in these infants is incompletely formed. Hypospadias may be accompanied by chordee, a condition in which fibrotic tissue causes the penis to curve downward. These conditions are later corrected by surgery.

Parents are very concerned about any abnormalities of the genitalia. If the meatus is abnormally positioned, they need an explanation of the condition and why the infant should not be circumcised. The foreskin may be needed for later plastic surgery to repair the defect.

Integumentary System
Skin

The newborn's skin is fragile and shows marks easily, especially in infants with fair coloring. Because the skin is so sensitive, reddened areas and rashes may develop during the early days of life. The nurse should examine every inch of skin surface carefully during the initial assessment and at the beginning of each shift. Marks should be documented and explained to parents, who may be worried and need emotional support.

Color. The skin color should be pink or tan. Red, thin skin occurs in preterm infants. Redness (ruddy color or plethora) in the full-term infant may indicate polycythemia. Acrocyanosis is common during the first day as a result of poor peripheral circulation. The infant's mouth and central body areas should not be cyanotic at any time. Blanching the skin over the nose or chest shows the presence of jaundice. Jaundice is abnormal during the first day of life but common during the first week.

A greenish–brown discoloration of the skin, nails, and cord results if meconium was passed in utero. The discoloration may indicate the infant was compromised at some time

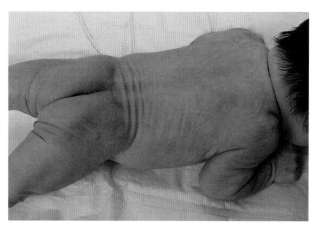

FIG. 21.13 Lanugo is abundant on this slightly preterm infant.

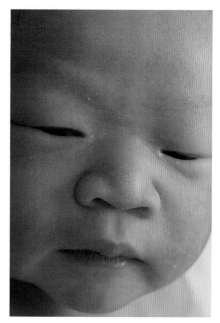

FIG. 21.14 Milia.

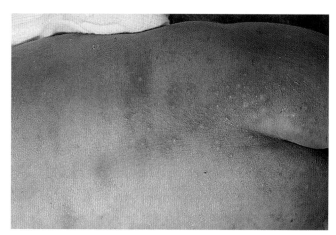

FIG. 21.15 Erythema toxicum. (From Hurwitz, S. (1993). *Clinical pediatric dermatology* (2nd ed., p. 13). Philadelphia: Saunders.)

before birth, and it is more common in the postterm infant. These infants should be watched for other complications such as respiratory difficulty.

Harlequin color change. Harlequin coloration is a clear color division over the body with one side deep pink or red and the other half pale or of expected color. The cause is vasomotor instability, and it is usually transient and benign.

Mottling (Cutis marmorata). Mottling is a lacy, red or blue pattern from dilated blood vessels under the skin. It is usually normal from vasomotor instability, occurring when the infant is exposed to cold, stressed, or overstimulated. If persistent, it may indicate a chromosomal abnormality.

Vernix caseosa. Vernix caseosa, a thick white substance that resembles cream cheese, provides a protective covering for the fetal skin in utero. The full-term infant has little vernix left on the body except small amounts in the creases. A thick covering of vernix may indicate a preterm infant, and a postterm infant may have none at all. Yellow-tinged vernix may result from elevated bilirubin in utero, and green-tinged vernix is caused by meconium staining.

Lanugo. Lanugo is fine, soft hair that covers the fetus during intrauterine life (Fig. 21.13). As the fetus nears term, the lanugo becomes thinner. The term infant may have a small amount of lanugo on the shoulders, forehead, sides of the face, and upper back. Dark-skinned infants often have more lanugo than infants with lighter coloring, and their darker hair is more visible. Lanugo is assessed as part of the gestational age assessment.

Milia. Milia are white cysts, 1 to 2 mm in size, caused by sebaceous gland secretions, which disappear without treatment (Tappero, 2021). They occur on the face over the forehead, nose, cheeks, and chin (Fig. 21.14).

Erythema toxicum. The nurse notes the presence of erythema toxicum—red, blotchy areas with white or yellow papules or vesicles in the center (Fig. 21.15). It is commonly called *flea bite rash* or *newborn rash* and resembles small bites or acne. The rash occurs in as many as 70% of newborns. It appears during the first 24 to 48 hours after birth and can continue for several days (Gardner & Niermeyer, 2021). It is most common over the face, back, shoulders, and chest. The condition does not result from infection but should be

differentiated from a pustular rash caused by staphylococcal infection or vesicles from herpes simplex.

Birthmarks. The nurse inspects all areas of the skin for birthmarks or other changes. The size, color, location, elevation, and texture of all birthmarks should be carefully documented. All marks should be explained, as follows, to parents, who are often concerned:

- Mongolian spots are bluish–gray marks that resemble bruises on the sacrum, buttocks, arms, shoulders, and other areas (Fig. 21.16). Mongolian spots occur most frequently in newborns with dark skin, such as Black, Asian, Native American, and Hispanic newborns (Gardner & Niermeyer, 2021; Kibbi, 2019). Although they usually disappear after the first few years of life, some continue into adulthood.
- A nevus simplex is also called a *salmon patch, stork bite,* or *telangiectatic nevus* (Fig. 21.17). It is a flat, pink discoloration from dilated capillaries that occurs on the eyelids,

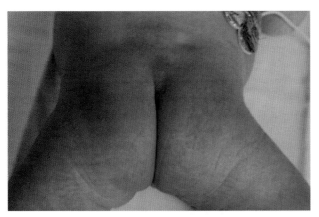

FIG. 21.16 Mongolian spots.

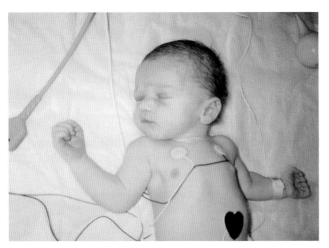

FIG. 21.17 Nevus simplex, salmon patch, or stork bite.

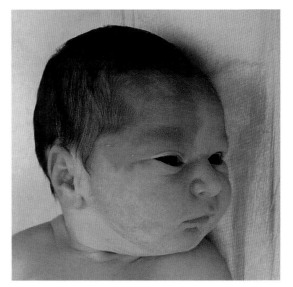

FIG. 21.18 Port-wine stain (nevus flammeus).

just above the bridge of the nose, or at the nape of the neck. The color blanches when the area is pressed and is more prominent during crying. The lesions disappear by 2 years of age, although those at the nape of the neck may persist.
- Nevus flammeus (port-wine stain) is a permanent, flat, pink to dark reddish–purple mark that varies in size and location and does not blanch with pressure (Fig. 21.18). The lesion may darken and may become nodular as the child gets older. If it is large and in a visible area, it can be lightened by laser surgery, which is often begun in infancy. Lesions located over the forehead and upper eyelid may be associated with Sturge–Weber syndrome, a serious neurologic condition.
- Nevus vasculosus (strawberry hemangioma) consists of enlarged capillaries in the outer layers of skin. It is dark red and raised with a rough surface, giving a strawberry-like appearance. The hemangioma usually is located on the head. It may be present at birth or develop by 6 months of age. After growing larger for 6 months, the hemangioma regresses over several years and disappears. No treatment is necessary unless it becomes infected or ulcerated.
- Café-au-lait spots are permanent, light-brown areas that may occur anywhere on the body. Although they are harmless, the number and size are important. Six or more spots or spots larger than 0.5 cm are associated with neurofibromatosis, a genetic condition of neural tissue.

Marks from delivery. The nurse inspects the infant for marks that may have occurred from injury or pressure during labor or birth.
- Bruises may appear on any part of the body where pressure occurred during birth. Bruising or petechiae of the face may be present if the cord was wrapped tightly around the neck during birth (nuchal cord). Bruising on the head may result from use of a vacuum extractor.
- Petechiae, pinpoint bruises that resemble a rash, may appear on the back, face, and groin. They result from increased intravascular pressure during the birth process. Widespread or continued formation of petechiae may indicate infection or a low platelet count.
- A small puncture mark is present on the newborn's head if a fetal monitor scalp electrode was attached. The area should scab and heal normally but is observed for signs of infection.
- Forceps marks occur over the cheeks and ears where the instruments were applied. Their size, color, and location are carefully documented. Asymmetry or lack of movement of the face may indicate injury of the facial nerve.

Other skin assessments. The nurse records other aspects of the skin that may indicate abnormalities. Localized edema may be caused by trauma from birth. Generalized edema shows a more serious condition such as heart failure. Peeling of the skin is expected in full-term newborns. Excessive amounts of peeling may indicate a postterm infant.

Documentation. All marks, bruises, rashes, and other abnormalities of the skin should be recorded in the nurses' notes. The location, size, color, elevation, and texture of each mark are described. Subsequent changes in appearance from previous descriptions also are noted on the chart.

The nurse may not always know the proper name for each type of mark on the infant's skin.

When in doubt about the name of a mark, a description is sufficient. For example, a nevus simplex (stork bite) might be described as a "flat, pink area 1 × 2 cm in size over nape of the neck, which blanches with pressure."

Breasts

The nurse notes the placement of the nipples and looks for extra (supernumerary) nipples, which may appear on the chest or in the axilla. Occasionally, the breasts become engorged and secrete a small amount of white fluid (sometimes called *witch's milk*) a few days later. This condition is caused by maternal hormones and resolves within a few weeks without treatment. The breasts should not be expressed or manipulated because this could cause infection.

Hair and Nails

The hair on the full-term infant should be silky and soft, whereas hair on the preterm infant is woolly or fuzzy. The nails come to the end of the fingers or beyond. Very long nails may indicate a postterm infant. A green–brown staining of the nails may occur if the infant passed meconium before birth. It is a sign of possible fetal distress (Table 21.2).

ASSESSMENT OF GESTATIONAL AGE

The gestational age assessment is an examination of the newborn's physical and neurologic characteristics to determine the number of weeks from conception to birth. It is important because neonates born before or after term and those whose size is not appropriate for gestational age are at increased risk

for complications. Although the gestational age may be calculated from the mother's last menstrual period and by ultrasonography during the pregnancy, the date of the last menstrual period is not always accurate, and ultrasonography is not always performed.

Because the times of development for various fetal characteristics are known, the presence or absence of these characteristics can help estimate gestational age. The estimated age then can be compared with the newborn's weight, length, and head circumference to determine whether the neonate is large, appropriate (average), or small in size for gestational age.

Assessment Tools

The New Ballard Score (Fig. 21.19) is often used to assess gestational age based on neuromuscular and physical characteristics. It is designed to assess gestational age from 20 to 44 weeks and provides accurate information within 2 weeks. It is most accurate when performed within 12 to 20 hours of birth (Arshpreet, 2017). A score is given to each assessment, and the total score is used to determine the gestational age of the infant. The New Ballard Score is described in the following section.

Neuromuscular Characteristics

Posture. The posture and degree of flexion of the extremities are scored before disturbing the quiet infant (Fig. 21.20).

TABLE 21.2· Summary of Newborn Assessment

Normal	Abnormal (Possible Causes)	Nursing Considerations
Initial Assessment		
Assess for obvious problems first. If infant is stable and has no problems that require immediate attention, continue with complete assessment.		
Vital Signs		
Temperature		
Axillary: 36.5°C–37.5°C (97.7°F–99.5°F). Axilla is preferred site.	Decreased (cold environment, hypoglycemia, infection, CNS problem). Increased (infection, environment too warm).	Decreased: Institute warming measures and check in 30 min. Check blood glucose. Increased: Remove excessive clothing. Check for dehydration. Decreased or increased: Look for signs of infection. Check radiant warmer or incubator temperature setting. Check thermometer for accuracy if skin is warm or cool to touch. Report abnormal temperatures to provider.
Pulses		
Heart rate 120–160 bpm (100 sleeping, 180 crying). Rhythm regular. PMI at third to fourth intercostal space, left midclavicular line. Brachial, femoral, and pedal pulses present and equal bilaterally.	Tachycardia (respiratory problems, anemia, infection, cardiac conditions). Bradycardia (asphyxia, increased intracranial pressure). PMI to right (dextrocardia, pneumothorax). Murmurs (normal or congenital heart defects). Dysrhythmias. Absent or unequal pulses (coarctation of the aorta).	Note location of murmurs. Report abnormal rates, rhythms and sounds, pulses.

TABLE 21.2 Summary of Newborn Assessment—cont'd

Normal	Abnormal (Possible Causes)	Nursing Considerations
Respirations		
Rate 30–60 (average 40–49) per min.	Tachypnea, especially after the first hour (respiratory distress).	Mild variations require continued monitoring and usually clear in early hours after birth.
Respirations irregular, shallow, unlabored.	Slow respirations (maternal medications).	If persistent or more than mild, suction, give oxygen, call physician, and initiate more intensive care.
Chest movements symmetric.	Nasal flaring (respiratory distress).	
Breath sounds present and clear bilaterally.	Grunting (respiratory distress syndrome).	
	Gasping (respiratory depression).	
	Periods of apnea more than 20 seconds or with change in heart rate or color (respiratory depression, sepsis, cold stress).	
	Asymmetry or decreased chest expansion (pneumothorax).	
	Intercostal, xiphoid, or supraclavicular retractions or seesaw (paradoxical) respirations (respiratory distress).	
	Moist, coarse breath sounds (crackles, rhonchi) (fluid in lungs).	
	Bowel sounds in chest (diaphragmatic hernia).	
Blood Pressure		
Varies with age, weight, activity, and gestational age.	Hypotension (hypovolemia, shock, sepsis).	Report abnormal BP readings.
Average systolic 65–95 mm Hg, average diastolic 30–60 mm Hg.	BP ≥ 20 mm Hg higher in arms than legs (coarctation of the aorta).	Prepare for intensive care if BP is very low.
Measurements		
Weight		
Weight 2500–4000 g (5 lb., 8 oz to 8 lb., 13 oz).	High (LGA, maternal diabetes).	Determine cause.
Weight loss up to 7%–10% in early days.	Low (SGA, preterm, multifetal pregnancy, medical conditions in mother which affected fetal growth).	Monitor for complications common to cause.
	Weight loss above 10% (dehydration, feeding problems).	
Length		
48–53 cm (19–21 inches).	Below normal (SGA, congenital dwarfism).	Determine cause.
	Above normal (LGA, maternal diabetes).	Monitor for complications common to cause.
Head Circumference		
32–38 cm (13–15 inches).	Small (SGA, microcephaly, anencephaly).	Determine cause.
Head and neck are approximately one-fourth of infant's body surface.	Large (LGA, hydrocephalus, increased intracranial pressure).	Monitor for complications common to cause.
Chest Circumference		
30–36 cm (12–14 in).	Small (SGA).	Determine cause.
Is 2 cm less than head circumference.	Large (LGA).	Monitor for complications common to cause.
Posture		
Flexed extremities move freely, resist extension, return quickly to flexed state.	Limp, flaccid, "floppy," or rigid extremities (preterm, hypoxia, medications, CNS trauma).	Seek cause, report abnormalities.
Hands usually clenched.	Hypertonic (neonatal abstinence syndrome, CNS injury).	
Movements symmetric.	Jitteriness or tremors (low glucose or calcium).	
Slight tremors on crying.	Opisthotonos, seizures, stiff when held (CNS injury).	
"Molds" body to caretaker's body when held, responds by quieting when needs met.		
Breech: Extended, stiff legs.		

Continued

TABLE 21.2 Summary of Newborn Assessment—cont'd

Normal	Abnormal (Possible Causes)	Nursing Considerations
Cry		
Lusty, strong.	High-pitched (increased intracranial pressure). Weak, absent, irritable, catlike "mewing" (neurologic problems). Hoarse or crowing (laryngeal irritation).	Observe for changes, report abnormalities.
Skin		
Color pink or tan with acrocyanosis. Vernix caseosa in the creases. Small amounts of lanugo over shoulders, sides of face, forehead, upper back. Skin turgor good with quick recoil. Some cracking and peeling of skin. Expected variations: Milia. Skin tags. Erythema toxicum ("flea bite" rash). Puncture on scalp (from electrode). Mongolian spots. Harlequin color (normal transient autonomic imbalance).	**Color:** Cyanosis of mouth and central areas (hypoxia). Facial bruising (nuchal cord). Pallor (anemia, hypoxia). Gray (hypoxia, hypotension). Red, sticky, transparent skin (very preterm). Ruddy (polycythemia). Greenish–brown discoloration of skin, nails cord or vernix (possible fetal compromise, postterm). Mottling (normal or cold stress, hypovolemia, sepsis). Jaundice (pathologic if first 24 hr.). Yellow vernix (elevated bilirubin in utero) Thick vernix (preterm). **Delivery marks:** Bruises on body (pressure), scalp (vacuum extractor), or face (cord around neck). Petechiae (pressure, low platelet count, infection). Forceps marks. **Birthmarks:** Mongolian spots. Nevus simplex (salmon patch, stork bite). Nevus flammeus (port-wine stain). Nevus vasculosus (strawberry hemangioma). Café-au-lait spots ($\geq$6 larger than 0.5 cm (neurofibromatosis). **Other:** Excessive lanugo (preterm). Excessive peeling, cracking (postterm). Pustules or other rashes (infection). "Tenting" of skin (dehydration).	Differentiate facial bruising from cyanosis. Central cyanosis requires suction, oxygen, and further treatment. Report jaundice in first 24 hr. or more extensive than expected for age. Watch for respiratory problems in infants with meconium staining. Look for signs and complications of preterm or postterm birth. Record location, size, shape, color, type of rashes and marks. Differentiate Mongolian spots from bruises. Check for facial movement with forceps marks. Watch for jaundice with bruising. Point out and explain normal skin variations to parents.
Head		
Sutures palpable with small separation between each. Anterior fontanel diamond-shaped, 4–6 cm, soft, and flat. May bulge slightly with crying. Posterior fontanel triangular, 0.5–1 cm. Hair silky and soft with individual hair strands. Expected variations: Overriding sutures (molding). Caput succedaneum or cephalohematoma (pressure during birth).	Head large (hydrocephalus, increased intracranial pressure) or small (microcephaly). Widely separated sutures (hydrocephalus) or hard, ridged area at sutures (craniosynostosis). Anterior fontanel depressed (dehydration, molding), full or bulging at rest (increased intracranial pressure). Woolly, bunchy hair (preterm). Unusual hair growth (genetic abnormalities).	Seek cause of variations. Observe for signs of dehydration with depressed fontanel; increased intracranial pressure with bulging of fontanel and wide separation of sutures. Refer for treatment. Differentiate caput succedaneum from cephalohematoma and reassure parents of normal outcome. Observe for jaundice with cephalohematoma.
Ears		
Ears well-formed and complete. Area where upper ear meets head even with imaginary line drawn from outer canthus of eye. Startle response to loud noises. Alerts to high-pitched voices.	Low-set ears (chromosomal disorders). Skin tags, preauricular sinuses, dimples (may be normal or associated with anomalies). No response to sound (deafness).	Check voiding if ears abnormal. Look for signs of chromosomal abnormality if position abnormal. Refer for evaluation if no response to sound.

TABLE 21.2 Summary of Newborn Assessment—cont'd

Normal	Abnormal (Possible Causes)	Nursing Considerations
Face		
Symmetric in appearance and movement. Parts proportional and appropriately placed.	Asymmetry (pressure and position in utero). Drooping of mouth or one side of face, "one-sided cry" (facial nerve injury). Abnormal appearance (chromosomal abnormalities).	Seek cause of variations. Check delivery history for possible cause of injury to facial nerve.
Eyes		
Symmetric. Eyes clear. Transient strabismus. Scant or absent tears. Pupils equal, react to light. Alerts to interesting sights. Doll's-eye sign, red reflex present. Expected variations: May have subconjunctival hemorrhage or edema of eyelids from pressure during birth.	Inflammation or drainage (chemical or infectious conjunctivitis). Constant tearing (plugged lacrimal duct). Unequal pupils. Failure to follow objects (blindness). White areas over pupils (cataracts). Setting-sun sign (hydrocephalus). Yellow sclera (jaundice). Blue sclera (osteogenesis imperfecta).	Clean and monitor any drainage; seek cause. Reassure parents that subconjunctival hemorrhage and edema will clear. Report abnormalities.
Nose		
Both nostrils open to air flow. May have slight flattening from pressure during birth.	Blockage of one or both nasal passages (choanal atresia). Malformations (congenital conditions). Flaring, mucus (respiratory distress).	Observe for respiratory distress. Report malformations.
Mouth		
Mouth, gums, tongue pink. Tongue normal in size and movement. Lips and palate intact. Sucking pads. Sucking, rooting, swallowing, gag reflexes present. Expected variations: Precocious teeth, Epstein's pearls.	Cyanosis (hypoxia). White patches on cheeks or tongue (candidiasis). Protruding tongue (Down's syndrome). Diminished movement of tongue, drooping mouth (facial nerve paralysis). Cleft lip or palate or both. Absent or weak reflexes (preterm, neurologic problem). Excessive drooling (tracheoesophageal fistula, esophageal atresia).	Check oxygen saturation and apply oxygen for cyanosis. Expect loose teeth to be removed. Obtain order for antifungal medication for candidiasis. Check client for vaginal or breast candidiasis infection Report anomalies.
Feeding		
Good suck/swallow coordination. Retains feedings.	Poorly coordinated suck and swallow (prematurity). Duskiness or cyanosis during feeding (cardiac defects). Choking, gagging, excessive drooling (tracheoesophageal fistula, esophageal atresia).	Breastfeeding: assist with latch on. Feed slowly. Stop frequently if difficulty occurs. Suction and stimulate if necessary. Refer infants with continued difficulty.
Neck and Clavicles		
Short neck, turns head easily side to side. Infant raises head when prone. Clavicles intact.	Weakness, contractures, or rigidity (muscle abnormalities). Webbing of neck, large fat pad at back of neck (chromosomal disorders). Crepitus, lump, or crying when clavicle or other bones palpated, diminished or absent arm movement (fractures).	Fracture of clavicle more frequent in large infants with shoulder dystocia at birth. Immobilize arm. Look for other injuries. Refer abnormalities.
Chest		
Cylinder shape. Xiphoid process may be prominent. Symmetric. Nipples present and located properly. Expected variation: May have engorgement, white nipple discharge (maternal hormone withdrawal).	Asymmetry (diaphragmatic hernia, pneumothorax). Supernumerary nipples. Redness (infection).	Report abnormalities.

Continued

TABLE 21.2   Summary of Newborn Assessment—cont'd

Normal	Abnormal (Possible Causes)	Nursing Considerations
Abdomen/Elimination		
Rounded, soft.	Sunken abdomen (diaphragmatic hernia).	Report abnormalities.
Bowel sounds present within 15 min after birth.	Distended abdomen or loops of bowel visible (obstruction, infection, enlarged organs).	Assess for other anomalies if only two vessels in cord.
Liver palpable 1–2 cm below right costal margin.	Absent bowel sounds after first hour (paralytic ileus).	Tighten or replace loose cord clamp.
Skin intact.	Masses palpated (kidney tumors, distended bladder).	If stool and urine output abnormal, look for missed recording, increase feedings, report.
Three vessels in cord.	Enlarged liver (infection, heart failure, hemolytic disease).	
Clamp tight and cord drying.	Abdominal wall defects (umbilical or inguinal hernia, omphalocele, gastroschisis, exstrophy of bladder).	
Meconium passed within 24 hr.	Two vessels in cord (other anomalies).	
Urine generally passed within 12–24 hr.	Bleeding (loose clamp).	
Expected variation: "Brick dust" staining of diaper (uric acid crystals).	Redness, drainage from cord (infection).	
	No passage of meconium (imperforate anus, obstruction).	
	Lack of urinary output (kidney anomalies) or inadequate intake amounts (dehydration).	
Genitals		
Female		
Labia majora dark, cover clitoris and labia minora.	Clitoris and labia minora larger than labia majora (preterm).	Check gestational age for immature genitalia.
Small amount of white mucous vaginal discharge.	Large clitoris (ambiguous genitalia).	Report anomalies.
Urinary meatus and vagina present.	Edematous labia (breech birth).	
Expected variations: Vaginal bleeding (pseudo menstruation).		
Hymenal tags.		
Male		
Testes within scrotal sac, rugae on scrotum, prepuce nonretractable.	Empty scrotal sac (cryptorchidism).	Check gestational age for immature genitalia.
Meatus at tip of penis.	Testes in inguinal canal or abdomen (preterm, cryptorchidism).	Report anomalies.
	Lack of rugae on scrotum (preterm).	Explain to parents why no circumcision can be performed with abnormal placement of meatus.
	Edema of scrotum (pressure in breech birth).	
	Enlarged scrotal sac (hydrocele).	
	Small penis, scrotum (preterm, ambiguous genitalia).	
	Urinary meatus located on upper side of penis (epispadias), underside of penis (hypospadias), or perineum.	
	Ventral curvature of the penis (chordee).	
Extremities		
Upper and Lower Extremities		
Equal and bilateral movement of extremities.	Crepitus, redness, lumps, swelling (fracture).	Report all anomalies, look for others.
Correct number and formation of fingers and toes.	Diminished or absent movement, especially during Moro reflex (fracture, nerve injury, paralysis).	
Nails to ends of digits or slightly beyond.	Polydactyly (extra digits).	
Flexion, good muscle tone.	Syndactyly (webbing).	
	Fused or absent digits.	
	Poor muscle tone (preterm, neurologic injury, hypoglycemia, hypoxia).	
Upper Extremities		
Two transverse palm creases.	Single transverse palmar crease (STPC; normal or Down's syndrome).	Report all anomalies, look for others.
	Diminished movement (injury).	
	Diminished movement of arm with extension and forearm prone (Erb–Duchenne paralysis).	

TABLE 21.2 Summary of Newborn Assessment—cont'd

Normal	Abnormal (Possible Causes)	Nursing Considerations
Lower Extremities		
Legs equal in length, abduct equally, gluteal and thigh creases and knee height equal, no hip "clunk." Normal position of feet.	Ortolani and Barlow tests abnormal, unequal leg length, unequal thigh or gluteal creases (developmental dysplasia of the hip). Malposition of feet (position in utero, talipes equinovarus).	Report all anomalies, look for others. Check malpositioned feet to see if they can be gently manipulated back to normal position.
Back		
No openings observed or felt in vertebral column. Anus patent. Sphincter tightly closed.	Failure of one or more vertebrae to close (spina bifida), with or without sac with spinal fluid and meninges (meningocele) or spinal fluid, meninges, and cord (myelomeningocele) enclosed. Tuft of hair over spina bifida occulta. Pilonidal dimple or sinus. Imperforate anus.	Report abnormalities. Observe for movement below level of defect. If sac is present, cover with sterile dressing wet with sterile saline. Protect from injury.
Reflexes		
See Table 21.1.	Absent, asymmetric, or weak reflexes.	Observe for signs of fractures, nerve injury, or injury to CNS.

BP, Blood pressure; *bpm,* beats per minute; *CNS,* central nervous system; *LGA,* large for gestational age; *PMI,* point of maximum impulse; *SGA,* small for gestational age.

Preterm neonates have immature flexor muscles and little energy or muscle tone. Therefore they have extended, limp arms and legs, which offer little resistance to movement by the examiner. Flexor tone improves as the gestational age increases, and it moves in a cephalocaudal manner down the infant's body. Full-term infants hold their arms close to the body with the elbows sharply flexed. The legs should be flexed at the hips, knees, and ankles. Posture is scored from 0 for a limp, flaccid posture to 4 if the newborn demonstrates good flexion of all extremities. The legs of infants who were in a frank breech position may be more extended than flexed even when they are full term.

Square window. The square window sign is elicited by flexing the hand at the wrist until the palm is as flat against the forearm as possible with gentle pressure (Fig. 21.21). The angle between the palm and forearm is measured. If the palm bends only 90 degrees (which is the extent of flexion in the adult wrist and looks like a square window), the score is 0. The gestational age of the infant is probably 32 weeks or less. The more mature the neonate, the smaller the angle until the palm folds flat against the forearm at term, the result of maternal hormones at the end of pregnancy.

Arm recoil. Full-term infants resist extension of the arms. In testing for arm recoil, the nurse holds the neonate's arms fully flexed at the elbows for 5 seconds, then pulls the hands straight down to the sides (Fig. 21.22). The hands are quickly released, and the degree of flexion is measured as the arms return to their normally flexed position. Preterm infants may move the arms slowly or not at all and receive a score of zero. Somewhat older infants have a sluggish recoil, with only partial return to flexion. If the arms move briskly to an angle of less than 90 degrees at the elbows, the score is 4.

Popliteal angle. To measure the popliteal angle, the newborn's lower leg is folded against the thigh, with the thigh on the abdomen (Fig. 21.23). With the thigh still flexed on the abdomen, the lower leg is straightened just until resistance is met. Continued pressure causes the infant to further extend the leg and results in an inaccurate score. The angle at the popliteal space when resistance is first felt is scored on a scale of 0 (if the leg can be fully extended) to 5 (if the angle at the popliteal space is less than 90 degrees). The preterm infant extends the leg farther than the full-term infant. The leg may extend with little resistance if the infant was in a frank breech position at birth.

Scarf sign. For the scarf sign, the nurse grasps the infant's hand and brings the arm across the body to the opposite side, keeping the shoulder flat on the bed and the head in the middle of the body (Fig. 21.24). The position of the elbow in relation to the midline of the infant's body is noted. The infant receives a score of 0 if muscle tone is so poor the arm wraps across the body like a scarf, with the elbow beyond the edge of the body. A top score (4) shows the elbow fails to reach the midline.

Heel to ear. The heel-to-ear assessment is similar to the measurement of the popliteal angle. In this case, however, the nurse grasps the infant's foot and pulls it straight up alongside the body toward the ears while the hips remain flat on the surface of the bed (Fig. 21.25). When resistance is felt, the position of the foot in relation to the head and the amount of flexion of the leg are compared with the diagrams. Increasing maturity is identified by the level of resistance and flexion. Record the position when resistance is first felt because the neonate may relax the leg if pressure continues. This assessment also may be inaccurate in infants who were in a breech position at birth.

Physical Characteristics

Skin. The skin is assessed for color, visibility of veins, peeling, and cracking. The very preterm infant's skin is translucent because it is thin and has little subcutaneous fat beneath the surface. The skin is red, sticky, and fragile, with easily

NEWBORN MATURITY RATING & CLASSIFICATION

ESTIMATION OF GESTATIONAL AGE BY MATURITY RATING
Symbols: X - 1st Exam   0 - 2nd Exam

NEUROMUSCULAR MATURITY

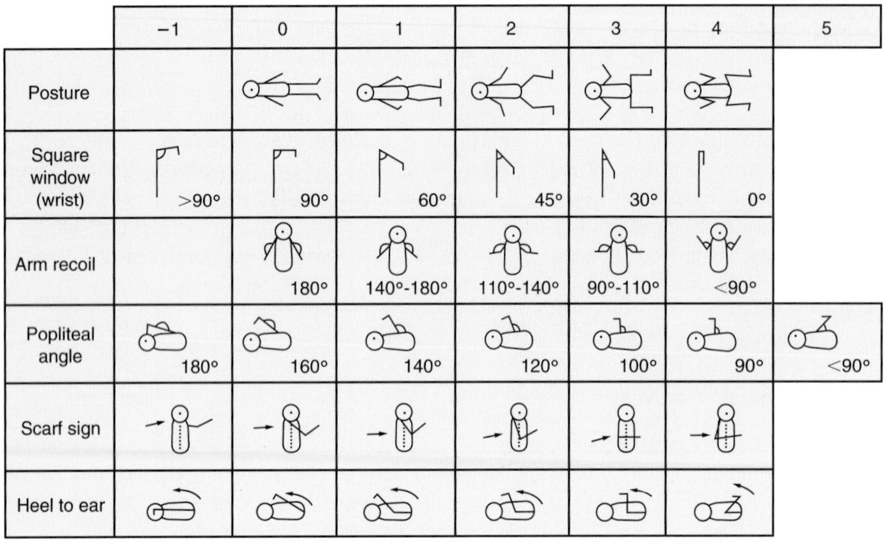

	−1	0	1	2	3	4	5
Posture							
Square window (wrist)	>90°	90°	60°	45°	30°	0°	
Arm recoil		180°	140°-180°	110°-140°	90°-110°	<90°	
Popliteal angle	180°	160°	140°	120°	100°	90°	<90°
Scarf sign							
Heel to ear							

Gestation by Dates _____ wks

Birth Date _____ Hour _____ am pm

Apgar _____ 1 min _____ 5 min

MATURITY RATING

score	weeks
−10	20
−5	22
0	24
5	26
10	28
15	30
20	32
25	34
30	36
35	38
40	40
45	42
50	44

PHYSICAL MATURITY

Skin	Sticky friable transparent	Gelatinous red, translucent	Smooth pink, visible veins	Superficial peeling &/or rash, few veins	Cracking pale areas rare veins	Parchment deep cracking no vessels	Leathery cracked wrinkled
Lanugo	None	Sparse	Abundant	Thinning	Bald areas	Mostly bald	
Plantar surface	Heel-toe 40-50 mm:−1 <40 mm:−2	>50 mm no crease	Faint red marks	Anterior transverse crease only	Creases ant. 2/3	Creases over entire sole	
Breast	Imperceptible	Barely perceptible	Flat areola no bud	Stippled areola 1-2 mm bud	Raised areola 3-4 mm bud	Full areola, 5-10 mm bud	
Eye/Ear	Lids fused loosely:−1 tightly:−2	Lids open pinna flat stays folded	Sl. curved pinna; soft; slow recoil	Well-curved pinna; soft but ready recoil	Formed & firm instant recoil	Thick cartilage ear stiff	
Genitals (male)	Scrotum flat, smooth	Scrotum empty faint rugae	Testes in upper canal rare rugae	Testes descending few rugae	Testes down good rugae	Testes pendulous deep rugae	
Genitals (female)	Clitoris prominent labia flat	Prominent clitoris small labia minora	Prominent clitoris enlarging minora	Majora & minora equally prominent	Majora large minora small	Majora cover clitoris & minora	

SCORING SECTION

	1st Exam=X	2nd Exam=O
Estimating Gest Age by Maturity Rating	_____ Weeks	_____ Weeks
Time of Exam	Date _____ Hour _____ am pm	Date _____ Hour _____ am pm
Age of Exam	_____ Hours	_____ Hours
Signature of Examiner	_____ M.D.	_____ M.D.

FIG. 21.19 New Ballard Score. (From Bristol-Myers Co., Evansville, IN. From Ballard, J. L., Khoury, J. C., Wedig, K., Wang, L., Eilers-Walsman, B. L., & Lipp, R. (1991). New Ballard Score, expanded to include extremely premature infants. *Journal of Pediatrics, 19*(3), 417–423.)

visible veins. In the mature newborn, the skin is thicker and the color is paler. Few veins are visible, usually over the chest and abdomen (see Fig. 21.24). At term, vernix is present only in the creases.

The full-term infant exhibits some peeling and cracking of the skin, especially around areas with creases, such as the ankles and feet. The postmature infant has deeply cracked skin, which appears as dry and thick as leather. Peeling becomes even more apparent during the hours after birth as the skin loses moisture.

Lanugo. Lanugo appears at 20 weeks of gestation and increases in amount until 28 weeks (see Fig. 21.13), when it begins to disappear. Most is shed by 33 to 36 weeks (Verhave, et al., 2020). A small amount may remain over the upper back

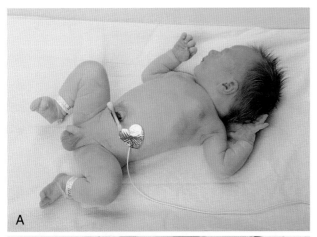

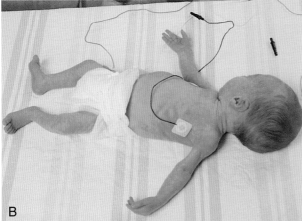

FIG. 21.20 Posture in newborns. A, The healthy full-term infant remains in a strongly flexed position. B, The preterm infant's extremities are extended.

and shoulders, on the ears, or on the sides of the forehead. The infant receives a score based on the amount of lanugo present on the back.

Plantar surface. Plantar creases begin to appear at 28 to 32 weeks of gestation and cover the entire foot by term (Jyothsna et al., 2018; Fig. 21.26). Although the creases are only red lines near the toes at first, they gradually spread down toward the heel and become deeper. The plantar creases should be assessed during the early hours after birth because creases appear more prominent as the infant's skin begins to dry. For the very preterm infant, the length of the foot is measured to help determine gestational age.

Breasts. The nipples, areolae, and size of the breast buds are assessed and scored. In very preterm infants, the structures are not visible. Gradually they grow larger and the areolae become raised above the chest wall. The breast buds enlarge until they are approximately 1 cm at term. To determine their size, the nurse places a finger on each side and measures the diameter (Fig. 21.27). Use of the thumb and forefinger may cause excess tissue to be drawn together, resulting in an inaccurate score.

Eyes and ears. The eyelids are fused until about 26 weeks of gestation (Gardner & Goldson, 2021). When the ear is assessed, the incurving and thickness of each pinna are rated (Fig. 21.28). At about 34 weeks of gestation, the upper pinnae, which have been flat, begin to curve over. The incurving continues around the ear until it reaches near the earlobe at 40 weeks of gestation (Tappero, 2021).

The amount of cartilage present in the ears is a more accurate guide to gestational age than the incurving of the pinnae because of individual differences in ear shape. As cartilage is deposited in the pinnae, the ears become stiff and stand away

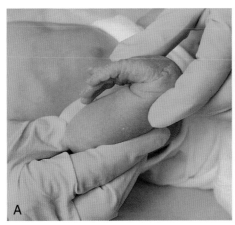

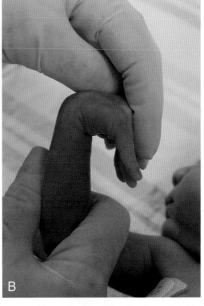

FIG. 21.21 The square window sign is performed on the arm without the identification bracelet. The nurse flexes the wrist and measures the angle. **A,** Infant near full term. **B,** Preterm infant.

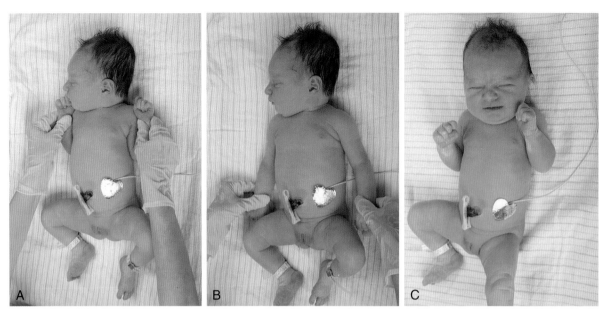

FIG. 21.22 **Arm recoil.** A, Arms flexed. B, Arms extended. C, Recoil for the full-term infant.

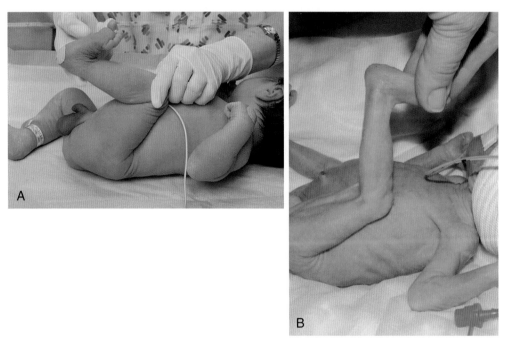

FIG. 21.23 The popliteal angle is measured by flexing the thigh against the abdomen and extending the lower leg to the point of resistance. A, Full-term infant. B, Preterm infant.

from the head. The ear is folded longitudinally and horizontally to assess the resistance and speed with which the ear returns to its original state. In newborns less than 34 weeks of gestation, the ear has little cartilage to keep it stiff. When folded, it remains folded over or returns slowly. In the term neonate, the ear springs back to its original position immediately.

Genitals. In the female infant, the relationship in size of the clitoris, labia minora, and labia majora is noted (Fig. 21.29). In the preterm infant, the labia majora are small and separated, and the clitoris and labia minora are large by comparison. As the infant nears term, the labia majora enlarge until the clitoris and labia minora are completely covered. Because the size of the labia majora is affected by the amount of fat deposited, the infant who is malnourished in utero may have genitalia with an immature appearance.

In the male infant, the location of the testes and the rugae on the scrotum are assessed (Fig. 21.30). The testes originate in the abdominal cavity and begin to descend at 28 weeks of gestation. By 37 weeks of gestation, they are located high in the scrotal sac, and they are generally completely descended by term. Rugae cover the surface of the scrotum by 40 weeks

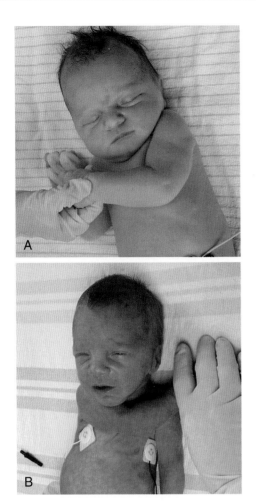

FIG. 21.24 **Scarf sign.** The nurse determines how far the arm will move across the chest and observes the position of the elbow when resistance is felt. A, Full-term infant. B, Preterm infant. (Note the many visible veins in the preterm infant and the absence of visible veins in the full-term infant.)

of gestation (Tappero, 2021). Once the testes are completely down into the scrotum, the scrotum appears large and pendulous.

Scoring

As each part of the gestational age assessment is performed, the infant's response is matched with the diagrams and descriptions on the assessment tool. The total score is compared with the corresponding gestational age. It is important to understand one or two characteristics alone are not enough to assign a gestational age. It is the total score of all assessed characteristics that determines the gestational age.

A difference of 2.5 points is necessary to change the gestational age by 1 week. Therefore, slight variations in the scores of examiners are not likely to cause significant differences in the outcome of the examination.

Gestational Age and Infant Size

The appropriateness of the neonate's size for gestational age is determined by plotting the weight, length, head circumference, and gestational age on a graph of intrauterine

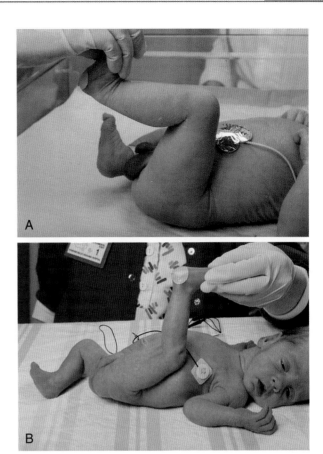

FIG. 21.25 **Heel-to-ear assessment.** The nurse grasps the foot and brings it up toward the ear. The score is recorded when resistance is felt. A, Full-term infant. B, Preterm infant.

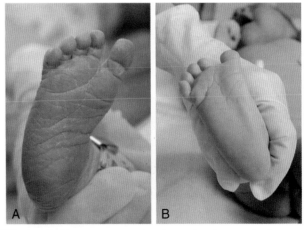

FIG. 21.26 Plantar creases begin to develop at the base of the toes and extend to the heel. A, The postterm infant has deep creases. B, The preterm infant has few creases on the entire foot.

development. This score determines how well the infant has grown for the amount of time spent in the uterus. An infant may be small, large, or of appropriate size for gestational age. The infant whose size is appropriate for gestational age falls between the 10th and 90th percentiles on the graph.

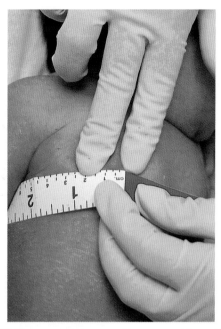

FIG. 21.27 The nurse places a finger on either side of the breast bud and measures the size. In the full-term infant, breast tissue is raised and the nipple is easily distinguished from surrounding skin. (Note the peeling skin.)

The large-for-gestational-age (LGA) infant is above the 90th percentile, and the small-for-gestational-age (SGA) infant is below the 10th percentile.

Further Assessments

When an infant's gestational age or measurements fall outside the expected range, the nurse monitors for complications. Specific complications are common to preterm, postterm, SGA, and LGA infants. For example, pregnancy complications may cause a poorly functioning placenta and an SGA infant. LGA infants are also prone to complications.

ASSESSMENT OF BEHAVIOR

Assessment of the infant's behavior helps determine intactness of the CNS and provides information about the ability to respond to caretaking activities. Because behavior differs at various times after birth, the nurse should be aware of the periods of reactivity and the six different states of behavior so nursing care can be adapted appropriately.

Periods of Reactivity

During the first and second periods of reactivity, newborns may have elevated pulse and respiratory rates, low temperatures, and excessive respiratory secretions. Careful observation is important at this time but usually can be done unobtrusively so parents can continue to enjoy the newborn. During the time between the first and second periods of reactivity, newborns cannot be awakened easily and are not interested in feeding.

Behavioral Changes

Nurses assess the infant's behavior and alert the physician to abnormalities. Assessment includes the six different behavioral states: quiet sleep, active sleep, drowsy, quiet alert, active alert, and crying. Movement between states should be smooth and not abrupt. The Brazelton Neonatal Behavioral Assessment Scale is often used when detailed knowledge about the infant is needed. In addition to assessing behavioral states, the scale analyzes other aspects of the newborn's behavior, such as orientation, habituation, self-consoling behaviors, social behaviors, and the appropriateness of the amount of time in each of these activities.

Orientation

The nurse notes the infant's orientation (ability to pay attention) to interesting visual or auditory stimuli. It is most prominent during the quiet alert state. Infants focus their eyes and turn their heads toward a stimulus in an attempt to prolong

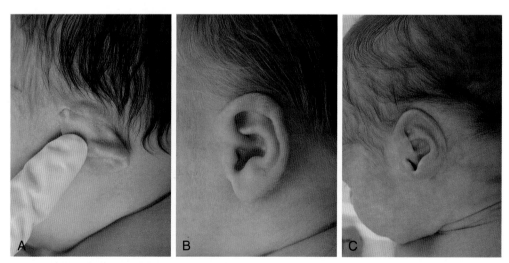

FIG. 21.28 Ear Maturation. A, The nurse folds the ears and notes how quickly they return to position. B, Ears in the full-term infant are well formed and have instant recoil. C, In the preterm infant, ears show less incurving of the pinna and recoil slowly or not at all.

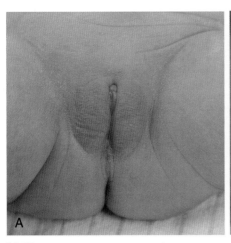
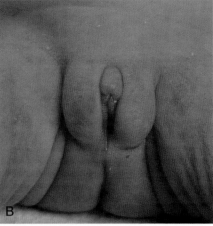

FIG. 21.29 **Female Genitals.** As the female matures, the labia majora cover the labia minora and clitoris completely; in the preterm infant, these structures are not covered. **A,** Near-term infant. **B,** Preterm infant.

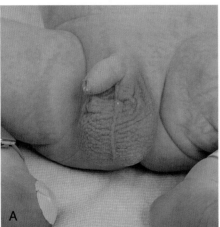
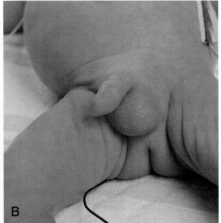

FIG. 21.30 **Male Genitals.** A, The full-term infant has a pendulous scrotum with deep rugae. B, In the preterm infant, the testes may not be descended and rugae are few.

contact with it. Preterm and ill neonates have less ability to orient to stimuli.

Habituation

The infant's response to a visual, auditory, or tactile stimulus is an important assessment. Generally, the first response of a healthy newborn to an interesting stimulus, such as a brightly colored object or bell, is a period of alertness. If the stimulus is disturbing, such as a bright light flashed in the eyes, the infant startles and attempts to escape by averting the eyes.

Infants gradually stop responding to continued unpleasant stimuli. This gradual habituation allows them to ignore the stimuli and save energy for physiologic needs. Newborns may display a dull, drowsy state or fall into a deep sleep. Those who seem unresponsive in a bright, noisy environment may be in a state of habituation. The preterm infant or one with damage to the CNS may not be able to habituate.

Self-Consoling Activities

Newborns are able to console themselves for short periods. Self-consoling activities include bringing their hands to their

mouth, sucking on their fists, listening to voices, and watching objects in the environment. Infants who are ill, preterm, or exposed to drugs prenatally have less ability to console themselves.

Parents' Response

The parents' growing ability to respond to the infant's behavioral cues should be noted. The nurse can point out the infant's behavioral changes to facilitate attachment and help the parents learn to interpret the infant's cues. The methods the parents use to meet the infant's needs during different behavior states also are noted.

? KNOWLEDGE CHECK

10. When should the first voiding occur? How often do infants void?
11. What is the nurse's responsibility regarding marks on the newborn's skin?
12. Why is the gestational age assessment important?
13. How do the periods of reactivity affect nursing care?

SUMMARY CONCEPTS

- Nurses assess newborns immediately after birth to detect serious abnormalities. If no problems are detected with a quick assessment, a more comprehensive examination is performed after parent-infant attachment and initiation of breastfeeding.
- Assessment of cardiorespiratory status includes history, airway, color, heart sounds, pulses, and blood pressure.
- Because they are safer, axillary temperatures are preferred to rectal temperatures.
- Molding of the head is expected during birth and may cause the head to appear misshapen. Caput succedaneum (localized swelling from pressure against the cervix) or a cephalohematoma (bleeding between the periosteum and the bone) may be present.
- Measurements are an important way to learn about growth before birth. Abnormal measurements alert the nurse to complications that may occur.
- Reflexes are an indication of the health of the central nervous system. Asymmetry or retention of reflexes beyond the time when they should disappear is abnormal.

- Early signs of hypoglycemia include jitteriness, poor muscle tone, respiratory distress, sweating, low temperature, and poor suck.
- In performing heel sticks to obtain blood samples, the nurse should choose the site carefully to avoid injury to the bone, nerves, or blood vessels of the heel.
- The initial feeding provides information about the neonate's ability to coordinate sucking, swallowing, and breathing and tolerance to feeding.
- Newborns pass the first stool within 24 hours of birth. Absence of stool for 48 hours may indicate an obstruction.
- The newborn's first void occurs within 12 to 48 hours. Infants may void only one or two times during the first 2 days and at least six times daily by the fourth day.
- Marks on the skin should be documented, including location, size, color, elevation, and texture. Because marks can be upsetting, they should be explained to the parents.
- The gestational age assessment provides an estimate of the infant's age from conception. It alerts the nurse to possible complications related to age and size.

Clinical Judgment and Next Generation NCLEX® Examination Style Questions

1. A newborn male was born 4 hours ago by spontaneous vaginal birth after an uncomplicated pregnancy and labor to a 29-year-old primigravida. **Use an "X" to indicate whether each of the following assessment findings are expected (normal), common variation (usually normal or transient), or unexpected (abnormal).**

Assessment Finding	Expected/ Normal	Common Variation	Unexpected/ Abnormal
Acrocyanosis			
Substernal retraction			
Faint audible murmur			
Respiratory rate 48			
Apical heart rate 134			
Jitteriness			
Nasal flaring			
Large bluish pigmented areas on buttocks			
Small white cyst on the face			

2. A client with no prenatal care and unknown last menstrual period (LMP) delivers a 7 lb. 6 oz. male. **Place an "X" to indicate if the assessment finding is associated with a preterm, term, or postterm newborn.**

Assessment Finding	Preterm	Term	Postterm
Tightly flexed posture			
Abundant lanugo			
Parchment-like skin with deep cracking			
Flat areola with no breast tissue palpable			
Plantar creases on anterior $2/3$ of sole of foot			

REFERENCES

Abramowski, A., Ward, R., & Hamdan, A. H. (2020). Neonatal hypoglycemia. In *StatPearls*. StatPearls Publishing. https://www.ncbi.nlm.nih.gov/books/NBK537105/.

Alden, K. R. (2018). Physiologic and behavioral adaptations of the newborn. In S. E. Perry, D. L. Lowdermilk, K. Cashion, K. R. Alden, E. F. Olshansky, & M. J. Hockenberry (Eds.), *Maternal child nursing care* (6th ed., pp. 462–479). Elsevier.

American Academy of Pediatrics & American College of Obstetricians and Gynecologists (AAP & ACOG). (2017). *Guidelines for perinatal care.* (8th ed.).

Arshpreet, D. (2017). Validity of modified Ballard score after 7 days of life. *International Journal of Medical Research and Health Sciences, 6*(7), 79–83. https://www.ijmrhs.com/medical-research/validity-of-modified-ballard-score-after-7-days-of-life.pdf.

Azevedo, I. G., Holanda, N. S. O., Arrais, N. M. R., Santos, R. T. G., Araujo, A. G. F., & Pereira, S. A. (2019). Chest circumference in full-term newborns: How can it be predicted? *BMC Pediatrics,* *19,* 341. https://doi.org/10.1186/s12887-019-1712-3.

Ballard, J. L., Khoury, J. C., Wedig, K., Wang, L., Eilers-Walsman, B. L., & Lip, R. (1991). New Ballard Score, expanded to include extremely premature infants. *Journal of Pediatrics, 19*(3), 417–423.

Blackburn, S. T. (2018). *Maternal, fetal, and neonatal physiology: A clinical perspective* (5th ed.). Elsevier.

Bush, D., Juliano, C., Laitman, B. M., Londino, A., & Spencer, C. (2019). A comprehensive multidisciplinary approach to the evaluation of the neonatal airway. *Current pediatric reports* (7), 107–115. https://doi.org/10.1007/s40124-019-00199-0.

Churchman, L. (2021). Apnea. In M. T. Verkaln, M. Walden, & S. Forest (Eds.), *Core curriculum for neonatal intensive care nursing* (6th ed., pp. 417–424). Elsevier.

Crumley, N. (2020). *Thermometers 101: How to check temperature during COVID-19 pandemic. American Academy of Pediatrics.* https://www.aappublications.org/news/2020/11/01/parentplus-thermometers110120.

Dionne, J. M., Bremner, S. A., Baygani, S. K., Batton, B., Ergeneckon, E., Bhatt-Mehta, V., Dempsey, E., Kluckow, M., Koplowitz, L. P., Apele-Freimane, D., Iwami, H., Klein, A., Turner, M., & Rabe, H. (2020). Method of blood pressure measurement in neonates and infants: A systematic review and analysis. *The Journal of Pediatrics.* https://www.jpeds.com/article/S0022-3476(20)30286-9/fulltext.

Gardner, S. L., & Goldson, E. (2021). The neonate and the environment impact on development. In S. L. Gardner, B. S. Carter, M. Enzman-Hineset al., et al. (Eds.), *Merenstein & Gardner's handbook of neonatal intensive care* (9th ed., pp. 93–136). Elsevier.

Gardner, S. L., & Niermeyer, S. (2021). Immediate newborn care after birth. In S. L. Gardner, B. S. Carter, M. Enzman-Hineset, et al. (Eds.), *Merenstein & Gardner's handbook of neonatal intensive care* (9th ed., pp. 93–136). Elsevier.

Hibiya-Motegi, R., Nakayama, M., Matsuoka, R., Takeda, J., Nojiri, S., Itakura, A., Koike, T., & Ikeda, K. (2020). Use of sound-elicited fetal heart rate accelerations to assess fetal hearing in the second and third trimester. *International Journal of Otorhinolaryngology, 133.*

Horwood, A. M. (2019). Typical and atypical development of ocular alignment and binocular vision in infants—The background. *American Academy of Ophthalmology.* https://www.aao.org/disease-review/typical-atypical-development-of-ocular-alignment-b.

Hurwitz, S. (1993). *Clinical pediatric dermatology* (2nd ed.). Saunders.

Jyothsna, B., Srinivas, M., Priya, I., Motvani, N., & Sunitha, Sridevi. (2018). Gestational age correlation by last menstrual period, ultrasonography and new Ballard score. *International Journal of Contemporary Medical Research, 5*(7), 2454–7379.

Kibbi, A. G. (2019). *Congenital dermal melanocytosis (Mongolian spot).* Medscape. https://emedicine.medscape.com/article/1068732-overview#a6.

Krause, L. (2019). *Single transverse palmar crease.* Healthline. https://www.healthline.com/health/simian-crease.

Mersch, J. (2021). Physical growth in newborns. *Emedicinehealth.* https://www.emedicinehealth.com/physical_growth_in_newborns/article_em.htm#how_long_is_the_newborn_period.

National Institute for Health. (2021). Cranial sutures. Retrieved In *MedlinePlus* from https://medlineplus.gov/ency/article/002320.htm#:~:text=The%20posterior%20fontanelle%20usually%20closes,infant's%20brain%20growth%20and%20development.

Niermeyer, S., & Clarke, S. B. (2021). Care at birth. In S. L. Gardner, B. S. Carter, M. Enzman-Hineset, et al. (Eds.), *Merenstein & Gardner's handbook of neonatal intensive care* (9th ed., pp. 67–92). Elsevier.

Nyp, M., Brunkhorst, J. L., Reavey, D., & Pallotto, E. K. (2021). Fluid and electrolyte management. In S. L. Gardner, B. S. Carter, M. Enzman-Hineset, et al. (Eds.), *Merenstein & Gardner's handbook of neonatal intensive care* (9th ed., pp. 407–430). Elsevier.

Patnana, S. R., & Selb, P. M. (2018). *Coarctation of the aorta clinical presentation.* eMedicine. https://emedicine.medscape.com/article/895502-clinical#b4.

Rauch, K. (2021). *Why are my eyes changing color? American Academy of Ophthalmology.* https://www.aao.org/eye-health/tips-prevention/why-are-my-eyes-changing-color.

Rivers, K. (2019). *Ear tags and preauricular pits in newborns: A common birth defect. Nabta Health.* https://nabtahealth.com/ear-tags-and-preauricular-pits-in-newborns-a-common-birth-defect/.

Rohan, A. J. (2021). Newborn physical assessment. In K. R. Simpson, P. A. Creehan, N. O'Brien-Abel, C. K. Roth, & A. J. Rohan (Eds.), *Perinatal nursing* (5th ed., pp. 578–607). Wolters Kluwer.

Stewart, L. S., & Rodgers, E. (2020). *Assessment and care of the term newborn transitioning into extrauterine life. Nurse Key.* https://nursekey.com/assessment-and-care-of-the-term-newborn-transitioning-to-extrauterine-life/.

Tamai, J. (2020). *Developmental dysplasia of the hip. Medscape.* https://emedicine.medscape.com/article/1248135-overview.

Tappero, E. (2021). Physical assessment. In M. T. Verkaln, M. Walden, & S. Forest (Eds.), *Core curriculum for neonatal intensive care nursing* (6th ed., pp. 99–130). Elsevier.

Urology Care Foundation. (2021). *What are undescended testicles (cryptochordism)? Urology Care Foundation.* https://www.urologyhealth.org/urology-a-z/c/cryptorchidism.

Verhave, B. L., Nassereddin, A., & Lappin, S. L. (2020). *Embryology, lanugo. StatPearls.* https://www.ncbi.nlm.nih.gov/books/NBK526092/.

Verklan, M. T. (2021). Adaptation to extrauterine life. In M. T. Verkaln, M. Walden, & S. Forest (Eds.), *Core curriculum for neonatal intensive care nursing* (6th ed., pp. 99–130). Elsevier.

Care of the Newborn

Lisa Wallace

The role of the nurse in ongoing assessments and care of the newborn in the birth facility is to help the newborn and parents have a successful transition after birth. The nurse identifies and responds to changes in the condition of newborns as they adapt to life outside the uterus, keeps infants safe, and teaches parents how to provide care. Nurses often receive questions from parents about care of infants after discharge. Infant home care for the first 12 weeks of life is discussed. Detailed information about ill or older infants can be found in pediatrics textbooks.

INPATIENT CARE

EARLY CARE

Early care after birth involves assignment of Apgar scores (Table 15.4) and assessment and stabilization of the infant as necessary. Once the infant's condition is stable, and they have had the opportunity to bond with the parents, prophylactic medications are given. Ongoing assessments continue during this time, including temperature, heart rate, respiratory rate and character, skin color, muscle tone, level of consciousness, and activity level. These assessments should be documented every 30 minutes until the newborn is stable for 2 hours (American Academy of Pediatrics & American College of Obstetricians and Gynecologists [AAP & ACOG], 2017). If abnormalities are noted, the provider is notified, and the infant is assessed more frequently. High-risk neonates and those experiencing difficulty with normal respiratory or cardiac transition to extrauterine life should have vital signs monitored continuously to detect early changes and provide appropriate interventions (Kumar et al., 2020).

Because of blood and amniotic fluid on the infant's skin from birth, the nurse wears gloves during all contact with the infant until the bath is completed. After the bath, gloves are necessary only when contact with body fluids may occur.

Administering Vitamin K

Vitamin K is given to neonates because they cannot synthesize it in the intestines without bacterial flora. This places them at risk for hemorrhagic disease of the newborn. One dose of vitamin K intramuscularly after birth prevents bleeding problems until the infant is able to produce vitamin K in sufficient amounts. Although the injection is usually given after the first feeding, it can be delayed up to 6 hours after birth (Centers for Disease Control and Prevention [CDC], 2019) (Procedure 22.1; Drug Guide: Vitamin K_1 [Phytonadione]).

Providing Eye Treatment

Infants also receive prophylactic treatment to prevent ophthalmia neonatorum, conjunctivitis, which is most often caused by *Neisseria gonorrhoeae* acquired from the birth canal. Because this infection can cause blindness if not treated promptly, most states mandate prophylactic treatment within 1 to 2 hours of birth, regardless of mode of birth (Fig. 22.1; Drug Guide: Erythromycin Ophthalmic Ointment). Erythromycin 0.5% is the only commercially available and approved agent in the United States to prevent gonococcal ophthalmia neonatorum (U.S. Preventive Task Force, 2019; AAP & ACOG, 2017). Topical antibiotics are not effective against chlamydia, which often occurs with gonorrhea (AAP & ACOG, 2017).

1. Perform hand hygiene.
2. Wash the infant's thigh if the bath has not yet been given. *Wear gloves and perform hand hygiene when complete.*
3. Compare the Medication Administration Record (MAR) to the infant's wrist/ankle band. *Note: the band will have the mother's name, date and time of birth, and sex of the baby.*
4. Verify provider's order and MAR.
5. Prepare medication for injection. Use a 1-mL syringe and a ⅝-inch, 25-gauge needle. If the medication is in a glass ampule, use a filter needle to draw it up. Remove the filter needle and place a 25-gauge needle on the syringe to give the injection.
6. Put on gloves.
7. Verify the infant, compare the wrist/ankle band to the MAR.
8. Locate the correct site. The best site for newborn intramuscular injections is the vastus lateralis muscle. Divide the area between the greater trochanter of the femur and the knee into thirds. Give the injection in the middle third of the muscle, lateral to the midline of the anterior thigh. *Note: The gluteal muscles are not used until a child has been walking for at least a year. These muscles are poorly developed and dangerously near the sciatic nerve.*

9. Stabilize the leg firmly while grasping the thigh between the thumb and fingers.
10. Cleanse the area with an alcohol or facility antiseptic wipe. Continue to hold the leg to prevent contamination of the site due to movement.
11. Insert the needle at a 90-degree angle. Inject the medication.

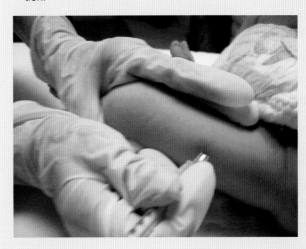

12. Withdraw the needle and apply gentle pressure to the site with small gauze pad.
13. Place safety shield on needle and discard the needle and syringe in the appropriate place; comfort the infant.
14. Perform hand hygiene and document the medication administration.

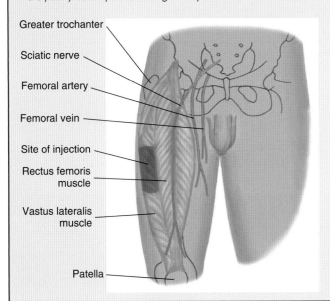

Greater trochanter
Sciatic nerve
Femoral artery
Femoral vein
Site of injection
Rectus femoris muscle
Vastus lateralis muscle
Patella

DRUG GUIDE

Vitamin K₁ (Phytonadione)

Classification
Fat-soluble vitamin, antihemorrhagic.

Other Names
AquaMEPHYTON, Konakion, Mephyton.

Action
Promotes the formation of factors II (prothrombin), VII, IX, and X by the liver for clotting; provides vitamin K, which is not synthesized in the intestines until intestinal flora necessary for vitamin K production are established.

Indication
Prevention or treatment of vitamin K–deficiency bleeding (hemorrhagic disease of the newborn).

Neonatal Dosage and Route
0.5 to 1 mg (0.25 to 0.5 mL of solution containing 1 mg/0.5 mL) given once intramuscularly after birth for prophylaxis. May be delayed for breastfeeding at birth.

Absorption
Readily absorbed after intramuscular injection; effective within 1 to 2 hours; metabolized in the liver.

Adverse Reactions
Erythema, pain, and edema at injection site; anaphylaxis; hemolysis; or hyperbilirubinemia, especially in a preterm infant or when a large dose is used.

Nursing Considerations
Protect the drug from light until just before administration to prevent decomposition and loss of potency. Observe all infants for signs of vitamin K deficiency (ecchymoses or bleeding from any site). Verify administration of vitamin K has been completed before a circumcision is performed.

DRUG GUIDE

Erythromycin Ophthalmic Ointment

Classification
Antibiotic.

Other Name
Ilotycin ophthalmic ointment.

Action
Inhibits protein synthesis in bacteria; bacteriostatic.

Indications
Prophylaxis against the organism *Neisseria gonorrhoeae;* helps prevent ophthalmia neonatorum in infants from maternal gonorrheal infections; required by law for all infants, even if there is no known infection.

Neonatal Dosage and Route
A "ribbon" of 0.5% erythromycin ointment, 1 cm (0.4 inch) long, is applied to the lower conjunctival sac of each eye within 1 to 2 hours of birth, after breastfeeding.

Adverse Reactions
Burning, itching; irritation may result in chemical conjunctivitis lasting 24 to 48 hours; ointment may cause temporary blurred vision.

Nursing Considerations
Do not rinse. Excess ointment may be wiped from the outer eye after 1 minute. Observe for irritation.

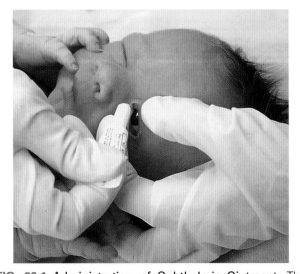

FIG. 22.1 Administration of Ophthalmic Ointment. The nurse wears gloves and gently cleans the eyes of blood or vernix. Then, placing a finger and thumb near the edge of each lid, the nurse gently presses against the periorbital ridges to open the eyes, avoiding pressure on the eye itself. The tube is held horizontally as a ribbon of ointment is squeezed into each conjunctival sac from the inner canthus to the outer canthus. The tube should not touch any part of the eye. Use a new tube for each infant.

Because the ointment may temporarily blur the infant's vision, parents may wish to delay treatment for a short time during initial bonding. It may be delayed until the end of the first hour after birth or after the first breastfeeding (U.S. Preventive Task Force, 2019; AAP & ACOG, 2017).

Some infants develop a mild inflammation a few hours after prophylactic treatment. Any discharge from the eyes, especially if purulent, should alert the nurse to the possibility of infection. A culture may be ordered, and the drainage should be removed with sterile saline and a cotton ball. Additional antibiotic treatment will be needed in cases of known infections.

APPLICATION OF THE NURSING PROCESS: CARDIORESPIRATORY STATUS

The transition from fetal life to neonatal life may include temporary problems in cardiorespiratory status.

Assessment

Assess the newborn for signs of difficult transition. Note the rate and character of the heart rate, pulses, respirations, and breath sounds. Look for signs of respiratory distress, including tachypnea, retractions, flaring of the nares, pallor or cyanosis, grunting, seesaw respirations, and asymmetry of chest movements. Check blood pressure, if indicated.

Identification of Client Problems

Fluid from the lungs must be removed by absorption or drainage from the respiratory passages after birth. This does not happen immediately and may cause a temporary problem during the early hours after birth. A common client problem is difficulty clearing the airway because of excessive secretions.

Planning: Expected Outcomes

The expected outcomes for this client problem are as follows. The newborn will:
1. Maintain a patent airway as evidenced by a respiratory rate within the normal range of 30 to 60 breaths per minute.
2. Show no signs of respiratory distress (retractions, grunting, nasal flaring).

Interventions

Positioning and Suctioning Secretions

Position the infant on the back with the head in a neutral position or to the side. Wipe the mouth and nose with a towel. Bulb suctioning should be used only when the infant is having difficulty clearing the airway (AAP & ACOG, 2017; Aziz et al., 2020). When bulb suctioning is indicated, suction the mouth first and then nose because newborns tend to gasp when the nose is suctioned, risking aspiration of mucus or fluid in the mouth (Aziz et al., 2020). Then suction the nose gently and only if necessary. Suctioning is traumatic to the delicate tissues and may cause edema of the nasal passages.

Keep the bulb syringe in the crib near the infant's head, where it is available if needed quickly. Teach both parents how to use the bulb syringe correctly, including cleaning after use. (Procedure 22.2). Send the syringe home with the infant so parents can use it if the infant experiences a problem.

NURSING PROCEDURE 22.2   Using a Bulb Syringe

1. Perform hand hygiene and put on gloves.
2. Position the infant's head to the side.
3. Compress the bulb before inserting it into the mouth. *Do not compress the bulb while it is in the infant's mouth, or secretions in the bulb will be expelled back into the mouth.*
4. Gently insert the tip of the syringe into the side of the infant's mouth between the gums and the cheek. Do not insert it straight to the back of the throat (*to avoid stimulating the gag reflex, regurgitation, or vagal response*).
5. Release the bulb slowly while it is in the infant's mouth. Remove from the baby's mouth and empty it by compressing several times before using again.
6. Turn the baby's head to the other side and repeat on the opposite side.
7. Suction the nose, only if necessary, after the mouth is suctioned.
8. Suction the nose gently and avoid unnecessary suction. Compress the syringe, place the tip at the entrance of the nostril, and release slowly.
9. Remove from the baby's nostril. Empty the syringe by compressing several times. Repeat in the other nostril if necessary.

10. Clean the bulb syringe after use with soapy water, rinse well, and allow to air dry to prevent bacterial growth.

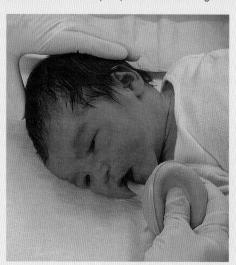

If mechanical suctioning is necessary to remove deeper secretions, choose a small catheter to avoid damaging the tissues of the respiratory tract. Suction for no more than 5 seconds at a time, using minimal negative pressure to avoid trauma, laryngospasm, and bradycardia. Apply suction only as the catheter is being withdrawn.

Providing Continuing Care

Continue monitoring the infant for problems throughout the stay in the birth facility. By the second period of reactivity, the infant may be alone with the parents. Although nurses know that regurgitation, gagging, and brief episodes of cyanosis are normal during this time, these may be very frightening to the parents.

Teach the appropriate responses to the behaviors common to this phase. Assess the parents' ability to use the bulb syringe and their comfort with its use. Remind them to use the bulb syringe and call for help, if needed. Check frequently to see if the infant is having difficulty.

Evaluation

The newborn has little difficulty clearing the airway after the first few hours of life. The expected outcomes are met if the following occur:

- The respiratory rate is between 30 and 60 breaths per minute.
- The infant shows no signs of respiratory distress.

APPLICATION OF THE NURSING PROCESS: THERMOREGULATION

Because any neonate may have difficulty with thermoregulation, the nurse should identify problems and intervene to prevent complications related to this vital function.

Assessment

Assess the newborn's temperature shortly after birth and then according to agency policy. Axillary temperatures are preferred and less invasive. Generally, the temperature is assessed every half hour until it has been stable for 2 hours. It is checked again at 4 hours and then every 8 to 12 hours or according to agency policy. Assess the temperature more often if it is abnormal.

Identification of Client Problems

Ineffective temperature maintenance is a common problem for newborns because of their immature compensation for changes in environmental temperature.

Planning: Expected Outcome

The expected outcome for this problem is as follows.

The infant will maintain an axillary temperature within the normal range of 97.7 to 99.5°F (36.5 to 37.5°C).

Interventions

Interventions for this problem include prevention, restoring thermoregulation, and performing expanded assessments.

Preventing Heat Loss

Preparing the Environment Before Birth. Begin preventive measures before the infant is born. Prepare a neutral thermal environment with a radiant warmer available and ready in case it is needed at birth. Check the radiant warmer to ensure it is functioning properly. Turn it on early enough to warm the bed before the birth. Prewarm blankets, caps, and any other items that will be used for the care of the newborn. This ensures excess oxygen and glucose are not used to maintain body temperature.

Providing Immediate Care. Immediately after birth, place the infant on the mother's abdomen to provide warmth from skin-to-skin (STS) contact or under a radiant warmer to counteract the cool temperature of the birth environment. Routine assessment and care can be performed while the infant is STS, and breastfeeding can begin if both are stable. Infants placed STS immediately after birth are more likely to have stable temperatures (Aziz et al., 2020).

Dry the wet infant quickly with warm towels to prevent heat loss by evaporation. Pay particular attention to drying the hair because the head has a large surface area and hair that remains damp increases heat loss. Remove towels or blankets as soon as they become wet and replace them with dry, warmed linens. Cover the head with a prewarmed cap when the infant is not under a radiant warmer. Do not use a hat when the infant is under the warmer because it interferes with transfer of heat to the infant's head.

If infant is placed under a radiant warmer, it is important to prewarm the mattress prior to use, if time allows. After placing infant under the radiant warmer, attach the sensor with gel to the infant's abdomen over a nonbony, unbruised area with intact skin (such as around the liver or lower left abdomen) (Lynn, 2019). Set the **servocontrol** to 36.5°C (Gardner & Cammack, 2021). This setting regulates the heat from the warmer to maintain the infant's skin temperature at the normal level. The sensor also displays the infant's temperature continuously. Check frequently (at least hourly) to see if the infant's skin temperature is increasing as expected and monitor for probe attachment.

Providing Ongoing Prevention. Warm objects that will come in contact with the infant to avoid conduction of heat away from the infant's body. Pad cool surfaces such as scales or circumcision restraint boards with warm blankets before placing infants on them. Warm stethoscopes and clothing before using them. Before touching the infant, wash your hands in warm water.

To prevent heat loss by radiation in cold weather, position the newborn's crib or incubator away from exterior walls or windows of the building. These sources of heat loss are easily overlooked when the objects and air around the infant seem warm, but infants may lose heat to objects not in close contact with them. Keep this possibility in mind when positioning cribs in clients' rooms, which are often short of space. Place the crib away from windows or doors, if possible. Avoid areas with drafts such as those near hall doors or air conditioners. Keep traffic low around radiant warmers because movement increases air currents, causing heat loss by convection. When assessing or caring for newborns, avoid exposing more of their bodies than necessary. Remove clothing and blankets only from areas being assessed. Keep the upper part of the infant's body covered when changing diapers. Wrap newborns in blankets, and place a stockinette or insulated hat on the infant to prevent heat loss from the large surface area of the head.

Restoring Thermoregulation

If an infant with a previously normal temperature develops a low temperature, institute nursing measures to assist thermoregulation immediately. First, look for obvious causes. The blankets around the infant may have come loose or the infant's diapers or clothing may have become wet. The room may be too cold, or the crib may have been placed near the air conditioner. These causes can be corrected easily.

A slight drop in temperature may only require placing the infant, dressed in just a diaper and hat, next to the bare skin of one of the parents. This STS contact is very effective in using the parent's body heat to warm the infant. Place a warm blanket over both parent and infant.

If STS contact is not possible, add extra clothing. Use two blankets, each wrapped separately around the infant, to increase insulation of heat by trapping air between the layers. Place another blanket over the infant in the crib and a hat on the infant's head. Warm linens in a warmer before use.

A greater drop in the infant's body temperature or a temperature that has not improved within an hour of using STS contact requires additional measures. Place the infant under a radiant warmer for a short time. For an infant with a markedly decreased temperature, set the temperature control on the warmer to warm the infant slowly. Gradually increase the temperature until the infant's temperature is within the normal range. Warming the infant too rapidly can cause complications such as apnea (Gardner & Cammack, 2021).

Performing Expanded Assessments

Expanded assessments are necessary whenever the body temperature decreases in a newborn. Assess the respiratory rate and observe for signs of respiratory distress because nonshivering thermogenesis increases the need for oxygen. Because the cold infant uses more glucose to produce heat, test the blood glucose when the temperature is abnormal, following agency protocol.

Ingestion of warm colostrum or breast milk helps warm the infant. Notify the physician or nurse practitioner if the infant does not respond to these measures. Place the infant under a radiant warmer or in an incubator for close observation until the temperature stabilizes.

Evaluation

When the infant's body temperature has been maintained within the normal range for several hours, the infant can be considered stable. Continue to monitor thermoregulation throughout the stay.

? KNOWLEDGE CHECK

1. Why are prophylactic medications given to all newborns?
2. How can nurses prevent heat loss in newborns?

APPLICATION OF THE NURSING PROCESS: BLOOD GLUCOSE

Assessment

Assess all infants for risk factors and signs of hypoglycemia. Perform screening tests for blood glucose according to the symptoms and agency policy.

Identification of Client Problems

Definitions of hypoglycemia vary. Most facilities consider infants to be hypoglycemic when the glucose level is below 40 to 45 mg/dL (milligrams per deciliter) or the value according to agency policy. These infants have the potential for injury because of decreased blood sugar levels.

Planning: Expected Outcomes

Hypoglycemia requires an interprofessional approach between the nurse and the provider. The nursing plan of care will reflect both dependent and independent nursing functions. Agency protocols usually allow the nurse to intervene for hypoglycemia and then notify the provider of the infant's response. Planning revolves around the nurse's role, including the following:
1. Assessing for signs of hypoglycemia
2. Notifying the provider of signs of hypoglycemia or following hospital protocol for infants with hypoglycemia and then notifying the provider
3. Intervening to minimize hypoglycemia

Interventions

Maintaining Safe Glucose Levels

Follow agency policy and provider orders regarding feeding infants with low glucose levels. A common practice is to feed the newborn if the glucose screening shows 40 to 45 mg/dL or less to prevent further depletion of glucose. Infants with severe hypoglycemia may need intravenous treatment to provide glucose rapidly.

For most infants, breastfeeding or giving formula is sufficient. Glucose water is not recommended for newborns because the rapid rise in glucose results in increased insulin production, causing a further drop in blood glucose. Milk (breast milk is optimum, but formula is appropriate if the infant will not be breastfed) provides a longer-lasting supply of glucose.

Assist with feeding the infant. Explain the need for prompt feeding with hypoglycemia.

Repeating Glucose Tests

Until blood glucose is stable, closely observe newborns who have shown signs of hypoglycemia. Repeat glucose screenings may be performed according to agency policy. Keep the physician or nurse practitioner aware of the newborn's status. If the blood glucose does not remain at an adequate level, other causative factors are investigated. The infant may be transferred to an intensive care nursery for more treatment, including intravenous feedings, until the blood glucose is stabilized.

Providing Other Care

Watch for signs of other complications. Infants who do not have enough glucose may experience a drop in temperature, which could lead to respiratory distress as oxygen is used for nonshivering thermogenesis. The parents will be distressed over the multiple heel sticks their infant must endure. Explain the importance of maintaining adequate blood glucose and why the tests and frequent feedings are necessary. Discuss the plans for blood testing and criteria for discontinuing it.

Evaluation

In evaluating collaborative interventions for hypoglycemia, note the infant's response to interventions and the presence or absence of continued signs of hypoglycemia. Most agency protocols identify a target blood glucose above 45 to 50 mg/dL prior to feeds during the first 48 hours after birth.

APPLICATION OF THE NURSING PROCESS: BILIRUBIN

Because elevated bilirubin is common in newborns, be alert to situations that require intervention.

Assessment

Assess for jaundice by blanching the infant's skin on the nose or sternum and visually inspecting the skin and sclera for any yellowish appearance at least once a shift (every 8 to 12 hours) along with vital signs. If present, determine how far down the body the jaundice extends. Because visual assessment of jaundice is unreliable to determine the degree of hyperbilirubinemia accurately, obtain transcutaneous bilirubin (TCB) or total serum bilirubin (TSB) measurement in any jaundiced infant. TCB is less invasive and painful compared with TSB. Compare the results with what is expected for the infant's age on the BiliTool (see Chapter 20, Fig. 20.7) and previous results.

Identification of Client Problems

Physiologic jaundice does not occur until at least 24 hours after birth and often not until 72 to 96 hours of age. The average length of stay for a new family following a birth is 2 to 3 days; therefore, hyperbilirubinemia may not occur until after discharge. The newborn has a potential for jaundice because of the parents' lack of knowledge about hyperbilirubinemia.

Planning: Expected Outcomes

The expected outcomes for this problem are as follows:
1. Parents will identify methods for preventing or reducing jaundice.
2. Parents will seek treatment if jaundice develops or worsens after discharge.

Interventions

Determine which infants are at increased risk for hyperbilirubinemia. Most health care facilities require at least one TCB just prior to discharge. Others may perform one screen at 24 hours and a second screen on the day of discharge.

Explain the significance of jaundice to parents and show them how to assess for color changes in the skin. Answer parents' questions about blood tests, phototherapy, and other care.

Discuss the importance of adequate feedings to stimulate passage of stools and prevent high levels of bilirubin. If a newborn is feeding poorly, determine the reasons and intervene appropriately. Help parents wake sleeping infants to feed, encourage them to spend extra time with the infant with a poor suck, and explain the appropriate amount to give at each feeding. Explain giving water to jaundiced infants does not stimulate stool excretion and should be avoided.

If the infant is breastfeeding, evaluate the infant's suck and the client's understanding of positioning and other techniques. The breastfed baby should be fed at least 8 to 12 times each 24 hours for adequate lengths of time. Assist clients having difficulty to ensure infants are feeding well before discharge. Refer to a lactation consultant if needed.

Instruct parents to contact their care provider if they see an increase in jaundice or if the infant is not eating well, not voiding at least six times daily by the sixth day, or not producing stools appropriately (at least one stool per day for formula-fed infants and at least four stools daily for breastfed infants).

Stress the importance of making and keeping follow-up appointments with the infant's health care provider. Offer written materials about jaundice for the parents to take home.

Continue to check the infant for jaundice during early clinic or home visits. Reinforce teaching about identification of jaundice and importance of feedings and stooling. Answer questions that have occurred to parents since discharge from the birth facility.

If an infant develops true breast milk jaundice, explain it to the parents. Discontinuation of breastfeeding for 1 or 2 days will be very concerning to the parents. Reassure them the milk is adequate and not harmful to the infant. Help maintain milk supply by using a breast pump during the time the infant is taking formula.

Evaluation

With proper nursing observation and parent teaching, infants with hyperbilirubinemia are identified early to allow for appropriate treatment and prevention of injury. Parents are able to discuss signs, prevention, and management of jaundice at home.

KNOWLEDGE CHECK

3. What should the nurse do when an infant shows signs of hypoglycemia?
4. What are some interventions for preventing jaundice in newborns?

ONGOING CARE

A complete assessment is necessary every 8 hours or according to birth facility policy, but the nurse should always watch for signs of change in the newborn's condition. Vital signs are assessed more often if they are abnormal. The infant is weighed once daily, and weight loss or gain is documented.

Skin Care

The skin should be assessed for new marks or changes in old ones. To assess skin turgor, the nurse pinches a small area of skin over the chest or abdomen and notes how quickly it returns to its normal position. The return should be immediate in the newborn, with no "tenting." Skin that remains tented is an indication of dehydration.

Bathing

For decades, newborns in the United States have been bathed as soon after birth as possible, once the temperature was stable. However, in 2013, the World Health Organization (WHO) published recommendations that included delaying the newborn bath for 6 to 24 hours following birth (WHO, 2013). Research has supported this recommendation, citing decreased rates of hypothermia and hypoglycemia and increases in STS time with the parents, parent participation in the bath, and rates of breastfeeding when the initial bath is delayed (Chamberlain et al., 2019; DiCioccio et al., 2019; Mardini et al., 2020; Warren et al., 2020). For the term neonate without complications, the Association of Women's Health, Obstetric and Neonatal Nurses (AWHONN, 2018) recommends a delay of at least 6 hours and axillary temperature greater than or equal to 36.8°C on two consecutive assessments prior to bathing.

The infant may be bathed by immersion in a tub or swaddled in a blanket then immersed in a tub. Studies have shown tub bathing does not increase infection or decrease cord healing. When swaddled, only the body part being bathed is removed from the blanket. Infants maintain their temperatures better during tub bathing than during sponge bathing. To be kept warm, infants should be immersed in water that covers their shoulders. Water temperature should be approximately 38°C (104°F), and the room temperature should be 26 to 28°C (78.8 to 82.4°F) (AWHONN, 2018; New, 2019).

If a sponge bath is given, it should be done with the infant under the radiant warmer to help maintain the infant's temperature. The bath should be performed quickly and the infant thoroughly dried to prevent heat loss by evaporation. While shampooing the hair, the nurse should comb through the hair to remove dried blood.

Regardless of the type of bath, the infant should be rewarmed afterward. STS contact with the parent is the preferred method to rewarm the baby. If this is not possible, the infant should be placed under the radiant warmer with the servo control connected and set at 36.5°C until the hair is dry and the temperature returns to the previous level. Once warm, the infant can be dressed and wrapped in two warm blankets, with a warm cap on the infant's head, and removed from the warmer or STS contact with the parent. The temperature should be rechecked within 1 hour to ensure the infant is maintaining thermoregulation adequately.

Encouraging parent participation in the bath or bathing the infant in the presence of the parents allows the nurse to point out infant characteristics in addition to teaching parents the bath procedure and safety precautions. After the initial bath, the infant may not receive another full bath during the stay in the birth facility. The skin is cleansed at diaper changes and to remove regurgitated milk. Clear water or a mild soap solution is used, according to agency policy.

Cord Care

The cord should be checked for bleeding or oozing during the early hours after birth. The cord clamp should be securely fastened with no skin caught in it. Purulent drainage or redness or edema at the base indicates infection. The cord begins to dry shortly after birth. It becomes brownish black within 2 to 3 days and falls off within approximately 10 to 14 days. A few drops of blood may occur with umbilical stump separation.

Evidence-based practice guidelines show cleaning the cord with water when necessary and keeping it clean and dry is the best method of cord care (AAP, 2020; AWHONN, 2018). This natural treatment of cords may shorten the time to cord separation and does not lead to increased infections. The diaper is folded below the cord to keep the cord dry and free from contamination by urine. The cord clamp is removed about 24 hours after birth if the end of the cord is dry (Fig. 22.2). Although the base of the cord is still moist, there is no danger of bleeding if the end is dry and crisp.

Cleansing the Diaper Area

Because contact with body fluids is likely, it is important to wear clean gloves while changing diapers. Meconium is very thick and sticky and can be difficult to remove from the skin. Plain water or mild soap solutions may be used for cleaning the diaper area. If commercial diaper wipes are used, they should be free of detergent and alcohol (AWHONN, 2018).

Assisting with Feedings

The nurse should ensure the infant is eating well and parents understand their chosen feeding method. This is particularly important for breastfeeding infants. A short period of observation at the start of feedings followed by another check during the feedings will help the nurse identify any problems that may have developed. Lactation consultants may provide additional consultation or support for clients who are having difficulty with latch.

Positioning for Sleep

Parents need to understand how to position infants properly. Placing infants in the prone position for sleep is associated with an increased risk for sudden infant death syndrome (SIDS). The AAP Task Force on Sudden Infant Death Syndrome (2016) and Moon (2021) recommend parents be taught to place infants on their back for sleep because this position is associated with the lowest rate of SIDS. It is important for nurses to model correct positioning for sleep for parents by positioning the newborn on his or her back to sleep at the birth facility.

Parents should also be taught to use a firm sleep surface without bumper pads and avoid loose or soft bedding, which might interfere with breathing. Sack-like sleepers, which take the place of blankets, are available. The infant should not sleep in a bed or on a couch with another person (Fig. 22.3). However, placing the infant's bed in the parents' room is recommended up to the first year of life. Giving a pacifier when putting the infant to

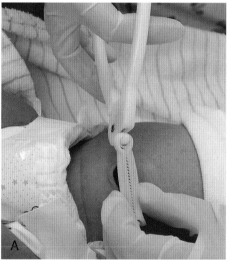

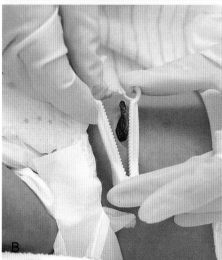

FIG. 22.2 The cord clamp is removed when the end of the cord is dry and crisp. The clamp is cut (A) and separated (B).

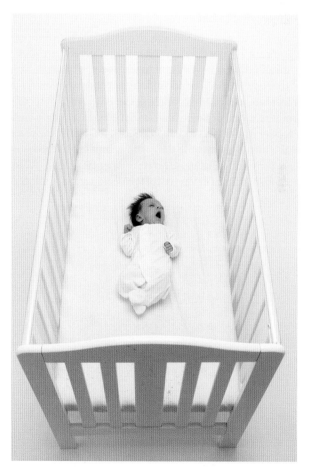

FIG. 22.3 A safe crib has a firm mattress without pillows, blankets, sheep skins, bumper pads, or stuffed toys. The infant is placed on his or her back and is dressed in a sleeper, not covered with blankets, quilts, or comforters. The baby should not sleep on an adult bed, a couch or chair, or with another person. (Courtesy of iStock.)

sleep is also recommended, but this may be delayed for 1 month in infants who are breastfeeding to help establish breastfeeding. Overheating during sleep should be avoided (Moon, 2021).

Positioning and Head Shape

Infants who spend long periods in the supine position may develop flattening or asymmetry of the back of the head (positional **plagiocephaly**). This occurs because the bones are not fully developed and can be molded by positioning.

To prevent flattening of the head, infants should be placed on the abdomen several times each day while they are awake. This "tummy time" is an opportunity for play and interaction with the parents. It is essential for infants to be supervised at all times when in the prone position, and they should be moved to the supine position if they fall asleep.

Protecting the Infant

Safeguarding the infant is a major nursing role. Primary ways nurses protect newborns are by (1) ensuring infants always go to the correct parents, (2) taking precautions to prevent infant abductions, (3) preventing infections or recognizing early signs, and (4) preventing infant falls.

Identifying the Infant

Methods to identify the infant, parent(s), and in some cases a significant support person other than a parent, are used to ensure an infant is never given to the wrong person.

Electronic devices or identification bands with imprinted numbers are used. The electronic device is designed to set off an alarm if removed or the infant is taken beyond a certain area of the facility. The devices or bands are used to identify the parents and the infant at any time the infant is brought to the parents after a period of separation, however brief (Fig. 22.4). All staff should follow the facility protocol for identification of infants.

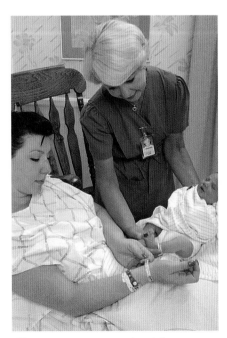

FIG. 22.4 The nurse unwraps the infant to compare the infant's identification band with the parent's band.

Other methods to identify infants include taking footprints of the infant and a fingerprint of the client or photographs of the infant. Birthmarks or other distinguishing features are carefully documented in the nurses' notes.

Preventing Infant Abduction

An essential nursing role is protecting the infant from abduction (kidnapping). Between 1964 and November 2020, 329 infants were abducted; 140 from health care facilities, 142 from homes, and 47 from other places (National Center for Missing & Exploited Children, n.d.).

Newborns are often abducted by women who are familiar with the birth facility and its routines. They usually visit more than one agency several times to learn the routines so they can impersonate birth facility staff to gain access to a newborn. They often know the layout of the facility and the locations of exits well.

The profile of the abductor is a woman of childbearing age, often overweight, who may want an infant to solidify her relationship with her partner. She may be pretending to be pregnant, appear pregnant, have had a previous pregnancy loss, or be unable to have a child of her own. Although the woman plans the kidnapping, she waits for an appropriate opportunity to take any infant available. She may wear a uniform to impersonate hospital staff and tell the parents she is taking the baby to have a test performed (National Center for Missing & Exploited Children, n.d.). Many precautions are necessary to protect infants from abduction (Box 22.1). Additional information about abduction is available for parents and professionals at the National Center for Missing & Exploited Children website: https://www.missingkids.org/theissues/infantabductions.

Preventing Infection

Because the newborn has a limited ability to combat infection, prevention is of utmost importance and constitutes a major part of parent teaching.

Many nursing actions help prevent infection. At the beginning of their shift, nurses wash their hands and arms thoroughly. Throughout the day, hand hygiene according to agency policy is important before and after touching any infant.

To avoid cross-contamination, each infant's supplies are kept separate from those used for other infants. Supplies in drawers or cupboards of each crib unit should be used only for that infant.

The nurse should instruct parents and visitors to wash their hands before touching infants. Parents should be instructed to discourage visitors with colds or other infections from visiting at the birth facility or during the early weeks at home.

Nurses should be vigilant for signs of infection during assessment and care of the infant. These signs are often different from those in the older infant or child and may be subtle. Instead of a fever, the infant's temperature may decrease. The infant may feed poorly, be lethargic, or have periods of apnea without obvious cause. Any unexplained change in behavior should be recorded and investigated. The same holds true, of

BOX 22.1 Precautions to Prevent Infant Abductions

All personnel should wear picture identification that is easily visible at all times. No one without appropriate identification should handle or transport infants.

Enlist parents' help in preventing kidnapping. Teach them to allow only hospital staff with proper identification to take their infants from them.

Teach parents and staff to transport infants only in their cribs and never by carrying them. Question anyone carrying an infant outside the room.

Question anyone with a newborn near an exit or in an unusual part of the facility.

Be suspicious of anyone who does not seem to be visiting a specific client, asks detailed questions about facility routines, asks to hold infants, or behaves in an unusual manner.

Be suspicious of unknown people carrying large bags or packages, which could contain an infant.

Respond immediately when an alarm signals a remote exit has been opened or an infant has been taken into an unauthorized area.

Never leave infants unattended. Teach parents infants should be observed at all times. Infants may be taken into the bathroom with the mother, if necessary. Suggest the nursing staff take care of the infant if the client wants to nap or feels unwell and no family members are present.

If infants need to be moved to another area, take one infant at a time. Never leave an infant in the hall while the nurse is in another room. Never leave an infant unsupervised.

When infants are in client rooms, position the crib away from the doorways, preferably on the side of the bed opposite the door.

Protect codes, card keys, and identification badges, which allow entrance to maternity units or nurseries so unauthorized people cannot use them. Report lost access devices to security immediately.

When a parent or family member comes to a nursery or nurses station to take their infant, always match the infant and adult identification. Never give an infant to anyone who does not have the correct identification.

Alert hospital security immediately of any suspicious activity.

Suggest parents do not place public announcements or signs in their yard, which might alert an abductor a new baby is in the home.

KNOWLEDGE CHECK

5. How can the nurse prevent a baby being given to the wrong parent?
6. What can nurses and parents do to prevent infant abductions?
7. What is the most important method of preventing infection in newborns?

Circumcision

In the United States, circumcision is one of the most common surgical procedure performed on males by pediatric surgeons (Munevveroglu & Gunduz, 2020). It is the removal of the prepuce (foreskin), a fold of skin that covers the glans penis. Although it can be retracted easily for cleaning in the older child, the prepuce may not be fully retractable until about 5 years of age or later (AAP, 2017). The prepuce should never be forcibly retracted in any infant because trauma and adhesions can result.

Circumcision is a controversial issue, and parents may have questions about choosing it for their son. The current AAP policy states the health benefits of circumcision outweigh the risks of the procedure, but the benefits are not so great it should be recommended as a routine for all newborns. Parents should have access to circumcision if they choose it for their infants (AAP Task Force, 2012a).

Reasons for Choosing Circumcision

The major benefits of circumcision are it reduces penile cancer, urinary tract infections in the first year of life, human immunodeficiency virus (HIV) infection, and transmission of other sexually transmitted diseases (AAP Task Force, 2012b; Warees et al., 2021). Some parents choose circumcision for religious, cultural, or social reasons. Some parents want their son to look like his circumcised father or peers. Others think circumcision is an expected part of newborn care, and some do not realize they have a choice in the matter.

Lack of knowledge about care of the prepuce leads to some circumcisions. Poor hygiene may increase the risk for infections and other problems. Teaching parents and children about proper care of the uncircumcised penis can prevent complications related to inadequate cleanliness.

Reasons for Rejecting Circumcision

Parents decide against circumcision for various reasons. Some parents believe the incidence of conditions more common in uncircumcised males is too low to warrant the pain and risks associated with surgery. Others believe having the infant circumcised to look like the father or peers is cosmetic surgery and therefore unnecessary. These parents especially object to subjecting their son to pain during and after surgery. Circumcision is less often practiced by families from Asian, Hispanic, and Native American cultures. It is less common in Latin American, European, and Caribbean countries (Morris et al., 2016; World Population Review, 2021).

Parents may be concerned about removing the prepuce, which serves to protect the glans. The glans is more prone

course, for the more obvious signs of infection such as drainage from the eyes, cord, or circumcision site.

Preventing Infant Falls

Infant falls are another concern. They are most likely to happen when the infant is being fed, especially at night. An exhausted or medicated parent may doze off during the feeding, loosening their hold on the infant who then slips from their arms. Parents should be instructed to place their newborn in the crib or request a family member to help watch the newborn while they sleep. Health care staff should be educated to round on clients frequently, assess the safety of the environment for the baby, offer to help as needed, and encourage parents to place infants in their cribs when the parent becomes sleepy.

to irritation from constant exposure to urine and rubbing against diapers when unprotected by the prepuce.

Complications of circumcision are rare but include hemorrhage and infection. Removal of too much or too little of the prepuce, an unsatisfactory cosmetic result, urinary retention, stenosis or fistulas of the urethra, adhesions, necrosis, or other injury to the glans penis also may occur.

Only healthy newborns should undergo circumcision. The preterm or sick infant should not be circumcised until he is healthy enough to tolerate the procedure. For the repair of anatomic abnormalities of the penis such as hypospadias or epispadias, an intact prepuce may be needed for use in plastic surgery.

Pain Relief

To decrease pain experienced during the procedure, newborns should receive pharmacologic and nonpharmacologic pain relief (AAP Task Force, 2012b; Munevveroglu & Gunduz, 2020). A combination of methods such use of an oral sucrose solution, topical agents (EMLA cream, topical lidocaine cream), or local nerve block may be used (Warees et al., 2021). The dorsal penile nerve block (anesthetic injected into the dorsal penile nerve) is a safe method to eliminate pain during circumcision. It has been found to be more effective than other methods of pain relief. EMLA cream may be applied at least 1 hour before the procedure to anesthetize the skin, but it is less effective than anesthetic injection and requires a longer waiting period before it is effective. Pediatric acetaminophen may be given throughout the first day for postprocedure pain, not to exceed five doses (Ogundoyin et al., 2019).

Nonpharmacologic pain relief methods include pacifiers, oral sucrose, soothing music, recordings of intrauterine sounds, decreased lights, and talking softly to the infant. All have shown some success in reducing an infant's pain responses to circumcision but are not as effective as anesthetics. Pain and pain management in newborns is discussed further in Chapter 24.

Methods

The Gomco (Yellen) clamp (Fig. 22.5), Mogen clamp (Fig. 22.6), and PlastiBell (Fig. 22.7) are three devices used for performing circumcisions. In all methods, the prepuce is first separated from the glans with a probe and incised to expose the glans.

Nursing Considerations

Assisting in Decision Making. Ideally, parents decide about circumcision early in pregnancy on the basis of a careful consideration of risks and benefits. Although the physician is responsible for explaining the risks and benefits of circumcision to parents, the nurse may be asked to answer questions or clarify misconceptions.

Although nurses generally teach parents of circumcised infants how to care for the penis, they may not think about providing teaching for parents who decide against circumcision. Proper care of the intact penis should be included in the teaching plan for these parents and should be discussed with parents who are undecided about the procedure as well.

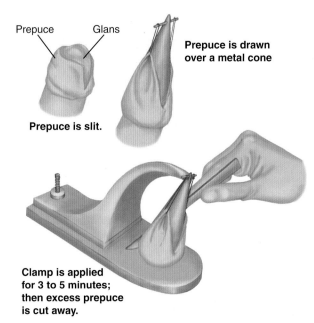

FIG. 22.5 Circumcision Using the Gomco (Yellen) Clamp. After separating the prepuce from the glans, the physician pulls the prepuce over a cone-shaped device that rests against the glans. A clamp is placed around the cone and the prepuce and tightened to provide enough pressure to crush the blood vessels. This prevents bleeding when the prepuce is removed after 3 to 5 minutes.

CLIENT EDUCATION

How to Care for the Uncircumcised Penis

Wash your baby's penis daily and when soiled diapers are changed. Do not retract the foreskin because it does not separate from the glans (or end of the penis) until about 5 years of age.

Occasionally, gently pull back on the foreskin to see how much separation has occurred. However, *never* force the foreskin to retract because it would be painful and might cause bleeding, infection, and adhesions.

As your son gets older and is able to take care of himself, teach him to wash under the foreskin by gently pulling it back as far as it retracts easily. This should become a part of his daily bath.

Providing Care during Circumcision. As with any surgical procedure, informed consent from parents is necessary before a circumcision is performed. The nurse sees that the consent has been signed, the infant is stable, and vitamin K has been given to prevent excessive bleeding. The physician is informed of any problems that might impair the infant's ability to withstand circumcision.

Although no longer routine, some facility protocols or provider orders may direct the nurse to withhold feedings for 2 to 4 hours prior to the procedure to decrease the risk of regurgitation and possible aspiration while the infant is restrained in the supine position. The nurse gathers equipment and supplies before the procedure. A bulb syringe should be placed nearby in case suction is necessary.

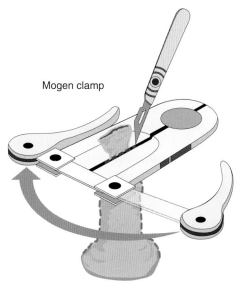

Mogen clamp

FIG. 22.6 Circumcision Using the Mogen Clamp. After separating the prepuce from the glans, the physician pulls the prepuce over the glans of the penis. The clamp is placed just beyond the tip of the glans, crushing the blood vessels. This prevents bleeding when the prepuce is removed. (From HowStuffWorks.com. © [2008] HowStuffWorks.com. All rights reserved. Used under license.)

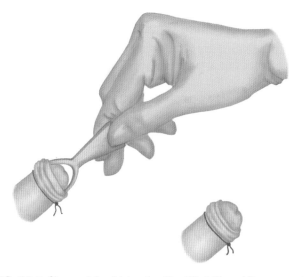

FIG. 22.7 Circumcision Using the PlastiBell Ring. After separating the prepuce from the glans, the physician places the PlastiBell, a plastic ring, over the glans, draws the prepuce over it, and ties a suture around the prepuce and the PlastiBell ring. This prevents bleeding when the excess prepuce is removed. The handle is removed, leaving only the ring in place over the glans.

When the physician and equipment are ready, the infant is placed on the circumcision board. (Fig. 22.8). A warm blanket is placed under the infant, and a surgical drape provides warmth and maintains sterility. A heat lamp or radiant warmer helps prevent cold stress.

The nurse should comfort the infant during the procedure. The physician administers the anesthesia. The nurse may provide a pacifier or sucrose, talk to the infant, or play soft music or recordings of intrauterine sounds to help distract the infant from pain.

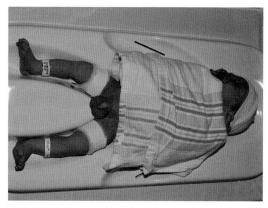

FIG. 22.8 The infant is placed on the circumcision board just before the procedure is begun.

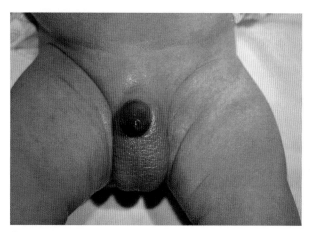

FIG. 22.9 An infant with a recently circumcised penis. (Courtesy Cheryl Briggs, RNC, Annapolis, MD.)

Evaluating Pain. Nurses should evaluate the infant's pain with one of the pain scales available for use with newborns. An example is the Neonatal Inventory Pain Scale (NIPS) (Lawrence et al., 1993). This scale measures facial expression, crying, breathing pattern, muscle tone of the extremities, and state of arousal. The infant's pain responses should be measured before, during, and after the procedure.

Providing Postprocedure Care. The infant should be removed from the restraints immediately after the circumcision is completed. If a Gomco or Mogen clamp was used, the nurse squeezes petroleum jelly on the circumcision site to prevent the diaper from sticking to it. A small piece of gauze may be placed over the area. Petroleum jelly should not be used with a PlastiBell because it may cause the ring to be displaced. The diaper is attached loosely to prevent pressure. The infant should be comforted and returned to his parents, who may be anxious about their son. Breastfeeding will provide comfort.

The nurse watches carefully for signs of complications after the circumcision (Fig. 22.9). The wound is checked frequently for bleeding during the first few hours after the procedure. If excessive bleeding occurs, pressure is applied to the site. The nurse notifies the physician, who may apply Gelfoam or epinephrine or may suture the small blood vessels. Even a small amount of blood loss may be significant in an infant, who has a small total blood volume.

Noting the first urination after circumcision is important because edema could cause obstruction. If the infant goes home before voiding, the parents are instructed to call the physician if the baby does not urinate within 6 to 8 hours.

⚡ SAFETY CHECK

Signs of complications of circumcision include the following:
Bleeding more than a few drops with first diaper changes
Failure to urinate
Signs of infection: fever or low temperature, purulent or foul-smelling drainage
Displacement of the PlastiBell ring

Teaching Parents. Because circumcision is often performed on the day of discharge, the parents take over care of the site. Each time the site is checked for bleeding, the nurse should show the parents the amount of blood on the diaper to help them understand how much to expect. The normal yellowish exudate that forms over the site should be described and differentiated from purulent drainage. Signs of complications should be discussed thoroughly with parents.

CLIENT EDUCATION

How to Care for the Circumcision Site

Observe the circumcision site at each diaper change and check the amount of bleeding. Call the physician if more than a few drops of blood are present with diaper changes on the first day or any bleeding thereafter.

Continue to apply petroleum jelly to the penis with each diaper change for the first 4 to 7 days or as directed by your pediatrician. If a PlastiBell ring was used, do not use petroleum jelly because it might make the ring fall off too soon.

Keeping the circumcision site clean is important for healing. Squeeze warm water from a clean washcloth over the penis to wash it. Pat gently to dry the area. Fasten the diaper loosely to prevent rubbing or pressure on the incision site.

Expect a yellow crust or scab to form over the circumcision site. This is a normal part of healing and should not be removed. The scab will fall off within 7 to 10 days. If a PlastiBell ring was used, the plastic rim will fall off in 7 to 10 days (Soltany & Ardestanizadeh, 2020). If it does not fall off by then or falls off sooner, notify your physician. Watch for signs of infection such as fever or drainage, which smells bad or has pus in it. *Call your physician if you suspect any abnormalities.* The circumcision site should be fully healed in approximately 10 days.

❓ KNOWLEDGE CHECK

8. What are the reasons parents decide for or against circumcision?
9. What information do parents need about care of the intact and circumcised penis?

Immunization

Immunization for hepatitis B is now included with other routine childhood vaccinations. Newborns of clients with acute or chronic hepatitis B infection (hepatitis B surface antigen [HBsAg]-positive) may become infected from exposure at birth. Infected infants have a very high chance of developing chronic infection, which may later cause cancer or other serious liver disease.

These infants should receive both the vaccine and hepatitis B immune globulin (HBIG). HBIG provides passive immunity against hepatitis to protect infants until they develop their own antibodies and should be given within 12 hours of birth (CDC, 2021d). The vaccine promotes antibody formation to protect infants from further exposure to the disease. The rest of the vaccine series is given in the health care provider's office or in a clinic.

Newborns of uninfected clients also receive hepatitis B vaccine. It is often given during the stay in the birth facility but may also be given later in the pediatrician's office. The CDC (2021d) recommends stable newborns weighing more than 2000 g should receive the first hepatitis B vaccine within 12 hours of birth. Parents should be referred to their pediatrician for two more doses of the vaccine after discharge (see Drug Guide: Hepatitis B Vaccine; Drug Guide: Hepatitis Immune Globulin [HBIG]).

Newborn Screening Tests

Prompt identification and treatment of infants with conditions that can affect their survival or long-term health is essential. Stable newborns are screened after 24 hours of age or prior to hospital discharge. Newborns may be screened for critical congenital heart defects, hearing, metabolic, hematologic, and genetic disorders. Each state determines which specific tests are performed before discharge from the birth facility. Parents are provided information prior to each test. Infants identified by these tests may need repeat screening or more complex diagnostic testing.

Critical Congenital Heart Defect Screening

Congenital heart defects are a leading type of birth defects. Although many are identified soon after birth, some are not easily detected. It is essential for critical congenital heart defects (CCHDs) be identified early after birth to prevent injury or death. All stable, alert newborns should be screened after 24 hours of age but before discharge (AAP Section on Cardiology and Cardiac Surgery Executive Committee, 2012). A motion-tolerant pulse oximeter is used on the right hand and either foot to measure oxygenated hemoglobin in the blood. An oximetry reading of 95% or less in either extremity or 3% or more absolute difference between the upper and lower extremity requires further testing (Fig. 22.10).

Hearing Screening

Approximately 1 to 2 of every 1000 infants are born in the United States each year with hearing impairment. Infants begin learning language within the first 6 months of life

DRUG GUIDE

Hepatitis B Vaccine

Classification
Vaccine.

Other Names
Engerix-B, Recombivax HB.

Action
Immunization against hepatitis B infection.

Indications
Prevention of hepatitis B in exposed and unexposed infants.

Neonatal Dosage and Route
Recombivax HB
5 mcg.

Engerix-B
10 mcg.
   The first dose of hepatitis B vaccine is given to newborns before hospital discharge. The second dose of vaccine is given at age 1 to 2 months. The third dose is given at 6 to 18 months (at least 16 weeks after the first dose).

Infants of HBsAg-Negative Clients
The usual routine is followed.

Infants of HBsAg-Positive Clients
The vaccine is given within 12 hours of birth along with hepatitis B immune globulin (HBIG), which is given at a different site. The usual routine is followed for the rest of the series. The infant should be tested for HBsAg and antibody to HBsAg after completing three doses of vaccine.

Infants of Clients Whose HBsAg Status Is Unknown
The vaccine is given within 12 hours of birth, and the client is tested. If the HBsAg test is positive, the infant should receive HBIG as soon as possible and no later than 1 week of age. The usual routine is followed for the rest of the series. Give intramuscularly in the anterolateral thigh.

Absorption
Absorbed slowly; not affected by maternal antibodies.

Contraindications:
Hypersensitivity to yeast.

Adverse Reactions
Pain or redness at site, fever, fatigue, headache.

Nursing Considerations
If the solution is in a vial, shake well before preparing. Give vaccine within 12 hours of birth to infants of infected clients. Do not inject intravenously or intradermally. Obtain parental consent before administering.

DRUG GUIDE

Hepatitis B Immune Globulin (HBIG)

Classification
Immune globulin.

Other Names
HBIG, Hep-B-Gammagee, HyperHEP.

Action
Provides antibodies and passive immunity to hepatitis B.

Indications
Prophylaxis for infants of hepatitis B surface antigen–positive clients.

Neonatal Dosage and Route
0.5 mL within 12 hours of birth if possible but no later than 1 week of age; given intramuscularly in the anterolateral thigh; should not be given intravenously.

Absorption
Absorbed slowly.

Contraindications
None known.

Adverse Reactions
Pain and tenderness at the site, urticaria, anaphylaxis.

Nursing Considerations
Do not shake or give intravenously. Hepatitis vaccine series should begin within 12 hours of birth. Give injections of vaccine and immune globulin at separate sites.

(National Institute on Deafness and Other Communication Disorders [NIDCD], 2020).

Because early detection and treatment can prevent or reduce developmental delays and help the child communicate better, auditory screening of all newborns within the first month is recommended. Infants who do not pass the screening should be rescreened, and if they still do not pass, they should have audiologic and medical evaluations by no later than 3 months of age (NIDCD, 2020).

A goal of *Healthy People 2030* is to increase the proportion of newborns who are screened for hearing impairment by age 1 month to a target of 97% and increase initiation of audiologic evaluation by age 3 months to 79.2% (Office of Disease Prevention and Health Promotion [ODPHP], 2020).

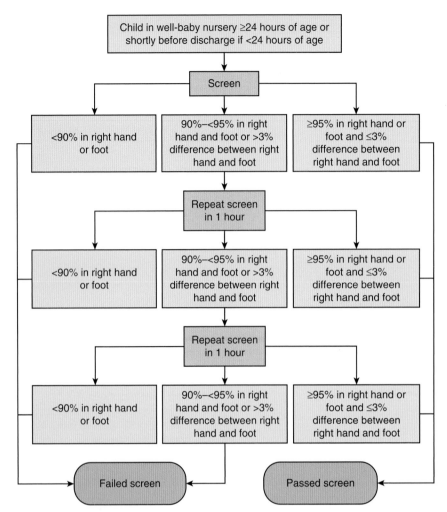

FIG. 22.10 Congenital Heart Disease Screening Algorithm. (Kemper, A. R., Mahle, W. T., Martin, G. R., Cooley, W. C., Kumar, P., Morrow, W. R., Kelm, K., Pearson, G. D., Glidewell, J., Grosse, S. D., Lloyd-Puryear, M., Howell. R. R. (2011). Strategies for implementing screening for critical congenital heart disease. *Pediatrics, 128*(5), e1-8. As depicted in Centers for Disease Control (2020). Congenital heart defects information for healthcare providers.)

To accomplish this goal, a screening test is usually given to infants before discharge from the birth facility.

Otoacoustic emissions and acoustic brainstem response tests are used for screening. The tests can be done while the infant sleeps. The nurse ensures infants receive screening and explains the testing to the parents. An infant who fails the first screening is often retested in the birth facility. Parents of infants referred for further testing after discharge need more explanation and emotional support.

Other Screening Tests

Blood tests to screen for metabolic, hematologic, or genetic disorders are also performed. With early identification and treatment, infants with these conditions may avoid severe intellectual disability or other serious problems. Common disorders often included are phenylketonuria (PKU), hypothyroidism, galactosemia, hemoglobinopathies such as sickle cell disease and thalassemia, and congenital adrenal hyperplasia.

The screening tests are easy and inexpensive. The heel is warmed, a few drops of blood collected, and the specimen is sent to the state laboratory for processing (see Chapter 21, Procedure 21.3). The tests are performed at 24 to 48 hours after birth. Parents and the newborn's provider receive results. Further testing is necessary to confirm any abnormalities.

Parents may have questions for the nurse about the purpose of the tests. A pamphlet with information about the tests may be given to parents. Nurses often refer to the tests as "PKU tests," but they should call them "screening tests" instead to emphasize a number of conditions are included.

Tests performed within the first 24 hours of life are less sensitive than those performed after 24 hours. Infants tested before age 12 to 24 hours should have repeat tests at age 1 to 2 weeks so disorders are not missed because testing was done too early (Health Resources & Services Administration, 2021).

Phenylketonuria. PKU is a genetic condition in which the infant cannot metabolize the amino acid phenylalanine, which is common in protein foods such as milk. Although some phenylalanine is essential to growth, accumulations of it can result in severe intellectual disability. Treatment should be started immediately once a positive result is obtained (National Health Service, 2019). PKU is treated with a special low-phenylalanine diet, in which the amount of the amino acid is carefully regulated.

Congenital Hypothyroidism. Congenital hypothyroidism occurs when the thyroid does not produce enough thyroid hormones, which affect the entire body. Symptoms in an untreated infant include a hoarse cry, large fontanel and tongue, slow reflexes, abdominal distention, lethargy, and feeding problems and can lead to intellectual disability. Infants may have no signs in the early weeks, but early treatment with thyroid hormones is necessary to ensure normal growth and intellectual function.

Galactosemia. Absence of the enzyme necessary for the conversion of the milk sugar galactose to glucose causes galactosemia. The condition results in damage to the liver, increased susceptibility to infection, intellectual disability, and other developmental problems. Treatment includes a diet free of lactose and galactose. Long-term complications such as delayed growth and neurologic impairment may occur even with treatment.

Hemoglobinopathies. Hemoglobinopathies include sickle cell anemia, thalassemia, and other disorders. The conditions are most often found in infants of African, Mediterranean, Indian, or South and Central American background. The hemoglobinopathies cause chronic anemias, sepsis, and other serious conditions.

Congenital Adrenal Hyperplasia. The term *congenital adrenal hyperplasia* refers to a group of disorders with an enzyme defect that prevents adequate adrenal corticosteroid and aldosterone production and increases production of androgens. Infants may have ambiguous genitalia or masculinization of female infants at birth. Salt-wasting crisis with low sodium and glucose and high potassium levels may occur within the first week of life. Treatment is administration of corticosteroids and mineralocorticoids for the remainder of the child's life.

Other Conditions. Screening also may be performed for maple syrup urine disease, biotinidase deficiency, homocystinuria, cystic fibrosis, and other conditions. Each of these conditions can be accurately diagnosed in newborns so treatment can begin early. Knowing many conditions are included in testing allows the nurse to explain its importance to the parents.

APPLICATION OF THE NURSING PROCESS: PARENTS' KNOWLEDGE OF NEWBORN CARE

Parents often feel anxious about taking over total care of their newborn. Postpartum clients dealing with exhaustion and physiologic changes from childbirth may have difficulty remembering the extensive information they are given. Therefore, finding creative teaching methods is especially important. The nurse should use every contact with the parents as an opportunity for further teaching.

Assessment

Assess parents' changing learning needs throughout the birth facility stay. Consider the postpartum client's and infant's physical conditions and any special concerns the parents may have.

Determine the learning needs of experienced parents. They may be unaware of information that has changed since the birth of the last infant. Concerns about helping other children adjust to the newborn may be especially important.

Assess the partner's learning needs and plans for involvement in infant care. Determine whether there are cultural dictates about the partner's participation in infant care. They often have many questions and are eager to learn about care of their infant.

Identification of Client Problems

In general, newborns are healthy; nursing care is wellness-oriented. Client problems center around parent education. Most parents are ready to improve their knowledge of infant care in anticipation of discharge.

Planning: Expected Outcomes

The primary expected outcomes for this teaching opportunity are as follows.

Before discharge the parents will:
1. Identify their own information needs and seek assistance from nurses to meet those needs.
2. Correctly demonstrate infant care.
3. Express confidence in their ability to meet their infant's needs.

Interventions
Setting Priorities

Because of the short time available for teaching, set priorities when determining what to teach. After assessing the parents' learning needs, make a teaching plan with them. Use a topic list to help them point out major concerns regarding infant care to ensure effective use of the teaching time. Begin by discussing their most pressing concerns to decrease anxiety so they can concentrate on the information. Then proceed to other subjects.

Using Various Teaching Methods

Use a variety of teaching methods to increase effectiveness, make the subject more interesting, and increase retention of the material. Use verbal and written methods, demonstrations, and return demonstrations. Parents often learn best by seeing skills performed correctly and then practicing them while the nurse gives suggestions. To increase the likelihood parents will follow instructions, explain the rationale for each point made during teaching sessions.

Use audiovisual materials, including pamphlets, magazines, television programs, and internet sites. Highlight the most important areas in written material, discuss the programs with the new parents, and clarify information, as necessary, to reinforce learning.

Many parents use the internet to obtain information about child care. Suggest they look for websites provided by well-known organizations such as the AAP (https://www.healthychildren.org). Warn them to be wary of sites with unclear sources or information that seems contrary to generally accepted knowledge. Suggest they have their health care provider confirm the validity of the information if they are unsure about it. Commend parents for their interest in obtaining information to increase their parenting skills.

Texts to cell phones are another source of information. One source that provides tips for infant care during the first year is Text4baby (https://www.text4baby.org) from the National Healthy Mothers, Healthy Babies Coalition (NORD).

Modeling Behavior

Most parents watch closely when nurses handle infants. Nurses model parenting behavior by the way they hold, care for, and talk to infants. Modeling is particularly important for the parents with no experience in infant care.

Use every opportunity during general care to point out infant characteristics and behavior states and to model how to calm crying infants. Teach parents to use progressive consoling interventions such as talking to the infant, folding the infant's arms across the chest, holding, swaddling, and facilitating sucking of the infant's finger or a pacifier. Point out the different behavior states and how to help infants move to a more awake state for feeding. Instruct parents to intervene before infants reach the point of frantic crying.

Teaching Intermittently

Plan teaching in small segments that are interspersed with infant care. Check the parents' understanding often. Encourage them to take over various tasks until they are performing all of the infant's routine care. Use a checklist of major teaching topics to ensure all important areas are covered (Box 22.2).

BOX 22.2 Major Teaching Topics

Newborn characteristics and behavior
Use of bulb syringe
Breastfeeding
  Frequency, length, positioning, latch, supply and demand, supplementing, potential problems
Formula feeding
  Frequency, amount, positioning, avoiding propping, types of formula, formula preparation
Burping
Cord care
Care of the penis, uncircumcised or circumcised
Holding and positioning
Sleep pattern and position
Elimination patterns
Bathing and skin care
Clothing
Signs of problems
Taking a temperature
Infant safety
Abusive head trauma (shaken baby syndrome)
Car seat use

Including the Partner

Identify partners who would like to participate in the care of their infants but hesitate because they lack experience. Offer them the same teaching given to inexperienced parents. Give praise liberally to increase confidence when the partners practice their new infant care skills.

Documenting Teaching

Document all teaching performed and the evaluation of the parents' abilities to carry out infant care. This information shows other nurses what teaching has been completed and what is still needed. It also provides legal proof teaching was completed before discharge.

Providing for Follow-Up Care

If the client and infant will be seen by a clinic or home visit nurse, provide information about unmet learning needs. Reinforcement then can be provided at a time when memory has improved after the stress of birth.

Give as much information as possible in written form so parents can refer to it later if they have concerns. Also, provide telephone numbers they can call for further help. Offer written information in the parents' primary language, if possible. Even if they speak English as a second language, they may prefer to read the information in their native language.

Remind parents about timing of follow-up care. Suggest they schedule the appointment before they leave the birth facility.

Incorporating Cultural Considerations

Consider the family's cultural beliefs about childcare when teaching. Asian parents may be uneasy when caregivers are too complimentary about the baby or casually touch the infant's head. Mexican parents, however, may prefer a person who compliments the infant and touches the infant to ward off the *mal ojo* or "evil eye" (Bell et al., 2020). Cord care may also differ in various cultures.

Ask the parents who will be helping them care for the baby to determine family members who should be included in the teaching. This varies according to the culture and availability of the traditional caregiver. In addition to the partner, the mother of one of the parents is often the major support person.

Elicit questions during the discussions. However, be aware clients from some cultures will not ask questions. Other clients may be too shy or uneasy about their limited English. When questions are not asked, discuss questions often asked by other parents.

Evaluation

Ongoing evaluation of parents' learning is necessary throughout the birth facility stay and during the follow-up home, clinic, or office visits. Determine whether the parents think their questions have been answered and if they can demonstrate important aspects of infant care safely and correctly. As they learn more caregiving skills, they should verbalize more confidence in their abilities.

CLIENT EDUCATION

Techniques of Infant Care

This guide is written in language the nurse might use when teaching parents about infant care. Adapt the subjects to meet the needs of individual parents.

Handling the Infant

Head Support

An infant's head is the heaviest part of the body. Infants are unable to support the head when held in an upright position for the first few months of life. You should place one hand behind the infant's head to support it when you pick up or carry the baby.

Positions

Most parents hold the infant in the cradle position. For the "football" position, support the baby's head in the palm of your hand with the body held along your arm and supported against your side (see Chapter 23, Fig. 23.4). This position allows one hand to be free when washing the baby's hair or breastfeeding.

The shoulder hold is good for burping the baby. Or sit the baby on your lap, and support the head and chest with one hand while gently patting or rubbing the infant's back with the other hand. This allows you to see the baby's face in case of spit-ups.

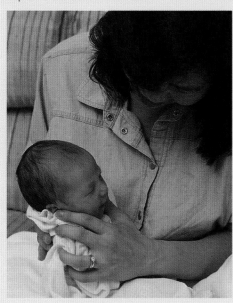

Always place your baby on his or her back for sleep. This position is recommended by the American Academy of Pediatrics because it helps prevent sudden infant death syndrome (SIDS), the sudden unexplained death of an infant. The baby should sleep on a firm mattress and have no loose blankets or pillows in the bed. The crib or bassinet should be in the parents' room up until 1 year of age. The baby should not sleep with anyone else. You may use a pacifier when you put the baby down to sleep. If you are breastfeeding, you can wait 1 month to fully establish breastfeeding and then give the baby a pacifier.

Place your baby on the abdomen for play when the infant is awake and will be observed. This "tummy time" helps the infant develop muscles in the back and neck and prevents flattening of the back of the head. If the infant becomes sleepy, change the position to lying on the back for safety during sleep.

Wrapping

Young infants seem to feel secure when wrapped firmly in a blanket (swaddled). Fussy babies often respond well to swaddling. To swaddle the infant, turn down one corner of a blanket and position the baby's head over the edge. Fold one side of the blanket over the body and arm. Bring the lower corner up, and fold it over the chest. Then bring the other side around the infant, and tuck it underneath snugly.

Normal Body Processes

Breathing

Newborns normally breathe about 30 to 60 times a minute. Their breathing is irregular and may vary from loud to very soft. Sneezing is normal and not likely to be from a cold unless there are other signs.

Using a Bulb Syringe

Use the bulb syringe if the infant has excessive mucus in the mouth or nose or spits up milk. Be very gentle, and use the bulb only if necessary. Squeeze the bulb before you gently insert the tip into the side of the mouth. Do not aim it to the back of the mouth because the baby might gag. Always suction the mouth before the nose. Extra mucus is common in the first days of life but is usually not a problem thereafter.

Clean the bulb with soap and water. Rinse and dry well before using again.

Call 9-1-1 if the baby's skin becomes blue or the baby stops breathing for more than 15 seconds, or has difficulty breathing. Call your provider for yellow or green drainage from the nose.

Regulating Temperature

Newborns have difficulty regulating their body temperature. If they become cold, they need more calories and oxygen than when they are warm. Dress your baby as you would like to be dressed. Add a light receiving blanket, except in very hot weather.

Using a Thermometer

Check your baby's temperature during illness. Place the thermometer in the pit of the arm so the bulb does not stick out the other side of the arm. Hold the arm firmly over the thermometer. Read it according to the manufacturer's directions. Call your physician if the baby has a temperature higher than 38.0°C (100.4°F) or lower than 36.5°C (97.7°F).

Urine Output

Your baby will have at least one or two wet diapers a day during the first day or two and at least six wet diapers a day by the sixth day. Counting the number of wet diapers helps you know if the baby is getting enough milk. *Call your baby's doctor if the baby has no wet diapers for more than 12 hours.*

Stool Output

Breastfed infants pass at least four soft, seedy stools, which have a sweet–sour odor and are mustard yellow each day.

Continued

Formula-fed infants pass one to several stools each day, which are pale yellow to light brown and formed. Babies are not constipated when they turn red and seem to strain when passing a stool. Constipated stools are dry with small, hard pieces like marbles.

Diarrhea

Babies with diarrhea pass more frequent stools, which are greener and more liquid than usual. There may be a *water ring*, an area in the diaper where the watery stool has been absorbed, sometimes around an area of more solid stool. Call your physician if the infant passes more than two diarrhea stools because serious dehydration can occur very quickly in infants.

Skin Care

A number of normal marks occur on the newborn's skin. A normal newborn rash called *erythema toxicum* resembles small insect bites or pimples. Small whiteheads called *milia* are normal and disappear without treatment. Do not squeeze them, or they may become infected. Newborns have dry, peeling skin, which will be soft after peeling. Lotions or creams are unnecessary and may cause irritation.

Cord

Clean the cord with plain water, if necessary, and keep it dry. Fold the diaper below it so it is not wet by urine. The cord generally falls off in about 10 to 14 days. Some care providers suggest waiting for the cord to fall off before tub bathing, but others allow tub baths. Check with your health care provider. When the cord detaches, there may be a few drops of blood or a slight odor, which is normal. Notify your physician if you see more bleeding or signs of infection, such as redness, drainage, or a foul odor.

Diaper Area

Clean the diaper area with each diaper change. For girls, separate the labia (folds) and remove all stool. Wipe the diaper area from front to back. Wiping back and forth may move stool into the vagina or urethra and cause an infection. For boys, wash under the scrotum to help prevent rashes. Changing the diaper frequently, avoiding commercial diaper wipes, and using absorbent diapers may help prevent diaper rash. If the diaper area becomes red, change the diaper more often. Leaving the diaper off to expose the area to air is also helpful. Petroleum jelly or a barrier-type zinc oxide ointment may be used. If redness persists, ask your baby's doctor for suggestions.

Bathing

Because infants are washed as needed after they spit up and with diaper changes, baths are not necessary every day. Partners often enjoy giving the infant a bath and make this their special time with the baby.

Sponge Baths

Before the bath, gather all the supplies: a container or sink for warm water, washcloth, towel, baby shampoo, and clean clothes. Soap is not necessary for the young infant, but, if used, it should be gentle and nonalkaline to protect the natural acids of the infant's skin.

Give the bath in a room that is warm and free of drafts. Bathe the baby on a safe surface at a comfortable height for you. If you use a counter, pad it with blankets or towels.

Never leave the infant alone on an unprotected surface, even for a moment. Keep one hand on the infant at all times to prevent falls. Avoid answering the phone during bath time to avoid distractions. If you must leave the room, take the baby along or place the baby in the crib.

Before fully undressing the baby, use the football position to shampoo the baby's head. Although the fontanel or "soft spot" may seem delicate, it is covered with a tough membrane and is not injured by washing. Pulse movements in the fontanel are normal. Dry the hair well to prevent heat loss.

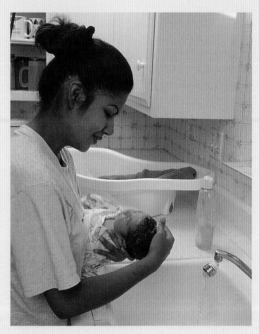

Keep the baby warm by uncovering only the area you are washing. Wash and dry one part of the baby's body at a time. Wash the face with clear water. Use a separate clean area of the washcloth to wipe across each eyelid and around each eye. Use a washcloth to clean in and around the ears, where milk may accumulate. Do not use cotton-tipped swabs in the infant's ears or nose, because injury may occur if the baby moves suddenly.

To clean the neck folds, put one hand under the baby's shoulders and lift slightly to cause the head to drop back enough so the creases in the neck can be washed. Clean the diaper area last.

Tub Bath

For a tub bath, use a plastic tub or a clean sink. Pad the bottom with a towel or foam pad to make it more comfortable and prevent the infant from slipping. Place enough warm water in the tub to cover the shoulders to prevent chilling. Wash the baby's face and hair before placing the baby in the tub. Keep the infant dressed until after the hair is washed to prevent chilling.

It is not unusual for infants to be frightened when they are first put into the water. To help your baby adjust to this new experience, talk softly and calmly while holding the baby securely.

Keep the bath short so the baby does not get cold. Dry quickly, dress, and wrap the infant in two blankets for a short while to help the baby maintain heat.

CLIENT EDUCATION—cont'd

Feeding

See Chapter 23 for information on breastfeeding and formula feeding.

Behavior

Knowing the different behavioral states of infants helps you learn about your baby's individual characteristics.

Sleep Phases

During quiet sleep the infant sleeps soundly with quiet breathing and little movement. Your baby will not be disturbed by noises from appliances or other children at this time. In active sleep, the baby moves or fusses while still asleep. During the drowsy state, the baby is beginning to wake but may go back to sleep if not disturbed. However, if it is time for feeding or other activities, talk softly to help the baby awaken.

Awake Phases

The quiet alert state is a good time for infant stimulation and "play time." The quiet alert state lasts only a short time, and infants often need a break from interaction. Signs of overstimulation are present if the infant turns the head away; begins to cough, sneeze, hiccup, or spit up; or becomes fussy. They show the infant needs a short quiet time.

The active alert or "fussy" phase is a time when the infant may show hunger, discomfort, or fatigue. With intervention the baby may move back to the quiet alert state or eat and then go to sleep. If you do not intervene, the baby soon moves to the crying state.

The baby may use self-consoling measures such as sucking on a finger. However, if these efforts are not effective, parents should comfort the infant quickly. Babies who cry too long may not respond at first to care activities. A few minutes of rocking and holding close may be necessary before the infant settles down.

Socialization

Infants are social beings who enjoy contact with people. The baby should be part of family life. Use an infant seat or carrier to keep the baby near you and the rest of the family. Infants enjoy watching the human face. Hold your baby close, and talk to your baby to provide social stimulation.

Stimulation

Babies respond best to gentle stimulation and enjoy a variety of types. They enjoy music that is not too loud. They focus their eyes best at a distance of 8 to 12 inches. Items such as mobiles should be placed within this range. Newborns especially like black and white geometric figures and bright colors. Infants respond to gentle stimulation when they are in the quiet alert state. Do not try to use stimulation techniques with a fussy infant. Overstimulation causes the baby to be irritable and have difficulty going to sleep.

? KNOWLEDGE CHECK

10. What are some important considerations in planning parent teaching?
11. What immunization may be performed at the birth facility?
12. Why is it important to perform screening tests on infants' blood as close to discharge as possible? For which infants is retesting important?

DISCHARGE AND NEWBORN FOLLOW-UP CARE

Discharge

Although state and federal legislation allows postpartum clients and infants to stay in the birth facility for 48 hours after vaginal birth and 96 hours after cesarean birth, some families choose to go home earlier. The time of discharge varies according to the wishes and needs of the parents and the primary caregiver's assessment of conditions of both clients.

Discharge is considered when term newborns who are appropriate for gestational age have normal physical examination results and show they are making the transition from fetal to neonatal life without difficulty. Infants should have stable vital signs for the 12 hours before discharge, passed urine and stool, have no excessive bleeding at the circumcision site and have fed successfully at least twice. The assessment of an actual feeding session by a qualified caregiver should be documented in the medical record. In addition, newborn laboratory and screening tests and evaluation for sepsis should have been completed based on risk factors. Hepatitis B vaccine should have been given or plans for administration made (AAP & ACOG, 2017). The infant's parents, family members, and caregivers should have all appropriate vaccinations such as a recent Tdap (tetanus, diphtheria, and pertussis) vaccine, influenza vaccine during flu season, and so on. The article "Vaccines for Family and Caregivers" (https://www.cdc.gov/vaccines/pregnancy/family-caregivers.html) provides information on appropriate vaccinations. Newborn screening tests for metabolic, hearing, and critical congenital heart defect should be completed and appropriate follow-up arrangements made (AAP & ACOG, 2017).

If infants have significant jaundice, it should be evaluated and treated appropriately, and plans for follow-up after discharge should be made. The parents should have received teaching about infant care and should demonstrate knowledge, ability, and confidence to provide adequate care to the newborn. An appropriate infant car seat should be available at discharge. Family, environmental, and social risk factors should have been assessed and plans made to safeguard the infant as necessary. The family should have an adequate support system and have plans for continued care from a health care provider and telephone numbers with instructions to follow in the event of complications or emergencies. A phone number for nonemergency questions and concerns should also be provided. The appointment for the first follow-up visit for the newborn should be scheduled. If this is not possible before discharge, the parents should have instructions to schedule an appointment (AAP & ACOG, 2017).

Follow-Up Care

Care after discharge from the birth facility is very important. The AAP recommends follow-up by a health care professional be provided within 48 hours for all newborns who are taken home from the birth facility less than 48 hours after birth (AAP & ACOG, 2017). All healthy newborns should be evaluated within 48 to 72 hours after hospital discharge or 3 to 5 days after birth (Taylor & Parekh, 2020). This care can be provided in the home, clinic, or office (AAP & ACOG, 2017).

HOME CARE OF THE INFANT

In the birth facility, parents often receive more information about care of the newborn than they can absorb. This may leave them inadequately prepared to cope with the multiple demands of early parenting. Family members, once the primary source of support for new parents, frequently live far away, and parents must rely on friends, health care personnel, child care classes, television, books, magazines, and the internet for information. Nurses are ideal sources of assistance in these situations and can also help parents evaluate the validity of information they receive from nonprofessional sources.

Care After Discharge

Various programs have been instituted to provide after-discharge care for postpartum clients and infants. They may include parenting and childbirth classes or nursing contact with the family in the home, in the clinic, or by telephone.

Home Visits

The home visit is ideally scheduled during the first 24 to 72 hours after discharge. This timing allows early assessment and intervention for problems in nutrition, jaundice, newborn adaptation, and parent-infant interaction. Nurses may visit low-risk mothers and infants or may follow high-risk infants after discharge from the neonatal intensive care nursery (Fig. 22.11). Visits usually last 60 to 90 minutes to allow enough time for assessment and teaching. Home visits are expensive and are not available in all areas, but they do provide the most comprehensive care.

Visits to Low-Risk Families

During the home visit, the nurse performs a physical examination of the postpartum client and the infant. Family adaptation to the addition of a new member and the adequacy of the parents' support system is also assessed. Reinforcement of the teaching that was begun at the birth facility is important. A feeding session should be observed, especially if the infant is breastfeeding. The nurse may take blood for metabolic screening if the infant went home too early to have had reliable testing in the birth facility. Safety in the home is often discussed, and questions about infant care and general parenting are answered.

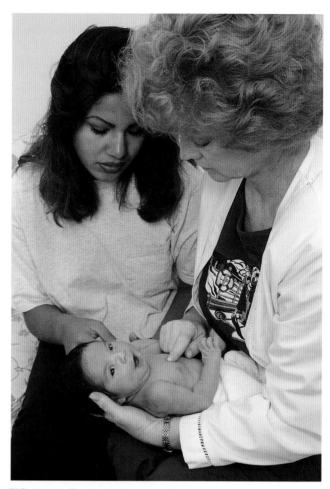

FIG. 22.11 During the home visit, the nurse performs a complete assessment of the infant. Here, the nurse shows how to blanch the skin to check for jaundice and discusses what the parents should do if they see jaundice in the baby.

Home visits provide reassurance for parents and may increase parents' confidence and competence in self and infant care. The visits are especially valuable in recognizing jaundice and intervening before bilirubin levels become dangerously high. When jaundice is found, the nurse can discuss the implications and check the TCB level or draw blood for testing serum bilirubin levels. Appropriate care, including hydration and phototherapy, is discussed, as necessary.

Feeding is an area of concern for many parents, especially when the baby is breastfeeding. When the nurse helps the parents cope with problems, the infant's intake may increase. Increased intake leads to greater bilirubin excretion, which may help avoid the need for phototherapy.

Visits to Families with High-Risk Infants

High-risk infants often need special care after discharge. Parents may be very anxious about assuming the care of an infant who has had a prolonged hospitalization. Many hospitals have programs that enable parents to take over their infant's care gradually before discharge.

A nurse may visit the home before the infant's discharge to help the family plan for accommodating the equipment and the type of care the infant needs. The home is checked for the availability of electricity, heat, and a telephone. If the family has a technology-dependent infant, the nurse verifies they have notified the utility companies and have battery backup to ensure no disruption of services occurs.

After the infant is discharged, nursing visits can help the family maintain the infant's health and decrease the need for rehospitalization. Components of each visit vary according to the infant's needs. The nurse provides assessment of the infant and the parents' caregiving ability in addition to necessary teaching and nursing care.

Medically fragile infants may require home treatment with mechanical ventilation, oxygen therapy, or apnea monitors. Parents may have to perform such nursing skills as tracheostomy care, tube feedings, suctioning, and care of intravenous sites. They often have concerns about feeding the infant, which may differ greatly from feeding a healthy full-term infant. Follow-up telephone calls from nurses between visits help families adapt to the needs of these infants and may also decrease the need for rehospitalization.

Infants with complications often need more frequent visits to the pediatrician or nurse practitioner or are rehospitalized during the early months after birth. Common problems include respiratory illness, infections (gastroenteritis, sepsis, urinary tract infections, otitis media), and need for surgery. These parents need information on preventive measures and care of the infant with an acute illness.

General Considerations in Home Visits

The nurse making a home visit is a guest of the family and should adapt nursing care to the home setting. The needs of other family members should be considered.

Careful planning before the visit is essential. The nurse calls to schedule the visit at a time convenient for the family. Setting priorities based on the needs identified by the nurse and the family is important. Strong communication skills and the ability to quickly develop rapport facilitates accomplishment of mutual goals. A brief social interaction may be beneficial at the beginning of the visit to develop a trusting relationship. The purpose of the visit should be explained and the family's expectations and desires discussed.

The nurse should be aware of any cultural practices affecting the family's view of care. In patriarchal cultures, the father is the head of the family and teaching should be performed through him. In some cultures, one or both grandmothers are important influences in the care.

After the visit, additional visits may be planned or the family may be given a telephone number to call to receive further help, if needed. The results of the assessments, teaching, nursing care, referrals, and plans for follow-up should be recorded. Copies of the record usually are sent to the primary caregiver. If problems are identified that need to be discussed with the primary care provider, a report is made.

Outpatient Visits

Outpatient visits may be provided in a pediatrician's office or in a birth facility clinic. Assessment and care are essentially the same as those provided for home visits. A feeding session is often observed for the lactating client so the nurse is able to assess and provide assistance as needed.

The advantage of outpatient visits is the nurse does not have to travel to the home and can see more clients each day, thereby reducing the cost of the service. Assessment of the home setting and family interaction, however, is not possible. Clinic visits usually last 30 to 45 minutes.

Telephone Counseling

Telephone counseling may be provided during follow-up calls to discharged clients or when parents call "warm lines" for help with problems or questions. The major disadvantage is the nurse cannot perform an in-person assessment of the postpartum client, baby, or home environment and must rely on the caller to present an accurate picture of the situation.

Follow-Up Calls

Follow-up calls are placed by nurses in the first few days after discharge. The nurse asks a series of questions to assess the physical condition of the postpartum client and infant and to identify any needs or problems. All families may receive calls or only those considered at risk for problems. If problems are discovered, the nurse may schedule another call or a home visit or refer the family to the primary care provider.

Warm Lines

Warm lines, also called *help lines* or *information lines*, provide parents with an opportunity to ask a nurse questions arising from the daily challenges of parenting. Warm lines are used for troubling, but not emergency, situations. The service should be available 24 hours a day and should be staffed by qualified nurses. Parents often call about infant feeding, breastfeeding concerns, postpartum blues, and basic care of the postpartum client and infant. Calls last about 15 to 20 minutes. The nurse answers the caller's questions and assesses for other problems. The nurse may call back later to find out if the issue has been resolved.

Telephone Techniques

Nurses caring for clients by telephone should understand telephone counseling techniques. They need special education in telephone communication and triage.

Telephone triage involves determining the existence of and solution to a serious problem. The nurse should be skilled at soliciting information to identify problems and determining the priority of the problems identified.

The nurse should help the caller describe the major concerns, which may not be those discussed first. "What worries you most?" may help the caller focus on the most important problems. Although most problems discussed are concerns about normal infants, the nurse should be alert for "red flags," which signal serious situations needing immediate referral.

The client should be allowed enough time to avoid feeling hurried. Lay terminology should be used and questions asked to elicit detailed description of the problems. Parents should be reassured their questions are valued so they do not feel hesitant to ask what they may see as a "silly" question.

An emergency situation (such as respiratory difficulty, bleeding). Tell the parent to call 9-1-1 or take the infant to a hospital emergency department immediately. Call back in 5 minutes to ensure parents did seek help.

Illness (fever, dehydration, change in feeding or behavior, unusual rashes).

Severe feeding problems (infant may become dehydrated or jaundiced or may fail to thrive).

Problem has been present for longer than usual or usual remedies are ineffective (e.g., prolonged crying or sleeping, rash is spreading).

Parent's affect seems inappropriate for situation (extremely emotional with apparently minor situation or unconcerned when situation could be serious).

Note: Callers should be referred to the primary health care provider or the hospital emergency department, if necessary, when a serious problem may be present. Being overcautious is preferable. Refer parents to the primary care provider early rather than miss a serious situation.

Guidelines and Documentation

When nurses give care by telephone, they should have written protocols and policies that provide guidelines for care to ensure all who perform this service provide clients with similar information. A list of common questions can be compiled to help nurses give appropriate information when parents call about a problem.

Parents should always be told when and how to seek more care if problems are not resolved. If the infant seems ill, referral to the pediatrician or hospital emergency department is most appropriate. The nurse's judgment, based on education, expertise, and experience, determines how helpful the service is to clients.

All calls should be documented so accurate records are available for future reference. The nurse may use a checklist or a simple written description of the call. Documentation should include identifying information for the caller, reason for the call, problems described, advice given, and any referrals given. A copy of the information is sent to the primary caregiver to provide continuity of care.

KNOWLEDGE CHECK

13. Where do parents obtain information about caring for their infant during the early weeks after birth?
14. What are some ways in which nurses offer follow-up services to new parents?

INFANT EQUIPMENT

Generally, parents obtain most of their baby equipment before the infant is born, but nurses may receive questions in the weeks after the birth. Although nurses should not recommend specific brand names of equipment, their guidance about features and safety is helpful.

Safety Considerations

Parents should understand few, if any, pieces of equipment are essential for newborns. Infants sleep in padded dresser drawers and designer cribs with equal comfort. Safety is the most important consideration.

New equipment sold in the United States is generally safe because manufacturers are required to follow certain governmental standards for safety. A ruling by the U.S. Consumer Protection Safety Commission (2010) banned the sale of cribs with a side rail, which drops down. Other changes included in the ruling have made cribs more durable and safer for infants. The U.S. Consumer Product Safety Commission (n.d.) recommends avoiding the use of cribs more than 10 years old.

Safety risks associated with purchasing second-hand or after-market furniture or equipment from individuals or online marketplaces/websites, which may be faulty or recalled, should be discussed with parents. They can check with the Consumer Product Safety Commission (CPSC) for a list of recalled products at https://www.cpsc.gov. Older equipment should be checked carefully to ensure all parts are strong and working properly (Box 22.3). All nuts, screws, bolts, and hooks should be checked periodically to ensure they are tight.

Car Safety Seats

Child safety seats for cars are essential to reduce injury and death to infants and children when accidents occur. An infant carried by an adult while in a car is never safe. Legislation has been passed in all 50 U.S. states requiring restraint of infants and young children in car seats when they are riding in automobiles.

Laws vary with regard to when and at what weight or height an infant or child can move from one type of car seat to another. The current recommendation from the AAP is rear-facing seats be used for infants until they have reached the highest weight or height allowed by the car seat manufacturer, usually about 2 years of age (AAP, 2021c).

Discharge teaching should include information about state car seat laws and the change in the age at which infants can move to a forward-facing seat. Infants should be placed in a rear-facing car seat when they are discharged from the hospital. The seat should recline at approximately a 45-degree angle (Fig. 22.12). Blankets or bolsters placed at the head, along the sides, and between the legs may improve the fit but should be used per manufacturer recommendations or guidelines. Blankets and bolsters should not be placed under the infant.

Car seats should be installed per vehicle and car seat manufacturer instructions (Box 22.4). Helpful information from the AAP is available at https://www.healthychildren.org.

Preterm infants less than 37 weeks old and small infants less than 2500 g may need a special car seat. These infants should have a Car Seat Challenge Test (CSCT) prior to discharge. The parents are asked to bring their car seat to the hospital to test the infant's response to being placed in the seat. During testing, the infant's vital signs and oxygen level are monitored (Jensen, et al., 2018). Infants who have respiratory compromise in car seats may need to use special seats

BOX 22.3 Safety Considerations for Infant Equipment

Cribs

Cribs that meet the current Consumer Protection Safety Commission guidelines should be used for infants.

If parents choose to use an older crib, an immobilizer should be added to prevent drop sides from moving. The crib should be checked frequently to be sure hardware is secured tightly and no loose, missing, or broken parts are present.

The crib mattress should fit snugly with only one finger able to fit into the space between the mattress and the sides of the crib. More room could allow the infant to become wedged in the space and possibly suffocate. The mattress should be firm. The crib should contain no loose bedding, pillows, or stuffed animals because they increase the risk for suffocation. Parents should be cautioned about marketing photos, which may display unsafe practices to attract sales (such as bumper pads or stuffed animals).

Crib toys or mobiles should be firmly attached, with no straps or strings within the infant's reach. Mobiles should be removed when the infant can reach them.

Cribs should be placed away from hanging cords of blinds or drapes, which could become wrapped around an active infant.

Cribs should be placed away from windows.

Other Equipment

Paint used to refurbish infant equipment should be marked "lead-free" and "safe for children's equipment" to prevent lead poisoning.

All parts should function properly: Highchair trays should stay firmly in place, latches should remain fastened, and so on. The frame and basic construction of all equipment should be sturdy.

All moving parts should be examined carefully to see whether little fingers could get caught or whether the infant could trigger a catch, which would cause the equipment to become unsafe.

Safety straps for infant seats, swings, changing tables, high chairs, or other equipment must be in good condition. Straps should fit around the infant but not be long enough for the infant could become entangled.

Automatic swings should have legs that are stable so the swing does not tip over. Note how difficult it is to put the infant into the swing and remove the infant from the swing safely.

All toys should be examined carefully for parts that can be removed and swallowed. Small toys should have a diameter of more than 3.5 cm (1⅜ inches) and be at least 6.35 cm (2½ inches) long to prevent the infant from choking on them.

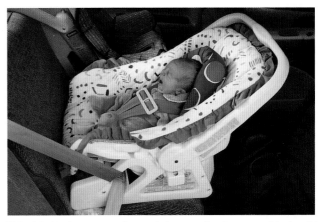

FIG. 22.12 A car seat for an infant under 2 years old should face the rear of the car. Note the clip, which holds the straps together for a snug fit.

BOX 22.4 Safety Considerations for Infant Car Seats

Use only car seats that are approved for use in automobiles. Seats designed for use in the home do not provide adequate protection in a car.

Use car seats that are appropriate for the infant's age and size. Place the seat in the back seat of the car, in the center if possible, and never where an air bag is installed.

Use a rear-facing car seat placed in the back seat until your baby reaches the highest height and weight recommended by the manufacturer, usually about 2 years of age. Never place the baby in the front seat of a car.

Follow the manufacturer's directions for fastening the seat in the car and the infant in the car seat. Recheck the restraint straps each time the seat is used.

To ensure proper fit, place your infant in the seat in their clothing, no heavy or thick jackets, additional bunting, or blanket wraps. If necessary, a coat or blanket can be wrapped around the baby, over the buckled harness strap.

Blankets or bolsters placed at the head, along the sides, and between the legs may improve the fit but should be used per manufacturer recommendations or guidelines.

Be certain the straps are tight enough to prevent the infant from getting out of the restraints or turning over in the seat. Infants who turn over can suffocate in the padding of the seat.

Be certain the infant cannot become caught with the straps tightly around the neck.

Use car seats only in an automobile. Do not place them on a soft surface such as a bed, where they might turn over and suffocate the infant.

Do not place car seats on surfaces from which they might fall, for example, grocery carts.

Never leave infants alone in a car, even for a few minutes. They could be kidnapped or injured in an accident involving the car even though it is parked. Cars quickly become very warm, and the infant could become dangerously overheated. To avoid "forgetting" the infant is in the car, use available cell phone apps or simple reminders, like putting one shoe or your purse in the back seat with the infant.

or beds designed specifically for preterm or low-birth-weight infants.

In many agencies, nurses are not allowed to install car seats for parents. Some agencies have technicians on site who have special training to help parents determine whether car seats are correctly installed. Car seat fitting stations are available in some areas to determine whether car seats are used properly and to provide teaching for parents. A list of such stations is available at https://www.nhtsa.dot.gov/cps/cpsfitting/index.cfm. Further information about proper use of car seats, recall of seats, and a rating system of car seat brands is available on the internet from sources such as the National Transportation Safety Board at https://www.nhtsa.gov.

❓ KNOWLEDGE CHECK

15. What advice can the nurse offer to parents about the safety features of equipment used for infants?
16. What should the nurse teach parents about buying and using a car seat?

EARLY PROBLEMS

Crying

Crying is a major parental concern during the early weeks after birth. Crying increases from birth and peaks at approximately 2 to 3 months of age and may last up to 5 hours a day. It usually decreases by 5 to 6 months (National Center on Shaken Baby Syndrome, n.d.). Babies may also cry more in the late afternoon or evening. Crying is most frustrating to parents when they cannot find the cause for it. Infants cry for many reasons, including hunger, discomfort, fatigue, overstimulation, and boredom. Parents often can identify the problem on the basis of the type of sound made during crying. Sometimes no specific cause can be determined.

When the cause for crying is not obvious, some parents are afraid responding may spoil the infant. If the infant stops crying when picked up, their concern may increase. However, changing the infant's position may help gas move in the intestines, relieve tired muscles, or distract the infant by changing the scenery, bringing about a temporary end of crying.

Infants cannot signal they have unmet needs in any other way but by crying and are not spoiled when parents meet their needs. In fact, their needs should be met in a consistent and prompt manner for the development of trust to occur. Infants who are frequently placed STS have shown increased self-control at 1 year of age and positive long-term outcomes, such as increased education, decreased criminal behaviors or drug addiction, and decreased aggression (Widström et al., 2019). Therefore parents should be taught the importance of consistently and quickly answering infant cries and the use of STS contact for comforting the newborn.

Some families develop creative methods for dealing with crying infants. Others benefit from a nurse's suggestions about appropriate techniques to use.

CLIENT EDUCATION

Techniques to Relieve Crying in Infants

Treating Common Causes

Hunger—Try feeding the infant if it has been more than 30 minutes since the last feeding. A bubble of air may have caused a feeling of fullness too soon during the last feeding. The infant may be experiencing a "growth spurt" and need more frequent feedings for a day or two to provide necessary nutrients for rapid growth. However, avoid overfeeding the baby because that may cause discomfort.

Air bubbles—Fussy infants may need more frequent burping during and after feedings compared with other infants. Try burping during crying spells because the infant may swallow air.

Diapers—Although most infants do not mind wet or soiled diapers, they may become cold or their skin may be irritated when diapers are not changed frequently enough.

Clothing—Check the infant's clothing for anything that could cause discomfort. Look for stiff seams, scratchy tags, or elastic that is too tight.

Warmth—Be sure the infant is warm enough, but not too warm. The abdomen should feel warm even if the hands and feet are slightly cool. Dress a newborn as warmly as an adult would want to be dressed, but add a receiving blanket. Infants who are overdressed rarely perspire but often cry because of their discomfort.

Overstimulation—Too many visitors handling the infant or too much noise and commotion in the household may be overstimulating the infant. Holding the infant in a quiet environment, rocking, or walking with the infant may be helpful.

Quieting Techniques

Rocking—The gentle motion of rocking, reminiscent of intrauterine life, is often soothing for infants.

Automatic swings—The continued motion of automatic swings may be helpful. Be sure they move smoothly and are not noisy. Getting the baby into and out of the swing should be easy to avoid awakening the infant. All parts of the body should be supported. Small infants may need padding with blankets for safety and comfort. Observe the baby throughout the time in the swing.

Walking, jiggling, swaying—Sometimes, newborns prefer a particular style of motion. Rocking sideways with the infant held in an upright position is helpful for some infants, whereas others prefer vertical rocking. Taking a walk outside with new sights and sounds may provide distraction.

Skin-to-skin contact (STS)—Remove the baby's clothes and leave just the diaper. Place the baby against the parent's bare skin and cover both with a blanket. This STS contact is often soothing to a young infant.

Swaddling—Wrap the infant snugly. This is comforting because infants are used to restricted activity in the uterus. Swaddling is especially helpful during the first few weeks after birth.

5Ss Technique—A combination of soothing techniques includes *swaddling* with the infant in the *side* or stomach position, making *shushing* sounds while *swinging* the baby in the arms, and having the baby *suck* on a pacifier has been found to be calming for babies (Rocha et al., 2020).

Stroller rides—The motion of a stroller may be soothing to some infants. The ride can be inside or outside the house. A parent can move a stroller back and forth with one foot while eating meals. The stroller should allow the infant to lie down rather than sit. Padding the stroller may increase comfort.

CLIENT EDUCATION—cont'd

Techniques to Relieve Crying in Infants

Car rides—Some infants go to sleep in a moving car. A short ride may put the infant to sleep. The infant may stay asleep when carried into the house.

Music—The sound of a parent singing or humming may be reassuring to the infant. Some newborns respond well to a music box, radio, or CD. Soft music with a steady beat or classical music may be particularly effective.

White noise—Background noise sometimes puts infants to sleep by diffusing other noises. A radio set on low volume, a clock ticking, an indoor fountain, a fan, or the sound of a dishwasher, dryer, vacuum cleaner, or shower may be effective. Recordings of sounds heard in utero are available.

Heat—A blanket warmed in the clothes dryer for a few minutes held against the infant's skin may be soothing. (Take care not to burn the infant's skin.) Do not use a heating pad. Be sure the infant is well secured and watched at all times.

Bathing—Although older infants love baths, young infants may not yet have reached that stage. However, giving a bath may be a distraction for both parent and infant, and the infant may fall asleep after the bath.

Infant carriers or packs—Front carriers are designed for the young infant and may be especially helpful during crying episodes. A parent's warm body, soothing voice, and gentle swaying motion can often put an infant to sleep. At the same time, the parent can accomplish other tasks. Backpacks should be used only for older infants who are able to support the head well.

Pacifiers—Parents may find pacifiers useful for an irritable infant. The infant may be comforted by sucking even though not hungry.

Position changes—Try varying the infant's position. Laying the infant prone across a parent's lap (or over a warmed blanket) may help expel gas. Placing the infant in the supine position and gently flexing the knees on the abdomen may also help.

Massage—Gentle massage may be soothing for some infants. Massage of the abdomen may help infants with colic.

Taking turns—Ask your partner to take turns comforting the baby. This provides each partner with a chance to rest, and sometimes a different approach is effective.

Colic

Description

Colic is characterized by the "rule of threes" with irritable crying in the late afternoon or evening for no obvious reason for 3 hours or more a day, at least 3 days a week, and lasting at least 3 weeks (Gordon et al., 2019). It occurs in 10% to 20% of infants under 3 months of age. Colic begins at 2 to 3 weeks, peaks at 6 to 8 weeks, and ends at 3 to 4 months of age (Gordon et al., 2019). Some infants continue to have colic until 6 months of age. The infant is in good health, eats well, and gains weight appropriately despite the daily crying episodes. Both breastfed and formula-fed infants have colic.

Infants with colic cry as though in pain, draw their knees onto the abdomen or rigidly extend the legs, and may pass flatus. The crying is intense and may last until the infant falls asleep, exhausted. Because crying causes so much parental distress and may interfere with bonding or be a factor in parenting disorders or child abuse, nurses should find ways to provide support to parents of infants with colic.

Although many theories have been investigated, the cause of colic remains unknown. Allergies to cow's milk or to substances in the breastfeeding mother's diet, abnormal intestinal peristalsis, gastrointestinal tract or nervous system immaturity, feeding techniques such as overfeeding, and parental stress have all been considered. The cause is probably a combination of factors. Actual disease states should be ruled out before a diagnosis of colic can be made.

Interventions

Nursing interventions include using therapeutic communication to help parents express their frustrations and teaching techniques for coping with the problem. Parents should be encouraged to talk about their feelings and should be reassured colic is temporary and does not indicate poor parenting. They often feel inadequate because of their failure to manage the problem and guilty if their frustration develops into anger.

The nurse should explain it is not abnormal to have ambivalent feelings or even anger toward the infant. It is essential to take time away from infant care to rest and recoup energy needed to cope with the demands of a crying infant. Parents should leave the infant with a babysitter for short periods or take turns consoling the infant to provide breaks from the crying.

The techniques listed in "Client Education: Methods to Relieve Crying in Infants" may temporarily alleviate crying caused by colic, but generally no technique gives prolonged relief. Feeding the infant in an upright position and burping frequently may help relieve discomfort caused by swallowed air. Use of the "five S's" technique may be helpful (Daelemans et al., 2018), and administration of *Lactobacillus reuteri* DSM 17938 (a probiotic) has been shown to decrease crying by 50% in breastfed babies (Daelemans et al., 2018). Chamomile tea is often given to infants because it has an antispasmodic effect. Any herbs the parents uses should be checked with the health care provider to ensure they are safe. Simethicone, an antiflatulent, has not been found effective, although some parents have reported it helps (Daelemans et al., 2018).

A quiet environment, a calm approach, and a fairly regular schedule may help some infants with colic. Increasing the time spent carrying the infant often results in some improvement. Parents should be assured that spoiling does not result from responding to the infant's cries.

THERAPEUTIC COMMUNICATIONS
Coping with Crying

Linda tells her nurse, Daniel, about her daughter, Rebecca, who has been having crying spells every day lasting 4 hours or longer. Linda looks tired and worried. Rebecca, age 4 weeks, eats well, shows good weight gain, and is developing appropriately for her age.

Linda: It seems like all I do is try to stop Rebecca's crying. I can't get anything else done.

Daniel: You spend a lot of time trying to find ways to comfort her. *(Paraphrasing to encourage the mother to continue.)*

Linda: I've tried everything! I rock her, walk with her, feed her, and change her. We go for car rides and put her in her swing, but nothing works for long. She just starts crying again.

Daniel: It's so frustrating when nothing seems to work! *(Reflecting mother's feelings shows that the nurse is trying to understand.)*

Linda: Sometimes I wonder if I was cut out to be a mother. I never thought it would be like this.

Daniel: Being a mother is so much harder than you expected that sometimes you aren't sure you made the right choice. *(Reflecting the content of what the mother said helps her focus and shows acceptance.)*

Linda: But I really do love her. I just don't know how to help her. I must be a terrible mother *(becomes teary).*

Daniel: Parents often feel guilty when they can't find a way to help an upset baby. Yet we really don't know all the reasons why babies cry. You've tried very hard to help Rebecca. Maybe we can work together to think of some other techniques to use. *(Gives reassurance that what the mother is feeling is normal, then offers information and further help.)*

Linda: I'd love that. It worries me to have Rebecca so unhappy. What else can I do for her?

One possible result of crying in infants is abusive head trauma (AHT), formerly known as *shaken baby syndrome.* AHT results from blunt trauma or shaking an infant vigorously enough to cause the soft tissue of the brain to bounce against the skull. Subdural or subarachnoid hemorrhage, retinal hemorrhage or detachment, skull and other fractures, and damage to the spinal cord may result. The infant may show little sign of external trauma.

AHT is a leading cause of physical abuse leading to death of children less than 5 years of age in the United States (CDC, 2021b). The highest risk is infants less than 1 year of age. AHT causes death in 25% of babies who are shaken violently. The primary cause of AHT is inconsolable crying in an infant (CDC, 2021b).

Nurses can help prevent AHT by making parents aware of the danger in shaking infants and by helping parents learn methods to cope with infant crying and their own anger, which may result from it. Parents are encouraged to share information about the dangers of AHT with other caregivers.

Birth facilities often include pamphlets and other information on AHT with discharge teaching. Various educational programs have been held in hospitals, middle and high schools, daycare facilities, and other community centers to increase the public awareness of the problem. Further information on AHT may be found at internet sites such as the National Center on Shaken Baby Syndrome at https://www.dontshake.org/.

KNOWLEDGE CHECK

17. Why should parents respond to crying without fear of spoiling the infant?
18. How can nurses help parents of crying infants?

Sleep
Parents
During the early months after birth, parents often wonder whether they will ever get a full night's sleep again. Because they are often up during the night, they should try to make up for lost sleep at other times. If one of the parents is not employed, that parent may be able to sleep during the day when the infant naps. If both parents are working, they can alternate responsibility for night or early morning feedings. When mothers are breastfeeding, fathers can change the diaper, bring the infant to the mother for night feedings, and settle the infant back in bed when the feeding is finished. This allows the mother more time to sleep and lets the father share the middle-of-the-night care.

Infant Sleep Patterns
Although many newborns sleep 16 to 17 hours per day, there is wide variation in the amount of time infants spend sleeping. Infants sleep less deeply than adults and spend 50% of their sleep time in rapid eye movement (REM) sleep (AAP, 2013; AAP, 2021a). During this type of sleep, they sometimes make noises loud enough to wake parents in the same room, and they move about as if awakening. Going to them at this time is likely to wake them, but they may return to quiet sleep if left alone.

Infants should be positioned on the back for sleep. The nurse should explain the prone position has been associated with SIDS. No pillows or soft stuffed animals should be placed in the crib because they could cause suffocation (see Fig. 22.3)

Sleeping through the Night
Parents are often confused about when infants should sleep through the night. Newborns are not ready to sleep through the night during the early weeks of life because of their neurologic immaturity. Pennestri et al. (2018) found 62.4% of parents reported their infants slept at least 6 consecutive hours by 6 months of age. By 12 months of age, 72.1% reported 6 hours or more at a time. Once infants establish longer sleep patterns, they often awaken at night again when they are teething or ill. Therefore, parents can expect to be awakened frequently during the early years. Parents should be taught methods of helping their infants achieve longer sleep periods at night.

CLIENT EDUCATION

How to Help Infants Sleep through the Night

Allow infants to fall asleep at bedtime on their own instead of always rocking or feeding the infant. If rocking is used, place the infant into the bed when the infant is drowsy but not fully asleep. This may help the infant go back to sleep after awakening in the night even when alone.

Allow the infant who wakes during the night to cry for a few minutes before responding. The infant may not be completely awake and often returns to sleep if left undisturbed. However, once the infant is awake, respond quickly to meet the infant's needs.

Keep night feedings for feeding only. Avoid unnecessary activity, or the infant may learn to think of this as a playtime.

Use a soft light that provides only the amount of light essential for care.

Give night feedings in the infant's room to further avoid stimulation.

Keep sounds subdued. Soft music or humming may help the infant return to sleep, but talking should be kept to a minimum.

Keep night feedings short, and put the infant back to bed immediately.

Change diapers before beginning the feeding to avoid awakening the infant after feeding.

As infants near 12 weeks, when longer sleep times are more likely, try patting them on the back instead of feeding.

COMMON QUESTIONS AND CONCERNS

Dressing and Warmth

The infant should be dressed as the parents would like to be dressed, with a receiving blanket added. The abdomen should be checked to see if the infant is warm enough. The infant's hands and feet may be slightly cooler than the rest of the body but should not be mottled or blue. The infant's head should be kept warm because many thermal skin sensors are located in the scalp. A hat is appropriate if the infant is outside when it is cold or windy.

Stool and Voiding Patterns

Formula-fed infants generally pass at least one stool each day. Breastfed infants may pass a stool after every feeding or, occasionally in the older infant, only one stool every 2 to 3 days. Infants may get red in the face and appear to be straining when having a bowel movement, but this is normal behavior and does not indicate constipation. Stools that are dry, hard, and marble-like indicate constipation.

Watery stools indicate diarrhea. A watery stool is absorbed into the diaper with little or no solid material left at the surface. A "water ring" remains on the diaper, showing where the liquid was absorbed. Diarrheal stools occur more frequently compared with the infant's normal stool pattern and are greenish from bile moving quickly through the intestines. Diarrhea can be serious because life-threatening dehydration develops rapidly. Infants should be taken to the pediatrician or nurse practitioner for treatment.

The infant should have at least six wet diapers by the sixth day of life. If there are fewer voidings, feedings should be assessed. The baby should be nursing 8 to 12 times daily, and the formula-fed infant should be fed 6 to 8 times each day.

Smoking

Many parents quit smoking before or during pregnancy but may not realize preventing infant exposure to smoke is just as important after birth as before. Infants exposed to smoke from parents' cigarettes are more likely to develop frequent respiratory tract problems. Parental smoking is a risk factor in SIDS. Smoke absorption by infants occurs even when smoking is done in another room. Parents who continue to smoke should do so outside the house and away from the infant.

Eyes

Parents can remove small amounts of mucus that accumulate in the corners of the eyes with a damp, clean washcloth, using a separate section for each eye. A large amount of mucus, redness, or excessive tearing indicates an infection or a blocked lacrimal duct. The infant should be seen by the pediatrician or nurse practitioner.

Transient **strabismus**—misalignment or deviation of one or both eyes—is sometimes called "crossing" of the eyes. Although the condition is normal for the first 2 to 3 months, it can be frightening to parents. The nurse should reassure them it will end after the first few months, when the infant gains control of the small muscles of the eye. It does not indicate the infant will have later problems.

Baths

Bathing, cord care, and care of the circumcision site are discussed earlier. If the infant is washed well at diaper changes and when milk is regurgitated, bathing the child every day is not necessary. Bathing should be a time for infant stimulation and parent-infant interaction. It can be done at any time of the day that is convenient for parents.

Nails

Nails should be cut straight across with either blunt-ended scissors or clippers. Pressing down on the skin at the fingertip makes it easier to avoid cutting the skin. Nail edges can be carefully smoothed with an emery board. Some parents prefer to cut nails while the infant is sleeping. Others have someone else hold the baby's hand steady while cutting nails. Nails grow rapidly and may need trimming once a week.

Sucking Needs

Parents often have questions about pacifiers and thumb sucking or finger sucking. All infants have an urge to suck, although the amount of sucking needed varies with individual infants. Some infants seem satisfied by feedings, but others suck their fingers or a pacifier even when not hungry. The AAP recommends the use of pacifiers for sleep and to help prevent SIDS. Use may be delayed 3 to 4 weeks until breastfeeding is well established in infants (National Institutes of Health, n.d.).

Parents may be concerned sucking on a pacifier or thumb will cause the teeth to become maloccluded. The nurse should reassure them sucking that is not all day long, or on an upside down pacifier, and ends before the secondary teeth begin to erupt is unlikely to cause malocclusion (Schmid et al., 2018).

In some infants, nonnutritive sucking increases because the time they spend sucking during feedings is too short. Breastfed infants should be allowed to continue sucking at the breast long enough to meet basic sucking needs. A short time of sucking after the end of feeding generally satisfies the infant's sucking needs and increases production of milk. For formula-fed infants, bottle nipples should have small holes and be replaced every couple of months before they get soft.

When infants use a pacifier, parents should be instructed to examine it often to see if it is in good condition. Cracked, torn, or sticky nipples or nipples that can be pulled away from the shield should be discarded. Pacifiers should be replaced every month or two because they may come apart as they deteriorate and cause aspiration of parts. The shield on the pacifier should be large enough that it cannot be pulled into the mouth. Pacifiers should not have any decorations, which might come off and cause a choking hazard.

Pacifiers should be kept clean by frequent washing, and parents should buy several so a clean one is always available when needed. Pacifiers should never be placed on a string around the infant's neck. The string could become tangled tightly around the neck and cause strangulation. Clips with a short band to attach pacifiers to the infant's clothing without danger are available, or several pacifiers can be placed in the bed for the infant to find.

Some parents find one advantage of pacifier use is the infant gives it up more quickly than a thumb or finger because it is not so easily accessible. Parents who resort to the use of a pacifier as the first response when the infant is fussy are likely to reinforce its use and increase dependence on it. Pacifiers used only after other causes of distress are ruled out may be given up sooner by the infant. Because the need for nonnutritive sucking begins to diminish between 4 and 6 months of age, pacifier use may begin to decrease at that time with parents' help.

Common Rashes

Diaper Rash (Diaper Dermatitis)

Diaper rash occurs as a result of prolonged exposure of skin to wetness, urine, feces, and friction against the diaper. A rash is more likely to develop when infants begin to sleep for longer periods and the time between diaper changes increases. Another cause may be sensitivity to commercial disposable wipes or components of paper diapers.

Diaper rash is primarily treated by keeping the diaper area clean and dry. The nurse should instruct the parents to change diapers as soon as they are wet or soiled. They should gently wash the perineum with mild soap and warm water but should avoid excessive washing or scrubbing. If commercial wipes are used, they should be free of alcohol, perfumes, or preservatives. Removing the diapers and exposing the perineum to warm air helps healing.

Applying a thin layer of zinc oxide or petrolatum may speed healing and help prevent recurrence. Vigorous rubbing to remove the skin barrier product is not necessary. Gentle cleansing to remove the soiled layer of barrier in the skin folds is adequate. Low-potency corticosteroid preparations may be necessary for severe cases. Talc-based powders should not be used because they can cause pneumonia if they get into the infant's lungs.

Secondary infection of diaper rash with organisms such as *Candida albicans* or *Staphylococcus* is common. When infection occurs, severe rash, pustules, or crusted areas may appear. The infant should be taken to a pediatrician or nurse practitioner for treatment. Antifungal or antibiotic creams may be necessary for infections.

Miliaria (Prickly Heat)

Although most common during hot weather, **miliaria**, or prickly heat, develops in infants who are too warmly dressed in any weather. It may also occur in infants with a fever. This rash results from occlusion and inflammation of the sweat (eccrine) glands. It has a red base with papules or clear vesicles in the center.

Treatment involves cooling the infant by removing excess clothing or by giving a soothing lukewarm bath. The condition clears quickly with removal of the cause, and ointments or other skin preparations should be avoided. The nurse should discuss the appropriate amount of clothing with parents when infants develop prickly heat.

Seborrheic Dermatitis (Cradle Cap)

Seborrheic dermatitis is a chronic inflammation of the scalp or other areas of the skin characterized by yellow, scaly, oily lesions. It sometimes results when parents do not wash the anterior fontanel for fear they will hurt the infant.

Treatment is application of oil or shampoo to the area to help the lesions soften and then removal with a comb or soft brush before shampooing the head. The nurse should teach parents how to shampoo the scalp and explain they will not injure the fontanel by normal gentle shampooing. The scalp should be rinsed well to remove all soap, which otherwise may cause irritation. A persistent problem may be treated with hydrocortisone cream or special shampoos recommended by the pediatrician or nurse practitioner.

Feeding Concerns

Breastfeeding, formula feeding, and weaning are discussed in Chapter 23. This section addresses only regurgitation and introduction of solid foods.

Regurgitation

Infants often regurgitate ("spit up") because they may eat more than the stomach can easily hold and because the immature lower esophageal sphincter allows the stomach contents to flow into the esophagus easily. "Wet burps" result when air is trapped under the stomach contents. As the air is expelled, a small amount of milk comes with it.

The nurse should teach parents to differentiate normal spitting up from vomiting, which is a sign of illness. Regurgitation may occur frequently but is usually only a small amount at a time. Vomiting may involve the entire feeding, and it is expelled forcefully. Parents should always seek treatment for the infant with projectile vomiting, in which the vomitus is expelled with such force it travels some distance.

If an infant has frequent regurgitation, place the infant in a more upright position during and for a short time after feedings. Small, more frequent feedings also may help. Some infants swallow excessive air because they feed rapidly. Nurses can instruct parents to feed infants before they get too hungry and to stop often for burping. If the hole in a bottle nipple is too small, an infant may swallow the air around the nipple. Enlarging the nipple hole slightly with a hot needle may prevent this. The hole should not be too big or the flow of milk may be too fast and cause choking.

The infant who has excessive regurgitation or vomiting should be referred for follow-up with the pediatrician or nurse practitioner.

Introduction of Solid Foods

Infants do not need solid foods until 6 months of age. It is recommended infants should have only breast milk for the first 6 months (AAP, 2021b). Some parents introduce solids earlier in the hope the infant will sleep longer at night. This is seldom successful because the infant receives no more calories from the small amounts of solids taken than from breast milk or formula. When infants are started on solids, they drink less milk, thus replacing a food that meets their nutrient needs well with a food that is poorly digested.

The **extrusion reflex**, in which infants push the tongue out against anything that touches it, continues until approximately 4 to 6 months of age (Duryea & Fleischer, 2021). This makes feeding a younger infant difficult because the infant pushes almost all of every spoonful out of the mouth. The nurse should explain the problems involved with early introduction of solid foods and encourage parents to wait until the infant is physiologically ready, at 6 months of age. The concerns that made the parents consider changing the feeding routine should also be discussed.

> ### ❓ KNOWLEDGE CHECK
>
> 19. How can parents prevent or treat diaper rash?
> 20. When should infants begin solid foods?
> 21. How can a parent differentiate between regurgitation and vomiting?

Growth and Development
Anticipatory Guidance

Parents often have questions about normal patterns of growth and stages of development. Nurses provide anticipatory guidance about these areas to help parents develop realistic expectations about infants' abilities at various ages.

Growth and Developmental Milestones

A brief summary of the changes which can be expected during the infant's first 12 weeks is included here. More in-depth information is found in pediatrics textbooks. The nurse should emphasize to parents guidelines are only averages, the range of normal is often broad, and individual differences are expected.

Growth proceeds at a predictable rate in normal infants, and steady increases are reassuring. The weight lost after birth is usually regained by 14 days of age. In the first 3 months, the average infant gains approximately 1 oz (30 g) each day and 2 lb (0.9 kg) per month.

The anterior fontanel closes by 18 to 24 months of age; the posterior fontanel closes by 2 months of age (Tappero, 2021). The lacrimal glands begin producing tears about 2 weeks of life, so tears are scant or absent until about 1 to 3 months of age (Gill, 2020).

Parents are especially interested in the Moro, grasp, and rooting reflexes. The nurse should point out their gradual disappearance helps prepare the infant to learn new skills such as voluntary grasping or turning over, which are impossible if the reflexes continue. The infant gradually develops more control of the heavy head and has less bobbing or head lag by the end of the third month.

Infants are social beings. They stare at objects of interest and focus best within a range of 8 to 10 inches as newborns (American Optometric Association [AOA], n.d.). By 8 weeks, infants can focus on a face of a person and at 3 months follow objects with their eyes (AOA, n.d.). A social smile begins, they turn their head in response to voice, and they begin to making "cooing" sounds at 2 months (CDC, 2021a). Infants can support their head independently by 4 months and reach for a toy with one hand. At 6 months, they can sit unsupported and begin to walk by 1 year (CDC, 2021a).

Accident Prevention

Knowing what infants can do helps prevent accidents. In the first 3 months after birth, they are totally helpless. Although they can communicate their needs through crying, someone must be available at all times to care for them. Parents should be taught the dangers of leaving the infant on any unprotected surface, even for seconds. In a short time, an infant can wiggle from the middle to the edge of a large bed and fall.

If parents must turn away, they should keep one hand on an infant lying on an unprotected surface. Infants should never be left, even for an instant, in even 1 inch of water because of the danger of drowning. Parents should turn the telephone off or take it with them and ignore the doorbell while bathing the infant. If they must leave the room, parents should take the infant out of the water and with them.

As infants learn to grasp objects with increasing accuracy (4 months), parents should be certain nothing that could be swallowed or otherwise cause harm is within the infant's reach. Help parents think ahead to the time when the infant will be crawling and walking and make plans for how they will "child-proof" their home.

Well-Baby Care
Well-Baby Checkups

Well-baby checkups are an opportunity for the pediatrician or nurse practitioner to assess the infant's growth and development, answer questions about feeding and infant care, observe for abnormalities, and give immunizations. These checkups may be provided by a private practitioner or in a well-baby clinic where examinations and immunizations are free or at reduced cost. Infants are usually taken to their first checkup between 48 hours and 2 weeks after discharge from the birth facility. The first year of life, they generally receive well-baby checkups at 1, 2, 4, 6, 9, and 12 months of age (AAP, 2021d). Anticipatory guidance is a major part of well-baby visits. Safety is discussed as parents are taught about skills infants will soon develop that might place them in danger.

Immunizations

Nurses often receive questions about the need for immunizations for uncommon diseases, such as diphtheria, which parents have never seen. Parents may consider a condition such as varicella (chickenpox) to be a harmless childhood illness. When they do not understand the need for immunizations, parents may be reluctant to have their infants undergo painful procedures.

The nurse should explain to parents the importance of immunizations, briefly describing the serious illnesses that are prevented by immunizations. Discuss the age at which each immunization is given and when boosters are needed. Because recommendations for immunizations change from time to time, parents should be referred to their pediatrician for the latest information. Parents may go to the https://www.cdc.gov or https://www.aap.org as sources offering information for parents as well as professionals.

In the United States, national health objectives for the year 2030 include maintaining or reducing the number of unvaccinated children under 2 years of age (ODPHP, 2020). Maintaining a high level of immunization is important to prevent the rise of communicable diseases, as has happened in the past when a resurgence of measles occurred in many U.S. communities.

KNOWLEDGE CHECK

22. How can parents use their knowledge about infant development to prevent accidents in the first 12 weeks of life?
23. What is the purpose of well-baby checkups?
24. Why are immunizations important?

Illness

Parents have many questions about illnesses in the infants. They have concerns about how to recognize an illness and when to call the pediatrician or nurse practitioner.

Recognizing Signs

Parents may need help in recognizing signs of illness in infants (Box 22.5). The nurse should explain any time the infant appears sick or parents think something is wrong with the infant, they should call the pediatrician or nurse practitioner. Office staff is usually educated to help parents determine whether the infant is sick enough to need an appointment.

Calling the Pediatrician or Nurse Practitioner

When calling the health care provider about an illness, parents should prepare by writing down the information about the illness to avoid forgetting something. They should have the name and telephone number of a pharmacy available in case a prescription drug is needed, and they should be ready to write down instructions (Box 22.6).

Office staff members are usually able to answer questions on the telephone about common concerns and simple illnesses. They can help determine whether an infant should be seen by the health care provider, but parents should be assertive in asking for an appointment if they believe one is needed. Parents should immediately identify emergencies so the staff can act accordingly.

BOX 22.5   Common Signs of Illness in Infants

Axillary temperature above 38°C (100.4°F)
Vomiting all of a feeding more than once or twice in a day
Watery stools or significant increase in number of stools over what is normal for the infant
Blisters, sores, or rashes which are unusual for the infant
Unusual changes in behavior: listlessness or sleeping much more than usual, irritability, or crying much more than usual
Coughing, frequent sneezing, runny nose (occasional sneezing is not a problem)
Pulling or rubbing at the ear, drainage from the ear

BOX 22.6   Calling the Pediatrician or Nurse Practitioner

Write down pertinent information before calling. Have your pharmacy name and telephone number handy, along with a pen and paper to write down instructions.

1. Give the infant's name and age first.
2. Describe the illness or problem.
   a. When did it start?
   b. How often does it occur (e.g., the number of times the infant vomits or passes stool)?
   c. How does this compare with the infant's normal patterns?
   d. What does it look like (e.g., appearance of rash, color and consistency of stools)?
3. Describe any fever.
   a. How high is it? (Take the axillary temperature.)
   b. How long has the fever been present?
   c. Has it been higher than it is now?
4. Describe other signs of illness.
   a. Has eating behavior changed?
   b. Have sleep patterns changed?
5. Describe the infant's behavior.
   a. Does the infant seem sick? How?
   b. Is the infant irritable, lethargic, acting differently from normal? How?
6. Describe what has been done so far to treat the condition (e.g., medicines, herbs) and the results.
7. Discuss other relevant information.
   a. Is there a similar illness in family members?
   b. Was the infant treated recently for a similar or different illness?
   c. Is the infant given any other medications?

Knowing When to Seek Immediate Help

Parents should take the infant to the pediatrician or to a hospital if signs of dyspnea are present. An infant from birth to 3 months of age should not have a sustained respiratory rate above 60 breaths per minute. If retractions, cyanosis, or extreme pallor is present, parents should get immediate help. If respiratory difficulty occurs suddenly in an infant who is well, the infant may have aspirated a feeding or small object. Parents should call the emergency medical services (EMS). Nurses should encourage all parents to take classes in cardiopulmonary resuscitation.

If an infant's respiratory rate is below 30 breaths per minute, parents should stimulate the infant and see if the respirations increase and stay within the normal range of 30 to 60 breaths per minute. If the respiratory rate continues to be below normal, the infant should be seen by a pediatrician, by a nurse practitioner, or at a hospital.

Parents should call the pediatrician if the infant is hard to arouse and keep awake. The infant could be semicomatose and showing signs of a central nervous system disease such as meningitis or encephalitis.

Learning about Sudden Infant Death Syndrome

SIDS is the abrupt death of an infant younger than 1 year of age that is unexplained by history, autopsy, or examination of the scene of death. SIDS, unknown causes, and accidental suffocation/strangulation while in bed are all grouped under the larger category of sudden unexpected infant deaths (SUID) (CDC, 2021c). In the United States, approximately 3500 to 3600 infants die of SUID each year. In 2018, 1300 infants died of SIDS (CDC, 2021c).

SIDS occurs in apparently healthy infants during sleep and more often in male infants. It peaks in infants who are 1 to 4 months of age, and 90% of SIDS cases occur before 6 months of age (Pacheco, 2021). Non-Hispanic Black and American Indian/Alaska Native infants are at an increased risk for SUID (CDC, 2021c).

There have been many studies, but the cause of SIDS remains unknown. Sleeping in the prone position; sleeping on a soft surface; overheating; maternal smoking or drug use during or after pregnancy; young maternal age; low socioeconomic status; late or no prenatal care; prematurity, low birth weight, and male gender; and prenatal exposure to nicotine, alcohol, and illicit drugs have been associated with SIDS. Risk for SIDS is increased when infants sleep in the same bed with another person; on adult beds or sofas; or with pillows, stuffed toys, or loose bedding; or become overheated during sleep. Bed-sharing with a parent is controversial and not recommended at this time (CDC, 2021c).

The current recommendation is a healthy infant be placed in the supine position for sleep because the prone position may increase the risk for upper airway obstruction, rebreathing of expired air, and hyperthermia (AAP Task Force on Sudden Infant Death Syndrome, 2016; CDC, 2021c) A national goal for the year 2030 is to reduce the number of SIDS deaths by increasing the number of infants who are put to sleep on their backs to at least 88.9% (ODPHP, 2020).

Approximately 20% of SIDS cases occur when the caregiver is not the parent (ChildCare Education Institute, 2018). Parents should ensure all caregivers of their child are aware of the risk associated with the prone position and follow the guidelines.

Nurses should teach parents about the AAP recommendations for the supine position for sleep and give parents educational material about the position. It is important for nurses to model this behavior in addition to teaching about it. For suggestions on modifying some risk factors, see the CDC website: https://www.cdc.gov/sids/Parents-Caregivers.htm.

CLIENT EDUCATION

How to Help Prevent Sudden Infant Death Syndrome

The following are suggestions that may help prevent sudden infant death syndrome (SIDS):

Always place the baby on his or her back for sleep, whether for naps or at night. Never allow the infant to be placed on the abdomen or side for sleep.

Ensure all other caregivers (babysitters, daycare workers, relatives) position the baby on the back for sleep.

The infant's sleep surface should be firm. Do not put the baby to sleep on a couch, armchair, soft mattress, or waterbed.

Do not let the baby sleep with any other person, whether an adult or a child.

If you feed your infant while you are in bed, put the baby back into the infant's bed when you are ready to sleep.

The infant's bed should be placed in the parent's room until at least 6 to 12 months of age.

Do not put any loose bedding, comforters, quilts, pillows, bumper pads, sheepskins, positioning devices, stuffed toys, or any soft items in the baby's bed.

Dress the baby in pajamas, sleepers, or a sleep sack instead of using blankets.

If blankets are used, place them no higher than the baby's waist and tuck the edges under the mattress to prevent blankets from covering the infant's face.

Do not let the infant get overheated. Dress the baby appropriately.

Consider giving the baby a pacifier for sleep. If you are breastfeeding, wait until the baby is 1 month old and breastfeeding is well established before giving the pacifier for sleep, if you wish. If the pacifier falls out during sleep, it is not necessary to reinsert it.

Do not smoke during or after birth or let anyone smoke around your baby.

Avoid alcohol and illicit drug use during pregnancy or after birth.

If possible, breastfeed your baby, because breastfeeding has been found to protect infants from SIDS.

To prevent flattening of the head, several times each day place your baby on his or her abdomen for "tummy time" when the baby is awake and you can watch the baby. This also helps develop the muscles of the baby's upper body.

Do not let infants sleep routinely in sitting devices such as car seats, strollers, and swings because infants may slump enough to obstruct the airway.

Parents may be concerned about abnormalities in head shape, which may occur in some infants from sleeping on the back. Flattening of the head may result from prolonged lying in the supine position. This can be prevented by the parents placing the infant in the prone position on a firm surface during awake periods several times a day while watching the infant.

Parents should be taught the importance of "tummy time" to help develop the shoulder muscles as well as prevent plagiocephaly. The prone position helps the infant develop neck, shoulder, and arm muscles. Toys placed within reach can help infants focus and begin to reach for objects. The position also helps the infant attain developmental milestones such as rolling over and crawling.

Infants tend to look toward the center of the room or the door when in their beds. Placing the infant at alternating ends of the crib often influences the direction of turning the head and distributes pressure more evenly. Avoiding prolonged time in car seats or other seats and holding the baby in an upright position some of the time may also help. Infants who develop flattening of the head should spend very little time in infant seats, swings, or car seats because these put pressure on the back of the head.

Because parents often have many concerns about SIDS, therapeutic communication techniques may assist them to talk about their fears. They may need reassurance the chance of any one infant will experience SIDS is small. When parents have experienced loss of an infant from SIDS, they need appropriate counseling. One organization which provides this is First Candle, https://www.firstcandle.org.

? KNOWLEDGE CHECK

25. When should immediate help be sought for an infant?
26. What should nurses teach parents about SIDS?

SUMMARY CONCEPTS

- Prophylaxis against vitamin K–deficiency bleeding (hemorrhagic disease of the newborn) and ophthalmia neonatorum is necessary shortly after birth. It is provided by an injection of vitamin K and use of erythromycin ophthalmic ointment.
- Newborns may need help with clearing the airway. Positioning, wiping secretions from the nose and mouth or suctioning, and close observation may be necessary.
- Nurses can prevent heat loss in newborns by keeping them dry and covered, avoiding contact between newborns and cold objects or surfaces, and keeping newborns away from drafts and exterior windows and walls.
- The nurse should identify actual or potential hypoglycemia and intervene appropriately.
- Important interventions for jaundice are to assess for its presence, ensure the infant is feeding well, and explain the condition to the parents.
- Parents should be taught to place infants supine for sleep to prevent sudden infant death syndrome. Infants should have supervised periods of lying prone while awake each day.
- The nurse should prevent mistaken identification of infants by checking the parents' and infant's identification whenever they have been separated.
- Parents and nurses should work together to prevent infant abductions. Parents should know how to identify hospital staff. Nurses should be alert for suspicious behavior.
- Infection can be best prevented by scrupulous handwashing by staff and all who come in contact with newborns.
- Reasons parents may choose circumcision include decreased risk of certain conditions, religious reasons, parental preference, or lack of knowledge about care of the foreskin.
- Parents reject circumcision because of a belief that uncommon conditions do not necessitate surgery and pain in infants and concerns about the complications that can occur.
- Risks of circumcision include hemorrhage, infection, unsatisfactory cosmetic effect, urinary retention, urethral stenosis or fistulas, adhesions, necrosis, injury to the glans, and pain during and after surgery.
- Infants who are circumcised should have pain relief provided. Dorsal penile nerve block along with nonpharmacologic methods of pain relief such as oral sucrose is often used.
- Parents of uncircumcised infants should be taught not to retract the foreskin until it becomes separated from the glans later in childhood.
- Parents of circumcised infants should be taught signs of complications and how to care for the area.
- Every nursing contact with parents should be used as an opportunity to teach.
- Screening tests are commonly performed to rule out cardiac and hearing abnormalities, phenylketonuria, hypothyroidism, galactosemia, congenital adrenal hyperplasia, and hemoglobinopathies.
- Nurses assist parents after discharge by way of home or clinic visits and telephone calls.
- Careful planning, good communication skills, and knowledge of cultural practices are necessary during home visits.
- Outpatient visits include the same assessment and teaching as home visits but do not allow the nurse to assess the home. They are, however, more cost-effective.
- Telephone calls after discharge from the birth facility are less expensive than home or clinic visits but do not allow the nurse to assess the client or home environment in person.
- All equipment, particularly older, used articles, should be checked by parents for safety.
- Infants should use a rear-facing car seat until they have reached the greatest weight and height recommended by the manufacturer, usually about 2 years of age. Older children need car seats that face forward. All should be placed in the back seat of the car.
- Crying is a major source of concern for parents. They should be reassured infants are not spoiled by prompt attention to their needs.

- Colic—crying without obvious cause which lasts 3 or more hours a day—usually occurs in the afternoon or evening and often disappears after 3 to 4 months. The cause is unknown, and infants with colic grow and develop normally.
- The nurse can help prevent abusive head trauma (shaken baby syndrome) by teaching parents not to shake their baby and helping them cope with crying.
- Diaper rash may be caused by prolonged exposure to wet and soiled diapers or sensitivity to substances in diapers or disposable wipes. The rash can become infected.
- Solid foods should be started at 6 months of age when the extrusion reflex is gone and solids can be digested by infants.

- Well-baby checkups are important for assessment of growth and development and to provide guidance and immunizations. Immunizations safeguard infants and communities from spread of communicable diseases.
- Parents should learn signs of illness in the infant and when immediate medical care is necessary. They should seek immediate medical attention if infants have respiratory difficulty or are difficult to arouse from sleep.
- The nurse should teach parents about current knowledge about SIDS and that the cause remains unknown. Parents should be taught to safe sleep practices for their newborn.

Clinical Judgment and Next-Generation NCLEX® Examination-Style Questions

1. **Choose the most likely options for the information missing from the statement below by selecting from the lists of options provided.** A term newborn is rapidly born by spontaneous vaginal delivery and placed directly on the mother's abdomen. This practice is known as _____1_____. This intervention benefits the newborn by promoting: _____2_____, _____3_____, and _____4_____.

Options for 1	Options for 2, 3, and 4
Bonding	Temperature regulation
Skin-to-skin contact	Iron stores
En face position	Blood glucose regulation
Engrossment	Breastfeeding
	Sensory development
	Meconium passage

2. A 19-year-old G1P1 and newborn are being admitted to the mother-baby unit 2 hours after birth. The pregnancy complicated only by a breech presentation. The 7 lb, 14 oz female was born via cesarean due to breech presentation with epidural anesthesia at 39^2 weeks of gestation and has transitioned without complications. Apgar scores were 9 and 9. She was put to breast following birth, latched on with assistance, and nursed well.

Assessment:
Heart rate: 150 beats/minute
Respiratory rate: 38 breaths/minute, bilateral breath sounds (BBS) equal with slight crackles
Temperature: 36.3°C (97.4°F) axiallary (Ax)
Color: pink with blue hands and feet
Activity: sleeping
Muscle tone: flexed
Which of the following are appropriate nursing actions to address the priority problem? Choose all that apply (CATA)
A. Place the newborn skin-to-skin with a parent
B. Provide oxygen
C. Notify the provider
D. Suction the baby for residual lung fluid
E. Place the newborn on a preheated radiant warmer in the mother's room

F. Position the baby in a head down position
G. Take the baby to the observation nursery or NICU for closer monitoring
H. Notify the lactation consultant for assistance with latch on

3. **Choose the most likely options for the information missing from the statement below by selecting from the lists of options provided.** Following admission assessments of both clients, the nurse provides critical parent teaching for infant safety. Parent teaching to decrease the risk of infant abduction includes ___1___, ___2___, and ___3___. Promotion of newborn thermal regulation includes teaching the parents ___4___, ___5___, and ___6___. ___7___ and ___8___ are included in parent teaching to decrease the risk of newborn airway obstruction.

Options for 1, 2, 3	Options for 4, 5, 6	Options for 7, 8
Matching ID bands are required for staff to give the newborn to an adult.	Change the baby's clothing or linens if they become wet.	Position the baby on the stomach after feeding
Facility staff may need to remove the baby from the room, but they do not need to take the bassinet every time.	Swaddle the baby or place in a sleeping sac when the baby is not skin-to-skin with the parent.	If the baby spits up, turn to the side, wipe the face and mouth with a clean cloth, and suction gently with the bulb syringe if needed.
Place the baby's bassinet away from the door to the room, preferably on the opposite side of the client's bed.	The baby only needs to wear the cap if the baby gets cold.	When using the bulb syringe, suction the mouth first, then the nose.
As long as the door to the room is closed, it's OK to leave the sleeping baby in the bassinet in the room while the client showers, even if there is no one else there.	Skin-to-skin contact is only used when the baby is cold and needs to be rewarmed.	
Do not allow anyone without the appropriate picture ID to take the baby out of the room.	Safe skin-to-skin positioning requires that the baby's face is visible and the nose and mouth are uncovered.	

4. Three days later, the nurse is providing discharge instructions. **The parents are taught to notify the provider for which of the following? CATA**
   A. Temperature greater than 100.4°F (axillary) or less than 97.7°F (axillary)
   B. Spitting up after feedings
   C. Two or more green or watery stools
   D. Six to eight wet diapers per day
   E. Sleeping for more than 6 hours without waking
   F. Drops of blood when umbilical cord falls off
   G. Redness or yellowish drainage from the umbilical cord
   H. Yellow tinge to skin or eyes

REFERENCES

American Academy of Pediatrics. (2013). *Stages of newborn sleep.* https://www.healthychildren.org/English/ages-stages/baby/sleep/Pages/default.aspx.

American Academy of Pediatrics. (2017). *Care for an uncircumcised penis.* https://www.healthychildren.org/English/ages-stages/baby/bathing-skin-care/Pages/Care-for-an-Uncircumcised-Penis.aspx.

American Academy of Pediatrics. (2020). *Umbilical cord care.* https://www.healthychildren.org/English/ages-stages/baby/bathing-skin-care/Pages/Umbilical-Cord-Care.aspx.

American Academy of Pediatrics. (2021a). *Sleep.* https://www.healthychildren.org/English/ages-stages/baby/sleep/Pages/default.aspx.

American Academy of Pediatrics. (2021b). *Infant food and feeding.* https://www.aap.org/en/patient-care-pages-in-progress/healthy-active-living-for-families/infant-food-and-feeding/.

American Academy of Pediatrics. (2021c). *Car seats: Information for families.* https://www.healthychildren.org/English/safety-prevention/on-the-go/Pages/Car-Safety-Seats-Information-for-Families.aspx.

American Academy of Pediatrics. (2021d). *AAP schedule of well child visits.* https://www.healthychildren.org/English/family-life/health-management/Pages/Well-Child-Care-A-Check-Up-for-Success.aspx.

American Academy of Pediatrics Section on Cardiology and Cardiac Surgery Executive Committee, Mahle, W. T., Martin, G. R., Beekman, R. H., Morrow, W. R., Rosenthal, G. L., Synder, C. S., Minich, L. L., Mital, S., Towbin, J. A., & Tweddell, J. S. (2012). Endorsement of health and human services recommendation for pulse oximetry screening for critical congenital heart disease. *Pediatrics, 129*(1), 190–192. https://doi.org/10.1542/peds.2011-3211.

American Academy of Pediatrics (AAP) Task Force on Circumcision. (2012a). Circumcision policy statement. *Pediatrics, 130*(3), 585–586. https://doi.org/10.1542/peds.2012-1989.

American Academy of Pediatrics (AAP) Task Force on Circumcision. (2012b). Male circumcision. *Pediatrics, 130*(3), e756–e785. https://doi.org/10.1542/peds.2012-1990.

American Academy of Pediatrics Task Force on Sudden Infant Death Syndrome. (2016). SIDS and other sleep-related infant deaths: Updated 2016 recommendations for a safe infant sleeping environment. *Pediatrics, 138*(5), e20162938. https://doi.org/10.1542/peds.2016-2938.

American Academy of Pediatrics & American College of Obstetricians and Gynecologists (AAP & ACOG). (2017). *Guidelines for perinatal care* (8th ed.).

American Optometric Association. (n.d.). Infant vision: Birth to 24 months of age. https://www.aoa.org/healthy-eyes/eye-health-for-life/infant-vision?sso=y.

Association of Women's Health, Obstetric and Neonatal Nurses (AWHONN). (2018). *Evidence-based clinical practice guideline: Neonatal skin care* (4th ed.).

Aziz, K., Lee, H. C., Escobedo, M. B., Hoover, A. V., Kamath-Rayne, B. D., Kapadia, V. S., Magid, D. J., Niermeyer, S., Schmolzer, G. M., Szyld, E., Weiner, G. M., Wyckoff, M. H., Yamada, N. K., & Zaichkin, J. (2020). Part 5: Neonatal resuscitation 2020 American Heart Association guidelines for cardiopulmonary resuscitation and emergency cardiovascular care. *Pediatrics, 147*(Suppl. 1), e2020038505E. https://doi.org/10.1542/peds.2020-038505E.

Bell, A. J., Arku, Z., Bakari, A., Oppong, S. A., Youngblood, J., Adanu, R. M., & Moyer, C. A. (2020). 'This sickness is not hospital sickness': A qualitative study of the evil eye as a source of neonatal illness in Ghana. *Journal of Biosocial Science, 52*(2), 159–167. https://doi.org/10.1017/S0021932019000312.

Centers for Disease Control and Prevention (CDC). (2019). *Vitamin K.* https://www.cdc.gov/breastfeeding/breastfeeding-special-circumstances/diet-and-micronutrients/vitamin-k.html.

Centers for Disease Control. (2020). *Congenital heart defects information for healthcare providers.* https://www.cdc.gov/ncbddd/heartdefects/hcp.html.

Centers for Disease Control and Prevention. (2021a). *Milestones.* https://www.cdc.gov/ncbddd/actearly/milestones/index.html.

Centers for Disease Control and Prevention. (2021b). *Preventing abusive head trauma.* https://www.cdc.gov/violenceprevention/childabuseandneglect/Abusive-Head-Trauma.html.

Centers for Disease Control and Prevention. (2021c). *Sudden unexpected infant death and sudden infant death syndrome.* https://www.cdc.gov/sids/data.htm.

Centers for Disease Control and Prevention. (2021d). *Hepatitis B.* https://www.cdc.gov/vaccines/pubs/pinkbook/hepb.html.

Chamberlain, J., McCarty, S., Sorce, J., Leesman, B., Schmidt, S., Meyrick, E., Parlier, S., Kennedy, L., Crowley, D., & Coultas, L. (2019). Impact on delayed newborn bathing on exclusive breastfeeding rates, glucose and temperature stability, and weight loss. *Journal of Neonatal Nursing, 25*(2), 74–77. https://doi.org/10.1016/j.jnn.2018.11.001.

ChildCare Education Institute. (2018). New course from ChildCare Education Institute on protecting infants: Reducing the risk of SIDS and shaken baby syndrome. *ChildCare Education Institute.* https://www.globenewswire.com/news-release/2018/06/12/1520046/0/en/New-Course-from-ChildCare-Education-Institute-on-Protecting-Infants-Reducing-the-Risk-of-SIDS-and-Shaken-Baby-Syndrome.html.

Daelemans, S., Peeters, L., Hauser, B., & Vandenplas, Y. (2018). Recent advances in understanding and managing infantile colic. *F1000Research, 7*(F1000 Faculty Rev), 1426. https://doi.org/10.12688/f1000research.14940.1.

DiCioccio, H. C., Ady, C., Bena, J. F., & Albert, N. M. (2019). Initiative to improve exclusive breastfeeding by delaying the newborn bath. *JOGNN, 48*(2), 189–196. https://doi.org/10.1016/j.jogn.2018.12.008.

Duryea, T. K., & Fleischer, D. M. (2021). Patient education: Starting solid foods during infancy (Beyond the basics). *UpToDate.* https://www.uptodate.com/contents/starting-solid-foods-during-infancy-beyond-the-basics.

Gardner, S. L., & Cammack, B. H. (2021). Heat balance. In S. L. Gardner, B. S. Carter, M. Enzman-Hines, & S. Niermeyer (Eds.), *Merenstein & Gardner's handbook of neonatal intensive care* (9th ed., pp. 137–164). Elsevier.

Gill, K. (2020). *When do babies start crying tears? Healthline parenthood.* https://www.healthline.com/health/baby/when-do-babies-get-tears.

Gordon, M., Gohil, J., & Banks, S. S. (2019). Parent training programmes for managing infantile colic. *Cochrane Database of Systematic Reviews, 12*(12), CD012459. https://doi.org/10.1002/14651858.CD012459.pub2.

Health Resources & Services Administration. (2021). *Newborn screening process: When does newborn screening happen?* https://newbornscreening.hrsa.gov/newborn-screening-process.

Jensen, E. A., Foglia, E. E., Dysart, K. C., Aghai, Z. H., Cook, A., Greenspan, J. S., & DeMauro, S. B. (2018). Car seat tolerance screening in the Neonatal Intensive Care Unit: Failure rates, risk factors, and adverse outcomes. *The Journal of Pediatrics, 194*, 60–66.e1. https://doi.org/10.1016/j.jpeds.2017.11.010.

Kemper, A. R., Mahle, W. T., Martin, G. R., Cooley, W. C., Kumar, P., Morrow, W. R., Kelm, K., Pearson, G. D., Glidewell, J., Grosse, S. D., & Howell, R. R. (2011). Strategies for implementing screening for critical congenital heart disease. *Pediatrics, 128*(5), e1–e8. https://doi.org/10.1542/peds.2011-1317.

Kumar, N., Akangire, G., Sullivan, B., Fairchild, K., & Sampath, V. (2020). Continuous vital sign analysis for predicting and preventing neonatal diseases in the twenty-first century: Big data on the forefront. *Pediatric Resuscitation, 87*(2), 210–220. https://doi.org/10.1038/s41390-019-0527-0.

Lawrence, J., Alcock, D., McGrath, P., Kay, J., MacMurray, S. B., & Dulberg, C. (1993). The development of a tool to assess neonatal pain. *Neonatal Network, 14*(5), 59–62.

Lynn, P. (2019). *Skill 2-2: Regulating temperature using an overhead radiant warmer. Taylor's clinical nursing skills: A nursing process approach* (5th ed., pp. 131–135). Wolters Kluwer.

Mardini, J., Rahme, C., Matar, O., Khalil, S. A., Hallit, S., & Khalife, M. F. (2020). Newborn's first bath: Any preferred timing? A pilot study from Lebanon. *BMC Res Notes, 13*, 430. https://doi.org/10.1186/s13104-020-05282-0.

Moon, R. Y. (2021). How to keep your sleeping baby safe: AAP policy explained. *American Academy of Pediatrics.* https://www.healthychildren.org/English/ages-stages/baby/sleep/Pages/A-Parents-Guide-to-Safe-Sleep.aspx.

Morris, B. J., Wamai, R. G., Henebeng, E. B., Tobian, A. A., Klausner, J. D., Banerjee, J., & Hankins, C. A. (2016). Estimation of country-specific and global prevalence of male circumcision. *Population Health Metrics, 14*(4). https://doi.org/10.1186/s12963-016-0073-5.

Munevveroglu, C., & Gunduz, M. (2020). Postoperative pain management for circumcision; Comparison of frequently used methods. *Pakistan Journal of Medical Sciences, 36*(2), 91–95. https://doi.org/10.12669/pjms.36.2.505.

National Center for Missing & Exploited Children. (n.d.). The issues: Infant abduction. Guidelines on prevention of and response to infant abductions. https://www.missingkids.org/theissues/infantabductions.

National Center on Shaken Baby Syndrome. (n.d.). The period of purple crying. https://www.dontshake.org/purple-crying.

National Health Service. (2019). *Phenylketonuria.* https://www.nhs.uk/conditions/phenylketonuria/.

National Institute on Deafness and Other Communication Disorders. (2020). *Your baby's hearing screening.* https://www.nidcd.nih.gov/health/your-babys-hearing-screening.

National Institutes of Health. (n.d.). Ways to reduce the risk of SIDS and other sleep-related causes of infant death. https://safetosleep.nichd.nih.gov/safesleepbasics/risk/reduce.

New, K. (2019). Evidence-based guidelines for infant bathing. Research Review. https://www.researchreview.co.nz/getmedia/0a9e5190-b8ac-419f-8f44-43b8e5ba8c4b/Educational-Series-Evidence-based-guidelines-for-infant-bathing.pdf.aspx?ext=.pdf.

Office of Disease Prevention and Health Promotion. (2020). *Healthy people 2030.* https://health.gov/healthypeople.

Ogundoyin, O. O., Olulana, D. I., Lawal, T. A., & Kumolalo, F. O. (2019). Comparing pain control using oral acetaminophen versus dorsal penile block in neonatal circumcision. *Annals of Pediatric Surgery, 15*(1). https://doi.org/10.1186/s43159-019-0002-z.

Pacheco, D. (2021). Sudden infant death syndrome (SIDS) and sleep. *Sleep Foundation.* https://www.sleepfoundation.org/baby-sleep/sudden-infant-death-syndrome#:~:text=Age%3A%20Infants%20younger%20than%20six,between%20one%20and%20four%20months.

Pennestri, M., Laganière, C., Bouvette-Turcot, A., Pokhvisneva, I., Steiner, M., Meaney, M. J., Gaudreau, H., & Mavan Research Team. (2018). Uninterrupted infant sleep, development and maternal mood. *Pediatrics, 142*(6), e20174330. https://doi.org/10.1542/peds.2017-4330.

Rocha, C. R., Verga, K. E., Sipsma, H. L., Larson, I. A., Phillipi, C. A., & Kair, L. R. (2020). Pacifier use and breastfeeding: A qualitative study of postpartum mothers. *Breastfeeding Medicine, 15*(1), 24–28. https://doi.org/10.1089/bfm.2019.0174.

Schmid, K. M., Kugler, R., Nalabothu, P., Bosch, C., & Verna, C. (2018). The effect of pacifier sucking on orofacial structures: A systematic literature review. *Progress in Orthodontics, 19*(1), 8. https://doi.org/10.1186/s40510-018-0206-4.

Soltany, S., & Ardestanizadeh, A. (2020). The study of the factors affecting the time of ring fall off in circumcision using Plastibell. *Journal of Family Medicine and Primary Care, 9*(6), 2736–2740. https://doi.org/10.4103/jfmpc.jfmpc_1261_19.

Tappero, E. (2021). Physical assessment. In M. T. Verkaln, M. Walden, & S. Forest (Eds.), *Core curriculum for neonatal intensive care nursing* (6th ed., pp. 99–130). Elsevier.

Taylor, A., & Parekh, J. (2020). Follow-up care of the healthy newborn. In *American Academy of pediatrics: Textbook for Pediatric Care.* https://pediatriccare.solutions.aap.org/chapter.aspx?sectionid=139978717&bookid=1626.

United States Consumer Product Safety Commission (n.d.). Safe sleep—cribs and infant products information center. https://www.cpsc.gov/SafeSleep.

United States Consumer Product Safety Commission. (2010). *CPSC approves strong new crib safety standards to ensure a safe sleep for babies and toddlers.* https://www.cpsc.gov/Newsroom/News-Releases/2011/CPSC-Approves-Strong-New-Crib-Safety-Standards-To-Ensure-a-Safe-Sleep-for-Babies-and-Toddlers.

U.S. Preventive Services Task Force. (2019). Ocular prophylaxis for gonococcal ophthalmia neonatorum: US Preventative Services Task Force reaffirmation recommendation statement. *JAMA*, *321*(4), 394–398. https://doi.org/10.1001/jama.2018.21367.

Warees, W. M., Anand, S., & Rodriguez, A. M. (2020). Circumcision. *StatPearls*. https://www.ncbi.nlm.nih.gov/books/NBK535436/.

Warren, S., Midodzi, W. K., Newhook, L. A., Murphy, P., & Twells, L. (2020). Effects of delayed newborn bathing on breastfeeding, hypothermia and hypoglycemia. *JOGNN*, *49*(2), 181–189. https://doi.org/10.1016/j.jogn.2019.12.004.

Widström, A. M., Brimdyr, K., Svensson, K., Cadwell, K., & Nissen, E. (2019). Skin-to-skin contact the first hour after birth, underlying implications and clinical practice. *Acta paediatrica*, *108*, 1192–1204. https://doi.org/10.1111/apa.14754.

World Health Organization. (2013). Recommendations on postnatal care of the mother and newborn – 2013. *World Health Organization*. https://www.who.int/publications/i/item/9789241506649.

World Population Review. (2021). *Circumcision by country 2021*. https://worldpopulationreview.com/country-rankings/circumcision-by-country.

Infant Feeding

Allison L. Scott

OBJECTIVES

After studying this chapter, you should be able to:

1. Identify the nutritional and fluid needs of the infant.
2. Compare the composition of breast milk with that of formula.
3. Describe the impact of not breastfeeding for most clients and their infants.
4. Name the two primary contraindications to breastfeeding.
5. Explain important factors in choosing a method of infant feeding.
6. Explain the physiology of lactation.
7. Describe nursing management and anticipatory guidance of initial and continued breastfeeding.
8. Describe nursing assessments and interventions for common problems in breastfeeding.
9. Describe nursing assessments, anticipatory guidance, and interventions in formula feeding.

Breastfeeding benefits the environment and society. Breast milk is always available at the right temperature and is ready to feed, even in emergency situations. Due to the overwhelming evidence of the benefits as the normative method of infant feeding and reference against which infant nutrition is considered, the American Academy of Pediatrics (AAP), American College of Obstetricians and Gynecologists (ACOG), National Association of Pediatric Nurse Practitioners (NAPNAP), and the World Health Organization (WHO) recommend exclusive breastfeeding, or human milk, for the first 6 months of life and continued breastfeeding for at least 1 to 2 years (AAP, 2012; ACOG, 2019; Busch et al., 2018; WHO, 2020). The AAP and United States Department of Agriculture (USDA) recommends iron-fortified formula during the first year of life, when human milk is unavailable (AAP, 2018; USDA, 2020).

Support for breastfeeding by health care professionals promotes protection against a variety of infant and maternal diseases and improves dental health and neurodevelopmental outcomes of children (AAP, 2021). Nurses should partner with other health care workers and advocates to ensure that any social, cultural, economic, or educational barriers to breastfeeding are minimized (Association of Women's Health, Obstetric and Neonatal Nurses [AWHONN], 2015). Nurses play a key role in promoting and supporting informed decision making on infant feeding choice. This role requires knowledge of the newborn's nutritional needs and effective management to meet optimal health outcomes.

NUTRITIONAL NEEDS OF THE NEWBORN

Calories

Infants are generally capable of regulating their food intake to consume sufficient calories to meet energy and growth needs. The estimated energy requirements during infancy are based on this rationale (Box 23.1) (USDA, 2019). Caloric needs vary and are influenced by age, body size, growth rate, physical activity, and ambient (environmental) temperature. The infant must consume sufficient calories to meet energy needs, prevent the use of body stores, and provide for growth (Box 23.2).

Breast milk and infant formula contain 20 kilocalories per ounce (kcal/oz). During the early days after birth, infants may lose up to 10% of their birth weight (Hagan et al., 2017; Rohan, 2021). This loss is a result of normal excretion of meconium and extracellular water during newborn diuresis, especially if a large amount of IV fluid was administered during labor (Walker, 2017). Cesarean section delivery has also been identified as a risk factor for higher newborn weight loss (Miyoshi et al., 2020; Thulier, 2017; Walker, 2017). Newborns have a small stomach capacity and may fall asleep before feeding adequately or may sleep through feeding times in the early days of life. The average physiologic stomach capacity in the first 10 days of life for a full-term newborn is 2 mL/kg on day one, increasing to 24 mL/kg on day 10 (Walker, 2017). Nurses and other health care providers should consider weight loss in their feeding assessment but should also consider the quality of a directly observed breastfeeding session, the infant's output, and other clinical factors such as prematurity and jaundice risk.

Infants should be evaluated for feeding problems if weight loss exceeds 10% of birth weight or if weight loss continues beyond 3 days of age. Data indicates weight loss of 7% but less than 10% during the first week of life may be a normal phenomenon among breastfed newborns (DiTomasso & Paiva, 2018; Mujawar & Archana, 2017). This information should be explained to parents.

Nutrients

Macronutrients needed by the newborn are provided by carbohydrates, proteins, and fats in breast milk or formula. Full-term neonates digest simple carbohydrates and proteins well. Complex carbohydrates and fats are less well-digested because of the lack of pancreatic amylase and lipase in the newborn.

Water

The newborn needs larger amounts of fluid in relationship to size than the adult because infants lose water more easily from the skin, kidneys, and intestines, particularly extracellular fluid. Breast milk or infant formula supplies the infant's fluid needs. Breast milk is composed of approximately 90% water and can meet the fluid needs of the infant without water supplementation. Additional water is unnecessary, even in hot climates.

BREAST MILK AND FORMULA COMPOSITION

Breast Milk

Breast milk is species-specific (made for human infants) and is the reference point on which to compare necessary infant nutrition. The nutrients in breast milk are proportioned appropriately for the neonate and vary to meet the newborn's changing needs, so breast milk will change slightly in composition depending on the infant's age. Breast milk provides protection against infection and is easily digested, particularly the protein which is digested and absorbed more efficiently than the protein in infant formula (USDA, 2019). Maternal immunoglobulins, leukocytes, antioxidants, fat-digestive enzymes, and hormones important for growth are present in breast milk but are not available in formula.

Changes in Composition

The composition of breast milk changes in three phases: **lactogenesis** (the production of milk) stages I, II, and III.

Lactogenesis I. Lactogenesis I begins during pregnancy, around 16 weeks of gestation, and continues during the early days after giving birth. At this time, the breasts secrete **colostrum**—a thick, yellow milk. Colostrum is higher in protein, fat-soluble vitamins, and some minerals than mature milk. It is lower in carbohydrates, fat and lactose. It is rich in immunoglobulins, especially secretory immunoglobulin A (IgA), which helps protect the infant's gastrointestinal (GI) tract from infection. When the infant is first born, breast milk supplies antibodies (mainly IgA) until the immune system begins to take over weeks later. This supports early initiation of exclusive breastfeeding when possible (Janzon et al., 2019). Colostrum helps establish the normal flora in the intestines, and its laxative effect speeds the passage of meconium. Colostrum is sometimes referred to as "liquid gold" because of its many benefits (Maaks et al., 2021).

Lactogenesis II. Lactogenesis II begins 2 to 3 days after birth as the drop in placental hormones and increased prolactin levels trigger transition of milk. **Transitional milk**, milk that gradually changes from colostrum to mature milk, appears over about 10 days (Maaks et al., 2021). The amount of milk increases rapidly as the milk "comes in." Immunoglobulins and proteins decrease and lactose, fat, and calories increase. The vitamin content is approximately the same as that of mature milk.

Lactogenesis III. **Mature milk** replaces transitional milk during lactogenesis III, typically by week two. Because breast milk is bluish and not as thick as colostrum, some clients think their milk is not "rich" enough for their infants. Nurses should explain the normal appearance of breast milk to clients. Mature milk contains approximately 20 kcal/oz and nutrients sufficient to meet the infant's needs. It continues to provide immunoglobulins and other antibacterial components. Properties of mature milk will continue to change as the infant grows, perfectly meeting the infant's nutritional needs (Maaks et al., 2021). Discussions of breast milk and its contents refer to mature milk unless otherwise stated.

Nutrients

The nutrients provided in breast milk are present in the amounts and proportions needed by the infant, and with rare exception, it is the ideal food for human infants.

Protein. The concentrations of amino acids in breast milk are suited to the infant's needs and ability to metabolize them. Breast milk is high in cysteine and taurine, which is important for bile conjugation and brain development. High-quality proteins in breast milk are digested and absorbed more efficiently than in formula because it has a high whey-to-casein ratio, especially in early lactation (Maaks et al., 2021).

By contrast, formula has a higher ratio of casein to whey, which results in formula-fed babies having firmer stools with a large amount of the protein in formula not digested (Maaks et al., 2021). Cow's milk, one the most common allergens, is recognized by the body's immune system, and reactions may occur to this protein found in formula. Because breast milk is made for the human infant, it seldom causes an allergic response. However, antigenic food proteins in the maternal diet may pass into the milk and elicit clinical reactions in already-sensitized infants. Foods causing a reaction are difficult to identify, but those that are most likely to trigger an allergic response in an infant are those from dairy sources, shellfish, peanuts, and tree nuts (Rajani et al., 2020). Studies have been unable to determine whether avoiding eating common allergens impacts the likelihood of the infant developing food allergies. Current recommendations are to avoid excluding any foods routinely from the maternal diet unless there is evidence that food is causing symptoms of intolerance. The exception is moderate caffeine (no greater than 2 cups) consumption, especially in the first 2 months due to difficulty in the infant metabolizing caffeine (Maaks et al., 2021).

Carbohydrate. Lactose is the major carbohydrate in breast milk and is highly concentrated. It improves absorption of calcium, an important role due to the relatively low level of calcium in breast milk, and provides energy for brain growth (Maaks et al., 2021).

Fat. Various lipids (fat) compose the second greatest percentage of the components of breast milk. They are the most variable component, comprising 30% to 50% of the calories in breast milk (Maaks et al., 2021). The fat in breast milk is more easily digested by the newborn than that in cow's milk. The amount of fat in breast milk varies daily during the feeding and between feedings. Hindmilk, the milk produced at the end of the feeding is higher in fat than foremilk, the milk produced at the beginning of the feeding. Hindmilk produces satiety and helps the infant gain weight. You can think of hindmilk as the "dessert" after a nutritious meal.

Cholesterol and essential fatty acids such as the long-chain polyunsaturated fatty acids (LC-PUFAs), docosahexaenoic acid (DHA), and arachidonic acid (ARA) are present and play an important role in retinal and brain development. DHA and ARA have been added to some infant formula but little evidence is present regarding long-term outcomes being equal to those found in breastfed infants (Janke, 2021; Lien et al., 2017; Walker, 2017).

Vitamins. Levels of vitamins A, E, K, B_1, B_2, B_6, and C are adequate in breast milk; however, the vitamin D content of breast milk may be inadequate. Therefore, daily supplementation with 400 international units (IU) is recommended within the first few days of life (Maaks et al., 2021). Exclusively breastfed infants who are not exposed to the sun and those with dark skin are particularly at risk for insufficient vitamin D. Infants receiving formula supplementation or only infant formula do not need added vitamin D.

The presence of water-soluble vitamins in breast milk varies according to the client's intake. The infant of a vegan client may need supplementation with vitamin B_{12}.

Minerals. The casein protein in cow's milk interferes with iron absorption. Although low levels of iron are present in breast milk, the absorption is highly efficient with 49% absorbed in contrast to 4% from formula (Maaks et al., 2021).

The full-term infant who is exclusively breastfed maintains iron stores for the first 4 to 6 months of life (USDA, 2019). Generally, iron is added when the infant begins eating solids. Preterm infants may need iron supplements earlier. All formula-fed infants should receive iron-fortified formula (USDA, 2019).

Sodium, calcium, and phosphorus levels are higher in cow's milk than in human milk. This difference could cause an excessively high renal solute load if formula is not diluted

properly. Fluoride supplements are recommended for exclusively breastfed infants starting at 6 months of age to improve dental health, if the local water source contains less than 0.3 parts per million of fluoride (USDA, 2019).

Enzymes. Breast milk contains enzymes that aid in digestion. The amount of pancreatic amylase necessary for digestion of carbohydrates is low in the newborn but present in breast milk. Breast milk also contains lipase to increase fat digestion.

> ### KNOWLEDGE CHECK
>
> 1. Why do most newborns lose weight after birth and what weight loss warrants further evaluation?
> 2. What are the differences among colostrum, transitional breast milk, and mature breast milk?
> 3. How does breast milk compare with commercial formulas in composition, including protein content? How does this effect elimination?

Infection-Preventing Components

Although vitamins and minerals are provided by both breast milk and infant formula, only breast milk contains bioactive factors, or those that protect against infection, including immunoglobulins and bifidus factor, which promotes the growth of *Lactobacillus bifidus,* leading to optimal intestinal flora (USDA, 2019). This helps protect the infant from GI infections.

Leukocytes present in breast milk also help protect against infection. Macrophages are the most abundant and secrete lysozyme and lactoferrin. Lysozyme is a bacteriolytic enzyme that acts against gram-positive and enteric bacteria. Lactoferrin is a protein that binds iron in iron-dependent bacteria, preventing their growth. It also makes the iron in milk absorbed more easily (Walker, 2017).

Antibodies or immunoglobulins are present in highest amounts in colostrum but also are present throughout lactation. Higher levels occur when the infant is born prematurely. Lymphocytes in the milk produce secretory IgA, which helps prevent viral or bacterial invasion of the intestinal mucosa, resulting in fewer intestinal infections. Breast milk provides several tiers of protection against pathogens, resulting in protection from a number of acute and chronic diseases, even after discontinuation of breastfeeding (Walker, 2017). Infants who are breastfed have a decreased incidence of respiratory and GI problems, otitis media, asthma, diabetes, some cancers, childhood obesity, sudden infant death syndrome (SIDS), and necrotizing enterocolitis (AAP, 2021).

Effect of Maternal Diet

The fatty acid, linoleic acid, and some micronutrients, including fat-soluble vitamin content of breast milk, can be influenced by the client's diet and the stage of lactation. However, there is no evidence that breast milk composition is strongly influenced by the nutritional value of maternal daily food consumption (Bzikowska-Jura et al., 2018). Maternal nutritional needs include a balanced diet with a daily caloric intake of 300 extra calories over prepregnancy recommendations and water intake of approximately 3.4 L/day (Maaks et al., 2021). There is no "list of foods to avoid" based on the evidence.

Formulas

Commercial formulas are produced to replace or supplement breast milk. They are sometimes called "breast milk substitutes" or "artificial breast milk" because manufacturers must adapt them to correspond to the components in breast milk as much as possible. However, an exact match is impossible, and although formula provides adequate nutrition, it cannot provide the important immunologic components of breast milk and thus does not provide direct protection against illness. No brand of formula is superior for all infants, but iron-fortified formulas are recommended (Centers for Disease Control and Prevention [CDC], 2021a). Table 23.1 outlines various types of commercial formulas available.

TABLE 23.1 Specialized Infant Feeding Guidelines*: Formula Selection

Formula	Products	Indications	Contraindications	Main Features
Conventional cow's milk	Enfamil Infant Similac Advance Similac Sensitive	Healthy infants born >34 weeks gestational age	Cow's milk protein allergy	Protein: Intact cow's milk proteins (casein and whey)
Partially hydrolyzed	Enfamil Gentlease Good Start Gentle Good Start Soothe Similac Total Comfort	Note: marketed as intolerance formulas; not truly hypoallergenic Good Start Gentle: FDA approved for use in reducing risk of atopic dermatitis in high-risk infants	Cow's milk protein allergy	Protein: cow's milk proteins partially hydrolyzed into small peptides Note: Good Start and Similac: 100% whey
Extensive hydrolyzed	Alimentum, Nutramigen, Pregestimil	Hypoallergenic and used in cow's milk and soy protein allergy, protein maldigestion, or fat malabsorption	Severe cow's milk protein allergy	Protein: cow's milk proteins extensively hydrolyzed. Increased likelihood of tolerating whole cow's milk at age 1 year
Thickened	Enfamil A.R. Similac for Spit Up	Uncomplicated GERD Note: decreased efficacy when used with proton-pump inhibitor medications (e.g., Prilosec, Prevacid)	Premature infants <38 weeks GA Do not concentrate above 24 kcal/oz	Protein: intact cow's milk proteins Note: contains rice starch, which thickens upon contact with stomach acid Formulation maintains appropriate nutrient composition as opposed to adding cereal to formula
Soy	Enfamil Prosobee Good Start Soy Similac Soy Isomil	Vegan diet Family preference Galactosemia (Isomil and Prosobee powder only)	Prematurity Colic Constipation Cow's milk protein-induced enteropathy	Protein: soy protein isolates Note: all soy formulas are lactose free
Free amino acid	EleCare Infant (Abbott) Neocate Infant (Nutricia) PurAmino (Mead Johnson)	Cow's milk and soy protein allergy Multiple food protein allergies GERD Short bowel syndrome Malabsorption Eosinophilic esophagitis Galactosemia Note: limited availability and expensive		Protein: synthetic free amino acids Fat: EleCare and Neocate: 33% MCT oil Note: mixing ratios differ from standard formulas; refer to manufacturer's instructions
Low mineral	Breast milk Similac PM 60/40 (Abbott)	Impaired renal function Neonatal hypoglycemia		Protein: intact cow's milk proteins Note: breast milk's efficient absorption rate results in a naturally low mineral content Similac PM 60/40: Iron supplementation may be needed

TABLE 23.1	Specialized Infant Feeding Guidelines*: Formula Selection—cont'd			
Formula	Products	Indications	Contraindications	Main Features
Postdischarge premature	EnfaCare (Mead Johnson) Neosure (Abbott)	Birthweight >2000 g (4.5 lb) and <34 weeks GA Can be used until 1-year corrected age Contraindications: full-term infants and FTT infants due to the risk of hypervitaminosis and hypercalcemia		Protein: intact cow's milk proteins Note: provides 22 kcal/oz at standard dilution

FDA, U.S. Food and Drug Administration; *FTT*, failure to thrive; *GA*, gestational age; *GERD*, gastroesophageal reflux disease; *MCT*, medium-chain triglyceride.

*These are general guidelines; not intended for use in the treatment of a specific clinical condition or without medical supervision.

From Maaks, D. L., Starr, N. B., Brady, M. A., Gaylord, N. M., Driessnack, M., & Duderstadt, K. (2021). *Burn's pediatric primary care* (7th ed.). Elsevier. Modified from *Oregon Academy of Nutrition and Dietetics.* https://www.eatrightoregon.org/opnpg/page/pediatric-nutrition-resources.

Cow's Milk

Unmodified cow's milk (whole milk, low-fat milk, or fat-free milk) is not recommended for infants under 12 months of age. It contains high concentrations of protein and minerals, which can stress immature kidneys, and lacks essential fatty acids, vitamin C, iron, zinc, and other nutrients and may even cause iron-deficiency anemia (AAP, 2018).

Modified cow's milk is the source of most commercial formulas. Manufacturers specifically formulate it for infants by reducing protein content to decrease renal solute load. Saturated fat is removed and replaced with vegetable fats. Vitamins and other nutrients are added to simulate the contents of breast milk. Formula with added iron should be used for all infants receiving formula due to iron deficiency and its association with poor cognitive development (USDA, 2019).

Formulas for Infants with Special Needs

Soy formula may be given to infants with galactosemia or lactase deficiency but have no advantage over cow's milk–based formulas for healthy infants. Use of soy formula is not recommended for colic or a preterm infant with a birth weight less than 1800 g (USDA, 2019). Protein hydrolysate formulas (protein is extensively broken down) are better tolerated by infants with allergies and malabsorption disorders. Amino acid formulas are used for allergic infants who do not thrive on hydrolyzed protein formulas.

The preterm infant may require a more concentrated formula with more calories in less liquid. Human milk fortifiers can be added to breast milk to increase calories for preterm infants, but this is not done routinely. Lactose-free formula uses primarily glucose instead of lactose for infants who do not tolerate lactose. Low-phenylalanine formulas are needed for infants with phenylketonuria (PKU), a deficiency in the enzyme to digest phenylalanine found in standard formulas.

NURSING EDUCATION AND SUPPORT IN CHOOSING A FEEDING METHOD

Nurses should encourage breastfeeding as the best method of feeding most infants. An assessment of infant feeding knowledge, beliefs, and cultural influences should be done by the nurse. Unless there is a rare circumstance that contraindicates breastfeeding, nurses should provide patient and family education on the risks of formula feeding and the benefits of breastfeeding. This patient education should begin early in pregnancy. However, nurses should be supportive of the client's chosen method once a fully informed decision has been made.

Most clients determine infant feeding preference during pregnancy. Macro-level factors such as media broadcasting, infant formula marketing, and breastfeeding legislation interact with micro-level factors including hospital staff and policies, workplace policies and support, and cultural norms to influence maternal infant feeding decision. Clients with a support system are more likely to begin breastfeeding and continue longer than those without a perceived support system. The client's partner and the baby's grandmothers are often important influences in determining whether they breastfeed. Involvement of the partner in infant care is important in some families, and some may think it is possible mainly with feedings. Nurses can suggest other ways partners can participate in infant care, for example, holding, rocking, and bathing infants. Educating family members about the importance of breastfeeding and risks of formula feeding may lead to their encouragement and support as well.

The health care system itself and well-meaning but misinformed health care providers are one of the biggest barriers to successful breastfeeding (WHO/United Nations Children's Fund [UNICEF], 2020). Encouragement from the client's health care provider may be a powerful influence in the client choosing to breastfeed (Newton & Stuebe, 2021). The support the client receives from the nursing staff plays a significant part in the comfort felt with the feeding method chosen. Clients who do not feel confident in their ability to breastfeed before they leave the birth facility are less likely to continue breastfeeding if they encounter difficulties at home.

Culture

Cultural influences may dictate decisions about how to feed the infant. Clients in the lowest poverty ratio have much lower breastfeeding initiation rates than those in the highest poverty ratio (66% vs. 91%) (Spatz, 2018). Those with the lowest breastfeeding rates include clients who are non-Hispanic Black. Among all infants, Black infants have significantly lower rates of breastfeeding at 3 months of age (58%) than White infants (72%) (Beauregard et al., 2019). Some clients may think formula feeding is the preferred method in the United States because it is available in birth facilities and is widely accepted as an infant feeding norm. They also may think breastfeeding is inferior to formula feeding and consider formula a way to help their infants grow larger and become stronger. Nurses must emphasize the normalcy of breastfeeding and the risks of formula feeding and encourage these clients to continue their cultural tradition of breastfeeding.

Nurses should be particularly watchful for ways to help clients from other cultures who wish to breastfeed but fail to do so because of lack of information or support. Nurses should first examine their own biases about breastfeeding. They should then practice culturally competent care by asking families about their cultural practices and beliefs about breastfeeding and helping find ways for the family to both honor their culture and successfully breastfeed.

Employment

The need to return to roles outside the home soon after giving birth may cause concern about feeding methods. Unfortunately, returning to work or school is a major cause of discontinuation of breastfeeding, attributing to a sharp decline in breastfeeding at 3 months. The client may choose to directly breastfeed while not at work and then express milk for the baby to be fed while working. The initial plan may include feeding formula from the beginning, plan a short period of breastfeeding before weaning the infant to formula, or use a combination of breastfeeding and bottle feeding with breast milk or formula.

The nurse should encourage clients to continue to breastfeed, even if not exclusive, when they return to work and point out the potential risks of only formula-feeding. The increased incidence of illness in formula-fed infants means clients are more likely to miss work to care for a sick infant. This is a disadvantage for the employer, as well as the non-breastfeeding family.

Nurses who provide practical information about breastfeeding and working, use of breast pumps, and storage of breast milk help a client continue breastfeeding for a longer period. Pamphlets and books for the working breastfeeding client are particularly helpful. Referral to a lactation consultant can provide continued education and support after the client goes home.

Other Factors

Other factors also may influence a parent's feeding decision. Knowledge and past experience with infant feeding are important. Public shaming may be an issue for some clients who are concerned about breastfeeding in public situations. According to the CDC *SummerStyles Survey* (2021c), only

---

BOX 23.3 Impact of Not Breastfeeding

For the Infant
Allergies are more likely to develop.
Not receiving the immunologic properties of breast milk increases the risk for infections.
Increased incidence of necrotizing enterocolitis and respiratory tract, ear, urinary tract, and gastrointestinal tract infections.
Increased incidence of diabetes, asthma, obesity, some cancers, sudden infant death syndrome.
Formula's nutritional and immunologic properties do not change according to the infant's needs.
Formula is not as easily digested, and nutrients are not as well absorbed.
Protein, fat, and carbohydrate do not occur in the most suitable proportions in formula.
Formula can be improperly and potentially dangerously diluted.
Formula can be contaminated and can be affected by water supply.
Formula is more easily overfed.
Constipation is more common.

For the Mother
Formula feeding does not release oxytocin. Oxytocin enhances uterine involution.
Loses more blood because of earlier return of menses.
Resumes ovulation earlier.
Increased incidence of some cancers.
Receives less rest while feeding.
A balanced maternal diet that improves healing is less likely.
Less frequent skin-to-skin contact can be detrimental to bonding.
Inconvenient—bottles to wash and formula to buy, prepare, or heat.
Expensive—cost of formula and bottles and time spent in preparation.
Infant is more likely to be ill, increasing medical care costs.
Working mothers miss more days of work to care for sick infants.
Travel more difficult—bottles to prepare, carry, refrigerate, and warm.

68% of respondents agreed that a person should have the right to breastfeed in public spaces.

Those who live in rural areas or the southeastern United States have lower breastfeeding rates compared with clients in other parts of the United States (CDC, 2020a). Younger clients, age 20 to 29 years, are less likely to breastfeed than clients age 30 and above (CDC, 2020a). Obese clients, with a body mass index (BMI) of 30 or greater, are less likely to initiate breastfeeding and less likely to breastfeed for 6 months (Lyons et al., 2019).

Breastfeeding

Parents choose breastfeeding because, in almost all cases, it is the best choice for the health of the client and the infant (Box 23.3 presents the impact of not breastfeeding). It has been increasingly recognized that formula feeding can never fully equal breastfeeding in terms of providing for the infant's optimal health, growth, and development.

The AAP recommends that infants receive only breast milk for the first 6 months after birth. Breastfeeding should continue until the infant is at least 12 months old, with the addition of complementary foods (AAP, 2012). Breastfeeding and support to initiate breastfeeding in the first hour of life and breastfeed on-demand are recommended by the WHO (WHO, 2020).

Social and Economic Benefits

A goal set by the U.S. Department of Health and Human Services (DHHS) for the year 2030 is for at least 42.4% of infants to be breastfed exclusively through 6 months and 54.1% at 1 year of life (DHHS, 2020). Suboptimal breastfeeding (less than recommended) is estimated to result in roughly 2600 maternal deaths yearly (mostly due to increase lifetime risks for heart attacks, breast cancer, and diabetes in clients who do not follow breastfeeding recommendations) and over 700 pediatric deaths (mainly necrotizing enterocolitis and SIDS) (Newton & Stuebe, 2021). Research estimates that if 90% of U.S. families followed the recommended breastfeeding guidelines to breastfeed exclusively for 6 months and continue breastfeeding until at least 12 months, $2.45 billion in reduced medical and other costs could be saved (USDA, 2019). According to the WHO (2020), over 820,000 children's lives could be saved yearly among those 5 years old and younger if all children were optimally breastfed until 23 months.

The CDC (2020a) reports that in 2017, 84.1% of infants initiated breastfeeding; however, at 6 months, only 58.3% of mothers were breastfeeding, and at 12 months the rate was 35.3% breastfeeding. These statistics show a gradual but steady increase over previous years, but continued improvement is needed.

In an effort to promote breastfeeding, UNICEF, the WHO, and the U.S. Surgeon General advocate that birth facilities become designated through the Baby Friendly Hospital Initiative. Guidelines to becoming certified as a baby-friendly hospital emphasize education of staff and parents about breastfeeding, early initiation of breastfeeding, demand feedings, rooming-in, no pacifiers, and avoidance of formula unless medically indicated. In 2020, 27.96% of births in the United States occurred in certified baby-friendly hospitals (Baby Friendly, USA, 2020).

Contraindications to Breastfeeding

Only two primary (and permanent) contraindications to breastfeeding exist. Infants diagnosed with galactosemia (galactose 1-phosphate uridyltransferase deficiency) and clients in the United States who have human immunodeficiency virus (HIV) cannot breastfeed (AAP, 2021). Breastfeeding is *not* contraindicated in infants born to clients with hepatitis C virus, who are febrile, who are carriers of cytomegalovirus (CMV), who smoke tobacco (although it should be discouraged), or who are COVID-19 positive (AAP, 2021; CDC, 2021b). A few unusual circumstances may require temporary

cessation of breastfeeding including maternal diagnosis of cancer and its treatment; herpetic lesions on the client's nipple, areola, or breast (expression of breast milk is allowed); or maternal use of illicit drugs, especially cocaine and phencyclidine (PCP) (Maaks et al., 2021). Maternal use of cannabis is currently being studied and needs further research. It is recommended to abstain when lactating and if unable to abstain, avoid breastfeeding within 1 hour of inhaled use to decrease infant's risk of exposure (Ordean & Kim, 2020).

Formula Feeding

Parents choose formula feeding for many reasons. Some clients are embarrassed by breastfeeding, seeing their breasts only in a sexual context. Many clients have few relatives or friends who have had breastfeeding experiences. Cultural views, beliefs, and customs also influence infant feeding decision. Rarely, a client must take medications that might harm the infant or has had breast surgery that resulted in nerve intervention and disruption of the milk production cycle. Some parents choose formula feeding instead of breastfeeding due to a lack of understanding and education about the two methods. It is important for the nurse to provide infant feeding information, based on the evidence, to allow an informed decision. Formula feeding provides the best alternative to breast milk when the client cannot or chooses not to breastfeed and pasteurized donor breast milk is unavailable.

Combination Feeding

Some parents prefer a combination of breastfeeding and formula feeding. Unless medically indicated, it is best to delay giving bottles or formula until lactation has been well established when the infant is 3 to 4 weeks of age. Giving formula to breastfeeding infants may lead to a decrease in breastfeeding frequency and milk production, making successful breastfeeding less likely (ACOG, 2021a). Nurses can inform parents who wish to combination feed of the option of expressing breast milk so that the baby can bottle feed breast milk instead of formula, to ensure an adequate milk supply. If parents choose to both breastfeed and formula feed after being fully educated, however, the nurse should be supportive so the client and infant receive the benefits of partial breastfeeding.

> **KNOWLEDGE CHECK**
> 4. What factors that help prevent infection are present in breast milk?
> 5. What are the primary contraindications to breastfeeding?
> 6. What factors influence a client's choice of feeding method?

BREASTFEEDING

The anatomy and physiology of the breast are discussed in Chapter 3, and breast changes occurring in pregnancy are discussed in Chapter 6 (see Figs. 3.8 and 6.3).

Breast Changes during Pregnancy

Breast changes begin early in pregnancy in preparation for the production of milk. The ductal system elongates and expands into the adipose tissue in response to estrogen. Mammary glands are developed sufficiently by 20 weeks' gestation to produce milk, but production is inhibited by high estrogen and progesterone levels. Rapid decrease of these high levels shortly after birth allow milk production to occur as prolactin levels rise (Alex et al., 2020).

Milk Production

The process of lactation completes the reproductive cycle. Milk is produced in the alveoli of the breasts through a complex process by which substances from the client's bloodstream are reformulated into breast milk. Thus, amino acids, glucose, lipids, enzymes, leukocytes, and other materials are used to manufacture the nutrients needed by the infant. Milk ejection is stimulated via sensory nerves in the areola and nipple through suckling by the infant (Lawrence, 2022).

Hormonal Changes at Birth
Prolactin

At birth, loss of placental hormones results in increasing levels and effectiveness of prolactin and activates milk production. The tactile stimulation of **suckling** and the removal of colostrum or milk causes continued increased levels of prolactin. Prolactin, from the anterior pituitary gland, is secreted at the highest levels with suckling and during the night (Walker, 2017). Levels are high during the early months and then gradually decrease until weaning.

Oxytocin

Oxytocin increases in response to nipple stimulation and causes the **milk-ejection reflex** or **let-down reflex**, release of milk from the alveoli into the ducts. During feeding, the milk-ejection reflex occurs several times. Some clients have a tingling sensation of the breast when the let-down occurs.

When clients see, hear, or think about their infants, they often have an increase in oxytocin, resulting in let-down of milk, causing milk to drip or spurt from the breasts (Fig. 23.1). Pain or lack of relaxation can inhibit oxytocin release. Oxytocin also causes the uterine contractions clients may feel at the beginning of breastfeeding sessions. These contractions are beneficial because they hasten involution of the uterus and can decrease postpartum bleeding.

Continued Milk Production

The amount of milk produced depends primarily on adequate stimulation of the breast and removal of the milk by suckling or a breast pump, which causes production of prolactin. The concept of "demand and supply" is important for providers and parents to understand. The level and amount of infant suckling directly affects prolactin release and thus milk production, especially early in the initiation of lactation.

If milk (or colostrum) is not removed from the breasts, components in the milk cause feedback that decreases prolactin secretion and milk production. The milk in the ducts is absorbed, the alveoli become smaller, the cells return to a resting state, and milk production decreases. The nurse

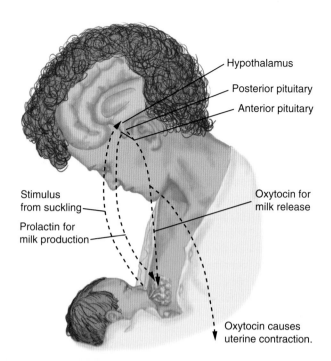

FIG. 23.1 Effect of Prolactin and Oxytocin on Milk Production. When the infant begins to suckle at the breast, nerve impulses travel to the hypothalamus, causing the anterior pituitary to secrete prolactin to increase milk production. Suckling causes the posterior pituitary to secrete oxytocin, producing the let-down reflex, which releases milk from the breast. Oxytocin also causes the uterus to contract, which aids in involution.

should encourage breastfeeding in the first hour of life and frequent nursing thereafter to ensure establishment of supply. Breast size does not correlate with milk production volume.

KNOWLEDGE CHECK

7. What is the effect of suckling on the let-down reflex and milk production?
8. Explain the concept of demand and supply for breast milk production.

APPLICATION OF THE NURSING PROCESS: BREASTFEEDING

Assessment

Assess both the client and the infant during the breastfeeding process. Various scoring tools have been developed to assess breastfeeding, but none are completely satisfactory. One method often used is the LATCH breastfeeding assessment tool (Table 23.2). The tool incorporates both client and infant assessment, including maternal comfort level while feeding. Breastfeeding with a correct latch seldom produces nipple pain. The "C" in LATCH assesses maternal comfort level and

TABLE 23.2 The Latch Scoring Tool*

	0	1	2
L Latch	Infant too sleepy or reluctant No sustained latch achieved	After repeated attempts is able to sustain latch and suck Must hold nipple in infant's mouth Must stimulate infant to suck	Grasps breast Tongue down Lips flanged Rhythmic sucking
A Audible swallowing	None	A few with stimulation	Spontaneous and intermittent <24 hours old Spontaneous and frequent >24 hours old
T Type of nipple	Inverted	Flat	Everted (with or without stimulation)
C Comfort (breast or nipple)	Engorged cracked, bleeding, large blisters, or bruises Severe discomfort	Filling Reddened or small blisters or bruises Mild to moderate discomfort	Soft Nontender
H Hold (positioning)	Full assist (staff holds infant at breast)	Minimal assist (e.g., elevate head of bed; place pillows for support) Teach one side; client does other side Staff holds and then client takes over	No assist from staff Client able to position or hold infant

*The nurse can use the LATCH scoring system to assess and document the need for assistance with breastfeeding. Each assessment area is scored 0 to 2. A score of 7 or less indicates the client needs more assistance in feeding.
Modified from Jensen, D., Wallace, S., & Kelsay, P. (1994). LATCH: A breastfeeding charting system and documentation tool. *Journal of Obstetric, Gynecologic, and Neonatal Nursing, 23*(1), 27–32. Reprinted with permission of Sage Publications.

nipple tenderness, bruising, redness, or cracking should be an indicator of a poor latch.

Maternal Assessment

Breasts and Nipples. Assess the condition of the breasts and nipples and the client's knowledge about breastfeeding to determine the need for assistance. Assess all clients regardless of past breastfeeding experience. The breasts should be examined during pregnancy to identify flat or inverted nipples, which can make an effective latch much more difficult to achieve (Fig. 23.2). The nipple should protrude, not retract, when the tissue behind the nipple is compressed between the thumb and forefinger. If retraction occurs, this indicates an inverted or flat nipple that may cause milk transfer issues due to a poor latch (Walker, 2017). The use of a two-piece plastic disk with vented dome, or breast shell, during the third trimester may help improve flat nipples. Care must be taken to avoid prolonged periods of wearing the breast shell to avoid potential areolar edema and tissue damage (Walker, 2017).

During lactation, especially in the first few days, nipples should be assessed for redness, bruising, fissures, or bleeding. The presence of any of these nipple abnormalities or nipple pain indicates the need for an evaluation of breastfeeding technique by the nurse or lactation consultant.

Engorgement is congestion and increased vascularity, edema from obstruction of lymphatic drainage, and accumulation of milk as lactation is established. Engorged

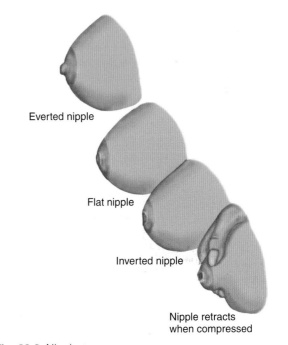

Fig. 23.2 Nipple types.

breasts may be hard and tender, with taut, shiny skin. Note any redness, tenderness, and lumps within the breasts. Engorged breasts may not be seen until after discharge from the birth facility.

THERAPEUTIC COMMUNICATIONS
Anxiety about Breastfeeding

Brianna gave birth to her second baby, Luis, by cesarean birth. She tells her nurse, Chela, that she breastfed her first infant for a week and then switched to bottle feeding because she did not have enough milk. Luis is a sleepy baby but does nurse at times. Brianna's breasts are engorged, and her nipples are sore.

Brianna: I really wanted to nurse Luis, but I don't know if it's worth the effort. My breasts hurt, and I don't know if he's getting enough milk. I probably should just use the bottle again.

Chela: You sound really discouraged! *(Reflecting the feelings expressed.)*

Brianna: When I couldn't nurse my daughter, I was so disappointed. I had this "Mother Earth" view of the kind of mother I was going to be. But the baby wouldn't stop crying, so I went to the bottle.

Chela: That must have been hard for you! *(Reflecting the feelings expressed.)*

Brianna: It was awful, and now it looks like I'm going to fail again. Luis won't nurse half the time, and I'm going home this afternoon.

Chela: And you're worried about what's going to happen at home. *(Seeking clarification of the mother's concerns.)*

Brianna: What if he won't nurse at home? I don't know what to do!

Chela: Breastfeeding isn't always easy. Mothers and babies both have to learn the process, and that takes time and a lot of patience. Luis seems hungry now—would you like to try again? I'll stay with you, help you find a comfortable latch, and answer your questions. *(Offering realistic encouragement and assistance in techniques.)*

Brianna: That would be great! Maybe I'll get the hang of this yet! *(By allowing Brianna to express her feelings of discouragement and disappointment before beginning to teach, the nurse learns how important breastfeeding is to Brianna and how best to go about teaching her. Brianna feels accepted, even though she is discouraged.)*

Infant Feeding Behaviors

Before initiating a breastfeeding session, assess the infant's readiness for feeding (Box 23.4). Young infants should not be put on a rigid feeding schedule but fed when indicating hunger cues. The infant should be awake and hungry. Trying to feed an infant in a deep sleep period is frustrating to both client and infant. Sucking on the hands, rooting when the cheek or side of the mouth is touched, smacking the lips, and hand-to-mouth movements are common hunger cues. Feeding should begin before crying, which is a late sign of hunger. Crying infants must be calmed before they are ready to feed. Continue to assess for problems throughout the feeding.

Identification of Client Problems

Clients with and without experience often need assessment of feeding and information to have a successful breastfeeding experience. A client's confidence in their breastfeeding ability may be an important determinant of their success. Therefore

BOX 23.4　Hunger Cues in Infants

Licking or sucking movements
Lip smacking
Rooting
Hand-to-mouth movements
Sucking on the hands
Increased activity
Crying (a late sign)

nurses should help clients increase their confidence and help prevent early weaning. Lack of understanding of breastfeeding techniques and confidence in using them are common client problems that may lead to breastfeeding challenges.

Planning: Expected Outcomes

The expected outcomes are:
1. The infant will breastfeed using nutritive suckling and swallowing before discharge.
2. The client will demonstrate correct breastfeeding techniques (such as positioning and latch) without nipple pain during feeding before discharge.
3. The client will verbalize satisfaction and confidence with the breastfeeding process before discharge.

Interventions

Interventions are focused on the teaching the nurse should provide all breastfeeding clients and their support persons. Inexperienced parents may need detailed teaching. Experienced parents often need only a review or clarification about techniques they have used previously.

Assisting with the First Feeding

Nurses are encouraged to keep babies in uninterrupted skin-to-skin contact after birth and then help begin breastfeeding when infants show feeding cues, ideally within the first hour after birth. This assumes both client and infant are in stable condition. Research shows mother-infant skin-to-skin contact increases the rate of exclusive breastfeeding (Karimi et al., 2020). During this first hour after birth, infants are in an alert state and receptive to feed. Early breastfeeding provides stimulation for milk production and improves suckling and maternal confidence. Feeding at this time also helps increase early bonding and maternal confidence in the ability to breastfeed.

Teaching Feeding Techniques

Position of the Client and Infant. Both the client and the infant must be positioned properly for optimal breastfeeding. Make the client as comfortable as possible before the feeding begins. Special equipment is not necessary, but pillows and having the client's feet elevated may encourage a comfortable position. Provide privacy and prevent interruptions so the client can concentrate on learning techniques.

There is no "right" way to position the infant, but the way the client positions the infant can influence successful breastfeeding. The cradle, football (or clutch), cross-cradle holds and the side-lying position are commonly used (Figs. 23.3 to 23.6).

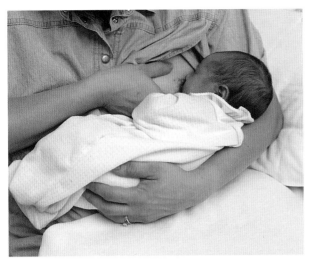

FIG. 23.3 For the cradle hold, the client positions the infant's head at or near the antecubital space and level with the nipple, with the arm supporting the infant's body. The other hand is free to hold the breast. Once the infant is positioned, pillows or blankets can be used to support the client's arm, which may tire from holding the baby.

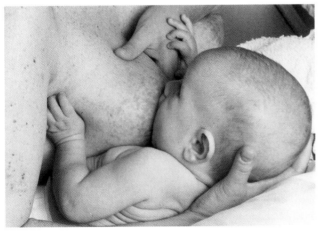

FIG. 23.4 For the football or clutch hold, the client supports the infant's head and neck in the hand, with the infant's body resting on pillows alongside the client's hip. This method allows the client to see the position of the infant's mouth on the breast, helps control the infant's head, and is especially helpful for clients with heavy breasts. This hold also avoids pressure against an abdominal incision.

The infant's head and body should directly face the breast. If the infant must turn the head to reach the breast, swallowing is difficult. The neck should be slightly extended. The infant's body should be aligned so the ear, shoulder, and hips are in a straight line.

Position of the Client's Hands. The client's hand position is also important. Using either a "C" (Fig. 23.7) or a "U" position, the hand gently shapes the breast so the client's fingers and thumb are parallel to the baby's mouth. Fingers should be behind the areola so the baby has plenty of room to latch onto as much breast tissue as possible.

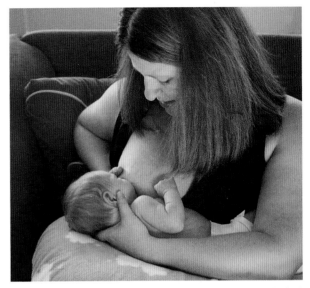

FIG. 23.5 The cross-cradle or modified cradle hold is helpful for infants who are preterm or have a fractured clavicle. The client holds the infant's head with the hand opposite the side on which the infant will feed and supports the infant's body with the arm across the lap. The other hand holds the breast. The client can guide the infant's head to the breast and see the mouth on the breast during the feeding.

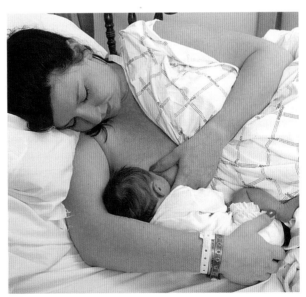

FIG. 23.6 The side-lying position avoids pressure on episiotomy or abdominal incisions and allows the client to rest while feeding. Lying on the side with the lower arm supporting the head or placed around the infant. Pillows behind the back and between the legs provide comfort. The upper hand and arm are used to position the infant on the side at nipple level and hold the breast. When the infant's mouth opens to nurse, the client draws the infant closer to insert the nipple into the mouth. A small blanket or towel can be placed over an abdominal incision to protect it from infant movement.

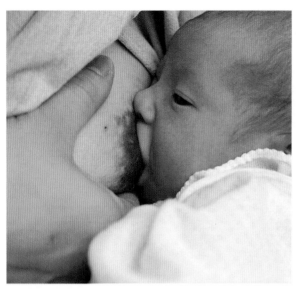

FIG. 23.7 "C" Position of Hand on Breast. The hand is positioned so that the thumb is on top of the breast while the fingers support the breast from below. Note the flaring of the infant's lips.

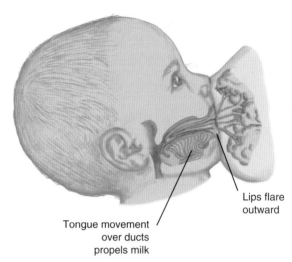

Lips flare outward

Tongue movement over ducts propels milk

FIG. 23.8 Position of the Infant's Mouth While Suckling. When the nipple and areola are properly positioned in the infant's mouth, the gums compress the areola instead of the nipple. The tongue is between the lower gum and breast. The infant's lips are flared outward.

The client should support their breast in place for the first few weeks if the weight of the breast makes it difficult for the infant to hold on to it. For large-breasted clients, a rolled receiving blanket or hand towel can be used under the breast prior to latching. As the infant becomes more adept at breastfeeding, the client no longer needs to hold the breast.

Although parents worry about the infant's ability to breathe while breastfeeding, indenting the breast tissue near the infant's nostrils is unnecessary. This might cause improper positioning of the nipple in the infant's mouth, interfere with the grasp of the nipple, or interfere with milk flow. Bringing the infant's hips closer to the client and lifting the body to a more horizontal position are usually sufficient if there is concern about the infant's ability to breathe while breastfeeding.

Latch-On Techniques. Teach the client techniques to help the infant latch on to the breast. Helping clients and babies achieve a comfortable latch is a key nursing intervention in the first few days postpartum because correct latch is key to preventing nipple trauma and promoting optimal milk transfer. The infant should be awake and hungry. Undressing the baby and placing skin-to-skin with the client can help a sleepy infant awaken or calm an upset infant.

Eliciting Latch-On. After positioning the infant to face the breast, instruct the client to hold the breast so the nipple brushes downward against the infant's lips. A hungry infant usually opens the mouth, but some need a minute of stroking the area around the mouth. The breast should not be inserted until the infant's mouth is opened widely, or the infant will compress the end of the nipple, causing pain, trauma, and little milk flow.

When the infant's mouth is wide open with the tongue down and forward over the gum, the client should latch the baby asymmetrically by aiming the nipple toward the roof of the baby's mouth, then quickly bring the infant close so the

infant can latch on to the areola with the chin touching the breast first. The infant should always be brought to the client's breast, not the client to the infant. To ensure correct latch, instruct the client to wait until the infant opens the mouth as though yawning or taking a bite out of an apple. This visual may help the client understand correct latch technique.

Position of the Mouth. Assess the position of the infant's mouth on the breast (Fig. 23.8). The infant's lips should be flanged or curved outward and the nose should be touching the skin of the breast. This prevents the infant from sucking on the nipple only, which leads to sore nipples and possible insufficient milk production. It also places the infant's gums over the ducts so the milk is released into the mouth as the gums compress the breast. The nurse should assess whether most of the areola on the underside is covered by the baby's mouth; some of the areola on the top side may be visible. When the infant detaches from the breast, the nipple should look elongated but never creased or blanched. For more details on a good latch, refer to womenshealth.gov at https://www.womenshealth.gov/breastfeeding/learning-breastfeed/getting-good-latch.

Suckling Pattern. Teach the parents about the infant's suckling pattern. During **nutritive suckling (sucking)**, the infant sucks with smooth, continuous movements with occasional pauses to rest. The infant may swallow after each suck or may suck several times before swallowing. **Nonnutritive sucking**, in which little or no milk flow is obtained, often occurs when the infant is falling asleep. A fluttery or choppy motion of the jaw not accompanied by the sound of swallowing indicates nonnutritive sucking.

Parents often wonder whether their infants are actually receiving milk from the breast. Point out the sound of swallowing when it occurs. A soft "ka" or "ah" sound indicates the infant is swallowing colostrum or milk. In the first few weeks, the client may not feel the milk ejection reflex (tingling in the breast), but rapid swallowing and/or milk dripping from the other breast indicates the reflex has occurred.

Short pauses are normal during breastfeeding. Gentle breast massage can help the baby transfer more milk with less effort and stay awake and involved in the feeding. In addition, gently stroking the baby's back or hands and feet may keep a sleepy baby awake to feed.

Removal from the Breast. Teach the client to remove the infant from the breast by inserting a finger in to the corner of the infant's mouth between the gums to break the suction. Then remove the breast quickly before the infant begins to suck again.

Frequency of Feedings. Breastfeeding is most successful when babies are not on a rigid feeding schedule, but are instead allowed to feed as frequently and for as long as they show feeding cues (fed on demand). Most babies need to feed 8 to 12 times per day, but these feedings may not be evenly spaced. Frequent feedings are especially important in the early days after birth, while lactation is being established and the infant's stomach capacity is small.

An infant may vary in the length of feedings and time between each feeding. Several feedings close together (sometimes called "cluster feedings") are followed by a longer interval between feedings. Cluster feedings may occur on the second or third night at home or in later weeks when an appetite spurt occurs in the infant (Academy of Breastfeeding Medicine [ABM], 2017a). An infant's frequent need to nurse may cause the client to think the milk supply is inadequate, when, in fact, it may be normal. Nurses should provide clients with anticipatory guidance about frequent nighttime feedings and should encourage daytime maternal rest.

Length of Feedings. Early feedings were once limited to only a few minutes per breast to prevent sore nipples; however, improper positioning, rather than time at breast, is the usual cause of nipple trauma. When feedings are too short, infants receive little or no colostrum or milk. It may take as long as 5 minutes for the milk-ejection (let-down) reflex to occur during the early days after birth.

Generally, clients can allow infants to set the length of feedings. Parents should be taught to note the quality of a breastfeeding session instead of the length. The infant should suckle vigorously for a certain period with swallowing noted. Gentle breast massage and infant stimulation can help keep a baby in a nutritive sucking pattern. When choppy, nonnutritive suckling without the sound of swallowing occurs, the client should burp the infant and complete the feeding at the other breast. When the infant is satisfied, the suckling pattern will slow greatly and the infant's hands typically are completely open and relaxed.

Variations in feeding length will occur, especially in the first week. Average intake of colostrum in the first 48 hours is 2 mL to 15 mL per feed (ABM, 2017a). Feeding time increases as needed by the infant over the next few days. Teach the client that longer feedings do not cause sore nipples if the infant is positioned properly. Prolonged feeding of over 45 minutes typically means the infant is sleepy and may lead to slow weight gain due to calorie use during feeding. In the first

2 weeks, a newborn should not nurse longer than 4 hours at night without breastfeeding (USDA, 2019).

Explain the differences between **foremilk**, the watery first milk that quenches the infant's thirst, and **hindmilk**, which comes at the end of the feeding. Hindmilk is richer in fat, more satisfying, and leads to weight gain. Feeding for too short a time prevents the infant from getting the hindmilk and decreases weight gain. Therefore, the client should continue feeding on the first side as long as the infant nurses vigorously before burping and continuing on the other breast. Clients should alternate the breast offered first at each feeding to provide equal stimulation of the breasts.

Determining Sufficient Milk Supply. One of the main reasons for early weaning to formula is parents' perception of insufficient milk supply. Clients with positive attitudes toward breastfeeding and confidence that they will produce enough milk are less likely to wean early because of perceived insufficiency of milk. The nurse should include education on signs of adequate milk transfer (infant getting enough milk). An exclusively breastfed infant is likely consuming enough milk when the following are present:

Suggest that the client count the number of wet and soiled diapers to help determine whether the infant is receiving enough milk. A simple chart can be used to record the quality and total number of feedings per day along with the number of voids and stools each day.

Weight gain is the most reliable sign of breastfeeding success. After the initial weight loss following birth between day one and four, infants generally gain approximately 20 to 30 g (0.7 to 1 oz) each day during the first 6 months (USDA, 2019).

Common causes of decreased milk supply include ineffective suckling by the infant, feedings that are infrequent or too short, maternal fatigue, low maternal thyroid function, preterm or late preterm infants, and some medications, including oral contraceptives containing estrogen. Intervene appropriately if any common causes are present.

Although clients were once taught to drink large quantities of liquids to maintain milk supply, fluid intake sufficient to satisfy their thirst and to keep their urine light yellow is adequate.

When the breasts are soft and large amounts of milk are not present during the first few days, the client may believe little or no breast milk is present. This may influence the client to give formula before or after the feeding, decreasing milk production. Teach clients who need to increase milk supply to feed more often and to hand express or use a breast pump after feedings.

If problems persist, refer the client to a lactation consultant. Lactation professionals are often available in the birth facility and in the community. They can help with breastfeeding techniques and special problems.

The nurse should include education on signs of adequate milk transfer (infant getting enough milk). An exclusively breastfed infant is likely consuming enough milk when the following are present (see Client Education).

CLIENT EDUCATION

Is My Baby Getting Enough Milk?

Your baby is probably getting enough milk if:

You hear the baby swallow frequently during feedings. It sounds like a soft "ka" or "ah" sound.

You see nutritive suckling—a smooth series of suckling and swallowing with occasional rest periods. This is different from short, choppy sucks, which occur when the baby is falling asleep and not getting milk.

Once your milk has increased, your breast is getting softer during the feeding. (However, your breasts do not have to be hard [engorged] for you to have enough milk.)

You can see milk in the baby's mouth or dripping from your breast occasionally.

You feed your baby 8 to 12 times every 24 hours. More milk is produced when you nurse more often. (Keep track, at first, by writing down the quality and number of feedings each day.)

Your baby has at least one or two wet diapers per day for the first 2 days after birth, at least three or four wet diapers a day by day 3, and at least six wet diapers per day by day 4. Disposable diapers are very absorbent, and knowing whether they are wet is sometimes hard. If you are unsure, place a tissue or cotton ball inside the diaper to show even small amounts of urine. Urine should be light yellow, not dark yellow.

Your baby has at least three bowel movements per day by day 3 and four bowel movements per day after that time. The bowel movements transition in color over the first week from black tarry (meconium stool) to brown or brownish–green to yellow, seedy, loose stool.

Your baby seems satisfied after feedings. (An occasional fussy time is not unusual and does not mean that the baby is not getting enough to eat.)

Well-baby checkups show that your baby is gaining weight. Weight gain is the most important indicator of sufficient milk intake (note that on the initial visit on day 2 to 5, weight loss is expected).

Getting Help from Family. Partners often feel there is nothing they can do to help the client during breastfeeding. Give suggestions on how the partner can be involved. For example, helping the client recognize early hunger signs. Partners can prepare the infant for feeding by changing the diaper and calming the infant. Assisting with positioning the infant so both client and baby are comfortable and burping the infant after feedings are other methods of support. Caring for other children, preparing meals, and helping with housework can help clients get more rest.

Increasing Confidence. Use every opportunity to offer praise and reinforcement of the client's ability to breastfeed the infant. Point out the infant's positive response to the client's handling and feeding. Mention the improvements made in recognizing hunger cues, positioning, latch-on, and other aspects of care. The nurse's support and encouragement will help the client feel more confident with each feeding and may lead to a longer duration of breastfeeding.

Providing Resources. Clients who stop breastfeeding before they originally planned often cite nipple pain, problems with latch-on, belief that their milk supply was insufficient, and need to return to work as their reasons. Providing information for local resources such as lactation consultants, La Leche League (https://www.llli.org), and other breastfeeding resources in their area may help them continue breastfeeding. Providing written material and internet resources such as https://www.kellymom.com/category/bf/ or https://www.womenshealth.gov/breastfeeding may also be helpful. Specific resources with cultural considerations may also be helpful. For example, breastfeeding resources for people of color:

- Black Mothers' Breastfeeding Association: https://black-mothersbreastfeeding.org
- It's Only Natural: https://www.womenshealth.gov/its-only-natural
- ROBE: Reaching Our Brothers Everywhere: https://breast-feedingrobe.org

Evaluation

Evaluation of interventions should be continued throughout the birth facility stay and during the postpartum period after discharge. Before discharge, the infant should be feeding well with nutritive sucking and audible swallowing at least 8 to 12 times per day. Parents should be taught to evaluate feeding by monitoring for a comfortable latch, listening for the infant to swallow while feeding, and watching the baby for signs of satiety. The client should correctly demonstrate feeding techniques and voice satisfaction and confidence with breastfeeding. Satisfaction and confidence are major determinants of whether breastfeeding will continue at home.

? KNOWLEDGE CHECK

9. How can the nurse help the client establish breastfeeding during the initial feeding sessions?
10. What should the nurse teach the client about frequency and quality of feedings?

COMMON BREASTFEEDING CONCERNS

Clients may be discharged from the birth facility before problems arise; therefore, nurses should teach them how to prevent and treat common concerns. When the client seeks help for problems that developed after discharge, the nurse should ask what has been tried to solve the problem and whether any complementary or alternative therapies have been tried. The safety of any therapy should be determined. Herbs may have been used to promote milk production. Research on the use of these therapies is inadequate; therefore, the parent should be referred to a health care provider for information before using any substances because some may be harmful.

Problems may be divided into those originating with the infant and those pertaining to the mother.

Infant Problems

Infant problems require prompt attention to ensure successful breastfeeding.

⚡ SAFETY CHECK

Infant signs of breastfeeding problems are as follows:
Falling asleep after feeding for less than 5 minutes
Refusal to breastfeed
Tongue thrusting
Smacking or clicking sounds
Dimpling of the cheeks
Failure to open the mouth widely at latch-on
Lower lip turned in
Short, choppy motions of the jaw
No audible swallowing
Use of formula

Sleepy Infant

During the first few days after birth, infants often sleep longer than expected or fall asleep at the breast after feeding for only a short time. They may be tired from the birth process and may not recognize or respond appropriately to hunger.

The nurse should show clients how to arouse sleepy infants for breastfeeding (see "Client Education: Solutions to Common Breastfeeding Problems").

When the infant falls asleep during feedings, the nurse should evaluate whether the infant has fed adequately, should be awakened to feed longer, or should be fed again sooner than usual. Nurses should emphasize gentle wake-up techniques. The client should avoid techniques that are excessively irritating to the infant, because feeding should be associated with pleasurable sensations. Infants who continue to be excessively sleepy or nurse poorly need further evaluation. Poor feeding may be an early sign of a complication such as sepsis (see Chapter 25).

Nipple Confusion

Nipple confusion (or nipple preference) may occur when an infant who has been fed by bottle confuses the tongue movements necessary for bottle feeding with the suckling of breastfeeding. Some infants may refuse to breastfeed or use tongue movements that push the breast out of the mouth.

Movements of the mouth and tongue are different in breastfeeding and bottle feeding. During breastfeeding, the infant uses suction to hold the nipple in place near the soft palate. The tongue cups around the nipple and areola with the tip over the lower gum. With each compression of the lower jaw, the tongue presses against the breast, causing the milk to move forward from the ducts and into the infant's mouth.

To feed from a bottle, infants must push the tongue over the nipple to slow the flow of milk and prevent choking. This constant flow can be demonstrated by noting the steady drip of milk when a bottle is held upside down. The infant's lips are relaxed because there is no need to hold the nipple in place. If the infant uses the same thrusting tongue motion and relaxed lips while breastfeeding, the breast may be pushed out of the mouth.

Nurses should discourage the use of bottles or formula during the first 2 weeks of life, unless supplementation is medically necessary. It reduces breastfeeding time, which decreases prolactin secretion and therefore milk production. The increased time between feedings limits breast stimulation and may lead to engorgement.

Pacifier use while breastfeeding has not been determined to shorten breastfeeding in randomized controlled trials. It may be wise to avoid using pacifiers in the first 2 weeks with infants having severe difficulty breastfeeding (Hermanson & Astrand, 2020).

Suckling Problems

Suckling problems may occur when the nipple is poorly positioned in the infant's mouth. Dimpling of the cheeks and smacking or clicking sounds may indicate the infant is sucking on the tongue or nipple only. Some infants do not open their mouths widely enough and suck on the end of the nipple.

Inserting a gloved finger into the infant's mouth helps assess suckling. The motion of the tongue should be felt as the infant sucks and should be a drawing in type motion. The infant who is thrusting the tongue may have an issue needing evaluation by a lactation consultant or professional trained in tongue-tie or suck dysfunction.

Infant Complications

Infant complications may be minor and cause minimal interference with breastfeeding or may prevent the infant from breastfeeding for a long period.

Jaundice. Jaundice (hyperbilirubinemia) in the infant does not necessarily interfere with breastfeeding but may make them sleepy and more difficult to keep awake at the breast.

Infants receiving phototherapy should not be supplemented with water, which may decrease the intake of breast milk. Decreased intestinal motility from insufficient milk intake allows reabsorption of bilirubin through the intestinal wall into the bloodstream, increasing the work of the immature liver. Frequent breastfeeding increases the number of stools, which aids in bilirubin excretion and provides adequate intake of protein and fluid. If supplementation is needed, donor breast milk is the preferred choice.

Prematurity. If the preterm infant cannot breastfeed immediately after birth, the client needs encouragement and instruction on how to express breast milk. The nurse should provide assistance in hand expression within the first 1 to 2 hours after delivery and then in the use of a breast pump to establish and maintain the milk supply. Breast pumping should be initiated within the first 6 hours of separation to maximize long-term milk supply. Breast milk offers immunologic and nutritional benefits and is adapted to the preterm infant's needs. Formula use is associated with necrotizing enterocolitis, a serious complication of prematurity, so providing breast milk to a preterm infant can be lifesaving. It also helps the client feel more involved with infant care while the baby has to remain in the hospital.

The client can express milk and take it to the nursery for the infant's feedings. The nurse should provide sterile containers for the client to take home and provide special nursery requirement instructions. The containers should be labeled with the infant's name and the date and time the milk was pumped.

Some preterm infants or those with breastfeeding problems respond well to the use of supplementary feeding devices. These consist of a container of milk with a small plastic feeding tube attached to the breast. When the infant begins to breastfeed, milk is drawn from both the container and the breast, increasing the infant's intake and motivation to continue suckling. As the infant gains weight and feeding ability increases, use of the device is gradually decreased until it can be discontinued completely.

Late preterm infants, born between 35- and 36-weeks' gestation, may have difficulty feeding. Although they may look like full-term infants, their suck–swallow coordination is often immature, and they are at higher risk for hyperbilirubinemia and poor weight gain (ABM, 2016a). Ideally, a lactation specialist should be consulted, especially if weight gain is very poor by day 3 to 5 of life. Weight checks should be done weekly until the infant reaches 40 weeks of postconceptional age (ABM, 2016a).

Illness and Congenital Defects

Infant illness and congenital defects such as a cleft palate may cause breastfeeding problems. If the client is not able to nurse the infant at first, assistance may be needed to maintain lactation until breastfeeding is possible. Referral to support groups can be particularly helpful. Some groups focus on particular congenital defects, and others focus on breastfeeding infants with special problems.

Maternal Concerns

Early nursing intervention can help the client overcome common breast problems.

Common Breast Problems

Engorgement, nipple trauma, flat or inverted nipples, plugged ducts, and **mastitis** (infection of the breast) are common problems involving the breasts.

Engorgement. Many clients experience a temporary swelling or fullness of the breasts, which is most common day 3 to 5 after giving birth when the production of milk begins to increase or the milk "comes in" (ACOG, 2021a). Vascular and lymphatic compression occur from the distention of the alveolar ducts with milk, and severity varies from mild to severe (ACOG, 2021a). A history of breast surgery or lumpectomy increase the incidence of engorgement (ABM, 2016b). Engorgement may lead to nipple trauma, mastitis, and even the discontinuation of breastfeeding.

Engorgement may become a problem if feedings are delayed, too short, or infrequent. Engorged breasts become edematous, hard, and tender, making feeding and even movement painful. The areola may become so hard that the infant cannot compress it for feeding. An engorged areola causes the nipple to become flat, making it more difficult for the infant to draw it into the back of the mouth.

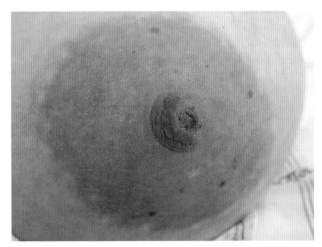

FIG. 23.9 Note the cracked area on this nipple.

Nurses help prevent engorgement by assisting clients to begin breastfeeding early and to feed frequently. Encouraging breastfeeding with all infant feeding cues, even at night, ensures that the breasts are emptied regularly. The use of water and formula should be discouraged, as should *frequent pumping during engorgement*, as this may lead to oversupply.

> ### ⚡ SAFETY CHECK
>
> Maternal signs of breastfeeding problems are as follows:
> Hard, tender breasts
> Painful, red, cracked, blistered, or bleeding nipples
> Flat or inverted nipples
> Localized edema or pain in either breast
> Fever, generalized aching, or malaise

Nipple Pain. Although nipple pain is common during early breastfeeding, it should not be persistent and should never be severe enough to cause premature weaning (ABM, 2016c). Discomfort for 1 minute or less may occur at the beginning of feedings because of tissue stretching and suction on the ductules before they fill with milk. Traumatized nipples that appear red, cracked, blistered, or bleeding are never normal (Fig. 23.9). The most common cause of nipple pain is suboptimal positioning. Other sources of pain include disorganized latch/suck, ankyloglossia (tongue-tie), and breast pump trauma/misuse (ABM, 2016c).

Flat and Inverted Nipples. Nipple abnormalities should be identified during pregnancy, if possible, but interventions can begin after birth, if necessary. Nipple rolling just before feeding helps flat nipples become more erect so the infant can grasp them more readily (Fig. 23.10). A breast pump used for a few minutes before feedings or a breast shield may help draw out inverted nipples.

Plugged Ducts. Although the exact cause of occlusion of a lactiferous duct is unknown, engorgement, missed feedings, or a constricting bra may be involved. Localized edema and tenderness are present, and a hard area may be palpated. A tiny, white area may be present on the nipple. Massage of the

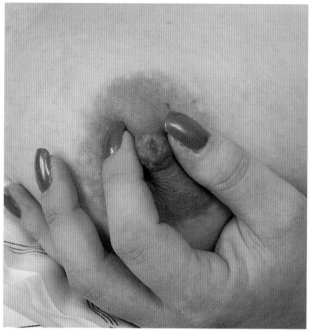

FIG. 23.10 Rolling helps flat nipples become erect in preparation for latch-on.

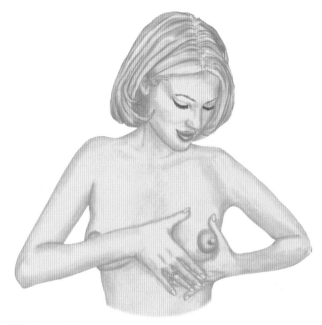

FIG. 23.11 To massage the breasts, the client places hands against the chest wall with the fingers encircling the breasts. Then gently slides the hands forward until the fingers overlap. The position of the hands is rotated to cover all breast tissue. Massaging with the fingertips in a circular motion over all areas of the breast is also helpful.

area (Fig. 23.11), frequent breastfeeding, heat application, and using varied breastfeeding positions are helpful. A plugged duct may progress to mastitis if not treated promptly. Mastitis involves localized pain accompanied by fever, generalized aching, and malaise.

Illness in the Mother

It is rarely necessary for a client to stop breastfeeding when ill. If breastfeeding must be temporarily stopped because of the client's condition or the medications administered, the nurse should help the client hand express or use a breast pump until breastfeeding can be resumed. Abrupt weaning may lead to mastitis. Human milk has been shown to be protective against COVID-19, and breastfeeding should not be interrupted (Spatz et al., 2021).

Medication Transfer to Breast Milk

Most medications taken by the client are compatible with breastfeeding. Some may interfere with milk production.

Therefore, both prescription and certain over-the-counter medications should be approved by the health care provider. In many cases, another medication can be substituted for one that adversely affects the infant. If the medication will be harmful to the infant, the client should pump and discard the milk while taking the medication. Once the medication clears the bloodstream, the client may resume breastfeeding. Some medications may not reach the infant in harmful amounts if taken after a feeding or at night when there is a longer time between feedings. Clients who take methadone or buprenorphine for opiate addiction are allowed to breastfeed because only minimal amounts of the drugs pass to breast milk (ACOG, 2021b). The U.S. National Library of Medicine has a website for information about medications during lactation at https://www.ncbi.nlm.nih.gov/books/NBK501922/.

CLIENT EDUCATION

Solutions to Common Breastfeeding Problems

Problem: Sleepy Infant
An infant is sleepy at feeding time or falls asleep shortly after beginning feeding.

Prevention
Look for signs your baby is ready to wake up, such as movement of the eyes through closed eyelids, small twitches of the face, sucking movements, stretching, and increased movements of the entire body.

Gently awaken your baby when you see those signs. Talk to the infant, gently move the infant's arms and legs, and play with the infant for a short time before beginning the feeding. Unwrap the baby's blankets and change the diaper. Swaddling infants by wrapping them tightly with blankets is a calming technique that often helps them sleep. Leave the blanket and shirt off as you begin the feeding with the baby skin-to-skin against your chest.

Continued

CLIENT EDUCATION—cont'd

Solutions

If your baby goes to sleep during the feeding and has fed for just a few minutes, try the following:

Undress the baby (except for the diaper) and place the infant against your skin (if you have not done this already).

Rub the baby's hair or back gently, stroke around his or her mouth, or shift the baby's position slightly to see if he or she will wake up.

Remove the baby from the breast. Rub the infant's back to bring up bubbles of air that may cause a sensation of stomach fullness. Rubbing the back also stimulates the central nervous system and arouses the baby.

Change the diaper.

Express a few drops of colostrum onto the nipple. The baby tastes the colostrum when the nipple is offered and often resumes suckling.

Wipe the face gently with a lukewarm washcloth to help the infant wake up.

If your baby cannot be aroused with a few of these gentle techniques, a longer sleep period may be needed. Let the infant remain skin-to-skin with you for another half hour, then begin again. Watch for signs the baby is in a lighter phase of sleep and can be awakened more easily.

Problem: Nipple Confusion

Artificial nipples require different movements of the infant's tongue, lips, and jaw than breastfeeding and may cause difficulties with correct latch and suckling at the breast.

Prevention

Avoid all bottles for the first 2 weeks unless absolutely necessary. If the baby has a medical need for extra breast milk, consider using a supplemental nursing system, spoon or cup feeding, or an oral syringe.

Solution

Stop all bottle feeding and limit pacifier use so the baby becomes accustomed to suckling from the breast instead of the bottle. Nurse more often to stimulate milk production and help the baby learn what to do. The use of skin-to-skin by the mother may also help with latch.

Problem: Latch-On Difficulty

The infant sucks on the end of the nipple or fails to open his or her mouth widely enough.

Prevention

Do not insert the breast into the infant's mouth until the infant opens the mouth widely with the tongue down and forward (like biting into an apple).

Bring the baby to the breast with your nipple pointed toward the roof of the baby's mouth and the baby's chin touching your breast first. The baby should have more breast tissue from underneath the breast than from on top (asymmetric latch).

Solutions

Stop the feeding and start again if there is persistent nipple pain, you see dimples in the infant's cheeks, or hear smacking, slurping, or clicking sounds. Short, choppy movement of the jaw means the infant is going to sleep or has finished feeding.

If you believe the infant should nurse longer, awaken the infant and begin again.

Problem: Engorgement

The client's breasts are hard and tender from engorgement.

Prevention

Room-in with your baby so you can respond to feeding cues. Breastfeed the infant with all feeding cues, usually at least 8 to 12 times in a 24-hour period. Do not give bottles during the day or night because this increases the risk for engorgement. Waiting even 4 hours between feedings may increase the risk for engorgement, but frequent breastfeeding often can prevent it.

Solutions

To reduce edema and pain, apply warm packs just before feeding and cold packs to the breasts between feedings (ABM, 2016b). Taking a warm shower while using breast massage may also be used. Use commercial cold packs or make inexpensive cold packs from frozen washcloths, packages of frozen vegetables, or plastic bags filled with crushed ice. Cover cold packs with a washcloth before applying to the skin. A disposable diaper with crushed ice placed between the layers also may be used.

Treatments such as cool cabbage leaves applied to the breast between feedings are inexpensive, although evidence for their use is not conclusive (ABM, 2016b).

Massage the breasts before and during feedings to stimulate the let-down reflex so the baby can nurse more easily.

If the areola is engorged and hard, making it difficult for the baby to latch on, express a little milk by hand or with a breast pump. Or apply gentle pressure on the areola to move some swelling back into the breast and soften the areola to allow the infant to latch on. As soon as the areolae are soft, begin to feed.

Increase skin-to-skin contact and feed more often, such as every 1.5 to 2 hours.

Wear a well-fitting bra for support during the day and at night for comfort.

Take prescribed pain medication just before feedings to make you more comfortable.

Problem: Sore Nipples

The nipples are sore and may be cracked, blistered, or bleeding.

Prevention

Position the baby at the breast in an asymmetric latch with enough of the breast in the mouth that the nipple is not compressed between the baby's gums during breastfeeding (there should be no compression or creasing of the maternal nipple).

Avoid engorgement by breastfeeding frequently. Express enough milk to soften the areola if engorgement makes the areola too hard for the infant to grasp.

Vary the position of the baby to change the areas of pressure on the nipple.

Do not use soap on the nipples because it removes the protective oils and causes drying.

If you use breast pads for leaking milk, remove them when they become wet to prevent irritation of the skin. Avoid pads with plastic linings that retain moisture. Use a handkerchief or pieces of cotton cloth as inexpensive, washable substitutes for commercial breast pads.

CLIENT EDUCATION—cont'd

Solutions

The cause of the soreness must be identified in order to resolve sore nipples.

Problem: Flat or Inverted Nipples

The client's nipples are flat or inverted, and the baby has difficulty drawing them into his or her mouth.

Prevention

Some clients find wearing breast shells in the bra helps make the nipples protrude. These may be used in the last 6 weeks of pregnancy during the daytime.

Solutions

Just before beginning breastfeeding, roll the nipple between your thumb and forefinger to help it protrude (see Fig. 23.10).

Use a breast pump for a few minutes just before feedings. Put the baby to your breast immediately after the pump causes the nipple to become erect. The normal suckling process usually causes the nipple to stay erect.

In some situations, a nipple shield may be used with the help of a lactation consultant to assist the infant to achieve a correct latch. Recent research indicates there is no impact on milk production or milk transfer when used properly (Coentro et al., 2021).

KNOWLEDGE CHECK

11. What wake-up techniques should the nurse teach the client of a sleepy infant?
12. How does sucking from a bottle differ from suckling from the breast?
13. What help can the nurse offer the client with engorged breasts?
14. How should the nurse advise the client with sore nipples regarding management?

Previous Breast Surgery/Procedures

Clients who have had surgery for breast reduction, augmentation, or other conditions may have difficulty with lactation. The ability to produce and transfer milk to the nipple depends on the surgical technique used and the amount of tissue involved. Surgery may disrupt the neural pathways, ducts, and blood supply. Some clients can breastfeed without problems.

Clients with pierced nipples should not have difficulty with breastfeeding. They should remove the rings or studs before feeding the infant.

Employment

Federal law requires employers allow reasonable time to express breast milk while working up to the infant's first birthday. This law, called "Break Time for Nursing Mothers," is part of the Fair Labor Act of 2010 (U.S. Department of Labor, n.d.). Mothers must be provided with a private space, other than a bathroom, if the employer has more than 50 employees.

The mother will need to procure a breast pump. The expense of a pump is covered under most insurance plans, as required by the Affordable Care Act (ACA) (DHHS, 2017).

Milk Expression and Storage

When milk expression is needed, the nurse helps the client use hand expression (Fig. 23.12) or a breast pump (Fig. 23.13).

Hand Expression. Hand expression can be performed without other equipment and is often a more effective way to collect colostrum. It also can be used in emergency situations when a client is separated from the baby and may be done without electricity or a pump. Hand expression or manual pumps are also useful for the client who wants to save breast

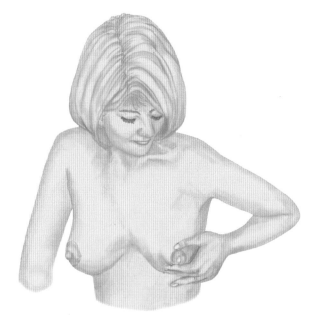

FIG. 23.12 To express milk from the breast, the client places the hand just behind the areola, with the thumb on top and the fingers supporting the breast. The tissue is pressed back against the chest wall; then the fingers and thumb are brought together and toward the nipple. This compresses the ducts and causes milk to flow. The action is repeated to simulate the suckling of the infant. Moving the hands around the areola allows compression of all areas and increases removal of milk from the breast. Compression should be gentle to avoid trauma. Application of heat and massage before expression increase the flow of milk.

milk for another feeding occasionally or whose areolae are so engorged the infant cannot grasp them.

Use of a Breast Pump. The client who plans to pump for a prolonged period should use an electric breast pump. Battery-operated pumps are small, portable, and relatively inexpensive for short-term use. Large electric hospital-grade pumps can be rented for home use. They are more efficient than hand pumps or battery-operated pumps and are indicated when the client plans to pump for a long time. A double pump allows the client to pump both breasts at once, saving time and increasing milk production.

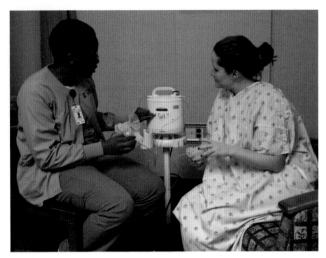

FIG. 23.13 The nurse helps the client use an electric breast pump.

Clients who cannot breastfeed their infants should be instructed in the use of the breast pump as soon as possible after birth, but at least within the first 6 hours (Spatz, 2018). Pumping should occur as often as the infant would nurse with a goal of eight or more pumping sessions in a 24-hour period (Spatz, 2018).

The client should wash their hands before using the pump and before preparing the pumped milk for storage or feeding. Breast massage and application of heat before pumping help initiate the flow of milk. Massaging the breast during pumping may increase the volume of milk obtained at each session. Pumping after the first morning feeding often produces the greatest volume. Relaxation during pumping increases volume, but tension or discomfort may reduce the output. Pumping should begin with the pump on the lowest setting. A pumping session typically lasts for about 10 to 15 minutes per breast (or 15 minutes if pumping both sides simultaneously), but length and milk production varies so pumping should last as long as comfortable and milk production continues (USDA, 2019). The pump should be cleaned according to the manufacturer's instructions after each use.

Milk Storage. Milk should be stored in clean (sterile for a hospitalized infant) glass or rigid polypropylene containers with a tight cap (CDC, 2019). A nipple should not be used to cover the container during storage because the hole allows passage of organisms, which can contaminate the milk.

Fresh unrefrigerated breast milk should generally be used within 4 hours of pumping. Under very clean conditions using it within 6 to 8 hours is acceptable. It may be stored in a refrigerator at 4°C (39°F) or below for up to 4 days and frozen for up to 12 months in a freezer at −17°C (0°F) or below. Milk that is fresh or has been refrigerated rather than frozen should be used as much as possible so the leukocytes are available for the infant (CDC, 2019).

Breast milk can be thawed and warmed by holding the container under running water. Cool water should be used first to defrost it; then the milk can be warmed by placing it under warm running water or in a bowl of warm water. It also can be thawed in the refrigerator and used within 24 hours. It should not be refrozen. Slow thawing in the refrigerator causes less fat loss than using warm water (ABM, 2017b).

Milk should not be heated in a microwave because the microwave heats unevenly. The infant might be burned because the container may be cool but the milk may have hot spots. Thawed breast milk should be gently inverted a few times to mix the foremilk and hindmilk. Milk that is not finished in one feeding should be discarded within 2 hours. A summary of storage and preparation of breast milk is found in Fig. 23.14.

Breastfeeding after Multiple Births

Clients who have more than one newborn have many questions about breastfeeding and need help and support from nurses and family members to be successful. Explain the milk supply adjusts to the demand and the client can produce enough milk for both infants. Breastfeeding each baby 8 to 12 times per day to build up the milk supply is important. If the infants cannot breastfeed at first, the client will need help hand expressing and using a breast pump.

If the client decides to feed two infants simultaneously, the nurse helps position them in the football (clutch) hold, cradle hold, or a combination of both. Encourage the client to eat well, get enough rest, and ask for help from family and friends.

CLIENT EDUCATION

Breastfeeding after the Birth of More than One Infant

Ensuring Adequate Milk Production
Because the amount of milk produced depends on the amount of suckling the breasts receive, mothers can produce enough milk for more than one baby. Breastfeeding each baby frequently (8 to 12 times per day) helps build up the milk supply. Production of milk may be more evenly stimulated if you alternate breasts for each infant, especially if one baby has a weaker suck.

Using a Breast Pump
If your infants are not ready for breastfeeding, use hand expression and a breast pump to build up your milk supply and provide milk for them until they are ready to nurse. Follow the recommended guidelines for pumping.

If one baby is ready to breastfeed before the other(s), nurse the baby and pump your breasts after each feeding to stimulate milk production. An alternative is to nurse the infant on one breast and use a breast pump on the other at the same time.

Feeding Simultaneously or Individually
You can feed each baby separately or feed two infants at once. Simultaneous breastfeeding shortens feeding times, but both infants must be awake at once. You may need help positioning the infants at first. Individual feeding can be done without help and on each infant's own schedule, but a larger portion of your day will be spent feeding.

Keeping Track
Keep track of the frequency and quality of each infant's feedings. Record the number of wet diapers and bowel movements each infant has each day. You can assign each infant one breast without changing to the opposite breast, if you choose. Clients often alternate the breast each infant nurses from at each feeding to keep stimulation of the breasts similar. Alternating breasts every 24 hours may be easier to remember.

STORAGE AND PREPARATION OF BREAST MILK

BEFORE EXPRESSING/PUMPING MILK

Wash your hands well with soap and water.

Inspect the pump kit and tubing to make sure it is clean.

Replace moldy tubing immediately.

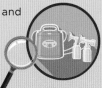

Clean pump dials and countertop.

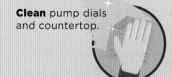

STORING EXPRESSED MILK

Use breast milk storage bags or clean food-grade containers with tight fitting lids.

Avoid plastics containing bisphenol A (BPA) (recycle symbol #7).

HUMAN MILK STORAGE GUIDELINES

TYPE OF BREAST MILK	STORAGE LOCATIONS AND TEMPERATURES		
	Countertop 77°F (25°C) or colder *(room temperature)*	**Refrigerator** 40 °F (4°C)	**Freezer** 0 °F (-18°C) or colder
Freshly Expressed or Pumped	Up to **4 Hours**	Up to **4 Days**	Within **6 months** is best Up to **12 months** is acceptable
Thawed, Previously Frozen	1–2 Hours	Up to **1 Day** *(24 hours)*	**NEVER** refreeze human milk after it has been thawed
Leftover from a Feeding (baby did not finish the bottle)	Use within **2 hours** after the baby is finished feeding		

FIG. 23.14 CDC infographic

Continued

STORE

Label milk with the date it was expressed and the child's name if delivering to childcare.

Store milk in the back of the freezer or refrigerator, not the door.

Freeze milk in **small amounts of 2 to 4 ounces** to avoid wasting any.

When freezing leave an inch of space at the top of the container; breast milk expands as it freezes.

Milk can be stored in an insulated cooler bag with frozen ice packs for **up to 24 hours** when you are traveling.

If you don't plan to use freshly expressed milk **within 4 days**, freeze it right away.

THAW

Always thaw the oldest milk first.

Thaw milk under lukewarm running water, in a container of lukewarm water, or overnight in the refrigerator.

Never thaw or heat milk in a microwave. Microwaving destroys nutrients and creates hot spots, which can burn a baby's mouth.

Use milk **within 24 hours** of thawing in the refrigerator *(from the time it is completely thawed, not from the time when you took it out of the freezer)*.

Use thawed milk **within 2 hours** of bringing to room temperature or warming.

Never refreeze thawed milk.

FEED

Milk can be **served cold, room temperature, or warm.**

To heat milk, place the sealed container into a bowl of warm water or hold under warm running water.

Do not heat milk directly on the stove or in the microwave.

Test the temperature before feeding it to your baby by putting a few drops on your wrist. It should feel warm, **not hot.**

Swirl the milk to mix the fat, which may have separated.

If your baby did not finish the bottle, leftover milk should be used **within 2 hours.**

CLEAN

Wash disassembled pump and feeding parts in a clean basin with soap and water. **Do not wash directly** in the sink because the germs in the sink could contaminate items.

Rinse thoroughly under running water. Air-dry items on a clean dishtowel or paper towel.

Using clean hands, store dry items in a clean, protected area.

For extra germ removal, sanitize feeding items daily using one of these methods:

- clean in the dishwasher using hot water and heated drying cycle *(or sanitize setting).*
- boil in water for 5 minutes *(after cleaning).*
- steam in a microwave or plug-in steam system according to the manufacturer's directions *(after cleaning).*

June 2019

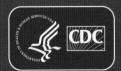

Centers for Disease Control and Prevention
National Center for Chronic Disease Prevention and Health Promotion

FOR MORE INFORMATION, VISIT:
https://bit.ly/2dxVYLU

296657-B

FIG. 23.14, cont'd

Weaning

Weaning is a personal decision and is the process of switching a baby's diet from breast milk to other foods and drinks (CDC, 2020b). There is no one "right" time to wean the infant. The AAP suggests exclusive breastfeeding for at least 6 months and then to add complementary foods and continue to breastfeed until the baby is at least 1 year old and as long after that as both mother and baby desire (AAP, 2012). The nurse should provide information so parents can make informed decisions about weaning and should support parents once their decision is made. Explaining that even a short period of breastfeeding offers the infant many advantages.

Parents may need help in planning a slow weaning process to help avoid engorgement and allow the infant to become accustomed to a bottle or cup gradually. If they are not in a hurry to wean, they may allow the infant to take the lead. Omitting one breastfeeding session a day and waiting several days or a week before omitting another will allow the client and the infant to adjust to the change more easily. Weaning too rapidly increases the risk for plugged ducts or mastitis. Infants who are weaned before 12 months of age should be given iron-fortified formula instead of cow's milk (CDC, 2020b).

CLIENT EDUCATION

How to Wean from Breastfeeding

Deciding When to Wean
Breastfeeding protects both your health and the health of your baby, and this protection is stronger the longer your baby breastfeeds. You can continue to breastfeed as long as both you and your baby wish. Only you and your baby can make the decision about when to wean. Before you decide to begin weaning, evaluate the reasons for continuing breastfeeding or beginning weaning.

How to Proceed
Gradual weaning is best for both you and your baby. Abrupt weaning can lead to engorgement and mastitis for you and can be upsetting for both you and your baby. You both need to get used to this change slowly.
Replace one breast milk feeding daily with a bottle of infant formula (for infants under 12 months of age) or a cup of fortified cow's milk (for a child older than 12 months of age).
Omit a middle of the day feeding first. Begin with the feeding in which the baby seems least interested, and then gradually eliminate others.
Wait several days before eliminating another feeding. This allows time for your milk production to adjust and the baby to accept the changes.
Eliminate the baby's favorite feedings last. Many infants are particularly fond of morning and bedtime feedings.
Expect your infant to want to nurse again when tired, ill, or hurt during the weaning process. This is sometimes called "comfort breastfeeding." A few minutes of breastfeeding may be all that is necessary to comfort the baby.

Home Care

Some infants have not breastfed well by the time of discharge from the birth facility, placing them at risk for failure to gain weight, dehydration, and hyperbilirubinemia. Problems with engorgement and sore nipples are more likely to occur after discharge. The infant should be seen by the physician or other health care provider 3 to 5 days after birth or within 48 hours of discharge and again at 2 to 3 weeks of age to assess for any problems that might occur after discharge (AAP & ACOG, 2017).

The nurse can provide reassurance regarding milk production when signs of adequate breastfeeding are present, such as adequate weight gain and normal expected output for age. Parents should be taught growth spurts may occur periodically during the first year of life and may cause the infant to temporarily nurse longer or more frequently (USDA, 2019).

Guidance for dealing with breastfeeding problems can be continued after discharge by referring the client to lactation consultants or organizations such as La Leche League, a support group that provides assistance to breastfeeding clients. La Leche League groups are available in most communities and are available on their website (https://www.llli.org). Support groups also may be provided by the birth facility.

KNOWLEDGE CHECK

15. What teaching should be included for the client who plans to work and breastfeed?
16. What should the client know about weaning?

FORMULA FEEDING

When parents make an informed decision to formula feed, they should be given appropriate guidance on its use. Parents who are formula feeding need to be taught how to safely prepare, handle, and feed formula to mitigate some of the risks of this feeding method.

Formula Supplementation

Avoid use of formula supplementation in the hospital unless there are medical indications. Avoidance of supplements of any kind during the first 72 hours is a nursing care quality measure supported by WHO and UNICEF (2020). Supplements may lessen the success of breastfeeding because they decrease feeding from the breast and decrease milk production (Spatz, 2018; ABM, 2017a). Teach parents supplementing with formula will not necessarily result in their getting more sleep during the night. Breastfed infants do not need water or glucose water because they will interfere with adequate intake of breast milk.

Formula Gift Packs

The AAP and WHO enacted the International Code of Marketing of Breast Milk Substitutes in 1981 and recommend against direct marketing to parents and giving formula gift packs at hospital discharge because this practice may lead to an expectation in some clients that formula will be necessary (Romo-Palafox et al., 2020). The United States is just one of six countries that has not enacted any provisions of the code, despite lack of scientific evidence supporting the accuracy of some claims found on formula products, such as DHA fortification and brain development (Romo-Palafox et al., 2020).

APPLICATION OF THE NURSING PROCESS: FORMULA FEEDING

Assessment

Assess both the client and the infant during the feeding process.

Parent's Knowledge

Assess the parent's knowledge of formula feeding. Ask whether they have fed an infant before and whether they have questions. Observe the technique during the initial and subsequent feedings. Note how the parent holds the infant and the bottle, and evaluate the burping technique to identify potential problem areas.

Infant Feeding Behaviors

Point out infant feeding cues, which are the same regardless of how infants are fed. Waiting until the infant is frantic may result in a feeding taken too fast, with excess swallowing of air or choking. Assess the way the infant sucks to identify problems.

Identification of Client Problems

Because improper formula preparation and feeding techniques could harm the infant, the parents' lack of understanding of formula preparation and feeding techniques is a potential client problem that could lead to a potential for negative outcomes.

Planning: Expected Outcomes

The client will demonstrate correct techniques in holding the infant and bottle during feedings and will correctly describe how to prepare formula and the frequency of feedings before discharge.

Interventions
Teaching about Formula

The parents must learn about types of formula available and how to prepare them.

Types of Formula. The provider prescribes the type of formula the client is to use. Infants should receive iron-fortified formula. Formula may be purchased in three different forms: ready-to-use formula, concentrated liquid formula, and powdered formula.

Ready-to-Use Formula. Ready-to-use formula is available in bottles to which a nipple is added or in cans to be poured directly into a bottle. It should not be diluted. The container should be shaken and the top of the can washed before opening and pouring it into a bottle. Although expensive, it is presterilized and practical when traveling, when there is difficulty in mixing formula, or if the water supply is in question. Refrigeration is not necessary until the container is opened. An open container should be refrigerated and used within 48 hours.

Concentrated Liquid Formula. Explain to the parents how to dilute concentrated liquid formula. Equal parts of concentrated liquid formula and water are mixed together and poured into a bottle to provide the amount desired for each feeding. Once again, the container should be shaken well and the top washed before opening. Opened containers should be stored in the refrigerator and used within 48 hours (USDA, 2019).

Powdered Formula. Use water from a safe source to mix infant formula and always measure the water first and then add the powder (CDC, 2021a). Usually, one level scoop of powder is added to each 60 mL (2 oz) of water in a bottle, but directions should be followed according to the manufacturer label instructions. Formula should be well mixed to dissolve the powder and make the solution uniform.

Because prepared formula is an ideal growth medium for pathogens, new formula should be prepared for each feeding and used immediately. Cronobacter is a rare but serious infection that can occur from powdered infant formula, so premature infants or those with a weakened immune system may be safer consuming nonpowdered forms of formula (CDC, 2021a).

⚡ SAFETY CHECK

Formulas must be properly diluted to prevent serious, possibly fatal, illness (such as fluid and electrolyte imbalance) and promote weight gain and growth in the infant. Too much water may not meet nutritional needs of the infant. Too little water may cause the kidneys and digestive system to work too hard and can cause dehydration (CDC, 2021a). It is essential that the instructions on the label be followed accurately. Many parents may not read labels because they are unaware of the different types of formula.

Ready-to-use preparations: Use as is without dilution.
Concentrated formulas: Dilute with equal parts of water.
Powdered formulas: Follow the label mixing directions.

Any prepared formula left at room temperature for more than 2 hours before feeding, should be discarded (CDC, 2021a).

Store unopened infant formula containers in a cool, dry place (not in a warm space such as the garage or in a vehicle).

Once the formula container is open, it should be used within 1 month (CDC, 2021a).

Never use formula after the "due date" on the container.

Discard any formula left in the bottle after a feeding as the infant's saliva can encourage bacterial growth.

Never use a microwave to prepare infant formula. The liquid can become overheated or develop "hot spots." This can lead to infant's having oral burns.

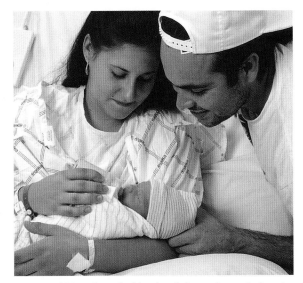

FIG. 23.15 This client holds the infant close during bottle feeding. The bottle is positioned such that the nipple is filled with milk at all times. The partner offers encouragement.

Equipment. Many different types of bottles and nipples are available. Parents may use glass or plastic bottles or a plastic liner that fits into a rigid container. Selection of type of bottles and nipples depends on individual preference. Although bisphenol-A (BPA) was once a concern, it is no longer used in baby bottles in the United States.

Preparation. Discuss preparation of formula with the parents. Instruct them to wash their hands. Infection may occur if the equipment, milk, or water used for preparation is contaminated. Emphasize the importance of following the directions on the label when mixing the formula. If water from a well is used, it should be tested for high levels of nitrates, which can be harmful to infants. The local health department can assist families in determining water safety.

Warming of infant formula should be done by holding the bottle under warm, running tap water or placing in a container of warm water and testing the formula's warmth on the inside of the wrist of the preparer (USDA, 2019). Only the amount to be given to the infant should be warmed.

Bottles and nipples can be washed in hot, sudsy water using a brush to clean well, then rinsed and allowed to air-dry. They also may be washed in a dishwasher. The formula and water are poured into the bottles, which then are capped.

Explaining Feeding Techniques

Positioning. Show the parents how to position the infant in a semiupright position such as the cradle hold. This allows them to hold the infant close in a face-to-face position. The bottle is held with the nipple kept full of formula to prevent excessive swallowing of air (Fig. 23.15). Placing the infant in the opposite arm for each feeding provides varied visual stimulation during feedings.

Burping. For the first few days, the infant should be burped or "bubbled" after every 15 mL (0.5 oz) of formula. Gradually,

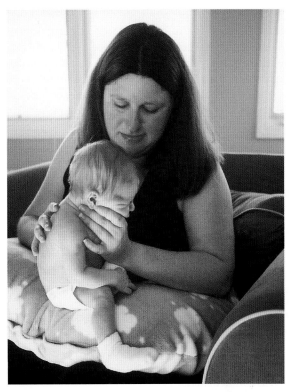

FIG. 23.16 The client burps the infant by holding the infant in the sitting position. Supporting the infant's head and chest with one hand and gently patting the back with the other hand.

the infant is able to take more formula before burping and should be burped halfway through feeding. Show the parents how to burp the infant over the shoulder or in a sitting position with the head supported while patting or rubbing the infant's back (Fig. 23.16).

Frequency and Amount. Instruct the parents to feed the infant every 3 to 4 hours but to avoid rigid scheduling and take cues from the infant. Hunger signs are the same as for breastfed infants. Teach the parents to begin feeding 15 to 30 mL (0.5 to 1 oz) at a time during the first 24 hours. Full-term infants may consume 2 to 3 oz of formula every 3 hours by day 3. Teach parents to increase the amount if the infant seems hungry and is not spitting up frequently (USDA, 2019).

Cautions. Sometimes, formula flow is too fast for infants. If this occurs, the infant may choke, gag, sputter, drool, or bite the nipple. Some infants suck without stopping to breathe frequently enough. To provide a rest period, the parent should tip the baby forward to stop the flow of milk. The following guidelines should be included to assist a parent in choosing the correct nipple size and ensure proper flow (USDA, 2019):

- The nipple should not be altered to increase or decrease the flow.
- When holding the bottle upside down, a few drops of milk should drip and then stop.
- Tailor the nipple size to the infant's needs and avoid a nipple hole that is too small or too large (increases the risk of choking).

Prolonged contact of teeth with milk promotes growth of bacteria and may lead to cavities once teeth erupt. Fluoride supplementation is determined by the water source and should be considered after the age of 6 months if unfluoridated water or premixed formula is used (CDC, 2021a).

Propping the bottle against a pillow or other object is never appropriate to feed an infant, due to the following possible problems (USDA, 2019):

- Propping the bottle increases the risk of choking due to liquid accidentally flowing into the lungs.
- Otitis media (middle ear infections) are more likely to occur due to the possibility of the fluid entering the middle ear and not draining properly (infants have horizontal Eustachian tubes).
- Overfeeding is more likely.
- Human contact is important during feeding for security and normal infant development.

Spitting Up. Young infants will often spit up small amounts, especially with burping. Sometimes spitting up can indicate overfeeding. As long as the infant is gaining weight and seems comfortable, spitting up is not a concern (USDA, 2019). If the infant forcefully vomits (projectile) or has blood or a dark green color in the vomit, the provider should be contacted immediately.

Weaning. The AAP recommends an infant be weaned from a bottle by 15 months of age. Infants bottle feeding longer than 18 months may be at higher risk for iron deficiency due to increased milk intake, a poor source of iron. This process can begin as early as 6 months of age, when a cup can be introduced (USDA, 2019). Night feedings should not continue past 12 months of age.

Infant Variations. Infants vary in their feeding preferences. Some infants drink from the bottle reluctantly. Although formula is usually given at room temperature, some infants take heated or cool formula better. The parent of a sleepy infant needs to use the same wake-up techniques described for the breastfeeding client.

Angling the tip of the nipple so it rubs the palate triggers the suck reflex in most infants. It may take patience and persistence to find the most effective techniques.

Evaluation

The parent should hold the infant and bottle correctly during feedings. They should be able to correctly describe formula preparation and the amount and frequency of feedings.

? KNOWLEDGE CHECK

17. What questions might a parent have about formula feeding?
18. Why should parents avoid propping bottles?

■ SUMMARY CONCEPTS

- Full-term breastfed infants need 85 to 100 kcal/kg (39 to 45 kcal/lb), and formula-fed infants need 100 to 110 kcal/kg (45 to 50 kcal/lb) daily. They may lose weight in the first few days after birth as a result of insufficient intake and normal loss of extracellular fluid and meconium.
- Lactogenesis I begins during pregnancy and continues after birth with the secretion of colostrum. Lactogenesis II begins 2 to 3 days after birth when transitional milk appears. Lactogenesis III is the time when mature milk replaces transitional milk.
- Colostrum is rich in protein, vitamins, minerals, and immunoglobulins. Transitional milk appears between colostrum and mature milk. Mature milk continues to provide immunoglobulins and antibacterial components.
- Breast milk has nutrients in proportions required by the newborn and in an easily digested form. Most commercial formulas are cow's milk adapted to simulate human milk but cannot fully replicate breast milk.
- Breast milk contains factors that help establish the normal intestinal flora and prevent infection. These include bifidus factor, leukocytes, lysozymes, lactoferrin, and immunoglobulins.
- A variety of commercial formulas are available. They include modified cow's milk formula, soy-based or hydrolyzed formulas, and formulas for preterm infants or those with special problems.
- The American Academy of Pediatrics recommends exclusive breastfeeding for the first 6 months and continued breastfeeding with the addition of complementary foods until the infant is 12 months old or longer, and thereafter, as long as mutually desired.
- Cow's milk should not be fed to infants during the first year of life.
- Factors that influence the parent's choice of feeding method include knowledge about each method, support from family and friends, cultural influences, and employment.
- Suckling at the breast causes release of oxytocin, which triggers the let-down reflex. It also causes the release of prolactin, which increases milk production.
- The principle of supply and demand applies to breastfeeding. Milk production increases when the infant feeds frequently. When breastfeeding ceases, prolactin is decreased, and eventually the alveoli of the breasts stop producing milk.
- Flat and inverted nipples should be identified during pregnancy. Creams and methods to toughen the nipples are not necessary.
- The nurse should assess the client's knowledge and the condition of the breasts and nipples. The LATCH score can be used to identify problems.
- The nurse can help the client establish breastfeeding by initiating early skin-to-skin contact, assisting with positioning the infant at the breast, and showing hand position to the client. The nurse should teach the client how to help the infant latch onto the breast, assess the position of

the mouth on the breast, and remove the infant from the breast.

- The parent should feed the infant with hunger cues 8 to 12 times per day, watching for nutritive sucking, audible swallowing, and infant satiety.
- Wake-up techniques for sleepy infants include unwrapping the blankets, placing the infant skin to skin, talking to the infant, changing the diaper, rubbing the infant's back, and expressing colostrum onto the breast.
- When infants suck from a bottle, they must push the tongue against the nipple to slow the flow of milk. When they suckle at the breast, they position the nipple far into the mouth so that the gums compress the areola.
- The nurse can help the client with engorged breasts by encouraging frequent nursing, application of warm compresses prior to nursing and cold compresses between feedings, massaging the breasts, and expressing milk to soften the areola.
- The nurse teaches the client with sore nipples how to check the positioning of the infant at the breast. The client should vary the position of the infant at the breast and apply breast milk and warm-water compresses to the nipples.
- Teaching for the client who plans to work and breastfeed includes expression of breast milk by hand or pump and proper storage of the milk.
- Clients who use formula need information about the types of formula available, correct preparation, and feeding techniques.
- Formula should be diluted exactly according to directions. It should not be heated in a microwave.
- Propping of bottles increases the risk of otitis media and infant choking.

Clinical Judgment and Next-Generation NCLEX® Examination-Style Questions

Infant Feeding Case Study

A nurse evaluates a 2-day-old infant born via cesarean delivery to a G1P1 24-year-old client at 39 weeks' gestation. The client labored for 14 hours prior to emergency cesarean for fetal distress. Apgars were 6 and 9. Birth weight = 7 lb, 1 oz (3.20 kg). No NICU stay was required, and the infant has been rooming-in with the client. The infant has been sleepy at the breast since the second breastfeeding with feedings averaging 10 minutes every 3 to 4 hours. When observing a breastfeeding, the client states, "My nipples are very tender most of the feeding and I do not think the baby is getting enough milk." Inspection of maternal nipples reveals slight cracking on the right side and nipple erythema. The infant presented with some jitteriness just prior to feeding but otherwise was alert and crying. The partner is present in the room.

1. **Highlight or place a check mark next to the assessment findings that require follow-up by the nurse or lactation consultant on the floor.**

Infant Assessment:
 Capillary glucose: 52 mg/dL
 Weight: 6 lb, 10 oz (3.005 kg)
 Skin: face, trunk, and extremities pink and dry with no rash
 Heart rate: 140
 Respiratory rate: 50
 Neuro: strong muscle tone and cry. All newborn reflexes intact, including sucking reflex

Maternal Assessment:
 Nipples appear flat but protrude slightly when stimulated. No inversion with pinch test.
 Right nipple with slight crack and redness; left nipple with slight redness.

Feeding Assessment:
 Client positions the baby slightly tilted toward the infant's back with the chin pointed downward and the hand supporting the posterior upper part of the head.
 Latch assessment: L = 1, A = 1, T = 2, C = 0, H = 0. Total score = 4

2. The nurse will teach the client the signs of hunger and encourage feeding the infant during this time. **Use an X to indicate which of the following infant behaviors indicate the infant is hungry and will most likely nurse successfully or are behaviors not related to signs of hunger (unrelated to feeding cues).**

Infant Behavior	Positive Hunger Cues	Unrelated to Feeding Cues
Jitteriness		
Lip smacking		
Hand-to-mouth movements		
Increased activity		
Moro reflex		
Sucking on hands		

3. The nurse is educating the parents of a 5-day-old term, formula-fed infant on formula amount needs. The infant weighs 6 lb, 14 oz (3.118 kg). The infant is eating every 4 hours in a 24-hour period. **Using the energy requirements during the first 3 months, choose which of the following would be the correct required caloric need per day if using full-term formula containing 20 cal/oz. (24-hour period). Round to the nearest one hundredth.**
A. 343 calories per day
B. 342.98 calories per day
C. 180 calories per day
D. 180.75 calories per day
Based on the above caloric needs, which of the following would be the correct amount (in ounces) the infant should be taking per feeding, based on eating every 4 hours in a 24 hour period? Round to the nearest tenth.
A. 3.25 oz
B. 2.45 oz
C. 2.86 oz
D. 2.14 oz

4. Indicate which nursing action/response listed in the far left column is appropriate for the client's question. Note that not all actions will be used.

Nurse's Action or Response	Client Question	Appropriate Nurse's Action or Response for Each Client Question
1. "Your baby's stomach is very small so your colostrum is sufficient for the first couple of days. During the first few days, infants often fall asleep at the breast but try to feed at least 8 times in a 24 hour period and watch for audible swallowing and at least 3–4 wet diapers by day 3"	"How do I keep my baby awake during a feeding?"	
2. "Vary the position of the baby every other feeding, avoid using soap on the nipples, and ensure the baby has a wide open latch as if it were taking a bite out of an apple"	"How do I tell if my baby is getting enough from my breast?"	
3. "Unwrap the baby and feed skin to skin. You can also remove the baby and rub the back"	"What can I do about my nipples being sore?"	

Nurse's Action or Response	Client Question	Appropriate Nurse's Action or Response for Each Client Question
4. "Longer feedings of 45 minutes or more indicate the baby is very hungry"	"After I go home, how do I know how long to feed my baby?"	
5. "Feedings will vary in length but generally, your baby will slow the suckling pattern greatly and his/her hands will be completely open and relaxed"		
6. "If you baby nurses at least 5 minutes and falls asleep, they should be getting enough milk"		
7. Use tea bags on the nipples and apply Vasoline or olive oil every few hours to the breast and nipple area.		

REFERENCES & READINGS

Academy of Breastfeeding Medicine (ABM). (2016a). ABM clinical protocol #10: Breastfeeding the late preterm infant (34 0/7 to 36 6/7 weeks gestation). *Breastfeeding Medicine*, *11*(10), 494–500.

Academy of Breastfeeding Medicine (ABM) Protocol Committee. (2016b). ABM clinical protocol #20: Engorgement. *Breastfeeding Medicine*, *11*(4), 159–163.

Academy of Breastfeeding Medicine (ABM) Protocol Committee. (2016c). ABM clinical protocol #26: Persistent pain with breastfeeding. *Breastfeeding Medicine*, *11*(2), 1–8.

Academy of Breastfeeding Medicine (ABM) Protocol Committee. (2017a). ABM clinical protocol #3: Hospital guidelines for the use of supplementary feedings in the healthy term breastfed neonate. *Breastfeeding Medicine*, *12*(3), 1–11.

Academy of Breastfeeding Medicine (ABM) Protocol Committee. (2017b). ABM clinical protocol #8: Human milk storage information for home use for full-term infants. *Breastfeeding Medicine*, *12*(7), 390–395.

Alex, A., Bhandary, E., & McGuire, K. P. (2020). Anatomy and physiology of the breast during pregnancy and lactation. In S. Alipour, & R. Omranipour (Eds.), *Diseases of the breast during pregnancy and lactation. Advances in experimental medicine and biology: 1252)*. Springer. https://doi.org/10.1007/978-3-030-41596-9_1.

American Academy of Pediatrics (AAP). (2012). Section on breastfeeding policy statement: Breastfeeding and the use of human milk. *Pediatrics*, *129*(3), e827–e841.

American Academy of Pediatrics (AAP). (2018). Why formula instead of cow's milk? https://www.healthychildren.org/English/ages-stages/baby/formula-feeding/Pages/Why-Formula-Instead-of-Cows-Milk.aspx.

American Academy of Pediatrics (AAP). (2021). *Breastfeeding overview*. https://services.aap.org/en/patient-care/breastfeeding/breastfeeding-overview/.

American Academy of Pediatrics & American College of Obstetricians and Gynecologists (AAP & ACOG). (2017). *Guidelines for perinatal care* (8th ed.).

American College of Obstetricians and Gynecologists (ACOG). (2019). *Breastfeeding your baby: Faq*. https://www.acog.org/womens-health/faqs/breastfeeding-your-baby.

American College of Obstetricians and Gynecologists (ACOG). (2021a). *Breastfeeding challenges*. ACOG Committee Opinion 820.

American College of Obstetricians and Gynecologists (ACOG). (2021b). *Opioid use and opioid use disorder in pregnancy*. ACOG Committee Opinion 771. Published 2012, reaffirmed 2021.

Association of Women's Health, Obstetric and Neonatal Nurses (AWHONN). (2015). Breastfeeding: An official position statement of the Association of Women's Health, Obstetric and Neonatal Nurses. *Journal of Women's Health, Obstetric and Neonatal Nurses*, *44*(1), 145–150.

Baby Friendly, USA. (2020). *Find facilities*. https://www.babyfriendlyusa.org.

Beauregard, J. L., Hamner, H. C., Chen, J., Avila-Rodriguez, W., Elam-Evans, L. D., & Perrine, C. G. (2019). Racial disparities in breastfeeding initiation and duration among U.S. infants born in

2015. *MMWR Morbidity Mortality Weekly Report, 68*, 745–748. https://doi.org/10.15585/mmwr.mm6834a3.

Busch, D. W., Sibert-Flagg, J. S., Ryngaert, M., & Scott, A. (2018). NAPNAP position statement on breastfeeding. *Journal of Public Health Care, 33*(1). https://doi.org/10.1016/j.pedhc.2018.08.011.

Bzikowska-Jura, A., Czerwonogrodzka-Senczyna, A., Olędzka, G., Szostak-Węgierek, D., Weker, H., & Wesołowska, A. (2018). Maternal nutrition and body composition during breastfeeding: Association with human milk composition. *Nutrients, 10*(10), 1379. https://doi.org/10.3390/nu10101379.

Centers for Disease Control and Prevention (CDC). (2019). *Storage and preparation of breast milk*. U.S. Department of Health and Human Services. https://www.cdc.gov/breastfeeding/pdf/preparation-of-breast-milk_H.pdf.

Centers for Disease Control and Prevention (CDC). (2020a). *Breastfeeding report card*. U.S. Department of Health and Human Services. https://www.cdc.gov/breastfeeding/data/reportcard.htm.

Center for Disease Control (CDC). (2020b). *Breastfeeding: Weaning*. U.S. Department of Health and Human Services. https://www.cdc.gov/nutrition/infantandtoddlernutrition/breastfeeding/weaning.html.

Center for Disease Control (CDC). (2021a). *Choosing an infant formula*. U.S. Department of Health and Human Services. https://www.cdc.gov/nutrition/InfantandToddlerNutrition/formula-feeding/choosing-an-infant-formula.html.

Centers for Disease Control and Prevention (CDC). (2021b). *Coronavirus disease (COVID-19) and breastfeeding*. U.S. Department of Health and Human Services. https://www.cdc.gov/breastfeeding/breastfeeding-special-circumstances/maternal-or-infant-illnesses/covid-19-and-breastfeeding.html.

Center for Disease Control (CDC). (2021c). *Public opinions about breastfeeding*. U.S. Department of Health and Human Services. https://www.cdc.gov/breastfeeding/data/healthstyles_survey/index.htm.

Coentro, V. S., Perrella, S. L., Lai, C. T., Rea, A., Murray, K., & Geddes, D. T. (2021). Impact of nipple shield use on milk transfer and maternal nipple pain. *Breastfeeding Medicine, 16*(3), 222–229. https://doi.org/10.1089/bfm.2020.0110.

DiTomasso, D., & Paiva, A. L. (2018). Neonatal weight matters: An examination of weight changes in full-term breastfeeding newborns during the first 2 weeks of life. *Journal of Human Lactation, 34*(1), 86–92. https://doi.org/10.1177/0890334417722508.

Hagan, J. F., Shaw, J. S., & Duncan, P. M. (Eds.). (2017). *Bright futures: Guidelines for health supervision of infants, children and adolescents* (4th ed.). American Academy of Pediatrics.

Hermanson, A., & Astrand, L. L. (2020). The effects of early pacifier use on breastfeeding: A randomized controlled trial. *Women and Birth, 33*(5), e473–e482. https://doi.org/10.1016/j.wombi.2019.10.001.

Janke, J. (2021). Newborn nutrition. In K. Simpson, P. Creehan, N. O'Brien-Abel, C. Roth, & A. Rohan (Eds.), *AWHONN's perinatal nursing* (5th ed., pp. 609–650). Wolters Kluwer.

Janzon, A., Goodrich, J. K., Koren, O., TEDDY Study Group, Waters, J. L., & Ley, R. E. (2019). Interactions between the gut microbiome and mucosal immunoglobulins A, M, and G in the developing infant gut. *mSystems, 4*(6), e00612–e00619. https://doi.org/10.1128/mSystems.00612-19.

Jensen, D., Wallace, S., & Kelsay, P. (1994). Latch: A breastfeeding charting system and documentation tool. *Journal of Obstetric, Gynecologic, and Neonatal Nursing, 23*(1), 27–32.

Karimi, F. Z., Miri, H. H., Khadivzadeh, T., & Maleki-Saghooni, N. (2020). The effect of mother-infant skin-to-skin contact immediately after birth on exclusive breastfeeding: A systematic review and meta-analysis. *Journal of the Turkish-German Gynecological Association, 21*(1), 46–56. https://doi.org/10.4274/jtgga.galenos.2019.2018.0138.

Lawrence, R. A. (2022). *Breastfeeding: A guide for the medical profession* (9th ed., pp. 58-92). Elsevier.

Lien, E. L., Richard, C., & Hoffman, D. R. (2017). DHA and ARA addition to infant formula: Current status and future research directions. *Prostaglandins, Leukotrienes and Essential Fatty Acids, 128*, 26–40. https://doi.org/10.1016/j.plefa.2017.09.005.

Lyons, S., Currie, S., & Smith, D. M. (2019). Learning from women with a body mass index (BMI) ≥30 kg/m2 who have breastfed and/or are breastfeeding: A qualitative interview study. *Maternal Child Health Journal, 23*(5), 648–656. https://doi.org/10.1007/s10995-018-2679-7.

Maaks, D. L., Starr, N. B., Brady, M. A., Gaylord, N. M., Driessnack, M., & Duderstadt, K. (2021). *Burn's pediatric primary care* (7th ed.). Elsevier.

Miyoshi, Y., Suenaga, H., Aoki, M., & Tanaka, S. (2020). Determinants of excessive weight loss in breastfed full-term newborns at a baby-friendly hospital: A retrospective cohort study. *International Breastfeeding Journal, 15*(19). https://doi.org/10.1186/s13006-020-00263-2.

Mujawar, N. S., & Archana, N. J. (2017). Hypernatremia in the neonate: Neonatal hypernatremia and hypernatremic dehydration in neonates receiving exclusive breastfeeding. *Indian Journal of Critical Care Medicine, 21*(1), 30–33. https://doi.org/10.4103/0972-5229.198323.

Newton, E. R., & Stuebe, A. M. (2021). Lactation and breastfeeding. In M. Landon, H. Galan, E. Jauniaux, D. Driscoll, V. Berghella, W. Grobman, S. Kilpatrick, & A. Cahill (Eds.), *Gabbe's Obstetrics: Normal and problem pregnancies* (8th ed., pp. 475–502). Elsevier.

Ordean, A., & Kim, G. (2020). Cannabis use during lactation: Literature review and clinical recommendations. *Journal of Obstetrics and Gynaecology, 42*(10), 1248–1253. https://doi.org/10.1016/j.jogc.2019.11.003.

Rajani, P. S., Martin, H., Groetch, M., & Jarvinen, K. M. (2020). Presentation and management of food allergy in breastfed infants and risks of maternal elimination diets. *Journal of Allergy and Clinical Immunology: In Practice, 8*(1), 52–67.

Rohan, A. J. (2021). Newborn physical assessment. In K. Simpson, P. Creehan, N. O'Brien-Abel, C. Roth, & A. Rohan (Eds.), *AWHONN's perinatal nursing* (5th ed., pp. 579–608). Wolters Kluwer.

Romo-Palafox, M. J., Pomeranz, J. L., & Harris, J. L. (2020). Infant formula and toddler milk marketing and caregiver's provision to young children. *Maternal and Child Nutrition, 16*, e12962. https://doi.org/10.1111/mcn.12962.

Spatz, D. L. (2018). Helping mothers reach personal breastfeeding goals. *Nursing Clinics of North America, 53*(2), 253–261. https://doi.org/10.1016/j.cnur.2018.01.011.

Spatz, D. L., Riccardo, D., Muller, J. A., Powell, R., Rigourd, V., Yates, A., Geddes, D. T., van Goudoever, J. B., & Bode, L. (2021). Promoting and protecting human milk and breastfeeding in a COVID-19 world. *Frontier in Pediatrics, 8*. https://doi.org/10.3389/fped.2020.633700.

Thulier, D. (2017). Challenging expected patterns of weight loss in full-term breastfeeding neonates born by cesarean. *Journal of*

Obstetric Gynecologic and Neonatal Nurses, 46(1), 18–28. https://doi.org/10.1016/j.jogn.2016.11.006.

U.S. Department of Agriculture (USDA). (2019). *Infant nutrition and feeding: A guide for use in the supplemental nutrition program for women, infants and children (WIC).* https://wicworks.fns.usda.gov/sites/default/files/media/document/Infant_Nutrition_and_Feeding_Guide.pdf.

U.S. Department of Agriculture (USDA). (2020). *Dietary guidelines for Americans: Executive summary.* https://www.dietaryguidelines.gov/sites/default/files/2021-03/DGA_2020-2025_ExecutiveSummary_English.pdf.

U.S. Department of Labor, Wage and Hour Division (n.d). *Break time for nursing mothers.* https://www.dol.gov/agencies/whd/nursing-mothers#:~:text=Federal%20law%20requires%20employers%20to,Section%207%20of%20the%20FLSA.

U.S. Department of Health and Human Services (DHHS). (2017). *Are breast pumps covered by the affordable care act?.* https://www.hhs.gov/answers/affordable-care-act/are-breast-pumps-covered-by-the-affordable-care-act/index.html.

U.S. Department of Health and Human Services (DHHS). (2020). *Healthy people 2030.* https://health.gov/healthypeople/objectives-and-data/browse-objectives/infants.

Walker, M. (2017). *Breastfeeding management for the clinician: Using the evidence.* Jones & Bartlett Learning.

World Health Organization (WHO). (2020). *Infant and young child feeding.* https://www.who.int/news-room/fact-sheets/detail/infant-and-young-child-feeding.

World Health Organization (WHO)/United Nations Children's Fund (UNICEF). (2020). *Protecting promoting and supporting breastfeeding: The baby-friendly hospital initiative for small, sick and preterm newborns.*

High-Risk Newborn: Complications Associated with Gestational Age and Development

Della Wrightson

OBJECTIVES

After studying this chapter, you should be able to:

1. Contrast characteristics of the preterm infant with those of the term infant.
2. Explain the special problems of the preterm infant and explain the nursing care for each.
3. Explain the complications that may result from premature birth.
4. Describe the implications of late preterm birth.
5. Describe the characteristics and problems of the infant with dysmaturity syndrome.
6. Explain the effects of fetal growth restriction.
7. Compare the problems of the large-for-gestational-age infant with those of the small-for-gestational-age infant.

Maternity nurses identify and begin care for the immediate needs of neonates with complications until nurses from the neonatal intensive care unit (NICU) can assume care. NICU nurses often attend births when complications of the newborn are expected.

CARE OF HIGH-RISK NEWBORNS

Nurses care for minor illness or conditions in the mother-baby unit or the normal newborn nursery, but more serious problems require intensive care in NICUs, specialized nurseries designed for that purpose.

Multidisciplinary Approach

The care of infants with problems at birth often involves collaboration among many different professionals. In the hospital setting, such professionals may include nurses, nurse practitioners, physicians with different specialties, respiratory therapists, laboratory personnel, and pharmacists. Care from social workers, physical therapists, feeding specialists, occupational therapists, and infant development experts may begin during the hospital stay and continue after the infant is discharged. Nurses often coordinate this care and explain or clarify it for parents.

PRETERM INFANTS

Preterm infants (also called *premature infants*) are born before the completion of 37 weeks' gestation (World Health Organization [WHO], 2018). Preterm infants can further be classified as **extremely preterm** (<28 weeks' gestation);

moderately preterm (28 to <34 weeks' gestation); or **late preterm** (34 to <37 weeks' gestation) (Shviraga & Hensley, 2021).

The word *preterm* is sometimes confused with the term **low birth weight (LBW)**, which refers to infants weighing 2500 g (5 lb, 8 oz) or less at birth and of any gestational age. **Very-low-birth-weight (VLBW)** infants weigh 1500 g (3 lb, 5 oz) or less at birth. **Extremely low-birth-weight (ELBW)** infants weigh 1000 g (2 lb, 3 oz) or less at birth. Although most of these infants are preterm, others are full term and have failed to grow normally while in the uterus, a condition called **fetal growth restriction (FGR)** or intrauterine growth restriction (IUGR).

Incidence and Etiology
Scope of Problem

Advances in technology have resulted in infant survival at much lower birth weights than ever before. Despite these advances, prematurity and its complications are the second leading cause of infant mortality in the United States. After steadily declining, the percent of live births that are preterm have been on the rise since 2015 (March of Dimes, 2020). In terms of the suffering of infants and their parents, lost potential, and medical expense, preterm birth is extremely costly. Infant mortality and morbidity rates increase as gestational age decreases.

Causes

The exact causes of preterm birth are not known, but all risk factors in pregnancy are potential causes (see Chapter 16, Box 16.1).

Prevention

Prevention of preterm birth is best accomplished by provision of adequate prenatal care for every pregnant woman to identify and treat risk factors as early as possible. Teaching women signs of preterm labor will encourage them to seek care early, maximizing treatment outcomes.

Characteristics of Preterm Infants

Characteristics of preterm infants vary, depending on gestational age. For example, the appearance and problems of infants born at 34 weeks of gestation are different from those of infants born at 26 weeks of gestation. Some characteristics, however, are common to all preterm infants.

Appearance

Preterm infants often appear frail and weak, and they have less developed flexor muscles and muscle tone compared with full-term infants. Their extremities are limp and offer little or no resistance when moved. Premature newborns typically lie in an extended position (see Chapter 21, Fig. 21.20). The infant's head is large compared with the rest of the body.

Preterm infants lack subcutaneous or white fat, which makes their thin skin appear red and translucent, with blood vessels being clearly visible. The nipples and areola may be barely perceptible, but vernix caseosa and lanugo may be abundant. Plantar creases are absent in infants younger than 32 weeks of gestation (see Chapter 21, Fig. 21.26).

The pinnae of the ears are flat and soft and contain little cartilage (see Chapter 21, Fig. 21.28). They lack the rolled-over appearance of the pinnae of a full-term infant. In the female infant, the clitoris and labia minora appear large and are not covered by the small, separated labia majora. The male infant may have undescended testes, with a small, smooth scrotal sac (see Chapter 21 Figs. 21.29 and 21.30).

Behavior

The behavior of preterm infants varies, depending on gestational age. It often differs from that of full-term infants because of the stress of having to adjust to extrauterine life before they are ready. Premature newborns may have poor development of flexion and little excess energy for maintaining muscle tone. They are easily exhausted by noise and routine activities. Their responses are varied, including lowered oxygenation levels and stress-related behavior changes. The cry may be feeble.

Assessment and Care of Common Problems

Because preterm infants are "unfinished" in their growth and development, they are prone to problems affecting all systems and body processes.

Problems with Respiration

Problems of the respiratory system are a major concern because preterm newborns have immature lungs but must go through the same processes as the full-term infant to begin breathing. The presence of surfactant in adequate amounts is of primary importance. Surfactant reduces surface tension in the alveoli and prevents their collapse with expiration. It allows the lungs to inflate with lower negative pressure, decreasing the work of breathing. Infants born before surfactant production is adequate develop respiratory distress syndrome (RDS). In addition, preterm infants have a poorly developed cough reflex and narrow respiratory passages, which increase the risk for respiratory difficulty.

Assessment. The infant's respiratory status should be observed constantly. The lungs are assessed for adventitious breath sounds or areas of absent breath sounds.

The nurse differentiates periodic breathing from apneic spells. **Periodic breathing** is the cessation of breathing for 5 to 10 seconds followed by 10 to 15 seconds of ventilation (Martin & Eichenwald, 2022). Changes in color or heart rate do not occur. Although periodic breathing sometimes occurs in term infants, preterm infants experience it more often.

Apneic spells involve absence of breathing lasting more than 20 seconds or less if accompanied by cyanosis, pallor, bradycardia, or hypotonia (Crowley & Martin, 2020). Apneic spells are common in preterm infants, increasing in incidence with lower gestational age. Apnea without an identified cause in a preterm infant is called *idiopathic apnea* or *apnea of prematurity* and generally improves as the infant matures. Episodes may occur along with periodic breathing, and the infant may require gentle tactile stimulation, bag and mask ventilation, medications, or assisted ventilation. Apnea should be investigated because it may be related to other conditions.

The nurse observes the effort required for breathing and the location and severity of retractions. Retractions are particularly noticeable in preterm infants, whose weak chest wall is drawn in with each inspiration. The excessive **compliance** (elasticity) of the chest cage during retractions occurs because the bones of the chest wall are very pliable. This may interfere with full expansion of the lungs.

Grunting may be an early sign of RDS. It closes the glottis and increases the pressure within the alveoli. This keeps the alveoli partially open during expiration and increases the amount of oxygen absorbed.

Nursing Interventions. Interventions focus on collaborating with other team members such as the respiratory therapist to manage technical equipment and facilitate removal of secretions.

Working with Respiratory Equipment. An oxygen hood may be used for infants who can breathe independently but need extra oxygen. The hood is a plastic dome that fits over the infant's head or over the head and upper body. The infant breathes the higher levels of oxygen within the hood, and the device does not interfere with access to the rest of the infant's body for care (Fig. 24.1).

Oxygen also may be given by nasal cannula to the infant who breathes well independently. After discharge, many preterm infants continue to receive oxygen via nasal cannula at home. Oxygen should be warmed to maintain body temperature and humidified to prevent insensible water loss and drying of the delicate mucous membranes.

Continuous positive airway pressure (CPAP) may be necessary to keep the alveoli open and improve expansion of the lungs. CPAP can be delivered via nasal prongs, a mask, or an endotracheal tube. The infant may need conventional mechanical ventilation when respiratory failure, severe apnea, bradycardia, or other conditions are present. High-frequency ventilation may be used to provide very fast respirations with

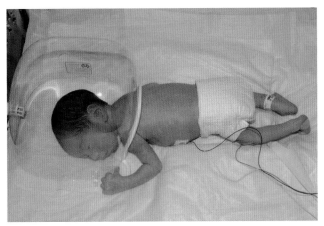

FIG. 24.1 The oxygen hood is one way of delivering oxygen to an infant who can breathe unassisted. (Courtesy Cheryl Briggs, RN.)

less pressure and volume. This helps decrease lung injury from pressure (barotrauma) and volume (volutrauma).

When oxygen is administered, the level of oxygen in the infant's blood should be monitored. Arterial blood may be drawn for testing oxygen levels. **Pulse oximetry** may also be used. This method is less invasive and provides continuous information about oxygen partial pressure (Po_2) levels through sensors attached to the skin. Nurses and respiratory therapists titrate oxygen, depending on the pulse oximetry or arterial oxygen levels, according to facility policy.

The nurse should observe the infant's increasing or decreasing dependence on breathing assistance and need for oxygen during activity such as handling, feeding, and linen changes. An increase in oxygen and/or other respiratory support settings may be needed during care activities.

Positioning the Infant. The prone and side-lying positions are not recommended for normal newborn infants because they are associated with an increased incidence of sudden infant death syndrome (SIDS). In the preterm infant, however, the prone position increases oxygenation and improves lung mechanics (Gardner, Enzman-Hines & Nyp, 2021).

The reason for prone positioning should be explained to parents. Supine positioning for sleep is begun as soon as the infant can tolerate it and before discharge so the infant can become accustomed to sleeping on the back before going home. The supine position often can be used at approximately 32 weeks' gestational age (Baessler et al., 2019). Before discharge parents should be taught the importance of supine positioning in preventing SIDS. It is important for nurses to model SIDS prevention by placing infants in the supine position as soon as infants are able and removing any soft, loose items from the bed because parents are more likely to mimic the conditions they saw in the hospital (Baessler et al., 2019).

Suctioning Secretions. The weak or absent cough reflex and very small air passages make the preterm infant's airways susceptible to obstruction by mucus. The nurse checks the suction equipment at the beginning of each shift to ensure that it is available and functioning properly at all times.

The infant is suctioned only as necessary. Suction should be gentle to avoid traumatizing the delicate mucous membranes.

Trauma could cause edema, decreasing the size of the air passages further and leading to more respiratory difficulty.

Suctioning also provides an entry for organisms and decreases oxygenation. The procedure causes changes in heart rate, blood pressure, and cerebral blood flow. Suction should be applied for only 5 to 10 seconds at a time. The mouth is suctioned before the nose because stimulation of the nares causes reflex inspiration that could cause aspiration of fluids in the infant's mouth. Increased oxygen should be provided before and after each suction attempt. To avoid harmful hyperoxia, the increase should be based on each infant's individual clinical response to suctioning and is rarely greater than 20%. A rest period should be provided after suctioning (Gardner, Enzman-Hines & Nyp, 2021).

Maintaining Hydration. Adequate hydration is essential to keep secretions thin so they can be removed by drainage or suction. If infants become dehydrated, secretions will become thick and viscous and could obstruct tiny air passages. Fluid intake should be increased, as ordered by the provider, if secretions seem to indicate even minimal dehydration.

? KNOWLEDGE CHECK

1. How does the appearance of a preterm infant differ from that of a full-term infant?
2. What factors contribute to respiratory problems in preterm infants?
3. What nursing responsibilities relate to care of preterm respiratory problems?

Problems with Thermoregulation

Although heat loss can be a thermoregulation problem for full-term infants, it is even more significant in preterm infants. Their skin is thin, with blood vessels near the surface, and little subcutaneous white fat for insulation. As a result, heat loss is rapid. The preterm infant's shorter time in the uterus allows less brown fat to accumulate before birth, impairing the infant's ability to produce heat.

Preterm infants have a larger head in proportion to body size compared with full-term infants. The preterm infant's extended extremities increase exposure to air and thus heat loss. Their body surface area in proportion to their body mass is larger than that of adults (Agren, 2020). The temperature control center of the brain of preterm infants is less mature and may be further impaired by asphyxia. These conditions all contribute to heat loss.

Complications from heat loss are more likely to develop in preterm infants. These include hypoglycemia, respiratory problems, metabolic acidosis, pulmonary vasoconstriction, impaired surfactant production, and more respiratory difficulty. In addition, calories used for heat production are unavailable for growth and weight gain.

Assessment. The infant's temperature is monitored continuously by a skin probe attached to the heat control mechanism of the radiant warmer or incubator. The probe should be placed on the upper right quadrant of the infant's abdomen, or as recommended by the manufacturer (Gardner & Cammack, 2021). The infant should not lie on the probe.

Temperatures should be maintained between 36.5 and 37.5°C (97.7 to 99.5°F) (Gardner & Cammack, 2021). The infant's skin temperature as shown on the bed or monitor should be recorded every 30 to 60 minutes initially and every 1 to 3 hours when the infant is stable. The axillary temperature should be compared with the heat control reading to ensure that the equipment is functioning properly.

Rectal temperatures should not be used in preterm neonates. Checking a core temperature is of little value in a neonate because it may not show a decrease until the infant has completely decompensated (Brand & Shippey, 2021).

Indications of hypothermia include poor feeding or intolerance to feedings in an infant who previously had little difficulty, irritability, lethargy, poor muscle tone, cool skin temperature, and mottled skin. Hypoglycemia and respiratory distress may be the first signs that the infant's temperature is low. A decrease in weight gain or weight loss may occur over time. Because temperature instability may be an early sign of infection, the nurse should assess for other evidence that infection may be present.

Being too hot (hyperthermic) may be just as detrimental to a preterm infant as being too cold. Overheating leads to an increase in the metabolic rate, with increased oxygen and glucose needs and insensible water losses. Children and adults compensate for being too warm by sweating. Preterm infants are unable to sweat and will need interventions to help dissipate heat. The most common causes of hyperthermia are iatrogenic (e.g., excessive blankets and clothing, warm room temperature, a loose skin temperature probe, or a radiant warmer without servo control). Nonenvironmental factors that may cause hyperthermia include sepsis, central nervous system injury, medication side effects, and dehydration.

CRITICAL TO REMEMBER

Signs of Inadequate Thermoregulation

General
Axillary temperature <36.5°C or >37.5°C (<97.7°F or >99.5°F)
Skin temperature <36.2°C or >37.2°C (<97.2°F or >99°F)
Poor feeding or feeding intolerance
Lethargy
Irritability
Weak cry or suck
Decreased muscle tone
Apnea

Hypothermia
Cool skin temperature
Mottled, pale, or acrocyanotic skin
Signs of hypoglycemia
Bradycardia
Poor weight gain, if chronic

Hyperthermia
Warm, flushed, or red skin
Tachycardia
Tachypnea
Seizures

Nursing Interventions. Maintenance of heat in preterm infants involves the same basic nursing care principles as for the full-term infant. These principles, however, should be adapted to meet the needs of the preterm infant.

Maintaining a Neutral Thermal Environment. A neutral thermal environment (NTE) is especially important to prevent the need for increased oxygen to maintain the infant's body temperature. The temperature necessary to maintain the NTE varies according to gestational age. Charts are available that indicate the appropriate temperature setting to maintain an NTE according to the infant's size and maturity.

The delivery room should be warm to decrease heat loss at birth. Immediately after birth, the infant is dried with warm towels and placed on the client's abdomen or a prewarmed radiant warmer for care, and a hat is put on the infant's head. Before infants are dried, those who are younger than 32 weeks of gestation (or up to 35 weeks if the baby is small for age or the environment is cool) are placed in a polyethylene bag or wrap that covers the body from the shoulders down. This prevents heat loss by evaporation during initial care and transfer to the NICU and is used until the infant's condition is stabilized. It also decreases insensible water loss. The infant should be placed on a chemical thermal mattress, which can provide heat for up to an hour after activation (Brand & Shippey, 2021).

Because they produce heat less effectively and lose more heat than larger or older preterm infants, smaller, less-mature infants need more warmth to maintain body heat. Radiant warmers or incubators are used until infants can maintain normal body temperature alone. Some devices convert from a radiant warmer to an incubator and back again to eliminate the need to move the infant from one device to another.

Infants needing many procedures are usually placed under an open radiant warmer to make it easier to see them and work with equipment. However, air currents around an unclothed infant can cause heat loss by convection despite the heat generated by the warmer. Doors near the warmer should be closed and traffic kept to a minimum to decrease convective heat loss. The infant should receive only warmed oxygen because thermal receptors in the face are very sensitive to cold. Cold oxygen could quickly lead to cold stress.

Equipment and caregivers should not come between the infant and the heat source, preventing heat from reaching the infant. A transparent plastic blanket over the infant allows heat from the warmer to pass across to the infant. The blanket decreases convective heat loss from exposure to drafts and insensible water loss while maintaining visibility of the infant's body.

Incubators are used for infants who do not need to be under radiant warmers. They have double walls to minimize radiant heat loss to the cooler outer walls. Warmed air circulating inside the incubator provides heat. Humidity should be added to decrease evaporative heat loss and insensible water loss, especially in very preterm infants. Incubators should be placed away from air-conditioning ducts or windows that may affect the incubator temperature. Alarms to detect high or low temperature should be turned on at all times.

When infants are in incubators, the nurse should keep portholes and doors closed as much as possible. A significant amount of heat is lost each time the incubator is opened, and it takes time to build up the heat again. When removed from the incubator for procedures or holding, infants should be wrapped in heated blankets and a hat applied. Incubator doors should be closed while the infant is outside to retain the heat inside. Infants should be placed under a radiant warmer or on a surface padded with warm blankets for procedures that cannot be performed inside the incubator. A heat lamp provides an alternative source of heat.

Although temperature regulation in preterm infants is usually provided in incubators until infants can maintain their own temperature, warmth is also provided when parents hold them. Adequate temperature is maintained in stable infants during skin-to-skin care (SSC).

Weaning to an Open Crib. Preparation of infants for moving to an open crib should begin early. When stable, infants can be dressed in a shirt, diaper, and hat while in the incubator. Clothing conserves heat and helps infants adjust to a different temperature on the face than the rest of the body. Infants who weigh about 1600 g (3 lb, 8 oz), have a consistent weight gain for 5 days, have no medical complications, and are tolerating feedings can begin gradual weaning from external heat (Gardner & Cammack, 2021).

Each NICU has its own protocol for the weaning process. The incubator temperature is usually decreased gradually. It is raised if the infant's temperature falls below the normal range. If the temperature remains stable, the process can continue the next day.

When the infant is ready for transfer to an open crib, double-wrapping with warm blankets helps insulate body heat. Sleep sacks (sleepers made of blanket material and closed at the bottom) are often used when infants are dressed. The temperature is assessed at gradually increasing intervals until the infant's temperature is stable and then may be monitored on a routine schedule. A blanket is added for a low temperature, but if the temperature does not rise to normal, the infant is returned to the incubator.

Nurses should observe infants carefully during the first few days after transfer to an open crib. Signs that may indicate inadequate thermoregulation include decreased weight gain, poor feeding, or increased requirement for oxygen.

Problems with Fluid and Electrolyte Balance

Preterm infants lose fluid very easily, and the loss increases with the degree of prematurity. The rapid respiratory rate and the use of oxygen increase fluid losses from the lungs. Their thin skin has little protective subcutaneous white fat and is more permeable than the skin of term infants. The large surface area in proportion to body weight and lack of flexion further increase transepidermal water losses. Radiant warmers raise insensible water losses by 40% to 50% compared with loss in an incubator (Gardner & Cammack, 2021). Heat from phototherapy lights causes even more fluid to be lost through the skin.

The ability of the kidneys to concentrate or dilute urine is poor, causing a fragile balance between dehydration and overhydration. Great differences in fluid needs occur, depending on variables such as the infant's size, gestational age, insensible water losses, and medical needs. Normal urinary output is 1 to 3 mL/kg/hour for preterm infants for the first few days. After 24 hours of life, output less than 0.5 mL/kg/hour is considered oliguria (Blackburn, 2018).

Regulation of electrolytes by the kidneys is also a problem. Preterm infants need higher intakes of sodium because the kidneys do not reabsorb it well. If they receive too much sodium, however, they may be unable to increase sodium excretion adequately and are susceptible to sodium and water overload.

Assessment. The nurse should be alert for fluid overload or deficit. Monitoring intake and output of fluids helps determine fluid balance. The infant's intake and output by all routes are carefully calculated. Parenteral fluids, feeding tube intake, medication, and oral fluids are included when measuring intake. Output from regurgitation, drainage tubes, stools, and urine should be measured. The nurse should also keep track of the amount of blood taken for laboratory tests because the loss can be substantial and the infant cannot make new blood fast enough.

Urine Output. There are several methods of measuring urine output. Plastic bags that adhere to the perineum are not suitable for the preterm infant because they may damage the fragile skin. Weighing diapers is less harmful to the infant. The weight of dry diapers is subtracted from the weight of wet diapers to determine the amount of urine excreted. One gram (1 g) is equivalent to 1 mL of urine. However, humidification may add moisture to the diaper, and a radiant warmer may cause evaporation of urine on the diaper. When precise measurement is essential, diapers can be fastened instead of being placed open under the infant.

Specific gravity should be checked to determine whether urine is more concentrated or dilute than expected. Urine is collected by placing gauze or a cotton ball at the perineum. The urine-specific gravity should range between 1.005 and 1.012 (Nyp et al., 2021).

Weight. Changes in the infant's weight can give an indication of fluid gain or loss, especially if the changes are sudden or greater than would be expected. The undressed infant should be weighed at the same time each day with the same scale. Very small infants are often placed in a bed with a scale so they are not disturbed for daily weighing. They may be weighed two to three times a day to monitor their fluid status more closely.

Signs of Dehydration or Overhydration. The nurse should observe for signs that indicate the infant has received too little or too much fluid.

CRITICAL TO REMEMBER

Signs of Fluid Imbalance in the Newborn

Dehydration
Urine output <1 mL/kg/hour
Urine specific gravity >1.012
Weight loss greater than expected
Dry skin and mucous membranes
Sunken anterior fontanel
Poor tissue turgor
Blood—Elevated sodium, protein, and hematocrit levels
Hypotension

Overhydration
Urine output >3 mL/kg/hour
Urine specific gravity <1.005
Edema
Weight gain greater than expected
Bulging fontanels
Blood—Decreased sodium, protein, and hematocrit levels
Moist breath sounds
Difficulty breathing

Nursing Interventions. Intravenous (IV) fluids should be carefully regulated using infusion control devices that administer fluid with a precision of 0.01 mL/hour to help prevent fluid volume overload (Nyp et al., 2021). IV medications should be diluted in as little fluid as is consistent with safe administration of the drug and should be considered when intake is measured. Starting IV lines on infants can be a difficult procedure. Once IV access is achieved, care should be taken to prevent infiltration.

IV sites should be assessed at least every hour for signs of infiltration; some solutions, if they infiltrate, cause extensive damage as a result of tissue sloughing. When identified, IV infiltrations require immediate intervention.

Many infants have central venous catheters or umbilical lines that should be assessed for infection and position changes. Small blood transfusions may be necessary to replace blood drawn for frequent laboratory tests.

Problems with the Skin

Preterm infants have fragile, permeable, easily damaged skin. They often have endotracheal tubes, IV lines, electrodes, and other equipment that should be maintained in place, but standard adhesive tape should not be used because it can be very damaging to the skin. Removal of adhesive tape may strip the epidermal layer of the skin, causing pain and increasing transepidermal water loss and the risk for infection. Preparations used to disinfect the skin before invasive procedures can injure fragile skin and may be absorbed. Diaper dermatitis, or diaper rash, is common in infants.

Assessment. The nurse should frequently assess the condition of the infant's skin and record any changes, using a valid and reliable tool. The infant's response to products used for cleansing and disinfection should be noted.

Nursing Interventions. Guidelines for evidence-based practice in care of the neonate's skin have been developed

by two prominent neonatal nursing organization: the Association of Women's Health, Obstetric and Neonatal Nurses (AWHONN) and the National Association of Neonatal Nurses (NANN) (AWHONN, 2018). Medical adhesives that effectively secure devices and monitoring equipment that cause the least injury to tissues should be used. Skin can be protected from adhesives by using silicone-based protective films.

Adhesives should be removed slowly and gently by pulling horizontally parallel to the skin. The interface between the adhesive and the skin should be wet with gauze or saline pledgets. Mineral oil, petrolatum, or silicone-based adhesive removers also can be used to wet the area. (AWHONN, 2018).

All disinfectants have potential risks when used on neonates. Aqueous chlorhexidine gluconate solutions are commonly used at this time. Povidone–iodine may injure the skin and may have toxic effects on the thyroid gland in premature infants. All disinfectants should be removed with sterile water or saline. Alcohol should not be used (AWHONN, 2018; Lund & Durand, 2021).

Cleansers with a pH of 5.5 to 7 may be used for bathing infants. Preterm infants usually should not be bathed every day. Warm water without soap should be used for infants younger than 32 weeks of gestational age for the first week after birth. Sterile water is not necessary unless there are concerns about the safety of tap water or there is a break in skin integrity (AWHONN, 2018; Lund & Durand, 2021). Stable preterm infants without umbilical IV lines may be immersed in water that covers the shoulders for bathing if there are no contraindications. Swaddled bathing, in which the infant is wrapped in a blanket and then immersed in water for bathing, also may be used. Tubs should be used by only one infant for the duration of hospital stay or cleaned well if used between infants.

Humidity in incubators should be regulated to reduce the drying effects of heat. Emollients can help reduce fissures in dry skin and transepidermal water loss. They are safe to use under radiant warmers and during phototherapy (AWHONN, 2018). The infant's skin should be observed for signs of infection.

Infants and their equipment should be positioned to avoid undue pressure on the skin. The most common cause of pressure-related injuries in neonates is from equipment. Skin breakdown may occur over any bony prominence but especially on the head, which has the largest body surface area. Frequent position changes are important but should be based on the infant's ability to tolerate changes. Alcohol-free skin protectant and pressure-reducing devices may help prevent skin breakdown (AWHONN, 2018).

Problems with Infection

Preterm infants are often exposed to situations that may cause infection. A prolonged stay in the hospital increases the likelihood of acquiring an infection from multiple exposures to organisms. Sepsis may occur in up to 25% of VLBW infants (Haslam, 2020). Many preterm infants have one or more episodes of sepsis during their hospital stay. Factors contributing to the high rate of infection include exposure to infection in utero, lack of adequate passive immunity from the transfer of immunoglobulin G (IgG) during the third trimester of pregnancy, and immature response to infection.

Infants are subject to invasive procedures such as insertion of IV lines and drawing of blood specimens. Peripherally inserted central catheters (PICCs) are commonly used for IV therapy. However, catheter-related bloodstream infections may occur, and special care is necessary when they are used. Infants often have central IV catheters that require sterile dressings. All dressing changes should be done under strict sterile technique.

Assessment. The nurse should be alert for signs of sepsis at all times (see Chapter 25).

Nursing Interventions. Handwashing is one of the most important aspects of preventing hospital-acquired infections. Nursing care involves scrupulous cleanliness and maintenance of the infant's skin integrity. Even normal flora on the hands of caregivers may cause sepsis. Therefore, parents and staff members should thoroughly wash their hands and arms before handling infants. No jewelry is worn in many units because of the possibility of it carrying organisms. Exposure to family and staff members who have contagious diseases should be prevented.

Early signs of infections should be identified and reported so treatment may begin immediately. The nurse carefully notes the infant's response to treatment because some organisms become resistant to antibiotics. Other nursing care for infection is discussed in Chapter 25.

Problems with Pain

Infants in the NICU undergo many painful procedures and treatments such as intubation, heel sticks, chest tube placement, venipuncture, and suctioning each day. Younger and sicker infants tend to need more interventions and suffer more pain-producing procedures compared with older, less-ill infants. It was once thought that newborns, particularly preterm infants, were neurologically too immature to feel pain. It is now recognized that preterm infants do feel pain and that pain stimuli cause physiologic and behavioral changes in infants (Blackburn, 2018).

Pain can have numerous untoward effects. For example, increases in intracranial pressure resulting from pain elevate the risk for intraventricular hemorrhage. Other risks include hypoxia, changes in metabolic rate, and adverse effects on growth and wound healing. Stress and pain in the newborn may alter pain thresholds and cause permanent changes in neural pathways (Blackburn, 2018). Tissue injury occurring early in development may lead to higher sensitivity to pain at the involved site and the surrounding areas (Gardner, Enzman-Hines & Agarwal, 2021).

The long-term effects of pain in the neonate are not yet fully understood. It is possible that repeated painful events may cause emotional, behavioral, and learning disabilities. The AAP and ACOG, (2017) recommend that pain be routinely assessed, painful procedures be minimized, and nonpharmacologic and pharmacologic therapies be used to prevent pain from minor procedures and eliminate pain from surgeries and major procedures in neonates.

Assessment. Because pain is the fifth vital sign, pain assessment is performed whenever vital signs are taken. In addition, the nurse should assess the infant's response to potentially painful stimuli and pharmacologic and nonpharmacologic interventions.

Assessment tools are available to evaluate physiologic and behavioral responses to pain in term and preterm infants. Some such as the Premature Infant Pain Profile (PIPP) are designed for term or preterm infants. This tool assesses gestational age and behavior states, heart rate, oxygen saturation, brow bulge, eye squeeze, and nasolabial furrow (lines from the edge of the nostrils to beyond the corners of the mouth) to assign a pain score (Gardner, Enzman-Hines & Agarwal, 2021).

CRITICAL TO REMEMBER

Common Signs of Pain in Infants

Increased or decreased heart and respiratory rates, apnea
Increased blood pressure
Decreased oxygen saturation
Color changes—red, dusky, pale
High-pitched, intense, harsh cry
Whimpering, moaning
"Cry face"
Eyes squeezed shut
Mouth open
Grimacing
Furrowing or bulging of the brow
Tense, rigid muscles or flaccid muscle tone
Rigidity or flailing of extremities
Sleep–wake pattern changes

Both physiologic and behavioral responses to pain occur. However, physiologic changes may be unpredictable and cannot be used alone to assess pain.

Infants who are intubated or too weak to cry have a "cry face," a facial expression of crying without the sound of a cry. Fewer than half of preterm infants experiencing painful stimuli respond with crying (Gardner, Enzman-Hines & Agarwal, 2021). Infants who have been exposed to prolonged or repeated pain may no longer be able to show behavioral changes even though they are experiencing pain. Critically ill or very immature infants also may not show pain responses in the same way that older, less sick infants do. Therefore, lack of response to a painful situation should not be perceived as absence of pain.

Parents often spend many hours with their preterm infants in the NICU setting. The nurse should involve them in assessing the infant's pain and encourage them to share their evaluation of the infant's response to relief measures. They may have questions the nurse can answer about the effects of pain and the measures used to treat it.

Nursing Interventions. Handling before a painful procedure should be minimized, if possible. Even positioning for procedures can be uncomfortable and upsetting. Therefore, other care should be performed at another time to allow the infant to rest before and after the procedure. Nurses should prepare infants for potentially painful procedures by waking them slowly and gently and using containment. **Containment** simulates the enclosed space of the uterus, prevents excessive and disorganized motor activity, and is comforting to infants. It involves keeping the extremities in a flexed position with swaddling, with positioning devices, or with the nurse's hands. The infant is in the supine or side-lying position with at least one of the infant's hands near the mouth for sucking. Containment is also called *facilitated tucking*. Facilitated tuck can help infants self-regulate. It is often used with other non-pharmacologic pain measures like nonnutritive sucking, oral sucrose, and breast milk/feeding and has been shown to be effective at lessening single, mild, procedural pain (Gardner, Enzman-Hines & Agarwal, 2021; Pillai Riddell et al., 2015; Hartley et al., 2015). If several things must be done together, the least traumatic should be performed first. The infant is often hypersensitive after a painful stimulus and may perceive other activities as painful (NANN, 2012).

Comfort measures help the infant cope with short-term, mild pain and reduce agitation. Nonnutritive sucking with a pacifier or the infant's hands is helpful but is effective only as long as the infant continues to suck. Sucrose placed on a pacifier or in the infant's mouth 2 to 3 minutes before a painful stimulus increases pain relief. Combining sucrose with non-nutritive sucking has been found to reduce pain in neonates when used before and during painful procedures (Gardner, Enzman-Hines & Agarwal, 2021; Peng et al., 2018; Johnston et al., 2017). Sucrose may not be appropriate, however, for very young preterm infants.

Talking softly, holding, rocking, and restraining the extremities to prevent flailing are other common methods of pain relief that may be used alone or with sucrose. Measures should be adapted according to the infant's responses. A combination of measures, such as SSC and breastfeeding, may increase effectiveness (Gardner, Enzman-Hines & Agarwal, 2021; Pillai Riddell et al., 2015; Johnston et al., 2017). SSC and breastfeeding also are used to reduce pain. They are a way for parents to be involved in helping relieve infant pain. The parent's voice and smell, which are familiar to the infant, are added to SSC to increase pain relief (Gardner, Enzman-Hines & Agarwal, 2021; Peng et al., 2018; Johnston et al., 2017).

Comfort measures alone are not enough for moderate to severe pain. The nurse should discuss the infant's pain with the primary care provider to ensure that medications are available for long-term and more severe pain. Opioids such as morphine and fentanyl can be tolerated by preterm infants. Nonnarcotic analgesics such as acetaminophen also may be used. Topical anesthesia can be used to reduce pain during some procedures.

Sedatives may be used for agitation in sick newborns but are not effective for pain and should not be used in place of analgesics. Regional or general anesthesia is given during surgery.

The nurse gives ordered medications before painful procedures and when indicated by pain assessments. The infant's response is carefully noted to determine the need to increase or decrease the dosage. Analgesics may be given continuously or on an as-needed basis. To be most effective, analgesics should be given before pain reaches its peak. To avoid inconsistent pain relief occurring with as-needed (PRN) dosing, pain medications are best given on a regular schedule or by continuous infusion (Gardner, Enzman-Hines & Agarwal, 2021).

> **❓ KNOWLEDGE CHECK**
>
> 4. How do nurses help infants adjust to the cooler environment of an open crib?
> 5. How does the nurse keep track of an infant's intake and output?
> 6. What special problems related to fluid balance, infections, and pain occur in preterm infants?
> 7. What nonpharmacologic measures can nurses use to manage pain in infants?

APPLICATION OF THE NURSING PROCESS: ENVIRONMENTALLY CAUSED STRESS

Preterm infants commonly have difficulty with stress from the NICU environment. Their parents may have difficulty with bonding. The effects of environmental factors on the preterm infant have led to developmentally supportive care. Developmental care keeps stressors in the environment to a minimum based on the infant's physiologic and behavioral responses.

In the past, the effects of exposing preterm infants to bright lights and a noisy environment were not well understood. Improvements have occurred, but noise continues to be a problem. Although the recommended noise level in NICUs is below 45 decibels, levels may range between 38 and 90 decibels or higher (Gardner & Goldson, 2021). Noise tends to be loudest during report and caregiver rounds and in areas where staff congregate, such as at entrances, sinks, and computer areas.

The sounds of ventilators, incubators, doors, people, and alarms from equipment and monitors can create a noise level that increases the risk for hearing loss and other complications. In addition, stimulation of any kind can cause increased energy expenditure by the preterm infant. Noise and even routine handling and nursing interventions are often accompanied by changes in heart rate, oxygen saturation levels, and behavior states.

Preterm infants undergo multiple assessments, procedures, and treatments that may cause frequent interruptions of sleep and may interfere with the development of normal sleep–wake cycles. Sleep disruption alters neuronal maturation and secretion of growth hormone and interferes with growth and development (Gardner & Goldson, 2021). Energy that must be directed toward coping with an overstimulating and stressful environment may be unavailable for normal growth and development.

Although touch is generally thought to be comforting to infants, it is often associated with painful events for preterm infants. This can cause them to develop touch aversion, a negative response to touch of any kind. They may cry, squirm, and recoil when touched, expecting that touch will lead to pain.

Assessment

Assess the amount of noise to which the infant is exposed. Determine how often interruptions occur and how the infant responds to different types of care.

Assess the infant's ability to tolerate activity and noise. Overstimulation results in changes in oxygenation and behavior. Behavioral indications of stress, also called *avoidance cues* or *avoidance behavior*, show the infant is seeking to escape the noxious stimuli. Observe for these signs and determine what situations cause them to occur or increase.

CRITICAL TO REMEMBER

Signs of Overstimulation in Preterm Infants

Oxygenation Changes
Blood pressure, pulse, and respiratory instability
Cyanosis, pallor, or mottling
Flaring nares
Decreased oxygen saturation levels
Apnea
Sneezing, coughing

Behavior Changes
Stiff, extended arms and legs
Fisting of the hands or splaying (spreading wide apart) of the
   fingers
Arching
Alert, worried expression
Turning away from eye contact (gaze aversion)
Regurgitation, gagging, hiccupping
Yawning
Fatigue signs

Identification of Client Problems

Preterm infants may have difficulty with multiple stimuli and have a potential for infant stress resulting from exposure to environmental overstimulation.

Planning: Expected Outcomes

The expected outcomes are the infant will do the following:
1. Show decreasing signs of overstimulation during routine activity as evidenced by fewer respiratory and behavioral changes during handling and increased periods of relaxed behavior or sleep.
2. Gradually show an ability to withstand more activity before signs of overstimulation occur.

Interventions

Interventions are focused on providing developmentally supportive nursing care that meets the preterm infant's ability to tolerate stimulation. Developmental care keeps stressors in the environment to a minimum based on the infant's physiologic and behavioral responses.

Scheduling Care

Schedule periods of undisturbed rest throughout the day to allow the infant to recover from treatments. Avoid waking the infant during the short quiet sleep phase. If the infant must be awakened for care, try to do it during an active period of sleep when the infant can be more easily aroused using quiet talking and gentle touch.

Arrange routine care to correspond with the infant's awake periods and avoid disturbing rest. Decrease the frequency of taking vital signs and performing other routine care as soon as possible. Even the handling involved in routine sponge bathing may cause stress in small infants.

Routine daily baths are unnecessary and should be avoided. Bathing every fourth day does not increase skin flora or pathogen counts. Bathing should be postponed until infants are physiologically stable (Spruill, 2021).

Cluster or group care so that several tasks are performed at once to allow for more rest between interruptions. However, keep clustered care short and be alert to the infant's signs of stress. Too many activities may be more than the infant can tolerate without rest. Clustered care may not be appropriate for preterm infants younger than 28 weeks of gestational age (Gardner & Goldson, 2021).

Provide short rest periods or "time out" periods for recovery within grouped activities or during long or painful procedures. Do not include painful procedures in a cluster of other care. Rest is needed before and after painful procedures.

An important nursing responsibility is managing the infant's care by coordinating activities of different health care workers.

Reducing Stimuli

Keep noise around the infant as low as possible. Place incubators away from traffic and congestion areas and avoid talking near the incubator. Use incubator covers to help lower sound inside the incubator. Set alarms, per facility policy, and respond quickly when they sound. Alarms should be audible but not disturbing to nearby clients. Open and close portholes and doors on incubators and cabinets quietly.

Do not place objects on top of the incubator or use it as a writing surface because it increases the noise inside. Teach parents and others to avoid tapping on the incubator. Soft classical music is sometimes used to help promote rest.

Lights that are on 24 hours a day in the nursery may interfere with the development of sleep cycles. Position the incubator so the infant is not facing bright lights and drape a blanket or incubator cover over the top and sides to decrease light and noise further. Use a dimmer switch to vary the intensity of lights, as needed. Reduce lighting at night to as low as possible to help promote rest, conserve energy for growth, and help development of circadian rhythms.

Some NICU have single rooms for each infant. This reduces noise and allows environmental stimuli to be adapted to each infant's individual needs. It also provides more privacy for visiting family members and may reduce hospital-acquired infections.

Promoting Rest

When possible, schedule "quiet periods" when lights and noise in the unit are kept to a minimum to promote rest. Rest periods should be at least an hour long to allow preterm infants to complete a sleep cycle (Spruill, 2021). Only emergency procedures should take place during rest times.

Contain the infant's arms and legs to promote flexion and reduce energy loss from flailing extremities. Containment also promotes quieting, improves physiologic stability, and reduces stress (Gardner & Goldson, 2021). Provide boundaries with rolled blankets or commercial positioning devices placed around the infant. For the side-lying and supine positions, arrange the infant's arms and legs in a flexed position, with the hands near midline to allow hand-to-mouth activity and sucking.

Stroking and gentle massage may be calming for stable preterm infants. It may help increase weight gain and improve development. It also can help involve parents in care of the infant. Not all types of touch are appropriate for smaller, more fragile infants; however, an appropriate option can be used to facilitate parent-infant interaction (Spruill, 2021).

Promoting Motor Development

Preterm infants may have musculoskeletal and developmental problems from prolonged immobilization and the effects of gravity on their immature neuromuscular system. Because the extensor muscles mature before the flexor muscles, the infant tends to remain in an extended, "frog-leg" position. Shoulder retraction, abduction and external rotation of the lower extremities, lateral flexion of the arms, neck hyperextension, and flattening of the sides of the head may be prevented by using correct positioning.

Reposition the infant every 2 to 3 hours or when other care is given. Change the position slowly because position changes may be stressful. When possible, position the infant with the extremities flexed and the hands placed in the midline and near the mouth to allow the infant to suck them for comfort. Use swaddling, blanket rolls, and commercial positioning devices to maintain flexion.

Individualizing Care

Although all NICU nurses are competent in caring for preterm infants, they have slightly different styles in approaching infants. When possible, the same nurse or nurses should be assigned to care for the infant. This allows the nurse to learn the infant's unique behavior and response to stress and allows the infant to get accustomed to the nurse's individual caregiving pattern. It is also very helpful to parents to relate with a small number of nurses who know their infant well.

The ability to tolerate stress varies with each infant. Adapt general care according to the infant's ability to tolerate it. Determine the infant's response to various stimuli, particularly those that cause adverse responses. Even positive stimuli such as soft music or talking quietly can cause overstimulation at times.

Infants often require extra energy to adjust to changes in care. Observe how well they tolerate changes such as moving from assisted to more independent breathing or introduction of new feeding methods. Increase rest periods during these times.

Communicating Infants' Needs

Use the nursing care plan and shift reports to inform other caregivers of techniques that are especially effective for certain infants. Tape laminated notes near the bedside as reminders of needs unique to each infant. Doing so also alerts the parents to the methods that nurses use to care for the infant. Explain all techniques to the parents and solicit their suggestions so they can participate in care appropriately.

Evaluation

As a result of interventions, the infant displays fewer and less frequent signs of overstimulation and shows an increasing tolerance to stimuli before signs appear.

APPLICATION OF THE NURSING PROCESS: NUTRITION

Preterm infants are born before full accumulation of nutrient stores has occurred or digestive capacity is achieved. The problem increases with decreasing gestational age.

Full-term newborns have reservoirs of calcium, iron, and other nutrients, but these are lacking in preterm infants. Fat stores are minimal or absent, and glucose reserves are used soon after birth. Hypoglycemia develops very quickly and should be prevented or treated promptly.

Preterm infants receiving enteral feedings need approximately 105 to 130 kcal/kg/day (Poindexter & Martin, 2020). This amount varies according to activity, illness, and other factors that may affect caloric need. These infants need more protein, iron, calcium, and phosphorus. The average healthy preterm infant should gain approximately 15 to 20 g/kg/day (Brown et al., 2021).

The gastrointestinal (GI) tract of preterm infants does not absorb nutrients as well as that of full-term infants. Although they digest protein well, preterm infants have insufficient bile acids and pancreatic lipase to absorb fat adequately. They have some lactase deficiency but rarely have lactose intolerance (Brown et al., 2021). Their smaller stomach capacity limits the volume preterm infants can tolerate at each feeding. They need more of many nutrients per kilogram than do full-term infants, and supplementation is necessary.

Assessment

Changes in feedings are often made according to the nurse's recommendations based on assessment of an infant's tolerance of feedings, readiness for change, and signs indicating complications.

Feeding Tolerance

Despite little evidence of its efficacy, measuring residual gastric feeding volumes has traditionally been done to determine the tolerance of a feeding by identifying how much of the feeding had been digested. Recently studies suggest routine monitoring of residuals, in infants with a normal abdominal assessment, increases the time to full enteral feedings (Riskin et al., 2017; Parker et al., 2019; Kadam & Devi, 2020), and the repeated negative pressure of the aspiration can damage the stomach lining (Li et al., 2014) without clearly identifying feeding intolerance. Alternative, noninvasive assessment measures can be used.

Measuring abdominal circumference (AC) prior to a feeding may be used as an assessment of feeding tolerance (Kaur et. al., 2015; Thomas et al., 2018). Providers should be notified of abnormal physical assessment findings such as emesis, abdominal discoloration or tenderness, or an AC that has increased by 1.5 cm or more. Placing the infant in a prone or right-side position after feeding can aid in gastric emptying and reduce residuals (Ameri et al., 2018; Yayan et al., 2018; Ceylan & Keskin, 2020).

Vomiting or frequent regurgitation may indicate the feedings are too large. Vomitus or residuals containing bile may be a sign of intestinal obstruction and may require surgery. Diarrhea may be caused by too rapid advancement of the feeding or intolerance to the type of formula.

Observe for signs of intestinal complications such as visible loops of bowel. Obtain objective data about abdominal distention by using a tape to measure abdominal girth per facility protocol. Place the tape directly above the umbilicus and record the placement to ensure consistency. Stools may be tested for reducing substances (which indicate malabsorption of carbohydrates) or occult blood if feeding intolerance is suspected. Report signs to the health care provider because they may be early indications of complications such as ileus, sepsis, obstruction, or necrotizing enterocolitis (NEC).

Readiness for Nipple Feeding

Preterm infants often are initially fed parenterally or by gavage. The ability to feed orally and the ability to gain weight are important milestones, as they are often among the criteria for discharge from the hospital. Coordination of sucking, swallowing, and breathing is a complex task for infants.

Preterm infants do not have the well-developed buccal sucking pads in the cheeks that term infants use to form a seal around the nipple for efficient sucking. The jaw is less stable, and the infant tires easily during oral feedings. The gag reflex may function poorly. The infant's respiratory status, other problems, and distractions in the environment can greatly affect feeding ability.

During gavage feedings, watch for signs that nipple feeding may soon be possible. These include rooting, respiratory rate below 60 breaths per minute, and increasing ability to tolerate holding and handling. Although sucking on the gavage tube, a finger, or a pacifier may be a sign of readiness, it is not enough. Infants should also have an intact gag reflex or they are more likely to aspirate feedings. Note whether the infant gags on the catheter or a gloved finger inserted into the mouth.

Most infants are ready to begin oral feedings when they reach 34 weeks' gestational age. Some are ready as early as 30 weeks, and others need until 36 weeks (Brown et al., 2021). At this age, many healthy preterm infants are able to coordinate sucking with swallowing and breathing and have a functional gag reflex. In addition, infants must have enough energy to feed orally without compromising oxygenation. Very weak infants expend too much oxygen, glucose, and energy when sucking and must continue to receive gavage feedings.

By 30 to 32 weeks, feeding readiness assessments should be initiated (NANN, 2013). When the infant begins to feed by nipple, assess coordination of suck, swallow, and breathing and observe for aspiration. Frequent choking, gagging, or cyanosis during feedings may indicate that the infant cannot coordinate all feeding movements well enough for nipple feeding. In many infants, signs of aspiration are minimal or absent; this is called *silent aspiration.*

Assess the respiratory rate before and during feedings. When the respiratory rate is more than 60 breaths per minute before feedings, gavage feed to prevent aspiration. During feedings observe for signs that the effort of nipple feeding requires too much energy and oxygen for the infant.

Identification of Client Problems

When the infant's nutritional needs are met by parenteral methods, the nursing care is collaborative. However, once the infant is able to breastfeed or take formula by bottle, many nursing interventions are involved. They include the potential for ineffective feeding because of uncoordinated suck and swallow as well as fatigue during feedings.

Planning: Expected Outcomes

The expected outcomes are that the infant will do the following:
1. Consume adequate amounts of breast milk or formula to meet nutrient needs for age and weight.
2. Gain weight as appropriate for age, generally 15 to 20 g/kg/day.

The actual amount of feedings and weight gain will vary according to the infant's gestational age and other conditions. Discuss what is appropriate for a particular infant with the physician or nurse practitioner.

Interventions
Administering Parenteral Nutrition

The nurse manages the administration of **total parenteral nutrition (TPN)**, the IV infusion of solutions containing major nutrients needed for metabolism and growth. It may be necessary for very immature infants because of respiratory problems, limited gastric capacity, surgery, or reduced peristalsis. It provides calories, amino acids, fatty acids, vitamins, and minerals in amounts adapted to the specific needs of infants. TPN is decreased as enteral feedings are increased, continuing until the infant is able to tolerate full enteral feedings.

Administering Enteral Feedings

Enteral feedings (feeding into the GI tract, orally or by feeding tube) are usually begun within the first few days with minimal enteral feedings, also called *trophic feedings.* These feedings are only a few milliliters of breast milk or formula given at a time. They stimulate development of the GI tract, enhance gut motility, decrease the need for parenteral nutrition, and decrease feeding intolerance (Poindexter & Martin, 2020). Bowel sounds should be present, there should be no significant abdominal distention, and infants should be in relatively stable condition. Mother's milk is preferred if it is available. Donor breast milk also may be used. Colostrum is especially high in immune agents to help prevent infection. Feedings are gradually increased according to the infant's tolerance.

Colostrum or breast milk also can be used for oral care of infants. It is applied to the infant's lips and inside of the mouth at care times with a sterile swab. It provides the immunologic benefits of breast milk before the infant can take feedings (Gardner, Lawrence & Lawrence, 2021).

Preterm infants need special formulas or fortified breast milk. These formulas are adapted to meet the need for easily digestible, concentrated nutrients in a smaller volume of fluid. Preterm infants may need formulas that have 24 kcal/oz or more (instead of 20 kcal/oz used for the full-term infant) to meet their requirements. Preterm formulas may contain added calories, protein, vitamins, minerals, and complex fatty acids. Other components may be added to meet individual needs. Breast milk fortifiers add needed nutrients to breast milk.

Administering Gavage Feedings

Gavage feedings are usually started before oral feedings for preterm infants (Procedure 24.1). A small, soft catheter is inserted through the nose or mouth every 2 to 3 hours for intermittent (bolus) feedings. An indwelling catheter also may be used to provide for intermittent or continuous feedings. Indwelling catheters stay in place up to 30 days.

Inserting the catheter at each feeding may be more traumatic than leaving it in place. Frequent oral placement may cause vomiting or increase infant aversion to oral stimuli, which may lead to difficulty with oral feedings later. Vagal stimulation during insertion may cause apnea and bradycardia. Nasal placement avoids aversive oral stimulation but may increase airway resistance by interfering with air flow through the infant's small nasal passages.

Intermittent bolus feedings provide a more normal feeding pattern with periodic stimulation of gastric hormones and enzymes. They should be given slowly over 30 to 60 minutes.

Continuous feedings may be better for infants with short-bowel syndrome, congenital heart disease, or intolerance to bolus feedings or those recovering from NEC (Brown et al., 2021). However, continuous feedings carry a higher risk for aspiration because the infant is not observed at all times during the feeding. In addition, bacteria counts in the milk or formula may become too high, and fats tend to adhere to the tubing during continuous feeding.

Feedings are gradually increased according to the infant's tolerance. Carefully observe the infant's response at each feeding to determine when the feeding type or amount can be changed. Parenteral nutrition continues until the infant is able to take adequate enteral feedings.

Pacifiers are often used during gavage feedings. Preterm infants have been exposed to noxious oral stimulation, such as intubation and suctioning. As a result, they may react negatively to any additional oral stimulation, which interferes with feedings. Providing a pacifier during gavage feedings gives positive oral stimulation and helps associate the comfortable feeling of fullness with sucking. Nonnutritive sucking increases later success in oral feedings and decreases behavior changes during feedings.

Nonnutritive sucking also can be provided by having an infant who is not ready for oral feeding suck on the postpartum client's emptied breasts as a way to prepare for feeding from the breast. Gavage feeding can be done at the same time to help infants associate the breast with the feeling of being fed. This may improve breastfeeding ability when the infant is ready to be fed at the breast (Kaya & Aytekin, 2017).

Administering Oral Feedings

Oral feedings should be cue-based (begun when the infants shows signs of physiologic and behavioral readiness to feed) rather than on a time schedule. Crying is a late hunger sign and may cause the infant to be too tired to eat. The frequency and volume of oral feedings are based on the infant's readiness and ability. Oral feedings may be offered at each feeding time if the infant shows positive feeding readiness signs (Fig. 24.2). Full oral feedings are reached faster using cue-based feedings (NANN, 2013; Gardner & Goldson, 2021). Cue-based feedings may help infants develop sleep–wake cycles and begin to self-regulate better.

CRITICAL TO REMEMBER

Nipple Feedings

Signs of Readiness for Nipple Feedings
Rooting
Sucking on gavage tube, finger, or pacifier
Ability to tolerate holding/handling
Respiratory rate <60 breaths per minute
Presence of gag reflex
Maintains quiet alert state for at least 10 minutes

Signs of Nonreadiness for Nipple Feedings
Respiratory rate >60 breaths per minute
No rooting or sucking
Absence of gag reflex

Adverse Signs during Nipple Feedings
Tachycardia
Bradycardia
Increased or decreased respiratory rate
Nasal flaring
Markedly decreased oxygen saturation level
Cyanosis, pallor
Apnea
Choking, coughing, sneezing, hiccoughs
Finger splaying—"Stop sign" hand
Gagging, regurgitation
Drooling, gulping
Falling asleep early in the feeding
Feeding time longer than 20 to 30 minutes

NURSING PROCEDURE 24.1   Administering Gavage Feeding

Purpose:

To feed infants who are unable to take the full feedings by nipple; may be used alone or along with nipple feedings.

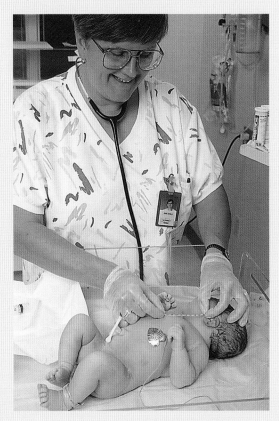

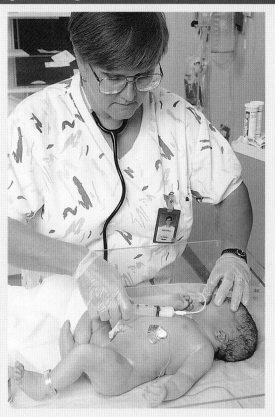

1. Wash hands. Gather equipment, including gavage catheter of proper size (4 to 8 French, depending on the size of the infant); measured container, 20 mL or larger; syringe; stethoscope; syringe pump, if appropriate; and extension tubing, if needed. Warm the breast milk or formula to room or body temperature. Check the chart to determine how previous feedings were tolerated. Add fortifier to breast milk, if ordered. *Having all materials ready helps the procedure go smoothly and avoids disturbing the infant or delaying feedings. Cold milk could interfere with thermoregulation. Information about previous feedings will help meet the infant's needs.*

2. Don gloves. If the parents are present, they may hold the infant in their arms or in SSC once the catheter is inserted. If the infant cannot be held, they may hold the infant's hands. *Feeding is important to the parents and helping increases their sense of involvement.*

3. Determine the length of catheter to insert. Measure from the tip of the nose to the base of the ear to halfway between the xiphoid process and the umbilicus. Mark the catheter at the proper point with a piece of tape or indelible ink. *The measured distance is equal to the distance from the mouth or nose to the stomach. The mark on the catheter shows whether the tube has moved out of place.*

4. For oral placement, insert the tube gently into the mouth until the mark on the tube is reached. For nasal placement, lubricate the tip with sterile water or lubricant. Gently insert into one nostril until premeasured mark is reached. Remove the catheter immediately if persistent coughing, choking, cyanosis, apnea, or bradycardia occurs. *Moistening or lubricating the tip allows easier passage. Gentle insertion prevents trauma. Signs may indicate that the catheter is entering the trachea instead of the esophagus. Stimulation of the vagus nerve may cause bradycardia or apnea.*

5. Check for placement according to hospital protocol. Attach a syringe to the catheter and gently aspirate stomach contents. Move or rotate the catheter slightly if the plunger does not withdraw easily. Check that the mark on the tube is in the same place whenever care is given and before feeds. *The pH shows if the aspirate is stomach contents. Radiography also may be used to verify placement (usually only if done for another reason). Use of force could traumatize the stomach lining if the end of the catheter is resting against it. Moving the catheter may draw it away from the stomach lining. Checking the tube marking ensures the tube is still in the correct place.*

6. Secure the catheter to the cheek with an adhesive dressing. Securing ensures the catheter will remain inserted to the proper point during the procedure.

Continued

NURSING PROCEDURE 24.1   Administering Gavage Feeding—cont'd

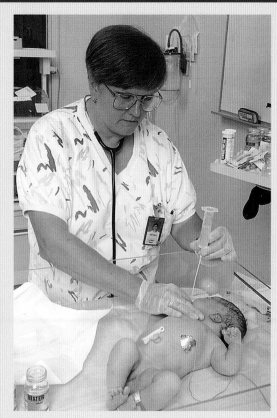

7. For gravity flow feedings, remove the plunger and attach the syringe to the feeding tube. Pour the correct amount of milk into the syringe. Raise or lower the syringe to increase or decrease the flow rate so the feeding moves slowly into the stomach over 30 minutes. *The higher the syringe, the faster the flow of solution and the greater the pressure. Feedings should be given slowly to prevent sudden distention or trauma from pressure, and from filling the stomach too fast.*

8. For timed or continuous feedings, place no more than a 2- to 4-hour supply of milk in a syringe. Set the pump to deliver the correct rate of flow. Change the equipment according to hospital policy. *Limiting the amount of feeding and changing equipment prevent excessive growth of bacteria in the milk or tubing. Infusion pumps deliver the feeding at a constant, measured rate.*

9. Give the infant a pacifier during the feeding. *The pacifier stimulates the sucking reflex, helps prepare the infant for nippling, is comforting, and helps the infant associate sucking with feeding.*

10. Burp the infant after feeding. *Air may be swallowed around the catheter and can cause the infant to regurgitate and aspirate.*

11. For intermittent feedings with a catheter that remains in place, flush the tube with the smallest amount of sterile water needed to clear the tube (1 to 2 mL) and close off the end when the feeding is completed. *This prevents clogging of the tubing. Closing the end prevents formula from coming back through the catheter.*

12. When the catheter is to be withdrawn, pinch it and remove quickly. *Pinching prevents drops of fluid from entering the trachea as the catheter is removed, and quick removal decreases irritation.*

13. Record time, type and amount of feeding given, and how the infant tolerated it. *Documentation allows monitoring of the infant's ability to tolerate feedings and meet nutritional needs.*

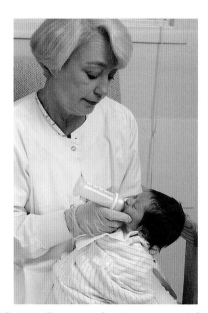

FIG. 24.2 The nurse feeds a preterm infant.

Feedings. Provide for maintenance of heat during feedings. When infants have stable temperature maintenance, wrap them in warm blankets and hold them for feedings. If thermoregulation is a problem, feed the infant in the radiant warmer or incubator.

Nipple feedings involve a greater expenditure of energy by the infant than gavage feedings. Allow for a period of rest before and after feedings. Use of a pacifier before feedings helps bring preterm infants to an alert state that enhances oral feeding success. Infants take feedings better if they are awake. Assess for signs of overstimulation and stress during feedings. If they occur, stop the feeding and let the infant rest. If the infant continues to show signs of stress, the feeding should be completed by gavage.

Choosing a Nipple. A variety of nipples for neonates are available. Packaging descriptions are often misleading to the actual nipple flow rate (Pados et al., 2019). Soft, high-flow nipples ("preemie" nipples) are more pliable than regular nipples and require less energy for sucking. However, they may deliver milk too rapidly, cause choking, and interfere with breathing between sucking bursts. Standard nipples are firmer and deliver the milk more slowly so the infant can control it more easily. Nipples are available in several sizes, including those for infants with a very small mouth.

Facilitating Breastfeeding

Breast milk is best for almost all infants and especially for preterm infants. The NANN Position Statement (NANN, 2015) states human milk and breastfeeding are essential components in care of critically ill newborns. The AAP (2017) recommends that all preterm infants receive human milk.

Explain to parents that the immunologic benefits of breast milk are particularly important to the preterm infant who did not receive passive immunity during fetal life. Human milk provides protection against infections and decreases the incidence of NEC (Gardner, Lawrence & Lawrence, 2021). Breast milk may stimulate the immune system and GI maturation. It is well tolerated, and the nutrients in it are more available than those in cow's milk formulas. Nutrients in breast milk are more easily digested, and breast milk provides antimicrobial components, enzymes, hormones, and growth factors important for the preterm infant. If the postpartum client's milk is not available, use of human donor milk should be encouraged (AAP, 2017).

Offer support and encouragement to parents who want to breastfeed. Contributing breast milk helps them realize they have something important to offer at a time when many believe there is little they can do for their baby. Many parents find this particularly rewarding and worth the effort involved. They may develop a sense of increased control when they are able to breastfeed and may take on more responsibility in infant care (Ikonen et al., 2015).

The client who plans to breastfeed needs help with maintaining lactation until the infant is mature enough to nurse. Assist with the use of a breast pump as soon as possible after birth and provide teaching regarding the need to pump at least five times a day for 20 minutes per pumping session or a total of at least 100 minutes per day (Hand & Noble, 2022).

Give the parents sterile containers to store the milk. Show how to label the milk and where to take it in the NICU. Discharge instructions should include storing the milk in a refrigerator if the infant will receive it within 24 hours or in a freezer if it will be more than 24 hours. If fortifiers will be added to the milk, explain the higher needs of the preterm infant so that the parents do not think something is wrong with the breast milk or that it is inadequate.

In some facilities, healthy preterm infants progress to breastfeeding from gavage feedings without using the bottle at all. This should be encouraged with eligible infants and parents who desire breastfeeding.

Ongoing support for the parents is important. Encourage their efforts in feeding, which may be difficult at first. Remind them that even full-term infants must learn how to breastfeed.

Clients who have not breastfed previously have to learn the basic techniques and also how to adapt them for the preterm infant.

Relaxation needed for feeding is difficult in the busy NICU. Provide as much privacy as possible, using a separate room or screens. Help the client feel comfortable holding the tiny infant and any attached equipment. The presence of a lactation consultant during initial breastfeeding sessions is very helpful.

Adapt breastfeeding teaching to the needs of a very small infant. Show how to use the football and cross-cradle holds, which allow visualization of the infant's face during latching on and throughout the feeding (see Figs. 23.4 and 23.5). A supplemental nursing system, a device that holds expressed breast milk in a bag with a small tube attached to the nipple, may be used to help infants receive more milk with less effort during early feedings. Feedings should begin gradually and progress similar to initial bottle feedings.

Make the same observations of the infant during breastfeeding as during bottle feeding. Signs of fatigue, bradycardia, tachypnea, or apnea may show lack of readiness for breastfeeding. Be sure the infant stays warm. The client's body heat will help maintain the infant's temperature during feedings. SSC is often started before the infant is able to breastfeed. As the infant becomes ready to breastfeed, SSC can be continued during the feeding.

Thin nipple shields may be used in the first few days of breastfeeding to help the infant latch on to the breast and remain latched. Instruct the client to pump at the end of each feeding because preterm infants may not suckle well enough to extract all milk from the breasts at first (Gardner, Lawrence & Lawrence, 2021).

Making Ongoing Assessments

Continually assess the infant for feeding readiness cues and the infant's responses to all feeding methods. Watch for signs of distress, especially when feedings are first initiated. Record the amount of breast milk or the amount of formula the infant takes by gavage or bottle and compare it with the amount needed to meet nutrient needs for the infant's age and weight.

Because accurate estimation of milk intake is difficult during breastfeeding, infants may be weighed on an electronic scale before and after feedings to determine intake. Both weights should be taken with the infant wearing the same clothing and before the diaper is changed after the feeding. The difference in the weights in grams equals the milliliters taken. This allows supplementary gavage feeding amounts to be calculated on the basis of the infant's oral intake of breast milk.

Note the infant's response to other stimuli during feedings. Some infants respond well to being talked to and rocked during feedings. Others become distracted by any noise, motion, or nearby activities.

Weigh the infant daily at the same time with the same scale. Record the length and head circumference each week.

Plot measurements on a growth chart for preterm infants and compare results with expected ranges. Weight increase not accompanied by increased length may be caused by edema and may be a sign of a complication such as congestive heart failure.

Observe changes in the infant's ability to take feedings. The suck and swallow coordination should gradually improve with maturity and practice. As the infant becomes more mature, less energy should be expended during the feeding sessions. The infant will take the feedings more quickly and show fewer signs of fatigue such as falling asleep during feedings.

Explain to the client that the infant's suck may still be too weak to adequately stimulate milk production. Pumping after feedings several times a day helps maintain the milk supply. The need to pump will lessen gradually as the infant nurses more vigorously.

Evaluation

If the expected outcomes have been met, the infant will consume adequate amounts of breast milk or formula to meet nutrient needs for age and weight and will gain weight as appropriate for age.

KNOWLEDGE CHECK

8. What can the nurse do for the infant at risk for stress from overstimulation?
9. How does the nurse assess feeding tolerance?
10. Why should the nurse allow the infant to set the pace of feedings instead of urging continuous sucking?
11. How can the nurse help the parents who choose breastfeeding for their preterm infant?

APPLICATION OF THE NURSING PROCESS: PARENTING

The birth of a preterm infant is generally unexpected and always emotionally traumatic to parents. Infants are often hurried to the NICU shortly after birth. Later, when parents go to the NICU, the infant is attached to an array of machines.

Parents cannot hold or feed the infant at first or offer any of the usual care that parents expect to give their infants. The infant may not be capable of common newborn behaviors such as making eye contact and grasping the parent's finger. When the infant's appearance and behavior are different from the parents' expectations, attachment may be delayed.

The extended hospitalization of the preterm infant causes separation of the parents from their newborn, produces emotional trauma, and disrupts family life. Parents must relinquish the role of primary caregiver during their infant's hospitalization. They may feel they are in the nurse's way and may state they do not feel like parents at all. Loss of the parental role is a major stressor for these parents.

Being unable to participate fully in the infant's care for a prolonged period hampers the parents' ability to learn their baby's unique characteristics, such as the way the infant responds to stress and the methods of consolation that work best. Separation delays the development of the parent-infant relationship and may impair bonding.

In addition, parents worry about the infant's condition and outcome. They need help in understanding the infant's condition and what can be expected to occur throughout the hospital stay. Nurses should evaluate the progress of attachment to assist parents to feel important in caring for their infant.

Assessment

Assess for signs of parental attachment on the first and subsequent visits to the NICU nursery. Expect parents to be fearful at first but more able to focus on the infant as they recover from the initial shock of preterm birth. Assess for common behaviors that show normal progression of attachment. These include talking about the infant in positive terms, making eye contact, pointing out physical characteristics, naming the infant, and calling the infant by name.

Parents should ask questions about the infant. When they are able to hold and participate in the care of the infant, observe for gradual increase in comfort and skill. The parents should smile and talk to the infant and verbalize increasing confidence in their caregiving abilities.

Watch for signs that bonding is not occurring as expected. These include failure to show usual attachment behaviors or a decrease in behaviors that were previously present. Parents who seem as interested in other infants in the NICU as in their own infant or talk about the infant in an impersonal way may be having difficulty. Note how often the parents make visits or calls to the NICU and changes that may indicate their need for support.

Determine whether there are other stressors in the parents' lives that may interfere with their ability to visit and form attachment to the infant. The financial need to return to work, lack of transportation, long distances, or the need to care for other children may prevent parents from visiting as often as they would like.

There is a growing body of literature suggesting traumatic childbirth experiences may result in higher levels of stress, which may lead to or contribute to posttraumatic stress disorder (PTSD) in the postpartum client. It may be worse if the infant is admitted to the NICU (Sharp et al., 2021; Ayers et al., 2016; Schecter et al., 2020). Being aware of the past trauma history and perceptions of the birth experience can help caregivers provide trauma-informed care (TIC) that may potentially prevent or lessen postpartum PTSD.

The premise of TIC is that a person is more likely than not to have a history of some type of trauma. The approach for health care providers is to recognize the trauma, to understand everyone will react differently, and to avoid retraumatization (Center for Health Care Strategies, 2021).

For the infant, a stay in the NICU, no matter how short, can be filled with potentially toxic stressors such as separation from parents, repeated painful procedures (often with little or no analgesia), interrupted sleep, periods of being NPO, and sensory overload. It is hypothesized these events have short- and long-term neurodevelopment consequences that may produce PTSD as the infant grows older. Although stress for the baby in the NICU cannot be eliminated, TIC may help the parents better cope with their own stressors, engage in supportive activities with their infant, and keep their infant's stress below toxic levels (Sanders & Hall, 2018; D'Agata et al., 2016).

Strategies NICUs can implement to support TIC include family-centered care and teaching, developmental and complementary care interventions, and psychosocial support and counseling for families (Sabnis et al., 2019; Sanders & Hall, 2018).

After the critical period in the early days after birth, healthy preterm infants become more stable. They still require specialized nursing care and hospitalization but gradually need fewer technologic interventions. They are sometimes called "growers" at this time. This is a time when parental participation in the infant's care should increase in preparation for discharge.

CRITICAL TO REMEMBER

Signs That Bonding May Be Delayed

Using negative terms to describe the infant
Discussing the infant in impersonal or technical terms
Failing to give the infant a name or to use the name
Visiting or calling infrequently or not at all
Decreasing the number and length of visits
Showing interest in other infants equal to that in their own infant
Refusing offers to hold and learn to care for the infant
Showing a decrease in or lack of eye contact
Spending less time talking to or smiling at the infant

Identification of Client Problems

For parents of preterm infants, an important client problem is the potential for inadequate development of parent-infant relationship resulting from lack of understanding of the infant's condition and separation from the infant.

Planning: Expected Outcomes

The expected outcomes are that the parents will do the following:
1. Demonstrate bonding behaviors, including visiting or calling frequently and interacting as appropriate for the infant's condition throughout the hospital stay.
2. Verbalize understanding of the preterm infant's condition and characteristics within 2 days.
3. Express gradually increasing comfort in participating in infant care throughout the hospital stay.

Interventions
Making Advance Preparations

Preparing for stressful situations such as preterm birth helps parents cope with the actual event. Parents at higher risk for

a preterm birth should visit the NICU before delivery. If the postpartum client is confined to bed, arrange for a nurse from the NICU to visit and establish a link with the nursery. The partner or another support person should tour the nursery and share the nursery environment with the client. Encourage the parents to ask questions.

Assisting Parents after Birth

After the birth, allow the parents to see and touch the newborn in the delivery room, even if only for a few moments, so they have a realistic idea of the infant's appearance and condition. This helps the bonding process that began in pregnancy to continue.

If possible, allow the primary support partner to watch the initial care in the NICU. Explain what is happening and why. This attention allows the partner to see the intense efforts made on behalf of the infant, increases confidence in the staff, and enables the partner to give the childbearer a full description later. Support the partner as well by using therapeutic communication during this difficult time.

If the infant must be transported to another facility, ask the transport team to visit the parents before leaving, if possible. The visit helps parents feel connected to their infant and to the staff providing care. Leaving photographs with the parents is another way of helping them bond even though the infant is not with them.

Supporting Parents during Early Visits

Take the parents to the NICU as soon as possible. If the childbearer is too ill to be with the infant, bring photographs. Before parents first visit the infant, prepare them for what they will see. Describe the equipment, the various attachments to the infant, and the purposes (Fig. 24.3). Explain how the infant will look and behave. Box 24.1 provides specific steps that the nurse can follow to help parents become familiar with the NICU setting.

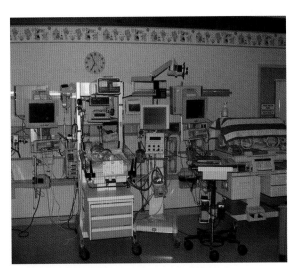

FIG. 24.3 An infant in the neonatal intensive care unit is surrounded by highly technologic equipment. This can be very frightening to parents at first. Preparation of parents before they visit is an important nursing responsibility.

BOX 24.1 Introducing Parents to the Neonatal Intensive Care Unit Setting

Before Parents Visit the Neonatal Intensive Care Unit

If possible, provide the parents with a tour of the NICU before the birth.

If a tour is not possible, describe the NICU environment. Include the noise of alarms, the busyness of the staff, and the number of people and sick infants.

Describe the equipment. Include ventilators, intravenous lines, feeding tubes, and monitors. Explain how they look and how they are attached to the infant. Keep the explanations simple, without technical details.

Show the parents photographs of their infant. This helps prepare them, but seeing photographs is not as overwhelming as seeing the infant in person.

Describe the infant. Include the size, lack of fat, breathing problems, and weak cry. Explain that no sound of crying can be heard if the infant is intubated. Include some personal aspects: "He's a real fighter" or "She makes the funniest faces during her feedings."

When Parents Visit the Neonatal Intensive Care Unit

Help the parents perform thorough handwashing, and explain the importance.

Stay with the parents during their visit. Having a familiar person nearby will help them feel more comfortable while they adjust to this unfamiliar environment.

Introduce them to their infant's nurse. Ask the NICU nurse to explain some of the care being provided for the infant.

Give parents printed information about the NICU so that they can take it home to read later. This includes visiting hours, telephone updates, availability of classes on preterm infant care, and support groups.

Tell the parents they will receive instruction on how to care for their infant in time. Encourage them to visit the infant as much as they can. Emphasize how important they are to their infant.

Offer realistic encouragement based on the infant's condition.

Provide an opportunity for the parents to express their concerns and feelings and ask questions.

NICU, Neonatal intensive care unit.

becoming attached to an infant who may not live. They need sensitive support from the nurse until they are ready to progress in their relationship with the infant.

THERAPEUTIC COMMUNICATIONS

Reassuring Parents during Visits to the Neonatal Intensive Care Unit

Shareen gave birth to a preterm infant, Valerie, at 28 weeks of gestation. Shareen is visiting the NICU for the first time the day after the birth. Andy, the nurse, has talked to her about what to expect and stays with her during the visit.

Shareen: Oh, she looks so tiny! I saw her for only a minute after she was born, and I didn't really get a good look. How can she ever survive when she's so small and covered with tubes?

Andy: So far, Valerie's doing very well. Her vital signs are stable, and she's holding her own. But it's frightening when she looks so small and vulnerable, isn't it? *(Offering realistic reassurance and reflecting Shareen's fearful feelings. Using infant's name to promote bonding.)*

Shareen: I stayed in bed like they told me to do to help my blood pressure. I thought she wouldn't be born so soon if I stayed in bed.

Andy: It must have been a shock, especially when you tried so hard to prevent it. *(Reflecting feelings and acknowledging that Shareen did what she could to prevent early birth.)*

Shareen: Now she's so tiny and so sick! She looks very different from what I expected.

Andy: Valerie's small, but babies her size grow very quickly. Would you like to touch her? *(Offering realistic reassurance and attempting to bring Shareen closer to her infant.)*

Shareen: Oh, I might hurt her. Maybe I should wait until she's bigger.

Andy: Even tiny babies like to have their parents touch them and talk to them. She listened to your voice all through your pregnancy, so it's familiar to her. Why don't you talk softly to her while I work with her? And I can tell you about all this equipment and what we are doing for Valerie. *(Emphasizing the parents' importance, involving them in care being given, and offering information about the infant's equipment and care.)*

At first, stay with the parents during visits. When they are comfortable, allow them time alone with the infant so they can interact in private. Answer questions and explain changes in the infant's condition and treatment. Expect to repeat explanations because stressed parents may not understand or remember what was said. Parents often do not know what questions to ask at first or are too overwhelmed to ask questions. In this situation, discuss questions that are common when parents first visit the NICU. Use therapeutic communication as the parents cope with their grief, guilt, and emotional turmoil.

Parents should touch the infant as soon as possible because touching helps promote attachment. They may be hesitant initially because of fear they will interfere with equipment. The smaller the infant, the more reluctant the parents may be. Some parents may hesitate to touch because they are afraid of

Show parents how to touch in ways appropriate for the infant, such as holding the infant's hand through the portholes of the incubator or touching the small areas of skin not encumbered by equipment. Explain that handling is kept to a minimum for physiologically unstable infants because it is too stressful to them. As the infant becomes more stable and mature, show parents which forms of touch work best with their infant. This helps parents feel more a part of the infant's plan of care.

Help the parents hold the baby as soon as possible. Parents often look forward to the opportunity to hold the baby as a positive sign of the infant's condition. Yet it is frightening, too, especially if the infant is attached to various kinds of equipment. Help the parents find a comfortable position for themselves and the infant and point out positive responses from the infant.

Providing Information

An important role of the nurse is providing accurate information to parents. Allow parents to express their concerns before beginning to teach. Encourage them to ask questions about all aspects of their infant's condition and care. Although some parents are not hesitant to ask questions, others may avoid asking for explanations or advocating for their need to care for their infants because they are afraid they might be seen as difficult or "demanding parents" (Gardner & Voos, 2021). Let the parents know their questions are welcome and do everything possible to give them the answers when they do ask questions. Give information about common concerns if the parents do not ask questions.

Explain the equipment used to care for the infant. Interpret the information obtained from monitors and the meanings of alarms. Clarify all nursing care, its purpose, and the expected response. Point out how preterm infants are similar to and different from full-term infants to help parents develop an accurate understanding of the infant's capabilities.

Offer realistic reassurance about the infant's condition, emphasizing positive aspects while being truthful. If the parents have misconceptions or did not understand a provider's explanations, clarify or ask the provider to go over specific information again. Translate medical terms into words the parents can understand. Avoid using medical abbreviations and acronyms. Repeat explanations, especially at first. Because of their emotional distress, parents are often unable to fully comprehend or remember what is said to them.

Use an interpreter if the parents do not understand English. Even if the parents speak English, if it is not their primary language, they may have difficulty understanding the information. Provide an interpreter as needed. Offer written information about NICU policies and procedures in the parents' language. Explanations about visiting hours, who can visit, routines for handwashing, and the role of parents can be reinforced in writing so they are available for later reading by overwhelmed parents.

Instituting Skin-to-Skin Care

Parents need to feel they can contribute to the care their infants receive. One way to do this is with SSC. SSC, also known as kangaroo care, is a method of providing direct skin contact between preterm infants and their parents. Begin SSC as soon as possible, if the parents are interested. Individual NICUs create guidelines for which infants may receive SSC and for its frequency and duration. Literature suggests there are few contraindications to SSC and it may be safely used and beneficial for infants weighing less than 1000 g, infants who are intubated, and infants with central or umbilical lines (Gardner & Goldson, 2021).

During SSC, the infant, wearing only a diaper and hat, is placed upright under the postpartum client's clothes between the breasts. A blanket is placed over them both (Fig. 24.4). Clients may breastfeed if they wish and if the infant is able. Partners are encouraged to participate in SSC (Fig. 24.5). The infant is monitored for changes in vital signs and behavior.

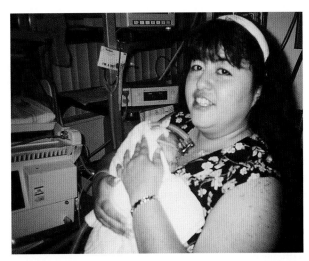

FIG. 24.4 This 27-week-gestation preterm infant is tucked under the parent's clothes against the skin for skin-to-skin care. Such care enhances bonding and has many other benefits for infants and parents.

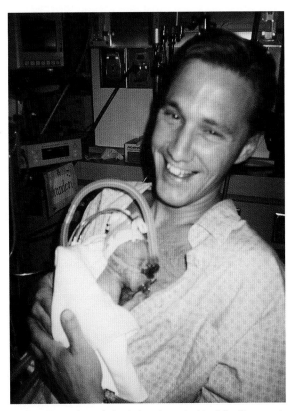

FIG. 24.5 Even though he is intubated, this 1 lb, 8 oz preterm infant goes to sleep against the parent's chest.

Explain the advantages of SSC to parents and elicit their participation. This method of care has been found safe for stable infants, even if intubated. It provides an opportunity for parents to participate in the infant's care and increases parental attachment. SSC provides developmental care that is so important for the preterm infant. It is associated with stability of vital signs, increased weight gain, shorter length of stay, more quiet sleep, and less crying. It also promotes thermoregulation and bonding (Spruill, 2021). SSC has also been found to be a nonpharmacologic way to relieve pain (Johnston et al., 2017).

The upright position of the infant against the parent's chest makes breathing easier. The containment of the extremities decreases purposeless movements that use valuable oxygen and calories. Breastfeeding is facilitated, and the infant has more alert periods and increased deep sleep. The contact with the parent's skin maintains the infant's body temperature. In addition, SSC enhances early and long-term parent-infant interaction and parental confidence and competence (Gardner & Goldson, 2021).

SSC also provides gentle stimulation. This includes tactile stimulation against the parent's skin, auditory stimulation as the infant listens to the parent's heartbeat and voice, and the vestibular stimulation of moving with the parent's breathing or rocking.

Provide privacy for parents interested in SSC. Assist them, following facility protocol, in transferring the infant from the bed, managing the attachments, and making the infant comfortable. Also, check to see that they are comfortable.

Facilitating Interaction

Preterm infants often have little facial expression and seldom make eye contact. Parents may feel rejected by the infant's lack of response or by negative responses during interactions. Explain the interaction that is so effective with full-term infants may be too stimulating for very young or sick preterm infants. Suggest forms of touch and interaction based on the individual infant's capacity. Quiet holding may be better until the infant is able to tolerate more stimulation.

Help parents understand the infant's behavior and cues. Teach them signs of overstimulation to help them adapt their interaction to meet the infant's needs. Explain these signs help protect the infant from overstimulation and show that the infant needs a quiet rest period without added stimulation. Discuss methods to avoid too much stimulation and to calm the infant. If several types of simultaneous stimulation (such as rocking, eye contact, and talking) cause signs of distress, suggest they stop one or more activities until the infant has had a rest period.

In learning to provide comfort care, parents may go through stages. At first they are afraid to touch the infant. They spend time just observing the infant before they feel comfortable enough to touch the infant. When they begin to participate in caregiving such as changing a diaper, their confidence grows. Parents become more confident in their ability to recognize when the infant is uncomfortable and their skill in comforting their infant.

Teach parents how to soothe infants when they show signs of stress. Explain containment and demonstrate how to do it. Placing the palm of the hand over the infant's chest or holding the infant's arms on the chest may help quiet the infant (Spruill, 2021). Show the parents how to position the infant with the hands near the mouth so the infant can

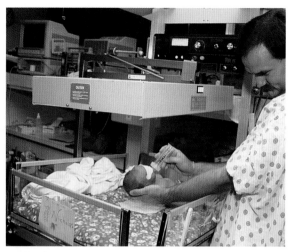

FIG. 24.6 To promote family bonding with the infant, parents are involved as much as possible in the care of their infant. This parent bottle feeds the infant who is in a radiant warmer.

suck on them as a self-comforting measure. As the infant is ready for more interaction, suggest appropriate types of stimulation.

Point out small signs of improvement and even minor strengths. Talk about normal preterm characteristics and emphasize individual traits that make this infant different from all others. The way the infant eats, reacts to sounds, or seems to get tangled in the monitor leads may help parents feel closer to their newborn.

Involve the parents in care of the infant as soon as possible to help them gain a sense of control (Fig. 24.6). Plan to change the linens in the incubator or radiant warmer when the parents are there so they can hold their infant, even if for only a few moments. Save baths and other routine caregiving for times when parents can be present and participate. Taking an axillary temperature is something a parent can be taught to do for even a critically ill infant that does not disturb the infant but fosters a feeling of contribution in the parent. As the infant's condition improves, parents can develop skill in caring for the tiny infant by changing diapers, feeding, and bathing.

Include other family or support system members by allowing them to visit with the parents (Fig. 24.7). Being able to see the infant in the hospital setting allows support system members to provide the parents with more realistic emotional support. Involve others in learning how to feed and care for the infant if they will be helping the parents after discharge.

In some facilities, parents, and in some cases grandparents, are not considered "visitors" and may come to the NICU at any time of the day or night. They may be asked to leave during reporting or be invited to stay and participate to help them feel more a part of the infant's care.

Web cameras are used in some NICUs to allow parents to see their infants from their homes or from the hospital room. A web camera is placed over the infant's bed, and parents use a computer to access a secure website to see their infant. The camera may be on continuously or only on at certain times. Parents can share the website with family and friends so they

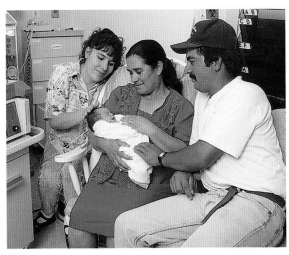

FIG. 24.7 The parents look on while the grandmother holds the infant in the neonatal intensive care unit.

can see the infant as well. While most families have positive experiences using this technology, for some, it may increase the stress and guilt of not being with their infant (Gibson & Kilcullen, 2020).

Increasing Parental Decision-Making

Parents should be considered an essential part of the health care team and given the information they need to take an active part in decisions made about the infant's treatment plan (Friedman et al., 2020). This is true even for decisions that seem insignificant to the staff (Baker, 2009). This knowledge will increase parents' feelings of control over a situation in which many parents feel they have little power.

As parents get to know the infant better, they become experts on the infant's response to various situations and caregiving activities. Their expertise should be recognized and respectfully considered in planning infant care. Although parents often feel like outsiders when first visiting the NICU, they can, in time, move into the role of partners with the NICU staff in caring for the infant.

Look for opportunities to praise parenting abilities. Point out positive ways the infant responds to the parents' touch and caregiving. Model methods to respond to behavioral cues and acknowledge parents when they respond to the infant's signals appropriately. Listen to their ideas about what works best for the infant and incorporate them if at all possible.

Alleviating Concerns

Invite parents to call the NICU at any time for information about their infant. This helps allay worry when parents wake up at night and wonder how the infant is doing. Phone calls are especially beneficial for parents unable to visit the infant because of distance or other reasons.

Parents also need support from others besides nursing staff. Put them in touch with parents of other preterm infants and refer them to support groups, parent-to-parent groups with veteran NICU parents, telephone support, educational

offerings, or counseling sessions. Tell them about internet sources such as https://www.preemieworld.com. Talking with others who have faced the same problems can be very comforting as parents compare notes and get practical suggestions from an experienced parent's point of view. Some agencies pair parents with a "buddy" who has had a similar experience and is from the same culture. Special programs may be available after discharge to provide parents with ongoing support and education. It is important to consider language and culture during this process.

Cultural practices should be incorporated into the care of the infant. Determine who in the family will make the decisions and who will be managing the infant's care. In some cultures, the father makes decisions, and the grandmother, rather than the mother, is the major caregiver. In these cases, it is essential that the right persons be included in appropriate teaching (Gardner & Voos, 2021).

Helping with Ongoing Problems

Parents may be unprepared for the inconsistent progress infants often make after surviving the risks of the early days. They expect steady progress once the infant can breathe independently and take feedings. However, complications such as NEC or sepsis can cause major setbacks at this time. To cope with a new crisis, parents need extensive support from the nurse. Use therapeutic communication techniques such as reflecting feelings to help them express and cope with their extreme disappointment. Give information about the infant's changing condition and what to expect in the days ahead.

Having a hospitalized child can be exhausting for the parents. Remind them to take breaks away from the infant, whether to go to the cafeteria for a meal or to go home and rest. As the infant's condition improves, parents may take more time away as they begin to prepare for discharge. Encourage them to do this while making sure they feel welcome to stay with the infant as much as they desire.

Parents with infants in a NICU may have problems with sleep disturbances and depressive symptoms. Be alert for signs of postpartum depression because fatigue and having an ill infant are factors that may lead to this condition (Gardner & Voos, 2021). One study found a 45% rate of depression in parents at the time of their high-risk infants' discharge from a NICU (Soghier et al., 2020). An additional study suggested NICU stress and depression had a negative, long-term impact on the parenting skills of mothers with infants born at less than 31 weeks of gestation (Gerstein et al., 2019).

Preparing for Discharge

Most preterm infants are discharged about the time of their expected birth. However, many infants may go home before their due date. It is important that the parents understand the expected hospital course.

Begin early to teach parents and other caregivers any special procedures, treatments, and medications that the infant will need after discharge. Observe the parents as they perform care until they are comfortable and can do it safely. Praise their efforts and provide hints to make the care easier. Provide written information about home care of the preterm infant.

Help the parents learn what is normal for their infant and how to recognize and respond to abnormal signs. Some hospitals have the parents spend a night or two "rooming-in" in a special parent room, where they assume full 24-hour care of the infant and still have help when they need it. This helps increase parents' confidence that they can care for the infant by themselves. It also allows staff to evaluate the parents' abilities to care for the infant.

Help the parents determine what adaptations they will need to make at home before discharge. Utility companies should be notified if the infant is considered medically fragile to ensure the family receives priority service in case of a power failure. Provision for emergency electricity such as batteries also should be arranged. Organize home nursing services, purchase of supplies, and delivery of special equipment before discharge, if needed.

Discuss what to expect with regard to care of the infant after discharge. Infants may require oxygen, cardiorespiratory monitoring, suctioning, gavage or gastrostomy (tube) feedings, or other treatments that parents will have to learn to perform. Many infants need feedings every 3 hours, day and night, to help them gain weight adequately. Feedings may be time-consuming, and parental fatigue resulting from sleep interruptions may be more than they expected, especially if they are parents of multiples.

Infants are accustomed to the noises of a nursery 24 hours a day and may not sleep well at first in a quiet home environment. Suggest parents play soft music and use a night light for the first week. They should gradually eliminate these aids to avoid conditioning the infant to their use. Visitors and noise or activity may be too much for the infant at first and should be limited.

Explore with parents what kind of help they might need to meet the everyday requirements of the infant and the rest of the family. Help them identify where they might find assistance from family and friends. Reassure them that friends and family often welcome opportunities to help.

The AAP and ACOG (2017) have recommendations of accomplishments that should occur before discharge, which include the following:

- Signs of readiness for discharge include a sustained pattern of weight gain, adequate maintenance of body temperature in an open bed, feeding without cardiorespiratory compromise, and stable cardiorespiratory function.
- Appropriate immunizations should have been given (or arrangements made to get them); car seat evaluation completed; metabolic screening performed; assessment of hearing, the eyes, hematologic status, and nutritional risks performed; and appropriate treatment plans completed before discharge.
- The family and home should have been evaluated. The family must have at least two members who demonstrate the ability to feed and provide all needed care, perform cardiopulmonary resuscitation, give medications, operate equipment, and show understanding of signs of problems and what to do about them.
- A primary care physician and other appropriate follow-up care should have been arranged.

Help parents form realistic expectations about the infant. For example, they should know that the infant will accomplish developmental tasks such as crawling and walking later compared with full-term infants. Parents should base their expectations on the infant's **corrected age** (corrected or developmental age is the chronologic age minus the number of weeks the infant was born early) rather than on chronologic age.

Assist the parents in planning how to integrate the new infant into the family. Meeting the needs of their other children, in addition to the new responsibilities of caring for the preterm infant, is a major source of worry. Listen to their concerns about their other children and encourage siblings who do not have infections to visit, if possible.

Help parents prepare siblings for what they will see and do when visiting. Siblings should touch or hold the infant, if possible, to help them bond. Taking photographs of the siblings with the infant will help them remember the visit.

Before discharge, a car seat challenge is often performed. Proper positioning with blanket rolls may be necessary because the infants may slump over, interfering with chest expansion. Some infants need car beds to allow them to ride in the recumbent position.

Evaluation

Expected outcomes are met if parents visit often and interact appropriately with the infant, express their understanding of and comfort with the infant's needs, and take an increasingly active role in the care of the infant. Parents and designated caregivers should be able to independently provide care before discharge.

KNOWLEDGE CHECK

12. How can the nurse help parents be comfortable with their preterm infant?
13. How should the nurse prepare parents for the discharge of their preterm infant?

COMMON COMPLICATIONS OF PRETERM INFANTS

Complications of prematurity increase as the infant's gestational age and birth weight decrease. Some complications that occur in full-term and preterm infants, such as hyperbilirubinemia, are discussed in Chapter 25. Complications most often associated with preterm birth are discussed here. Further information about each condition can be found in pediatric texts.

Respiratory Distress Syndrome

Respiratory distress syndrome (RDS) is a condition caused by insufficient production of surfactant in the lungs. It occurs most often in preterm infants under 28 weeks of gestation and increases as the gestational age decreases. Other risk factors for RDS include birth asphyxia, cesarean birth, multiple births, male sex, cold stress, and maternal diabetes because these conditions interfere with surfactant production. It is less frequent, however, when antenatal corticosteroids or chronic fetal stress, such as in heroin addiction, maternal hypertension, or prolonged rupture of membranes, causes the lungs to mature more quickly (Ahlfeld, 2020).

Pathophysiology

Surfactant is a phospholipid that lines the alveoli. Surfactant decreases surface tension to allow the alveoli to remain open when air is exhaled. It must be continuously produced as it is used. Sufficient surfactant is usually produced beginning at 34 to 36 weeks of gestation to prevent RDS (Gardner, Enzman-Hines & Nyp, 2021).

When too little surfactant is present, the alveoli collapse each time the infant exhales. The lungs become **noncompliant** or "stiff" and resist expansion. Noncompliant lungs require a much higher negative pressure for the alveoli to open with each inhalation. This results in severe retractions with each breath because the chest wall is very compliant. The weak muscles of the chest are drawn inward, placing pressure on the lungs that further interferes with expansion. Seesaw respirations also may occur.

As fewer alveoli expand, atelectasis, hypoxia, and hypercapnia occur. This causes pulmonary vasoconstriction and decreased blood flow to the lungs because of the high resistance within the pulmonary blood vessels. Persistent pulmonary hypertension can result in a return to fetal circulation patterns, with opening of the ductus arteriosus. Acidosis and alveolar ischemic injury further complicate the condition by interfering with surfactant synthesis.

Tests of amniotic fluid can detect lecithin, sphingomyelin, phosphatidylglycerol, and phosphatidylinositol, which are components of surfactant. These tests can predict whether the fetal lungs are mature enough for survival outside of the uterus. They are done before an elective induction or cesarean birth is performed on an infant younger than 38 weeks of gestation. The incidence and severity of RDS may be reduced by giving the pregnant client corticosteroids before birth.

Manifestations

Signs of RDS begin during the first hours after birth. They include tachypnea, tachycardia, nasal flaring, and cyanosis. Retractions of accessory muscles are common. They may be above or below the sternum and/or between or below the ribs. Audible grunting on expiration is characteristic. It results from air moving past a partially closed glottis, which helps maintain lung expansion; gas exchange during exhalation; and functional residual capacity. Breath sounds may be decreased, and crackles may be present.

Acidosis develops as a result of hypoxemia. Blood gases show increased carbon dioxide levels and decreased oxygen levels. Chest radiographs show the "ground glass" reticulogranular appearance of the lungs that is characteristic of RDS. Areas of atelectasis are present. Signs become worse, peak within 3 days, and then begin to improve gradually (Ahlfeld, 2020).

Therapeutic Management

Surfactant is instilled into the infant's trachea shortly after birth or as soon as signs of RDS become apparent. Doses are repeated, if necessary. Infants treated with surfactant have higher survival rates, although the incidence of other complications of prematurity such as bronchopulmonary dysplasia (BPD) is unchanged (Ahlfeld, 2020; Gardner, Enzman-Hines & Nyp, 2021).

Other treatment is supportive, including oxygen, continuous CPAP or mechanical ventilation, inhaled nitric oxide, correction of acidosis, IV fluids, and care of other complications. Antibiotics may be given because signs of neonatal pneumonia are similar to those of RDS (Lagoski et al., 2020). Low temperature and low glucose level may occur and should be treated promptly.

Nursing Considerations

The nurse observes for signs of developing RDS at birth and during the early hours after birth. Changes in the infant's condition are constantly assessed. Changes in ventilator settings may be necessary as the infant's ability to oxygenate increases. Observation for signs of common complications such as patent ductus arteriosus and BPD is important. The nurse should monitor the results of laboratory tests for abnormalities in blood gases and acid-base balance. Early signs of sepsis should be identified and reported. Other care is similar to general care for the preterm infant.

Bronchopulmonary Dysplasia (Chronic Lung Disease)

Bronchopulmonary dysplasia (BPD), also known as *chronic lung disease,* is a chronic condition in which damage to the infant's lungs requires prolonged dependence on supplemental oxygen. It occurs most often in infants younger than 32 weeks of gestational age and in one-third of VLBW infants. The diagnostic criteria for BPD include gestational age, the length of time on oxygen, and the amount of oxygen needed. The common definition of BPD is when an infant requires oxygen 28 days after birth (Bancalari & Jain, 2020).

Pathophysiology

BPD results from a combination of factors such as mechanical ventilation, high levels of oxygen, PDA, and infections that injure bronchial epithelium and interfere with alveolar development. The result is inflammation, atelectasis, edema, and airway hyperreactivity, thickening of the walls of the alveoli, and fibrotic changes (Bancalari & Jain, 2022).

Manifestations

The major sign of BPD is an increased need for or an inability to be weaned from respiratory support and oxygen. Other signs include inability to tolerate handling or care activities, tachycardia, tachypnea, retractions and nasal flaring, crackles, wheezing, respiratory acidosis, cyanosis, increased secretions, bronchospasm, and characteristic changes in the lungs on chest radiographs. Pulmonary edema and cardiac hypertrophy may occur (Gardner, Enzman-Hines & Nyp, 2021).

Therapeutic Management

Prevention includes administration of steroids to pregnant clients at risk of preterm birth to reduce noenatal RDS, minimizing exposure to oxygen and pressure with ventilation as much as possible, avoidance of fluid overload, and increased nutrition. Treatment is supportive, with antibiotics and bronchodilators as necessary, and gradual decreases in the amount of oxygen. Diuretics are given and fluids are restricted because infants are prone to fluid overload. Increased calories and protein are important. The infant may be discharged home with long-term oxygen therapy, and some need frequent rehospitalization during the first 2 years of life because of respiratory tract infections.

Intraventricular Hemorrhage

Intraventricular hemorrhage (IVH) is also called *germinal matrix hemorrhage* and *periventricular–intraventricular hemorrhage.* It is bleeding into and around the ventricles of the brain. Approximately 30% of preterm infants weighing less than 1500 g (3 lb, 5 oz) develop IVH (Mehan & Thomas, 2020). The first few days of life are the most common times for hemorrhage to occur. It may also occur in approximately 3.5% of term infants (Hall & Reavey, 2021).

Pathophysiology

IVH results from rupture of the fragile blood vessels in the germinal matrix, located around the ventricles of the brain. It is associated with increased or decreased blood pressure, asphyxia or respiratory distress requiring mechanical ventilation, and increased or fluctuating cerebral blood flow. Rapid blood volume expansion, hypercarbia, anemia, and hypoglycemia are other causes.

Hemorrhage is graded 1 through 4, according to the amount of bleeding. Grade 1 is a very small bleed at the germinal matrix. Grade 2 hemorrhage extends into the lateral ventricles without distention, and grade 3 causes distention of ventricles. Grade 4 hemorrhage causes ventricular dilation and extends into surrounding brain tissue. The condition is diagnosed by cranial ultrasound through the anterior fontanel.

Manifestations

Signs of IVH are determined by the severity of the hemorrhage. They may be subtle or remarkable, including lethargy, poor muscle tone, bradycardia, deterioration of respiratory status with cyanosis or apnea, drop in hematocrit, acidosis, hyperglycemia, tense fontanel, and seizures.

Therapeutic Management

Most hemorrhages take place in the first week. Ultrasonography performed at 7 days of age for preterm infants at risk for IVH shows 90% of hemorrhages (de Vries, 2020). If bleeding is found, serial ultrasonography may be performed to determine progression of the problem.

Treatment is supportive and focuses on maintaining respiratory function and dealing with other complications. Outcomes vary depending on the severity of the hemorrhage. Of preterm infants with an IVH, 50% have no neurologic complications (Ditzenberger, 2021). Hydrocephalus may develop from blockage of cerebrospinal fluid flow. A ventriculoperitoneal shunt (catheter leading from the ventricles of the brain to the peritoneal cavity) may be necessary to drain the fluid.

Nursing Considerations

Many aspects of care may increase cerebral blood flow and blood pressure. These include mechanical ventilation, suctioning, and excessive handling. Even crying and changing diapers may produce changes in cerebral blood flow. Therefore, the nurse should avoid situations that may increase the risk for IVH as much as possible. Handling is kept to a minimum, and pain and environmental stressors are reduced as much as possible. Developmental care has been found helpful. Nurses are alert for early signs of IVH. Nursing care includes daily measurement of the head circumference and observation for changes in neurologic status, which may be subtle.

Parents need assistance to cope with the diagnosis and their concerns regarding long-term implications. They should learn how to assess for signs of increasing intracranial pressure if their infant has IVH-induced hydrocephalus and understand that follow-up care may include periodic ultrasound examinations.

Retinopathy of Prematurity

Retinopathy of prematurity (ROP) is a condition in which injury to the blood vessels in the eye leads to growth of new blood vessels that abnormally develop and may result in visual impairment or blindness in preterm infants. It occurs in over 80% of infants born at less than 26 weeks' gestation (Fraser & Diehl-Jones, 2021).

Pathophysiology

The exact cause of ROP is unknown, but high levels of oxygen in the blood and prematurity are major risk factors. However, ROP develops in some infants who have never received supplementary oxygen. Many additional risk factors to developing ROP have been suggested, but clear evidence is lacking (Salmon, 2020; Kim et al., 2018).

In ROP, immature blood vessels in the eye are injured. After a period, new vessels proliferate, extending throughout the retina and into the vitreous humor of the eye in some infants. Fluid leakage and hemorrhages from the fragile vessels may cause scarring, traction on the retina, and retinal detachment. However, the progress of pathologic processes stops in more than 90% of infants, and there is little visual loss (Olitsky & Marsh, 2020).

Therapeutic Management

Infants with a birth weight of 1500 g (3 lb, 5 oz) or less or gestational age of 32 weeks or less and selected infants with a birth weight of 1500 to 2000 g (4 lb, 6.6 oz) or gestational age of more than 32 weeks with an unstable clinical course should be screened to detect changes of the eye. The frequency of repeat examinations is determined by the results of screenings.

Laser surgery to destroy abnormal blood vessels is the current treatment of choice. Intravitreal bevacizumab has been used in some cases and will have more study to determine its use in the future. Cryosurgery or reattachment of the retina also may be necessary (Olitsky & Marsh, 2020).

Nursing Considerations

The nurse should check the pulse oximetry readings frequently for any infant receiving oxygen. Oxygen should be titrated to keep oxygen saturation levels within prescribed limits. Extremes of high or low saturations should be avoided. Parents should be informed about ophthalmologic tests and receive an explanation of the results. Eye examinations can be very stressful to the infant and swaddling and rest periods should be provided as appropriate. Mydriatic eye drops given to dilate the eyes may cause hypertension, bradycardia, and apnea (Fraser & Diehl-Jones, 2021). If surgery is performed, the eye is assessed for drainage. Ice packs may be used for edema, and pain medication should be given. Support for parents is essential throughout the examinations and especially if damage to the eye is found. The importance of follow-up eye examinations after discharge should be stressed.

Necrotizing Enterocolitis

Necrotizing enterocolitis (NEC) is a serious inflammatory condition of the intestinal tract that may lead to cellular death of areas of intestinal mucosa. It occurs in 1% to 5% of infants admitted to NICUs (Greenberg et al., 2019). The mortality rate is 20% to 30% and is higher in infants who had surgical versus medical treatment. The ileum and proximal colon are the areas most often affected and survivors may have long-term GI problems (Kudin & Neu, 2020).

Pathophysiology

Although the exact causes are unknown, immaturity of the intestines is a major factor in preterm infants. The rate of NEC increases with decreasing gestational age. Previous hypoxia of the intestines may be a causative factor. The incidence of NEC is much higher after infants have received feedings.

Although minimal enteric feedings are thought to increase maturation of the intestines, feedings that are too early or increased too fast may cause NEC. When infants are fed, bacteria proliferate, and gas-forming organisms may invade the intestinal wall in some infants. Eventually, necrosis, perforation, and peritonitis may occur. Breast milk, which contains immunoglobulins, leukocytes, and antibacterial agents, may have a preventive effect on the development of NEC. Studies about using prenatal steroids, indomethacin, and probiotics to prevent NEC are mixed, with some showing less and others showing greater incidence (Greenberg et al., 2019).

Manifestations

Signs include increased abdominal girth caused by distention, increased gastric residuals, decreased or absent bowel sounds, loops of bowel seen through the abdominal wall, vomiting, bile-stained residuals or emesis, abdominal tenderness and discoloration, signs of infection, and occult blood in the stools. Respiratory difficulty may occur because of pressure from the distended abdomen on the diaphragm. Apnea, bradycardia, temperature instability, lethargy, hypotension, and shock also may be present. On radiographs, there may be loops of bowel dilated with air. The presence of air within the intestinal wall is characteristic of the condition. Free air in the peritoneum indicates that perforation has occurred, although perforation may occur without this sign.

Therapeutic Management

Breastfeeding should be encouraged, especially if the infant has risk factors for NEC. If maternal breast milk is not available, donor milk can be used.

Treatment of NEC includes antibiotics, discontinuation of oral feedings, continuous or intermittent gastric suction, and use of parenteral nutrition to rest the intestines. Surgery may be necessary if perforation or continued lack of improvement occurs. The necrotic area is removed, and an ostomy may be performed. Infants who have had large areas of bowel removed may develop short bowel syndrome with malabsorption and malnutrition.

Nursing Considerations

Nurses should encourage interested parents to provide breast milk for their infants because NEC is less likely to occur in breastfed infants. Early recognition of signs of NEC is essential to decrease mortality. Because nurses are constantly observing the infant, they often are able to detect the early, subtle signs that lead to prompt diagnosis. If one or more signs are noted, the nurse withholds the next feeding and notifies the provider.

Abdominal girth is measured, and IV fluids and parenteral nutrition must be managed. Intake and output are important because third-space fluid loss occurs when fluid moves from the intravascular spaces to the extracellular spaces. The infant should be positioned on the side to minimize the effects of pressure on the diaphragm from the distended intestines. During recovery, the nurse should observe for signs of feeding intolerance when feedings are resumed. Scar tissue may cause partial or complete bowel obstruction.

Short Bowel Syndrome

Short bowel syndrome (SBS) is a condition caused by a bowel that is shorter than normal. It is caused by congenital malformations of the GI tract or surgical resection that decreases the length of the small intestines.

Pathophysiology

When the bowel is too short, decreased mucosal surface area causes inadequate absorption of fluids, electrolytes, and nutrients. A loss of more than 50% of the small bowel may result in symptoms of generalized malabsorption or deficiencies of certain nutrients related to the region of bowel that has been removed (Shamir, 2020).

Manifestations

The most common symptoms of SBS are malabsorption, diarrhea, and failure to thrive. If the small bowel is 40 cm or more, the malabsorption may improve in time because the remaining bowel continues to grow and adapt in function.

Therapeutic Management

During surgery, every effort is made to preserve as much of the small bowel length as possible. After surgery, the child's fluid and electrolyte balance must be restored and stabilized. The mainstay of treatment for infants and children is nutritional support.

TPN is begun as the primary source of nutrition. It is formulated to meet the child's nutritional needs as well as promote weight gain and growth. Enteral nutrition is begun as soon as possible after surgery to allow the intestines to adapt to food.

Nursing Considerations

The nurse manages the infant's TPN and enteral feedings. TPN is generally infused through a central venous access device. Strict asepsis should be used when performing central line dressing changes and when administering TPN to prevent central line–associated bloodstream infections. Enteral nutrition is advanced slowly while corresponding adjustments are made to the composition of the TPN. The nurse carefully assesses and documents tolerance of enteral feedings noting any signs of dehydration, electrolyte imbalances, and nutritional deficits. Nonnutritive sucking is provided as well.

LATE PRETERM INFANTS

Infants born between 34 $^{0/7}$ and 36 $^{6/7}$ weeks of gestation are called **late preterm infants** because they have many needs similar to those of preterm infants. They are more stable than preterm infants but are physiologically and metabolically immature and have higher mortality and morbidity rates than full-term infants. In 2005 the AWHONN launched the multiyear Late Preterm Infant Initiative to develop evidence-based practice guidelines for care of the late preterm infant. Results of the study showed 46% of late preterm infants spent some time in a special care nursery. Hypothermia, hypoglycemia, feeding difficulties, hyperbilirubinemia, respiratory distress, and/or a need for a septic workup occurred in half of the infants studied (Cooper et al., 2012).

Incidence and Etiology

Late preterm births comprised 7% of births in 2017 (Huff et al., 2019). Contributing factors in late preterm birth include elective and medically indicated inductions and cesarean births, preterm labor, premature rupture of membranes, preeclampsia, multifetal pregnancies, obesity, assisted reproductive technology, advanced age of the childbearing client, and inaccurate estimate of gestational age before birth (Parsons & Jain, 2020).

Characteristics of Late Preterm Infants

Because late preterm infants often look like full-term infants, they may not be recognized as being preterm. However, they are physiologically immature. They are at risk for respiratory disorders, problems with temperature maintenance, hypoglycemia, hyperbilirubinemia, feeding difficulties, acidosis, and infection (such as respiratory syncytial virus) because of their immaturity (Gardner & Niermeyer, 2021; Huff et al., 2019). They are also at risk for long-term neurodevelopmental disorders as well as cognitive and behavioral problems (Parsons & Jain, 2020). They are more likely to be admitted to the NICU after birth and are at increased risk for rehospitalization after discharge.

Therapeutic Management

Therapeutic management varies according to the problems presented. Many interventions are similar to those for preterm infants discussed in this chapter.

Nursing Considerations
Assessment and Care of Common Problems

Late preterm infants may receive care similar to that for full-term infants, but, compared with full-term infants, these infants need closer monitoring for complications during the hospital stay. Nursing care is similar to that given to preterm infants in many aspects.

Thermoregulation. Once stable, normal newborns usually have their temperature checked only once every 8 to 12 hours. A late preterm infant may develop cold stress that is not noticed until signs appear or it is time for the next vital sign assessment. Therefore, nurses should be more vigilant in watching for thermal instability in these infants. The temperature, as well as other vital signs, should be checked every 3 to 4 hours for the first 24 hours and then every shift, depending on need and agency policy (Parsons & Jain, 2020). SSC is often used to keep infants warm. A radiant warmer or an incubator also may be used if the infant cannot maintain normal temperature.

Feedings. Late preterm infants may have immature suck and swallow reflexes, have shorter awake periods, and fall asleep during feedings before they have fed adequately (Mohan & Jain, 2018). They may have difficulty with latch when breastfeeding. Their low tone and weak suck may decrease the amount of milk they obtain with each suck. They have an increased caloric need and should be fed every 2 to 3 hours.

Feeding problems are common, and nurses should assess feeding sessions to ensure swallowing is occurring. Breastfeeding clients need special help see that infants are feeding well. Two key breastfeeding elements to be assessed and supported are protecting the client's milk supply and ensuring the infant is adequately gaining weight (Gardner, Lawrence & Lawrence, 2021). The football and cross-cradle holds are helpful in positioning these infants at the breast.

Urine and stool output are monitored as indications of adequate intake. Late preterm infants are at risk for hypoglycemia, and blood glucose measurements should be performed according to hospital protocol, especially during the first 24 hours. Because late preterm infants are at greater risk for breastfeeding-associated rehospitalization compared with term infants, lactation consultants should be involved in their care (Verklan, 2021; Cartwright et al., 2017).

Discharge. Late preterm infants often can be discharged at the same time as full-term infants. They should not be discharged earlier than 48 hours after birth. Before discharge, nurses should ensure infants are feeding adequately and have had normal vital signs for at least 12 hours. Bilirubin levels should be assessed before discharge (Parsons & Jain, 2020).

Teaching should include the need for keeping the infant warm. The infant should be kept away from drafts and dressed in one more layer than an adult would wear. Late preterm infants are subject to overstimulation. This may occur when parents take the baby home to an environment of many different stimuli. The nurse should teach signs of overstimulation and how to minimize them.

A car seat challenge should be conducted before discharge to ensure the infant can tolerate sitting in a car seat without bradycardia, apnea, or decreased oxygen saturation. The parents bring their own car seat for the test. Preterm and LBW infants should be observed in the car seat for 90 to 120 minutes (or more, if travel time to go home is longer) (Bull et al., 2018).

Parents should be taught signs of common complications such as jaundice or dehydration and what to do if they occur. Because some problems may not be noticeable at discharge, late preterm infants should have a follow-up visit with the health care provider 24 to 48 hours after discharge (Parsons & Jain, 2020).

POSTTERM INFANTS

Postterm infants are those who are born after the 42nd week of gestation. Their longer-than-normal gestation places them at risk for a number of complications.

Scope of the Problem

Globally, less than 10% of all pregnancies are considered posterm (Rampersand & Macones, 2021). In some cases, the fetus continues to be well supported by the placenta and is of normal size or is large for gestational age. Some grow to more than 4000 g (8 lb, 13 oz), placing them at risk for birth injuries or cesarean birth.

In other cases, placental functioning decreases when pregnancy is prolonged. If placental insufficiency is present, decreased amniotic fluid volume (oligohydramnios) and compression of the umbilical cord may occur. The fetus may not receive the appropriate amount of oxygen and nutrients and may be small for gestational age. This condition, called *dysmaturity syndrome,* occurs in about 20% of posterm pregnancies (Blickstein & Rimon, 2020).

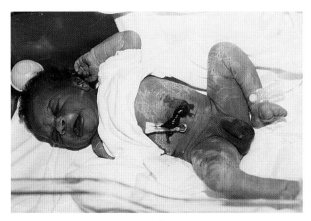

FIG. 24.8 The postmature infant has no vernix and dry, cracked, peeling skin.

When labor begins, poor oxygen reserves may cause fetal compromise. The fetus may pass meconium as a result of hypoxia before or during labor, increasing the risk for meconium aspiration at delivery (see Chapter 25). These infants are also at higher risk for asphyxia than are other infants. Posterm infants have a higher perinatal mortality rate than infants born at term.

Assessment

Most infants will be normal at birth. If the infant is large, the nurse should observe for injury and hypoglycemia. The infant with dysmaturity syndrome may be thin with loose skin and little subcutaneous fat. The umbilical cord is thin with little Wharton's jelly. There is little or no vernix caseosa, but the infant generally has abundant hair on the head and long nails. The skin is wrinkled, cracked, and peeling (Fig. 24.8). If meconium was present in the amniotic fluid, the cord, skin, and nails may be stained yellow green, indicating that meconium was present for some time.

Posterm infants should be assessed for hypoglycemia because of rapid use of glycogen stores. If loss of subcutaneous fat has occurred, the infant is at risk for low temperature.

Therapeutic Management

Therapeutic management focuses on prevention and symptomatic treatment. Expectant clients who are "overdue" are scheduled for tests of placental functioning, and labor is induced if signs of placental deterioration are discovered during fetal diagnostic testing. If the fetus cannot tolerate labor, a cesarean birth is necessary. Apgar scores less than 7 are more likely in posterm infants. In cases of meconium aspiration, respiratory support is needed at birth (see Chapter 25).

Nursing Considerations

The nurse's role is primarily one of prevention of complications, where possible, and monitoring of changes in status. During labor and delivery, the nurse responds appropriately to fetal heart rate decelerations, prepares for and assists in emergency delivery, and cares for respiratory problems at birth.

Signs of dysmaturity syndrome in infants are noted during the initial assessment. Respiratory problems may necessitate continued assessment and care. Infants with any indications of dysmaturity should be tested for hypoglycemia soon after birth and again an hour later or according to hospital policy. They need early and more frequent feedings to help compensate for the period of poor nutrition before birth.

Temperature regulation may be poor because fat stores were used for nourishment in utero. Providing extra blankets, assessing temperature frequently, and teaching parents about prevention of cold stress are important throughout the hospital stay. Polycythemia, resulting from hypoxia before birth, increases the risk for hyperbilirubinemia.

SMALL-FOR-GESTATIONAL-AGE INFANTS

Small-for-gestational-age (SGA) infants are those who fall below the 10th percentile in size on growth charts. They have failed to grow in the uterus as expected and have FGRs. Some infants who do not meet the definition for SGA may have FGR and fail to grow to full potential before birth for a variety of reasons. The terms SGA and FGR often are incorrectly used interchangeably. SGA infants may be preterm, full-term, or postterm. Infant mortality and morbidity increase steadily as growth restriction increases (Resnik, 2019).

Causes

Many risk factors may cause an infant to be SGA. Congenital malformations, chromosomal anomalies, genetic factors, multiple gestations, and fetal infections such as rubella or cytomegalovirus may cause FGR. Poor placental function resulting from aging of the placenta, small size, separation, or malformation may interfere with fetal growth. Illness in the expectant client, such as preeclampsia or severe diabetes, restricts uteroplacental blood flow and decreases fetal growth. Smoking, drug or alcohol abuse, and severe malnutrition in the expectant client also impair fetal growth.

Scope of the Problem

Infants affected with FGR have higher perinatal morbidity and a mortality rate that is 5 to 30 times that of infants who are not growth-restricted (Chu & Devaskar, 2020). Death may occur from asphyxia before or during labor because of poor placental functioning or from complications of congenital anomalies or prematurity.

Full-term SGA infants are subject to many of the same complications as those who are preterm or postterm. Problems tend to be greatest in infants who are preterm in addition to being SGA.

Low Apgar scores, meconium aspiration, and polycythemia are increased in the SGA infant. Hypoglycemia is common because of inadequate storage of glycogen in the liver. Although mature muscle tone enables the SGA infant to maintain better flexion than the preterm infant, SGA infants are prone to inadequate thermoregulation because subcutaneous white fat and brown fat stores have been used to survive in utero. If hypoglycemia develops, inadequate glucose is available for increased metabolism to produce heat, increasing the problem.

Characteristics of Small-for-Gestational-Age Infants

The appearance of the SGA infant varies, depending on whether the cause of growth restriction began early or late in the pregnancy. Variation occurs because growth restriction affects the weight first. If it continues, the length and then the head size eventually will be affected.

Symmetric growth restriction involves the entire body. It may be caused by congenital anomalies, genetic disorders, exposure to infections or drugs early in pregnancy, or normal genetic predisposition. Although the infant's weight, length, and head circumference are all below the 10th percentile, the body is proportionate and appears normally developed for size. The total number of cells as well as the cell size are decreased, and the infant may have long-term complications. These infants are often small throughout their lives. They have a higher rate of neonatal mortality. Approximately 20% to 30% of SGA infants have symmetric growth restriction (Chu & Devaskar, 2020).

Asymmetric growth restriction is caused by complications such as preeclampsia that begin in the third trimester and interfere with uteroplacental function. In asymmetric restriction, the head is normal in size but seems large for the rest of the body. Brain growth and heart size are normal. The length is normal, but the weight is below the 10th percentile for gestational age. The AC is decreased because the liver, spleen, and adrenals are smaller than normal (Chu & Devaskar, 2020).

The infant appears long, thin, and wasted. The dry, loose skin has longitudinal thigh creases from loss of subcutaneous fat. The infant has a sunken abdomen, sparse hair, a thin cord, and the facial appearance of being elderly. The anterior fontanel may be large with wide or overlapping cranial sutures. Most SGA infants have some "catch up" in growth, particularly in the first 2 years, if they are adequately nourished after birth (Mandy, 2020).

Therapeutic Management

Therapeutic management is focused on prevention, with good prenatal care to identify and treat problems early. When growth restriction cannot be prevented, ultrasound examination may permit early discovery of the condition. Serial nonstress tests and biophysical profiles help determine whether the infant should be delivered early, and preparation can be made for the expected complications at birth. Problems during and after birth are treated as they occur. They may include asphyxia, meconium aspiration, hypoglycemia, and polycythemia (Chu & Devaskar, 2020). SGA infants have a greater surface area and higher metabolic rate than infants who are appropriate for gestational age. This increases their risk for problems with temperature stability (Gardner & Cammack, 2021).

Nursing Considerations

Because the causes of growth restriction are so varied, care of the SGA infant should be adapted to meet the specific problems presented. When signs of growth restriction are present, the nurse should observe for complications that commonly accompany it. The general appearance and measurements give an indication of the type of growth restriction that has occurred. Measurements of the head, chest, length, and weight are below normal in the infant with symmetric growth restriction. If the restriction is asymmetric, the head circumference and length are normal, but the AC and weight are low.

The nurse should assess for hypoglycemia, especially in asymmetric, growth-restricted infants. The brain of the infant is normal and needs large amounts of glucose, but the liver is small and has inadequate stores of glycogen. Caloric needs are greater than for a normal infant, making early and more frequent feedings important. Temperature regulation and respiratory support are additional nursing concerns. Observation for jaundice is important in infants with polycythemia because a large amount of bilirubin may be released when the red blood cells break down.

LARGE-FOR-GESTATIONAL-AGE INFANTS

Large-for-gestational-age (LGA) infants are those who are above the 90th percentile for gestational age on intrauterine growth charts. They may have **macrosomia** (weigh more than 4000 to 4500 g [8 lb, 13 oz to 9 lb, 15 oz]) and are usually born at term, although they may be preterm or postterm. The preterm LGA infant may be mistaken for a full-term infant but has the same problems as other preterm infants.

Causes

Infants who are LGA may be born to multiparas, large parents, and clients with obesity (Fanaroff et al., 2020). Diabetes in the pregnant client also may cause increased size, as may hemolytic disease of the newborn (see Chapter 25).

Scope of the Problem

The LGA infant is more likely to go through a longer labor, suffer injury during birth, or need a cesarean birth. Shoulder dystocia may occur because the shoulders are too large to fit through the pelvis. Fractures of the clavicle or skull, injury to the brachial plexus or the facial nerve, cephalhematoma, subdural hematoma, and bruising occur more often in these infants than those of normal size. Congenital heart defects and a higher mortality rate also are more common (Fanaroff et al., 2020).

Therapeutic Management

Therapeutic management is based on identification of increased size during pregnancy by measurements of fundal height and ultrasound examination. Delivery problems may lead to use of vacuum extraction, forceps, or cesarean birth. Birth injuries and complications are treated as they arise.

Nursing Considerations

The nurse assists in a difficult delivery or cesarean birth resulting from dystocia when the infant is LGA. After birth the infant is carefully assessed for injuries or other complications such as hypoglycemia or polycythemia (see Chapter 25). Nursing care is geared to the problems presented.

KNOWLEDGE CHECK

14. What is the typical appearance of the infant with dysmaturity syndrome?
15. What special problems might a postmature infant have?
16. How are symmetric and asymmetric FGR different?
17. What problems may occur in infants who are LGA?

SUMMARY CONCEPTS

- Preterm infants differ in appearance from full-term infants. Some differences include small size, limp posture, red skin, abundant vernix and lanugo, and immature ears and genitals.
- The lungs of preterm infants may lack adequate surfactant, which interferes with expansion of the lungs, increasing the amount of energy necessary for breathing and leading to atelectasis.
- Other factors that may increase respiratory problems are poor cough reflex, narrow respiratory passages, and weak muscles.
- The prone position is used for preterm infants because it decreases breathing effort and increases oxygenation.
- Preterm infants are subject to cold stress because they have thin skin with blood vessels near the surface, little subcutaneous white fat or brown fat, a large surface area, a limp position, and an immature temperature control center.
- Maintaining a neutral thermal environment at all times for infants is important. The nurse should prevent drafts, use warmed oxygen, and keep incubator doors and portholes closed. When taken out of heating devices, the infant should be wrapped in warmed blankets and should wear a hat.

- Preterm infants are subject to increased insensible water losses and have difficulty maintaining fluid balance. Their kidneys do not concentrate or dilute urine as well as those of full-term infants. Intake and output should be carefully measured.
- The fragile skin of a preterm infant is easily damaged. Adhesives or chemicals that could injure the skin should be avoided. Special products designed to prevent injury to the skin should be used.
- Preterm infants are subject to infections because they did not recieve passive antibodies during fetal life, have an immature immune system, have fragile skin, and are subjected to many invasive procedures.
- The nurse should watch carefully for signs of pain and use comfort measures, containment, pacifiers, sucrose, breastfeeding, SSC, and medications to alleviate it.
- Infants demonstrate they are receiving too much stimulation by changes in oxygenation and behavior. The nurse should schedule care to allow rest periods, keep noise to a minimum, and teach parents how to interact with the infant appropriately.
- Preterm infants lack nutrient stores and need more nutrients but do not absorb them well. They lack coordination in sucking and swallowing and become fatigued easily.

- Signs indicating an infant may be ready for nipple feeding include rooting, sucking on a gavage catheter or pacifier, presence of gag reflex, and respiratory rate less than 60 breaths per minute.
- The nurse should teach clients who wish to breastfeed their preterm infants how to use a breast pump and store breast milk. Nurses provide privacy, give support and encouragement, explain the infant's behavior, and answer questions about breastfeeding.
- Nurses can increase parents' comfort with their preterm infant by providing information about the infant's condition and characteristics, the neonatal intensive care unit, equipment, and infant care. Spending time with parents during visits, offering therapeutic communication and realistic encouragement, and involving parents in care of the infant also help with bonding.
- Preparation for discharge should be started early in the infant's hospital stay. This allows parents to learn gradually and assume increasing responsibility in the care of the infant until they are comfortable with complete care.

- Common complications of preterm birth are respiratory distress syndrome, bronchopulmonary dysplasia, intraventricular hemorrhage, retinopathy of prematurity, necrotizing enterocolitis, and short bowel syndrome.
- Late preterm infants, born between 34 $^{0/7}$ and 36 $^{6/7}$ weeks, are at risk for respiratory, thermoregulation, and feeding problems, as well as hypoglycemia, hyperbilirubinemia, acidosis, and sepsis.
- Infants with dysmaturity syndrome may appear thin, with loose skin folds, cracked and peeling skin, and meconium staining. They may have respiratory difficulties at birth and suffer from hypoglycemia and inadequate temperature regulation.
- Infants with fetal growth restriction may be small for gestational age at birth. In symmetric growth restriction, the infant is proportionately small; in asymmetric growth restriction, the head and length are normal, and the body is thin.
- Large-for-gestational-age infants may have birth injuries such as fractures, nerve damage, or bruising as a result of their size. They may have hypoglycemia or polycythemia.

Clinical Judgment And Next-Generation NCLEX® Examination-Style Questions

1. A preterm infant, born at 30 weeks' gestation, was discharged from the hospital at 8 weeks of age. The newborn was seen by the pediatrician at 48 hours after discharge. The parents have many questions about the infant.

   For each client response, use an X to indicate whether the nurse's teaching was effective (helped the parents understand how to take care of a preterm infant), ineffective (did not help the parents understand how to take care of a preterm infant), or unrelated (not related to the discharge teaching of a preterm infant).

Client's Response	Effective	Ineffective	Unrelated
"My daughter is being fed every 3 hours, day and night."			
"We are keeping the home very quiet."			
"I have help from family and friends."			
"I am keeping the home warm and the baby wrapped in blankets to prevent getting cold."			
"We hold the baby four to five times a day."			
"Developmentally, my baby will crawl at a later time than normal."			

2. A client delivered a 23-week preterm infant 3 days ago. The client comes to see the infant each day, but does not touch the infant.

   Use an X to indicate whether the nursing actions listed below are indicated (appropriate or necessary), contraindicated (could be harmful), or nonessential (make no difference or are not necessary) for the client's care at this time.

Nursing Action	Indicated	Contraindicated	Nonessential
"Let the parents know their questions are welcome."			
"Continue to instruct the parents not to touch the infant as this could startle the baby and cause the heart rate to increase."			
"Use an interpreter as the parents do not understand English."			
"Explain the equipment used to care for the infant.			
"Teach the parents about skin-to-skin care and touching the baby's hand."			

REFERENCES & READINGS

Agren, J. (2020). Thermal environment of the intensive care nursery. In R. J. Martin, A. A. Fanaroff, & M. C. Walsh (Eds.), *Fanaroff and Martin's neonatal-perinatal medicine: Diseases of the fetus and infant* (11th ed., pp. 566–576). Elsevier.

Ahlfeld, S. K. (2020). Respiratory tract disorders. In R. M. Kliegman, J. W. St. Geme, N. J. Blum, S. S. Shah, R. C. Tasker, & K. M. Wilson (Eds.), *Nelson textbook of pediatrics* (21st ed., pp. 929–949). Elsevier.

Ameri, G. F., Rostami, S., Baniasadi, H., Aboli, B. P., & Ghorbani, F. (2018). The effect of prone position on gastric residuals in preterm infants. *Journal of Pharmaceutical Research International, 22*(2), 1–6. https://doi.org/10.9734/JPRI/2018/40433.

American Academy of Pediatrics (AAP), Committee on Nutrition, Section on Breastfeeding and Committee on Fetus and Newborn. (2017). Donor human milk for the high-risk infant: Preparation, safety, and usage options in the United States. *Pediatrics, 139*(1), e20163440. https://doi.org/10.1542/Peds.2016-3440.

American Academy of Pediatrics and American College of Obstetricians and Gynecologists (AAP & ACOG). (2017). *Guidelines for perinatal care.* (8th ed.).

Association of Women's Health, Obstetric and Neonatal Nurses (AWHONN). (2018). *Neonatal skin care: Evidence-based clinical practice guideline* (4th ed.). AWHONN.

Ayers, S., Bond, R., Bertullies, S., & Wijma, K. (2016). The aetiology of posttraumatic stress following childbirth: A meta-analysis and theoretical framework. *Psychological Medicine, 46*(6), 1121–1134. https://doi.org/10.1017/S0033291715002706.

Baessler, C., Capper, B., McMullen, S., & Smotrich, L. (2019). *Safe sleep guidelines.* National Association of Neonatal Nurses Newborn Safe Sleep Guideline. NANN.

Baker, B. (2009). Supporting the maternal experience in the neonatal NICU. *Newborn and Infant Nursing Reviews, 9*(2), 81–82. https://doi.org/10.1053/j.nainr.2009.03.002.

Bancalari, E. H., & Jain, D. (2022). Pathophysiology of bronchopulmonary distress syndrome. In R. A. Polin, S. H. Abman, D. H. Rowitch, W. E. Benitz, & W. W. Fox (Eds.), *Fetal and neonatal physiology* (6th ed., pp. 1703–1709). Elsevier.

Bancalari, E. H., & Jain, D. (2020). Bronchopulmonary dysplasia in the neonate. In R. J. Martin, A. A. Fanaroff, & M. C. Walsh (Eds.), *Fanaroff and Martin's neonatal-perinatal medicine: Diseases of the fetus and infant* (11th ed., pp. 1256–1269). Elsevier.

Blackburn, S.T. (2018). Maternal, fetal, & neonatal physiology: A clinical perspective (5th ed.). Elsevier.

Blickstein, I., & Rimon, O. F. (2020). Post-term pregnancy. In R. J. Martin, A. A. Fanaroff, & M. C. Walsh (Eds.), *Fanaroff and Martin's neonatal-perinatal medicine: Diseases of the fetus and infant* (11th ed., pp. 364–370). Elsevier.

Brand, M. C., & Shippey, H. A. (2021). Thermoregulation. In M. T. Verklan, M. Walden, & S. Forest (Eds.), *Core curriculum for neonatal intensive care nursing* (6th ed., pp. 86–98). Elsevier.

Brown, L. D., Hendrickson, K., Evans, R., Davis, J., & Hay, W. W. (2021). Enteral nutrition. In S. L. Gardner, B. S. Carter, M. Enzman-Hines, & S. Niermeyer (Eds.), *Merenstein & Gardner's handbook of neonatal intensive care* (9th ed., pp. 480–533). Elsevier.

Bull, M. A., Engle, W. A., & American Academy of Pediatrics (AAP), Committee on Injury, Violence, Poison Prevention and Committee on Fetus and Newborn. (2018). Safe transportation of preterm and low birthweight infants at hospital discharge. *Pediatrics, 123*(5), 1424–1429. https://doi.org/10.1542/peds.2009-0559. Published, 2009, reaffirmed 2018.

Cartwright, J., Atz, T., Newman, S., Mueller, M., & Demirci, J. R. (2017). Integrative review of interventions to promote breastfeeding in the late preterm infant. *Journal of Obstetric, Gynecologic, and Neonatal Nursing, 46*(3), 347–356. https://doi.org/10.1016/j.jogn.2017.01.006.

Center for Health Care Strategies. (2021). What is trauma informed care? traumainformedcare. https://www.traumainformedcare.chcs.org/what-is-trauma-informed-care/.

Ceylan, S. S., & Keskin, Z. (2020). Effects of two different positions on stress, pain and feeding tolerance of preterm infants during tube feeding. *International Journal of Nursing Practice*, e12911. https://doi.org/10.1111/ijn.12911.

Chu, A., & Devaskar, S. U. (2020). Intrauterine growth restriction. In R. J. Martin, A. A. Fanaroff, & M. C. Walsh (Eds.), *Fanaroff and Martin's neonatal-perinatal medicine: Diseases of the fetus and infant* (11th ed., pp. 260–273). Elsevier.

Cooper, B. M., Holditch-Davis, D., Verklan, M. T., Fraser-Askin, D., Lamp, J., Santa-Donato, A., Onokpsie, B., Soekem, K. L., & Bingham, D. (2012). Newborn clinical outcomes of the AHWONN late preterm infant research-based practice project. *Journal of Obstetric, Gynecologic, & Neonatal Nursing, 41*(6), 774–785. https://doi.org/10.1111/j.1552-6909.2012.01401.x.

Crowley, M. A., & Martin, R. J. (2020). Respiratory problems. In A. A. Fanaroff, & J. M. Fanaroff (Eds.), *Klaus and Fanaroff's care of the high-risk neonate* (7th ed., pp. 190–210). Elsevier.

D'Agata, A. L., Young, E. E., Cong, X., Grasso, D. J., & McGrath, J. M. (2016). Infant medical trauma in the neonatal intensive care unit (IMTN): A proposed concept for science and practice. *Advances in Neonatal Care, 16*(4), 289–297. https://doi.org/10.1097/ANC.0000000000000309.

de Vries, L. S. (2020). Intracranial hemorrhage and vascular lesions in the neonate. In R. M. Kliegman, J. W. St. Geme, N. J. Blum, S. S. Shah, R. C. Tasker, & K. M. Wilson (Eds.), *Nelson textbook of pediatrics* (21st ed., pp. 970–988). Elsevier.

Ditzenberger, G. (2021). Neurologic disorders. In M. T. Verklan, M. Walden, & S. Forest (Eds.), *Core curriculum for neonatal intensive care nursing* (6th ed., pp. 629–653). Elsevier.

Fanaroff, A. A., Lissauer, T., & Fanaroff, J. (2020). Physical growth: Physical examination of the newborn infant and the physical environment. In A. A. Fanaroff, & J. M. Fanaroff (Eds.), *Klaus and Fanaroff's care of the high-risk neonate* (7th ed., pp. 58–79). Elsevier.

Fraser, D., & Diehl-Jones, W. (2021). Ophthalmologic and auditory disorders. In M. T. Verklan, M. Walden, & S. Forest (Eds.), *Core curriculum for neonatal intensive care nursing* (6th ed., pp. 691–704). Elsevier.

Friedman, S. H., Thomson-Salo, F., & Ballard, R. (2020). Support for the family. In R. J. Martin, A. A. Fanaroff, & M. C. Walsh (Eds.), *Fanaroff and Martin's neonatal-perinatal medicine: Diseases of the fetus and infant* (11th ed., pp. 690–702). Elsevier.

Gardner, S. L., & Cammack, B. H. (2021). Heat balance. In S. L. Gardner, B. S. Carter, M. Enzman-Hines, & S. Niermeyer (Eds.), *Merenstein & Gardner's handbook of neonatal intensive care* (9th ed., pp. 137–164). Elsevier.

Gardner, S. L., Enzman-Hines, M., & Agarwal, R. (2021). Pain and pain relief. In S. L. Gardner, B. S. Carter, M. Enzman-Hines, & S. Niermeyer (Eds.), *Merenstein & Gardner's handbook of neonatal intensive care* (9th ed., pp. 273–333). Elsevier.

Gardner, S. L., Enzman-Hines, M., & Nyp, M. (2021). Respiratory diseases. In S. L. Gardner, B. S. Carter, M. Enzman-Hines, & S. Niermeyer (Eds.), *Merenstein & Gardner's handbook of neonatal intensive care* (9th ed., pp. 729–835). Elsevier.

Gardner, S. L., & Goldson, E. (2021). The neonate and the environment: Impact on development. In S. L. Gardner, B. S. Carter, M. Enzman-Hines, & S. Niermeyer (Eds.), *Merenstein & Gardner's handbook of neonatal intensive care* (9th ed., pp. 334–406). Elsevier.

Gardner, S. L., Lawrence, R. A., & Lawrence, R. M. (2021). Breastfeeding the neonate with special needs. In S. L. Gardner, B. S. Carter, M. Enzman-Hines, & S. Niermeyer (Eds.), *Merenstein & Gardner's handbook of neonatal intensive care* (9th ed., pp. 534–601). Elsevier.

Gardner, S. L., & Niermeyer, S. (2021). Immediate newborn care after birth. In S. L. Gardner, B. S. Carter, M. Enzman-Hines, & S. Niermeyer (Eds.), *Merenstein & Gardner's handbook of neonatal intensive care* (9th ed., pp. 93–136). Elsevier.

Gardner, S. L., & Voos, K. (2021). Families in crisis: Theoretical and practical considerations. In S. L. Gardner, B. S. Carter, M. Enzman-Hines, & S. Niermeyer (Eds.), *Merenstein & Gardner's handbook of neonatal intensive care* (9th ed., pp. 334–406). Elsevier.

Gerstein, E. D., Njoroge, W. F. M., Paul, R. A., Smyser, C. D., & Rogers, C. E. (2019). Maternal depression and stress in the neonatal intensive care unit: Associations with mother-child interactions at age 5 years. *The Journal of American Academy of Child & Adolescent Psychiatry*, 58(3), 350–358. https://dx.doi.org/10.1016%2Fj.jaac.2018.08.016.

Gibson, R., & Kilcullen, M. (2020). The impact of web-cameras on parent-infant attachment in the neonatal intensive care unit. *Journal of Pediatric Nursing*, 52, e77–e83. https://doi.org/10.1016/j.pedn.2020.01.009.

Greenberg, J. M., Haberman, B., Narendran, V., Nathan, A. T., & Schibler, K. R. (2019). Neonatal morbidities of prenatal and perinatal origin. In R. K. Creasy, R. Resnik, J. D. Iams, C. J. Lockwood, & T. R. Moore (Eds.), *Creasy & Resnik's maternal-fetal medicine: Principles and practice* (8th ed., pp. 1309–1333). Elsevier.

Hall, A. S., & Reavey, D. A. (2021). Neurologic disorders. In S. L. Gardner, B. S. Carter, M. Enzman-Hines, & S. Niermeyer (Eds.), *Merenstein & Gardner's handbook of neonatal intensive care* (9th ed., pp. 929–968). Elsevier.

Hand, I. L. & Noble, L. (2022). Premature infants and breastfeeding. In R. A. Lawrence, R. M. Lawrence, L. Noble, C. Rosen-Carole & A. M. Stuebe (Eds.), *Breastfeeding: A guide for the medical profession* (9th ed., pp.502–545). Elsevier.

Hartley, K. A., Miller, C. S., & Gephart, S. M. (2015). Facilitated tucking to reduce pain in neonates: Evidence for best practice. *Advances in Neonatal Care*, 15(3), 201–208. https://doi.org/10.1097/ANC.0000000000000193.

Haslam, D. B. (2020). Healthcare-acquired infections. In R. M. Kliegman, J. W. St Geme, N. J. Blum, S. S. Shah, R. C. Tasker, & K. M. Wilson (Eds.), *Nelson textbook of pediatrics* (21st ed., pp. 1005–1008). Elsevier.

Huff, K., Rose, R. S., & Engle, W. A. (2019). Late preterm infants: Morbidities, mortality, and management recommendations. *Pediatric Clinics of North America*, 66(2), 387–402. https://doi.org/10.1016/j.pcl.2018.12.008.

Ikonen, R., Paavilainen, E., & Kaunonen, M. (2015). Preterm infants' mothers' experiences with milk expression and breastfeeding: An integrative review. *Advances in Neonatal Care*, 15(6), 394–406. https://doi.org/10.1097/anc.0000000000000232.

Johnston, C., Campbell-Yeo, M., Disher, T., Benoit, B., Fernandez, A., Streiner, D., Inglis, D., & Zee, R. (2017). Skin-to-skin care for procedural pain in neonates. *Cochrane Database of Systematic Reviews*, 2, CD008435. https://doi.org/10.1002/14651858.CD008435.

Kadam, R., & Devi, V. (2020). Gastric residual volume as a measure of feed intolerance/necrotising enterocolitis in very low birth weight infants: An observational cohort study. *International Journal of Contemporary Pediatrics*, 7(2), 432–436. https://doi.org/10.18203/2349-3291.ijcp20200124.

Kaur, A., Kler, N., Saluja, S., Modi, M., Soni, A., Thakur, A., & Garg, P. (2015). Abdominal circumference or gastric residual volume as measure of feed intolerance in VLBW infants. *Journal of Pediatric Gastroenterology and Nutrition*, 60(2), 259–263. https://doi.org/10.1097/MPG.0000000000000576.

Kaya, V., & Aytekin, A. (2017). Effects of pacifier use on transition to full breastfeeding and sucking skills in preterm infants: A randomised controlled trial. *Journal of Clinical Nursing*, 26(13-14), 2055–2063. https://doi.org/10.1111/jocn.13617.

Kim, S. J., Port, A. D., Swan, P., Campbell, J. P., Chan, R. V. P., & Chaing, M. F. (2018). Retinopathy of prematurity: A review of risk factors and their clinical significance. *Survey of Ophthalmology*, 63(5), 613–637. https://doi.org/10.1016/j.survophthal.2018.04.002.

Kudin, O., & Neu, J. (2020). Neonatal necrotizing enterocolitis. In R. J. Martin, A. A. Fanaroff, & M. C. Walsh (Eds.), *Fanaroff and Martin's neonatal-perinatal medicine: Diseases of the fetus and infant* (11th ed., pp. 1571–1581). Elsevier.

Lagoski, M., Hamvas, A., & Wambach, J. A. (2020). Respiratory distress syndrome in the neonate. In R. J. Martin, A. A. Fanaroff, & M. C. Walsh (Eds.), *Fanaroff and Martin's neonatal-perinatal medicine: Diseases of the fetus and infant* (11th ed., pp. 1159–1173). Elsevier.

Li, Y.-F., Lin, H.-C., Torrazza, R. M., Parker, L., Talaga, E., & Neu, J. (2014). Gastric residual evaluation in preterm neonates: A useful monitoring technique or a hindrance? *Pediatrics and Neonatology*, 55(5), 335–340. https://doi.org/10.1016/j.pedneo.2014.02.008.

Lund, C., & Durand, D. J. (2021). Skin and skin care. In S. L. Gardner, B. S. Carter, M. Enzman-Hines, & S. Niermeyer (Eds.), *Merenstein & Gardner's handbook of neonatal intensive care* (9th ed., pp. 602–622). Elsevier.

Mandy, G. T. (2020). Infants with fetal (intrauterine) growth restriction. In L. E. Weisman (Ed.), *UpToDate. Infants with fetal (intrauterine) growth restriction - UpToDate*. https://www.uptodate.com/contents/infants-with-fetal-intrauterine-growth-restriction#:~:text=Infants%20with%20fetal%20growth%20restriction,with%20normal%20in%20utero%20growth

March of Dimes. (2020). *United States report card*. US_REPORTCARD_FINAL_2020.pdf https://marchofdimes.org.

Martin, R. J. & Eichenwald, E.C. (2022). Control of ventilation. In M. Keszler, & K. S. Gautham (Eds.), *Goldsmith's assisted ventilation of the neonate: An evidence-based approach to newborn respiratory care* (7th ed., pp. 33–38). Elsevier.

Mehan, S. L., & Thomas, C. W. (2020). Nervous system disorders. In R. M. Kliegman, J. W. St Geme, N. J. Blum, S. S. Shah, R. C. Tasker, & K. M. Wilson (Eds.), *Nelson textbook of pediatrics* (21st ed., pp. 913–925). Elsevier.

Mohan, S. S., & Jain, L. (2018). Late preterm infants. In C. A. Gleason, & S. E. Juul (Eds.), *Avery's diseases of the newborn* (10th ed., pp. 405–418). Elsevier.

National Association of Neonatal Nurses (NANN). (2012). *Pain assessment and management: Guideline for practice.* 3rd ed. https://apps.nann.org/store/product-details?productId=545" Newborn Pain Assessment and Management Guideline for Practice | NANN.

National Association of Neonatal Nurses (NANN). (2013). *Infant-directed oral feeding for premature and critically ill hospitalized infants: Guidelines for practice.* https://apps.nann.org/store/product-details?productId=1416099" Infant-Directed Oral Feeding for Premature and Critically Ill Hospitalized Infants | NANN.

National Association of Neonatal Nurses (NANN). (2015). *The use of human milk and breastfeeding in the neonatal intensive care unit. Position Statement #3065.* http://nann.org/uploads/About/PositionPDFS/1.4.3_Use%20%20of%20Human%20Milk%20and%20Breastfeeding%20in%20the%20NICU.pdf.

Nyp, M., Brunkhorst, J. L., Reavey, D., & Pallotto, E. K. (2021). Fluid and electrolyte management. In S. L. Gardner, B. S. Carter, M. Enzman-Hines, & S. Niermeyer (Eds.), *Merenstein & Gardner's handbook of neonatal intensive care* (9th ed., pp. 407–430). Elsevier.

Olitsky, S. E., & Marsh, J. D. (2020). Disorders of the retina and vitreous. In R. M. Kliegman, J. W. St. Geme, N. J. Blum, S. S. Shah, R. C. Tasker, & K. M. Wilson (Eds.), *Nelson textbook of pediatrics* (21st ed., pp. 3377–3385). Elsevier.

Pados, B. F., Park, J., & Dodrill, P. (2019). Know the flow. Milk flow rates from bottles nipples used in the hospital and after discharge. *Advances in Neonatal Care, 19*(1), 33–41.

Parker, L. A., Weaver, M., Murgas Torrazza, R. J., Shuster, J., Li, N., Krueger, C., & Neu, J. (2019). Effect of gastric residual evaluation on enteral intake in extremely preterm infants: A randomized clinical trial. *JAMA Pediatrics, 73*(6), 534–543. https://doi.org/10.1001/jamapediatrics.2019.0800.

Parsons, K. V., & Jain, L. (2020). The late preterm infant. In R. J. Martin, A. A. Fanaroff, & M. C. Walsh (Eds.), *Fanaroff and Martin's neonatal-perinatal medicine: Diseases of the fetus and infant* (11th ed., pp. 654–669). Elsevier.

Peng, H. F., Yin, T., Yang, L., Wang, C., Chang, Y.-C., Jeng, M.-J., & Liaw, J.-J. (2018). Non-nutritive sucking, oral breast milk, and facilitated tucking relieve preterm infant pain during heel-stick procedures: A prospective, randomized controlled trial. *International Journal of Nursing Studies, 77*, 162–170. https://doi.org/10.1016/j.ijnurstu.2017.10.001.

Pillai Riddell, R. R., Racine, N. M., Geniss, H. G., Turcotte, K., Uman, L. S., Horton, R. E., Ahola Kohut, S., Hillgrove, S. J., Stevens, B., & Lisi, D. M. (2015). Non-pharmacological management of infant and young child procedural pain. *Cochrane Database of Systematic Reviews Issue, 12*, CD006275. https://doi.org/10.1002/14651858.CD006275.pub3.

Poindexter, B. B., & Martin, C. R. (2020). Nutrient requirements/nutritional support in premature neonate. In R. J. Martin, A. A. Fanaroff, & M. C. Walsh (Eds.), *Fanaroff and Martin's neonatal-perinatal medicine: Diseases of the fetus and infant* (11th ed., pp. 670–689). Elsevier.

Rampersand, R., & Macones, G. A. (2021). Late and postterm pregnancy. In M. B. Landon, H. L. Galan, E. R. M. Jauniaux, D. A. Driscoll, V. Berghella, W. A. Grobman, S. J. Kilpartick, & A. G. Cahill (Eds.), *Obstetrics: Normal and problem pregnancies* (8th ed., pp. 548–554). Elsevier.

Resnik, R. (2019). Intrauterine growth restriction. In R. Resnik, C. J. Lockwood, T. R. Moore, Copel, & R. M. Silver (Eds.), *Creasy & Resnik's maternal-fetal medicine: Principles and practice* (8th ed., pp. 798–809). Elsevier.

Riskin, A., Cohen, K., Kugelman, A., Toropine, A., Said, W., & Bader, D. (2017). The impact of routine examination of gastric residual volumes on the time to achieve full enteral feedings in preterm infants. *The Journal of Pediatrics, 189*, 128–134. https://doi.org/10.1016/j.jpeds.2017.05.054.

Sabnis, A., Fojo, S., Nayak, S. S., Lopez, E., Tarn, D. M., & Zeltzer, L. (2019). Reducing parental trauma and stress in neonatal intensive care: Systematic review and meta-analysis of hospital interventions. *Journal of Perinatology, 39*(3), 375–386. https://doi.org/10.1038/s41372-018-0310-9.

Salmon, J. F. (2020). Retinal vascular diseases. In *Kanski's clinical ophthalmology* (9th ed., pp. 495–553). Elsevier.

Sanders, M. ,R., & Hall, S. L. (2018). Trauma-informed care in the newborn intensive care unit: promoting safety, security and connectedness. *Journal of Perinatology, 38*, 3–10. https://doi.org/10.1038/jp.2017.124.

Schecter, R., Pham, T., Hua, A., Spinazzola, R., Sonnenklar, J., Li, D., Papaioannou, H., & Milanaik, R. (2020). Prevalence and longevity of PTSD symptoms among parents of NICU infants analyzed across gestational age categories. *Clinical Pediatrics, 59*(2), 163–169. https://doi.org/10.1177/0009922819892046.

Shamir, R. (2020). Disorders of malabsorption. In R. M. Kliegman, J. W. St. Geme, N. J. Blum, S. S. Shah, R. C. Tasker, & K. M. Wilson (Eds.), *Nelson textbook of pediatrics* (21st ed., pp. 1987–2009). Elsevier.

Sharp, M., Huber, N., Ward, L. G., & Dolbier, C. (2021). NICU-specific stress following traumatic childbirth and its relationship with posttraumatic stress. *Journal of Perinatal and Neonatal Nursing, 35*(1), 57–67. https://doi.org/10.1097/JPN.0000000000000543.

Shviraga, B., & Hensley, J. G. (2021). Uncomplicated antepartum, intrapartum, and postpartum care. In M. T. Verklan, M. Walden, & S. Forest (Eds.), *Core curriculum for neonatal intensive care nursing* (6th ed., pp. 1–19). Elsevier.

Soghier, L. M., Kritikos, K. I., Carty, C. L., Glass, P., Tuchman, L. K., Streisand, R., & Frantantoni, K. R. (2020). Parental depression symptoms at neonatal intensive care unit discharge and associated risk factors. *Journal of Pediatrics, 277*, 163–169. https://doi.org/10.1016/j.jpeds.2020.07.040.

Spruill, C. T. (2021). Developmental support. In M. T. Verklan, M. Walden, & S. Forest (Eds.), *Core curriculum for neonatal intensive care nursing* (6th ed., pp. 172–190). Elsevier.

Thomas, S., Nesargi, S., Roshan, P., Raju, R., Mathew, S., P, S., & Rao, S. (2018). Gastric residual volumes versus abdominal girth measurement in assessment of feed tolerance in preterm neonates: A randomized controlled trial. *Advances in Neonatal Care, 18*(4), e13–e19. https://doi.org/10.1097/ANC.0000000000000532.

Verklan, M. T. (2021). Care of the late preterm infant. In M. T. Verklan, M. Walden, & S. Forest (Eds.), *Core curriculum for neonatal intensive care nursing* (5th ed., pp. 388–393). Elsevier.

World Health Organization. (2018). *Preterm Birth [Fact Sheet].* https://www.who.int/news-room/fact-sheets/detail/preterm-birth.

Yayan, E. H., Kucukoglu, S., Dag, Y. S., & Boyraz, N. K. (2018). Does the post-feeding position affect ... ic residue in preterm infants? *Breastfeeding Medicine, 13*(6), 43 ,–443. https://doi.org/10.1089/bfm.2018.0028.

High-Risk Newborn: Acquired and Congenital Conditions

Della Wrightson

In addition to the high-risk conditions related to gestational age discussed in Chapter 24, the newborn at risk may have acquired or congenital complications. Acquired conditions may be associated with prenatal complications or may occur at birth or shortly thereafter.

RESPIRATORY COMPLICATIONS

Respiratory distress is one of the most common problems of the neonate. It may be primary or secondary to conditions affecting the infant's ability to breathe. Complications affecting the respiratory system include transient tachypnea of the newborn, meconium aspiration syndrome, and persistent pulmonary hypertension of the newborn. The nurse is responsible for identification and evaluation of respiratory status at birth and throughout the hospital stay.

Neonatal Resuscitation

Although most newborns have no difficulty with breathing at birth, up to 10% require some help to begin respirations, and 1% require extensive resuscitative measures (Weiner, 2021). Therefore, all personnel involved in deliveries should know how to perform resuscitative measures. Courses in neonatal resuscitation are usually required of all staff members working with newborns, and many agencies expect these skills to be updated every 1 to 2 years. Before neonatal resuscitation, delivery personnel should ask four primary assessment questions: Is the baby term? Is the amniotic fluid clear? Is the baby breathing or crying? Is there good muscle tone? (Weiner, 2021).

All newborns should be considered at risk for needing neonatal resuscitation. Complications occurring during pregnancy or birth increase the infant's need for neonatal resuscitation.

Risk factors for neonatal resuscitation include factors affecting the pregnant client such as morbid obesity, diabetes, chorioamnionitis, blood loss, placental abnormalities, cord prolapse or tight nuchal cord, cesarean birth, cardiopulmonary disease, and hypertension. In addition, if the expectant client receives narcotics for analgesia shortly before birth, the infant's central nervous system (CNS) may be too depressed at birth to allow adequate spontaneous breathing. Newborn risk factors include abnormal lie, meconium, postterm birth, preterm birth, or intrauterine growth restriction (IUGR).

Once the newborn is delivered, the newborn should quickly begin to take their first breath. As soon as breathing begins, fluid is cleared from the alveoli in the lungs, and the pulmonary vasculature begins to expand. Sometimes, however, the newborn may have rapid respirations followed by cessation of respirations (primary apnea) and a rapid fall in heart rate. Stimulation, alone or with oxygen, may restart respirations. If breathing is not quickly established at birth, gasping respirations may resume weakly until the infant enters a period of secondary apnea. In secondary apnea, the oxygen levels in blood continue to decrease, the infant loses consciousness, and stimulation is ineffective. Resuscitative measures should be initiated immediately to prevent permanent injury to the brain or death.

Neonatal resuscitation begins by placing the newborn supine underneath a radiant warmer, drying the newborn, and stimulating and removing the wet towels. The baby should begin crying or have sustained breathing. If this does not occur, position the newborn's head to open the mouth/airway, clear the airway with a bulb suction or catheter, and begin positive pressure ventilation immediately (Weiner, 2021).

Chest compressions and medications are rarely needed during resuscitation. Nurses should be prepared for situations in which primary or secondary apnea may develop. Effective ventilation is the most important element in resuscitation (Weiner, 2021). Equipment should be readily available and functioning properly at all times so there is no delay in starting resuscitation. Nurses begin resuscitation measures as necessary and assist the physician or nurse practitioner with intubation, insertion of umbilical vein catheters, and administration of medications.

Maintenance of thermoregulation is very important throughout care. A warming pad may be placed under linens in the radiant warmer to provide extra heat. Infants less than 29 weeks of gestation may be placed in a polyethylene bag up to the neck before they are dried to reduce heat loss from evaporation. The bag also reduces stress from handling during drying. It is important to prevent hyperthermia when the bag is used with a chemical warming pad (Weiner, 2021).

Some infants may develop hypoxic-ischemic encephalopathy (HIE) after prolonged neonatal resuscitation. HIE is a cause of encephalopathy in term and the late preterm infant. This condition occurs when there is disruption of blood flow and oxygen to the brain. Typically, poor blood flow within the placenta causing chronic asphyxia over a period of time may promote HIE. Conditions in the pregnant client which contribute to HIE include morbid obesity, diabetes, hypertension, and uterine rupture. Fetal conditions include IUGR, placental abnormalities, cord prolapse, and blood loss. Therapeutic hypothermia has been used to improve neurologic outcomes for these infants. Infants should be 36 or more weeks of gestation, have evidence of an acute perinatal hypoxic-ischemic event, and be in a facility where the treatment can be initiated within 6 hours of birth (Weiner, 2021).

Once the infant is stabilized, the nurse continues to assess for changes. Infants requiring resuscitation at birth may have other complications such as hypoglycemia, feeding and thermoregulation problems, seizures, hypotension, pulmonary hypertension, metabolic acidosis, renal problems, and fluid and electrolyte imbalances. They need close monitoring and often need intensive nursing care.

Communication with the parents is a vital nursing function. They will be confused and frightened and will need explanation and realistic reassurance. Parents often need continued support after the crisis to talk about their fears and concerns.

Transient Tachypnea of the Newborn (Retained Lung Fluid)

Infants who experience **transient tachypnea of the newborn (TTN)** develop rapid respirations soon after birth from inadequate absorption of fetal lung fluid. Although the condition usually resolves within 24 to 48 hours, it is the most common respiratory cause of admission to a neonatal intensive care nursery (NICU; Greenberg et al., 2019).

Risk factors may include cesarean birth with or without labor, macrosomia, multiple gestation, excessive sedation of the pregnant client, prolonged or precipitous labor, male sex, and asthma in the pregnant client. Mild immaturity of surfactant

production also may be a factor. Infants are usually term or late preterm, although some may be preterm (Fraser, 2021; Greenberg et al., 2019).

Cause

Although the exact cause of TTN is unknown, it is thought to result from a delay in absorption of fetal lung fluid by the pulmonary capillaries and lymph vessels. This leads to decreased lung compliance and air trapping and produces signs similar to those of respiratory distress syndrome (RDS).

Manifestations

In TTN, tachypnea develops within a few hours of birth. Grunting, retractions, nasal flaring, and mild cyanosis also are present. Chest radiography demonstrates hyperinflation, perihilar streaking that shows engorged lymphatics, and the presence of fluid in the fissures between the lobes and in the pleural space. Unlike RDS, TTN typically resolves faster, causes less alveolar collapse, and results in the need for less supplemental oxygen (Fraser, 2021).

Therapeutic Management

Treatment is supportive and may include oxygen and continuous positive airway pressure (CPAP). Gavage feeding may be given when the respiratory rate is high to prevent aspiration and conserve energy. Because the signs are similar to those of RDS and sepsis, the infant is observed for those complications. Antibiotics may be given until sepsis is ruled out.

Nursing Considerations

The nurse may be the first person to see signs of TTN, especially if they are not apparent at birth. After identifying these signs, the nurse notifies the provider and carries out treatment. General nursing care is similar to that of the respiratory care of the preterm infant (see Chapter 24).

? KNOWLEDGE CHECK

1. What is the most important element in resuscitation?
2. What is the role of the nurse in care of the infant requiring resuscitation at birth?
3. How is TTN different from RDS?

Meconium Aspiration Syndrome

Meconium staining of amniotic fluid occurs in 10% to 15% of births. **Meconium aspiration syndrome (MAS)** is a condition in which there is obstruction, chemical pneumonitis, and air trapping caused by meconium in the lungs. It develops in 5% of those infants (Ahlfeld, 2020; Fig. 25.1). The condition occurs most often in infants who are postterm, small for gestational age (SGA), and/or compromised before birth by conditions such as placental insufficiency and cord compression (Crowley, 2020).

Causes

Although a normal fetus may pass meconium, MAS occurs most often when hypoxia causes increased peristalsis of

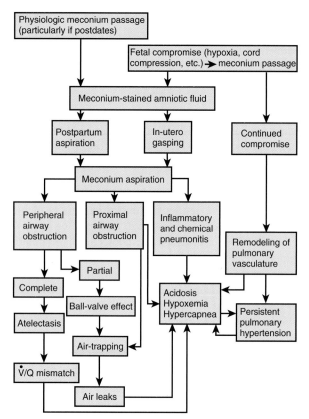

FIG. 25.1 Flow chart showing the effects of meconium aspiration syndrome. (From Wiswell, T. E., Bent, R. C. (1993). Meconium staining and the meconium aspiration syndrome: Unresolved issues. *Pediatric Clinics of North America*, 40:955–981.)

the intestines and relaxation of the anal sphincter before or during labor. MAS develops when meconium in the amniotic fluid enters the lungs during fetal life or at birth. It may be drawn into the lungs if gasping movements occur in utero, or the meconium in the upper airways may be pulled deep into the respiratory passages when the infant takes their first breaths after birth.

Obstruction of the airways may be complete or partial. Atelectasis may result if small airways are completely obstructed. In partial obstruction, air can enter but not escape from the alveoli. During inhalation, the bronchioles expand slightly as air flows into them past the meconium. During exhalation, the passages constrict, and meconium blocks the movement of air out of the lungs.

This ball-valve mechanism results in air trapping. The overdistended alveoli may develop an air leak, with escape of air into the pleural cavity (pneumothorax) or mediastinum (pneumomediastinum). Surfactant production may be inhibited, increasing respiratory distress. In addition, meconium is irritating to lung tissue and causes an inflammatory reaction and chemical pneumonitis.

Severe MAS develops in only a small number of newborns with meconium below the vocal cords. Meconium interferes with clearing of lung fluid and production of surfactant and causes pulmonary vasoconstriction that can result in return

to fetal circulation patterns. MAS may lead to persistent pulmonary hypertension.

Manifestations

If meconium in the amniotic fluid is minimal, respiratory problems usually do not develop. Nevertheless, more meconium may cause serious respiratory pathologic issues. Signs of mild to severe respiratory distress are present at birth, including tachypnea, cyanosis, retractions, nasal flaring, grunting, crackles, and, in severe cases, a barrel-shaped chest from hyperinflation. Radiography shows patchy infiltrates, atelectasis, consolidation, and hyperexpansion from air trapping. The infant's nails, skin, and umbilical cord may be stained yellow–green.

Therapeutic Management

Suctioning the infant's secretions as soon as the head is born has not been found to reduce the incidence of MAS. At birth, the vigorous infant (who has a heart rate more than 100 beats per minute [bpm], spontaneous respirations, and good muscle tone) does not need special suctioning and receives routine care. Infants with depressed respirations and muscle tone should be moved to a radiant warmer and suctioned with a bulb syringe. If the infant is not breathing or has a heart rate below 100 bpm after opening the airway, suctioning, and being dried and stimulated, positive pressure ventilation is required (Weiner, 2021).

Infants may need only warmed, humidified oxygen, or extensive respiratory support with mechanical ventilation may be required. High-frequency ventilation may be used. Surfactant lavage has been used in severe cases but is controversial (Gardner et al., 2021). Surfactant replacement therapy has been shown to improve gas exchange and to decrease the severity of respiratory illness (Fraser, 2021).

Ongoing management consists of supportive care to meet the problems presented. Infants with severe MAS who do not respond to conventional treatment may benefit from extracorporeal membrane oxygenation (ECMO). ECMO, which is available in some hospitals, oxygenates blood while bypassing the lungs, much like heart–lung machines used during heart surgery. It allows the infant's lungs to rest temporarily and recover.

Nursing Considerations

When meconium is noted in the amniotic fluid during labor, the nurse notifies the primary provider so that delivery care can be adapted as necessary. Nurses from the NICU and a neonatologist may be present for the birth. The nurse ensures that equipment such as oxygen and suction devices are functioning properly and assists with care at birth. After the infant's birth, nursing care is adapted to the problems presented. Although meconium is sterile, lung injury promotes the growth of bacteria. Infants should be closely observed for infection, which may further complicate the condition. Nursing attention to respiratory status, thermoregulation, and decreased stimulation is important.

Persistent Pulmonary Hypertension of the Newborn

Persistent pulmonary hypertension of the newborn (PPHN) is a condition in which pulmonary vasoconstriction occurs after birth and elevates vascular resistance of the lungs. Normal changes to neonatal circulation are impaired as a result. For this reason, the condition is also called *persistent fetal circulation.*

Causes

PPHN occurs most often in infants who are term or postterm. The cause may be abnormal lung development, use of nonsteroidal antiinflammatory drugs (NSAIDs) or selective serotonin reuptake inhibitors (SSRIs) by the pregnant client, or it may be unknown. It is often associated with hypoxemia and acidosis from conditions such as asphyxia, MAS, sepsis, polycythemia, diaphragmatic hernia, and RDS (Ahlfeld, 2020).

Inadequate oxygenation results in constriction, instead of the normal dilation, of the pulmonary artery and small pulmonary vessels, which causes increased vascular resistance in the lungs. The elevated pulmonary vascular resistance causes a rise in pressure on the right side of the heart. This results in a right-to-left shunt of unoxygenated blood that flows through the foramen ovale. In addition, unoxygenated blood from the pulmonary artery flows through the ductus arteriosus to the aorta. Thus, blood bypasses the lungs, as occurs during fetal circulation. Metabolic acidosis causes more pulmonary vasoconstriction, making the condition even worse.

Manifestations

Infants with PPHN develop signs within the first 12 hours after birth. Tachypnea, respiratory distress, and progressive cyanosis often become worse with handling. Oxygen saturation and partial pressure of oxygen in arterial blood (PaO_2) are decreased, $PaCO_2$ is increased, and acidosis is present. Other signs may result from associated conditions. An echocardiogram demonstrates right-to-left shunting through the foramen ovale and ductus arteriosus.

Therapeutic Management

Management involves treating the underlying cause of poor oxygenation and relieving pulmonary vasoconstriction. Respiratory therapy goals are to eliminate hypoxemia. Drug therapy may be used to cause pulmonary vasodilation and support blood pressure and perfusion. Sedation, high-frequency ventilation, and surfactant therapy may be necessary. Inhaled nitric oxide may be given to dilate pulmonary vessels. ECMO therapy may be lifesaving if conventional therapies are unsuccessful.

Nursing Considerations

Nursing care is similar to care of other infants with severe respiratory disease. Because infants become hypoxic with activity and other stimuli, handling and noise are kept to a minimum. Cold stress increases the metabolic rate and need for oxygen and causes additional pulmonary vasoconstriction.

Therefore, the nurse should pay particular attention to maintaining the infant's temperature. Assessment for hypoglycemia, hypocalcemia, anemia, and metabolic acidosis is important.

KNOWLEDGE CHECK

4. Which infants are most likely to have meconium staining of the amniotic fluid?
5. Why is there resistance of blood flow into the lungs in PPHN?

Hyperbilirubinemia (Pathologic Jaundice)

Jaundice is a common concern in the care for neonates. Conjugation of bilirubin and physiologic jaundice are discussed in Chapters 20, 21 and 22. This discussion focuses on nonphysiologic or pathologic jaundice.

When the total serum bilirubin (TSB) level is greater than 5 to 6 milligrams per deciliter (mg/dL), cutaneous jaundice appears (Kaplan et al., 2020). Jaundice is considered abnormal or nonphysiologic when the TSB rises more rapidly and to a higher level than is expected or stays elevated for longer than normal. Charts showing the expected rise and fall of bilirubin according to the age of the infant in hours are used to determine the degree of risk and which infants need treatment for rising TSB level.

Nonphysiologic jaundice may be seen in the first 24 hours of life. It is a concern because it may lead to **bilirubin encephalopathy**, the acute manifestation of bilirubin toxicity. This may lead to **kernicterus**, the chronic and permanent result of bilirubin toxicity. In this condition, bilirubin deposits cause yellowish staining of the brain, especially the basal ganglia, cerebellum, brainstem, and hippocampus. It is more likely to occur in infants who have suffered hypoxemia, respiratory acidosis, infection, or other injury that impairs the blood–brain barrier and allows unconjugated bilirubin to enter the brain (Marcdante & Kliegman, 2019).

Although bilirubin encephalopathy and kernicterus are rare today because of improved treatment measures, the mortality and morbidity rates among affected infants are high. Those who survive may suffer from cerebral palsy, cognitive impairment, hearing loss, or more subtle long-term neurologic and developmental problems. The exact level at which bilirubin encephalopathy develops is not known. The toxic level may not be the same for all infants. It occurs at lower TSB levels and is more severe in infants who have complications, who are preterm or late preterm, or who have lower birth weight than full-term healthy infants.

Causes

In the past, the most common cause of pathologic jaundice was hemolytic disease of the newborn caused by Rh incompatibility between the blood of the pregnant client and that of the fetus. The incompatibility occurs when the Rh-negative pregnant client forms antibodies in response to the Rh-positive blood of the fetus entering the client's circulation (see Chapter 10). Antibodies may have developed during a previous pregnancy or after injury, abortion, amniocentesis, or a transfusion of Rh-positive blood. The antibodies cross the placenta, attach to fetal red blood cells (RBCs), and destroy them. The result is hemolytic disease of the fetus and newborn (HDFN), agglutination and hemolysis of fetal erythrocytes.

Infants with HDFN are anemic from destruction of RBCs. Severely affected infants may develop **hydrops fetalis**, a severe anemia that results in heart failure and generalized edema. Intrauterine fetal transfusions may be given. After birth, phototherapy and exchange transfusions are used to prevent kernicterus. Use of Rho(D) immune globulin (RhoGAM) to prevent the Rh-negative client from forming antibodies against Rh-positive blood has greatly decreased the incidence of erythroblastosis fetalis.

ABO incompatibility also causes pathologic jaundice. It is more common but less severe than Rh incompatibility. People with type O blood have natural antibodies to type A and B blood. In a pregnant client, these antibodies cross the placenta and cause hemolysis of fetal RBCs. Nevertheless, the destruction is much less severe than with Rh incompatibility and causes milder signs. This is because most of the antibodies are immunoglobulin M (IgM), which does not cross the placenta. Some of the antibodies are immunoglobulin G (IgG), which does cross the placenta and can cause RBC destruction but usually at a lower rate (Kaplan et al., 2020).

Other causes of nonphysiologic jaundice include infection, hypothyroidism, glucuronyl transferase deficiency, polycythemia, glucose-6-phosphate dehydrogenase deficiency, and biliary atresia. Infants of diabetic mothers are more likely to develop nonphysiologic jaundice, especially if they have macrosomia. Any condition that causes destruction of erythrocytes, impairment of the liver, or delay in passage of meconium may result in elevated bilirubin levels.

Therapeutic Management

The focus of therapeutic management is prevention of bilirubin encephalopathy and kernicterus. The cause is determined by history and diagnostic tests to identify infections or blood abnormalities. During pregnancy, an Rh-negative client will have blood drawn for an indirect Coombs' test to identify the presence of antibodies against fetal blood. If the antibodies are present, additional testing may be performed to evaluate fetal status (see Chapter 10).

When an infant is jaundiced, the infant's blood type and a direct Coombs' test are performed. A positive Coombs' test indicates that antibodies from the pregnant client attached to the fetal RBC's during pregnancy. TSB levels are monitored closely to detect changes that indicate treatment should be initiated or changed. The health care provider considers the bilirubin level as well as other factors such as gestational age and presence of other risk factors to determine whether therapy is appropriate for an individual infant.

Nurses assess infants for changes in jaundice. Nevertheless, visual inspection for jaundice is not an accurate way of determining actual bilirubin levels. Because taking blood samples for TSB measurement is painful and expensive, other noninvasive tests may be used. Transcutaneous bilirubinometers are hand-held devices that allow screening of the transcutaneous bilirubin (TcB) level. When the sensor on the device is placed against the infant's skin, the amount of bilirubin in the tissues is measured. This noninvasive test allows for frequent estimates of the TSB level without discomfort to the infant, but it may not be accurate in preterm infants, in infants receiving phototherapy, or in those with high skin melanin levels (Kamath-Rayne et al., 2020).

Phototherapy

Phototherapy is the most common treatment for jaundice and involves placing the infant under special fluorescent lights. During phototherapy, bilirubin in the skin absorbs the light and changes into water-soluble products, the most important of which is lumirubin. These products do not require conjugation by the liver and can be excreted in bile and urine. Because preterm infants are more vulnerable to bilirubin toxicity, phototherapy is begun at lower TSB levels than for full-term infants.

Phototherapy can be delivered in several ways. A bank of fluorescent lamps or "bili" lights can be placed over the infant who is in an incubator or under a radiant warmer to maintain heat or in an open crib. The infant wears only a diaper to ensure maximal exposure of the skin to the lights. The diaper is removed if the TSB is becoming dangerously high. The eyes are closed and patches placed over them to protect them from injury (Fig. 25.2). The lights are placed above the infant at a distance determined by the type of bulb used. More than one bank of lights may be used if the bilirubin level is very high. Bilirubin levels are checked frequently to determine the effectiveness of treatment and when it can be discontinued.

Other options for phototherapy include light-emitting diodes (LEDs), halogen lamps, and fiberoptic phototherapy blankets. As with fluorescent lights, the LED device is placed over the infant. It is long-lasting, does not generate excessive heat, and decreases insensible water loss. The halogen spotlight is used alone or with other lamps. The infant can be swaddled with the fiberoptic phototherapy blanket against the skin. With the blanket, the parents may hold the infant without interfering with therapy. Nevertheless, the blanket is not as effective alone as the other methods. To increase its effectiveness, the blanket may be placed under the infant when phototherapy lights are used. Additionally, there are phototherapy platforms or beds with lights underneath the surface where the infant is laying.

The side effects of phototherapy include frequent, loose, green stools that result from increased bile flow and peristalsis. This causes more rapid excretion of the bilirubin but may be damaging to the skin and result in fluid loss. A 25% increase in fluid intake is needed during phototherapy (Kaplan et al., 2020). A macular skin rash may occur in some infants. *Bronze baby syndrome,* a grayish–brown discoloration of the skin and urine, occurs in some infants with cholestatic jaundice. The rash and color changes disappear gradually when phototherapy is completed. Hypo- or hyperthermia may also occur.

When phototherapy is discontinued, a rebound TSB level increase of 1 to 2 mg/dL is normal. Therefore, the TSB should be monitored for at least 24 hours to see that it does

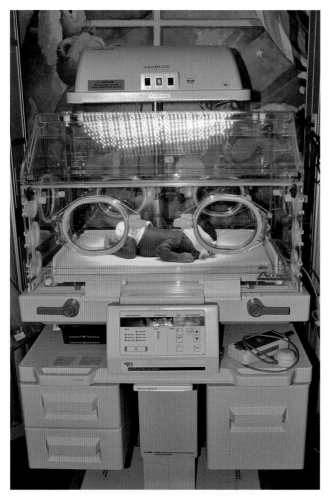

FIG. 25.2 An infant receiving phototherapy is wearing eye patches to protect the eyes.

not become excessively high. Explain the expected elevation to parents and that the health care provider may order additional blood tests after discharge.

Exchange Transfusions

Exchange transfusions are seldom necessary but are performed when phototherapy cannot reduce dangerously high bilirubin levels quickly enough. This treatment removes maternal antibodies, unconjugated bilirubin, and antibody-coated (sensitized) RBCs. It provides fresh albumin with binding sites for bilirubin and helps correct severe anemia. When an immediate transfusion is needed for Rh incompatibility, type O, Rh-negative blood cross-matched against the postpartum client and infant is used. In ABO incompatibility, type O–packed RBCs with type AB plasma are used so there are no anti-A or anti-B antibodies present to destroy the erythrocytes (Ramasethu, 2020).

Procedure. During the exchange transfusion, small portions of blood are removed from the infant and replaced with an equal amount of donor blood. The volume of blood exchanged is described as partial, single, or double. Double volume exchanges are most commonly used for neonatal exchange transfusions. At the end of the procedure,

approximately 85% of the infant's RBCs will have been replaced and the bilirubin level reduced by 45% or less (Jacquot et al., 2020).

When the bilirubin level in blood decreases, bilirubin from tissues moves into plasma. This may increase the level of bilirubin in the blood to 60% of the pre-exchange level (Kamath-Rayne et al., 2021). This rebound elevation of bilirubin level may necessitate repeat transfusions, but phototherapy is generally adequate to resolve it.

Complications. Complications that may occur from exchange transfusions include electrolyte and acid-base imbalance, hypocalcemia, hypomagnesemia, hypoglycemia, hyperkalemia, infection, cardiac dysrhythmias, necrotizing enterocolitis, bleeding, thrombosis, thrombocytopenia, and air embolism. Samples of blood are analyzed for a complete blood cell (CBC) count, bilirubin and calcium levels, and other tests as needed before and after the exchange.

Role of the Nurse. The nurse's role during exchange transfusion is to prepare equipment, assess the infant during and after the procedure, and keep accurate records. A cardiac monitor is attached to the infant, and warmth is provided by a radiant heater. The nurse also should clarify any misunderstandings that the parents may have about the treatment and help allay their anxiety.

APPLICATION OF THE NURSING PROCESS: HYPERBILIRUBINEMIA

Assessment

Assess the level of jaundice at least every 8 hours by blanching the skin (pressing the skin over a bony prominence) to see the color in the area before blood returns. Evaluate the skin color in good light with phototherapy lights turned off because they distort the skin color. In infants with dark skin, assess the color of the palate and mucous membranes of the mouth and the conjunctivae. Determine the areas of the body affected by jaundice and document carefully to use for comparison during future assessments. Jaundice begins at the head and moves down the body as the bilirubin level rises. Monitor the TSB and TcB levels for change because visualization of jaundice is a subjective assessment and the color in the skin may be affected by phototherapy.

Assess for risk factors that might further increase bilirubin levels. Note temperature fluctuations, hypoglycemia, and infection. Determine the infant's oral intake and number of stools.

Identification of Client Problems

In addition to the possibility of increasing bilirubin levels, the infant receiving phototherapy is at risk for associated problems. These potential problems include injury caused by the light, temperature instability, changes in fluid and nutrition status, and damage to the retina.

Planning: Expected Outcomes

Nurses can intervene to prevent situations that might cause further increases in bilirubin. They should also protect the infant from injury caused by the light during phototherapy. The expected outcome for this diagnosis is that the infant will have no injury resulting from increased bilirubin levels or exposure of the skin or eyes to phototherapy lights.

Interventions

Interventions are designed to prevent situations that might cause injury to the infant from rising bilirubin levels or effects of treatment.

Maintaining a Neutral Thermal Environment

Prevent situations such as cold stress or hypoglycemia, which could result in increased fatty acids in blood caused by acidosis. Acidosis would decrease the availability of albumin-binding sites for unconjugated bilirubin. Prevent cold stress at birth and during all care by maintaining the infant in a neutral thermal environment. Check the infant's axillary temperature every 2 to 4 hours to identify an early decrease before it becomes a problem. Dress the infant in warmed clothes and blankets on removal from phototherapy lights.

Prevent elevation of the infant's temperature from exposure to the heat of the "bili" lights. Position the lights according to the manufacturer's guidelines to prevent overheating. Use a skin probe when the infant is in an incubator or radiant warmer to maintain the appropriate environmental temperature, and monitor the settings to be sure they are correct for the infant's needs.

Providing Optimal Nutrition

Ensure the infant receives feedings as prescribed. Breastfeeding should not be stopped because the infant is receiving phototherapy. Provide extra support and teaching to breastfeeding clients. Frequent feedings prevent hypoglycemia, provide protein to maintain the albumin level in the blood, and promote gastrointestinal (GI) motility and prompt removal of bilirubin from the intestines.

Avoid offering water because the infant may take less milk, which is more effective in promoting stooling and removal of bilirubin from the intestines. If breastfeeding must be supplemented, use formula instead of water. Weigh the infant at least daily, and monitor intake and output to identify dehydration early and intervene appropriately.

Protecting the Eyes

Provide patches to protect the eyes from retinal damage from the phototherapy lights. Patches should be used with all phototherapy methods, not just overhead lights. Close the infant's eyes before placing the patches to avoid abrasions to the cornea. Check the position of the patches at least every hour. Infants often wiggle enough to push the patches above or below the eyes, leaving them exposed. The edges of the patches can press too hard on the eyes or compress the nose and interfere with breathing. Turn off the lights and observe for skin irritation around or under the patches at least every 4 hours. Explain to the parents it is normal for the yellow color under the patches to be deeper than in areas that have been exposed to the lights.

Enhancing Response to Therapy

Position the lights the proper distance from the infant. Lights too close may burn the skin. Lights too far away from the infant will not be effective in reducing jaundice. Halogen lights should be placed farther away from the infant than other lights to prevent burning. Follow the manufacturer's instructions about light placement. Although phototherapy increases insensible water loss from the skin, avoid the use of creams or lotions on the infant's skin that might cause burning.

Use a light meter to check the level of irradiance (energy output) to be sure the apparatus is functioning appropriately and to determine whether the bulbs need to be replaced. Check laboratory reports of TSB levels to determine the effectiveness of treatment and when it can be discontinued.

Expose as much skin as possible to the light. Remove all of the infant's clothing except a diaper. Turn the infant frequently to expose all areas evenly and prevent irritation of the skin from lack of position change. If a fiberoptic blanket is used, check the position of the blanket frequently. Infants sometimes need to be repositioned so that the blanket remains in contact with the skin.

Detecting Complications

Observe for other complications. Although bilirubin encephalopathy is rare today, monitor for signs that indicate its presence. These include lethargy, increased or decreased muscle tone, poor feeding, decreased or absent Moro reflex, high-pitched cry, opisthotonos, and seizures (Kamath-Rayne et al., 2021). Note the presence of rashes or changes in the color of the skin. Inform parents that they are not harmful and will disappear when phototherapy is discontinued.

Teaching Parents

Explain care to parents, who may be frightened to see their infant in an incubator with the infant's eyes covered. Explaining the causes of jaundice and the purpose of phototherapy will decrease their worry. Removing the infant from phototherapy for feeding and interaction with the parents for periods up to an hour at a time does not significantly decrease the effectiveness of phototherapy (Kamath-Rayne et al., 2021). In addition, allowing the parents to hold their baby increases their opportunity for attachment. Explain the importance of minimizing further interruptions to phototherapy.

When the infant is discharged, give the parents written and verbal information about jaundice. Teach them how to assess for further jaundice, signs of complications, and when to call the health care provider. Emphasize the need to keep follow-up laboratory work and visits to the health care provider so any increases in jaundice or other problems can be identified and treated early. Explain that most infants have no further problem with jaundice.

Although sunlight is known to reduce bilirubin level, caution the parents against putting the infant in direct sunlight. The infant might be sunburned or have temperature instability and is exposed to unnecessary ultraviolet light from the sun.

Evaluation

No signs of injury should be present. The infant's eyes will not have been exposed to the phototherapy lights, and the skin should not be harmed. Laboratory reports should show a steady decrease in serum bilirubin levels.

? KNOWLEDGE CHECK

6. How can kernicterus be prevented?
7. How can the nurse help reduce bilirubin levels in infants receiving phototherapy?

INFECTION

Nurses should be constantly alert for signs of infection in newborns. As many as 10% of infants develop infections during the first month of life (Haslam, 2020).

Transmission of Infection

Newborns can acquire infections before, during, or after birth. Vertical infection is acquired before or during birth from the pregnant client. Organisms such as those causing rubella, cytomegalovirus infection, syphilis, human immunodeficiency virus (HIV) infection, and toxoplasmosis may pass across the placenta and cause infection during pregnancy. During labor and birth, organisms in the vagina, such as group B *Streptococcus* (GBS), herpes, and hepatitis, may enter the uterus after rupture of membranes or infect the infant during passage through the birth canal.

Horizontal infection occurs after birth, acquired from hospital staff members or from contaminated equipment (health care–associated infections) or from family members or visitors. An example is staphylococcal infections associated with central venous catheters. Some of the most common infections and their effects on the neonate are listed in Table 25.1.

Sepsis Neonatorum

Infection that occurs during or after birth may result in sepsis neonatorum, a systemic infection from bacteria in the bloodstream. Newborns are particularly susceptible to sepsis because their immune systems are immature and react more slowly to invasion by organisms. Newborns, and especially preterm infants, have fewer antibodies and are unable to localize infection as well as older children. This inability allows the infection to spread easily from one organ to another. In addition, the blood–brain barrier is less effective in preventing the entrance of organisms, and CNS infection may result.

Causes

Common causative agents of neonatal sepsis include bacteria, such as GBS, *Escherichia coli*, coagulase-negative *Staphylococcus*, *Staphylococcus aureus*, and *Haemophilus influenzae*, and fungi, such as *Candida albicans* (Rudd, 2021). Sepsis may be divided into early-onset and late-onset sepsis, according to when signs of disease begin. Early-onset sepsis is acquired during birth, often from complications of labor such as prolonged rupture of membranes, prolonged labor,

or chorioamnionitis (also known as "Triple I"). Infants show signs within the first 3 days of life (Pammi et al., 2021). It is a rapidly progressive multisystem illness with high mortality and morbidity rates. Pneumonia and meningitis are commonly present.

Late-onset sepsis is most common after the first week of life (Pammi et al., 2021). It is acquired during or after birth, before or after hospital discharge. Preterm birth is a major risk factor, along with the invasive procedures required by these infants, and serious long-term effects may occur.

Therapeutic Management

Diagnostic Testing. Neonatal sepsis may be confused with other illnesses. For example, GBS pneumonia has the same initial symptoms as RDS. Diagnostic testing helps identify sepsis and the organisms responsible.

A CBC count with differential may show decreased total neutrophils, increased bands (a form of immature neutrophils), an increased ratio of immature neutrophils to total neutrophils, and decreased platelets. Elevated levels of leukocytes are normal in newborns, but a sudden rise or fall in leukocyte levels compared with previous results is abnormal. The presence of elevated IgM levels in cord blood or shortly after birth indicates that infection was acquired in utero because this immunoglobulin does not cross the placenta. It often indicates transplacental infection.

The C-reactive protein (CRP) level, a sign of an inflammatory process, may be elevated. Serial tests of CRP are often performed to check for rise and then fall as infection improves. Cultures of blood, urine, any skin lesions, and cerebrospinal fluid may be obtained. Cultures of the nasopharynx, umbilical cord, and gastric aspirate usually show colonization with organisms but not infection. Chest radiography helps differentiate between RDS and sepsis. Blood glucose levels should be checked because they may be unstable (high or low) in sepsis.

Recent work on improving antibiotic stewardship has led to the growing use of sepsis calculators to predict the probability of early-onset sepsis based on maternal history and the clinical picture of the infant (Pammi et al., 2021).

Treatment. Infants who develop signs of infection are treated with broad-spectrum antibiotics, given intravenously, until culture and sensitivity results are available. Continued antibiotic therapy is based on culture results. Commonly used antibiotics include ampicillin, aminoglycoside, and cephalosporins. Vancomycin also may be used (Pammi et al., 2021).

Other care is supportive to meet the infant's specific needs. The infant may require oxygen or mechanical ventilation. Fluid balance maintenance and monitoring of the blood pressure and hourly urine output are important. Shock, hypoglycemia or hyperglycemia, electrolyte imbalances, and problems in temperature regulation are potential complications.

Nursing Considerations

Assessment

Risk Factors. The nurse should identify infants at risk for infection. Prematurity and low birth weight are the most

TABLE 25.1   Common Infections in the Newborn[a]

Transmission	Effect on Newborn	Nursing Considerations
Viral Infections		
Cytomegalovirus		
Transplacental, during birth, in breast milk	Most asymptomatic at birth. SGA, FGR, enlarged liver, CNS abnormalities, jaundice, learning impairment, hearing loss, purpura, chorioretinitis, microcephaly, seizures. May have no signs for months or years.	Diagnosed by urine or pharyngeal culture. May shed virus in saliva and urine for months or years. Antiviral drug therapy may be used but has toxic effects and is not recommended routinely. Treatment supportive.
Hepatitis B		
Usually during birth through contact with maternal blood Also transplacental and from breast milk	Asymptomatic at birth. LBW, prematurity. Most become chronic carriers. Risk for later liver cancer.	Wash well to remove all blood before skin is punctured for any reason. After cleaning, administer HBIG and hepatitis B vaccine to prevent infection. May breastfeed if infant receives vaccine and HBIG.
Herpes		
Usually during birth through infected vagina or ascending infection after rupture of membranes Transplacental rarely Transmission highest with primary infection	Clusters of vesicles, temperature instability, lethargy, poor suck, seizures, encephalitis, jaundice, purpura. Death or severe neurologic impairment is high with disseminated infection. High mortality rate if untreated.	Contact precautions. Obtain specimens of lesions for culture. Antiviral drugs given to the pregnant client during pregnancy and to infant after birth. May breastfeed if no lesions on the breasts.
Human Immunodeficiency Virus and Acquired Immunodeficiency Syndrome		
Transplacental, during birth from infected blood and secretions, or from breast milk Transmission rate much lower if the pregnant client receives antiretroviral drugs during pregnancy and labor, and birth is by cesarean before rupture of membranes	Asymptomatic at birth; signs usually apparent at 12–24 mo. Enlarged liver and spleen, lymphadenopathy, failure to thrive, pneumonia, persistent *Candida* and bacterial infections, diarrhea, meningitis, septic joints.	Diagnosis may be delayed because of antibodies from the pregnant client. Some early tests available. Wash early to remove blood before skin is punctured. Treat with antiretroviral drugs and prophylaxis against other infections. Advise against breastfeeding.
Rubella		
Transplacental	Spontaneous abortion, asymptomatic or FGR, cataracts, cardiac defects, deafness, microcephaly, cognitive impairment. Injury greatest if infected in first trimester.	Contact precautions. Infant may shed virus for 1 year after birth. Diagnosed by presence of antibody and virus. Treatment supportive.
Varicella-Zoster Virus (Chickenpox)		
Transplacental	Congenital varicella syndrome (skin scarring, limb hypoplasia, CNS and eye abnormalities, death), rash. Highest incidence between 13 and 20 wk of gestation. Severe effects with maternal infection between 5 days before and 2 days after birth.	Varicella immune globulin for pregnant client exposed in pregnancy or for infants of clients infected just before or after delivery. It modifies but does not prevent infection. Acyclovir to treat. Strict isolation precautions for postpartum clients and infants with lesions.
Other Infections		
Group B Streptococcal Infection		
During birth or ascending after rupture of membranes	Sudden onset of respiratory distress in infant usually well at birth, temperature instability, pneumonia, shock, meningitis. May have early or late onset.	Early identification essential to prevent death. Antibiotic treatment of infected clients during labor has decreased neonatal infection. Antibiotics given to infected infants.

TABLE 25.1   Common Infections in the Newborn[a]—cont'd

Transmission	Effect on Newborn	Nursing Considerations
Gonorrhea		
Usually during birth	Conjunctivitis (ophthalmia neonatorum), with red, edematous lids and purulent eye drainage. May result in blindness if untreated.	All infants receive prophylactic treatment. Erythromycin eye ointment is most common. Infected infants are treated with IV antibiotics.
Chlamydia		
During birth	Conjunctivitis 1–2 wk after birth, pneumonia at 4–11 wk, otitis media, bronchiolitis.	Treated with oral azithromycin or erythromycin. Topical treatment of conjunctivitis is not effective.
Candidiasis		
During birth	White patches in mouth (thrush) that bleed if removed. Rash on perineum. May be systemic in preterm or LBW.	Administer nystatin drops or cream and teach parents how to administer them. Assess postpartum client for vaginal or breast infection. medications for systemic infection.
Toxoplasmosis		
Transplacental	Asymptomatic or FGR, LBW, preterm, thrombocytopenia, enlarged liver and spleen, jaundice, cerebral calcifications, encephalitis, seizures, microcephaly, hydrocephalus, chorioretinitis. Signs may not develop for years.	Consider in infants with FGR. Confirmed by serum tests. Treatment: Spiramycin during pregnancy, pyrimethamine, sulfadiazine, and folic acid for 1 yr for infant.
Syphilis		
Transplacental	Asymptomatic or spontaneous abortion, stillbirth, enlarged liver and spleen, jaundice, hepatitis, anemia, rhinitis, pink- or copper-colored peeling rash, pneumonitis, osteochondritis, CNS involvement.	Diagnosed by blood and CSF testing. Treated with penicillin.

CNS, Central nervous system; *CSF,* cerebrospinal fluid; *FGR,* fetal growth restriction; *HBIG,* hepatitis B immune globulin; *IV,* intravenous; *LBW,* low birth weight; *SGA,* small-for-gestational-age.
[a]Standard precautions for infection control apply to all clients and are not listed in this table.

important risk factors. Infants of clients who have rupture of membranes longer than 12 to 18 hours also have an increased risk for infection. Other risk factors for sepsis include prolonged or difficult labor, signs of infection in the pregnant client before or during labor, chorioamnionitis (Triple I), and foul-smelling amniotic fluid (Rudd, 2021). The nurse should identify clients known to be GBS-positive and those who show signs of infection so they can be treated with antibiotics during labor to reduce risk to the infant.

Every infant in the NICU is at risk for health care–associated infections. These infants have complications or conditions such as prematurity that make them more susceptible to infection. The risk for infection increases as gestational age and birth weight decrease. Preterm infants have not received antibodies from the pregnant client that help protect them from infection. In addition, they sometimes spend prolonged periods in the NICU, where they are exposed to many invasive procedures such as use of intravenous (IV) catheters and endotracheal tubes, which increase their risk for infection. NICU infants may develop abnormal flora that may be carried by personnel from one infant to another and may be resistant to usual drug

therapy. Catheter-related bloodstream infections are a significant problem in NICUs (Srinivasan & Evans, 2018).

Signs of Infection. In the newborn, early signs of infection are not as specific or obvious as those in the older infant or child. Instead, they tend to be subtle and could indicate other conditions. Temperature instability may occur. Only 50% of infected newborns have an axillary temperature above 37.8°C (100°F; Haslam, 2020).

Respiratory problems are common, and changes may occur in feeding habits or behavior. The nurse may identify the early, subtle changes in behavior that could indicate sepsis. Experienced nurses may have a feeling that the infant is not doing well even before specific signs of infection are present. When this occurs, the nurse expands the assessment and watches carefully for the development of other signs. Early identification and treatment are important because infants can develop septic shock with little warning.

Nursing Interventions

Preventing Infection. Although it is not always possible to prevent infection, every effort should be made. Careful and frequent hand hygiene is the most important aspect of infection prevention. The nurse should practice and teach

CRITICAL TO REMEMBER

Signs of Sepsis in the Newborn

General Signs
Temperature instability (usually low)
Nurse's or parents' feeling that the infant is not doing well
Rash

Respiratory Signs
Tachypnea
Respiratory distress (nasal flaring, retractions, grunting)
Apnea

Cardiovascular Signs
Color changes (cyanosis, pallor, mottling)
Tachycardia
Bradycardia
Hypotension
Decreased peripheral perfusion (decreased peripheral pulses, capillary refill greater than 3 seconds)
Edema

Gastrointestinal Signs
Decreased oral intake
Vomiting
Diarrhea
Abdominal distention
Hypoglycemia or hyperglycemia

Neurologic Signs
Decreased or increased muscle tone
Lethargy
Jitteriness
Irritability
Full fontanel
High-pitched cry

Signs That May Indicate Advanced Infection
Jaundice
Evidence of hemorrhage (petechiae, purpura, pulmonary bleeding)
Anemia
Enlarged liver and spleen
Respiratory failure
Shock
Seizures

parents to perform good handwashing or to use hospital-provided hand disinfectants before and after touching any infant. Equipment should be disinfected according to hospital protocols. Meticulous sterile technique should be used during invasive procedures. Invasive procedures should be kept to the lowest number possible.

The skin is delicate in the newborn, particularly so in preterm infants. Handling and trauma to the skin should be minimized as much as possible to prevent skin breakdown and infection.

Precautions should be taken to avoid transmission of infection to other infants. This is accomplished with hand hygiene, separation of each infant's supplies, and standard precautions

for infection control. These techniques should be conscientiously performed by all who come in contact with the infant. Parents should be taught about all infection control measures so that they can help protect their infants.

Placing the infant in an incubator provides a physical separation between infected and well infants, similar to placing adults in isolation in private rooms. In addition, the nurse can observe the infant in an incubator more easily.

Providing Antibiotics. The nurse is responsible for obtaining or helping obtain specimens for laboratory analysis and checking that other tests ordered by the provider are completed. Laboratory tests will help determine the type and duration of antibiotics prescribed.

Because the signs of infection are nonspecific and the disease can be fatal, physicians may order antibiotics before an actual diagnosis is made for infants who are at high risk or show early signs. Broad-spectrum IV antibiotics are given after samples for culture and sensitivity are taken and before the results are available. Continued antibiotic therapy is specific to organisms found on culture. The nurse should be knowledgeable about the antibiotics used and possible side effects.

The nurse starts IV fluids and ensures that medications are administered as scheduled. If more than one antibiotic is ordered, the timing of administration should be coordinated to increase effectiveness. Antibiotics usually are continued for 10 to 14 days for sepsis and 21 days for meningitis (Rudd, 2021).

Providing Other Supportive Care. Infants may be critically ill and need intensive nursing care. Care includes giving oxygen or other respiratory support, as needed. Fluid balance maintenance, monitoring of vital signs, and hourly urine output measurements are important. IV or gavage feeding may be necessary if the infant is unable to take oral feedings.

Infants with sepsis may have additional problems. They may be premature or have other transplacentally acquired infections. In addition, the nurse should be alert for signs of complications such as disseminated intravascular coagulopathy (DIC).

Supporting Parents. Nurses provide support to parents of newborns with sepsis and help them understand their infant's illness and treatment. The infant with sepsis often appears healthy at birth but suddenly becomes critically ill. Parents experience feelings of shock, fear, and disappointment when their apparently healthy newborn is suddenly moved to the NICU or the preterm infant they thought was making good progress may suddenly develop a life-threatening illness. Parents benefit from a chance to talk about their feelings with an understanding nurse who can explain the infant's treatment and care. Keeping the parents informed and involving them in care are essential.

INFANT OF A DIABETIC MOTHER

Scope of the Problem

The infant of a diabetic mother (IDM) faces many risks that depend on the type of diabetes affecting the pregnant client and how well it is controlled. The neonatal mortality rate is greater than five times that of infants born to clients without diabetes. Congenital anomalies are three to five times greater if the diabetes was present before the pregnancy and was not

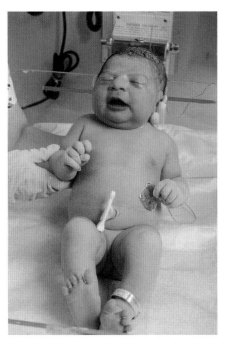

FIG. 25.3 Macrosomia is common in infants of clients with diabetes.

well controlled (Sheanon & Muglia, 2020). Cardiac, urinary tract, GI, neural tube, and skeletal anomalies are most frequent. Cardiomegaly is common and may lead to heart failure. The incidence of anomalies is decreased with good control of diabetes before conception and during the early weeks of gestation when fetal organs are being formed (Blickstein et al., 2020).

Insulin acts as a growth hormone. The accelerated protein synthesis and the deposit of fat and glycogen in fetal tissues can result in macrosomia (Fig. 25.3). Strict control of the pregnant client's blood glucose level reduces the risk for macrosomia (Rosene-Montella, 2020). Infants with macrosomia are at risk for trauma during birth, including fracture of the clavicles from shoulder dystocia, cephalohematoma, and facial nerve and brachial plexus injury.

When the pregnant client is hyperglycemic, large amounts of amino acids, free fatty acids, and glucose are transferred to the fetus. Insulin does not cross the placenta because the molecules are too large. The excessive glucose received by the fetus causes the fetal pancreas to secrete large amounts of insulin and leads to hypertrophy of the islet cells. Hypoglycemia may occur after birth when the supply of glucose from the client is no longer available but the infant's high insulin production continues.

Infants of clients with long-term diabetes and vascular changes may have fetal growth restriction (FGR), which is also known as IUGR, instead of macrosomia because of decreased placental blood flow. Hypertension occurs more often in clients with diabetes and further compromises uteroplacental blood flow.

The IDM has a higher risk for asphyxia and RDS. RDS occurs because increased levels of insulin block the effect of cortisol on stimulation of lung maturation and surfactant production may be delayed (Moore, Hauguel-DeMouzon, & Catalano, 2019). Other complications for which the IDM is

at risk include hypocalcemia as a result of decreased parathyroid hormone production. Magnesium levels may also be low.

Polycythemia may occur as a response to chronic hypoxia in utero. It may cause hyperbilirubinemia when the large number of RBCs break down after birth. In addition, IDMs are more likely to be born prematurely.

Characteristics of Infants of Diabetic Mothers

The IDM with macrosomia is different from other large-for-gestational-age (LGA) infants. The infant's size results from fat deposits and hypertrophy, particularly of the liver, spleen, and heart (Blinkstein et al., 2020). The length and head circumference are generally within the normal range for gestational age. Other LGA infants do not have enlargement of the organs and tend to be long, with large heads to match the rest of their bodies. IDMs have a characteristic appearance. The face is round, the skin is often red (plethoric), and the body is obese. The infant has poor muscle tone at rest but becomes irritable and may have tremors when disturbed. The SGA IDM is similar to infants who are SGA from other causes but is more likely to have congenital anomalies.

Therapeutic Management

Therapeutic management includes controlling the client's diabetes throughout pregnancy to decrease complications in the fetus and newborn (see Chapter 10). If the infant is large, there may be shoulder dystocia or cephalopelvic disproportion, and a cesarean birth may be required. Immediate care of respiratory problems and continued observation for complications determine treatment.

Nursing Considerations
Assessment

The IDM is assessed for signs of complications, trauma, and congenital anomalies at delivery and during the early hours after birth. Respiratory problems may be apparent at birth or may develop later. The initial assessment may reveal injuries. For example, an infant who cries when an arm is moved or fails to move an arm may have a fractured clavicle or nerve injury.

Hypoglycemia occurs in 15% to 25% of infants born to clients with diabetes (Sheanon & Muglia, 2020). It may be present without observable signs. The most frequent sign of low blood glucose is jitteriness or tremors. Diaphoresis is uncommon in newborns but may occur with hypoglycemia. Rapid respirations, low temperature, and poor muscle tone are also common. Because these signs are not specific for hypoglycemia, the nurse should be alert for other complications, particularly if signs continue after feeding.

Nursing Interventions

The nurse assesses glucose levels according to hospital policy. Because these infants are at risk for hypoglycemia, they should have a blood glucose screen done shortly after birth and be monitored more frequently than other infants. Glucose levels reach the lowest point in the first few hours after birth and begin to improve by 3 to 6 hours. Glucose levels of less than 40 to 45 mg/dL measured with a bedside glucometer should be reported and verified by laboratory analysis (Garg & Devaskar, 2020). Infants should be fed early to prevent hypoglycemia and immediately if low blood glucose occurs to prevent further decreases; 40% oral dextrose gel, massaged into the cheek, may be used as a supplement to feeding infants with transient hypoglycemia. Gavage feeding may be used if the infant does not suck well or if respirations are rapid. The glucose level is rechecked in 30 to 45 minutes. Infants who are symptomatic, have glucose levels that are not maintained with feedings and oral dextrose gel, or whose condition does not allow enteral feedings need IV glucose to maintain glucose balance and prevent injury to the brain.

The nurse should be alert for signs of other complications that occur in IDMs. RDS or other respiratory complications may develop. Cold stress, which increases the need for oxygen and glucose, could increase respiratory problems and exacerbate hypoglycemia. Infants with polycythemia need adequate hydration to prevent sluggish blood flow to vital organs and ischemia. Hypocalcemia may be suspected if tremors continue and the blood glucose concentration is normal.

Providing support to parents is important. Up to 35% of IDMs may have neurologic or developmental complications (Rozance et al., 2021). The nurse should work with the infant and the parents to ensure feedings are adequate. Parents may have many questions for the nurse. They may not understand why their infant, who appears fat and healthy to them, needs close observation and frequent blood tests. The pregnancy may have been difficult and the client may feel guilty, even if good diabetic control was maintained. Ample opportunity for discussion of feelings and information about the care of the infant is important.

> ### ⓘ KNOWLEDGE CHECK
>
> 8. What is the role of the nurse in caring for the infant with sepsis?
> 9. Why are IDMs more likely to develop macrosomia?
> 10. Why are IDMs at risk for hypoglycemia after birth?

POLYCYTHEMIA

In polycythemia, infants have a venous hematocrit greater than 65% or a hemoglobin greater than 22 g/dL (Letterio et al., 2020). The increased viscosity of the blood causes resistance in the blood vessels and decreases blood flow. Blood flow to all organs is impaired. Organ damage from ischemia and venous thrombosis may result along with neurologic and developmental problems (Diehl-Jones & Fraser, 2021). Polycythemia also may result in hyperbilirubinemia as the excessive RBCs break down after birth.

Causes

Polycythemia may occur when poor intrauterine oxygenation causes the fetus to compensate by producing more erythrocytes than normal. It is more common in infants who are postterm, LGA, or SGA or have FGR. It also occurs in infants of clients who smoke, have hypertension or diabetes. Delayed cord clamping or a transfusion from one twin to another also may cause the condition.

Manifestations

Most infants have minimal or no signs of polycythemia. Symptomatic infants may have a plethoric color, lethargy, irritability, poor tone, and tremors. Abdominal distention, decreased bowel sounds, poor feeding, hypoglycemia, and respiratory distress also may be present. Hyperbilirubinemia occurs as RBCs are broken down.

Therapeutic Management

Treatment is primarily supportive. Infants who are asymptomatic are observed and receive increased hydration. A partial exchange transfusion may be performed if the hematocrit is above 65%; however, the long-term benefits of the procedure are unclear (Jacquot et al., 2020). Blood is replaced with normal saline to decrease the total number of RBCs. Phototherapy is used to treat the jaundice.

Nursing Considerations

Monitoring of bilirubin levels is important to determine whether phototherapy is necessary. Infants should be hydrated adequately to prevent dehydration that would slow already sluggish blood flow and increase ischemia to vital organs. If an exchange transfusion is performed, the nurse assists and monitors for complications.

HYPOCALCEMIA

Hypocalcemia is a total serum calcium concentration of less than 7 mg/dL. It is divided into early-onset (in the first 72 hours of age) and late-onset (1 week of age) forms (Nyp et al., 2021).

Causes

Early-onset hypocalcemia occurs most often in IDMs and in infants with asphyxia, prematurity, and delayed nutrition. Late-onset hypocalcemia is caused by hypoparathyroidism, malabsorption, low magnesium levels, extensive diuretic therapy, and rickets (Nyp et al., 2021).

Manifestations

Signs of hypocalcemia include irritability, jitteriness, poor feeding, high-pitched cry, muscle twitching, apnea, seizures, and electrocardiographic changes. It is often asymptomatic.

Therapeutic Management

Laboratory testing of serum calcium levels determines the presence of the problem. IV calcium gluconate is given if feeding alone does not raise the calcium level. A cardiac monitor is necessary when IV calcium is given because bradycardia can occur.

Nursing Considerations

The nurse should be alert for signs of hypocalcemia. IV calcium should be administered slowly and stopped immediately if bradycardia or dysrhythmia develops. The IV site should be assessed frequently because infiltration can cause necrosis and ulceration.

PRENATAL DRUG EXPOSURE

Substance abuse affects the fetus at any time during pregnancy. Most drugs readily cross the placenta and cause a variety of problems. The effects of substance abuse on pregnancy, the fetus, and the neonate are discussed in Chapter 11. This section includes nursing care for infants with **neonatal abstinence syndrome (NAS)**, a disorder in which infants exposed to drugs before birth demonstrate signs of drug withdrawal.

Identification of Drug-Exposed Infants

Substance abuse by a pregnant client may be identified before the infant is born, but some infants are born to clients whose substance use is not known to the health care professionals caring for them. A history of minimal or no prenatal care or the client's behavior during labor may cause nurses to suspect substance abuse. When there is any reason to suspect drug use, the infant is observed closely for signs of prenatal drug exposure.

NAS occurs in infants who have suffered prenatal opiate exposure sufficient to cause withdrawal signs after birth. Pregnant clients who use heroin are generally switched to methadone or buprenorphine during pregnancy to decrease the incidence of wide variations in the drug dosage, which is harmful to the fetus. These clients usually receive better prenatal care, and their infants have a higher birth weight than those exposed to heroin. Nevertheless, infants may still undergo withdrawal after birth.

NAS is also seen in some infants exposed to other drugs such as amphetamines and antidepressants. Methamphetamine exposure results in lethargy, irritability, high-pitched cry, and hypertonicity in infants.

SSRIs and other antidepressants taken during pregnancy also result in NAS behaviors (Jackson et al., 2021). Signs of drug exposure usually begin during the first 24 to 72 hours after birth but may not occur for up to 2 weeks depending on the specific drug, the dose, and the time of the client's last use (Jackson et al., 2021). Use near the time of delivery causes a later onset but more severe signs of withdrawal.

◎ NURSING PROCEDURE

Applying a Pediatric Urine Collection Bag

PURPOSE: To collect a nonsterile urine specimen from an infant.

1. Wash hands and obtain needed equipment. Include pediatric urine collector, washcloth and towel, diaper, sterile specimen cup, and clean gloves. *Gathering equipment allows the procedure to be completed efficiently.*

2. Apply gloves. Wash and dry the genitalia. Dry the skin completely. *Removal of gross contaminants prevents contamination of the specimen. The bag adheres to a clean, dry surface best.*

3. Remove the paper covering on the posterior adhesive tabs of the bag first. To apply to female infants, gently hold the skin taut at the perineum. Fold the bag in half and apply smoothly over the perineum, extending the tabs to the side. For male infants, place the penis and scrotum (if small enough) inside the bag and apply the posterior adhesive tabs to the perineum. If the scrotum will not fit in the bag easily, apply the tabs smoothly over the scrotum. *Covering the perineum with the posterior tabs first helps ensure a smooth fit at this area, where leakage of urine may occur in the female infant especially, and prevents contamination with feces. Care in application prevents losing the specimen.*

4. Remove the paper covering on the anterior adhesive tabs, and apply to cover the genitalia. Be sure that there are no wrinkles in the tabs. *Wrinkles allow openings for urine to leak out of the bag.*

5. Cut a slit in the diaper, and gently pull the bag through the slit. Apply the diaper loosely. *Cutting a slit in the diaper allows for visualization of the bag. Placing the diaper too tightly over the bag might pull against the adhesive, causing trauma to the skin and providing an opening through which the specimen is lost.*

6. Check the bag for urine frequently and gently remove the bag as soon as urine is present. Transfer the urine to a specimen cup by removing the tab over the hole in the bottom and pouring. The specimen also can be aspirated with a syringe after cleaning the puncture site with alcohol. *This step ensures removal of the bag before urine loosens the adhesive and prepares the specimen to be sent to the laboratory for analysis.*

7. Clean the genitalia and observe for irritation. *This removes urine and adhesive from the skin.*

8. Place the specimen in a biohazard bag and label it. Transport the specimen to the laboratory or refrigerate it, if necessary. Record the date and time of urine collection, and the amount, color, and appearance of urine in the infant's chart. *This ensures proper disposition of the specimen.*

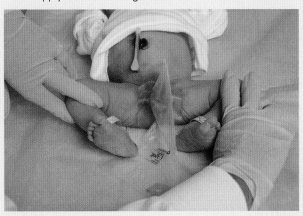

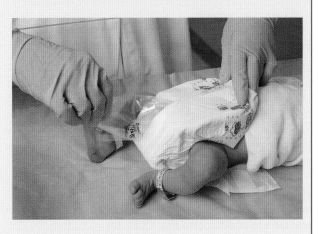

Polydrug use, along with use of alcohol and cigarettes, is common. This makes it difficult to determine which substance led to individual effects. Signs differ according to the drug or combination of drugs used but often include neurologic and GI abnormalities. Some infants with prenatal drug exposure show no abnormal signs at all.

Infants with NAS may be irritable and have hyperactive muscle tone and a high-pitched cry. Although they have tremors, the blood glucose level is normal. Infants appear hungry and suck vigorously on their fists but have poor coordination of suck and swallow. Frequent regurgitation, vomiting, and diarrhea are common. Infants are restless, and their excessive activity coupled with poor feeding ability results in failure to gain weight. Seizures may occur.

The Finnegan Neonatal Abstinence Score System and the Lipsitz Tool have been used for decades to determine the number, frequency, and severity of behaviors that indicate NAS. The score is used when considering whether drug therapy to alleviate withdrawal signs is needed and to determine dosage. Behaviors are generally scored every 2 to 4 hours until low scores are obtained consistently. It is important that all nurses are able to use the scoring tool consistently to provide optimal treatment for the infant. Recently the *Eat, Sleep, Console (ESC)* model of care for NAS infants has gained popularity as a simpler tool that focuses on the functional aspects of NAS that may be treated by nonpharmacologic means (Grossman et al., 2018). The success of ESC in limiting medication use and shortening the infant's hospital stay may depend on the parent's or caregiver's involvement and their ability to room-in with their infant (Dodds et al., 2019). Congenital anomalies and other effects of prenatal drug exposure may be apparent at birth. FGR and prematurity are common. Infants are more likely to have respiratory problems at birth, jaundice, or sudden infant death syndrome. Infants with fetal alcohol syndrome have a characteristic appearance.

When drug exposure is suspected, a urine specimen is collected for analysis. Drugs or their metabolites are present in the newborn's urine for various lengths of time. Some drugs last several days because the infant's immature liver and kidneys delay excreting them, whereas others disappear very soon. Therefore, it is important to obtain the first urine output from the infant, if possible (Procedure 25.1). Meconium analysis may detect drug exposure as far back as the second trimester (D'Apolito, 2021). A hair sample or a segment of umbilical cord is tested in some facilities.

Therapeutic Management

Because many signs of drug exposure are similar to the signs for other conditions, testing may be performed to rule out other causes. Sepsis, hypoglycemia, hypocalcemia, and neurologic disorders are possible causes for the infant's problems. In addition, the infant may have been exposed to infections such as hepatitis or sexually transmitted diseases during the pregnancy or at birth.

Therapeutic management includes dealing with the complications common to drug-exposed infants during and after birth. Respiratory problems and those related to prematurity are treated as for other infants. Many infants will require drug

---

CRITICAL TO REMEMBER

Signs of Intrauterine Drug Exposure[a]

Behavioral Signs
Irritability
Jitteriness, tremors, seizures
Muscular rigidity, increased muscle tone
Restless, excessive activity
Exaggerated Moro reflex
Prolonged high-pitched cry
Difficult to console
Poor sleeping patterns
Yawning

Signs Relating to Feeding
Exaggerated rooting reflex
Excessive sucking
Uncoordinated sucking and swallowing
Frequent regurgitation or vomiting
Diarrhea
Weight loss

Cardiovascular and Respiratory Signs
Nasal stuffiness, sneezing
Tachypnea, apnea
Retractions
Tachycardia

Other Signs
Hypertension
Fever
Diaphoresis
Excoriation
Mottling

[a]Some infants with prenatal drug exposure have no abnormal signs at all, or signs may be delayed.

---

therapy to manage their withdrawal symptoms; however, no evidence-based standard for pharmacologic treatment of NAS exists. Medications commonly used include oral morphine and methadone. Phenobarbital may be used for polydrug exposure. Buprenorphine and clonidine also have been used when first-line treatment has been unsuccessful (D'Apolito, 2021). Medication dosage is gradually tapered until the infant no longer needs it. Although these drugs help relieve the signs of withdrawal, all have side effects that may be undesirable.

Because the infant's suck and swallow are uncoordinated, gavage or IV feeding may be required. Some infants need more than the normal caloric requirements because of their excessive activity. The specific calories needed for each infant will be prescribed by the health care provider.

Involvement by social services in and out of the hospital is important to deal with the long-term effects of the drugs, placement of the infant after hospitalization, and follow-up of the parent or other caregiver to help provide for the infant's needs.

Nursing Considerations

The infant who has been exposed to drugs prenatally needs special care to cope with drug withdrawal. Care is focused on minimizing withdrawal symptoms, encouraging feeding, promoting rest, and, if possible, enhancing parental attachment.

Feeding

Feeding can be difficult and time-consuming. The poor suck and swallow coordination of drug-exposed infants interferes with caloric intake, yet their excessive activity increases their caloric needs.

Assessment. Infants often suck frantically on their fists or a nipple but are unable to coordinate feeding behaviors well. The nurse should assess the infant's ability to suck and swallow with breathing. Changes in the frequency and amount of regurgitation, vomiting, or the length of time it takes infants to finish feedings should be noted.

Nursing Interventions. Gavage feedings may be necessary to conserve the infant's energy and prevent aspiration if the infant is excessively agitated, is unable to suck and swallow adequately, or has rapid respirations. The infant's excessive activity, poor sleeping, vomiting, and diarrhea increase the caloric need. The infant may need as many as 150 to 215 calories per kilogram (cal/kg) each day (D'Apolito, 2021). Formula with 24 calories or more per ounce instead of the usual 20 calories per ounce may be used. More frequent feedings may be needed, as well.

Distractions during feedings can be prevented by choosing a quiet, low-activity area of the nursery for feedings. Infants should be swaddled to prevent the startling that occurs when drug-exposed infants are handled. Stimuli such as rocking and talking should be kept to a minimum during feedings.

Rest

The excessive activity and poor sleep patterns of drug-exposed neonates interfere with their ability to rest.

Assessment. The infant's muscle tone, tremors, and tendency for excessive activity with and without being disturbed should be assessed. The degree of tremors and stimuli that increase or decrease irritability are important. The nurse also keeps track of the number of hours the infant sleeps after each feeding.

Nursing Interventions. Keep stimulation of the drug-exposed infant to a minimum, especially at first when the infant is excessively irritable. Position the crib in the quietest area of the nursery or, ideally, a private room. Place a sign nearby to remind others of the need for quiet near the infant. The number of different types of stimulation should be kept to a minimum and adapted to each infant's needs. Reduce noise and bright lights as much as possible. If the infant shows signs of overstimulation, stop all activity briefly to allow a rest.

Swaddling the infant in a flexed position helps prevent startling and agitation. Placing the excessively agitated infant in a dark, quiet room may be necessary. As the infant shows the ability to withstand stimulation, add new types of stimuli gradually, one at a time. Some infants respond well to soft music, which has the added advantage of masking other environmental sounds.

Organize nursing care to reduce handling and disturbances. Cluster care activities to avoid unnecessary interruptions yet provide rest periods if signs of stress occur. A calm approach and slow, smooth movements during care help avoid startling the infant. A pacifier for nonnutritive sucking also helps quiet the infant.

Skin abrasions from excessive activity and rubbing of the face, elbows, and knees may increase discomfort and agitation. Cover the infant's hands with mittens or the end of the shirtsleeves to help prevent facial scratching. Diaper rash from frequent diarrhea also may occur. Skin breakdown should be prevented, if possible, and treated promptly if it occurs. Placing the infant in the prone position promotes better sleep for some infants, but supine positioning should be used as soon as possible.

Bonding

When prenatal drug use is known or suspected, many hospitals require a 3- to 7-day observation period to monitor for appearance of withdrawal symptoms. If the infant is transferred to another unit for observation and the postpartum client is discharged from the hospital without the baby, bonding is jeopardized. Many parents do not understand the need for this observation period because they mistakenly think that if they are using prescription medication, or switched from heroin to methadone or buprenorphine, their infant will not suffer from withdrawal.

When an infant tests positive for drugs, child protective services become involved. The client's ability to safely care for the infant may need to be assessed by social services or a court. The client may be required to enter a drug rehabilitation program before obtaining custody of the infant. After hospital discharge, the infant may be cared for by family members approved by the court, in a foster home, or in an institution. The client will most likely gain custody of the infant eventually if the court-ordered treatment is completed. Attachment to the infant should be encouraged.

Assessment. The frequency of visits and the response to the infant may give an indication of the client's apparent interest in the baby. Although some clients who abuse substances are uninterested in their infants, for others, the infant provides a reason to attempt to overcome their addiction. Bonding behaviors such as calling the infant by name and smiling at the infant should be noted.

Nursing Interventions. Child neglect, abuse, and failure to respond appropriately to infant signals and cues are associated with alcohol and drug abuse. Because the client may become the infant's primary caregiver, it is essential that nurses do whatever they can to enhance bonding. Helping the client feel welcome during visits with the infant poses a challenge. It is sometimes easy to be judgmental and difficult to be accepting of the client whose behavior has been harmful to the infant. Yet a friendly approach will encourage visits to the infant and improve receptiveness to teaching from the nurse.

Promote bonding by encouraging the client to participate actively in infant care during visits. Communication of the nurse's belief that the client can provide care to the infant may result in an increase in client confidence and encourage active participation in the required rehabilitation to regain custody of the newborn.

Participation in infant care also provides an opportunity for the nurse to assess the client's infant care skills and identify areas for additional discussion of the newborn's needs. Also, it gives the nurse an opportunity to demonstrate parenting skills. Many parents who use drugs have not had good parenting role models and do not know how to care for an infant. Frequent positive feedback about the client's participation is also important.

Provide the same teaching given to all new parents, as well as special techniques necessary to meet the needs of drug-exposed infants. Teach about the newborn's unique characteristics and help the client gradually assume more of the infant's care.

Teach the parents that infants are easily overstimulated. These infants cannot tolerate simultaneous visual and tactile stimulation. Signs of overstimulation in drug-exposed infants have some similarities with those for the preterm infant. In addition, some infants cannot tolerate more than brief periods of interaction. They may not make eye contact, or they may avert their eyes after 30 to 60 seconds of social interaction. Cuddling and soothing to console the infant may not elicit the same response in these infants as in other infants. Teach the parents that the infant responds poorly to everyone, so they do not think that the infant is rejecting them.

Parents of a drug-exposed infant may experience feelings of rejection, frustration, and even hostility when the infant stiffens while being held, cries after being fed, or looks away. Explain that drug-exposed infants are easily stressed because of the decreased stability of their CNS. Emphasize that the infant needs gentle handling. Also explain that crying indicates a need, not a spoiled infant.

Demonstrate comfort measures that work best for the infant. These infants are often comforted when they are snugly swaddled in a flexed position with their hands brought to midline. Holding the swaddled infant close to the parent's body may increase comfort. Some infants are consoled with slow, rhythmic, vertical or horizontal rocking movements. Placing them in a front pack as the nurse or parent moves around may also be comforting.

When the infant is nearing discharge, explain that sleep problems will probably continue at home. The infant should sleep in a quiet room because normal household noises will disturb the drug-exposed infant more than other infants (Jackson et al., 2021).

Cocaine, amphetamines, heroin, and other drugs pass into breast milk. Trying to breastfeed an infant with poorly developed feeding skills may be too much stress for the client who is trying to recover from addiction. Therefore, those who are likely to continue drug use after delivery should be discouraged from breastfeeding.

Clients taking methadone may be allowed to breastfeed if they are not taking other drugs that are contraindicated. Methadone and buprenorphine have been found to be at very low levels in breast milk and may result in lower pharmacologic treatment doses and duration (Jackson, et al., 2021).

Breastfeeding assistance should be given to women who are interested because of the advantages of breast milk over formula and because it may facilitate bonding.

Provide information and referral to any special programs available to help parents learn stimulation techniques appropriate for drug-exposed infants. Some withdrawal signs may continue for 2 to 6 months, and the parents need to know how to cope with them (Jackson, et al., 2021). If the client is unable or not allowed to care for the newborn after discharge, the same interventions can be used to help the person who will take over care of the infant.

CLIENT EDUCATION

Measures to Prevent Frantic Crying in a Drug-Exposed Infant

Swaddle the infant with the hands brought to the midline.
Provide a pacifier.
Slowly and smoothly rock in a vertical or horizontal motion with the infant held upright.
Coo softly and gently.
Place the infant over your shoulder and gently stroke the back.
Keep the room fairly dark because some infants are particularly sensitive to light.
Avoid simultaneous auditory and visual stimuli.
Curtail stimulation if the infant shows signs of stress (yawning, sneezing, jerky movements, or spitting up).

KNOWLEDGE CHECK

11. How can the nurse deal with the inability to rest in infants with prenatal exposure to drugs?
12. How can the nurse promote bonding when there has been prenatal drug abuse?

PHENYLKETONURIA

Phenylketonuria (PKU) is a genetic disorder that causes CNS injury from toxic levels of the amino acid phenylalanine in blood. The incidence is 1 in 15,000 (Taylor et al., 2018). Severe cognitive impairment occurs in untreated infants and children. In the United States all newborns are screened for this condition before or shortly after discharge from the birth facility. Positive screening tests are followed by other testing to confirm the diagnosis.

Causes

PKU is caused by a deficiency of the liver enzyme phenylalanine hydrolase, which is necessary to convert phenylalanine to tyrosine for use. It is an autosomal recessive disorder.

Manifestations

Signs of untreated disease may begin with digestive problems and vomiting and later progress to seizures, musty odor of the urine, and severe cognitive impairment. Older children have eczema, hypertonia, hyperactive behavior, cognitive impairment, and hypopigmentation of the hair, skin, and irises.

Therapeutic Management

Treatment is a low-phenylalanine diet that should start immediately after the diagnosis is made and continue throughout life to avoid irreversible neurologic damage (Kliegman et al., 2020). Clients with PKU who are not following the diet closely need to return to it before they conceive and throughout pregnancy to prevent abnormalities in the fetus. Infants with PKU receive a special formula low in phenylalanine, and low-protein foods are introduced when solids are started. Small amounts of phenylalanine are allowed because it is a necessary amino acid. Early and continued treatment is necessary to prevent or minimize cognitive impairment.

Nursing Considerations

The nurse should be sure that all newborns are screened for PKU at the appropriate time in the birth facility. Screening performed before 24 hours of age should be repeated because the infant may not yet have consumed enough protein for the test to be accurate.

The nurse assists parents in regulating the diet to meet the infant's changing phenylalanine needs. Parents may need to talk about their feelings regarding the difficulty of following the diet for their children. They can be reassured that good control helps avoid long-term neurologic problems. Nevertheless, below normal intelligence and behavioral difficulties may occur (Kliegman et al., 2020).

CONGENITAL ANOMALIES

Approximately 2% of newborns have a major malformation at birth (Mitchell, 2020). Congenital anomalies are the leading cause of deaths in the first year of life. Some infants have more than one anomaly, which may be part of a syndrome or result from unrelated causes. Although congenital anomalies generally are treated in the pediatric setting, they are often identified soon after birth. Common congenital anomalies are noted in Box 25.1.

BOX 25.1   Common Congenital Anomalies

Gastrointestinal Tract

Cleft Lip and Palate

These are among the most common congenital anomalies. They occur together or separately on one or both sides.

Lip—Minor notching of the lip or complete separation through the lip and into floor of nose.

Palate—Only the soft palate or division of the entire hard and soft palate. Both genetic and environmental factors are included in the causes.

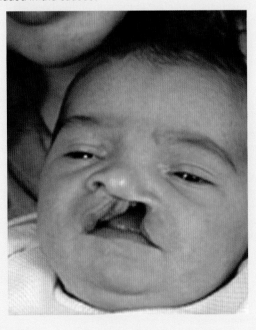

Assessment

Severe clefts are obvious at birth.

Palpate the hard and soft palate of all neonates during initial assessment.

Therapeutic Management

Lip surgery is usually performed by 3 months to enhance appearance and parental bonding.

Further surgery may be needed at 4 to 5 years.

Palate surgery is usually done by 1 year to minimize speech problems.

Long-term follow-up is necessary for orthodontia, speech therapy, and treatment of possible hearing problems.

Nursing Considerations

The degree of the cleft determines the approach to feeding.

Experiment to find methods that work best for individual infants. Try:
1. Breastfeeding (soft breast tissue fills in a small cleft of the lip or palate)
2. Nipples with enlarged hole
3. Compressible bottles
4. Special longer nipples
5. Special assistive devices

Feed the infant in the upright position because milk enters nasal passages through the palate, causing an increased tendency to aspirate.

Feed slowly with frequent stops to burp because infants tend to swallow excessive air.

Wash away milk curds with water after feeding.

Help the parents deal with their disappointment over the infant with an obvious anomaly. Show them before and after pictures of plastic surgery.

Reinforce the physician's explanation of plans for surgery.

Teach parents feeding techniques. Let them observe at first, then take over gradually.

Prevent infections. Infants are especially susceptible to respiratory tract and ear infections, which can delay surgery. Ear infections may lead to hearing loss.

Emphasize the need for long-term follow-up. Refer to agencies that help with the expense of long-term care and to support groups for help and emotional support from other parents.

Continued

BOX 25.1   Common Congenital Anomalies—cont'd

Esophageal Atresia and Tracheoesophageal Fistula

In **esophageal atresia (EA)** the esophagus is most commonly divided into two unconnected segments (atresia) with a blind pouch at the proximal end. If the distal end is connected to the trachea, it causes **tracheoesophageal fistula (TEF)**. The cause is a failure of normal development during the fourth week of pregnancy.

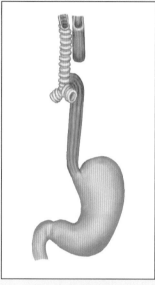

Assessment

Watch for EA when polyhydramnios occurs because the excessive fluid may be caused by fetal inability to swallow amniotic fluid.

Observe for other defects that may occur.

Signs vary by the type of defect.

Suspect EA in infants with excessive frothy drooling and needing suction more often than usual, when regurgitation occurs from secretions that pool in a blind pouch, and when a catheter will not pass into the stomach.

If a fistula connects the distal esophagus and the trachea, the stomach becomes distended with air from the trachea. Gastric secretions may be aspirated into the lungs, causing a severe inflammatory reaction.

Therapeutic Management

Diagnosis is confirmed by symptoms and radiography.

Esophageal suctioning should be used for the upper pouch, and a gastrostomy tube is placed.

Surgery involves ligation of the fistula and anastomosis of the esophageal segments. If the separation is large, surgery may be done in stages to allow growth.

Long-term follow-up is needed for esophageal reflux and dilation of strictures that may form at the surgical site.

Nursing Considerations

Observe all infants carefully during the first feeding for respiratory difficulty or other signs.

Prevent aspiration by maintaining the infant in a semiupright position to prevent reflux of gastric fluids.

Maintain suction equipment.

Care after surgery involves low-pressure ventilation, chest tubes, parenteral nutrition, and gastrostomy feedings.

Omphalocele and Gastroschisis

Both of these anomalies are caused by congenital defects in the abdominal wall.

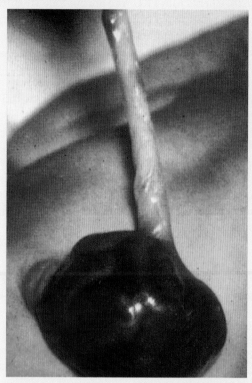

In **omphalocele**, the intestines protrude into the base of the umbilical cord. Other anomalies often occur with omphalocele.

Gastroschisis is a defect to the side of the abdomen through which the intestines protrude. They are not covered by peritoneum or skin and float freely in the amniotic fluid.

Assessment

Diagnosis is made by prenatal measurement of elevated alpha-fetoprotein level and by prenatal ultrasound and is obvious at birth.

Therapeutic Management

A gastric tube is placed to decrease air in the stomach. Gastric suction, parenteral nutrition, and antibiotics are necessary.

Surgery is performed as soon as the infant is stable. A Silastic silo (pouch) may be used to replace the intestines gradually over a period of days to prevent pressure on the other organs. The abdomen is closed when the contents have been replaced in the abdominal cavity.

Nursing Considerations

Place the infant's torso into a sterile plastic bag or cover the intestines with Silastic or warm sterile saline dressings wrapped with plastic immediately after birth to reduce heat and water loss.

Observe for respiratory distress from increased intraabdominal pressure.

Prevent infection and trauma.

Position to avoid pressure on the intestines.

BOX 25.1 Common Congenital Anomalies—cont'd

Diaphragmatic Hernia

The diaphragm fails to fuse during gestation. A large or small part of the abdominal contents moves into the chest cavity, usually on the left side.

If the herniation is large enough, the lungs may fail to develop (hypoplastic lungs). When gas fills the bowel, further pressure on the heart and lungs results.

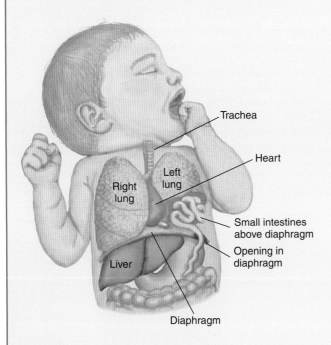

Trachea
Heart
Left lung
Right lung
Small intestines above diaphragm
Opening in diaphragm
Liver
Diaphragm

Assessment

Mild to severe respiratory distress may occur at birth, with breath sounds diminished or absent over the affected area, and barrel chest. The heartbeat may be displaced to the right. Bowel sounds are heard in the chest.

The abdomen may be scaphoid (concave). The condition may be diagnosed prenatally by ultrasound or by radiography after birth.

Therapeutic Management

Fetal surgery may be performed.

An endotracheal tube is placed for mechanical ventilation and a gastric tube for decompression of the stomach.

Surgery to replace the intestines and repair the defect is performed when the infant is stable.

Extracorporeal membrane oxygenation (ECMO) or inhaled nitric oxide may be used.

Nursing Considerations

Avoid bag and mask ventilation to minimize distention of the stomach and bowels.

Position the infant on the affected side to allow the unaffected lung to expand. Elevate the head to decrease pressure on the heart and lungs. Assist with ventilation and monitor respiratory status.

Continue to monitor respiratory status after surgery to determine whether lung function will be adequate.

Central Nervous System

Neural Tube Defects

Folic acid supplements in pregnancy help prevent neural tube defects, especially if they are taken before conception and in early pregnancy.

Spina bifida is failure of the vertebral arch to close. *Spina bifida occulta* is failure of the vertebra to close, usually without other anomalies. It is seen by a dimple on the back, which may have a tuft of hair over it.

Meningocele is protrusion of meninges and spinal fluid through the spina bifida, covered by skin or a thin membrane. Because the spinal cord is not involved, paralysis does not occur.

Myelomeningocele is protrusion of a membrane-covered sac through the spina bifida. The sac contains meninges, nerve roots, the spinal cord, and spinal fluid. The degree of paralysis depends on the location of the defect. The infant also may have hydrocephalus, or it may develop after surgery.

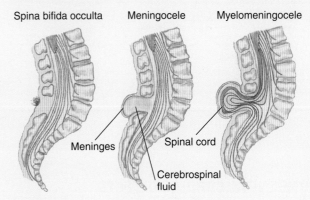

Spina bifida occulta   Meningocele   Myelomeningocele

Meninges   Spinal cord   Cerebrospinal fluid

Assessment

Prenatal diagnosis by elevated alpha-fetoprotein level or ultrasound.

Note the position and covering of the defect at birth.

Observe movement below the defect to determine the degree of paralysis.

Examine for a relaxed anus and dribbling of stool and urine.

Check for other anomalies.

Therapeutic Management

Fetal surgery may be performed.

Surgery is performed for meningocele and myelomeningocele as soon as possible to prevent infection.

A shunt is placed to divert cerebrospinal fluid if hydrocephalus develops.

Antibiotics are given to prevent infection.

Long-term follow-up is necessary, with physical therapy and other care as needed.

Nursing Considerations

Place the infant's torso in a sterile plastic bag or cover the defect with a sterile saline dressing and plastic to prevent drying.

Handle the infant carefully, and position prone or to the side to prevent trauma to the sac.

Continued

BOX 25.1   Common Congenital Anomalies—cont'd

Observe for signs of infection. Keep free of contamination from urine and feces.

Inspect the sac for intactness before surgery.

Every shift, check for increasing head circumference, bulging fontanels, separation of sutures, intermittent apnea, and other signs of increased intracranial pressure to identify early hydrocephalus.

The mother should take increased folic acid before and during future pregnancies to reduce the risk for a recurrence.

Congenital Hydrocephalus

This is a problem with absorption or obstruction to the flow of cerebrospinal fluid in the ventricles of the brain, causing compression of the brain and enlargement of the head.

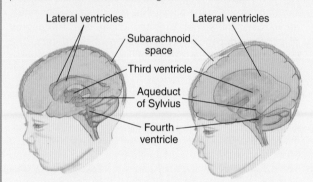

Assessment

The fontanel is full or bulging, and sutures may be separated.

The head is enlarged, especially in the frontal area.

Irritability and poor feeding occur.

The setting-sun sign is apparent (sclera visible above the pupils of the eyes).

Therapeutic Management

Surgery, most often with a ventriculoperitoneal shunt to drain fluid into the peritoneal cavity.

Will need revision as the child grows.

Nursing Considerations

Measure head circumference daily.

Prevent pressure areas.

Observe for signs of infection and intracranial pressure.

Teach parents how to care for the shunt and to observe for signs of increased intracranial pressure.

CONGENITAL CARDIAC DEFECTS

Approximately 0.8% of newborns have congenital heart defects. The defects are discovered by 1 week of age in 40% to 50% of infants and by 1 month of age in 50% to 60% of infants. Congenital heart defects are the leading cause of death from congenital anomalies (Bernstein, 2020). Genetics, teratogens, maternal diabetes, and rubella are known to be possible factors.

Classification of Cardiac Defects

Cardiac defects are generally categorized according to whether cyanosis results from the defect and by the pattern of blood flow. Some of the most common defects are illustrated in Fig. 25.4.

Acyanotic Defects

In acyanotic conditions, an obstruction of blood flow from the ventricles or a defect that causes increased flow of blood to the lungs occurs. Both increase the work of the heart. In addition, congestion in the lungs may eventually cause increased resistance of the pulmonary vessels and pulmonary hypertension. Infants are prone to respiratory tract infections because of the pulmonary congestion and increased work of the heart and lungs. Growth is slowed, and the infant fatigues easily. The heart may fail from overwork. Patent ductus arteriosus is an example of this group.

Cyanotic Defects

In cyanotic defects, blood flow to the lungs decreases, or venous blood and oxygenated blood are mixed in the systemic circulation, or both, decreasing the oxygen carried to the tissues and resulting in cyanosis. When venous blood from the right side of the heart flows through an abnormal opening to the left side of the heart, it is called a *right-to-left shunt*. Although the heart and lungs work harder, adequate oxygenation may be impossible, resulting in hypoxia of the major organs. Infants usually have serious problems from birth. They grow poorly, have frequent infections, and are easily fatigued. Heart failure may be an early complication. Transposition of the great vessels is an example of a cyanotic heart defect.

The presence of cyanosis depends on the severity and combination of defects and the child's ability to compensate. Some infants with cyanotic heart disease may be pink, and some with acyanotic heart defects may develop cyanosis. Because of this potential change in classification, further classification by blood flow is helpful.

Left-to-Right Shunting Defects

These heart defects allow blood to flow from the higher pressure of the left side of the heart to the right side or from the aorta to the pulmonary artery. This increases blood flow to the lungs and is called a *left-to-right shunt*. It causes some

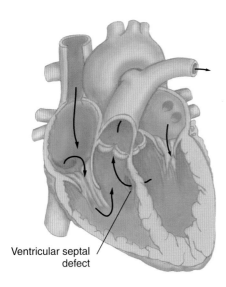

A

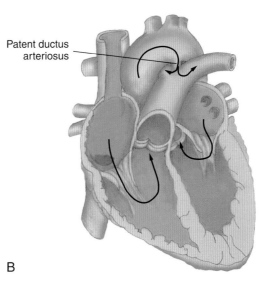

B

Ventricular septal defect is the most common type of congenital heart defect. It occurs alone or with other defects. The opening in the septum ranges from the size of a pin to very large. Many small defects close spontaneously. When the pressure in the left ventricle increases after birth, oxygenated blood is shunted through a large ventricular septal defect into the right ventricle and then recirculated to the lungs (a left-to-right shunt). Increased pulmonary resistance may cause pulmonary hypertension, hypertrophy of the right ventricle, and heart failure. Surgery is necessary for a large ventricular septal defect and increasing symptoms.

Patent ductus arteriosus is a failure of the ductus arteriosus to close after birth. Blood flows from the higher pressure of the aorta to the pulmonary artery and the lungs (left-to-right shunt). It is most common in the preterm infant. Symptoms vary from none to early congestive heart failure. Prostaglandins cause vasodilation and may interfere with closure of the ductus arteriosus. Indomethacin or ibuprofen lysine, prostaglandin inhibitors, may be effective in causing closure. Surgical ligation is used when necessary. Devices to close the defect nonsurgically are also used.

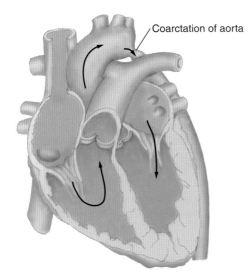

C

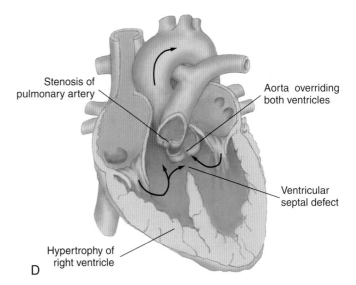

D

In *coarctation of the aorta,* blood flow is impeded through a constricted area of the aorta near the ductus arteriosus, increasing pressure behind the defect. The blood pressure is higher in the upper extremities than in the lower extremities. Carotid, brachial, and radial pulses are bounding, but pulses in the legs are weak or absent. The increased pressure in the left ventricle causes hypertrophy from the added workload. Congestive heart failure may result.

Tetralogy of Fallot has four characteristics: a ventricular septal defect, aorta positioned over the ventricular defect, pulmonary stenosis, and hypertrophy of the right ventricle. Cyanosis occurs if venous blood from the right ventricle flows through the septal defect and into the overriding aorta and blood flow to the lungs is diminished because of the narrowed pulmonary valve. The amount of right-to-left shunting and cyanosis varies according to the degree and position of each defect.

FIG. 25.4 Common Congenital Heart Defects. A, Ventricular septal defect. B, Patent ductus arteriosus. C, Coarctation of the aorta. D, Tetralogy of Fallot.

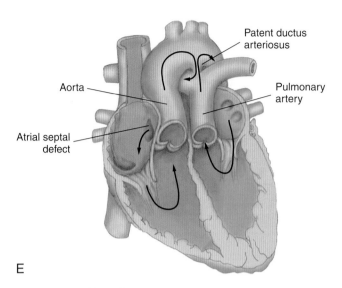

In *transposition of the great arteries,* the positions of the aorta and the pulmonary artery are reversed. The aorta carries venous blood from the right ventricle back to the general circulation. The pulmonary artery returns oxygenated blood from the left ventricle to the lungs. Unless there is another source for mixing oxygenated and venous blood, the infant cannot survive. A septal defect, open foramen ovale, or patent ductus arteriosus may be present. Prostaglandins may be given to keep the ductus open, and surgical correction is performed.

FIG. 25.4, cont'd E, Transposition of the great arteries.

oxygenated blood to be sent to the lungs instead of to the rest of the body, increasing the work of the right side of the heart and the lungs. Congestive heart failure and pulmonary hypertension may result. Examples are ventricular septal defects and patent foramen ovale.

Defects with Obstruction of Blood Outflow

In defects with obstruction of blood flow, a decrease in the blood flow through a vessel or valve occurs because of stenosis (narrowing). This adds to the work of the heart, causes hypertrophy of the heart or major blood vessels, and may lead to heart failure. Coarctation of the aorta and stenosis of the pulmonary or aortic valves fit into this classification.

Defects with Decreased Pulmonary Blood Flow

An impairment in the flow of blood from the right side of the heart to the lungs, combined with abnormal openings between pulmonary and systemic circulations, occurs in defects with decreased pulmonary blood flow. Systemic hypoxemia causes cyanosis. An example is tetralogy of Fallot.

Cyanotic Defects with Increased Pulmonary Blood Flow

These defects allow survival only if a mixing of venous and oxygenated blood in the heart occurs. There is increased blood flow to the lungs and mixing of venous and oxygenated blood in the systemic circulation. Transposition of the great vessels is an example of this type of defect.

Manifestations

Congenital heart defects may present obvious signs at birth or may not become apparent until later, when changes from fetal to neonatal circulation are completed. Some infants have no difficulty for months or years, but others experience early heart failure. The most common indications of cardiac problems are cyanosis, heart murmurs, tachycardia, and tachypnea.

Cyanosis

Cyanosis is a major sign of cardiac anomaly when it is not a result of respiratory disease. If the cyanosis is caused by mixing of oxygenated and unoxygenated blood, giving oxygen will not improve the infant's color. Cyanosis increases with crying, feeding, or other activity. Pallor, mottling, or a gray color may be present in infants who do not have cyanosis.

Heart Murmurs

Murmurs may sound like clicks, machinery, rumbling, swishing, or other muffled noises. It takes much practice to detect heart murmurs accurately. Although many infants have a temporary murmur until the fetal structures are closed, all abnormal sounds should be referred to the provider.

Tachycardia and Tachypnea

Tachycardia and tachypnea may occur any time the heart and lungs must work harder to provide sufficient oxygen to the body. Therefore, they are present in both respiratory conditions and cardiac conditions. They increase in congestive heart failure.

Other Signs

Fatigue and tachypnea may interfere with the infant's ability to eat. Infants may feed slowly and take small amounts. They may fall asleep before the feeding is finished because of the effort required for sucking. As a result, weight gain may be slow. Although diaphoresis is uncommon in the newborn, it may appear during feedings in the infant with a heart defect.

CRITICAL TO REMEMBER

Common Signs of Cardiac Anomalies

Cyanosis increasing with crying
Pallor
Murmurs
Tachycardia
Tachypnea
Dyspnea
Choking spells
Poor intake, falling asleep during feedings
Diaphoresis

Therapeutic Management

Therapeutic management involves diagnosis of the specific defect and supportive and surgical treatment, as indicated. Various tests such as echocardiograms and cardiac catheterizations confirm the diagnosis. The decision for surgery depends on the status of the infant and whether surgery can be delayed safely. Palliative surgery may be performed to partially correct a defect or make another defect to allow greater amounts of oxygenated blood to get to the systemic circulation.

Oxygen and drugs such as digitalis, diuretics, potassium supplements, and sedatives may be prescribed for the infant. Prostaglandins may be given to prevent the ductus arteriosus from closing in those cases in which keeping it open will increase the flow of oxygenated blood in the infant's body.

Nursing Considerations

Nursing care is focused on assessing for changes in condition and reducing the infant's need for oxygen. The need for rest is especially important, and the infant's response to all activity is evaluated. Infants with rapid respirations are at risk for aspiration and may need feeding by gavage. Oxygen may be increased during feedings or other exertion, but only enough oxygen to maintain saturation levels adequately should be used. Frequent rest periods are provided by clustering small amounts of nursing care.

Feedings with increased calories may be used to promote nutrition and weight gain. Accurate intake and output measurement are necessary. Maintaining a neutral thermal environment is important to avoid increasing oxygen need.

Support of the parents and education about the infant's condition and expected treatment are essential. The physician may use drawings to help parents understand the defect and plans for surgery. The nurse verifies the parents' understanding and provides additional teaching, as necessary. The parents are taught techniques for accurate administration of medications because the range between the therapeutic and toxic dosage of the drugs is narrow. Parents may be referred to support groups for families of children with heart anomalies.

SUMMARY CONCEPTS

- All newborns should be considered at risk for needing resuscitation. All personnel involved in deliveries should know how to perform resuscitative measures.
- In transient tachypnea of the newborn, respiratory difficulty in infants is caused by failure of fetal lung fluid to be absorbed completely. It usually resolves spontaneously with supportive care.
- In meconium aspiration syndrome, meconium in amniotic fluid enters the lungs before birth during gasping movements or is drawn in during the first breaths after birth, causing obstruction, air trapping, and inflammation.
- The nurse's role in meconium aspiration is to notify caregivers when meconium is discovered in amniotic fluid, prepare equipment, assist with intubation if necessary, and observe for further respiratory difficulty, infection, and other problems.
- Persistent pulmonary hypertension is a condition in which pulmonary vascular resistance remains high after birth and right-to-left shunting of blood occurs, causing severe respiratory difficulty.
- Nonphysiologic jaundice appears in the first 24 hours of life. Bilirubin levels rise faster and to higher levels than in physiologic jaundice. If untreated, it may result in injury to the brain.

- The nurse's role in phototherapy is to decrease situations such as cold stress or hypoglycemia that might further elevate bilirubin levels, ensure that lights are used properly, protect the eyes, observe for excessive fluid loss or skin impairment, ensure adequate oral intake, and teach parents.
- Infection can be transmitted to the neonate from the client during pregnancy or birth or from the parents, family members, visitors, or agency staff after birth.
- Infection in neonates is a problem because their immune system is immature, infection spreads easily, and the blood–brain barrier is less effective.
- The infant of a diabetic mother may have congenital anomalies, may be large or small for gestational age, and may suffer from respiratory distress syndrome, hypoglycemia, hypocalcemia, and polycythemia.
- Nursing responsibilities in caring for the infant with a diabetic mother include early identification and follow-up of complications, monitoring of blood glucose levels, ensuring early and adequate feedings, and support of the parents.
- Infants with polycythemia have increased viscosity of blood that may cause thromboemboli, stroke, hyperbilirubinemia, and other complications.

- Infants with prenatal exposure to drugs may have behavioral and feeding abnormalities. They may have difficulty interacting or bonding with their parents or caregivers and fail to gain weight.
- Nursing care for infants with neonatal abstinence syndrome includes obtaining accurate neonatal abstinence syndrome scores; decreasing stimuli from lights, noise, and handling; increasing feeding abilities; and fostering the parents' attachment to and ability to care for the infant.
- Infants with phenylketonuria should be on a low-phenylalanine diet to prevent severe intellectual disability.
- Congenital heart defects include left-to-right shunting defects, defects with obstruction of blood outflow, defects with decreased pulmonary blood flow, and cyanotic defects with increased pulmonary blood flow.

Clinical Judgment and Next-Generation NCLEX® Examination Style Questions

A 32-week infant was born to a 28-year-old G1 P0. The pregnancy was complicated by uncontrolled diabetes and prolonged rupture of membranes. The maternal blood type is O-. The infant weight was 6 pounds 2 ounces or 2857 grams. The baby is breastfeeding. Baby's blood type is A+. The nurse is assessing the infant 12 hours after birth.

1. **Place an X to indicate whether the assessment findings below are expected (finding within the usual limits or parameters), a common variation (finding that may or may not indicate and abnormality), or unexpected (finding that is abnormal and could be harmful) for the infant at this time.**

Assessment	Expected	Common Variation	Unexpected
Heart rate 150 bpm			
Jittery activity			
Pink mucous membranes			
Yellow tint to skin			
High-pitched cry			
Breastfed 10 minutes on both breasts			
Fontanels are soft with edema			

Assessment	Expected	Common Variation	Unexpected
Total serum bilirubin is 6 mg/dL			
Dark pink mark on the back of the neck			

2. **Choose the most likely option from the list of options below to fill in the blank.**

The baby's history of 32 weeks' gestation, prolonged rupture of membranes, and maternal history of diabetes puts this baby at risk for developing _____1_____ jaundice and _____2_____. Additional assessment and interventions the nurse may include are _____3_____, _____4_____, _____5_____.

Option 1, 2	Option 3, 4, 5
pathologic	Remove eye patch from eye during feeding
nonpathologic	Provide skin-to-skin
hypoglycemia	Assess glucose via heel stick
hyperglycemia	Place supine wrapped in blanket in crib
kernicterus	Turn infant frequently in the warmer
cold stress	Assess temperature every 2 hours
dehydration	Assess for ketonuria

REFERENCES & READINGS

Ahlfeld, S. K. (2020). Respiratory tract disorders. In R. M. Kliegman, J. W. St. Geme, N. J. Blum, S. S. Shah, R. C. Tasker, & K. M. Wilson (Eds.), *Nelson textbook of pediatrics* (21st ed., pp. 929–949). Elsevier.

Bernstein, D. (2020). Epidemiology and genetic basis of congenital heart disease. In R. M. Kliegman, J. W. St. Geme, N. J. Blum, S. S. Shah, R. C. Tasker, & K. M. Wilson (Eds.), *Nelson textbook of pediatrics* (21st ed., pp. 2367–2371). Elsevier.

Blickstein, I., Perlman, S., Hazan, Y., & Shinwell, E. S. (2020). Pregnancy complicated by diabetes mellitus. In R. J. Martin, A. A. Fanaroff, & M. C. Walsh (Eds.), *Fanaroff and Martin's neonatal-perinatal medicine: Diseases of the fetus and infant* (11th ed., pp. 304–311). Elsevier.

Crowley, M. A. (2020). Neonatal respiratory disorders. In R. J. Martin, A. A. Fanaroff, & M. C. Walsh (Eds.), *Fanaroff and Martin's neonatal-perinatal medicine: Diseases of the fetus and infant* (11th ed., pp. 1203–1230). Elsevier.

D'Apolito, K. (2021). Perinatal substance abuse. In M. T. Verklan, M. Walden, & S. Forest (Eds.), *Core curriculum for neonatal intensive care nursing* (6th ed., pp. 38–53). Elsevier.

Diehl-Jones, W., & Fraser, D. (2021). Hematologic disorders. In M. T. Verklan, M. Walden, & S. Forest (Eds.), *Core curriculum for neonatal intensive care nursing* (6th ed., pp. 568–587). Elsevier.

Dodds, D., Koch, K., Buitrago-Mogollon, T., & Horstmann, S. (2019). Successful implementation of the Eat Sleep Console model of care for infants with NAS in a community hospital. *Hospital Pediatrics,* 9(8), 632–638. https://doi.org/10.1542/hpeds.2019-0086.

Fraser, D. (2021). Respiratory distress. In M. T. Verklan, M. Walden, & S. Forest (Eds.), *Core curriculum of neonatal intensive care nursing* (6th ed., pp. 394–416). Elsevier.

Gardner, S. L., Enzman-Hines, M., & Nyp, M. (2021). Respiratory diseases. In S. L. Gardner, B. S. Carter, M. Enzman-Hines, & S. Niermeyer (Eds.), *Merenstein & Gardner's handbook of neonatal intensive care* (9th ed., pp. 729–835). Elsevier.

Garg, M., & Devaskar, S. U. (2020). Disorders of carbohydrate metabolism in the neonate. In R. J. Martin, A. A. Fanaroff, & M. C. Walsh (Eds.), *Fanaroff and Martin's neonatal-perinatal medicine: Diseases of the fetus and infant* (11th ed., pp. 1584–1610). Elsevier.

Greenberg, J. M., Haberman, B., Narendran, V., Nathan, A. T., & Schibler, K. R. (2019). Neonatal morbidities of prenatal and perinatal origin. In R. Resnik, C. J. Lockwood, T. Moore, M. F. Greene, J. A. Copel, & R. M. Silver (Eds.), *Creasy & Resnick's maternal-fetal medicine: Principles and practice* (8th ed., pp. 1309–1333). Elsevier.

Grossman, M. R., Lipshaw, M. J., Osborn, R. R., & Berkwitt, A. K. (2018). A novel approach to assessing infants with neonatal abstinence syndrome. *Hospital Pediatrics*, 8(1), 1–6. https://doi.org/10.1542/hpeds.2017-2018.

Haslam, D. B. (2020). Epidemiology of infections. In R. M. Kliegman, J. W. St. Geme, N. J. Blum, S. S. Shah, R. C. Tasker, & K. M. Wilson (Eds.), *Nelson textbook of pediatrics* (21st ed., pp. 996–1005). Philadelphia, PA: Elsevier.

Jackson, J., Knappen, B., & Olsen, S. L. (2021). Drug withdrawal in the neonate. In S. L. Gardner, B. S. Carter, M. Enzman-Hines, & S. Niermeyer (Eds.), *Merenstein & Gardner's handbook of neonatal intensive care* (9th ed., pp. 250–272). Elsevier.

Jacquot, C., Mo, Y. D., & Luban, N. L. C. (2020). Blood component therapy for the neonate. In R. J. Martin, A. A. Fanaroff, & M. C. Walsh (Eds.), *Fanaroff and Martin's neonatal-perinatal medicine: Diseases of the fetus and infant* (11th ed., pp. 1476–1503). Elsevier.

Kamath-Rayne, B. D., Froese, P. A., & Thilo, E. H. (2021). Neonatal hyperbilirubinemia. In S. L. Gardner, B. S. Carter, M. Enzman-Hines, & S. Niermeyer (Eds.), *Merenstein & Gardner's handbook of neonatal intensive care* (9th ed., pp. 662–691). Elsevier.

Kaplan, M., Wong, R. J., Burgis, J. C., Sibley, E., & Stevenson, D. K. (2020). Neonatal jaundice and liver disease. In R. J. Martin, A. A. Fanaroff, & M. C. Walsh (Eds.), *Fanaroff and Martin's neonatal-perinatal medicine: Diseases of the fetus and infant* (11th ed., pp. 1788–1852). Elsevier.

Kliegman, R. M., St. Geme, J. W., Blum, N. J., Shah, S. S., Tasker, R. C., & Wilson, K. M. (2020). Defects in metabolism of amino acids. In R. M. Kliegman, J. W. St. Geme, N. J. Blum, S. S. Shah, R. C. Tasker, & K. M. Wilson (Eds.), *Nelson textbook of pediatrics* (21st ed., pp. 695–739). Elsevier.

Letterio, J., Pateva, I., Petrosiute, A., & Ahuja, S. (2020). Hematologic and oncologic problems in the fetus and neonate. In R. J. Martin, A. A. Fanaroff, & M. C. Walsh (Eds.), *Fanaroff and Martin's neonatal-perinatal medicine: Diseases of the fetus and infant* (11th ed., pp. 1416–1475). Elsevier.

Marcdante, K. J., & Kliegman, R. M. (2019). Anemia and hyperbilirubinemia. In K. J. Marcdante, & R. M. Kliegman (Eds.), *Nelson Essentials of Pediatrics* (8th ed., pp. 247–254). Elsevier.

Mitchell, A. L. (2020). Congenital anomalies. In R. J. Martin, A. A. Fanaroff, & M. C. Walsh (Eds.), *Fanaroff and Martin's neonatal-perinatal medicine: Diseases of the fetus and infant* (11th ed., pp. 489–513). Elsevier.

Moore, T. R., Hauguel-DeMouzon, S., & Catalano, P. (2019). Diabetes in pregnancy. In R. Resnik, C. J. Lockwood, T. Moore, M. F. Greene, J. A. Copel & R. M. Silver (Eds.), *Creasy & Resnick's maternal-fetal medicine: Principles and practice.* (8th ed., pp. 1067–1097). Elsevier.

Nyp, M., Brunkhorst, J. L., Reavey, D., & Pallotto, E. K. (2021). Fluid and electrolyte management. In S. L. Gardner, B. S. Carter, M. Enzman-Hines, & S. Niermeyer (Eds.), *Merenstein & Gardner's handbook of neonatal intensive care* (9th ed., pp. 407–430). Elsevier.

Pammi, N., Brand, M. C., & Weisman, L. E. (2021). Infection in the neonate. In S. L. Gardner, B. S. Carter, M. Enzman-Hines, & S. Niermeyer (Eds.), *Merenstein & Gardner's handbook of neonatal intensive care* (9th ed., pp. 692–728). Elsevier.

Ramasethu, J. (2020). Exchange transfusions. In J. Ramasethu, & S. Seo (Eds.), *MacDonald's atlas of procedures in neonatology* (6th ed., pp. 383–393). Lippincott, Williams, & Wilkins.

Rosene-Montella, K. (2020). Common medical problems in pregnancy. In L. Goldman, & A. I. Schafer (Eds.), *Goldman-Cecil medicine* (26th ed., pp. 1575–1588). Elsevier.

Rozance, P. J., McGowan, J. E., Price-Douglas, W., & Hay, W. W., Jr. (2021). Glucose homeostasis. In S. L. Gardner, B. S. Carter, M. Enzman-Hines, & S. Niermeyer (Eds.), *Merenstein & Gardner's handbook of neonatal intensive care* (9th ed., pp. 431–458). Elsevier.

Rudd, K. M. (2021). Infectious diseases in the neonate. In M. T. Verklan, M. Walden, & S. Forest (Eds.), *Core curriculum for neonatal intensive care nursing* (6th ed., pp. 588–616). Elsevier.

Sheanon, M. N., & Muglia, L. J. (2020). The endocrine system. In R. M. Kliegman, J. W. St. Geme, N. J. Blum, S. S. Shah, R. C. Tasker, & K. M. Wilson (Eds.), *Nelson textbook of pediatrics* (21st ed., pp. 982–985). Elsevier.

Srinivasan, L., & Evans, J. R. (2018). Health-care associated infections. In C. A. Gleason, & S. E. Juul (Eds.), *Avery's diseases of the newborn* (10th ed., pp. 566–580). Elsevier.

Taylor, J. A., Wright, J. A., & Woodrum, D. (2018). Newborn nursery care. In C. A. Gleason, & S. E. Juul (Eds.), *Avery's diseases of the newborn* (10th ed., pp. 312–331). Elsevier.

Weiner, G. M. (Ed.). (2021). *Textbook of neonatal resuscitation* (8th ed.). American Academy of Pediatrics and American Heart Association.

26

Family Planning

Susan A. Angelicola

OBJECTIVES

After studying this chapter, you should be able to:

1. Discuss the nurse's role in contraceptive counseling and education.
2. Explain factors a couple should consider when choosing a method of contraception.
3. Explain the mechanism of action, advantages, disadvantages, side effects, and teaching needed for methods of family planning.
4. Explain why informed consent is important for contraception.
5. Compare and contrast contraceptive needs at both ends of the reproductive spectrum, in adolescence and perimenopause.

Family planning involves choosing if and when to become pregnant. It includes **contraception**—the prevention of pregnancy—as well as methods to achieve pregnancy. Thinking about goals for having or not having children and how to achieve those goals is important for all clients of childbearing age. Nurses should ask about such goals at each patient encounter and tailor conversations about contraception specific to these goals and desires. Each encounter is a valuable opportunity for this conversation. This chapter focuses on techniques used to avoid pregnancy. Chapter 27 describes methods used by couples having difficulty attaining pregnancy.

If both partners are fertile, approximately 85% will become pregnant over the course of a year without using contraception (Trussell & Aiken, 2018). Therefore, those who wish to avoid or control the timing of pregnancies should practice effective contraception.

Approximately 43 million women in the United States are fertile and sexually active and do not currently desire a pregnancy. Of those women, 70% are practicing contraception (Alan Guttmacher Institute [AGI], 2020). However, they may not be using contraception consistently.

Unintended pregnancies are those that are unwanted or are mistimed, occurring in clients who may wish to become pregnant at a time in the future but not at the time their pregnancies occur. The ability to delay and space childbearing is crucial to clients' social and economic advancement. A client's ability to obtain and effectively use contraceptives has a positive impact on their education and workforce participation, as well as on subsequent outcomes related to income, family stability, mental health and happiness, and children's well-being (Sonfield et al., 2013).

In the United States in 2013, 43% of pregnancies were unintended (U.S. Department of Health and Human Services [DHHS], 2020). Although this is an improvement from the previous 51%, it is still much higher than most industrialized nations. This rate remains the same in 2021. A *Healthy People 2030* goal is to decrease the number of unintended pregnancies to 36.5% (DHHS, 2020).

Because contraceptive methods available are most often the responsibility of the female client, the woman often chooses the type of contraception used. During a client's reproductive lifetime, the needs for contraception evolve. Most clients use a variety of methods before they reach menopause. Because the average woman in the United States bears only two children, she must make contraceptive decisions for more than 30 years. Many of those years occur after she has completed childbearing and is highly motivated to avoid further pregnancy.

INFORMATION ABOUT CONTRACEPTION

Common Sources

Clients often obtain information about contraception from friends, relatives, the internet, social media, blogs, television, and magazines. They seek answers to practical questions about side effects, effectiveness, comfort, and partners' responses.

The information they receive, however, is often incomplete or incorrect when their source is not a qualified health care professional. Clients frequently turn to nurses in outpatient ambulatory office settings, birth settings, and even social settings for accurate information about family planning.

Role of the Nurse

The nurse's role in family planning is that of caregiver, counselor, educator, and even health care provider. To fulfill this role, nurses need current, correct information about contraceptive methods and should share this information with clients who seek their advice.

Unintended pregnancies may occur less often if clients had adequate ongoing education and reevaluation regarding their chosen method. The initial teaching that accompanies selection of the contraceptive technique may be insufficient to meet the client's needs. Reinforcing teaching and providing an opportunity to ask questions after initial use can help ensure that the client is using the method correctly and is satisfied with the method. A client is more likely to use contraception if they have received counseling directed toward their own needs instead of general information about contraception. Therefore, the nurse should provide individualized family planning information to clients in every situation in which it would be appropriate.

Nurses should feel comfortable discussing contraception and be sensitive to the client's concerns, feelings, and culture. When discussing family planning, the client's preferences take priority. Care should be taken that nurses do not introduce their own biases toward or against specific methods. The focus of counseling should be tailored to the reproductive life plan goals of the client and partner (Fig. 26.1).

Counseling about contraception should include the following:

- Types of contraception available, both reversible and permanent
- Risks and benefits of each and determination of which methods may not be safe or effective based on health status or concurrent medication use

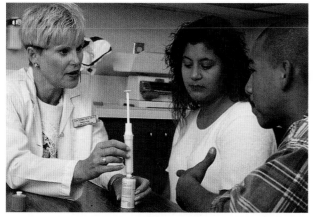

FIG. 26.1 Success of contraception is more likely when both the client and the partner are involved in discussions. The nurse demonstrates filling a foam applicator.

- How to ensure proper use of each method to maximize effectiveness
- What to do if an error is made
- Emergency contraception (EC)—specifically access and instruction
- Backup methods and when they should be used
- What to do if the client wishes to change methods
- Questions and concerns

CONSIDERATIONS WHEN CHOOSING A CONTRACEPTIVE METHOD

The perfect contraceptive method does not exist. Each has advantages and disadvantages (Table 26.1). Clients change contraceptive methods as circumstances in their lives change and in response to dissatisfaction with side effects or other traits of their current contraceptive (Table 26.2). Clients often try several methods before finding a satisfactory one. Some clients have an interval of using no contraception before beginning a new method, even though they do not wish to become pregnant.

Of clients who practice contraception, 72% currently use reversible methods, primarily oral contraceptives (OCs), the patch, the injectable, and the vaginal ring, long-acting reversible contraceptives (LARC) such as an intrauterine device (IUD) or the implant, and condoms (Kavanaugh & Jerman, 2018). The most popular methods of contraception in the United States since 1982 are OCs and female sterilization (Daniels & Abma, 2018). However, the most popular methods are often not right for every client. Nurses can help clients weigh the factors involved in choosing a family planning method. Careful consideration of all factors can help a client choose the safest method that best meets current needs.

Safety

The safety of a contraceptive method is a primary consideration and is unique to each client's health status. Chronic medical conditions or social practices such as tobacco use may make certain methods unsafe. For example, combined oral contraceptives should not be used by clients who have had a thromboembolic event such as deep vein thrombosis or stroke, because estrogen increases the risk for recurrence and associated morbidity and mortality. It is imperative for nurses who provide contraceptive counseling to be well versed in the Centers for Disease Control and Prevention's (CDC; 2016a) *US Medical Eligibility Criteria for Contraceptive Use* (US MEC) and *US Selected Practice Recommendations for Contraceptive Use* (US SPR), most recently published in July 2016; however, it is important to understand the potential risk associated with use of contraceptives, even hormonal contraception, is generally safer than the risk of pregnancy.

Protection from Sexually Transmitted Infections

No contraceptive (other than abstinence practiced perfectly) is 100% effective in preventing sexually transmitted infections (STIs). The risk for exposure to STIs should be discussed

TABLE 26.1 Advantages and Disadvantages of the Most Common Contraceptive Methods

Method	Advantages	Disadvantages
Sterilization	• Ends concern about contraception. • Tubal sterilization performed during or right after childbirth or between pregnancies. • Vasectomy performed in physician's office with local anesthesia. • Low long-term cost.	• No protection against STIs. • Reversal is difficult and expensive, and it may be unsuccessful. • Potential complications as in any surgery. • Vasectomy requires another contraceptive method until semen is free of sperm.
Intrauterine device or intrauterine system	• Unrelated to coitus. • In place at all times. • Low long-term cost. • Effective for 3–10 years. • Decreases dysmenorrhea and menstrual blood loss. • Some clients become amenorrheic. • Copper IUD may also be used for EC.	• No protection against STIs. Can be expelled. • Potential side effects or complications: change in bleeding patterns including menorrhagia, infection near time of insertion, ectopic pregnancy, spontaneous abortion if pregnancy occurs, perforation.
Progestin implant	• Unrelated to coitus. • Provides 3-year protection. • Safe during lactation. • Body weight has no effect.	• No protection against STIs. • Major side effect is irregular bleeding.
Progestin injections (Depo-Provera)	• Unrelated to coitus. • Avoids need for daily use. • May cause amenorrhea with continued use. • Requires use only every 12 weeks.	• No protection against STIs. • Must remember to repeat every 12 weeks. • Causes temporary decrease in bone density. • Effect on peak bone mass and osteoporosis unknown. • Side effects similar to those of other progestin contraceptives.
Oral contraceptives	• Taken at a time unrelated to coitus. (See Table 26.4.)	• No protection against STIs. • Must be taken daily at or near same time. • May cause side effects and complications. (See Table 26.4.)
Emergency contraception	• Helps prevent pregnancy after unprotected coitus or birth control failure. • Most available without prescription	• No protection against STIs. • Ideally must be taken within 3 days of unprotected intercourse. • May cause nausea.
Transdermal contraceptive patch	• Unrelated to coitus. • Requires only weekly application. • Regulates menstrual cycles.	• No protection against STIs. • Must apply on the right day. • May be less effective for clients over 90 kg (198 lb). • May cause skin irritation. • Other side effects similar to those of OCs. • Higher risk for VTE.
Vaginal contraceptive ring	• Unrelated to coitus. • In place for 3 weeks at a time. • No fitting required.	• No protection against STIs. • Must remember when to remove and when to insert. • Side effects include headache, expulsion, vaginitis, vaginal discomfort or discharge, and others similar to those of OCs.
Barrier All methods	• Avoid use of systemic hormones. • Offer some protection against STIs.	• Most coitus-related (must be used just before coitus). • May interfere with sensation. • Contraindicated for allergies to components of spermicide or latex.
Chemical (spermicide)	• Quick and easy. • No prescription needed. • Inexpensive per single use. • Provides lubrication.	• Films and suppositories must melt to be effective. • Effective time less than 1 hour. • No douching for 6 hours. • May be messy. • May cause irritation. • New application needed for repeated intercourse.

TABLE 26.1 Advantages and Disadvantages of the Most Common Contraceptive Methods—cont'd

Method	Advantages	Disadvantages
Condom	• Quick and easy. • No prescription needed. • Best protection available for STIs. • Low cost per single use. • Can be carried discreetly. • Vaginal condoms increase client's control over contraceptive use and protection from STIs.	• Interferes with spontaneity. • Must be checked for expiration date and holes. • Can break or slip off. • Can be used only once. • Female condoms may seem unattractive or cumbersome.
Sponge	• Available over the counter. • Can be inserted several hours before coitus. • Effective for repeated intercourse. • No prescription needed.	• No protection against STIs. • Must remain in place for 6 hours but no more than 30 hours total. • May cause irritation. • Risk for toxic shock syndrome if used too long or during menstruation.
Diaphragm	• Can be inserted several hours before coitus. • Provides some protection from STIs. • Can remain in place up to 24 hours.	• Requires education on proper use. • May be difficult to insert or remove for some clients • Added spermicide necessary for repeat coitus. • Possibility of toxic shock syndrome with prolonged use or use during menses. • Bladder infection may occur. • Must remain in place at least 6 hours after coitus.
Cervical cap	• Smaller than diaphragm and may fit clients who cannot use a diaphragm. • No pressure against bladder. • Less noticeable and requires less spermicide than diaphragm. • Provides some protection from STIs. • Can remain in place 48 hours.	• Initially expensive. • Requires health care provider to fit. • Requires education on proper use. • Added spermicide needed for repeat coitus. • Possibility of toxic shock syndrome. • Must remain in place at least 6 hours after coitus.
Natural Family Planning		
All methods	• Inexpensive. • No drugs or hormones. • Help client learn about the body. • Can be combined with barrier methods to increase effectiveness. • Acceptable in most religions. • May be used to help achieve pregnancy.	• No protection from STIs. • Requires high motivation and extensive education. • Abstinence necessary for large part of each cycle. • High risk for pregnancy from error. • Many factors may change ovulation time.

EC, Emergency contraception; *IUD,* intrauterine device; *OCs,* oral contraceptives; *STI,* sexually transmitted infection.

when counseling clients about contraceptive choices. The male condom is inexpensive and offers the best protection available. It should be used whenever there is a risk for STI exposure, when a woman engages in high-risk sexual behaviors, or if one partner may have an STI, and even when another form of contraception is practiced or during pregnancy.

Effectiveness

The importance of avoiding pregnancy must be considered when choosing a contraceptive method. A client may wish to delay pregnancy for a time but would accept if pregnancy occurs earlier. Other clients may be extremely upset about an unintended pregnancy.

How well the method prevents pregnancy includes efficacy and effectiveness:

1. The ideal, perfect, or efficacy rate refers to *perfect, consistent* use of the method with every act of intercourse. Failures are caused by a problem with the method itself rather than with the use of the method.

2. The typical, actual, or user effectiveness rate is most useful because it refers to the occurrence of pregnancy under *typical* use of the method. Failure is presumably the result of incorrect or inconsistent use of the technique.

The difference between the two rates shows how forgiving a method is—that is, how likely pregnancy is to occur if the use is occasionally imperfect. For example, in 100 women using combined hormonal contraceptives (COCs) in 1 year, perfect use results in 0.3 pregnancies but typical use results in 9 pregnancies. The typical failure rate is more meaningful when counseling women and their partners (Table 26.3). When comparing different methods, the same method of analysis should be used.

Effectiveness is highly correlated to accuracy of use. It drops greatly when the user does not understand how

TABLE 26.2   Percentage of Clients Continuing Use at 1 Year

Method	Clients Who Continue Use at 1 Year (%)
Implant	89
Intrauterine devices	
Mirena	80
Copper T 380A (ParaGard)	78
Depo-Provera	56
Oral contraceptives	67
Contraceptive patch	67
Vaginal ring	67
Condoms	
Male	43
Female	41
Diaphragm	57
Sponge	36
Spermicides, gel, foam, films, suppositories (used alone)	42
Natural family planning (all types)	47
Withdrawal	46

Data from Trussell, J., Aiken, A. R. (2018). Contraceptive Efficacy. In R. A. Hatcher, A. L. Nelson, & J. Trussell, C. Cwiak, P. Cason, M. S. Policar, A. Edelman, A. R. A. Aiken, J. Marrazzo, & D. Kowal (Eds.), *Contraceptive technology* (21st ed., p.844). Ardent Media.

to use the method or when an error is made. The failure rate commonly decreases after the first year of use as experience with the method leads to more accurate use. Combining two less reliable methods, for example, a condom and a spermicide, increases effectiveness. LARCs, including IUDs and the contraceptive implant, are the most effective reversible methods and do not require intervention by a client or the partner to be effective (American College of Obstetricians and Gynecologists [ACOG], 2021b).

Acceptability

The effectiveness of a method should be balanced against its acceptability to the couple. For example, permanent sterilization is an extremely effective method but is unacceptable to couples planning to have children or expand their family at a later time. Concern or experienced side effects or religious/cultural objections may influence the choice for less effective methods. A client or the partner may be concerned about using certain contraceptives because of perceived or feared side effects such as weight gain.

A chemical contraceptive such as a spermicide or the sponge may be "messy" and unacceptable or may cause vaginal irritation. Clients of any age who are not comfortable touching their bodies, specifically genitalia, may be unlikely

TABLE 26.3   Percentage of Clients Experiencing an Unintended Pregnancy During the First Year of Typical Use of Contraception

Method	Pregnancies during First Year of Typical Use (%)
Sterilization	
Male	0.15
Female	0.5
Contraceptive implant (Nexplanon)	0.1
Intrauterine devices	
Copper T 380A (ParaGard)	0.8
Skyla	0.4
Kyleena	0.2
Liletta	0.1
Mirena	0.1
Depo-Provera	4
Transdermal contraceptive patch	7
Vaginal contraceptive ring	7
Oral contraceptives	7
Condoms	
Male	13
Female	21
Diaphragm with spermicide	17
Sponge	
Nulliparous women	14
Parous women	27
Natural family planning (all types)	23
Coitus interruptus (withdrawal)	20
Spermicides, gel, foam, films, suppositories (used alone)	21
No contraceptive use	85

Data from Trussell, J., Aiken, A. R. (2018). Contraceptive Efficacy. In R. A. Hatcher, A. L. Nelson, & J. Trussell, C. Cwiak, P. Cason, M. S. Policar, A. Edelman, A. R. A. Aiken, J. Marrazzo, & D. Kowal (Eds.), *Contraceptive technology* (21st ed., p.844). Ardent Media.

to accept methods that involve inserting a device into the vagina or assessing the cervical mucus.

Convenience

Convenience is another important factor in choosing a contraceptive method. If the client perceives the contraceptive as difficult to obtain or use, time consuming, or too much "bother," it is less likely to be used consistently even if the level of motivation to avoid pregnancy is very high. The education received about the method may affect perception of its convenience. Clients who are knowledgeable about their family planning method are less likely to think the contraceptive is difficult to use.

Methods used weekly, monthly, or over many years, instead of daily or with each act of intercourse are more convenient and likely to lead to better compliance. Potential inconveniences include breakthrough bleeding (spotting between periods) common with some methods or needing to visit the health care provider's office for a prescription or injection.

The desire to avoid monthly menstruation also should be considered. Some clients prefer extended cycles with several months between menses or to avoid menstrual periods altogether. Extended or continuous use of OCs, the patch, and the ring may be used to achieve this goal. Further, the hormone implant or injection, or IUDs may also lead to *amenorrhea* (absence of menstruation) in some clients. Other clients may prefer to have a monthly period so they feel reassured of not being pregnant.

Education Needed

Clients may fail to use contraception because they do not understand their risk for pregnancy. They also may not be familiar with the variety of methods available or the risks and benefits of the different types. Some methods such as condoms involve very little education, whereas others require more guidance. Clients using natural family planning methods need extensive education about body changes that indicate ovulation to practice these methods successfully.

Benefits

Some methods have special benefits that should be discussed. For example, OCs have many noncontraceptive benefits such as reduction in acne, decreased bleeding during periods, and decreased menstrual cramps, as well as reduction in risk for ovarian and uterine cancer. Natural family planning methods, barrier methods, and the copper IUD offer freedom from exposure to hormones. Condoms provide better protection against bacterial sexually transmitted infections (STIs) such as chlamydia and viral STIs such as HIV compared with other contraceptives.

Side Effects

Some methods of contraception have bothersome side effects that should be explained clearly in advance and when educating clients about the advantages and disadvantages of each method. When clients know what to expect, they often are more willing to tolerate the side effects and continue using the method, especially if they know common side effects do not pose a health risk or a decrease effectiveness.

Effect on Spontaneity

Contraceptive methods related to **coitus** (sexual intercourse) such as chemical or mechanical barrier methods, withdrawal, and periodic abstinence must be used just before or during sexual intercourse. They require skill and motivation and may be more likely to be used inconsistently or incorrectly. The fact these methods must be readily available and interrupt sexual activity increases the chance they will not be consistently used. Some couples remedy this problem by including application of the contraceptive device such as a condom as a part of foreplay. Others prefer methods such as OCs or LARCs that do not interrupt sexual activity.

Availability

Condoms and spermicides are readily available without prescriptions. They can be purchased anonymously at any time without a visit to a health care provider. This may be important to an adolescent who wants to hide their sexual activity or to clients who are embarrassed to discuss contraception with a health care provider.

Expense

The cost of family planning methods is important. Less effective contraceptives may be chosen by some couples to save money. These methods may be less expensive but also have higher failure rates.

The "per use" cost of methods can be compared with long-term expense. The price of condoms or spermicides is relatively low, but frequent use makes them expensive over a period of years. Couples may find them economical for occasional sexual intercourse or until they can access a more expensive method. Methods requiring periodic visits to a health care provider are potentially more costly than over-the-counter methods. However, the visits provide an opportunity for teaching and may enhance the effectiveness of the contraceptive. Such visits also provide an opportunity for health screening and discussion of other health concerns. LARC methods are very cost effective over a 3- to 10-year period because their failure rate is so low.

Publicly funded family planning clinics may provide free or low-cost contraceptives, as well as access to counseling about all contraceptive methods and follow-up services. However, clients who attend these clinics may have a long wait for appointment access and may see a different health care provider at each visit which can affect continuity of care. Family planning is covered by many state Medicaid programs and most insurance companies. As of September 2017, the Patient Protection and Affordable Care Act designates a list of preventive services that must be covered without out-of-pocket costs to the consumer. Those services include provision of all contraceptive methods approved by the U.S. Food and Drug Administration (FDA), along with sterilization procedures and contraceptive counseling to all women (Health Resources and Services Administration, 2022).

Preference

The client usually makes the final decision about their contraceptive method, and satisfaction with the choice is crucial. Consistent use of any method depends on whether it meets the needs of the client and their partner. If the client feels pressured to choose a certain method or if the chosen method fails to live up to their expectations, use is more likely to be inconsistent. The opinion of the client's partner, friends, or family members also may influence the choice of method.

Religious and Personal Beliefs

Religious or other personal beliefs affect the choice of contraceptives. Certain religions may not believe in the use of any contraceptives other than natural family planning.

Culture

Culture may influence the method chosen. Some cultures place a high value on large families and especially on male children. A female client may have more pregnancies than she might otherwise desire in an effort to have sons. Asian and Hispanic clients are often very modest and may not talk about sexuality with others. Clients of all cultures need to feel very comfortable with the nurse before talking about sexuality or contraception. Taking time to establish rapport and trust before discussing intimate or sensitive subjects is paramount.

Some cultures and religions restrict a client's activities during menstruation. Methods that cause increased bleeding or breakthrough bleeding as a side effect may not be acceptable to such women. If there is a cultural taboo against a female client touching the genital area, sponges, diaphragms, spermicides, the female condom, or the contraceptive ring would not be acceptable.

Other Considerations

Clients also consider factors other than those discussed previously when choosing a contraceptive. The length of time before a pregnancy is desired will determine whether a long-acting contraceptive is appropriate. The breastfeeding client must choose a method that will not reduce milk production or supply. The client at risk for acquiring or transmitting a STI should use condoms either alone or with another more effective method of preventing pregnancy.

Clients experiencing intimate partner violence are at an increased risk for reproductive coercion and potentially unintended pregnancy (Kusunoki & Barber, 2019). In addition, clients who have experienced pressured sex may avoid pelvic examinations, which may limit access to some contraceptives (Holt et al., 2020).

Informed Consent

Some methods have potentially dangerous adverse events. Every client should receive information about the chosen contraceptive method and its proper use, safety, its risks and benefits, and alternative methods available. The nurse should thoroughly document the client received and understands this information. Some methods requiring procedural intervention such as permanent sterilization and LARC method insertions require written consent.

KNOWLEDGE CHECK

1. Why does the female client usually choose the method of contraception a couple uses?
2. What is the role of the nurse in assisting clients with contraceptive decision making and use?
3. What are some important considerations in choosing a contraceptive method?
4. Which contraceptive methods require that the client sign an informed consent form?

ADOLESCENTS AND CONTRACEPTION

Among high school students in 2019, 38% had sexual intercourse, 27% had sexual intercourse in the previous 3 months, 46% did not use a condom the last time they had sex, and 12% did not use any method to prevent pregnancy (CDC, 2019). Although the rate of adolescent pregnancies has decreased in recent years, adolescent pregnancy is still a major problem. Because of the serious impact of pregnancy on adolescents, the U.S. *Healthy People 2030* goals include the following (DHHS, 2020):

- Increase the proportion of adolescent females at risk for unintended pregnancy who use most effective or moderately effective methods of contraception overall to 70.1%.
- Increase the proportion of adolescent females at risk of unintended pregnancy who use most effective or moderately effective methods of contraception at last intercourse to 36.8%.

Adolescent Knowledge

Many adolescents have little knowledge about their own anatomy and physiology, including how and when conception occurs. They are likely to learn about contraception from other teenagers, who may pass on incorrect information. Adolescents have higher failure rates and poor rates of continuation with short-acting contraception (ACOG, 2021a).

Misinformation

Misinformation and erroneous beliefs about contraception are common among teens. As a result, adolescents may not seek highly effective contraception such as LARCs. It is the nurse's responsibility to educate teens about safe and available choices and distinguish any misplaced fears or misinformation.

Teenagers may *douche* (insert a solution into the vagina) after intercourse to "wash away the sperm" and prevent pregnancy. However, douching is ineffective because sperm may enter the cervix very soon after ejaculation. **Coitus interruptus** (withdrawal) is used by some teenagers, but it is unreliable. It requires more control over timing of ejaculation than many adolescent boys have; it is important to educate

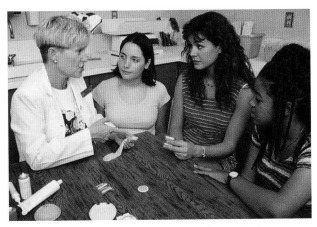

FIG. 26.2 Although many adolescents choose oral contraceptives, the nurse emphasizes the need to use condoms for protection against sexually transmitted infections. Demonstrating with actual contraceptives increases understanding.

adolescents there is a small amount of sperm present in the preejaculate fluid that may result in a pregnancy.

Risk-Taking Behavior

Adolescents often have a feeling of invincibility. They are more likely than adults to take risks in sexual activity because they believe their chances of becoming pregnant are low. They often do not plan intercourse and therefore are not prepared with contraceptives. This behavior may lead to increased exposures to STIs and pregnancy risk.

Some adolescents have ambivalent feelings about becoming pregnant. Although they do not plan to become pregnant, they do not have a firm commitment to avoid pregnancy during their teenage years. Discussing how pregnancy may affect them and their life goals may help determine their true feelings about becoming pregnant.

Counseling Adolescents

Nurses who counsel adolescents about sexuality should be sensitive to their feelings, concerns, needs, and different communication styles (Fig. 26.2). If they have negative feelings about adolescent sexuality, these opinions must be put aside.

For an adolescent to seek information about contraception, they must admit that the client is, and plans to continue to be, sexually active. The client may be afraid to ask about contraception because they do not want anyone to know they are sexually active (such as with the use of a parent's health insurance) or the client fears they will be lectured or judged about their behavior. The client's need for secrecy may cause them to miss appointments for family planning. The nurse should be adept at determining the adolescent's needs and reassure the client's visits are confidential and what is discussed will not be shared with others.

Each contact with the health care system provides an opportunity for counseling. Visits to a health care provider for well checkups, minor illnesses, or pregnancy testing provide such opportunities. If an adolescent thinks they might be pregnant but the pregnancy test result is negative, the client should be asked about their desire to become pregnant. The

client may be particularly interested in pregnancy prevention at that time. The nurse can assess the adolescent's use of contraception and the adequacy of the client's knowledge and can provide information and resources as appropriate.

Although nurses should encourage adolescents to discuss contraception with their parent or another trusted adult, many teenagers will forgo contraception rather than talk to their parents about it. Therefore, they need other reliable sources of information. Schools have helped increase birth control use among adolescents by offering information about family planning and prevention of STIs.

Contraceptive services also are available on some school campuses. School nurses and classroom discussions supply information about abstinence, as well as contraception. Encouragement to delay becoming sexually active and discussion of the effect pregnancy might have and ways to remain abstinent are included. Some family planning clinics are open after school, during evenings, and on weekends and have staff who are especially skilled in working with adolescents.

The pelvic examination, a source of great anxiety for many young clients, is not necessary for a prescription for or provision of most forms of contraception in healthy clients and may be postponed. Adolescents and young clients who forgo speculum or pelvic examinations may be tested for chlamydia and gonorrhea from a urine sample, without an invasive examination. During the first counseling visit, the adolescent should receive information about all appropriate contraceptive methods. Taking this extra time to explain different methods helps dispel misinformation and allays the common concerns of adolescents about potential adverse health effects of contraceptives. It also helps the teenager feel comfortable in the clinic setting and with the nurse.

Because of the client's youth and possible lack of knowledge about anatomy and physiology, the adolescent often needs more extensive teaching than does the older client. Liberal use of audiovisual materials such as pictures, anatomic models, and samples of various methods helps the young adult understand the information more easily. For example, giving the client a patch, a vaginal ring, and a condom to manipulate or showing the client the packet of pills they will be using are important aids.

Using understandable terminology is especially important when teaching adolescents. The nurse should know street terms for body parts and sexual intercourse because they may be the only words that are familiar to the teenager.

Adolescents are most successful when they choose contraceptive methods that are easy to use and seem unrelated to coitus. The most popular contraceptives for adolescents are OCs and condoms (Trussell & Aiken, 2018). Teenagers often choose OCs because they are safe, have few contraindications, seem unrelated to sex, and are not difficult or messy. In addition, they increase bone density, regulate menses, reduce menstrual flow and cramping, and may decrease acne (Cwiak & Edelman, 2018).

Adolescent clients may, however, be quite inconsistent with daily pill ingestion. A method such as a ring used once a month or a patch used once a week may be more useful. Use of LARCs is particularly effective in adolescents and is recommended by the ACOG (2018) as first-line contraception for adolescents.

Teens are more likely than older clients to discontinue any method for side effects such as spotting. Their concerns should be taken seriously, and attempts should be made to alleviate side effects. Otherwise, they are likely to stop using the method, often without notifying their health care provider, with pregnancy a possible result. They should understand all aspects of management of their contraceptive method and when a backup method is necessary.

Adolescents may use condoms alone to prevent pregnancy and STIs, especially at the beginning of a relationship or with casual partners. With long-term partners, they may discontinue condom use and use only hormonal methods. Some may use condoms, with or without hormonal methods, only if they have casual partners or if they are very concerned about both pregnancy and STIs.

Condom use should be encouraged to prevent STIs, even when another contraceptive method is used (see Fig. 26.2). Discussing perceived barriers to using condoms helps dispel misconceptions about pregnancy and STIs. Some young clients may be uneasy about asking their partners to use condoms. Discussing how to negotiate condom use with a partner can be particularly helpful. Teaching should include signs of STIs and what to do if they should occur, in addition to the current CDC recommendation of annual screening for chlamydia and gonorrhea for all sexually active women ages 24 and under. Using condoms and an OC or LARC method provides highly effective contraception along with protection from STIs and should be encouraged.

CONTRACEPTION USE IN PERIMENOPAUSAL CLIENTS

Pregnancy is uncommon after the age of 50 years. However, perimenopausal clients may continue to ovulate as long as they have regular menstrual periods, and some ovulate even when indications of menopause are present. Therefore, contraceptive counseling regarding the continued use of contraception until a client is 12 months past the last period is important for these clients.

Fertility begins to decline when female clients reach 35 to 40 years, but they are still at risk for an unintended pregnancy. In fact, more than 30% of pregnancies in clients over the age 35 years are unintended (Black & Nelson, 2018). Therefore, the nurse should offer contraceptive counseling whenever possible. Permanent sterilization is a very common method used by female clients who are older than 30 years. Healthy, nonsmoking clients in their forties can use COCs (ring, patch) to provide contraception and regulate the irregular bleeding that often accompanies perimenopause. Clients who smoke and are over the age of 35 years should not use estrogen-containing contraceptives (CDC, 2016b). Barrier methods, progestin-only contraception such as the contraceptive injection, progestin-only OCs, or LARC methods are safe choices for the perimenopausal clients who may smoke or

have other health conditions that make other methods potentially unsafe.

Perimenopausal clients should have regular physical examinations to identify any conditions or change in health status that would necessitate a change of contraceptive method.

KNOWLEDGE CHECK

5. What are some erroneous beliefs about contraception commonly held by adolescents?
6. Why might teenagers be hesitant to seek contraceptive information?
7. How can the nurse increase effectiveness in teaching adolescents about contraception?
8. What considerations are necessary in contraception for perimenopausal clients?

METHODS OF CONTRACEPTION

Permanent Contraception

Sterilization, both male and female, provides nonreversible, permanent contraception and is the most commonly used method of contraception in the United States (Hou & Roncari, 2018). Couples considering sterilization need counseling to ensure they understand all aspects of the procedure and its permanence. When this procedure is planned immediately after childbirth, the decision should be made well before labor begins and ideally during the third trimester of pregnancy. Future marriage, divorce, or death of a child may cause couples to regret their decision.

Complications of sterilization are similar to those of any surgery, such as hemorrhage, infection, and anesthesia complications. Although pregnancy is rare after sterilization, the risk for failure should be discussed. Pregnancies occurring after tubal sterilization are more likely to be ectopic.

Tubal Sterilization

Fallopian tube surgery/tubal sterilization is widely used throughout the world. The procedure involves cutting, occluding, or removing the fallopian tubes to prevent fertilization and can be performed at any time. Many couples choose surgical tubal sterilization at the time of a cesarean birth or before hospital discharge after a vaginal birth. The first 48 hours after vaginal birth is an optimal time for the surgery because the fundus is located near the umbilicus and the fallopian tubes are directly below the abdominal wall. When performed after childbirth, regional (spinal or epidural) anesthesia is most commonly used. Interval fallopian tube surgery, not associated with childbirth, is generally performed as outpatient surgery under general anesthesia.

Interval sterilization is usually performed in one of three ways. A mini-laparotomy incision may be made near the umbilicus in the postpartum period or just above the symphysis pubis at other times. Surgery also can be performed through a laparoscope inserted via a small incision. The third method is performed during other surgery, generally with cesarean birth. With each method, the surgeon blocks the tubes with clips, bands, or rings and removes the fallopian tubes or uses electrocoagulation to destroy a portion of the tubes. If portions of the tubes are removed, they are sent for pathologic examination to ensure the tissues are actually fallopian tubes. Surgical tubal ligation is approximately 99.5% effective (Hou & Roncari, 2018).

After sterilization, the client avoids intercourse, strenuous exercise, or lifting heavy objects for 1 week. Mild analgesics may be needed for pain. The client should call a health care provider if there is a fever over 38°C (100.4°F), fainting, severe pain, or bleeding or discharge from the incision sites (Hou & Roncari, 2018).

Vasectomy

Vas surgery/vasectomy, male sterilization, involves making a small incision or puncture in the scrotum to cut, tie, cauterize, or remove a section of the vas deferens, which carries sperm from the testes to the penis. After vasectomy, sperm no longer pass into the semen.

Although performed less frequently than female sterilization, vasectomy is a very popular method of contraception. It involves a lower morbidity rate and has a lower failure rate compared with tubal sterilization. Because it can be performed in a physician's office using a local anesthetic, it may be less expensive as well. Vasectomy is approximately 99.9% effective.

After surgery the man rests and then wears a scrotal support for 48 hours. He applies ice to the area for 4 hours and takes a mild analgesic, if needed. He should avoid bathing for 24 hours. Strenuous activity should be avoided for 1 week. The health care provider should be notified of fever, severe pain, bleeding or discharge at the site, swelling greater than twice the normal size, or a painful nodule (Hou & Roncari, 2018).

Ejaculation may be resumed in 1 week, but the man is not sterile at that time (Hou & Roncari, 2018). Sperm may be present in the ductal system, distal to the ligation of the vas deferens, and the man may be able to impregnate a woman until sperm are no longer present in the semen. The couple should understand that complete sterilization may not occur for 3 months or more. The man should submit a semen specimen for analysis at 8 to 16 weeks to be sure that sperm are no longer present.

Long-Acting Reversible Contraceptives
Intrauterine Devices

Intrauterine devices are long-acting contraceptives inserted into the uterus to provide continuous pregnancy prevention. The Copper T 380A (ParaGard) and the levonorgestrel intrauterine systems (LNG-IUS, or Mirena, Kyleena, Skyla, and Liletta) are all shaped like the letter "T" (Fig. 26.3). ParaGard is effective for 10 years, Mirena is effective for 7 years, Liletta is effective for 6 years, Kyleena is effective for 5 years, and Skyla is effective for 3 years. IUDs are more effective than any other contraceptive method except Nexplanon and male sterilization.

IUDs can be inserted at any time the client is not pregnant and does not have an active STI, such as chlamydia or gonorrhea, or pelvic infection. Insertion immediately after

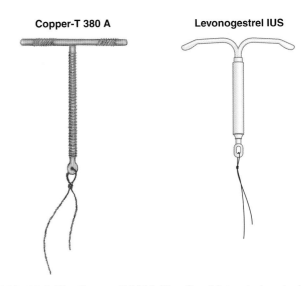

FIG. 26.3 The Copper T 380A (ParaGard) intrauterine device (IUD) and the levonorgestrel intrauterine system (LNG-IUS or Mirena). Currently, IUDs are considered a very safe method for preventing pregnancy.

childbirth and delivery of the placenta is considered safe but does confer a higher risk of expulsion (Eggebroten, 2017). Insertion during lactation is considered safe but has a higher risk of uterine perforation (Dean & Schwarz, 2018). ParaGard is effective immediately, and no backup is required. If Mirena, Kyleena, Skyla, or Liletta are inserted within 5 days of the start of the last menses, no backup contraceptive is needed. If it is inserted later, a backup contraceptive should be used for 7 days (CDC, 2016b). Fertility returns promptly when the device is removed. ACOG recommends increased usage of IUDs in women of all ages and regardless of previous pregnancy history because they provide long-term, cost-effective contraception lowering the risk for unintended pregnancy (ACOG, 2021b). A large proportion of clients have free or low-cost access to IUDs because of the Affordable Care Act.

IUDs are growing in popularity, but some clients, and those from whom they receive advice, still may be concerned about the safety of using an IUD. Although safety was a concern with very different, early models in the 1970s, IUDs are considered extremely safe at this time. IUDs are convenient long-term, highly effective continuous contraceptive methods and eliminate the need to take pills, have injections, or perform other tasks on a daily basis or just before intercourse. IUDs can be safely used by some clients who cannot use estrogen-containing hormonal contraception.

Action. All IUDs create a sterile inflammatory response in the uterus that results in a spermicidal intrauterine environment. They do *not* cause abortion (Dean & Schwarz, 2018). Levonorgestrel, a progestin, is continuously released from the LNG-IUS devices (Mirena, Kyleena, Skyla, and Liletta), which also thickens cervical mucus and prevents transport of sperm into the endometrial cavity and fallopian tubes. Only a small amount of progestin is absorbed systemically, leading to lower blood levels than those in users of other progestin-containing contraceptives.

The copper-covered ParaGard produces a spermicidal intrauterine environment by the release of copper ions into the uterus. This makes the uterus inhospitable to sperm transport and viability.

Side Effects. Side effects include cramping and irregular bleeding after insertion. *Menorrhagia* (increased bleeding during menstruation) and *dysmenorrhea* (painful menstruation) are common side effects of the copper-containing IUD. Irregular bleeding or spotting may occur with any IUD in the early months and amenorrhea is more common with the LNG-IUS devices. The Mirena LNG-IUS may be used in clients who had menorrhagia before using an IUD as a nonsurgical way to manage heavy menstrual bleeding. If used for this indication, the device is effective for 5 years. Ibuprofen or another nonsteroidal antiinflammatory drugs may reduce bleeding and cramping. Some clients may require iron supplementation to treat anemia related to the heavy menses associated with ParaGard.

Complications include perforation of the uterus at the time of insertion, 1%, as well as expulsion, which occurs in 1% to 5% of users (Dean & Schwarz, 2018). Although the rate of ectopic pregnancies in IUD users is much less than that in clients not using contraceptives, pregnancies that do occur are more likely to be ectopic or result in spontaneous abortion or preterm birth. Clients with recent or recurrent pelvic infections, a history of ectopic pregnancy, bleeding disorders, or structural abnormalities of the uterus may not be safe or appropriate IUD candidates.

There is a small risk for infection from contamination at the time of insertion, and this can be mediated by strict sterile technique during insertion. The IUD should not be inserted if a client has mucopurulent cervical discharge (that is suspicious for STI) or a known current infection such as chlamydia, gonorrhea, or pelvic inflammatory disease.

Teaching. Teaching the client about side effects and what to expect in terms of potential change in bleeding patterns is very important. It is also an option for a client to check for the presence of the plastic IUD threads or strings protruding from the cervix. Expulsion, though uncommon, may occur during menses, especially a heavy menses. If unable to feel the strings of the IUD, a visit to the health care provider can determine if the device remains safely in place. Signs and symptoms of infection such as moderate to severe pelvic or vaginal pain, foul-smelling discharge, or fever should prompt a call to the health care provider. Any signs of pregnancy should be reported to rule out ectopic pregnancy or spontaneous abortion. If a pregnancy occurs with the IUD in situ, the location of the pregnancy should be determined (intrauterine or ectopic), and the IUD should be promptly removed (Dean & Schwarz, 2018).

❓ KNOWLEDGE CHECK

9. What information is important for couples choosing sterilization to understand?
10. What education is important for clients choosing an IUD?

Contraceptive Implant

The contraceptive implant Nexplanon is a single rod implant that is inserted subcutaneously into the upper inner arm with the use of a local anesthetic. It is 2-mm thick and 4-cm (1.6 in) long and releases progestin continuously to provide 3 years of contraception. It acts to inhibit ovulation, thickens cervical mucus to prevent sperm penetrability, and thins out the endometrium making it unfavorable for implantation. As with IUDs, increased use of the contraceptive implant is recommended by ACOG as a means of offering highly effective, long-acting, reversible contraception (ACOG, 2021b). Implants can be inserted at any time of the menstrual cycle, including immediately postpartum.

Side effects of the contraceptive implant include irregular menstrual bleeding, as with other progestin-only contraceptives, acne, and minimal weight gain. Bleeding is expected and not a sign of abnormality, but irregular bleeding is the most common reason for discontinuation of this method. Amenorrhea may occur with longer use. Fertility returns immediately, and pregnancy can occur at normal rates when the implant is removed (Nelson et al., 2018). The implant is often an appealing method for clients who desire long-acting contraceptives but who may fear the potential discomfort related to an IUD insertion.

Hormone Injections

Depo-Provera (medroxyprogesterone acetate [DMPA]) is an injectable progestin available in intramuscular (IM) and subcutaneous (SubQ) forms. It prevents ovulation for 15 weeks, although injections should be scheduled every 13 weeks (CDC, 2016b). It is convenient and contains no estrogen. The action and side effects are similar to those of other progestin contraceptives; however, weight gain occurs more commonly, and clients should be informed of this potential.

The IM form of Depo-Provera is given by deep IM injection. The SubQ form is given in the anterior thigh or abdomen; although not FDA approved, clients have the option to self-administer the SubQ form. The site should not be massaged after injection because massage accelerates absorption and decreases the period of effectiveness. No backup method of contraception is necessary after the first injection if it is given within 7 days of the beginning of a menstrual period. A backup method of contraception is used for 7 days if the first injection is given at another time or if the client is more than 2 weeks late returning for a subsequent injection (CDC, 2016b). It also can be given on the day it is prescribed if it is certain the client is not pregnant and they will use backup for the first week.

Menstrual irregularities are the major reason for discontinuation, and clients should be informed about this before beginning the method. Although spotting and breakthrough bleeding are common, amenorrhea occurs at 40% to 50% at 1 year and 80% at 5 years (Nelson et al., 2018). Other side effects include headaches, depression, hair loss, nervousness, decreased **libido** (sexual desire), breast discomfort, and depression.

Because it suppresses estrogen production, a decrease in bone density occurs with Depo-Provera. Although there is an increase in bone density after the drug is discontinued, the effect on peak bone mass and risk for osteoporosis is not known, although it is believed to be temporary and reversible (Scholes et al., 2005). Therefore, a current FDA "black box warning" states that Depo-Provera should not be used for longer than 2 years unless other methods of contraception are not suitable. It may be more of a problem for clients who begin the drug during adolescence or young adulthood; however, the World Health Organization considers the advantages of use of Depo-Provera in adolescents under age 18 years to generally outweigh the theoretical risk for bone density decrease (CDC, 2016b). Clients using this method should obtain adequate amounts of calcium and vitamin D from diet or supplementation and should increase weight-bearing exercises.

Depo-Provera can be started in the immediate postpartum period and will not have a negative impact on milk supply in lactating clients. The effectiveness is not changed by a client's weight. There is a potential delay in return to fertility after the drug is discontinued for up to 15 weeks after the last injection. Approximately 50% of clients who stop DMPA to get pregnant will become pregnant within 10 months of the last injection. DMPA does not affect long-term fertility (Nelson et al., 2018).

Oral Contraceptives

Oral contraceptives are drugs inhibiting ovulation. They are the leading reversible contraceptive method in the United States (AGI, 2020). They are available as COCs, which contain both estrogen and **progestin** (a natural or synthetic form of progesterone), and "minipills," which contain only progestin. Both types have much lower hormone levels than the original OCs from many decades ago, and therefore the risk for long-term side effects is decreased. If OCs are used perfectly, 3 clients in 1000 become pregnant in the first year.

Combination Oral Contraceptives

Estrogen and progestin combination pills (COCs) are the most commonly used oral contraceptives. COCs prevent pregnancy primarily by suppressing production of luteinizing hormone and follicle-stimulating hormone, thus inhibiting maturation of the follicle and ovulation. COCs also may cause thickening of cervical mucus, which prevents sperm from entering the upper genital tract. In addition, tubal motility is slowed and interferes with sperm and ova transport.

Monophasic or multiphasic dosages are available. Monophasic pills have estrogen and progestin content, which remains constant throughout all active hormone pills. With multiphasic pills, the estrogen dose and progestin levels may vary at different times of the cycle. Because the dosage changes throughout the phases, the pills must be taken in the proper order to maintain effectiveness.

Patterns of pill use vary. Most COCs are available in packets of 21 or 28 tablets. With 21-tablet packets, the client takes 1 pill daily for 3 weeks and then stops for 1 week, during which time a withdrawal bleed occurs. Packets of 28 tablets include 21 active tablets and 7 tablets made of an inert substance that the client takes during the fourth week. In some types, the "placebo" pills contain iron. The extra pills avoid disrupting the daily routine of taking pills. Some formulations contain 24 active tablets with only 4 inactive tablets. Clients using COCs have shorter, lighter withdrawal bleeding. Other COCs are designed to provide 84 days of active pills and 7 placebo pills or 7 pills with a just a small amount of estrogen—this allows clients to have menses only four times a year.

Some clients prefer continuous extended cycles in which menses is delayed or does not occur. Clients may wish to regulate their cycle for a special event or for preference of not having a withdrawal menses. These clients take two or more pill packs without taking the placebo pills for several packs or indefinitely. Breakthrough bleeding and spotting are a common occurrence with extended or continuous use, but this usually improves and lessens over time. A potential disadvantage is a client might not recognize an early pregnancy if it occurred. COCs can be used in the postpartum period, but according to the CDC should be avoided in the first 21 to 42 days postpartum because of the increased risk for thrombotic event (Cwiak & Edelman, 2018).

Progestin Only

Progestin-only pills (POPs) are taken daily with no hormone-free days. POPs are less effective at inhibiting ovulation but cause thickening of cervical mucus to prevent penetration by sperm. They also make the endometrial lining unfavorable for implantation. These pills avoid the side effects and risk factors associated with estrogen and are useful for clients who cannot safely take estrogen.

If a client misses any progestin only pills or does not take them at the same time each day, the chances of pregnancy increase. Another method of contraception should be used for the first 2 days of the first cycle unless the client starts the method during the first 5 days of the cycle or immediately after stopping another hormonal method. Backup contraception also should be used for 2 days if the client is more than 3 hours late in taking a pill or has vomiting or diarrhea (Raymond & Grossman, 2018). Breakthrough bleeding and higher risk for pregnancy have made POPs less popular than the COCs. Amenorrhea occurs in some clients.

Benefits, Risks, and Cautions. When OCs are chosen, the balance between benefits and risks must be weighed for each individual (Table 26.4). The method has many benefits in addition to safe, reliable contraception. COCs result in regular menses and decreased flow, premenstrual syndrome, and dysmenorrhea; reduced acne; and improved bone density. COCs also provide a lifetime risk reduction for ovarian and uterine cancer.

COCs should not be used by clients who have certain health conditions making the use of estrogen unsafe (see "Critical to Remember: Cautions in Using Combined Oral Contraceptives"). Smoking significantly increases complications for clients of all ages. Clients who smoke and are over the age of 35 years should not use estrogen-containing contraceptives (CDC, 2016a). Taking any COC increases the risk

TABLE 26.4 Potential Benefits, Disadvantages, and Risks of Oral Contraceptives

Benefits	Disadvantages	Risks*

• Unrelated to coitus
• Highly effective
• Regulates menstrual cycles and reduces dysmenorrhea, menstrual blood loss, and associated anemia
• Amenorrhea (may be seen as a disadvantage)
• Fertility usually returns within 3 months
• Decreased incidence of:
  • Premenstrual dysphoric disorder symptoms
  • Benign breast disease
  • Pelvic inflammatory disease
  • Salpingitis
  • Ectopic pregnancy
  • Ovarian, endometrial, and colorectal cancer
• Improves:
  • Acne
  • Endometriosis
  • Many premenstrual symptoms
  • Dysmenorrhea
  • Bleeding from fibroids (leiomyomas)
  • Bone mass (COCs only)
  • Hirsutism (excessive hair growth)
	• Must be taken every day near same time, especially POPs
	• Side effects may include:
	  • Breakthrough bleeding
	  • Nausea
	  • Headache
	  • Breast tenderness
	  • Amenorrhea (may be seen as an advantage)
	  • Chloasma
		• No protection against STIs
		• May increase risk of cervical cancer
		• Increased incidence of:
		  • Deep and superficial vein thrombosis
		  • Pulmonary embolism
		  • Myocardial infarction
		  • Stroke
		  • Hypertension
		  • Migraines
		  • Chlamydial infection
		  • Gallbladder disease

COC, Combined oral contraceptive; *POP,* progestin-only contraceptive pills; *STI,* sexually transmitted infection.
*Incidence of many risks is significantly reduced with low-dose oral contraceptives (OCs) presently used. Avoiding OC use in clients who smoke or have other risk factors lowers risk for cardiovascular disease significantly.
Data from Cwiak, C., & Edelman, A. (2018). Combined oral contraceptives. In R. A. Hatcher, A. L. Nelson, & J. Trussell, C. Cwiak, P. Cason, M. S. Policar, A. Edelman, A. R. A. Aiken, J. Marrazzo, & D. Kowal (Eds.), *Contraceptive technology* (21st ed., pp. 263–315). Ardent Media.

for venous thromboembolism (VTE), and therefore their use should be avoided in clients with risk factors for any thromboembolic event.

Hazards are decreased by careful screening for risk factors in each client and the nurse's familiarity of the CDC MEC. Obese clients may have a higher risk for thromboembolic problems, but this is not considered a contraindication to OC use. Evidence is inconsistent about whether body weight affects OC effectiveness (CDC, 2016a). Clients with diabetes of less than 20 years' duration, who do not smoke, and who are in good health may use OCs with adequate supervision of their condition (CDC, 2016a).

OCs provide no protection against STIs. All clients at risk for STIs should be counseled about the importance of condom use to prevent infection.

Side Effects. Approximately 33% of clients who do not wish to become pregnant discontinue COCs within the first year, usually because of side effects (Trussell & Aiken, 2018). Most side effects are minor and include signs and symptoms often seen in pregnancy. Using a different formulation of hormones may reduce some side effects. For example, decreasing the amount of estrogen helps relieve nausea and breast tenderness. Breakthrough bleeding occurs most often in the first 3 months and then generally improves. Often, a COC with a different level or type of hormones can be used to decrease

CRITICAL TO REMEMBER

Medical Conditions Precluding Use of Combined Oral Contraceptives

• History of or current thromboembolic disorder or condition
• Cerebrovascular or cardiovascular diseases
• Valvular heart disease with complications
• Estrogen-dependent cancer or breast cancer
• Benign or malignant liver tumors
• Hypertension (unless well-controlled by medication)
• Migraines with aura
• Diabetes longer than 20 years or with vascular or other organ involvement
• Major surgery with prolonged immobilization
• Systemic Lupus Erythematosus with + antiphospholipid antibodies
• Solid organ transplant with complications
• Suspected or known pregnancy

Data from A. L. Nelson & C. Cwiak (2018). Combined oral contraceptives. In R. A.. Hatcher, A. L. Nelson, J. Trussell, C. Cwiak, P. Cason, M. S. Policar, A. Edelman, A. R. A. Aiken, J. Marrazzo, & D. Kowal (Eds.), *Contraceptive technology* (21st ed., pp. 249–341). Ardent Media.

breakthrough bleeding. Some clients complain of weight gain while taking OCs, but studies have shown that OCs are mostly weight-neutral.

Teaching. Many unintended pregnancies result from failure to carefully follow instructions for the use of OCs. Education about proper use greatly increases effectiveness. Teaching should be extensive when the client first begins to use the OCs. Follow-up is necessary to ensure questions are answered and unanticipated problems resolved. Because the instructions can be complex, they should be written clearly and simply in the preferred language and at the appropriate reading level.

Teaching about when to start taking OCs is especially important. OCs can be started on any day of the menstrual cycle, as long as it is reasonably certain the client is not pregnant (Cwiak & Edelman, 2018). Methods of beginning COC use include the following:

- *Quick start:* The client takes the first pill on the day the pills are prescribed (if it is reasonably certain the client is not pregnant). A backup method is needed for the first 7 days of the first cycle unless the period started 5 days ago or less. This method is preferred because it provides immediate initiation and may improve continuation. It avoids a delay during which a pregnancy might occur.
- *First-day start:* The first pill is taken on the first day of the next menstrual period. No backup method is needed.
- *Sunday start:* The pills are begun on the first Sunday after menses begins. A backup method is used for the first 7 days of the first cycle.

The nurse should listen carefully to the client's concerns about side effects, some of which may be unfounded, and help the client find methods of management. When clients discontinue OCs because of the side effects, they may not use another contraceptive or may use one that is less effective and therefore risk becoming pregnant. Clients should be instructed to keep a backup contraceptive method or emergency contraception readily available in case the OCs are taken incorrectly or they decide to discontinue the OCs.

It is essential that nurses be honest about the side effects that may occur with all contraceptives. Teaching about temporary side effects may help the client endure them until they are no longer present. Clients should know spotting is a common side effect of many hormonal contraceptive methods, particularly in the beginning. Over time, spotting may diminish, or amenorrhea may develop. If changes in bleeding patterns or irregularity are unacceptable to the client, they should choose another contraceptive method.

Consistent Daily Ingestion. Maintaining a constant blood hormone level is critical for effectiveness especially with POPs. Therefore, the client must take the pills near the same time each day. Many clients make them a part of their daily routine, and others take their OCs with a meal to avoid nausea; it is most important the client pick a preferred time which will provide consistency. Breakthrough bleeding is more likely when a significant time variation occurs between doses.

Clients should understand that some pills must be taken in a certain order and that changing the order may decrease the effectiveness of the method. Illness may affect the blood hormone levels. A client who experiences severe vomiting or diarrhea within 24 hours of taking their OCs should be treated as if they had missed pills (Cwiak & Edelman 2018).

Missed Doses. Instructions for what to do with one or more missed doses should be provided. Clients who frequently miss OCs should be counseled about other contraceptive methods that do not require daily ingestion and might be more effective for them.

The client should follow instructions from the provider if they miss doses of the OC. Instructions may vary according to the type of OC used, the number of doses missed, and the time in the cycle the OC is missed. The client who misses pills early in the cycle is at higher risk for ovulating. See "Client Teaching: What to Do if an Oral Contraceptive Dose Is Missed" for an example of instructions.

CLIENT TEACHING
What to Do If an Oral Contraceptive Dose Is Missed

Instructions for missed oral contraceptives are as follows (CDC, 2016b).

General
Missing inactive tablets at any time will not increase the risk for pregnancy.

Combined Oral Contraceptives
One Missed Pill
- Take one active pill as soon as possible. Take the next dose at the usual time.
- Continue the pack as usual.
- No backup contraceptive is necessary.

Two or More Missed Pills in the First 2 Weeks
- Take two pills as soon as possible, then one tablet daily.
- Use backup contraception or avoid intercourse for the next 7 days.

Two or More Missed Pills in the Last Week of Active Pills
- Omit the hormone-free interval by finishing the hormonal pills in the current pack
- Start a new pack the next day once the current pack is completed
- Use backup contraception for 7 days if unable to start a new pack of pills

From Centers for Disease Control and Prevention. (2016b). U.S. Selected practice recommendations for contraceptive use, 2016. *Morbidity and Mortality Weekly Report,* 65(4), 1–66.

If a client misses a period and thinks a pregnancy may have occurred because of one or more missed doses, the client should take a pregnancy test immediately. Using another contraceptive method during this time is essential. However, there is no association between inadvertently taking OCs when pregnant and fetal complications.

Postpartum and Lactation. COCs increase the risk for VTE, and the immediate postpartum period is the time the risk of VTE is highest. Therefore, all postpartum clients should avoid COCs for 21 to 28 days after giving birth. Progestin-only OCs may be a better choice if a client wishes to use a hormonal contraceptive because these OCs are less likely to affect milk quantity or quality. There is no evidence of adverse effects on the infant, and no waiting period is required (CDC, 2016b).

Medications. OCs may interact with other medications, and the effectiveness of each may be changed. Some may increase or decrease estrogen or progesterone levels. OCs may interact with some anticonvulsants (which may be used for seizure disorder or psychiatric illnesses) antiretroviral drugs, and rifampin for tuberculosis. Over-the-counter drugs should also be considered. For example, St. John's wort, which some clients take for depression, interferes with OC effectiveness (Berry-Bibee et al., 2016). Because of these various interactions, the client should always tell all health care providers and the pharmacist about other drugs or supplements used.

Follow-Up. The only essential follow-up for clients who take OCs is yearly blood pressure measurement. It is not necessary to have yearly pelvic examinations, cervical cancer screening, or breast examinations to receive prescriptions for OCs. Clients using OCs should follow the same recommendations for screenings as those for clients who do not take OCs.

During the follow-up visit, the client's ability to remember to take a pill every day should be evaluated. Other methods should be discussed if remembering is a problem or if the client wants to change methods.

Return of fertility is rapid after the pills are discontinued (Cwiak & Edelman, 2018). A client may wish to wait until the menstrual cycle is reestablished before conceiving so that menstrual dating of a pregnancy is more accurate. The client should be advised to take folic acid for 2 to 3 months before becoming pregnant to help prevent neural tube defects in the fetus.

The client should report any signs of adverse reactions immediately. Use of the acronym ACHES may help the client remember signs that may indicate complications (Table 26.5).

Emergency Contraception

EC is a method to prevent pregnancy after unprotected intercourse. EC may be used after contraceptive failure such as a condom breaking during intercourse or when a client misses too many OCs. It also may be used after rape or in other situations in which contraceptives were used incorrectly or not at all.

Two types of emergency contraceptive pills are currently available for use in the US (Trussell et al., 2018):
- Ella, a single 30-mg ulipristal acetate (UPA) pill was approved by the FDA in 2020; Rx required
- Plan B One Step, a single 1.5-mg levonorgestrel pill replaced the two-dose product in 2009. Several generics are available including My Way, Take Action, Fallback Solo, Opcicon One-Step, and Aftera; no prescription (Rx) required. In 2013, a federal court decision declared LNG emergency contraception should be available to women and men of all ages without a prescription (FDA, 2013).

The progestin-only ECs work by delaying or inhibiting ovulation, thickening cervical mucus, and interfering with the function of the corpus luteum. The treatment is ineffective if implantation has already occurred, and it does not harm a developing fetus (Trussell, Cleland, & Schwarz, 2018).

Ella, UPA, requires a prescription for all ages. Ella acts to delay or block the surge of luteinizing hormone and ovulation. It also may inhibit implantation and requires a pregnancy test before use, because it may disrupt an early pregnancy (Trussell, Cleland, & Schwarz, 2018).

ECPs are most effective when taken within 72 hours of unprotected sex or contraceptive failure (Trussell, Cleland, & Schwarz, 2018).

COCs may also be used in larger-than-usual doses to prevent pregnancy. The number of tablets varies according to the specific COC used, and this method should only be used under the guidance and recommendation of a health care provider. This method may cause nausea, so clients are often advised to take an antiemetic before taking the pills.

Insertion of the Copper T 380A IUD within 5 days of intercourse also may be used and provides 99% effectiveness (Trussell, Cleland,& Schwartz, 2018). It has the added advantage of providing long-term (10 years) protection from pregnancy for those who choose this method.

Although EC is available, use is suboptimal. Many clients are unaware of the availability of EC, and those who are do

TABLE 26.5	ACHES: Warning Signs of Oral Contraceptive Complications	
	Warning Sign	**Possible Complication**
A	Abdominal pain (severe)	Mesenteric or pelvic vein thrombosis Benign liver tumor, gallbladder disease
C	Chest pain	Pulmonary emboli or myocardial infarction, coughing/shortness of breath
H	Severe headache	Stroke, migraine
E	Eye problems (complete or partial loss of vision), headache	Retinal vein thrombosis, stroke, migraine
S	Severe leg pain or swelling (calf or thigh), swelling, heat, redness	Deep vein thrombosis

The acronym ACHES can be used to help clients remember warning signs that may indicate complications when using oral contraceptives. Other signs include jaundice, a breast lump, and severe mood swings or depression. The client should contact the health care provider if any of these signs develops.
Source: Data from Cwiak, C., & Edelman, A. (2018). Combined oral contraceptives. In R. A. Hatcher, A. L. Nelson, & J. Trussell, C. Cwiak, P. Cason, M. S. Policar, A. Edelman, A. R. A. Aiken, J. Marrazzo, & D. Kowal (Eds.), *Contraceptive technology* (21st ed., p. 297). Ardent Media.

not always use it to prevent unintended pregnancies. Clients may not know how or where to get it. Information about EC and how to obtain it should be included whenever education about contraception is offered to clients in case they might later wish to use it.

Clients who need EC should receive counseling about their regular contraceptive method. They may not understand how to use their method correctly or may wish for information about other, more effective options. Because of the short time frame during which emergency contraception is effective, some health care providers encourage clients to purchase ECPs to have on hand and use at a later date if they should need it. Information about where EC can be obtained is available on the internet at www.NOT-2-LATE.com.

Transdermal Contraceptive Patch

The **transdermal contraceptive patch** releases small amounts of estrogen (ethinyl estradiol) and progestin (norelgestromin), which are absorbed through the skin to suppress ovulation and thicken cervical mucus. It also regulates menstrual cycles.

The contraceptive patch is as effective as OCs, or potentially may be more effective because it is used once a week instead of daily. A nonhormonal contraceptive should be used during the first week of use, unless the patch is started within the first 5 days of the menstrual period (CDC, 2016b). For most users, fertility returns quickly when discontinued, with hormone levels back to normal within 1 month of discontinuing the patch (Nanda & Burke 2018).

The patch is applied to clean, dry, nonirritated skin on the abdomen, buttock, upper outer arm, or upper torso, excluding the breasts. Areas where clothing such as straps or waistbands may rub the patch should not be used. The client should avoid using oils or lotions in the area because the patch may not stick. Adherence to the skin is good even in the shower or when exercising or swimming. The patch should not be cut or altered, and no more than one patch should be worn at a time.

A new patch is applied to a different site weekly on the same day of the week for 3 weeks and worn continuously for 7 days. Then the patch is removed for 1 week. During the patch-free week, the client will have a withdrawal bleed. After 7 patch-free days, a new patch is applied and begins the cycle again. Clients can have extended cycles without menses by using patches for several cycles or continuously.

Side effects include spotting, breast tenderness, headaches, and skin reactions. Other side effects and risks are similar to those for COCs. Limited evidence suggests the patch has been found to be less effective in clients who weigh more than 198 lb (90 kg) (Nanda & Burke, 2018).

The risk for VTE may be higher with patch use than with OC use because total exposure to estrogen is greater. However, epidemiologic data is limited, and the risk for VTE with patch use is less than that for pregnancy (Nanda & Burke 2018). As with all combined hormonal contraceptives, the risk of VTE should be discussed.

Because the patch must be applied only once a week, it may be easier than OC use for clients who have difficulty remembering to take a pill every day. However, it is visible on the skin, which may be a problem for adolescents or others who do not want their contraceptive use visible to others.

If a patch detaches, the client should try to reattach it. If it will not adhere again, it should be replaced with a new patch. The client should not use tape to keep it on, because the contraceptive is in the glue of the patch. No backup contraception is necessary. If the patch is off 2 or more days or the client is 2 or more days late in changing the first or second patch, the client should apply a new one and use backup for 7 days. If the client is 2 or more days late in changing the patch in the third patch week, a new one should be applied, the client should omit the patch-free week and start a new patch cycle (CDC, 2016b).

Contraceptive Vaginal Ring

The **vaginal contraceptive ring** is a soft, flexible vinyl ring inserted into the vagina and left in place for 3 weeks. The ring, which measures 5 cm (2 inches) in diameter and is 4 mm thick, releases small amounts of progestin and estrogen continuously to prevent ovulation (Fig. 26.4). The client removes the ring at the end of the third week, and withdrawal bleeding occurs. A new ring is inserted to begin the next cycle 1 week after the old ring was removed.

Although a prescription is required, no fitting or particular placement in the vagina is necessary. There is no need to think about contraception except twice a month when the ring is being placed or removed.

Clients must be comfortable self-inserting the device into the vagina. Placement and removal are quick and easy. Allowing a client to try placing the ring in the provider's office where help is available often increases confidence. For the client who does not want their contraceptive use known by others, the fact the ring is not visible to others may be appealing.

Use can begin during the first 5 days of the menstrual cycle, even if the client is still bleeding or on any other day. A backup contraceptive is necessary for the first 7 days of the first cycle if the ring is inserted on any day but the first 5 days of menses.

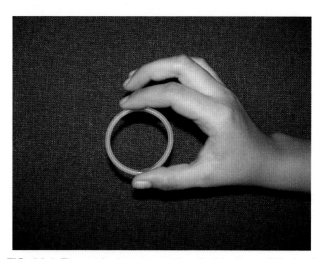

FIG. 26.4 The vaginal contraceptive ring) is 5 cm (2 inches) across and 4 mm thick.

The most common side effects are headaches, breast tenderness, and nausea—similar to those with COCs and the contraceptive patch. Other side effects include vaginitis, expulsion, or increased vaginal discharge or discomfort. Although some clients or their partners can feel the ring during intercourse, it is generally not a problem. Breakthrough bleeding is less common than with OCs. Clients who should not use hormonal contraceptives also should not use the vaginal ring.

The ring may be removed for up to 3 hours without loss of effectiveness. If 48 or more hours without the ring occurs in the first 2 weeks, the ring should be reinserted and a backup method used for 7 days. If the ring is out of the vagina for 48 or more hours in the third week, the client can leave it out and have a withdrawal bleed or insert a new ring, omit the ring-free week, and start a new cycle of ring use (CDC, 2016b). If the client desires extended cycles, the client can insert a new ring after the old one is removed and avoid the withdrawal bleeding.

A new contraceptive ring, Annovera, FDA approved in 2018, requires clients to use just one ring for an entire year. The regimen is the same with using the ring for 3 weeks and then removing for 1 week for the withdrawal bleed, but then reinserting the same ring for the next 3 weeks; this schedule continues for a full year.

KNOWLEDGE CHECK

11. What is the mechanism of action of oral contraceptives?
12. What is the most common reason clients discontinue the use of oral contraceptives?
13. What do clients taking OCs need to know about this contraceptive method?
14. How soon after unprotected intercourse should EC be used?

Barrier Methods

Barrier methods of contraception involve chemicals or devices preventing sperm from entering the cervix. The method may kill the sperm or place a temporary partition between the penis and the cervix. All barrier methods are coitus-related and may interfere with spontaneity. They avoid the use of systemic hormones, however, and provide some protection from STIs.

Chemical Barriers

Chemicals that kill sperm are called **spermicides** and are available in many forms. Creams and gels are generally used with mechanical barriers such as the diaphragm or the cervical cap. Foams, foaming tablets, suppositories, and vaginal film may be used alone or with another contraceptive. They are inserted deep into the vagina about 15 minutes before sexual intercourse so they are in contact with the cervix. Vaginal films and suppositories must melt before they become effective, which takes approximately 15 minutes. Spermicides are generally effective for less than 1 hour. They should be reapplied if intercourse is repeated. Women

should not douche for at least 6 hours after intercourse (Nelson & Harwood, 2018).

Spermicides are readily available without a prescription, inexpensive, and easy to use. Using spermicides increases lubrication, which decreases the risk for condom breakage. This is an advantage, especially during lactation or in menopause when vaginal secretions are decreased. Effectiveness is increased when spermicides are used with a mechanical barrier method.

Some clients and their partners think spermicides are messy and interfere with sensation during intercourse. Some clients also may experience a vaginal sensitivity to spermicide causing vaginal burning. Frequent use (two or more times a day) or sensitivity to the products may cause genital irritation, which could increase susceptibility to infections, including HIV infection. Spermicides do not protect against STIs and should not be used for that purpose.

Mechanical Barriers

Mechanical barriers are devices placed over the penis or the cervix to prevent passage of sperm into the uterus. They include the condom, sponge, diaphragm, and cervical cap.

Male Condom. Male latex condoms, the only male contraceptive device currently available, remain one of the most widely available and commonly used contraceptive method in the United States (Warner & Steiner, 2018). They cover the penis to prevent sperm from entering the vagina.

Condoms are most often made of latex and may be coated with a lubricant. Latex condoms provide the best protection available (other than abstinence) against STIs, including HIV infection. For this reason, condoms should be used during any possible exposure to an STI, even if another contraceptive technique is practiced or the client is pregnant.

People who are allergic to latex should avoid the use of latex condoms because severe reactions are possible. They may use polyurethane or natural membrane condoms instead. Polyurethane condoms are thinner than latex but may require lubrication to avoid breakage and are more likely to slip off. Natural membrane condoms do not prevent passage of organisms that may cause STIs.

Condoms are readily available, are inexpensive, and can be carried inconspicuously by the man or the woman. The typical failure rate can be decreased by combining condom use with another method such as a vaginal spermicide. Reservoir tips and water-based lubricants help prevent breakage. The slippage and breakage rate is very low with proper use.

Because condoms must be applied just before intercourse, some couples object to the interference with spontaneity. Others believe condoms interfere with sensation. Condoms may be affected by vaginal medications or certain lubricants, and they should not be used concurrently. Only water-based lubricants should be used for latex condoms because oil-based lubricants will cause deterioration of the latex.

CLIENT TEACHING

What Is the Proper Way to Use Male Condoms?

Although condoms are easy to use, proper use increases their effectiveness.

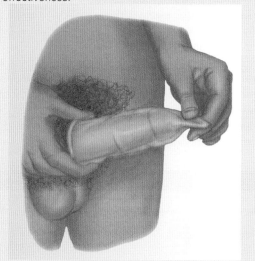

- Condoms are available in a variety of colors, textures, and materials, but those made of latex or polyurethane are most effective. Natural membrane condoms may help protect against pregnancy but not against sexually transmitted infections.
- Check the expiration dates on packages because condoms may deteriorate after 5 years. Open the package carefully and check the condom to see that it is not torn or damaged before using it.
- Lubrication may increase comfort for the client and reduce the risk for breakage. Use a water-soluble lubricant or a spermicide because oil-based products (such as petroleum jelly or baby oil) cause deterioration of latex condoms.
- Always apply the condom before there is any contact of the penis with the vagina.
- Squeeze the air out of the end of the condom, and leave half an inch of space at the tip as the condom is unrolled to the base of the erect penis. This space allows a place for sperm to collect and helps prevent breakage.
- Withdraw the erect penis from the vagina while holding the condom at the base so it does not slip off and no semen spills into the vagina.
- Use a new condom each time intercourse is repeated.

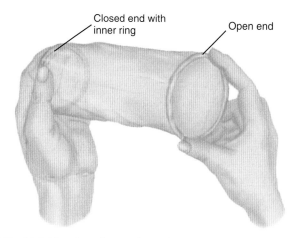

FIG. 26.5 The female condom. A client can protect themselves from sexually transmitted infections without relying on use of the male condom.

contraception for 24 hours without the need to add spermicide for repeated intercourse. It does not require a prescription, contains no hormones, is easy to use, and can be inserted just before intercourse or hours ahead of time (Nelson & Harwood, 2018).

To use the sponge, the client washes their hands and wets the sponge with about two tablespoons of water, squeezing the sponge until it becomes sudsy. The client then folds the sponge, with the concave ("dimple") area inside and the loop on the outside of the fold, and inserts it into the vagina. When the sponge is released, the "dimple" covers the cervix and helps keep the sponge in place during intercourse. To eliminate interference with spontaneity, some clients insert the sponge hours in advance when intercourse is anticipated.

Repeated intercourse does not require added spermicide or a new sponge. It should remain in place for at least 6 hours after the last intercourse. It is removed by inserting a finger into the loop and pulling slowly. The sponge should not be used during menstruation or left in the vagina for more than 24 to 30 hours because of an increased risk for toxic shock syndrome (Nelson & Harwood, 2018). It should not be used by clients with a history of toxic shock syndrome, and it does not protect against STIs. The sponge may cause irritation or be difficult to remove for some clients.

Diaphragm. The **Caya diaphragm** has essentially replaced earlier latex dome diaphragms that required fitting by a health care provider. It is a reusable (up to 2 years) lightweight silicone rubber device molded with a spring. It is a "one size fits most" device. The client places spermicidal cream or gel into the diaphragm and around the rim and then inserts it over the cervix. Because it covers the cervix, it prevents passage of sperm while holding spermicide in place for additional protection. It is available by prescription only (Nelson & Harwood, 2018).

Pressure on the urethra from a diaphragm may cause irritation and urinary tract infections. Voiding after intercourse may help prevent infections. An allergy to latex or a history of toxic shock syndrome precludes use. The diaphragm may be damaged by oil-based lubricants and some medications used for vaginal infections. It is not recommended for use in the first 6 weeks postpartum.

Female Condom. The female condom (FC2) is a synthetic rubber latex sheath inserted into the vagina. A flexible ring inside the closed end of the condom fits over or above the cervix. Another ring extends outside the vagina to partially cover the perineum (Fig. 26.5). The female condom is the first contraceptive device allowing a client some protection from STIs without relying on the male condom. Male and female condoms should not be used together because they may adhere to each other (Nelson & Harwood, 2018).

Sponge. The contraceptive sponge (Today) is a single use vaginal spermicide made of soft polyurethane that traps and absorbs semen and contains the spermicide nonoxynol-9. The sponge is approximately 5 cm (2 inches) in diameter and provides

Cervical Cap. The **cervical cap** (FemCap) is a cup-like device placed over the cervix to prevent sperm from entering. It is similar to the diaphragm but smaller and must be fitted by a health care provider. The flexible silicone cap is inserted over the cervix after placing spermicide on both sides. It stays in place by suction. The cap does not cause pressure on the bladder and can remain in place for 48 hours. The client must keep the FemCap in place for at least 6 hours after the last act of coitus (Nelson & Harwood, 2018). The nurse should teach the client to feel the cervix to check placement before and after intercourse because the cap can become dislodged. The cap has a loop to assist in removal. Caps should not be used during menses or in clients with a history of toxic shock syndrome. Cap sizes are based on whether the client has had past pregnancies and births.

Natural Family Planning Methods

Natural family planning methods, also called *fertility awareness* or *periodic abstinence methods,* use physiologic cues to predict ovulation so women can determine when conditions are favorable for fertilization (Table 26.6). These methods can help clients who wish to become pregnant (see Chapter 27) or avoid it.

Natural family planning helps clients learn about how their bodies change throughout the menstrual cycle. It is acceptable to most religious groups and avoids the use of drugs, chemicals, and devices. Couples must be highly motivated to use these methods because they must abstain from intercourse

---

CLIENT TEACHING

How to Use a Caya Diaphragm

- Follow instructions carefully when using your diaphragm. Skill at insertion and removal increases with practice.
- Plan to insert the diaphragm up to 6 hours before intercourse. Empty your bladder before insertion.
- Spread about a tablespoon of spermicidal cream or gel inside the dome and around the rim.

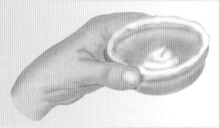

- Insert the diaphragm into the vagina with the spermicide toward the cervix. A squatting position or placing one foot on the tub or toilet seat makes insertion and removal easier.

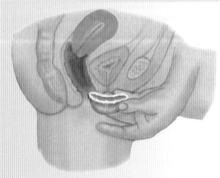

- Be sure that the front rim fits behind your pubic bone and that you can feel the cervix through the center of the diaphragm.

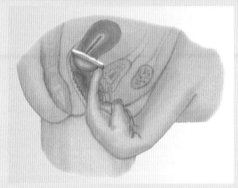

- If more than 6 hours passes between insertion and intercourse or if you have intercourse again, insert more spermicide into the vagina without removing the diaphragm.
- Leave the diaphragm in place for at least 6 hours after the last intercourse. Leaving it in place for more than 24 hours increases the risk for toxic shock syndrome.
- Using the diaphragm during menstrual periods increases the risk for toxic shock syndrome.
- Douching with the diaphragm in place is unnecessary and lessens the effectiveness.
- To remove the diaphragm, assume a squatting position and bear down. Hook a finger around the front rim to break the suction, and pull down.

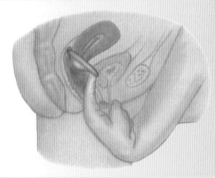

- Wash the diaphragm with mild soap and dry well after each use. Inspect it for holes by holding it up to a light or filling it with water. If you find a hole, use another contraceptive method and go to your health care provider for a new diaphragm.

TABLE 26.6 Natural Family Planning Methods

Method	Application	Comments
Calendar method	Subtract 18 days from shortest cycle and 11 days from longest cycle to determine fertile period.	*Example:* 28- to 32-day cycle = fertile between days 10 and 21.
Standard days method	Intercourse is safe only on days 1 through 7 and day 20 to the end of the cycle. Use a barrier method or abstain on days 8 through 19.	Ineffective if cycle length is shorter than 26 days or longer than 32 days.
Basal body temperature method	See "Client Teaching: How to Assess Cervical Mucus and Basal Body Temperature."	Avoid intercourse until night of third day after temperature rise. Unreliable if used alone. Affected by illness, lack of sleep, stress.
Cervical mucus (ovulation or Billings) method	Assess mucus at vaginal orifice daily. Avoid intercourse during menses and from time mucus appears until 4 days after clear, slippery, stretchy mucus ends.	Intercourse is safe only every other day, because semen interferes with assessment of mucus.
2-Day method	Check for mucus each day. Fertility is determined by presence of cervical mucus on current or previous day.	Intercourse is avoided if client notices any secretions at all.
Symptothermal method	Combine all other methods and assess weight gain, libido, bloating, and mittelschmerz.	Requires much education and motivation.

during as much as half the menstrual cycle. The method is very unforgiving, and errors in predicting ovulation may lead to pregnancy from intercourse during the fertile time. Some clients use the method to determine when they are fertile and use a barrier contraceptive at that time.

Calendar

The calendar method is based on the timing of ovulation approximately 14 days before the onset of menses. The couple must abstain or use another method during the days calculated to be fertile. The method may be unreliable because many factors such as illness or stress can affect the time of ovulation.

Standard Days Method

This method uses a digital platform to help keep track of the fertile and infertile days of each cycle. The client begins with the first day of menses. The method is designed for clients with cycles varying from 26 to 32 days in length but is ineffective for other clients. Days 8 through 19 are considered fertile days.

Symptothermal Method

The symptothermal method combines assessment of **basal body temperature (BBT**; body temperature at rest) and cervical mucus daily. In addition, symptoms occurring near ovulation, such as weight gain, abdominal bloating, **mittelschmerz** (pain on ovulation), and increased libido are noted. This increases awareness of when ovulation occurs and increases effectiveness. Some clients also use an electronic hormonal fertility monitor. It is designed for clients trying to become pregnant but also can be used by clients to avoid pregnancy by identifying fertile times.

Abstinence

Abstinence is avoidance of sexual intercourse and any activity that may allow sperm to enter the vagina. Although it is

the only completely effective method of preventing pregnancy and most STIs, abstinence requires perfect use to be effective. Depending on the time within the menstrual cycle it occurs, intercourse without the use of a contraceptive has up to an 85% chance of resulting in pregnancy over the course of 1 year. Most clients are not abstinent all of their reproductive lives, but many practice abstinence at various intervals. Some clients practice abstinence part of the time but have other methods available to use if they decide to become sexually active. Periodic abstinence is also practiced by clients using the natural family planning methods.

Nurses should support clients who choose to be abstinent. Sexual education programs in schools often include information on ways to maintain abstinence. Adolescents who choose abstinence need assistance to define their values and learn practical methods of reaching their goal. They need to consider just what this entails and when it might be challenging to maintain abstinence. Role playing often is used to help them work through what to do and say before it becomes necessary.

Abstinence has no cost, avoids the use of hormones, and has no side effects or medical risks. It is important users understand abstinence must include all forms of sexual contact, including oral and anal intercourse, to avoid exposure to most STIs. Clients using abstinence should know where to get information and contraception if they decide to become sexually active at a later time.

? KNOWLEDGE CHECK

15. How do barrier methods of contraception work?
16. What are the advantages and disadvantages of natural family planning methods?

Least Reliable Methods of Contraception

The methods of contraception discussed in the following section are not considered reliable but are used by clients who lack information about their risks and other options or who do not wish to use other methods for medical or personal reasons. The nurse needs to be familiar with these methods to help clients understand the risks involved.

Lactational Amenorrhea

Breastfeeding inhibits ovulation because suckling and prolactin interfere with secretion of gonadotropin-releasing hormone and luteinizing hormone. During lactation the ovarian response to follicle-stimulating hormone and luteinizing hormone may be altered. The frequency, intensity, and duration of suckling are very important in inhibiting ovulation.

Clients who breastfeed fully with no supplementary feedings may avoid ovulation and resumption of menstrual cycles. However, use of formula or solid foods decreases the frequency and duration of breastfeeding, increases the length of time between feedings, and reduces night feedings. This may lead to ovulation and a return of menses. The menstrual cycle generally resumes by 6 months, even in clients who breastfeed fully. Another method of contraception should be used by that time or earlier if menses has resumed or supplementary feedings are used.

Coitus Interruptus

Also called *withdrawal,* coitus interruptus is the removal of the penis from the vagina before ejaculation. The method requires great control by the client and may be unsatisfying to both partners. Even a client who wishes to use the method may misjudge the timing and withdraw too late. It is important to remember preejacaculate fluid may contain sperm and when spilled near the vaginal opening may enter the vagina and cause pregnancy.

APPLICATION OF THE NURSING PROCESS: CHOOSING A CONTRACEPTIVE METHOD

Contraceptive failure often occurs because clients lack knowledge about how to use their contraceptive methods correctly or choose methods unsuited to their needs. When contraception fails, the client is exposed to the physical, psychological, and social consequences of unintended pregnancy. Lack of understanding also may expose the client to unnecessary side effects, possible complications, or STIs.

CLIENT TEACHING

How to Assess Cervical Mucus and Basal Body Temperature

Cervical Mucus Assessment

Cervical mucus normally changes throughout the menstrual cycle. If you check the mucus each day, you can estimate when ovulation occurs. Before and after ovulation, the mucus is scant, thick, sticky, and whitish. It stretches less than 6 cm (2.3 inches). Just before and for 2 to 3 days after ovulation, cervical mucus is thin, slippery, and clear and is similar to raw egg white. It stretches 6 cm (2.3 inches) or more, a quality called *spinnbarkeit.* When this mucus is present, you have probably ovulated and could become pregnant.

Use a tissue to obtain a small sample of mucus each day from just inside the vagina. Note the following:

- The general sensation of wetness (around ovulation) or dryness (not near ovulation) on your labia.
- The appearance and consistency of the mucus: thick, sticky, and whitish, or thin, slippery, and clear or watery.
- The distance the mucus will stretch between the fingers.

The cervical mucus may be thicker if you take antihistamines. Vaginal infections, contraceptive foams or jellies, sexual arousal, and semen can make the mucus thinner even if ovulation has not occurred. Keep a record of the type of mucus present each day and anything that might affect it.

To use cervical mucus assessment as a method of contraception, avoid intercourse from the time secretions first occur until 4 days after the slippery mucus ends. Intercourse is safe only every other day when there is no mucus because semen interferes with mucus assessment.

Basal Body Temperature

BBT is the lowest, or resting, temperature of the body. It is assessed to detect the slight elevation in temperature that occurs near the time of ovulation. During the first half of the menstrual cycle, your temperature is lower than it is during the second half of the cycle. The BBT may drop slightly just before ovulation, but not all clients experience this fall in temperature.

Progesterone is secreted during the second half of the cycle, its level rising just after ovulation. This causes an increase in BBT. The BBT rises near ovulation and remains higher during the second half of the cycle. However, some clients do not have a temperature rise even when they ovulate. BBT remains higher if conception occurs and falls about 2 to 4 days before menstruation if conception does not occur.

An electronic thermometer digitally displays temperature in tenths of a degree. The thermometer should be placed under the tongue upon awakening each morning and before any activity. It should remain in place until the electronic signal sounds. Record the BBT on a chart.

Also note events that may alter your BBT, such as menstrual periods, intercourse, illness, or other occurrences. BBT may be altered by illness, restless or inadequate sleep (fewer than 6 hours), waking later than usual, traveling across time zones (jet lag), alcohol intake the evening before, sleeping under an electric blanket, or performing any activity before taking the temperature.

As a method to avoid pregnancy, intercourse should be avoided from the onset of the menstrual period until the night of the third day of elevated temperature. However, relying on cervical mucus is a better indicator of when intercourse is safe.

Assessment

Because contraception may be considered a private matter, approach it in a sensitive manner. Perform the assessment in a quiet area where interruptions are unlikely and confidentiality will be maintained.

Introducing the Subject

In the postpartum setting, introduce the subject by asking the client if they plan to have more children. Most clients indicate a desire to wait a certain period before the next pregnancy. Ask the client, "What method of family planning are you thinking about using now?" or "How did you feel about the method you used before pregnancy?" These questions may identify problems that the client has had with contraception in the past.

It is even helpful to mention contraceptive choice and provide educational materials in the late third trimester of pregnancy, so that by the time the postpartum visit occurs, the client will have had opportunity to think about contraceptive options.

Introduce the topic during well-checkups by asking about the client's current contraceptive method and if their needs have changed. In other settings, a client may make some reference to their contraceptive method. The nurse can respond by asking, "How do you like using (name method)?" This shows the nurse is interested if the client wishes to pursue the topic.

Determining the Client's Understanding

It is imperative to determine the client's understanding of the chosen contraceptive method and instructions for use. For example, ask where the client places the patch or if it is hard for the client to remember to take the OC each day. The client should know how to use the method effectively and what to do in special circumstances such as when there is a missed OC pill. Explore any misinformation, concerns, or problems clients may have with regard to effectiveness, technique, or common side effects of the method.

Assessing the Client's Satisfaction

Assess the client's satisfaction with the contraceptive. Clients may be unsure about their method in the early months until they gain comfort from repetitive use. Satisfaction and effectiveness increase with greater familiarity with the method. Side effects also affect satisfaction. They may be severe enough to cause the client to consider another method, or they may be relieved by simple techniques. Talking about side effects helps differentiate serious complications from minor effects and leads to a discussion of relief methods.

Assessing Appropriate Choices

If the client is considering a change in contraceptive method, assess factors that would help determine the best method. Include a history of medical conditions that might eliminate certain methods, childbearing history, cultural and religious beliefs, and intensity of the desire to prevent pregnancy. The client's ability to understand and follow complex directions may be important as well.

The couple's relationship is important in terms of contraceptive choice and protection against STIs. If the relationship is mutually monogamous and neither partner is infected, STIs may not be a risk. If there is a possibility that either member of the couple is infected or has more than one partner, condom use is essential, even if the client uses another type of contraceptive.

Frequency of coitus may help determine the best choice of contraception. For occasional sexual intercourse, a barrier method may be most satisfactory. If intercourse is frequent, the client may desire a method that is always in place, such as an IUD or a hormone implant. Explore any past experience with other methods, what they consider important, and individual preferences.

Identification of Client Problems

Inadequate knowledge about family planning is common. Many clients will have a need for teaching due to lack of understanding about contraceptive methods.

Planning: Expected Outcomes

Expected outcomes for this diagnosis are that the client will do the following:

- Correctly describe how to use the contraceptive method, including solving common problems.
- Describe common side effects, signs of complications, and correct follow-up.
- Report the client and partner are satisfied with their contraceptive method or explore choosing another method.

Interventions

Interventions involve teaching about contraceptive techniques and follow-up of problems that may interfere with the client's ability to effectively use the contraceptive.

Increasing Understanding of the Chosen Method

Educate the client about how the contraceptive method works, its effectiveness, advantages and disadvantages, common side effects and complications, and when to seek help or advice. Use demonstrations (such as applying a patch or inserting a vaginal ring) and return demonstrations for using the method. Give suggestions for managing side effects and common problems. Understanding common side effects and how to manage them often helps clients continue to use a method.

Teaching about Other Methods

Provide information about other forms of contraceptives, if the client wishes. Discuss characteristics of methods most important to the client's lifestyle. Compare other methods with the one the client is currently using. Talk about benefits, disadvantages, and risks so the client can make an informed choice. If a prescription, insertion, or injection is needed for a new method, discuss what may happen during the visit. Provide written information the client can take home to review and discuss with the partner, if the client wishes, before making a final decision.

Protecting Against Sexually Transmitted Infections

Address defense against STIs, particularly if the client is using a method that does not provide protection. A way to approach it might be to say, "The method you are using is very effective against pregnancy but does not protect you against diseases such as HIV infection that you might catch from a partner. If there is any chance that you or your partner might have sex with someone other than each other or that your partner might have an infection, you should protect yourself by using condoms along with your regular contraceptive."

Including the Client's Partner

Invite the client to include the partner in the discussions, if possible and appropriate. The partner may influence the client's choice of contraception and whether the client actually uses it and uses it correctly. If the partner understands the proper method of use, the client may be more cooperative and willing to help ensure contraceptive success.

Providing Ongoing Teaching

Instruct the client to contact the nurse or health care provider if they have any questions or difficulties. If the client chooses a new contraceptive, suggest they may wish to visit again in 1 to 2 months to discuss satisfaction with it. Make a note in the chart to discuss contraception at the next visit, even if the visit is for another reason.

Evaluation

The client should explain the contraceptive method, including ways to solve common problems and when to seek help for side effects or complications. At later visits, evaluate continued understanding, compliance with proper use, and satisfaction with the method. The client who wishes to change the contraceptive method should describe other contraceptives available and how they should be used. The client should choose a new method and, if necessary, visit a health care provider for further discussion, examination, or prescription.

SUMMARY CONCEPTS

- The average client must consider use of contraception for more than 30 years.
- The nurse helps clients with family planning by providing current, accurate information about contraception and assisting them to find methods that best meet their needs.
- Important issues in choosing contraceptives include safety, protection from STIs, effectiveness, acceptability, convenience, education needed, benefits, side effects, effect on spontaneity, availability, expense, preference, and religious and cultural beliefs.
- Because some methods have potentially serious complications related to procedural insertion, a written informed consent form may be necessary.
- Adolescents may lack knowledge about their own bodies, conception, and methods of contraception. Risk-taking behaviors are more common.
- Adolescents feel more comfortable talking about contraception with nurses who have an accepting attitude, provide extra time to teach, and use understandable terms and visual aids.
- The most successful methods of contraception for adolescents are those unrelated to coitus.
- Clients over 35 years who smoke and clients who have other risk factors should not use combined oral contraceptives.

- Sterilization offers permanent contraception. Female sterilization can be performed soon after childbirth or at any time. Male sterilization can be performed in a physician's office using local anesthesia. Surgery to reverse sterilization is possible but expensive and not always successful.
- Intrauterine devices and the contraceptive implant are very effective and safe for all clients regardless of age or parity.
- Hormonal contraceptives include implants, injections, oral contraceptives, emergency contraception, patches, and vaginal rings. Side effects and complications make these unsuitable for some clients.
- Oral contraceptives, the patch, and the ring may be used on a monthly basis, for extended cycles, or indefinitely to decrease menstrual periods.
- Emergency contraception helps protect against pregnancy if taken within 5 days after unprotected intercourse.
- Barrier methods may be chemical or mechanical. They kill or prevent sperm from entering the cervix and provide some protection against sexually transmitted infections.
- Natural family planning methods involve avoidance of coitus when physiologic cues suggest ovulation is likely. Clients and partners need high motivation and extensive education about their bodies to be successful with these methods.

Clinical Judgment and Next-Generation NCLEX® Examination-Style Questions

1. The nurse working in a family planning clinic is caring for a 30-year-old client, G0 T0 A0 L0, seeking a refill for oral contraceptive prescription at her annual check-up. **The nurse anticipates including the following warning signs of possible complications that can arise from oral contraceptive use as part of client education. (Select all that apply).**
   A. Abdominal pain
   B. Anorexia
   C. Crohn's disease
   D. Chest pain
   E. Heartburn
   F. Headaches
   G. Eye problems
   H. Electrolyte imbalance
   I. Swelling of calf or thigh
   J. Severe hearing loss

2. A 24-year-old female client is at the family planning clinic. After the visit with the advanced practice nurse, the client has decided to choose the transdermal contraceptive patch as a method of contraception. **What health teaching will the nurse share with the client?**
   (Select all that apply)
   A. "Apply the patch to clean, dry, nonirritated skin on the upper chest and lower abdomen."
   B. "Avoid using oils or lotions in the area of the patch."
   C. "A new patch is applied to a different site once a month."
   D. "The patch should be removed for 1 week."
   E. "Side effects of the patch include spotting, breast tenderness, or skin reactions."
   F. "If the patch falls off, you may replace and put a piece of tape on top of the patch."
   G. "If the patch is off for greater than 2 days, apply a new one and use a backup method."

REFERENCES & READINGS

Alan Guttmacher Institute. (2020). *Fact sheet: Contraceptive use in the United States.* http://www.guttmacher.org.

American College of Obstetricians and Gynecologists (ACOG). (2018). *Increasing access to contraceptive implants and intrauterine devices to reduce unintended pregnancy.* ACOG Committee Opinion No. 642. Published 2015, reaffirmed 2018.

American College of Obstetricians and Gynecologists (ACOG). (2019). *Emergency contraception.* ACOG Practice Bulletin No. 152. Published 2015, reaffirmed 2019.

American College of Obstetricians and Gynecologists (ACOG). (2021a). *Adolescents and long-acting reversible contraception: Implants and intrauterine devices.* ACOG Committee Opinion No. 735. Published 2018, reaffirmed 2021.

American College of Obstetricians and Gynecologists (ACOG). (2021b). *Long-acting reversible contraception: Implants and intrauterine devices.* ACOG Practice Bulletin No. 186. Published 2017, reaffirmed 2021.

Berry-Bibee, E. N., Kim, M. J., Tepper, N. K., Riley, H. E., & Curtis, K. M. (2016). Co-administration of St. John's wort and hormonal contraceptives: A systemic review. *Contraception, 94,* 668–677.

Black, A., & Nelson, A. L. (2018). Contraception in the later reproductive years. In R. A. Hatcher, A. L. Nelson, J. Trussell, C. Cwiak, P. Cason, M. S. Policar, et al. (Eds.), *Contraceptive technology* (21st ed., pp. 561–578). Ayers Company Publishers, Inc.

Centers for Disease Control and Prevention. (2016a). U.S. medical eligibility criteria for contraceptive use, 2016: Adapted from the World Health Organization Medical Eligibility Criteria for Contraceptive Use. 4th ed. In *MMWR Morbidity and Mortality Weekly Report* 65(3), 1–104.

Centers for Disease Control and Prevention. (2016b). U.S. Selected practice recommendations for contraceptive use, 2016. *Morbidity and Mortality Weekly Report,* 65(4), 1–66.

Center for Disease Control and Prevention. (2019). *Sexual risk behaviors can lead to HIV, STDs and teen pregnancy.* http://www.cdc.gov/healthyyouth/sexualbehaviors/.

Cwiak, C., & Edelman, A. (2018). Combined oral contraceptives. In R. A. Hatcher, A. L. Nelson, J. Trussell, C. Cwiak, P. Cason, M. S. Policar, et al. (Eds.), *Contraceptive technology* (21st ed., pp. 263–311). Ayers Company Publishers, Inc.

Daniels, K., & Abma, J. C. (2018). Current contraceptive status among women aged 15-49: United States, 2015-2017. *National Health Statistics Reports,* 173. https://cdc.gov/nchs/products/databriefs/db327.htm#:~:text=In%202015–2017%2C%2064.9%25—or%2046.9%20million%20of,among%20women%20aged%2040–49.

Dean, G., & Schwarz, E. B. (2018). Intrauterine devices. In R. A. Hatcher, A. L. Nelson, J. Trussell, C. Cwiak, P. Cason, M. S. Policar, et al. (Eds.), *Contraceptive technology* (21st ed., pp. 157–193). Ayers Company Publishers, Inc.

Eggebroten, J. L., Sanders, J. N., & Turok, D. K., (2017). Immediate postpartum intrauterine device and implant program outcomes. A prospective analysis. *American Journal of Obstetrics & Gynecology,* 217 (1), p51.e1–51.e7.

Health Resources & Services Administration. (2022). *Women's preventative services guidelines.* https://www.hrsa.gov/womens-guidelines-2016.

Hou, M. Y., & Roncari, D. (2018). Permanent contraception. In R. A. Hatcher, A. L. Nelson, J. Trussell, C. Cwiak, P. Cason, M. S. Policar, et al. (Eds.), *Contraceptive technology* (21st ed., pp. 459–510). Ayers Company Publishers, Inc.

Holt, H. K., Sawaya, G. F., El Ayadi, A. M., et al. (2020). Delayed visits for contraception due to concerns regarding pelvic examination among women with history of intimate partner violence. *Journal of General Internal Medicine,* 36(7), 1883–1889.

Kavanaugh, M. L., & Jerman, J. (2018). Contraceptive method use in the United States: Trends and characteristics between 2008 and 2014. *Contraception,* 97(1), 14–21.

Kusunoki, Y., & Barber, J. S. (2019). Intimate relationship dynamics and women's expected control over sex and contraception. *Contraception,* 100, 484–491.

Nanda, K., & Burke, A. (2018). Contraceptive patch and vaginal contraceptive ring. In R. A. Hatcher, A. L. Nelson, J. Trussell, C. Cwiak, P. Cason, M. S. Policar, et al. (Eds.), *Contraceptive technology* (21st ed., pp. 227–261). Ayers Company Publishers, Inc.

Nelson, A., & Harwood, B. (2018). Vaginal barriers and spermicides. In R. A. Hatcher, A. L. Nelson, J. Trussell, C. Cwiak, P. Cason, M. S. Policar, et al. (Eds.), *Contraceptive technology* (21st ed., pp. 367–394). Ayers Company Publishers, Inc.

Nelson, A. L., Crabtree, D., & Grentzer, J. (2018). Contraceptive implant. In R. A. Hatcher, A. L. Nelson, J. Trussell, C. Cwiak, P. Cason, M. S. Policar, et al. (Eds.), *Contraceptive technology* (21st ed., pp. 129–155). Ayers Company Publishers, Inc.

Raymond, E. G., & Grossman, D. (2018). Progestin-only pills. In R. A. Hatcher, A. L. Nelson, J. Trussell, C. Cwiak, P. Cason, M. S. Policar, et al. (Eds.), *Contraceptive technology* (21st ed., pp. 317–328). Ayers Company Publishers, Inc.

Scholes, D., Lacroix, A., Ichikawa, L., Barlow, W., & Ott, S. (2005). Change in bone mineral density among adolescent women using and discontinuing depot medroxyprogesterone acetate contraception. *Archives of Pediatric and Adolescent Medicine, 159*, 139–144.

Sonfield, A., et al. (2013). *The social and economic benefits of women's ability to determine whether and when to have children.* Guttmacher Institute.

Trussell, J., & Aiken, A. R. (2018). Contraceptive efficacy. In R. A. Hatcher, A. L. Nelson, J. Trussell, C. Cwiak, P. Cason, M. S. Policar, et al. (Eds.), *Contraceptive technology* (21st ed., pp. 829–927). Ayers Company Publishers, Inc.

Trussell, J., Cleland, K., & Schwarz, E. B. (2018). Emergency contraception. In R. A. Hatcher, A. L. Nelson, J. Trussell, C. Cwiak, P. Cason, M. S. Policar, et al. (Eds.), *Contraceptive technology* (21st ed., pp. 329–365). Ayers Company Publishers, Inc.

U.S. Department of Health & Human Services. (2020). *Healthy People 2030.*

U.S. Food and Drug Administration. (2013). *FDA News release: FDA approves Plan B One-Step emergency contraceptive without a prescription for women 15 years of age or older.* www.fda.gov.

Warner, L., & Steiner, M. J. (2018). Male condoms. In R. A. Hatcher, A. L. Nelson, J. Trussell, C. Cwiak, P. Cason, M. S. Policar, A. Edelman, A. R. A. Aiken, J. Marrazzo, & D. Kowal (Eds.), *Contraceptive technology* (21st ed., pp. 431–450).

Infertility

Susan A. Angelicola

OBJECTIVES

After studying this chapter, you should be able to:

1. Describe settings in which the nurse may encounter couples with infertility problems.
2. Explain factors that can impair a couple's ability to conceive.
3. Explain factors that may cause repeated pregnancy losses.
4. Specify evaluations that may be done when a couple seeks help for infertility.
5. Explain procedures and treatments that may aid a couple's ability to conceive and carry a fetus to viability.
6. Analyze ways in which infertility can affect a couple and family dynamics.
7. Summarize the nurse's role in caring for female and male clients experiencing problems with fertility.

Infertility nursing is a specialty, but general practice nurses also encounter couples who are seeking help or have had treatment for infertility in various settings. A nurse may be a source of information to friends and family if they personally have challenges conceiving. Nurses working in the perioperative area may care for these female or male clients during diagnostic or therapeutic procedures. Nurses in urology settings often see male clients who are being evaluated or treated for infertility. In the emergency department, nurses may care for female clients who are having a spontaneous pregnancy loss or a complication of an infertility procedure.

Nurses in antepartum, intrapartum, and postpartum settings often encounter clients with high-risk pregnancies or families who have a new baby after infertility therapy. In addition, parenthood after infertility may be particularly challenging, and nurses in pediatric and psychosocial settings may counsel families about parenting and changes in their personal relationships.

EXTENT OF INFERTILITY

The extent of infertility depends on its definition. Infertility is not an absolute condition but is a reduced ability to conceive. Infertility is defined as the inability to conceive after 1 year of unprotected intercourse (6 months if the client is older than 35 years of age) or the inability to carry a pregnancy to live birth. A more workable definition does not specify a time limit but recognizes that infertility is any involuntary inability to conceive when desired. The definition is commonly expanded to include couples who conceive but repeatedly experience pregnancy loss (pregnancy wastage) before the

fetus is viable. Couples with primary infertility have never conceived. Couples with secondary infertility may have conceived before but are unable to conceive again.

According to the Centers for Disease Control and Prevention (CDC, 2019), among women ages 15 to 49, 13.1% have impaired fertility, 8.8% are infertile, and 12.2% have used infertility services. Couples who delay childbearing until their mid to late 30s or later may feel pressured by the approaching end of their reproductive capacity. A female client without a male partner may seek infertility treatment before the end of her reproductive potential. For older couples, delay in achieving pregnancy or having a live birth may be more time sensitive than for younger couples, who—from an age perspective—have more time to pursue pregnancy and make treatment decisions. As technology advances and new methods of diagnosis and treatment emerge, couples may have more opportunities available to them during their infertility journey.

FACTORS CONTRIBUTING TO INFERTILITY

Conception depends on the normal reproductive function of each partner. For some couples, identification and treatment of infertility are simple, but others require complex evaluation and treatment. Some couples delay childbearing until their mid to late 30s, when a natural expected decline in fertility begins. Approximately 40% of infertility is related to male factor, 25% is related to irregular or abnormal ovulation, and 25% is related to more than one factor (American Society for Reproductive Medicine [ASRM], 2017).

Because some factors contributing to infertility remain unknown, treatment of an identified problem does not always result in a successful pregnancy. About 30% of infertile couples have unexplained infertility and never conceive despite having undergone all available treatments (ASRM, 2020a).

Male Infertility Factors

The test of a man's fertility is his ability to initiate pregnancy in a fertile female. Few absolute criteria exist to distinguish normal from abnormal male fertility, although an adequate number of sperm having normal structure and function must be deposited near the female's cervix. Abnormalities may exist with the sperm itself, or the ability to achieve or maintain an erection may be altered. There may also be problems with the ejaculation of **semen** or the seminal fluid that carries the sperm into the female's reproductive tract. One or more findings may be abnormal, and further complicating evaluation of a man's fertility are the normal daily variations in semen.

Abnormalities of the Sperm

Evaluation of the semen via a semen analysis may reveal that the man has **azoospermia** (sperm absent in semen) or **oligospermia** (decreased sperm in semen). According to the World Health Organization (WHO, 2021), normal sperm volume should be >1.5 million, total sperm count >39 million, and normal motility >32%. Liquefaction of the semen occurs within approximately 20 to 30 minutes, allowing motile sperm to move into the uterus without the seminal fluid. A sufficient number of normal sperm must move in a purposeful direction to reach the ovum in the fallopian tube. A semen analysis (Table 27.1) is used to evaluate whether the quantities and qualities of sperm and the seminal fluid are likely to result in successful conception, assuming the female partner is fertile. Abnormal sperm structure or movement may reduce fertility, regardless of the actual number of sperm (Fig. 27.1). Inflammatory processes in the man's reproductive organs may cause the sperm to clump, inhibiting their motility and fertilizing ability. Other sperm may have a normal appearance but may not be able to effectively penetrate the ovum.

Factors that can impair the number and function of the sperm include the following:
- Abnormal hormonal stimulation of sperm production
- Acute or chronic illness such as mumps, cirrhosis, or renal failure
- Infections of the genital tract
- Structural abnormalities such as a varicocele or obstruction of the ducts that carry sperm to the penis
- Exposure to toxins such as lead, pesticides, or other chemicals
- Therapeutic treatments such as antineoplastic drugs or radiation for cancer
- Excessive alcohol intake/tobacco intake
- Use of illicit drugs such as marijuana or cocaine
- An elevated scrotal temperature resulting from febrile illness, repeated use of saunas or hot tubs, wearing tight fitting undergarments, or sitting for prolonged periods

- Immunologic factors, produced by the man against his own sperm (autoantibodies) or by the woman, causing the sperm to clump or be unable to penetrate the ovum

Abnormal Erections

The inability to achieve or maintain an erection may reduce a male's ability to deposit sperm-bearing seminal fluid in the female client's upper vagina. Erections are influenced by physical and psychological factors. Central nervous system dysfunction, which may be caused by drugs, psychiatric disturbance, or chronic illness, can interfere with erections. Surgery and disorders affecting the spinal cord or the autonomic nervous system also may disrupt normal erectile function. Peripheral vascular disease, from cardiovascular disease or diabetes, reduces the amount of blood entering the penis and thereby reduces the ability to maintain an erection. Drugs such as antihypertensives or antidepressants may reduce the erection or shorten its duration.

Abnormal Ejaculation

Abnormal ejaculation prevents deposition of the sperm in the upper vagina to achieve pregnancy. **Retrograde ejaculation** is the release of semen backward into the bladder rather than forward through the tip of the penis. Conditions that may cause retrograde ejaculation are diabetes, neurologic disorders, surgery that impairs function of the sympathetic nerves, and drugs such as antihypertensives and psychotropics. Men who have suffered spinal cord injury may retain the ability to ejaculate, depending on the level of cord damage.

Anatomic abnormalities such as hypospadias (urethral opening on the underside of the penis) may cause deposition of semen near the vaginal outlet rather than near the cervix.

Excessive alcohol intake or use of some therapeutic or illicit drugs can adversely affect ejaculation as well as sperm number and function. Ejaculation may be slow, absent, or retrograde when a man takes drugs that affect neurologic coordination of this event. Premature ejaculation is usually related to psychological disorders such as performance anxiety or unresolved relationship conflicts.

Abnormalities of Seminal Fluid

The seminal fluid nourishes, protects, and carries sperm into the vagina until they enter the cervix. Only sperm enter the cervix; the seminal fluid remains in the vagina. Semen coagulates immediately after ejaculation but liquefies within 20 to 30 minutes, permitting forward progression of sperm. Seminal fluid that remains thick traps the sperm, impeding their movement into the cervix. The pH of seminal fluid is slightly alkaline to protect the sperm from the acidic secretions of the vagina. Adequate fructose, citric acid, and other nutrients must be present to provide energy for the sperm.

The specific abnormality found in the seminal fluid suggests the cause of the abnormality, such as obstruction or infection in a specific area of the genital tract. Seminal fluid that is abnormal in amount, consistency, or chemical composition suggests obstruction, inflammation, or infection. The presence of large numbers of leukocytes suggests infection.

TABLE 27.1   Selected Diagnostic Tests on Infertility

Test and Purpose	Nursing Implications
Male	
Semen Analysis Evaluates structure and function of sperm and composition of seminal fluid. Semen volume: ≥2 mL pH: 7.2–7.8 Sperm concentration: ≥20 million/mL Motility: ≥50% with normal forms Morphology: ≥30% with normal forms Viability: ≥50% live Liquefaction: Within 30 minutes Leukocytes (white blood cells): <1 million/mL	Explain purpose of semen analysis: Three or more specimens are usually collected over several weeks for improved accuracy. Explain to the man that he should collect the specimen by masturbation after a 2 to 7-day abstinence; semen may be collected in a condom if masturbation is unacceptable. Teach him to note the time the specimen was obtained so the laboratory can evaluate liquefaction of the semen. To maintain warmth, the specimen should be transported near the body and should arrive in the laboratory within 30 minutes.
Endocrine Tests Evaluate function of hypothalamus, pituitary gland, and response of testicles. Assays are made to determine testosterone, luteinizing hormone (LH), and follicle-stimulating hormone (FSH) levels. Additional tests may be done based on history, physical findings, and results of other tests.	Teach the man about the relationship between hypothalamic and pituitary function and sperm formation. LH stimulates testosterone production by Leydig cells of the testes, and FSH stimulates Sertoli cells of the testes to produce sperm.
Ultrasonography Evaluates structure of prostate gland, seminal vesicles, and ejaculatory ducts by use of a transrectal probe.	Teach the man that ultrasonography uses sound waves to evaluate these structures; no radiation is involved.
Testicular Biopsy An invasive test for obtaining a sample of testicular tissue; identifies pathology and obstructions.	Explain the purpose of the test; a local anesthetic is used, and there should be little discomfort. Ask the man questions to confirm that he understands the test.
Sperm Penetration Assay Evaluates fertilizing ability of sperm; assesses ability of sperm to undergo changes that allow penetration of a hamster ovum from which the zona pellucida has been removed. Infrequent use.	Explain the purpose of the test and that abnormal penetration of the hamster ovum does not necessarily mean that the sperm cannot fertilize a human ovum.
Female	
Ovulation Prediction Identifies the surge of LH, which precedes ovulation by 24–36 hours; improves ability to time intercourse to coincide with ovulation and identifies the absence of ovulation. Common prediction methods include commercial ovulation predictor kits and cervical mucus assessment (see "Client Education: What to Expect with Infertility Evaluation and Treatment"). Basal body temperature (BBT), or temperature at rest, may be used to identify if ovulation has occurred and the timing of intercourse in relation to probable ovulation.	Explain the purpose of the assessments. Teach the woman to follow the instructions on commercial ovulation predictor. Teach her how to do the basal body temperature and cervical mucus assessment if that is used. Teach her to indicate days on which she and her partner had intercourse to identify frequency during the menstrual cycle and intercourse near ovulation.
Ultrasonography Evaluates structure of pelvic organs. Evaluates cyclic endometrial changes. Identifies ovarian follicles and release of ova at ovulation. Evaluates for presence of ectopic or multifetal pregnancy.	Teach the woman that ultrasonography uses sound waves to evaluate these structures; no radiation is involved. Explain preparations needed for specific evaluations.
Hysterosalpingogram Gentle injection of contrast medium into the cervix while imaging the pelvis to visualize passage of the dye through the uterus and fallopian tubes.	Review purposes of the imaging test to determine whether the woman understands the procedure. Ultrasound imaging will use a different contrast medium from that used in radiographic imaging.

Data from World Health Organization (WHO). (2021). *WHO lab manual for the examination and processing of human semen.*

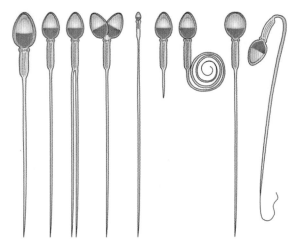

Fig. 27.1 Abnormal infertile sperm compared with a normal sperm on the left. (From Hall, J. E. [2016]. *Textbook of medical physiology* [13th ed.]. Elsevier.)

KNOWLEDGE CHECK

1. How is infertility defined? What is the difference between primary and secondary infertility?
2. What are normal characteristics of sperm and the seminal fluid that carries sperm into the vagina?
3. What problems in the male can occur with erectile dysfunction? With ejaculation of semen?
4. What can cause abnormalities in the sperm, ejaculation, and seminal fluid?

Female Infertility Factors

Female fertility depends on the following:

- Regular production of normal ova
- An open path from the cervix through the uterus and fallopian tube to permit fertilization and movement of the embryo into the uterus for implantation
- A uterine endometrium that supports the pregnancy after implantation

Disorders of Ovulation

Normal ovulation depends on delicately timed and balanced hormonal interactions between the hypothalamus and pituitary gland and on an ovarian response to cause maturation and release of an ovum. The hypothalamus secretes gonadotropin-releasing hormone (GnRH) beginning even before the obvious changes of puberty. GnRH stimulates the pituitary to release follicle-stimulating hormone (FSH) and luteinizing hormone (LH). FSH stimulates maturation of several follicles in the ovary. As the follicles mature, the ovary secretes estrogen to thicken the endometrium. About 24 to 36 hours before ovulation, a marked increase of LH level occurs, which stimulates final maturation and release of one ovum from its follicle. The other follicles regress permanently. The collapsed follicle from which the ovum was released, now called a *corpus luteum,* produces progesterone and estrogen, which further prepare the endometrium for implantation and nourishment of the fertilized ovum.

Ovulation can be disrupted by many factors, including the following:

- A dysfunction in the hypothalamus or pituitary gland that alters the secretion of GnRH, FSH, and LH
- Failure of the ovaries to respond to FSH and LH stimulation, preventing maturation and release of the ovum

Disruption of hormone secretion or of the ovarian or endometrial responses to hormone secretion can be caused by many factors, such as cranial tumors, stress, obesity, eating disorders, systemic disease, and abnormalities in the ovaries or other endocrine glands. Female clients with polycystic ovarian syndrome (PCOS) often have challenges conceiving, in addition to other problems from abnormal hormone and ovarian function. One percent of females experience premature ovarian insufficiency (POI), also known as *premature menopause,* before the age of 40. Autoimmune disorders, genetic disorders, and family history may play a role in the development of POI; however, most cases do not have an identifiable cause.

As a female approaches the end of her reproductive life, also known as the **climacteric**, ovulation and menstruation occur more irregularly as the pool of ova diminishes and fewer are available for successful fertilization. This is called a *decreased ovarian reserve.* Oocytes are produced only during prenatal life and are vulnerable to cumulative toxic effects of therapeutic drugs, abused substances, and environmental agents. In addition to normal aging and depletion of oocytes, factors that may impair normal ovulation include cancer chemotherapeutic agents, excessive alcohol intake, and cigarette smoking.

Female clients with ovulation disorders often have abnormal menstrual patterns because hormone levels do not permit regular and timely development and shedding of the endometrium. There may be absent, scant, or heavy menstrual periods. However, others may have no identifiable menstrual, ovarian, or hormonal disorders, and the inability to conceive may be the only complaint.

Abnormalities of the Fallopian Tubes

At least one patent fallopian tube is required for natural conception and implantation to occur (Fig. 27.2). Tubal occlusion may occur due to scarring and adhesions after reproductive tract infections. Infections such as chlamydia, gonorrhea, and other sexually transmitted infections (STIs) are responsible for many cases of infertility from tubal occlusion. Prevention or prompt treatment and eradication of pelvic and cervical infections can reduce the incidence of fallopian tube damage.

Endometriosis (uterine lining tissue growing and shedding outside the uterine cavity) may cause tubal adhesions, painful menstrual periods, and painful intercourse. Small lesions are unlikely to affect tubal function, but large lesions can distort tubal anatomy and lead to adhesions/scarring, tubal occlusion, and subsequent infertility.

Tubal obstruction may occur if adhesions develop after pelvic surgery, a ruptured appendix, peritonitis, or large ovarian cysts. In addition, the fallopian tubes and other reproductive organs may have congenital structural anomalies that disrupt normal function.

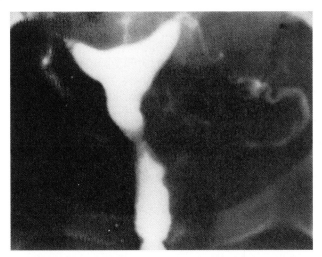

Fig. 27.2 A radiographic hysterosalpingogram evaluates patency of fallopian tubes. Contrast medium that was injected through the cervix spills out of the fallopian tubes into the peritoneal cavity if tubes are open. Sonohysterographic technique with ultrasound is becoming more common and uses contrast medium with hypoechoic effects. (From Gambone, J. C., & Rodi, I. A. [2015]. Infertility and assisted reproductive technologies. In N. F. Hacker, J. C. Gambone, & C. J. Hobel [Eds.], *Hacker & Moore's essentials of obstetrics and gynecology* [6th ed.]. Saunders.)

The conditions that cause obstruction may interfere with normal motility within the fallopian tube. Poor movement of the fimbriated (distal) end of the tube may prevent the ovum from being picked up at the ovarian surface after ovulation. Abnormal action of the cilia within the tube prevents normal transport of the ovum toward the uterine cavity.

Depending on the extent and location of the blockage, fallopian tube obstructions can prevent fertilization of the ovum or lead to an increased risk for ectopic pregnancy. Complete tubal occlusion prevents fertilizing sperm from reaching the ovum, and there will be a total inability to conceive, without the use of advanced techniques such as in vitro fertilization (IVF). Partial obstruction may diminish fertility and may result in a tubal ectopic pregnancy because sperm can reach the ovum to fertilize it but the embryo cannot reach the uterine cavity to implant.

Abnormalities of the Cervix

Estrogen levels from the ovary peak twice during the menstrual cycle, once before ovulation, and again about 1 week after ovulation. The first peak occurs about 2 days before ovulation and causes the woman's cervix to dilate slightly and produce a clear, thin, slippery mucus that is similar to egg white in consistency (**spinnbarkeit**). This mucus facilitates forward progression of sperm into the uterus and capacitation to prepare one sperm for fertilization. Low estrogen levels prevent development of this mucus and are usually associated with **anovulation** (menstrual cycles that occur irregularly without ovulation).

Polyps, cervical os scarring from past procedures for the treatment of cervical dysplasia, or cancer such as cryotherapy,

ablation, or conization may obstruct the female's cervix. Abnormal cervical mucus caused by estrogen deficiency, surgical destruction of the mucus-secreting glands, and cervical damage secondary to infection or other factors prevent normal capacitation and movement of the sperm through the cervix into the uterus and fallopian tubes for fertilization.

⍰ KNOWLEDGE CHECK

5. What factors can result in abnormal ovulation?
6. Why does a female with ovulation problems often have abnormal menstrual periods?
7. What are some causes of fallopian tube obstruction?
8. How do abnormalities of cervical mucus contribute to infertility?

Recurrent Pregnancy Loss

Early pregnancy loss is common—approximately 15% to 18% of pregnancies may end in first-trimester miscarriage. However, repeated losses may result from abnormalities in chromosomes, fetal structure, placenta, or maternal factors.

Abnormalities of the Fetal Chromosomes

Errors in the fetal chromosomes may result in spontaneous abortion, usually in the first trimester. Chromosomal abnormalities often severely disrupt development, and the embryo or fetus will not survive. Advanced maternal age–associated chromosome abnormalities in the ova increase spontaneous abortions and decrease live births in older female clients.

Most chromosome abnormalities are sporadic, occurring randomly. Others occur because one parent has a balanced chromosome translocation that is passed on to the offspring. The parent with the balanced translocation has a normal total amount of chromosome material, but the chromosome material is rearranged. When the chromosomes are divided during **gametogenesis** (development and maturation of sperm and ova), the resulting sperm or ovum may receive too much or too little chromosome material, or it may receive a balanced translocation like the parent. The sperm or ovum also may receive a normal chromosome complement with no translocation. (See Chapter 4 for more information about chromosome abnormalities that may affect fertility.)

Abnormalities of the Cervix or Uterus

Stenosis of the cervix or structural malformations of the uterine cavity may cause repeated loss of a normal embryo or fetus (Fig. 27.3). These malformations may prevent normal implantation of the fertilized ovum or normal prenatal growth of the placenta or fetus. Others may increase the risk for miscarriage or birth before fetal viability.

According to the CDC (n.d.), women who were exposed prenatally to diethylstilbestrol (DES), known as DES daughters, may have challenges with infertility and pregnancy completion. DES was used to prevent pregnancy complications and preterm birth until 1975 when the U.S. Food and Drug Administration (FDA) withdrew the drug from use. DES

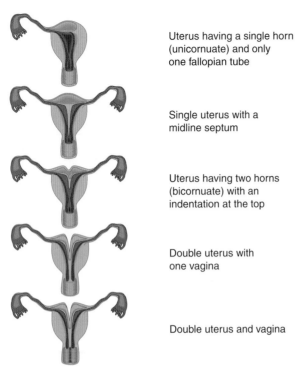

Uterus having a single horn (unicornuate) and only one fallopian tube

Single uterus with a midline septum

Uterus having two horns (bicornuate) with an indentation at the top

Double uterus with one vagina

Double uterus and vagina

Fig. 27.3 Types of uterine malformations that may cause infertility or repeated pregnancy loss.

daughters may have an increased risk of ectopic pregnancies, preterm birth, and infertility (CDC, n.d.). These female clients may be more likely to have uterine malformations or an **incompetent cervix** (will not remain closed). Painless and premature cervical dilation and shortening, often early in the second trimester, is characteristic in women with an incompetent cervix. Although the female may conceive, she may be unable to carry the pregnancy to viability. Cervical or uterine abnormalities and possibly hysterectomy may result from trauma associated with a previous birth or procedures for miscarriage.

Uterine myomas (benign fibroid tumors of the uterus) and adhesions may cause repeated fetal losses if they occur within the uterine cavity. These masses may alter the blood supply to the developing fetus or cause uterine irritability that results in preterm labor and birth. Myomas on the outer region of the uterus are often more obvious but will likely not cause the complications that myomas within the uterine cavity may cause.

Endocrine Abnormalities

Inadequate progesterone secretion by the corpus luteum (luteal phase defect) prevents normal thickening of the endometrium for implantation and establishment of the placenta. The embryo may not implant, or it may implant poorly. In other cases, the corpus luteum may develop and function properly but the female's endometrium may not respond to its progesterone secretion.

Uncontrolled or untreated hypothyroidism and hyperthyroidism may be associated with the inability to conceive and recurrent pregnancy loss. Poorly controlled diabetes can result in repeated pregnancy loss and many other complications of

pregnancy because of its effects on maternal blood glucose levels and the vascular system.

Immunologic and Thrombotic Factors

Immunologic factors are implicated in some cases of recurrent pregnancy loss, although not all are conclusively established. The embryo has antigens different from those of the mother and ordinarily would be rejected like any other foreign tissue. However, the mother's body normally blocks this rejection response and tolerates the developing baby. Some female's bodies respond inappropriately to the embryo, rejecting it as any other foreign tissue. These clients often have recurrent spontaneous abortions.

Clients with autoimmune disease such as systemic lupus erythematosus (SLE) are more likely to experience fetal loss. Pregnancy loss in these clients appears related to thrombosis or other damage in placental blood vessels. Clients with SLE often have other complications during pregnancy, such as exacerbation of their own symptoms, fetal heart block, nonreassuring fetal status on antepartum tests or labor monitoring, and fetal death.

Clients who have thromboembolic disorders, either inherited or acquired, may be more susceptible to pregnancy loss resulting from thrombosis. These clients may require anticoagulation throughout pregnancy and in the immediate postpartum period.

Environmental Agents

Some environmental agents have a well-established relationship to impairment of fertility and pregnancy loss. Others are believed to be damaging but do not show a conclusive link to pregnancy loss. In addition, the amount of exposure (dose) relates to the pregnancy outcome in most cases.

Examples of established toxins are ionizing radiation, alcohol, and isotretinoin (Accutane). Suspected or known toxins are numerous—for example, cigarette smoke, anesthetic gas, chemicals such as organic solvents or pesticides, and lead and mercury in occupational settings. These agents may be directly toxic to the embryo or fetus, causing its death, or they may interfere with the normal placental function necessary to sustain the pregnancy.

Infections

Infections of the reproductive tract are associated with general complications of pregnancy, and they also may be related to early pregnancy losses. These infections, such as chlamydia, are often asymptomatic, making their diagnosis and link to pregnancy loss difficult to establish.

> **? KNOWLEDGE CHECK**
>
> 9. How can anatomic abnormalities of the uterus or cervix cause the loss of a normal pregnancy?
> 10. What endocrine factors can cause repeated pregnancy loss?
> 11. What known immunologic factors may cause loss of a normal fetus?

EVALUATION OF INFERTILITY

Couples are often anxious for definitive therapy to achieve pregnancy, but a thorough assessment is essential for effective and financially sound treatment. Some tests, such as semen evaluation, must be repeated sequentially for an accurate analysis. Even a targeted, or focused, evaluation may be frustrating to many couples, especially those who are approaching advanced reproductive age. In addition, the usefulness and well-accepted normal values are not universally established for some tests, and other diagnostic tests are investigational. Despite many examinations and tests, infertility may remain unexplained in couples who seek care (ASRM, 2020a).

Women's health care and infertility providers use histories, physical examinations, and tests to identify a diagnosis and determine the best course of treatment. This often requires a series of steps and procedures, rather than one single treatment regimen.

The evaluation and care of infertile couples may involve numerous professionals: nurses, physicians specializing in reproductive medicine, gynecologists, genetic counselors, urologists, microsurgeons, embryologists, and ultrasonographers. In addition, general and specialized laboratory and radiologic facilities may provide diagnostic services. Nutrition counseling may be needed to support therapy. Because anxiety, depression, and relationship discord are common in couples experiencing infertility, psychological counseling should be offered to help the couple deal with associated personal and family issues. Nurses working in infertility settings often coordinate communication among the many providers and help the couple negotiate the maze of evaluation and treatment.

Preconception Counseling

Couples may be offered preconception counseling to help evaluate their risk for autosomal recessive disorders and birth defects and perhaps reduce their risk for bearing a child with an anomaly. Many female clients seeking infertility care are older than 35, an age at which having an infant with a chromosome defect increases. A thorough history and physical examination of both members of the couple, including their family histories, may identify increased risk for having a child with a single-gene defect. Preconception counseling also can help clients understand the importance of an adequate diet and avoidance of teratogens that can harm the developing fetus before pregnancy is confirmed.

History and Physical Examination

A thorough history and physical examination of each partner can help identify the appropriate diagnostic tests and therapy and identify risks for birth defects in the couple's offspring.

History

A reproductive history including the following is obtained for both the male and female:
- The female's menstrual pattern, including age of menarche, and menstrual characteristics (frequency, regularity, duration, amount of flow, presence of pain)
- Any pregnancies, complications, and their outcomes
- Contraceptive methods, past and present
- Previous fertility of the male or female with other partners
- Pattern of intercourse in relation to the female's cycles
- Length of time the couple has had intercourse without using contraception
- Exposure to potential toxins, including tobacco and illicit drug use
- Prescribed and over-the-counter medications
- Family history of multiple pregnancy losses, birth defects, or intellectual disability
- Home tests aiding in conception the couple has used, such as over-the-counter ovulation predictor kits
- Past surgeries, pelvic inflammatory disease, STIs, abnormal cervical cancer screening and treatment

The medical history, including childhood illnesses and surgery, and a history of exposure to toxins may give clues about the cause of infertility. The couple's past and present occupations may identify toxin exposure, stressors, or other adverse influences on reproduction. Investigation of their usual frequency and timing of intercourse may identify the need for a change to promote conception at the time of ovulation.

Physical Examination

Couples who seek evaluation of and management for infertility are often healthy. However, a thorough physical examination of each partner may identify endocrine disturbances, cranial tumors, or undiagnosed chronic disease. Examination of the reproductive organs may reveal structural defects, infection, masses, or other abnormalities. Chromosomal analysis or maternal blood clotting studies may be performed for couples experiencing recurrent pregnancy loss.

Diagnostic Tests

Each couple's evaluation is individualized but based on the history and physical examinations. Testing generally proceeds from tests that are less invasive and less expensive to more complex and expensive diagnostics. Simple evaluations can be done simultaneously, but more complex tests are often delayed until a need is established.

Early evaluation for the couple may include the following:
- Ovulation monitoring kit to identify if ovulation has occurred
- Evaluation of the cervical mucus to identify changes that occur with ovulation
- Hormone evaluations such as estrogen, progesterone, LH, FSH, antimüllerian hormone (AMH), and thyroid function
- Ultrasound imaging of internal reproductive organs
- Radiographic imaging (hysterosalpingogram) to visualize uterine cavity and patency of the fallopian tubes
- Semen analysis
- Testicular examination to include an ultrasound and/or a biopsy

Table 27.1 describes diagnostic tests that may be offered to an infertile couple and the nursing care associated with each.

THERAPIES TO FACILITATE PREGNANCY

Evaluation of the couple identifies whether therapy might improve their chances to conceive and complete a pregnancy. A variety of procedures may be used, depending on the couple's initial and ongoing evaluations and their personal choices. Some therapy is basic, such as timing intercourse to better coincide with ovulation. Other procedures may involve considerable expense, discomfort, or unpleasant side effects. Many infertile couples need a combination of treatments to improve their chances of conception.

Identification of appropriate infertility therapy is not always straightforward. Many factors should be considered, including the couple's history, medical evaluations, financial resources, ages, and other time constraints, as well as religious and cultural values. Simple treatments are indicated before more complex ones, but the needs of each couple are considered individually. More aggressive diagnostic testing and therapy may be appropriate if the female is approaching the end of her reproductive years or if it is determined that conception is unlikely to occur spontaneously.

Statistical success rates for various procedures often vary widely among facilities. Factors that affect a center's success rate for a procedure are numerous. For example, a referral center that is willing to help couples with long-standing infertility may have lower success rates than one that accepts only couples with less severe problems.

Pharmacologic Management

Hormones and other medications may be prescribed to either the male or female. A medication may be given to improve semen quality, induce ovulation, prepare the endometrium, or support the pregnancy once it is established. Medications may be given to treat infections or manage endometriosis. Others may help male clients for whom **erectile dysfunction** (also known as **impotence** or the consistent inability to achieve or maintain a sufficiently rigid penis) is the primary problem. Table 27.2 summarizes many of the medications used in infertility therapy.

Medications to induce ovulation may be prescribed for a female who does not ovulate or who ovulates erratically. Medications may be given to provide multiple ova if a female plans to have intrauterine insemination (IUI), IVF, gamete intrafallopian transfer (GIFT), or tubal embryo transfer. Clomiphene citrate (Clomid) or Letrazole are often used to stimulate follicle development. Human chorionic gonadotropin (hCG) can then be given to induce release of several ova. Human menopausal gonadotropin (hMG) may be injected in small regular pulses for pituitary insufficiency of LH and FSH, similar to use of an insulin pump.

CLIENT EDUCATION

What to Expect with Infertility Evaluation and Treatment

General

Both members of the couple are evaluated systematically to identify the most individualized and time- and cost-effective therapy.

Basic evaluations and therapies are completed before more complex efforts.

Evaluations and therapy proceed more quickly if the female is >35 years of age.

Costs may be partially covered by insurance; couples are advised to consult with their insurance carriers. The Patient Protection and Affordable Care Act does not cover infertility treatment.

Difficult decisions may be required at different times during evaluation and treatment. Decisions might include whether to proceed to more complex and expensive tests and therapies, to take a break from treatment, or to abandon treatment altogether. Infertility treatment can be stressful and time intensive, and it requires a substantial commitment to self-care.

Internet resources for infertility include the Centers for Disease Control and Prevention (https://www.cdc.gov), American Society for Reproductive Medicine (https://www.asrm.org), and Society for Assisted Reproductive Technology (https://www.sart.org).

Male Factor Infertility Evaluation

Semen analysis may be the first test because it is noninvasive, easy, and inexpensive. More than one sample may be needed for the best evaluation.

Depending on the male's medical history, physical examination findings, and semen analysis, other diagnostic tests may be done (hormone assay, an ultrasound of the reproductive organs, a biopsy of the testicles, and specialized tests of sperm function).

Corrective measures may include medications, surgery, and methods to reduce the scrotal temperature. A referral to a urologist may be necessary.

Female Factor Infertility Evaluation

The first evaluation usually is to determine whether and how regularly the female is ovulating. In addition to a detailed review of menstrual cycles and premenstrual physical changes, an ovulation predictor kit also may be helpful for the female to recognize and anticipate ovulation. Self-assessment of basal body temperature and cervical mucus also may be helpful. These assessments are often done at the same time as other tests.

Other common evaluations include pelvic ultrasound or x-ray imaging of the uterus and fallopian tubes (hysterosalpingogram). This examination helps to determine fallopian tube patency and normal architecture of the uterine cavity. As part of the evaluation, an operative procedure may be required (e.g., hysteroscopy, laparoscopy, laser surgery, and microsurgery).

Corrective measures depend on the problem identified. Examples include medications, surgery, and advanced reproductive techniques, such as in vitro fertilization.

DRUG GUIDE

Clomiphene Citrate (Clomid, Serophene) (Epocrates, 2021a)

Classification
Ovulation induction/estrogen receptor modulator

Action
Selectively binds to estrogen receptors in the hypothalamus, ovary, endometrium, and cervix. This results in estrogenic negative feedback inhibition to increase FSH and LH. FSH and LH stimulate maturation of the ovarian follicle, ovulation, and development of the corpus luteum.

Indications
Female infertility in which estrogen levels are normal, including polycystic ovary syndrome (PCOS)

Dosage and Route
Ovulation induction: first course: 50 mg PO daily for 5 days (usually days 3 to 7 of the menstrual cycle but can also use days 5 through 9). Second course: same dose and timing if ovulation occurred with first course but pregnancy did not occur. If ovulation did not occur, increase dose to 100 mg daily for the same 5 days. Some require up to 250 mg daily. A higher dose is not beneficial if ovulation is triggered with a lower dose.

Absorption
Readily absorbed from the gastrointestinal tract. Time to peak effect is 4 to 10 days after last day of treatment.

Excretion
Excreted in the feces and urine

Contraindications and Precautions
Pregnancy, liver disease, abnormal bleeding of undetermined origin, ovarian cysts, neoplastic disease. Therapy is ineffective in clients with ovarian or pituitary failure.
 The risk of twins with use of Clomiphene is 5% to 12%; the risk of triplets is <1%.

Adverse Reactions
Common:
Ovarian enlargement, vasomotor flushing, nausea, vomiting, breast tenderness, headache, abdominal distention, pelvic pain

Serious Reactions:
Thromboembolism, ovarian hyperstimulation syndrome, multiple gestation, severe visual disturbance, pancreatitis

Letrozole (Epocrates, 2021b)

Classification
Estrogen/androgen antagonist

Action
Inhibits androgen conversion to estrogen; this generates FSH and stimulates the ovary to grow more follicles.

Indications
Female infertility in which estrogen levels are normal

Dosage and Route
First course: 2.5 mg PO daily for 5 days (days 3 to 7 of menstrual cycle). Second course: same dose if ovulation occurred with the first dose but pregnancy did not occur. If ovulation did not occur, increase dose to 5 mg PO daily for the same 5 days.

Absorption
Excretion is primarily via urine.

Contraindications and Precautions
Pregnancy, liver disease, abnormal bleeding of undetermined origin, breastfeeding

Adverse Reactions
Common:
Hot flushes, arthralgia, flushing, asthenia, edema, headache, dizziness, fatigue, bone pain, nausea, cough, weight gain, constipation

Serious Reactions:
Anaphylaxis, severe skin reactions, hypertension, thromboembolism, stroke, angina, myocardial infarction (MI)
 The risk of twins with letrozole is <5%.

Nursing Considerations
Obtain an accurate history to determine whether the female has a history of liver dysfunction or abnormal uterine bleeding. Rule out the possibility of pregnancy. Teach the female to report abdominal distention, pain in the pelvis or abdomen, and visual disturbances. Instruct to avoid tasks requiring mental alertness or coordination because the drug can cause lightheadedness, dizziness, and visual disturbances. Instruct to stop taking clomiphene or letrozole and notify the provider if there is a suspicion of pregnancy. Teach the female client and partner that irritability, mood swings, and other symptoms similar to those in premenstrual syndrome may occur, but that these are temporary.

Ovulation induction, also known as *superovulation*, increases the risk for multiple births because several ova may be released and fertilized; however, this depends on the drug regimen. A serious complication of superovulation is *ovarian hyperstimulation syndrome*, which involves marked ovarian enlargement with exudation of fluid and protein into the client's peritoneal and pleural cavities. Adjustment of medication dosage and serial ultrasound examinations to determine the number of mature follicles reduce the occurrence of high-order multifetal pregnancy (triplets or more) and ovarian hyperstimulation syndrome.

Surgical Procedures

Minimally invasive endoscopic procedures may be used to correct obstructions in either the male or female. If disease is extensive and cannot be corrected via laparoscopy, the female may need a laparotomy to relieve pelvic adhesions and obstructions caused by endometriosis, infection, or previous surgical procedures. Laser surgical techniques may be used to reduce adhesions because they are minimally invasive, precise, and less likely to cause new adhesions. Correction of a **varicocele**, an abnormal dilation or varicosity, by ligating or embolizing the dilated vein may

TABLE 27.2 Selected Medications Used in Infertility Therapy

Drug	Primary Use
Bromocriptine (Parlodel); cabergoline (Dostinex)	Corrects excess prolactin secretion by anterior pituitary, improving gonadotropin-releasing hormone (GnRH) secretion, in turn, normalizing release of follicle-stimulating hormone (FSH) and luteinizing hormone (LH). These drug actions increase ovulation and support early pregnancy by stimulating progesterone secretion by the corpus luteum.
Chorionic gonadotropin, human (hCG; [Novarel, Pregnyl]); recombinant deoxyribonucleic acid (DNA) origin (r-hCG; [Ovidrel])	Used in conjunction with gonadotropins to stimulate ovulation in the female or sperm formation in the male. Stimulates progesterone production by corpus luteum.
Clomiphene citrate (Clomid) Letrozole (Femara)	Induction of ovulation in women who have specific types of ovulatory dysfunction. Drug increases frequency of GnRH secretion from the hypothalamus, thus increasing FSH and LH release, maturing the ovarian follicle, and causing release of the ovum.
FSH, recombinant DNA origin (follitropin [Gonal-F])	Stimulation of ovarian follicle growth; ovulation-induction gonadotropin.
GnRH antagonists (e.g., cetrorelix [Cetrotide], ganirelix [Antagon])	Reduces endometriosis; adjunct to drugs given to stimulate ovulation by suppressing LH and FSH, reducing ovarian hyperstimulation.
GnRH agonists (goserelin [Zoladex], leuprolide [Lupron], nafarelin [Synarel])	Stimulates release of FSH and LH from the pituitary gland in men and women who have deficient GnRH secretion by their hypothalamus. FSH and LH, in turn, stimulate ovulation in the female and stimulate testosterone production and spermatogenesis in the male.
Gonadotropins (Bravelle, Humegon, Pergonal, Repronex)	Induction of ovulation with human-derived FSH and LH; brands may differ in the proportions of FSH to LH; recombinant DNA preparations are becoming more common because of their greater purity.
LH, recombinant DNA origin	Replacement of LH via subcutaneous pump; promotes ability of mature ovarian follicle to rupture and luteinize when hCG is secreted.
Progesterone (parenteral or vaginal preparations)	Luteal phase support; prepares uterine lining and promotes implantation of embryo.
Metformin (Glucophage)	Adjunctive treatment for ovulation induction in women with polycystic ovary syndrome.
Erectile agents (sildenafil [Viagra], tadalafil [Cialis], vardenafil [Levitra])	Increase blood flow to the penis, improving erectile function.

Data from Lobo, R. A. (2015). Infertility. In R. A. Lobo, D. M. Gershenson, G. M. Lentz, & F. A. Valea (Eds.), *Comprehensive gynecology* (7th ed.). Mosby.

improve sperm quality and quantity, although there is not a consensus on its efficacy. Microsurgical techniques may be attempted for correction of obstructions in the fallopian tubes or male tubal structures.

Transcervical balloon tuboplasty is a minimally invasive method to unblock the fallopian tubes. A thin catheter is threaded through the cervix and uterus into the fallopian tube. The balloon is then inflated to clear the blockage.

Therapeutic Insemination

Therapeutic insemination may use either the partner's semen or that of a donor to overcome a low or absent sperm count. Donor insemination also may be used if the female's partner carries a genetic defect or if a female desires a biologic child without having a relationship with a male partner. Donor sperm is also used in same sex female couples who desire to become pregnant. IUI is a variation of therapeutic insemination that allows sperm to be placed directly into the uterus, thus bypassing the cervical mucus and reducing some immunologic incompatibilities. This process also removes many of the antibodies that interfere with sperm motility and ability to penetrate the ovum.

Sperm for therapeutic insemination or IUI are obtained from semen collected by masturbation or donation. The sperm are washed in laboratory solutions to remove prostaglandins that cause uterine cramping and then concentrated before insemination. Washing also removes many of the antibodies that interfere with sperm motility and ability to penetrate the ovum. If the male has retrograde ejaculation, he may take sodium bicarbonate 2 hours before obtaining the semen to render the urine alkaline. The urine is collected in a sterile container and washed with a medium to separate sperm from urine.

Male clients who donate semen for insemination are screened to reduce the risk for transmitting diseases or genetic defects. They are questioned about their personal and family health history, including genetic disorders or birth defects. Questions about their social habits and personality can disclose high-risk behaviors and give recipient parents information about potential traits of their child. Physical and laboratory examinations are performed to evaluate the man's general health, determine his blood type and Rh factor, and screen for infections such as STDs or human immunodeficiency virus (HIV). Carrier testing for specific genetic defects, such as cystic fibrosis, sickle cell anemia, and

Tay-Sachs diseases, reduces the risk for passing on these disorders. To reduce the risk for transmitting diseases that may not be apparent at the initial screening, donor semen is frozen and held for 6 months before use. The male is retested for diseases such as HIV several times during the 6 months.

Inadvertent **consanguinity** (blood relationship) can theoretically occur because half-siblings from two families may not know they were conceived with donor gametes. They may later conceive a child who shares a larger number of genes, both normal and abnormal, than the general population. For this reason, the number of sperm donations may be limited.

Egg Donation

Use of donor oocytes may be an option for some females who do not produce ova because of POI, who do not respond to ovarian stimulation, or whose ova are not successfully fertilized despite apparently normal sperm. It is less successful if used for female clients who have a chromosomal abnormality or who have received pelvic radiation due to prior cancer therapy.

As in use of donor semen, egg donation carries the risk for infecting the recipient and possibly the male partner of the recipient. The egg donor is routinely screened for genetic conditions and for hereditary problems that may exist in the donor or first-degree relatives (parent, sibling, child). Other tests may be available before conception such as chromosome analysis that may show fragile X-carrier status or an abnormal arrangement of chromosomes. Chromosome analysis may not indicate an abnormality in the female who donates the egg, but it may increase the possibility of an abnormality in the conceptus. Decisions about whether to pursue further available testing of the fetus should be made by the recipient.

Surrogate Parenting

A **pregnancy surrogate** may be required if the female is infertile or has a uterine abnormality, a prior hysterectomy, a medical condition for which a pregnancy would be contraindicated, or if unable to carry a fetus to live birth. The surrogate may supply the uterus only (**gestational carrier**), with the infertile couple supplying the sperm and ovum. Or the surrogate may be inseminated with the male partner's sperm and carry the fetus to birth, thus supplying both the genetic component and the gestational component. In addition, the surrogate who carries the child may form bonds with the fetus during the pregnancy. For these reasons, extensive interviews and counseling of both the infertile couple and the surrogate mother are required (American College of Obstetricians and Gynecologists [ACOG], 2019).

Money paid to the surrogate may raise ethical issues. Could a female who is fertile but in need of financial support feel compelled to provide her body for compensation? However, not compensating a female for the real physical and emotional risks of this undertaking can be construed as coercive. It also should be considered that the male/female partners will likely need to provide insurance coverage to the surrogate or gestational carrier.

Unfortunately, custody of the resulting child has been the issue in several court cases involving surrogate mothers. In 1986 the *Baby M* case, a female who was inseminated with the man's sperm refused to relinquish the baby as stated in the contract between the birth mother and the infertile couple. Ultimately, custody was awarded to the male providing the sperm and his spouse, but visitation rights were granted to the surrogate mother.

Custody issues when the birth mother is a gestational surrogate are clearer than when she also donates her ovum to the child. Courts have more often recognized the genetic parents as the legal parents and upheld the contracts between them and the gestational surrogate.

Assisted Reproductive Technologies

More than 1% of births in the United States each year are brought about by **assisted reproductive technologies (ARTs)**. The definition used by the CDC is specific: surgically removing eggs from a female's ovaries, combining them with sperm in a laboratory, and returning them to the female's body or donating them to another female. ART involves medical, surgical, laboratory, and micromanipulation techniques used with ova and sperm to improve the chance of conception. Simpler evaluations and other treatments often precede or accompany ART therapy. Annual National Summary and Fertility Clinic Success Rates are available in ART reports and resources at the https://www.cdc.gov/art/artdata/index.html.

In Vitro Fertilization

IVF may be done to bypass blocked or absent fallopian tubes, for male or female factor infertility, or for unexplained infertility in either the male or the female. The physician removes the ova by ultrasound-guided transvaginal retrieval, or occasionally laparoscopy, and mixes them with prepared sperm from the female's partner or a donor. The ova are examined to determine whether fertilization has occurred about 18 hours after addition of the sperm. The fertilized oocytes are then returned to the uterus or may be cultured for 48 to 96 more hours, allowing cell division for a total of 5 days (Fig. 27.4). The number of fertilized ova returned is individualized, but single embryo transfer lowers the rate of multiple births from the implantation of multiple embryos, without compromising success rates. Most centers use single embryo transfers as their standard of care. IVF is the most common of current ART procedures. IVF is also used for preimplantation genetic diagnosis. This procedure examines embryos for genetic or chromosomal abnormalities prior to implantation. It may be recommended for fertile couples who have a higher risk of an affected fetus due to their own chromosomal abnormality or ethnicity.

Embryo transfer (ET), combined with IVF (IVF-ET), has become more common. Gamete intrafallopian transfer (GIFT) and zygote intrafallopian transfer (ZIFT) are modifications in which sperm and ova are placed in open fallopian tubes. Variations of ZIFT include tubal embryo transfer (TET), also known as tubal embryo stage transfer (TEST), which places the conceptus in the fallopian tube later than GIFT. Ultrasound guidance targets the best location to obtain the ova. Intracytoplasmic sperm injection (ICSI) is a technique in which a single spermatozoon, obtained with

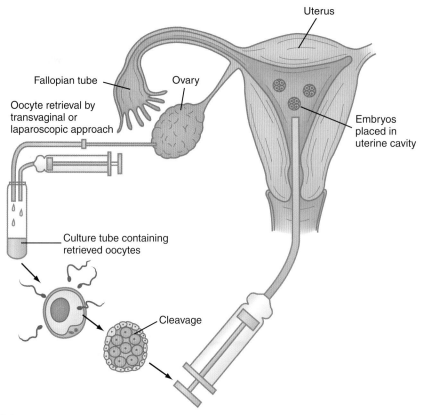

Fig. 27.4 In Vitro Fertilization. Multiple oocytes are obtained by using a transvaginal or laparoscopic approach. The retrieved oocytes are mixed with prepared sperm and incubated 1 to 2 days. Embryos are then transferred to the uterine cavity to allow implantation and continued development.

microsurgical techniques, is injected into the cytoplasm of an ovum (ASRM, 2020b).

Most ART procedures are done in an outpatient surgical setting. Each procedure begins with ovulation induction to permit retrieval of several ova to improve the likelihood of a successful pregnancy. Sperm are prepared and concentrated in a specialized laboratory as they are for therapeutic insemination.

Supplemental progesterone is given to the female to promote implantation and support the early pregnancy (luteal phase support). Because of the supplemental progesterone, the female will not have a menstrual period even if she is not pregnant. Transvaginal ultrasounds are used to identify whether one or more gestational sacs have implanted with IVF and to identify if an ectopic (tubal) pregnancy occurred after methods such as IUI, GIFT, or ZIFT.

IVF success rates vary among infertility centers. Not every ovum is successfully fertilized when IVF or its modifications are used, and embryos transferred to the uterus may not always implant. Although twins are the most common multifetal pregnancy, triplets or more may occur, raising issues related to the physical and emotional well-being of the female and babies.

Intrafallopian Transfer

The female must have at least one patent fallopian tube for GIFT to be an option. The procedure begins in a manner similar to that of IVF, with retrieval of multiple ova and washed sperm. The retrieved ova are drawn into a catheter that also carries prepared sperm. The mix of sperm and ova is injected into each fallopian tube through a laparoscope. Additional prepared sperm may be injected into the uterus through the cervix to improve the chance of successful fertilization. Progesterone is given as it is in IVF (Fig. 27.5).

Zygote Intrafallopian Transfer

ZIFT, often called *tubal embryo transfer (TET)*, is a hybrid of IVF and GIFT. The female's ova are fertilized outside the body, but the resulting fertilized ova are placed in the fallopian tubes and enter the uterus naturally for implantation. The female must have at least one patent fallopian tube.

Comparison of In Vitro Fertilization, Gamete Intrafallopian Transfer, and Tubal Embryo Transfer

The primary advantage of GIFT and ZIFT over IVF is that more people and religious groups may find GIFT and ZIFT more natural and therefore more acceptable than IVF. With IVF or ZIFT, evidence of fertilization exists before placement in the uterus or tubes. The GIFT and ZIFT procedures are more invasive, requiring a laparoscopy to place the gametes or fertilized ova in the distal fallopian tube. Tubal pregnancy may result if embryos cannot reach the uterine cavity to implant.

Intracytoplasmic Sperm Injection

Microsurgical techniques, combined with IVF, may help couples conceive despite severe male factor infertility. Men

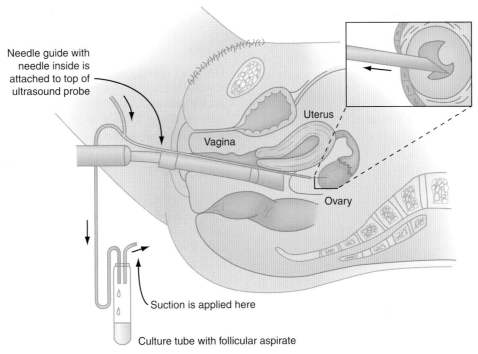

Needle guide with needle inside is attached to top of ultrasound probe

Uterus

Vagina

Ovary

Suction is applied here

Culture tube with follicular aspirate

Fig. 27.5 Gamete Intrafallopian Transfer (GIFT). Multiple ova aspirated from the ovary in this illustration are combined with washed sperm. The mixture of ova and sperm is then transferred directly to a fallopian tube.

who have obstructions to their epididymis or absence of an epididymis may be able to father children with the use of percutaneous or microsurgical sperm aspiration. The sperm are retrieved from the epididymis by percutaneous aspiration of a single spermatozoon with a small-gauge needle. Alternatively, a microsurgical incision may be made to aspirate the sperm if the percutaneous approach cannot be used. The sperm obtained are then used to fertilize ova by ICSI.

Preimplantation Genetic Testing

Couples with concerns about a specific genetic defect in the family may be offered preimplantation genetic testing of their fertilized ova. As in other types of prenatal screening, preimplantation genetic testing cannot rule out every potential abnormality in the offspring. Rather, the testing allows parents to make informed decisions about whether to implant the fertilized ova into the uterus. Prenatal screening of the fetus, if desired, is still recommended even if preimplantation genetic diagnosis has occurred and yielded normal results.

KNOWLEDGE CHECK

12. What elements are included in the history and the physical examination for an infertility workup?
13. What medications may be used to induce ovulation?
14. What screening tests are performed if donor sperm is used for therapeutic insemination or GIFT?
15. What are the differences in technique among IVF, GIFT, and ZIFT? What is done in ICSI?

EMOTIONAL RESPONSES TO INFERTILITY

Many couples desire natural childbearing. Even if they delay childbearing, many couples expect to have a child before the end of the woman's reproductive years. Those who chose childlessness earlier in life may reevaluate their decision as they age. If a couple does not achieve pregnancy or produce a living child as expected, the couple may experience psychological distress and a threat to their self-images. Either or both partners may feel like they have failed themselves or each other. Their marital and family relationships may be strained, and they may withdraw from relationships they previously found satisfying. Every couple is unique, and many reactions depend on the importance attached to having biologic children. Support and referrals for counseling may be indicated.

Assumption of Fertility

Most couples practice contraception for a number of years before they decide to become pregnant. They may wish to first establish careers and financial security or perhaps travel and live freely without the responsibility of a child. They usually assume they are fertile and take steps to avoid pregnancy until ready.

When pregnancy is desired, they discontinue contraception and assume pregnancy will occur within a few months. They may plan conception so the baby will be born at a certain time of year (such as not during the hottest weather) or to avoid major holidays.

Either or both partners may experiment with the role of parent as they anticipate pregnancy. They develop a heightened awareness of children and parenting. They may discuss issues such as full-time parenting by one partner, child care, and imminent lifestyle changes. They may begin acquiring toys and furnishings a child will need. Both partners may develop a fantasy child or a concept of what their baby will be like.

Growing Awareness of a Problem

As time goes on without successful conception, the couple may gradually become concerned about the inability to conceive. If the female partner is >35 years old, she may feel the urgency of her limited reproductive capacity. The plan to have a baby at a certain time of year is often replaced by the desire for a baby any time—and soon.

The couple may feel a shared loss of their future family not achieved or loss of the parenting role and ambition to become parents. The grief may be cyclic, with each passing cycle of not achieving pregnancy. The individual stress and stress as a couple is highest when infertility is endured for 2 to 5 years (Patel et al., 2018).

If family members are aware the couple is trying to conceive, they may become worried as the months pass without the longed-for announcement of a pregnancy.

Seeking Help for Infertility

Eventually, couples must decide whether to seek help conceiving. They may reach this point after only a few menstrual cycles or, at the opposite extreme, may never seek help. Many factors enter into their decision, such as their ages (especially in older female clients), how long they have been attempting conception, how much they desire a biologic child, how they regard adoption, and how they feel about a life without children.

Identifying the Importance of Having a Baby

Each partner may place a different priority on becoming pregnant. Conflicts may arise when one partner wants help conceiving sooner than the other. In addition, cultural or religious beliefs influence the way each feels about procreation and whether options such as assisted reproductive procedures or adoption are acceptable. The way in which the couple resolves these differences is crucial to the stability of the relationship.

Couples may differ in their reactions to infertility, although they are equally affected. If one partner has an abnormality causing infertility, there may be associated guilt and feelings of inadequacy. One member of the couple may be more invested emotionally than the other in the expansion of their family. It is crucial couples communicate these emotions; nurses can help facilitate this discussion.

Sharing Intimate Information

Evaluation and treatment for infertility require both partners reveal information about their sexual relationship, such as the frequency and timing of intercourse. This may be difficult for those who feel uncomfortable discussing their sexual relationship.

Considering Financial Resources

Financial concerns enter into the couple's decision about whether to seek treatment and how far to carry it. Techniques such as ovulation predictor kits are less expensive but have limited usefulness. Advanced techniques such as IVF are expensive and may have a low likelihood of success for some couples. Health insurance may or may not cover infertility treatment or may cover only certain procedures or medications. Investigational treatments are usually not covered. The drugs that must be taken to achieve pregnancy are often quite expensive. Expense and restricted coverage limit treatment choices for many couples. Those who seek and pursue infertility treatment may have greater financial resources than those who do not seek treatment.

Committing to Involvement in Care

Infertility evaluation and treatment require a great commitment from the couple in terms of time, emotional and physical energy, and money. Couples can be involved in this process for several years if they do not set a limit on when they want to stop. They participate daily as they do home assessments, take medications, and keep detailed records. The physical effects of drugs that induce ovulation and support conception can result in many side effects or adverse events. For infertility diagnosis and therapy to be most effective, couples should consider their ability and desire to be directly involved in the process over what may be a long time.

Reactions during Evaluation and Treatment

Couples undergoing infertility evaluation and treatment have different reactions to the process. Although early evaluations often result in simple treatment and quick response, a couple's reactions may change as treatment becomes more complex, demanding, and lengthy.

Influences on Decision-Making

If their evaluation shows a treatment or procedure may enable them to conceive, the couple must then decide whether to proceed. The decision-making process begins early and must be repeated during therapy if pregnancy does not occur. A complex array of factors enters into their decisions about beginning and continuing treatment or whether to end their pursuit of pregnancy. Although discussed separately, these factors interact dynamically as the couple makes each decision. The nurse helps them examine each factor and arrive at a decision that is best for them.

Social, Cultural, and Religious Values. Some medically appropriate options are not acceptable to every couple within their personal, social, cultural, and religious frameworks. Surrogate parenting, IVF, and therapeutic insemination (especially with donor sperm or egg) are not consistent with the personal or religious beliefs of some people. If a procedure offers the partners hope for a child but is incompatible with their beliefs, their choices are to use the technology despite their beliefs or be willing to accept childlessness. Adoption may be an alternative for some couples if the desire for a biologic child is not absolute. As in other decisions, couples must work out conflicting personal values about what therapy is acceptable.

Difficulty of Treatment. The couple must consider how difficult, risky, and physically and/or emotionally challenging therapy may be. The level of difficulty involves physical, psychological, geographic, and time factors. Employment constraints also may affect treatment decisions.

Several diagnostic tests and treatments for infertility involve invasive procedures or surgery. The person who undergoes the procedure should be the one who ultimately decides whether to do it. That person alone, with input from his or her partner, can decide whether the hope for a child is worth the risks and discomfort of the procedure.

Infertility treatment can be stressful. To reduce the stress, partners may abandon treatment completely or take a break for a few months from the constant preoccupation with conceiving. Female clients nearing or in their 40s often do not feel they have the luxury of skipping a treatment cycle.

Some couples encounter geographic difficulties if they must travel a long distance for therapy. Time stressors may be substantial, and one or both partners may spend many hours every week in pursuit of pregnancy. Employment constraints may be a barrier to infertility therapy because of the time required for treatment.

Probability of Success. Couples often have a biased interpretation of their statistical probability of success, especially when they begin treatment with a new procedure. For example, if a procedure has a 20% likelihood of success with each cycle, couples tend to expect they will be in the successful group rather than in the 80% who do not meet with success. As time goes by, however, they must weigh the likelihood of success of any therapy against financial concerns and their own willingness to accept the discomfort and difficulty associated with it. Again, the female's age imposes an inescapable limit.

Financial Concerns. Some couples, particularly those with ample resources and a strong desire for a biologic child, pursue expensive treatments and do so longer than others of more limited means, despite a low probability of success. Couples with financial limitations find they must abandon treatment sooner than they want. Other couples go heavily into debt, adding financial strain to the other stresses of treatment in their quest for a biologic child.

Psychological Reactions

A couple's initial reaction to infertility often is one of shock and sadness because the partners are usually healthy and did not expect to have problems conceiving. Their reactions vary according to how easily their infertility is alleviated, their personality and self-image, and the strength of their relationship.

Guilt. A partner having the only identified problem might feel he or she is depriving the other of children. This feeling may be compounded if the "normal" partner has children from another relationship. It may be difficult for this person to understand that not all factors affecting fertility are known and what seems like the problem of only one partner is often the couple's problem.

Either partner may feel guilty about past choices that now affect fertility. A female with adhesions resulting from a sexually transmitted infection may regret past sexual choices. The male who wanted to delay pregnancy longer than the female may feel guilty if age is now reducing her fertility.

Isolation. Infertile couples may withdraw from friends and relatives who have children to insulate themselves from painful reminders of their infertility. Some couples develop supportive relationships with others who are infertile, which somewhat diminishes their sense of isolation.

Depression. One or both partners may experience depression as their sense of competence and control over their bodies is challenged, especially if therapy is not successful quickly. They often feel as though they are on a roller coaster of hope alternating with despair when the female has her menstrual period each month. The couple may feel envy toward those who conceive easily.

Stress on the Relationship. Because infertility can challenge a person's identity and self-esteem, partners may find less satisfaction in their relationship.

The man may have difficulty ejaculating on demand for semen specimens, feeling others will judge his sexual function. The fact that semen samples are best obtained by masturbation in an office setting is unacceptable or uncomfortable to some men. Both partners may be stressed when intercourse must be scheduled to coincide with specific evaluations or ovulation. Intercourse can become a scheduled event more than an expression of intimacy. It may come to be associated with failure rather than fulfillment if a pregnancy is not forthcoming.

If sperm from an anonymous donor is used for therapeutic insemination or other techniques, the man may feel that his masculinity is further threatened. He does not want to deprive his partner of a child, but he may be ambivalent about use of sperm from a third party. He may have difficulty distinguishing between fatherhood as a biologic achievement and fatherhood as a relationship.

The couple may find their relationship strained if they disagree on which treatments are appropriate and how long they should be pursued. One partner may want to keep trying "one more month," and the other may want to abandon treatment. If they are considering adoption, their relationship again may be strained if they differ on whether to adopt and what kind of child they are willing to accept.

> ## KNOWLEDGE CHECK
>
> 16. What factors do couples consider when they are deciding whether to seek help for their infertility?
> 17. What factors should couples consider when they reach decision points during infertility evaluation and treatment?
> 18. What are possible psychological reactions to infertility?

OUTCOMES AFTER INFERTILITY THERAPY

After infertility therapy, three outcomes are possible. A pregnancy may occur and continue to a live birth, may end in pregnancy loss, or may not occur. If pregnancy loss occurs or if infertility therapy is unsuccessful, the couple must decide whether to continue treatments, pursue adoption, or remain a childless couple.

Pregnancy Loss after Infertility Therapy

Couples who suffer pregnancy loss after infertility therapy may interpret the experience with mixed feelings of loss and gain. Couples undergoing infertility evaluation and treatment often are aware of a pregnancy much earlier than fertile couples. If a spontaneous abortion occurs, they may grieve profoundly for what they achieved and then lost.

Yet despite their grief about the pregnancy loss, the couple may be encouraged because they have achieved a pregnancy. They may feel that if they succeeded once, they could become pregnant again. A miscarriage may give them the courage to continue or restart treatment.

If a pregnancy results in an ectopic pregnancy, the female may lose a fallopian tube, although earlier diagnosis reduces the risks for damage or loss of the affected tube. These couples may have an added threat to their fertility because of the increased risk for ectopic pregnancy in future conceptions.

Parenthood after Infertility Therapy

Couples who conceive experience varied emotions. If they have been disappointed before, they may be hesitant to be optimistic about this pregnancy. They will be happy but still anxious about whether they can bring the pregnancy to term and realize the dream of expanding their family. Pregnancy after infertility therapy is emotionally tentative for many infertile couples, especially those who have been trying to conceive for a long time or have lost a pregnancy. They may distance themselves from the reality of the pregnancy until much later in gestation than normally fertile couples.

The female has learned to sense and report every symptom and may interpret normal changes of pregnancy as a threat. If preterm labor occurs, this may stir greater anxiety in the previously infertile couple. The female may also assume that normal intermittent periods of decreased fetal movement are abnormal rather than sleep cycles of the fetus.

The previously infertile couple may find little support from those who do not understand their fear of investing in the pregnancy. Other infertile couples who have been a source of mutual support may either withdraw from the couple who achieve a pregnancy or rejoice in their success.

The parents' anxiety may be heightened during labor. They may be afraid something will go wrong at the last moment. Even after the birth of a healthy neonate, some parents need time to accept the fact that their baby is really alive and well.

Choosing Adoption

Not every couple who seeks treatment for infertility achieves a biologic pregnancy. Some couples discontinue treatment sooner than others, depending on their age and tolerance for the fatigue, stress, and expense. Some couples investigate adoption early in infertility treatment if a nonbiologic child is acceptable to them. A single parent may choose adoption. Agencies that coordinate international adoptions are often consulted.

Couples who consider adoption must confront their personal preferences, limitations, and prejudices. As much as they want a child, couples may be hesitant to adopt a child with special needs, one of a mixed or different race, or a group of siblings.

Some couples fear adopting a child because the female might then spontaneously become pregnant. Although pregnancy has been the goal for a long time, they may worry they would love their adopted child differently from their biologic child. If the couple plans to continue trying for a biologic child, they also must come to grips with this issue.

Couples who decide to adopt face further scrutiny of their personal lives. Agencies investigate their home, financial means (which may have been seriously drained), and fitness as parents. Once again, they may feel their personal competence is questioned. International adoptions often have many additional requirements that the couple does not encounter in their home country.

Couples who decide to adopt may have emotions similar to those who achieve a pregnancy. They may be slow to invest in the process emotionally because they expect disappointment again. In addition, the adopted child often arrives suddenly and unexpectedly. A delay in the adoption process may occur, bringing further uncertainty to the couple. Although they may have been waiting months for this happy event, the couple may have little time to adjust to the reality of their new roles as parents.

Menopause after Infertility

A woman or couple may decide when to stop unsuccessful infertility treatment, or natural biologic aging occur. After many attempts to conceive and carry a child to term, the ovarian reserve may be exhausted and she may become perimenopausal or menopausal.

> **? KNOWLEDGE CHECK**
>
> 19. If the partners become parents, either through birth or adoption, how might they react to parenthood?
> 20. What are the issues couples must face if they consider adoption?
> 21. What emotions do couples often experience if they lose a pregnancy after infertility treatment?

APPLICATION OF THE NURSING PROCESS: CARE OF THE INFERTILE COUPLE

Nurses may encounter couples facing infertility in many different settings and identify numerous nursing care needs.

Regardless of the setting, the nurse often addresses the couple's emotional needs associated with infertility evaluation, treatment, and outcomes of therapy.

Assessment

In many instances, infertile couples previously have had a positive self-image and feelings of competence about themselves. The diagnosis of infertility may alter this positive view. The nurse should be aware that these feelings may be present, regardless of the practice setting in which the couple is encountered.

The nurse should determine at what point the couple is in their infertility treatment journey. Couples who have just discovered they may have difficulty conceiving may be shocked yet optimistic that therapy will result in a baby. Other couples for whom simple treatments were unsuccessful may face shock again if the more complex treatments such as IVF or ICSI are recommended, particularly if these treatments may result in greater time commitments and financial hardship. Listen for remarks that are negative or expressing guilt or helplessness.

Evaluate the way infertility has affected the partners' relationship with each other. Are there conflicts or differences in values between the two? Observing their body language, such as eye contact, may provide clues about similarities and differences in their commitment to diagnosis and treatment. Ask them how their relationship has changed. Are they more or less satisfied with their relationship than they were before they had problems conceiving? How is each member of the couple adjusting to the situation?

Ask about support systems. Couples suffering from infertility often withdraw from old relationships yet do not form new supportive ones. Do others who are significant in the partners' lives know that they are trying to conceive? Are family members and friends supportive? Have they sought the counsel of a therapist trained in infertility? Ask whether they have encountered assumptions by others that infertility is the "fault" of one partner or the other. Are they subjected to questions that invade their privacy, such as "When are you two going to have a baby?"

Determine how the couple's culture or religion views infertility and the impact of these values on therapy. Are some therapies unacceptable to one or both partners? The partners may have differing views that can cause conflict during treatment, and they may need help work these out.

Determine how the couple is coping with the stresses of treatment. How much has infertility cost them in terms of time, money, and discomfort? Identify the successes and failures they have experienced as well as outcomes that have provided them hope or comfort. Their ages and potential decline in natural fertility may add another stressor that cannot be ignored in their decisions.

If the client is pregnant or has given birth recently or the couple has adopted a child recently, observe for high levels of anxiety in either or both parents. Assess them for negative behaviors and comments, such as reluctance to feel joy or a sense that they will "fail" again.

Identification of Client Problems

Infertility can result in a client feeling anxious, hopeless, and a sense of loss. An appropriate client problem is altered self-confidence resulting from a loss of control.

Planning: Expected Outcomes

Three expected outcomes are appropriate for this client problem during the early days of evaluation and decision-making. The outcomes may apply to the male, the female, or both partners. The person(s) will do the following:
- Express feelings about infertility and its evaluation and treatment.
- Explore ways to increase control within the situation of infertility.
- Identify aspects of self that are positive.

Interventions
Assist Communication

Therapeutic communication is the primary technique for assessment and intervention related to this client problem. Recognize either partner may be reluctant to express his or her feelings as openly as the other. A variety of communication techniques such as active listening and exploration may encourage the partners to express their feelings honestly. Provide privacy and acceptance of their feelings. Nurses should recognize the validity of the couple's views and emotions, even if they differ from the nurse's own feelings.

Encourage the partners to accept their feelings, both positive and negative. The partners may act elated because they believe they should feel happy, yet inside they are cautious and hesitant about becoming attached to their baby. Explain feelings are not right or wrong but simply exist. Opening the subject of negative feelings (fear of attachment) within a successful situation (pregnancy or birth) may be helpful to reinforce the normality of their emotions. This technique gives them the opportunity to talk about emotional reactions that they or others feel are inappropriate and might otherwise be reluctant to discuss.

Discuss possible differences in ways the couple communicates. For example, explain one may feel more comfortable than the other in talking about the problem and concerns about treatment. Explain these differences in communication style can cause misunderstandings because one partner believes that the other does not care as much about their problem. Encourage them to be open with each other for the best mutual support. Support groups provide another means for communication and ventilation of feelings among those who are most likely to understand what an infertile couple is experiencing.

Increase the Couple's Sense of Control

Explore how the couple has dealt with stressors in the past and how these techniques might be used to cope with the present crisis. A couple's pattern of dealing with stress in other parts of life is likely to carry over into infertility diagnosis and treatment and throughout pregnancy and parenthood. Reinforce positive coping skills such as learning more about infertility and the proposed therapy for it.

Couples who experience undue stress may benefit from relaxation techniques such as visualization and moderate exercise. Frequent strenuous exercise may reduce the female's ability to ovulate regularly. Although warm heat such as a hot tub is relaxing for some, it should be avoided because the high temperatures may inhibit spermatogenesis. In addition, the female could become pregnant with any cycle, and high maternal body temperatures may be associated with fetal anomalies.

Discuss behaviors that enhance the ability to handle stress and provide a good environment for a pregnancy that might occur. Reinforce healthy choices such as good nutrition and a balance between exercise and rest. Teach the couple ways to enhance general health if deficiencies are identified.

Explain any procedures and their purpose in language the couple can understand. Reinforce any medical explanations that may have been given. Encourage questions so the couple is fully informed. Have the partners restate what was explained to reduce misunderstandings.

Help the couple explore options at each decision point. The couple must decide the best course of action, but the nurse can help identify pros and cons of each choice so the partners can arrive at a decision appropriate for them. Be nondirective so the choices are theirs and do not reflect the biases of the nurse or other caregivers.

Reduce Isolation

Because couples often distance themselves from friends and family relationships they find painful, they may have little social support. Refer them to available support groups to provide emotional outlets, a sense of belonging, and a source of information.

Couples who achieve pregnancy or adopt a child may again find themselves isolated if infertile couples in their circle of support are no longer in the same stage or experience. Encourage them to take the initiative to reestablish ties with relatives and friends, who can be an important source of aid during pregnancy and child-rearing. Help them identify ways they can improve communication with these significant others. Remind them they have undergone significant shifts in self-image, which also have affected those around them.

Promote a Positive Self-Image

Because infertility work often is such a dominant factor in their lives, a continuing inability to conceive erodes the partners' perception of themselves. Explore with them other areas of competence and activities that make them feel good about themselves. Reinforce positive attitudes and self-evaluations. Encourage them to maintain activities such as hobbies, sports, or volunteer work. The career of either partner may be a source of stress that needs relief, or it may be an avenue that fosters a positive self-perception.

Encourage them to avoid activities that involve infants or children if these events make them sad. Help them identify the best way to cope with these activities if they do not want to avoid them.

Some people benefit from self-improvement activities such as continuing education courses or enhancement of appearance. Encourage these activities if they help the individuals feel better about themselves. If the activity might impair fertility treatments, such as strict dieting, also inform the person of this fact.

Evaluation

The goals established are achieved if the individual or both partners can do the following:

- Express their feelings about their situation, usually over time.
- Explore ways to increase personal control over their lives, as evidenced by expressing feelings of reduced helplessness and dependence.
- Identify one or more aspects of self that are perceived as positive and identify areas of competence.

SUMMARY CONCEPTS

- Nurses may encounter persons having infertility problems in a variety of settings other than infertility clinics, such as maternity and gynecology services, urology services, the perioperative area, and the emergency department. Friends and family members also see the nurse as an information resource about infertility care.
- About 20% of infertile couples have no identified problem that is explained by current evaluation techniques.
- Because many unknown factors in reproduction exist, identification and correction of problems in one or both partners does not necessarily resolve their infertility.
- A variety of structural and functional abnormalities may contribute to a couple's infertility. The male may have abnormalities of the sperm or the seminal fluid or with ejaculation. The female may have ovulation disorders, anatomic problems such as fallopian tube occlusion, or physiologic disorders such as hormone imbalances.
- A systematic evaluation of both partners, proceeding from basic to complex, identifies therapy that is most likely to

- be successful and cost-effective. The couple may decide to stop evaluation or therapy at any point.
- Infertility may be a crisis for the couple and often for the extended family. Either or both partners may think the inability to conceive represents a personal failure. They may have a variety of psychological reactions.
- Infertile couples must make choices at many points before and during evaluation and therapy. Some major factors that enter into their decisions involve personal, social, cultural, and religious values; difficulty of treatment; probability of success; financial resources; and age.
- The possible outcomes after infertility therapy may present new challenges to the couple and their families, such as unsuccessful therapy and the choice of whether to pursue adoption, pregnancy loss after infertility, and parenthood after infertility.
- Many nursing care needs may be identified as the couple negotiates infertility evaluation and treatment.

Clinical Judgment And Next-Generation NCLEX® Examination-Style Questions

1. A nurse working in an infertility clinic is caring for a 35-year-old female, G0 T0 A0 L0, diagnosed with an ovulation disorder. The client asks the nurse if there is anything she can do to recognize that ovulation is taking place to improve her ability to conceive.

For each client statement, use an X to indicate whether the nurse's explanation were effective (helped the client understand the instructions), ineffective (did not help the client understand the instructions), or unrelated (not related to the teaching). The nurse provides the following information.

Client's Statement	Effective	Ineffective	Unrelated
"The timing of ovulation can be affected by many factors."			
"Commercial ovulation kits are generally not effective as I am 35 years old."			
"When the cervical mucus becomes clear, thin, and slippery, I should be ovulating."			
"PCOS can cause anovulation."			
"Since I am 35 years old, I don't have many eggs left and will stop ovulating."			
"When using the basal body temperature method, my temperature rises just before ovulation."			
"I have a calendar to mark the dates of intercourse."			

2. A 40-year-old female presents to the infertility clinic. She provides a list of medications that she has received in the past for her infertility. **Choose the most likely options for the information missing from the table by selecting from the lists of options provided.**

Medication	Drug action
1	Stimulates the pituitary gland to produce LH and FSH
hCG	2
3	Given for clients with polycystic ovarian syndrome
Progesterone	4

Options for 1, 3

Baby aspirin
Clomiphene citrate (Clomid)
Bromocriptine (Parlodel)
Ganirelix (Antagon)
Metformin

Options for 2, 4

Works in conjunction with the antiphospholipid syndrome
Stimulates maturation of the ovarian follicle
Stimulates ovulation when used with gonadotropins
Suppresses LH and FSH
Provides luteal phase support

REFERENCES & READINGS

American College of Obstetricians and Gynecologists (ACOG). (2019). *Family building through gestational surrogacy.* ACOG Committee Opinion No. 660. Published 2016. reaffirmed 2019.

American Society for Reproductive Medicine (ASRM). (2017). *Quick facts about infertility.* www.reproductivefacts.org/faqs/quick-facts-about-infertilty/.

American Society for Reproductive Medicine (ASRM). (2020a). Evidence-based treatments for couples with unexplained infertility: A guideline. *Fertility and Sterility, 113*(2), 305–322.

American Society for Reproductive Medicine (ASRM). (2020b). *Intracytoplasmic sperm injection (ICSI).* https://www.asrm.org/topics/topics-index/intracytoplasmic-sperm-injection/.

CDC (n.d.). Known health affects for DES daughters. https://stacks.cdc.gov/view/cdc/55281.

CDC (2019). *Key statistics from the National Survey of Family Growth.* https://www.cdc.gov/nchs/nsfg/key_statistics/i-keystat.htm#infertility.

Epocrates version 21.3.0. (2021a). *Clomiphene. Epocrates Medical Information Editors.* https://www.epocrates.com.

Epocrates version 21.3.0. (2021b). *Letrozole. Epocrates Medical Information Editors.* https://www.epocrates.com.

Patel, A., Sharma, P., & Kumar, P. (2018). In cycles of dreams, despair and desperation. Research perspectives on infertility distress in patients undergoing fertility treatments. *Journal of Human Reproductive Science, 11*(4), 320–328.

World Health Organization (WHO). (2021). *WHO lab manual for the examination and processing of human semen.*

Women's Health

Suzanne White

OBJECTIVES

After studying this chapter, you should be able to:

1. Explain examinations and screening procedures recommended to maintain health.
2. Explain benefits of indicated immunization(s).
3. Explain benign disorders of the breast and discuss diagnostic procedures used to rule out breast cancer.
4. Describe the incidence, risks, pathophysiology, management, and nursing considerations related to malignant breast tumors.
5. Discuss cardiovascular disease in clients, including risk factors, signs and symptoms, and prevention measures.
6. Discuss common menstrual cycle disorders.
7. Explain premenstrual syndrome, management options, and nursing considerations.
8. Discuss medical termination of pregnancy in terms of procedures, possible complications, and follow-up care.
9. Describe the physical and psychological changes associated with menopause and options to alleviate uncomfortable changes.
10. Discuss measures to reduce severity of osteoporosis.
11. Describe the major disorders associated with pelvic relaxation in terms of cause, treatment, and nursing considerations.
12. Discuss the most common benign and malignant disorders of the reproductive tract in terms of signs and symptoms, management, and nursing considerations.
13. Describe care of the woman with an infectious disorder of the reproductive tract, including sexually transmitted infections, pelvic inflammatory disease, and toxic shock syndrome.

PREVENTIVE HEALTH CARE

There is an increasing demand for health care providers for biologic female clients as more is learned about health risks specific to this population including the need for preventive care. Certified nurse–midwives (CNMs) and women's health nurse practitioners (WHNPs) often provide basic preventive health care to nonpregnant biologic female clients. This chapter focuses on examinations and screening procedures recommended to maintain client health. It will include information as it relates to immunizations, benign and malignant disorders of the breast, cardiovascular disease, menstrual cycle disorders, premenstrual syndrome (PMS), medical termination of pregnancy, menopause, osteoporosis, pelvic floor dysfunction, common benign and malignant disorders of the reproductive tract, and infectious disorders of the reproductive tract.

NATIONAL EMPHASIS ON WOMEN'S HEALTH

Two national programs have had a major impact on the health of biologic female clients. The Women's Health Initiative (WHI) of the National Institutes of Health (NIH) was a major 15-year research program to address the most common causes of death, disability, and poor quality of life in postmenopausal clients: cardiovascular disease, cancer, and osteoporosis. Healthy People 2030 continues to have a health promotion and disease prevention agenda coordinated by the U.S. Department of Health and Human Services. For more information about these programs, see National Heart, Lung, and Blood Institute's (n.d.) website for women's health https://www.nhlbi.nih.gov/science/womens-health.

Healthy People 2030 Goals

Several Healthy People 2030 goals relate to the health of biologic female clients, and many address the goals in the WHI, as follows (U.S. Department of Health & Human Services, 2020a):

- Reduce the proportion of adults with obesity 20 years and older from 38.6% (2013–2016) to 36%.
- Reduce breast cancer deaths from 19.7 per 100,000 women in 2018 to no more than 15.3 per 100,000 women.
- Increase the proportion of females age 21 to 65 who receive a cervical cancer screening based on the most recent guidelines, from 80.5% in 2018 to 84.3%.
- Increase the proportion of adults who receive a colorectal cancer screening based on the most recent guidelines, from 65.2% in 2018 to 74.4%.

- Increase the proportion of cancer survivors who are living 5 years or longer after diagnosis from 64.1% in 2018 to 66.2%.
- Reduce pelvic inflammatory disease (PID) in adolescent and young females (aged 15 to 24 years) from 235.4 visits per 100,000 women in 2016 to 188.3 visits per 100,000.
- Reduce congenital syphilis from 23.3 per 100,000 live births in 2017 to no more than 21 per 100,000 live births.
- Reduce coronary heart disease deaths from 90.9 per 100,000 (2018) to 71.1 per 100,000.
- Reduce stroke deaths from 37.1 per 100,000 (2018) to 33.4 per 100,000.

HEALTH MAINTENANCE

Health maintenance refers to measures that can be taken for prevention or early detection of specific diseases. Unfortunately, many clients do not take advantage of recommended health maintenance procedures and choose to seek care only once a problem exists. For others, the only health care they receive comes from a gynecologist or nurse practitioner, often with their annual checkup. Therefore, it is important that those who provide health care for clients are familiar with principles of screening and counseling in areas that are not traditionally associated with gynecology, such as assessing risk factors for colon cancer and heart disease.

Health History

The client's health history often identifies actions taken to promote health. The health history identifies risk factors for a variety of conditions and may be obtained from sources such as questionnaires, interviews, and records. The focus of a health history depends on the client's age, but some topics should be discussed with all clients. Box 28.1 provides a summary of information to obtain. These topics include dietary intake, physical activity, habits, and sexual practices. Discussions of drugs should include long-term use of prescription and over-the-counter (OTC) medications. Additionally, illicit drugs should be discussed to provide the safest care for the client. Questions about use of **complementary and alternative medicine (CAM)** should be included in the client's history.

Many clients take herbal or other botanical preparations but do not mention them because they do not consider them drugs. The nurse should specifically ask about use of these preparations or any therapies the client may use in addition to medically prescribed interventions to obtain the most complete information for the medical history.

Family history identifies many risk factors that cannot be modified. A list of family members who had cancer, the type of cancer they had, and their ages when it was discovered provides important information about the client's risk for cancer, particularly breast and colon cancer.

A family history of heart disease is especially important when the client is postmenopausal because the level of estrogen, which provides some protection against coronary artery disease (CAD), decreases after menopause, and obesity may increase. If family history, obesity, or other factors increase

the client's risk for heart disease, a baseline electrocardiogram, stress test, and analysis of cholesterol and lipid profiles may be completed.

A psychosocial assessment helps caregivers determine the best way to teach the client health promotion behaviors.

BOX 28.1   Health History

Personal History
Demographic data (name, age, marital status or whether living with a partner)
Reason for seeking medical care (chief complaint)
Current and past state of health, previous surgeries
Height, weight, vital signs
Allergies (drugs, food, environmental allergens)
Medications, including the reason for taking (over-the-counter, prescribed, illicit)
Use of complementary or alternative therapies, such as herbal or botanical preparations, acupressure, and chiropractic treatment
Habits (smoking, use of alcohol, drugs)
Appetite, usual dietary intake
Exercise pattern (type, frequency, duration)
Patterns of elimination (current or chronic problems)
Sleep and rest patterns
Degree of stress and stress management techniques

Menstrual History
Age of menarche
Regularity, duration of menstrual cycle
Menstrual discomfort (time during cycles, intensity, relief measures)
Age at menopause, if applicable

Obstetric History
Gravida, para, length of gestation, weight of infant at birth
Labor experience, medical interventions, and method of delivery

Sexual History
Sexual activity (how many partners, age when first sexually active)
Method of contraception (satisfaction with method, adverse reactions, accuracy of use)
Previous sexually transmitted infection and treatment
Knowledge or practice of measures to protect self from sexually transmitted infections, including human immunodeficiency virus (HIV)

Family History
Cardiovascular problems (anemia, hypertension, clotting disorders, stroke, heart attacks)
Cancer (breast, uterine, ovarian, bowel, lung, other)
Osteoporosis

Psychosocial History
Primary language, additional languages spoken or understood, ability to read
Marital status, employment, occupation, education (relevant to determine financial, social, and emotional support)
Evaluation for possible domestic violence

Inquiry can help identify means of support and possible risks to well-being such as domestic (intimate partner) violence.

> ### 🕐 KNOWLEDGE CHECK
> 1. Why is a family history an important part of a health history?
> 2. What are some important psychosocial assessments in a health history?
> 3. What questions should be asked when taking a sexual history?

Physical Assessment

A complete physical examination is essential to detect general health problems and to identify positive aspects of health. (Refer to physical assessment textbook for a full explanation of the process of physical examination.) Blood pressure, temperature, pulse, respirations, and weight are measured at each visit. Height is taken at the initial examination and yearly. Loss of height, abnormal curvature of the vertebral column (dorsal kyphosis or scoliosis), and a thickening waistline in the absence of weight gain are important observations in identifying **osteomalacia** (softening of bones) or **osteoporosis** (increased spaces [porosity] of bone).

The heart is auscultated to determine rate and rhythm and detect heart murmurs or irregularities. Auscultation of the lungs identifies abnormal sounds suggesting the presence of fluid secondary to heart dysfunction or malignancy. The extremities are observed for varicosities or edema, and pedal pulses are palpated for strength and equality. Reduced sensation when palpating legs and feet may indicate circulation problems often associated with diabetes. The abdomen is palpated for tenderness, masses, or distention that may indicate the presence of benign or malignant tumors.

Additional assessments are necessary if the client is in a high-risk group. For instance, if there is a family history of diabetes mellitus, tests, such as a glucose tolerance test or hemoglobin A1C (Hgb A1C) may be indicated. Having a history of multiple sexual partners or a sexual partner with multiple contacts indicates testing for sexually transmitted infections (STIs), including human immunodeficiency virus (HIV) infection.

Preventive Counseling

Physical examination provides an excellent opportunity to counsel clients about preventive measures to promote health and well-being. Major preventable factors include being overweight and obese, physical inactivity, and smoking. Being overweight and obese are associated with numerous health problems including diabetes, hypertension, stroke, cardiovascular disease (CVD), and some cancers of the breast and reproductive organs. The prevalence of obesity was 42.4% in 2017 to 2018. Non-Hispanic Black adults (49.6%) had the highest age-adjusted prevalence of obesity, followed by Hispanic adults (44.8%), non-Hispanic White adults (42.2%) and non-Hispanic

Asian adults (17.4%). The prevalence of obesity was 40.0% among adults aged 20 to 39 years, 44.8% among adults aged 40 to 59 years, and 42.8% among adults aged 60 and older (Centers for Disease Control and Prevention [CDC], 2020a).

Client education and counseling regarding self-care measures to improve health should be offered. Positive health behaviors, such as adequate physical activity or making the decision to stop smoking, should be reinforced. Use of latex condoms should be emphasized for high-risk clients with multiple sexual partners or those whose partner has multiple sexual partners.

Client education about diet can improve nutritional concerns and improve overall health. For example, a weight reduction diet and increased physical activity can include measures to improve calcium intake to slow osteoporosis, lower cholesterol, and reduce the severity of diabetes.

The history or physical examination may identify other areas for client counseling. These include the dangers of malignant melanoma with repeated exposure to ultraviolet rays of the sun. In addition, counseling and referral for alcohol and other substance abuse may be required for some clients. Domestic violence issues may require counseling for the client dealing with this complex social problem.

Immunizations

Determining the need for immunizations is becoming more common at an annual well-client checkup. Immunization needs will vary with time of year, the client's age, and history of infections.

Influenza vaccine is offered during the fall and winter. The composition of annual flu vaccines must be determined well before the infections start to emerge so they may be more effective in 1 year compared with another year. Clients often do not realize that annual vaccines require about 2 weeks to become effective and can show signs of the infection if they have already acquired it at the time of their vaccination.

Hepatitis B vaccine may be offered if the client has not received previously. Rubella vaccine may be offered if the client has not had the infection or vaccine and is not pregnant. Pregnancy testing is done, and rubella immunization is delayed until after birth if pregnant.

Adults should receive a dose of tetanus and diphtheria (Td) every 10 years. One dose of tetanus, diphtheria, and acellular pertussis vaccine (Tdap) should be given to adults, ages 19 through 64, as a substitute for one of their Td immunizations. Tdap is especially important for health care professionals and anyone having close contact with an infant younger than 12 months. Pregnant clients should get a dose of Tdap during every pregnancy, to protect the newborn from pertussis (CDC, 2021).

Fear and misconceptions related to adverse effects from immunizations may become evident. The nurse should provide current education. Updated information about recommended immunizations is available at https://www.cdc.gov/vaccines/index.html.

DRUG GUIDE

Human Papillomavirus Quadrivalent Vaccine (Gardasil)

Classification
Vaccine against human papillomavirus (HPV), types 6, 11, 16, 18.

Indications
Gardasil 9 helps protect individuals ages 9 to 45 against the following diseases caused by 9 types of HPV: cervical, vaginal, and vulvar cancers in females; anal cancer; certain head and neck cancers, such as throat and back of mouth cancers; and genital warts in both males and females.

Dosage and Route
Intramuscular (IM) injection: Prefilled syringe of 0.5 mL of vaccine suspension.

Contraindications
Hypersensitivity to any component, including yeast.

Adverse Reactions
Headache is the most common adverse reaction. Others include fever, nausea, dizziness, pain, edema, itching, and bruising of the injection site. Fainting has occurred.

Nursing Considerations
Teach the client HPV vaccine is not a treatment for existing genital warts or cervical, vaginal, or vulvar cancers and regular cervical cancer screening should continue as recommended by gynecologic care provider. Cervical, vaginal, or vulvar cancers are not always caused by the HPV viral strains in this vaccine. Observation for 15 minutes after vaccine administration is recommended.

Gardasil 9 may be given as two or three shots. For persons 9 through 14 years of age, Gardasil 9 can be given using a two-dose or three-dose schedule. For the two-dose schedule, the second shot should be given 6 to 12 months after the first shot. If the second shot is given less than 5 months after the first shot, a third shot should be given at least 4 months after the second shot. For the three-dose schedule, the second shot should be given 2 months after the first shot and the third shot should be given 6 months after the first shot. For persons 15 through 45 years of age, Gardasil 9 is given using a three-dose schedule: The second shot should be given 2 months after the first shot, and the third shot should be given 6 months after the first shot. For more information about possible federal and manufacturer funding, see https://www.gardasil9.com.

KNOWLEDGE CHECK

4. What diseases may be prevented by HPV immunization?

SCREENING AND SELF-EXAMINATIONS

The value of screening procedures is based on two assumptions: (1) Prevention is better than cure, and (2) early diagnosis allows treatment while the pathologic process is most curable.

BOX 28.2 Risk Factors for Coronary Artery Disease

Cigarette smoking
Hypertension (including isolated systolic hypertension)
Unhealthy cholesterol levels
Diabetes mellitus
Overweight and obesity
Sedentary lifestyle
Poor nutrition, especially a diet high in saturated fat and cholesterol but low in fiber and fruit
Age older than 60
Postmenopause status
Family history of coronary artery disease

Data from American Heart Association. (2021). *Coronary microvascular disease (MVD).* https://www.heart.org/en/health-topics/heart-attack/angina-chest-pain/coronary-microvascular-disease-mvd.

Some screening procedures are recommended for all clients of reproductive age, including some screening procedures for early detection of breast cancer, as well as vulvar self-examination and screening for cervical cancer. Additional tests depend on the age, history, and risk assessment of the client and might include the following:

- Testing for STIs, such as gonorrhea, chlamydia, syphilis, and HIV
- Testing for rubella immunity, which is particularly important in the childbearing years, although the overall incidence of the disease is very low in the United States
- Tuberculosis skin testing or chest x-ray examination
- Cholesterol and other lipid profile testing for clients at risk for CVD (particularly important after menopause) (Box 28.2)
- Fasting glucose testing or Hgb AIC tests to identify development of diabetes, recommended every 3 years after age 45 or earlier if the client has high-risk factors such as family history or being overweight
- Urinalysis to detect signs of urinary tract infection (UTI)
- Thyroid function tests, which may be indicated if the client exhibits signs of thyroid dysfunction, such as heart palpitations and heat intolerance
- Serum testing for genes associated with specific cancers, such as the *BRCA1, BRCA2,* or *p53* genes associated with breast and some other cancers
- Serum testing for CA-125, a tumor marker that may be elevated with ovarian cancer
- Transvaginal ultrasonography, which may be recommended for clients who are at increased risk for malignant disorders of the reproductive tract
- Fecal occult blood test yearly
- Bone density test every 2 years starting at age 65; an earlier start to bone density screening may be recommended for clients at higher risk for osteoporosis
- A colonoscopy (every 10 years after age 45); a colonoscopy may be recommended more frequently if the client has a family history of colon cancer; every 3 years if presence of polyps or polyp removal

See Table 28.1 for a summary of recommended procedures.

TABLE 28.1 Screening Procedures

Procedure	Purpose
Breast self-awareness	To assess breasts so that clients become aware of their normal appearance and feel
Mammography with additional imaging, such as ultrasonography, as needed for ≥40–45 years (routine screening mammography)	To detect breast lumps before they become palpable, promoting long-term survival
Diagnostic mammograms and other imaging may be started at a younger age for clients having a higher risk for breast cancer or previous breast cancer or other disorders	
Cholesterol test	To detect blood levels that raise risk for heart disease; usually combined with additional tests for high-quality screening (lipid profile), such as triglyceride level, high-density (HDL), and low-density (LDL) lipoprotein (see Box 28.2)
Vulvar self-examination	To detect signs of precancerous conditions or infection
Pelvic examination	To confirm that no disease exists or for early detection if disease does exist
Pap test	To detect abnormal cervical cytology as early as possible
Rectal examination	To check for hemorrhoids and lesions and to evaluate sphincter control
Fecal occult blood test (FOBT)	To detect blood in stool, an early sign of colon cancer
Urinalysis	To screen for diabetes and urinary tract infections

Additional Procedures May Be Based on Risk Factors

Procedure	Risk Factors
Bone density every 2 years starting at age 65	
Begin bone density screening earlier than age 65 for high-risk clients	Family history, fracture history, estrogen deficiency, fall history, physically inactive, underweight, poor nutrition, tobacco or alcohol abuse, chronic steroid use, dementia, European or Asian ancestry
Sexually transmitted infection (STI) testing; human immunodeficiency virus (HIV) testing	Multiple sexual partners of the client or partner, history of STIs; seeking treatment for STIs, injection drug use, sexual partner who is HIV-positive or bisexual or injects drugs, recurrent or persistent episodes of infections such as candidiasis and herpes
Lipid profile	Diabetes, smoking, no estrogen use after menopause, family history of high cholesterol or coronary artery disease
Fasting glucose test	Overweight, history of gestational diabetes, family history of diabetes
Rubella antibodies	To determine immunity to rubella
Thyroid-stimulating hormone (TSH)	Signs or strong family history of thyroid disease
Blood tests to evaluate risk for reproductive cancers (see Box 28.9)	To determine the degree of higher risk influenced by genetic alterations, improving options for therapy
Transvaginal ultrasound examination	Family history of ovarian cancer
Sigmoidoscopy (every 5 years) or colonoscopy (every 10 years)	Family history of bowel cancer or older than age 50
Tuberculosis testing	To determine infection in a person at higher risk for tuberculosis

Screening for Breast Cancer

Because of the lack of evidence that indicates a clear benefit of physical breast examinations done by either a health professional or self-examinations performed by clients, the American Cancer Society (ACS) no longer recommends them. Still, all clients should be familiar with how their breasts normally look and feel and report any changes to a health care provider right away. Breast cancer that is found early, when it is small and has not spread, is easier to treat successfully. Getting regular screening tests is the most reliable way to find breast cancer early (ACS, 2021a).

Most clients have an average risk for breast cancer and should begin yearly mammograms at age 45. Clients should be able to start the screening as early as age 40 if desired and agreed upon by the health care providers regarding when to begin screening. At age 55, clients should have mammograms every other year, though those who want to continue having yearly mammograms should do so. Regular mammograms should continue for as long as the client is in good health. These guidelines are for those having an average risk for breast cancer. Clients who have a positive family history, a breast condition, or other reasons are considered high risk and should begin screening earlier and/or more often (Box 28.3).

BOX 28.3 Risk Factors for Breast Cancer

Being born female
Age: 55 years and older
Race: White clients are slightly more likely to develop breast cancer than African American clients although the gap between them has been closing in recent years. In clients under age 45, breast cancer is more common in African American clients. African American clients are also more likely to die of breast cancer at any age. Asian, Hispanic, and Native American clients have a lower risk of developing and dying from breast cancer.
Early menarche (<12 years), late menopause (>55 years)
Being taller
Having dense breast tissues
Having benign breast conditions
Personal history of breast cancer
Genetic risk factors
 Family history in first-degree relatives (mother, sister, daughter)
 Family history of other cancer
 Mutations in the BRCA1 and BRCA2 genes
 Mutations in other genes: CHEK-2 gene, ATM (ataxia-telangiectasia mutated) gene, PTEN gene
Previous irradiation of the chest area as a child or a young woman as treatment for another cancer (such as Hodgkin's disease or non-Hodgkin's lymphoma)
Previous abnormal breast biopsy results
 Atypical hyperplasia increases the risk four to five times
 Fibrocystic changes without proliferative changes do not change breast cancer risk
Exposure to diethylstilbestrol (DES)
Long-term hormone replacement therapy after menopause
Excessive alcohol consumption
Overweight or obesity
Physical inactivity
Not having given birth
Not having breastfed
Breast implants
Oral contraceptives

Data from American Cancer Society (ACS). (2021a). *Breast cancer risks and prevention.* https://www.cancer.org/cancer/breast-cancer/risk-and-prevention.html.

Despite the known value of mammography, many clients have never had a mammogram. Reasons for this include lack of a health care professional's recommendation, expense, fear that radiation exposure will cause cancer, fear of pain, and fear of a cancer diagnosis. Client education should emphasize mammography has minimal to nonexistent risks because very-low-dose radiation is used. Mammography is relatively expensive, but part of its cost is usually covered by health insurance, Medicaid, or Medicare. Screening mammograms may be offered by community agencies at low cost. Nurses should acknowledge brief discomfort may occur when the breast is compressed between two plates while the image is obtained. Scheduling the mammography after a menstrual period, when the breasts are less tender, reduces discomfort.

Vulvar Self-Examination

Vulvar self-examination should be performed monthly by clients older than 18 and by those younger than 18 who are sexually active. Vulvar self-examination is visual inspection and palpation of the external genitalia to detect signs of precancerous conditions or infections.

The client should sit in a well-lighted area and use a hand mirror to visualize the external genitalia. The client is taught to examine the vulva in a systematic manner, starting at the mons pubis and progressing to the clitoris, labia minora, labia majora, perineum, and anus followed by palpation. Reportable findings include the presence of any new moles, warts, or growths of any kind; ulcers; sores; changes in skin color; or areas of inflammation or itching. Increasing rates of human papillomavirus (HPV) are associated with increased incidence of vulvar intraepithelial neoplasia (VIN).

Pelvic Examination

The complete gynecologic assessment includes a pelvic examination. The client should schedule the examination between menstrual periods and should not douche or have sexual intercourse for at least 48 hours before the examination. Clients are also advised not to use vaginal medications, sprays, or deodorants that might interfere with interpretation of specimens that are collected.

The procedure is carefully explained before the examination. Have clients empty their bladders prior to the examination. Although pelvic examinations are relatively painless, some clients experience discomfort or emotional stress and welcome sensitive nursing support. Those having experienced genital mutilation (Box 28.4) require additional considerations. A pediatric vaginal speculum may be needed for these clients or other biologic females having a very small vaginal opening. Routine preventive pelvic examinations may be impossible for clients having an undersized opening left for drainage of urine and menstrual blood.

The pelvic examination is usually performed with the client in the lithotomy position, with a pillow under the head. The client may be placed in a semisitting position and offered a hand mirror to observe the external genitalia during examination to learn more about the genitalia. Partial draping is done to promote comfort and privacy. Older or medically compromised clients who cannot tolerate the lithotomy position may benefit from a side-lying position. The pelvic examination can also be done with the client in a semi-Fowler's position, with the knees bent and feet on the examination table, rather than using the stirrups and having the hips at the edge of the table. The paraplegic client having no control over lower extremities can usually be examined with the legs separated in a V shape without the knees being bent. Necessary equipment to be assembled before the examination begins includes gloves, speculum in several sizes, slides, cotton swabs, a fixative agent, and a Cytobrush and spatula for obtaining material for the cytology specimen or Pap test (see Cervical Cytology or Papanicolaou Test). A stool specimen may be obtained by the examiner during the rectal examination, and a slide for

BOX 28.4   Female Genital Mutilation

Female genital mutilation (FGM), sometimes called *female circumcision* or *female genital cutting,* is the ritual disfigurement and the partial or total removal of a girl's external genitalia or other injury to the external genitalia for cultural, religious, or other nontherapeutic reasons.

FGM involves the partial or total removal of external female genitalia or other injury to the female genital organs for nonmedical reasons. The practice has no health benefits for girls and women. It can cause severe bleeding and problems urinating, and later cysts, infections, and complications in childbirth, as well as increased risk of newborn deaths.

More than 200 million girls and women alive today have been cut in 30 countries in Africa, the Middle East, and Asia, where FGM is mostly carried out on young girls between infancy and age 15. FGM is a violation of the human rights of girls and women. The World Health Organization (WHO) is opposed to all forms of FGM and is opposed to health care providers performing FGM (medicalization of FGM).

Treatment of health complications of FGM in 27 high-prevalence countries costs 1.4 billion USD per year (WHO, 2020).

FGM may be done by a village practitioner using crude tools, such as knives, razor blades, broken glass, thorns, or scissors, and without anesthesia. Parents in more developed countries may obtain the procedure from a physician to ensure pain relief and sterility. However, the increasing trend for performance of FGM by health professionals is strongly discouraged.

FGM is considered a part of the coming-of-age ceremonies in some societies, and a girl may not be considered marriageable unless she has undergone the procedure. Some societies think the practice enhances female chastity and increases male sexual pleasure. Other societies consider the external female genitalia to be unsightly and dirty. Therefore they are removed to promote hygiene and the woman's attractiveness.

FGM is illegal and subject to criminal prosecution in several countries, including the United States.

Four major types of female genital mutilation exist (WHO, 2020):

- Clitoridectomy: partial or total removal of the clitoris and sometimes the prepuce that surrounds the clitoris
- Excision of part or all of the clitoris and the labia minora, with or without excision of the labia majora
- Infibulation: narrowing of the vaginal opening with the creation of a covering seal
- Other nonmedical practices of pricking, piercing, incising, scraping, and cauterizing the genitals

Health consequences may include the immediate results of severe pain, shock, hemorrhage, ulceration, urinary retention, and infection. Tetanus, bacterial sepsis, and human immunodeficiency virus infection are concerns if unsterile materials are used or if the vaginal opening is so small that anal intercourse is used as an alternative to vaginal intercourse. Infibulation may result in scar formation that causes dyspareunia, difficulty urinating, difficulty with menstruation, recurrent urinary tract infections, and infertility. Painful intercourse and reduced sexual sensitivity may have consequences on psychological health (WHO, 2020).

From World Health Organization. (2020). *Female genital mutilation. Published 2016, updated February 2020.* https://www.who.int/news-room/fact-sheets/detail/female-genital-mutilation.

this specimen should be available. Equipment for specimens to identify vaginal infections should be available.

External Organs

The pelvic examination is conducted systematically. The external organs are inspected for degree of development or atrophy of labia, distribution of hair, and character of the hymen. Any cysts, tumors, or inflammation of Bartholin's glands is noted. The urinary meatus and Skene's glands are inspected for discharge. Perineal scarring resulting from childbirth is noted.

Speculum Examination

A bivalve speculum of the appropriate size is used to inspect the vagina and cervix. The speculum is warmed with tap water and gently inserted into the vagina. Lubrication other than water or water-based lubricant on the cervix interferes with accurate cytology results. The size, shape, and color of the cervix are noted. Samples are taken for the Pap test. Routine testing for gonorrhea and chlamydia is common because of the increased incidence of these two sexually transmitted infections (STI). Additional samples of any unusual discharge are obtained for microscopic examination or culture.

Bimanual Examination

The bimanual examination provides information about the uterus, fallopian tubes, and ovaries. The labia are separated, and the gloved, lubricated index finger and middle finger of one hand are inserted into the vaginal introitus.

The cervix is palpated for consistency, size, and tenderness to motion. The uterus is evaluated by placing the other hand on the abdomen with the fingers pressing gently just above the symphysis pubis so that the uterus can be felt between the examining fingers of both hands. The size, configuration, consistency, and mobility of the uterus are evaluated Fig. 28.1.

Fallopian tubes are generally not palpated. Ovaries may be palpated between the fingers of both hands. Because ovaries atrophy after menopause, palpating the ovaries of a postmenopausal client may not be possible.

Cervical Cytology or Papanicolaou Test
Purpose

It is known that, in virtually all cases, changes occur in cells of the cervix before cervical cancer develops. These changes have variously been called *cervical intraepithelial neoplasia, dysplasia, squamous intraepithelial lesions (SILs),* and *carcinoma in situ.* Cervical cytology, or the Papanicolaou (Pap test) often combined with a test for HPV, is the most useful procedure for detecting precancerous and cancerous cells that may be shed by the cervix. It usually takes 3 to 7 years for high-grade changes in cervical cells to become cancer. Cervical cancer screening may detect these changes before they become cancer. Clients with low-grade changes can be

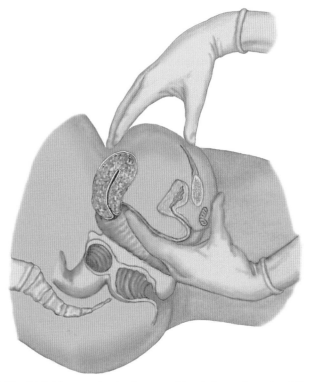

FIG. 28.1 Bimanual palpation provides information about the uterus, fallopian tubes, and ovaries.

tested more frequently to see if their cells go back to normal. Clients with high-grade changes can get treatment to have the cells removed (American College of Obstetricians and Gynecologists [ACOG], 2021).

Current Guidelines

According to the most recent guidelines from ACOG, clients aged 21 to 29 years should have a Pap test every 3 years. Clients aged 30 to 65 years should have a Pap test and an HPV test (cotesting) every 5 years. It is acceptable to have a Pap test alone every 3 years. Clients over age 65 who have had regular cervical cancer testing in the past 10 years with normal results should not be tested for cervical cancer. Once testing is stopped it should not be started again. Clients having a history of a cervical precancer should continue to be tested for at least 20 years after that diagnosis, even if testing goes past age 65. A client who has had their uterus and cervix removed for reasons not related to cervical cancer and who has no history of cervical cancer or precancer should not be tested. Some clients may require different screening schedules based on medical issues. Examples might include HIV infection, organ transplant, and exposure to diethylstilbestrol (DES) (ACOG, 2021).

Procedure

With the speculum blades open and the cervix in view, samples of the superficial layers of the cervix and endocervix are obtained. Samples are best obtained with a broom-type sampling device or a spatula and a Cytobrush.

Specimens obtained with the broom-type device, such as those in the liquid-based ThinPrep or AutoCyte tests for cervical cancer, are stirred into the liquid that preserves the cells for analysis. The liquid-based tests use image processing to select the slides that need additional preparation by a technician for best analysis.

Classification of Cervical Cytology

A great deal of variation existed in how cervical cytology findings were reported until recently. The Bethesda system was devised to offer standard terminology and give a narrative, descriptive diagnosis. It consists of three elements: (1) a statement of specimen adequacy, (2) a general categorization (normal or abnormal), and (3) a descriptive diagnosis regarding abnormal cytologic findings. Additional interpretations not related to cancer include presence of infecting organisms (such as *Trichomonas vaginalis*); changes that may be associated with inflammation, radiation, intrauterine contraceptives, or atrophy of the cervical cells.

Categories for epithelial cell abnormalities include the following:
- Atypical squamous cells of undetermined significance (ASCUS)
- Squamous intraepithelial lesion (SIL), which is subdivided into (1) low-grade SIL (including cellular changes of HPV) and (2) high-grade SIL (previously categorized as carcinoma in situ). High-grade SIL is more likely to become cancerous without definitive treatment.
- Squamous cell cancer

Glandular cell abnormalities are categorized as follows:
- Atypical glandular cells of unknown significance (AGCUS)
- Adenocarcinoma

The client's follow-up depends on the nature of the abnormality and whether it is persistent. Pap tests that have persistent ASCUS findings after a 3- to 6-month interval are also usually evaluated by colposcopy. Suspicious lesions are examined with colposcopy and biopsy.

Rectal Examination

The anus is inspected for hemorrhoids, inflammation, and lesions. The examiner's lubricated index finger is gently inserted, and sphincter tone is noted. A slide may be prepared to test for the presence of occult blood in stool.

High-sensitivity guaiac fecal occult blood testing (GFOBT) is a useful yearly screening measure for colorectal cancer beginning at age 50. The fecal immunochemical test (FIT) checks for hidden blood in the stool from the lower intestines. This test must be done every year (ACS, 2020a).

Special instructions are necessary to prevent false test results when the client is given materials for a GFOBT and include the following:
- Avoid aspirin and nonsteroidal antiinflammatory drugs (NSAIDs) such as ibuprofen or naproxen for at least 7 days before collecting the specimen.
- Avoid red meat, raw fruits and vegetables, horseradish, and vitamin C for 72 hours before testing.
- Collect a specimen from three consecutive stools.
- Return slides as directed within 4 to 6 days after the specimens are collected.

WOMEN'S HEALTH PROBLEMS

Cardiovascular Disease

CVDs include disorders of the heart and blood vessels, such as myocardial infarction (MI), congenital abnormalities, and stroke. Those discussed here primarily relate to diseases of the blood vessels, particularly CAD. The topic is extensive, and only an overview will be presented in this text. A medical–surgical text should be consulted for more extensive information about CVD and associated nursing care.

CVD is the leading global cause of death, accounting for more than 17.3 million deaths per year, a number that is expected to grow to more than 23.6 million by 2030. CVD is the number one killer of women, taking more lives than all forms of cancer combined. Non-Hispanic Blacks had a rate of 340.1 in 2008, which declined to 289.9 in 2018. Non-Hispanic Whites had a rate of 251.1 in 2008, which declined to 219.8 in 2018. American Indians/Alaskan Natives had a rate of 214.4 in 2008, which declined to 192.9 in 2018. Hispanics had a rate of 190.8 in 2008, which declined to 158.3 in 2018. Asian/Pacific Islanders had a rate of 156.5 in 2008, which declined to 127.5 in 2018.

Black adults are 32% more likely to die of CVD (American Heart Association [AHA], 2020a). Sometimes CVDs may be silent and progress undiagnosed until a client experiences signs or symptoms of a heart attack, heart failure, an arrhythmia, or stroke. Whereas some biologic female clients have no symptoms, others often experience symptoms with CVD that are atypical of biologic male clients: unusual fatigue, upper back pain, nausea and/or vomiting, loss of appetite, dizziness, palpitations, jaw pain, and neck pain. These may occur during rest, begin during physical activity, or be triggered by stress (AHA, 2020b).

Cerebrovascular accident or "stroke" affecting the arteries leading to and within the brain is the number five cause of death and a leading cause of disability in the United States. A stroke occurs when a blood vessel carrying oxygen and nutrients to the brain is either blocked by a clot or ruptures. As a result, circulation to part of the brain is compromised, and it becomes oxygen-deprived. If unresolved, the brain cells die. Stroke can be ischemic if a cerebral artery is blocked or hemorrhagic if a cerebral artery ruptures. Almost 90% of strokes are ischemic. Women in the 45- to 74-year age group have a lower mortality rate than men in this age group. However, women older than 85 years have a higher stroke mortality rate than men in their age group. Metabolic syndrome (abdominal obesity, dyslipidemia, hypertension, and hyperglycemia) doubles the stroke risk in women but does not affect the stroke risk in men. Migraine, particularly with an aura, is associated with risk for stroke in women younger than 45 and has been associated with increased CVD risk. Symptoms of ischemic stroke appear to have few gender differences. Traditional symptoms include arm and/or leg weakness and speech disturbance. Less common symptoms include facial weakness, loss of sensation in arm and/or leg, headache, and nonorthostatic dizziness (AHA, 2020b). Nurses should identify possible risk factors of the clients they care for and provide referrals if needed. The nurse should educate clients about risk factors and symptoms of CVD. An environment of collaborative and participatory care may help clients adopt health-promotion behaviors including weight control and exercise.

Risk Factors

Many risk factors exist for CVD including but not limited to hypertension, inadequate physical activity, being overweight and obese, and poor nutrition. Risk factors often contribute to development of other problems that further increase the risk for CVD, such as type 2 diabetes. Each risk factor may add to the risk for developing comorbidities.

Risk factors may be modifiable or nonmodifiable. Growing older is an example of a nonmodifiable risk factor as clients lose the protection from estrogen, secreted before menopause, on the blood vessels. Estrogen's protective effect delays onset of CVD, making most female clients older at the onset of the disease than male clients. See other risk factors listed in Box 28.2.

The leading modifiable cause of CVD is smoking. Cigarette smoking adds to the burden of heart, blood vessel, and respiratory disorders. Both systolic and diastolic blood pressure elevations are associated with CAD and other vascular disorders. Adequate control of hypertension reduces death and disability from MI, stroke, and other blood vessel disorders.

Dyslipidemia (abnormal fat and cholesterol levels) is more likely in all clients who do not get adequate exercise, adding further to the risk.

Prevention is the key to reducing death and illness from all CVDs among clients (AHA, 2020b).

Health Promotion Activities to Reduce the Risk for Coronary Artery Disease. Risks for CAD can be lowered with the following health promotion activities:

- Stop smoking
- Maintain a normal weight
- Maintain good nutrition
- Limit alcohol to one drink per day
- Control high blood pressure
- Exercise
- Control diabetes

To learn more about CVD and its prevention, visit the AHA website at https://www.heart.org.

Hypertension. People may be unaware of current definitions for the levels of blood pressure and do not seek the information because hypertension can be a disease that causes subtle damage over long periods. According to the current AHA guidelines, normal blood pressure is below 120/80 mm Hg. Clients with a systolic pressure of 120 to 129 and a diastolic pressure of less than 80 are said to have an elevated blood pressure. Clients with a systolic pressure of 130 or higher or a diastolic pressure of 80 or higher and that is elevated over time are said to have hypertension (AHA, 2020c). Lowering hypertension reduces the risk of CAD including stroke. Medication is often prescribed when lifestyle modifications fail to lower the blood pressure adequately. The Dietary Approaches to Stop Hypertension (DASH) diet plan was developed to lower blood pressure without medication in research sponsored by the National Institutes of Health, DASH. Early research indicates that following a DASH diet could lower blood pressure as well as first-line blood pressure medications, even with a sodium intake of up to 3300 mg/day. Since then, numerous studies have shown the DASH diet reduces the risk of many diseases, including some kinds of cancer, stroke, heart disease, heart failure, kidney stones, and diabetes (Mayo Clinic, 2019a). The DASH diet has been proven to be an effective way to lose weight and increase health promotion, and it can be viewed at https://dashdiet.org/default.html.

Diet and Glucose Control. Clients with diabetes have a relatively greater risk for CAD, so maintaining weight and glucose levels within normal limits is especially important. Good nutrition is the primary means to control the lipid profile. Dietary recommendations should be individualized, but general guidelines include limiting fat intake to a maximum of 30% of daily calories with no more than 10% of daily calories should come from saturated fat (found in foods such as meat, butter, cream, and cheese). It is recommended daily cholesterol intake should be less than 200 mg/day. Increasing evidence shows fish has cardiovascular benefits, and at least two servings per week is recommended. Eating a diet high in vegetables, fruits, and low-fat dairy products and limiting salt intake to under 6 g/day and alcohol to a maximum of one drink per day have shown to be beneficial at reducing blood pressure.

Physical Activity. Aerobic exercise helps control weight, blood pressure, lipid profile, and glucose level. It reduces body fat while increasing muscle mass and improving muscle tone, making it easier to maintain a healthy body weight or reduce weight if overweight or obese. Additionally, it reduces stress and depression. As described by the Physical Activity Guidelines for Americans, adults should engage in at least 150 minutes of moderate-intensity activity each week or 75 to 150 minutes per week of vigorous aerobic activity (U.S. Department of Health and Human Services [DHHS], 2020b).

Aspirin. Low-dose aspirin therapy each day has been shown to be beneficial to inhibit platelet aggregation, which can increase clot formation and lead to CAD. Some adults between ages 40 and 70 years at high risk of developing CVD and at low risk of bleeding may consider taking low-dose aspirin if they have experienced an MI, stroke, coronary stent, or coronary artery bypass graft surgery. Clients without these conditions or procedures and are older than 70 years, younger than 40 years, or at increased risk of bleeding because of a medical condition or medications should not take aspirin for primary prevention of heart disease (Peters & Mutharasan, 2020).

KNOWLEDGE CHECK

8. What are the symptoms of CAD, such as an MI, in biologic female clients?
9. List appropriate measures to reduce the risk for CAD.

DISORDERS OF THE BREAST

Benign Disorders of the Breast

Benign breast disease is an umbrella term for various nonmalignant lesions, such as tumors, trauma, mastalgia, and nipple discharge. These benign lesions are not usually associated with an increased risk for malignancy; however, McMullen et al. (2019) found an association up to 50% risk of developing breast cancer under certain histopathologic and clinical circumstances. A palpable mass upon clinical evaluation is evident in both benign and malignant breast conditions. Clinical findings include skin dimpling (peau de'orange), thickening, pain, and nipple discharge. The etiology of benign breast disease demonstrates a positive clinical association with biologically female clients receiving estrogen and antiestrogen treatment. The prevalence of benign breast lesions in postmenopausal women receiving estrogens and progestins for over 8 years is increased by 1.7-fold. During the WHI study, the combined use of estrogen and progestin correlated with a 74% risk of benign breast disease. The use of antiestrogens led to a 28% reduction in the prevalence of benign proliferative breast disease (Kour et al., 2019).

Fibrocystic Breast Changes

Fibrocystic breast disease is the most common benign type of breast disease and is diagnosed in millions of biologically female clients throughout the world. Hormonal factors dictate the function, evaluation, and treatment of this disease. Thickening of the normal breast tissue, or fibrosis, occurs in the early stages. Later, multiple cysts may develop and upon palpation are found to be a smooth, well-delineated nodules that are tender and movable. Nodules may be described as lumpy, rubbery, or rope-like and often vary in size, from less than 1 cm to several centimeters. Tissue specimens obtained by fine-needle aspiration (FNA) or from an open surgical biopsy are examined to identify the tissue type and any malignant changes. Signs and symptoms of fibrocystic breasts may include breast lumps or areas of thickening blending into the surrounding breast tissue, generalized breast pain or tenderness, breast lumps fluctuating in size with the menstrual cycle, green or dark brown nonbloody nipple discharge that tends to leak without pressure or squeezing, breast changes with similarity in both breasts, and monthly increase in breast pain or lumpiness from midcycle (ovulation) to just before the menstrual cycle.

Fibrocystic breast changes occur most often in clients in their twenties to fifties. It is rare for postmenopausal clients to experience fibrocystic breast changes unless they are on hormone therapy. Reportable findings include new breast lump or area of prominent thickening, continuous or worsening breast pain, breast changes that persist after menstrual cycle ends, or a previously evaluated breast lump that changes or grows in size (but now seems bigger or otherwise changed) (Mayo Clinic, 2020). If breast pain is severe for more than 6 months and disrupts daily activities, therapies such as tamoxifen, bromocriptine, or danazol can be options. Due to the recurrent nature and long duration of these symptoms, treatment for several months is necessary. Aspiration of cysts may relieve pain, with follow-up needed only if the cyst recurs or fluid aspirated is suspicious. Fluid from cysts aspirated for symptomatic relief does not require cytologic assessment. This evaluation is reserved for clinically evident lumps that resolve following the FNA procedure or where the cyst fluid appears macroscopically bloodstained (Malherbe & Fatima, 2021).

Fibrocystic breast changes may fall into the following three categories:

- Nonproliferative lesions
- Hyperplasia without atypical cells
- Atypical hyperplasia

Hyperplastic lesions with atypical cellular changes have an increased risk to become malignant, but most clients with fibrocystic breast changes do not have a greater risk for breast cancer.

Specific symptom relief for fibrocystic disease has not proved beneficial, but some methods may be worth trying. Wearing a support bra is a simple way to reduce pain from large breasts pulling on ligaments. Avoiding caffeine and other stimulants (coffee, tea, chocolate, and some soft drinks) reduces levels of methylxanthines, which may increase discomfort during the last half of the menstrual cycle. Oral contraceptives taken during the secretory phase (second half) of the menstrual cycle have been successful, but pain returns if the contraceptives are discontinued.

Fibroadenoma

Fibroadenomas are common benign tumors of the breast, and although they may occur at any age, they are most common during the teenage years and the twenties. Fibroadenomas are composed of both fibrous and glandular tissue. They are firm, freely mobile nodules that may or may not be tender when palpated. They are often described as feeling like a marble under the skin. Fibroadenomas do not change during the menstrual cycle. They are generally located in the upper, outer quadrant of the breast, and more than one is often present.

Treatment may involve careful observation for a few months to determine whether the mass is stable. FNA or core biopsy of the tumor is done if the mass continues to enlarge. The mass may be surgically removed and analyzed to rule out malignancy if results of other diagnostic tests are not conclusive (Mayo Clinic, 2019c).

Mammary Duct Ectasia

Mammary duct ectasia occurs when one or more milk ducts beneath the nipple widens. The duct walls thicken, and the duct may fill with fluid. The milk duct may become clogged with a thick, sticky substance. The condition often causes no symptoms, but some clients may have nipple discharge, breast tenderness, or inflammation of the clogged duct (periductal mastitis).

Mammary duct ectasia most often occurs in clients during perimenopause, around age 45 to 55 years, but can also occur after menopause. The condition often improves without treatment. If symptoms persist, antibiotics or surgery might be indicated to remove the affected milk duct (Mayo Clinic, 2019d).

Mammary duct ectasia initiates an inflammatory process resulting in the following:

- A firm or irregular mass near the areola
- Enlarged axillary nodes
- Nipple retraction and discharge

Intraductal Papilloma

Intraductal papillomas are benign, wart-like tumors that grow within the milk ducts of the breast. They are made up of gland tissue along with fibrous tissue and blood vessels called fibrovascular tissue. Solitary papillomas are single tumors that often grow in the large milk ducts near the nipple and are a common cause of clear or bloody nipple discharge, especially when it comes from only one breast. Solitary papillomas may be felt as a small lump behind or next to the nipple. Sometimes they cause pain. Papillomas may also be found in small ducts in areas of the breast farther from the nipple. In this case there are often several growths and are referred to as multiple papillomas. They are less likely to cause nipple discharge. In papillomatosis, there are very small areas of cell growth within the ducts, but they are not as distinct as papillomas.

Ductograms, which are x-rays of the breast ducts, are sometimes helpful in diagnosing papillomas. An ultrasound and/or mammogram may be obtained to learn more about the size and location of papillomas. If the papilloma is large enough to be felt, a biopsy may be done.

Having a solitary papilloma does not raise breast cancer risk unless it contains other breast changes, such as atypical hyperplasia. However, having multiple papillomas increases breast cancer risk slightly. The usual treatment is surgery to remove the papilloma and the part of the duct (ACS, 2019c).

Nursing Considerations

Nurses should acknowledge the anxiety that many clients experience when a breast disorder is discovered, realizing apprehension may continue while the client awaits a definitive diagnosis. Clients benefit from learning most breast disorders are benign. However, benign disorders do increase the risk for later occurrence of cancer. Clients should be encouraged to ask questions and share concerns regarding their diagnosis.

Diagnostic Procedures

Differentiating between benign and malignant breast disorders may require diagnostic procedures. Ultrasound examination can be used to discriminate fluid-filled cysts from solid tissue, which is more likely to be malignant. FNA biopsy can be done to remove fluid or small tissue fragments for analysis of the cells. Core biopsy uses a larger needle to obtain a cylinder of tissue from an area of questionable breast tissue. Open, or surgical, biopsy is performed to remove all or part of the lump of breast tissue if the following other conditions exist:

- Suspicious mass that persists through a menstrual cycle
- Bloody fluid aspirated from a cyst
- Failure of the mass to disappear completely after fluid aspiration
- Recurrence of the cyst after one or two aspirations
- Solid dominant mass not diagnosed as fibroadenoma
- Serous or serosanguineous nipple discharge
- Nipple ulceration or persistent crusting
- Skin edema and erythema suspicious for inflammatory breast carcinoma (IBC)
- Suspicious mammography or ultrasound findings
- Known or possible genetic abnormality that increases a client's risk for breast cancer

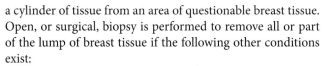

KNOWLEDGE CHECK

10. How is fibrocystic breast disease treated?
11. What diagnostic procedures are used to determine whether a breast disorder is benign or malignant?

Malignant Tumors of the Breast

Incidence

Breast cancer is the most common cancer in American biologic females, except for skin cancers. Currently, the average risk of a biologic female in the United States developing breast cancer sometime in their life is about 13%. This means there is a one in eight chance the client will develop breast cancer. The ACS estimates 281,550 new cases of invasive breast cancer will be diagnosed in biologic females, about 49,290 new cases of ductal carcinoma will be diagnosed, and about 43,600 of these clients will die of breast cancer (ACS, 2021b).

In recent years, incidence rates have increased by 0.5% per year. Breast cancer is the second leading cause of cancer death in biologic female clients (only lung cancer kills more each year).

Since 2007, breast cancer death rates have been steady in clients younger than 50 but have continued to decrease in older clients. From 2013 to 2018, the death rate decreased by 1% per year. These decreases are believed to be the result of earlier detection through screening and increased awareness, as well as better treatments. Breast cancer in biologic males is rare. The lifetime risk in biologic males is estimated to be 1 in 1000 (ACS, 2021b).

Overall, White clients are slightly more likely to develop breast cancer than African American clients, although the gap between them has been closing in recent years. In clients under age 45, breast cancer is more common in African American biologic female clients. African American clients are also more likely to die of breast cancer at any age. Asian, Hispanic, and Native American women have a lower risk of developing and dying from breast cancer (ACS, 2019a).

Risk Factors

Although the actual cause of breast cancer remains unknown, several factors are known to increase the risk for the development of breast and ovarian cancer or other diseases (see Box 28.3). Mutations in two genes (*BRCA1* and *BRCA2*) thought to be responsible for most cases of familial breast and ovarian cancer, including breast cancer in men, continue to be studied. Mutation of the *CHEK-2* gene has shown higher risk for development of breast cancer in both women and men. Mutation of the *p53* tumor suppressor gene has been associated with breast and other cancers. Study of genetic links to many types of cancers and nonmalignant diseases is ongoing. Because research has linked these and other genes to an increased risk for breast or other cancers, testing is offered to the biologic female having a higher risk or who has developed cancer at a younger age than expected (National Cancer Institute [NCI] & NIH, 2020).

Pathophysiology

Approximately 65% to 80% of breast cancers are infiltrating ductal carcinoma, which originates in the epithelial lining of the mammary ducts. The cancer becomes invasive when it is no longer confined to the duct and spreads to surrounding breast tissue. Another 10% to 14% of invasive breast cancers are infiltrating lobular cancer that originates in the milk-secreting pockets of breast tissue. Most breast cancers grow in irregular patterns and invade the lymphatic channels, eventually causing lymphatic edema and the dimpling of the skin that resembles an orange peel (**peau d'orange**). Several types of breast tumors may be present at the same time.

IBC has cutaneous findings with invasive involvement in the dermis. IBC is rare, occurring in 1% to 2% of biologic female clients and more likely to occur in younger or African American clients. IBC is aggressive and may manifest as a pink or red skin rash rather than a distinct lump that might show on imaging. Tenderness, itching, or breast edema may be present. These characteristics are typical of infection, so antibiotics are often prescribed. The client should promptly contact a health professional for follow-up testing if antibiotics do not quickly clear the infection to determine a treatment plan if needed.

Cancer cells are carried by the lymph channels to the lymph nodes, and 40% to 50% of clients have involvement of axillary lymph nodes at time of diagnosis. By the time the client consults a health care provider, breast cancer might have metastasized and is no longer confined to local tissue. Metastasis occurs when the malignant cells are spread by both blood and lymph systems to distant organs. Distant metastases include the lungs, liver, bones, and brain.

Staging

Once confirmation of malignancy occurs staging is necessary to determine the severity of the cancer and develop a treatment plan. Staging is based on the tumor, node, and metastasis (TNM) system used to describe the cancer's anatomic extent. Stages of breast cancer progress from stage 1, which indicates a small tumor without lymphatic involvement in the local area or metastases, to stage 4, which indicates spread to lymph nodes and metastases to distant organs. Staging is used to guide treatment and provide prognosis. The type of cancer cell, the presence of hormone receptors, and the proliferative rate of the breast cancer cells are important factors to consider when planning treatment.

Management

There are many medications and treatment procedures available to treat breast cancer with many more being studied. Some are classified as local treatments including surgery and radiation therapy, which are used to treat a specific tumor or area of the body. Medication treatments include chemotherapy, immunotherapy, or targeted therapy and are classified as systemic treatments because they can affect the entire body. The combination of therapies is individualized for each client. New techniques, medications, and management emerge frequently, and nurses should stay abreast of frequently emerging information.

Surgical Treatment

Curative Surgery. Curative or primary surgery is performed when breast cancer is located in one area. It is called "curative" because the purpose of the surgery is to remove all of the cancer completely. In this case surgery can be the main treatment. It may be used along with other treatments like chemotherapy or radiation therapy given before or after the operation, but surgery can also be used alone.

Surgery to Debulk Cancer. Debulking surgery is used to remove some, but not all, of the cancer. It's called debulking because the tumor being treated is a large, bulky object and might be located very close to important organs or tissues. Debulking can decrease the size of the tumor and is sometimes performed if entire tumor removal would result in damage to organs or tissues within close proximity. Often in the case of debulking, the surgeon might remove as much of the tumor as safely possible with a plan to treat the remainder with radiation, chemotherapy, or other treatments.

Palliative Surgery. Palliative surgery is used to treat problems caused by advanced cancer. Palliative surgery can be used with other treatments to correct a problem that's causing discomfort or disability. This type of surgery may also be used to treat pain when the pain is hard to control with medicine and can ease problems caused by cancer. Clients undergoing palliative surgery often feel better, however, because the cancer is usually in an advanced stage—it is not done to treat or cure the cancer itself.

Supportive Surgery. Supportive surgery is performed to assist clients to receive other types of treatment. For example, a vascular access device such as a Port-A-Cath® or Infusaport® is a thin, flexible tube that can be surgically placed into a large vein and connected to a small drum-like device that's placed just under the skin. A needle is put into the drum of the port to give treatments and draw blood, instead of putting needles in the hands and arms each time intravenous (IV) fluids, blood transfusions, or treatments are given.

Restorative (Reconstructive) Surgery. Reconstructive surgery is used for cosmetic purposes. It can also be used to restore the function of an organ or body part after surgery. Examples include breast reconstruction after mastectomy (surgical removal of one or both breasts). Breast reconstruction is often an option in breast cancer treatment, and the timing of reconstruction should be discussed with the client before surgical treatment. The prospect of having life-threatening breast cancer and simultaneously facing the loss of one or both breast may be overwhelming for many clients. Conversely, delayed reconstruction may give a client time to learn about the procedure, to heal from the mastectomy, and to explore and express emotions related to additional surgeries.

Several methods of breast reconstruction are performed. The tissue expansion method uses an empty silicone prosthesis fitted with a valve that can be accessed by percutaneous needle puncture. The bag is filled with saline in small increments to slowly expand the tissue. When the desired volume is attained, the incision is reopened, the device is removed, and the expander is exchanged for the appropriate implant. In some models, only the valve must be removed, and the expander serves as the permanent implant (ACS, 2019b).

Tissue flap procedures move autogenous tissue from the back, abdomen, or buttocks to create a breast mound. Although these procedures do not always involve implants of a foreign substance as the tissue expansion method does, they involve at least two incisions: one at the breast and one at the site of the client's donor tissue. Not all clients are candidates for muscle flap grafts, particularly those with diabetes or connective tissue disorders and those who smoke, because these procedures involve altering the blood supply to the transplanted tissue, with the possibility of poor wound healing for these clients (ACS, 2019b).

Preventive (Prophylactic) Surgery. Preventive or prophylactic surgery is performed to remove body tissue likely to become cancer, even though there are no signs of cancer at the time of the surgery. Sometimes a mastectomy or double mastectomy may be performed when the condition puts the client at high risk for developing breast cancer. The surgery is done to reduce breast cancer risk.

For example, some clients with a strong family history of breast cancer and have an inherited breast cancer gene (called *BRCA1* or *BRCA2*). Because the risk of breast cancer is very high, removing the breasts (prophylactic mastectomy) may be considered. This means the breasts are removed before cancer is found.

Adjuvant Therapy. Adjuvant therapy is supportive or additional therapy usually recommended after the surgical procedure. This includes radiation, chemotherapy, hormone therapy, and immunotherapy. The decision about adjuvant therapy is based on the client's age, stage of the disease, personal preference, and the hormone receptor status of the lesion. Radiation and chemotherapy are known to improve the chance of long-term survival, and one or both are usually recommended after surgical excision of the tumor. Research continues to determine the best uses for these adjuvant therapies when treating breast cancer.

Radiation Therapy. Radiation uses high-energy rays to destroy cancer cells remaining in the breast, the chest wall, and the underarm area after surgery. The lymph nodes above the clavicle and the internal mammary lymph nodes are also irradiated. Radiation may be used to reduce the size of a large tumor before surgery. A radiation oncologist directs use of radiation in cancer therapy. The skin in the treated area may have a reaction similar to sunburn. Lymphedema is more likely to occur if the axillary lymph nodes are treated or removed. A newer technology to limit the adverse effects of radiation on normal tissues while giving a maximum dose of radiation to the tumor site is intensity-modulated radiation therapy.

Chemotherapy. Chemotherapy drugs are designed to kill the proliferating cancer cells. The specific combination of drugs and the number of treatment cycles are individualized for factors such as type of cancer cells, the client's age, the hormone receptor status of malignant cells, whether the client is postmenopausal, and other important factors such as medications needed for nonmalignant disorders. Chemotherapy may both precede and follow tumor removal. Depending on the specific drugs, chemotherapeutics often destroy normal cells, especially rapidly dividing cells such as those in the mucosa, the blood cells, and the platelets. For this reason, the client often has sore, bleeding gums or other bleeding tendencies and may be more susceptible to infection during treatment. Loss of head and body hair or menstrual irregularities are common side effects during treatment. Anemia, with resulting fatigue, is common because erythrocyte production is impaired. Antiemetic drugs may be given to control nausea.

Hormone Therapy. Medications to reduce production of estrogen are prescribed because many breast tumors are estrogen and/or progesterone receptor–positive, meaning their growth is stimulated by estrogen. Estrogen receptor–positive tumors may occur in both premenopausal and postmenopausal clients. Risks and benefits of proposed estrogen-blocking medications are discussed with the oncologist, particularly in premenopausal clients because their estrogen and progesterone levels are coordinated with their menstrual cycles.

Tamoxifen is one of the oldest estrogen-blocking drugs given for breast cancer to prevent recurrence. However, tumors in some clients become resistant to tamoxifen, and the cells actually use the drug to stimulate growth. Laboratory values for calcium, cholesterol, and triglycerides may be elevated with tamoxifen.

Anastrozole (Arimidex), exemestane (Aromasin), and letrozole (Femara) are aromatase inhibitors that hinder production of estrogen because they block conversion of androgens to estrogen in postmenopausal clients. Aromatase inhibitors are being studied as alternatives to tamoxifen because they inhibit estrogen in a different way.

Raloxifene (Evista) is an estrogen modifier used to reduce osteoporosis by binding to estrogen receptors; therefore, this drug also blocks estrogen effects on the breast. Raloxifene lowers levels of low-density lipoproteins and cholesterol.

Immunotherapy. Trastuzumab (Herceptin) is a biological-based therapy targeting cell pathways promoting cancer growth. Some tumors produce excessive amounts of the HER-2 protein, promoting tumor cell growth. Trastuzumab blocks the effect of this protein to inhibit growth of the cancer cells. Research is ongoing into other immunotherapy for breast and other cancers.

Psychosocial Consequences of Breast Cancer

A diagnosis of breast cancer is a time of fear, concern, and stress for many clients. Often clients experience feelings of uncertainty when making treatment decisions. Because of the many complexities of breast cancer treatment, consultations with multiple members of the health care team is critical. Concerns expressed during treatment include fear of death, questions about quality of life, changes in body image, changes in sexuality, and possible side effects.

Breast cancer has psychological consequences not only for clients but also for their children, family, friends, and partners. Many clients experience sleep disturbances, eating disorders, and work-related issues. Client relationships may become strained, particularly in the areas of sexuality and communication.

Nursing Considerations

Nurses should include a psychosocial assessment as part of the nursing care plan and arrange for holistic care. Clients may depend on the nurse for emotional support and answers to questions. Clients should be encouraged to express feelings and emotions, and the nurse should convey a sense of empathetic understanding by quiet presence, touch, and attention to the client's concerns. Many clients feel a sense of loss of control and may be overwhelmed by their diagnosis and treatment plan. In addition to providing time and demonstrating genuine interest in client concerns, the nurse should use therapeutic communication techniques such as clarifying, paraphrasing, and reflecting feelings to encourage the client to participate in decisions about care.

For clients undergoing surgery, preoperative teaching should include significant others when possible. Client education should include the length of the hospital stay, dressings, drainage tubes, and appearance of incisions for procedures being planned. Specific exercises such as arm lifts and pulley exercises may be necessary to promote flexibility in surgical areas.

Lymphedema, caused by blocked drainage of the lymphatic system in the arm on the side of the mastectomy, is possible if most axillary lymph nodes are removed. Lymphedema may not occur for many years and is not anticipated for clients who do not require an extensive lymphatic tissue removal in the axilla. Compression arm sleeves, which are similar to thromboembolism deterrent (TED) hose, are an available treatment to control lymphedema if needed.

Discharge teaching focuses on self-care and the need for continued care and treatment. Some topics to be included are how to reduce the risk for wound infection, care of the arm on the affected side, side effects of postoperative and adjuvant medications, care of drains, and signs and symptoms that should be reported to the provider. Many clients will benefit from information about groups such as Reach to Recovery through the ACS (ACS, 2019d). The groups provide support, information, and guidance after mastectomy. Additional support groups may be associated with the hospital and oncology center. The internet may be a resource for community and online support groups. Printed information about local support groups is usually provided at discharge.

> **? KNOWLEDGE CHECK**
>
> 12. Why is staging for breast cancer important?
> 13. What is meant by *adjuvant therapy,* and why is it used?
> 14. When should the discussion with the client about breast reconstruction options occur and what methods are used for reconstruction?
> 15. What should preoperative teaching for breast cancer surgery include?
> 16. What should discharge planning following breast cancer treatment emphasize?

MENSTRUAL CYCLE DISORDERS

The four most common menstrual cycle disorders are absence of menses (**amenorrhea**), abnormal uterine bleeding, pain associated with the menstrual cycle, and cyclic mood changes, including PMS. Although most of the disorders are benign, all require comprehensive gynecologic assessment. Nurses should be knowledgeable about underlying processes, diagnostic procedures, and expected treatment to fulfill the basic core of nursing activities, which include client advocacy, education, and supportive counseling.

Amenorrhea

In addition to reproductive health, menstrual patterns can be an indicator of overall health and self-perception of well-being. Primary amenorrhea occurs when the client has not had their first menstrual period by age 15 or 3 years after breast development. Secondary amenorrhea occurs when the client has not had a menstrual period for 3 months or has had irregular menstrual periods for 6 months. Amenorrhea can be the result of primary ovarian insufficiency, hypothalamic or pituitary disorders, or other endocrine gland disorders. Abnormalities in the uterus, vagina, or hymen can obstruct the outflow of the menstrual flow. Congenital enzyme abnormalities may disable different aspects of the reproductive cycle.

Polycystic ovarian syndrome (PCOS) is caused by an imbalance of reproductive hormones primarily occurring in the ovaries. There are multiple cyst that are in the ovaries. The client may present with amenorrhea or irregular periods. Most clients with PCOS may present with infertility due to immature ovarian cysts. The cause is unknown, but the client will present with high levels of androgen and insulin. This causes anovulation male-pattern baldness or increase in facial, chest, and abdominal hair; insulin resistance leading to obesity; and type 2 diabetes.

A detailed history should be obtained to include information related to menarche (first menstrual period) and menstrual cycle patterns, eating and exercise habits, psychosocial stress, body weight changes, medication use, galactorrhea (flow of milk from breasts), and chronic illness. Additional

information might include neurologic symptoms and thyroid-related symptoms. The physical examination should include height, weight, and anthropometric measurements. Laboratory tests include a pregnancy test and serum follicle-stimulating hormone, luteinizing hormone, prolactin, and thyroid-stimulating hormone levels.

Medical management depends on the cause identified in a diagnostic workup. Treatment for amenorrhea should address the underlying cause and may be lifelong. Hormone therapy may reestablish regular menstrual periods if the cause is hormone imbalance. Clients with primary ovarian insufficiency may require hormone replacement therapy or contraceptives to maintain ovary function. Infertility services should be offered. Clients with polycystic ovary syndrome should undergo screening and intervention to identify a metabolic disorder and endometrial cancer risk.

However, some conditions cannot be successfully treated. For example, if the cause is reproductive tract or congenital anomalies, normal menses and fertility may not be possible, and psychological support becomes the most important therapy. Functional hypothalamic amenorrhea may indicate an eating disorder and decreased bone density.

Nursing Considerations

Nurses and other providers should care for clients with amenorrhea with sensitivity and emotional support (Klein et al., 2019). Client education includes teaching the importance of proper nutrition and healthy food choices. The nurse should provide information regarding the effect of physical activity on menstrual periods. Maintaining a healthy weight can reduce factors related to PCOS. Referral for psychological counseling may be necessary for clients having eating disorders or infertility. Providing a referral for an infertility support group such as RESOLVE may help with coping (RESOLVE, 2021).

Abnormal Uterine Bleeding

The normal menstrual cycle was described in Chapter 3. Abnormal uterine bleeding (AUB) includes prolonged or heavy bleeding (**menorrhagia**), intermenstrual bleeding that occurs irregularly and often between menstrual periods (**metrorrhagia**), or bleeding that occurs irregularly and more frequently (**menometrorrhagia**), which is essentially a combination of the other two terms. Complications of an unrecognized pregnancy, such as spontaneous abortion, should be considered when making the diagnosis. Many clients may show signs of anemia due to the heavy bleeding. In the postmenopausal client, AUB is abnormal and should be evaluated for malignancy.

Etiology

The most common causes of AUB include the following five basic categories:
1. Pregnancy complications, such as spontaneous abortion
2. Anatomic lesions, either benign or malignant, of the vagina, cervix, or uterus
3. Drug-induced bleeding, such as breakthrough bleeding that may occur in clients taking hormonal contraceptives

4. Systemic disorders, such as diabetes mellitus, uterine myomas (fibroids), and hypothyroidism
5. Failure to ovulate

Management

Evaluation of abnormal uterine bleeding may include a sensitive pregnancy test, coagulation studies, and tests to determine whether ovulation is occurring. Hormone and liver function tests, plus tests to determine whether the client is anemic, often are done. Ultrasonography or hysteroscopy may be used to look for polyps and check the condition of the uterine lining.

A common hormone treatment is progestin–estrogen combination oral contraceptives to suppress ovulation and allow a more stable endometrial lining to form. Surgical therapy may include dilation and curettage (D&C) to remove polyps or to diagnose **endometrial hyperplasia** (excess normal uterine lining cells), which may be treated with progesterone to suppress excess uterine lining. Hysterectomy may be performed if the uterus is enlarged because of fibroids or adenomyosis (benign invasive growth of the endometrium into the muscular layer of the uterus) and if the client does not want children. Laser ablation may be used to permanently remove the endometrial lining without hysterectomy. Many clients will need treatment for iron deficiency anemia. AUB is the most common symptom of endometrial cancer in postmenopausal women (Henry et al., 2020).

Nursing Considerations

Nurses should encourage clients to seek medical attention promptly when AUB occurs. Client education includes instructions to keep accurate records of bleeding episodes and amount of blood lost by counting feminine hygiene products used. Offering false reassurance is unwise, but providing information about diagnostic procedures, such as pelvic examination, Pap test, and pelvic ultrasound is beneficial.

KNOWLEDGE CHECK

17. How does primary amenorrhea differ from secondary amenorrhea in terms of onset?
18. What are possible causes of abnormal uterine bleeding and why should it not be ignored?

Cyclic Pelvic Pain

Cyclic pelvic pain should be distinguished from acute pelvic pain. Acute pelvic pain is sudden in onset and is not experienced with each menstrual cycle. It may indicate a serious disorder, such as ectopic pregnancy or appendicitis. Cyclic pelvic pain occurs repetitively and predictably in a specific phase of the menstrual cycle. The most common causes of cyclic pelvic pain are mittelschmerz, primary **dysmenorrhea** (painful menstruation), and **endometriosis** (tissue resembling endometrium outside uterine cavity). Secondary dysmenorrhea, or pelvic pain that is not cyclic, is usually related to pelvic pathologic processes.

Mittelschmerz

Mittelschmerz ("middle" pain) is pelvic pain occurring midway between menstrual periods at the time of ovulation. The pain results from growth of the dominant follicle within the ovary or rupture of the follicle and subsequent spillage of follicular fluid and blood into the peritoneal space. The pain is sharp and is felt on the right or left side of the pelvis. It generally lasts from a few hours to 2 days, and slight vaginal bleeding may accompany the discomfort. Generally, clients do not need medical treatment but require explanation of the discomfort and possible use of mild analgesics.

Primary Dysmenorrhea

Primary dysmenorrhea is menstrual pain without identified pathologic cause. Its onset is usually 1 to 3 years after menstruation begins, when ovulatory menstrual cycles are well established, and it is most common in young, nulliparous clients. Commonly called "cramps," primary dysmenorrhea causes significant loss of school or work hours. The pain begins within hours of the onset of menses, and it is spasmodic or colicky because of increased prostaglandins secreted at this time. It is felt in the lower abdomen but often radiates to the lower back or down the legs. Nausea, vomiting, loose stools, or dizziness may also occur. The duration of the pain is usually 48 to 72 hours.

Two recommended treatments of primary dysmenorrhea provide marked relief: oral contraceptives and prostaglandin inhibitors. Oral contraceptives decrease the amount of endometrial growth occurring during the menstrual cycle and thereby reduce the production of endometrial prostaglandins. For clients who do not wish to take oral contraceptives, prostaglandin inhibitors offer relief. The most effective prostaglandin inhibitors are NSAIDs such as ibuprofen (Motrin, Advil) and naproxen (Naprosyn, Anaprox). To be effective, the NSAID should be taken around the clock for at least 48 to 72 hours beginning when menstrual flow starts. Comfort measures such as rest and application of heat can supplement medical interventions.

Endometriosis
Pathophysiology

Endometriosis is defined as the presence of endometrial tissue outside the uterus on the ovaries, fallopian tubes, and other sites. The response of this tissue to the stimulation of estrogen and progesterone during the menstrual cycle is identical to the endometrial tissue within the uterus. The tissue continues to grow and proliferates during the follicular and luteal phases of the cycle and then sloughs during menstruation. However, the menstruation from endometriosis lesions occurs in a closed abdominal cavity, causing pressure and pain on adjacent tissue. In addition, prostaglandins secreted by the endometriosis lesions irritate nerve endings and stimulate uterine contractions, further increasing pain. Cyclic bleeding into the pelvic cavity can cause chronic inflammatory changes and may make conception and implantation difficult. The most common sites of endometriosis lesions are illustrated in Fig. 28.2.

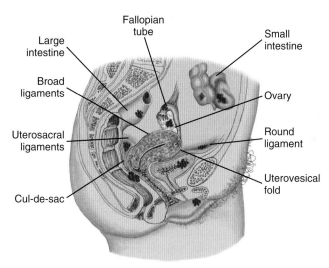

FIG. 28.2 Common Sites of Endometriosis.

The estimated incidence of endometriosis is about 5% to 10%, but the true prevalence is unknown. Some clients with significant endometriosis may be asymptomatic, and endometrial tissue is found on pelvic organs during an unrelated surgery. The cause remains unknown. One theory is the reflux of the menstrual flow through the fallopian tubes allows the endometrial cells to attach to nearby structures and proliferate, creating spots of endometrial tissue. Endometrial tissue has been found in distant sites such as the lungs, raising the possibility the cells are spread by blood circulation. Spread of the endometrial cells by the lymphatic system has been implicated. Endometriosis of the anterior abdominal wall has been found after a cesarean delivery near the incision line, leading to the theory that microscopic endometrial tissue may have been implanted during the cesarean and then stimulated to grow with later menstrual cycles. Endometriosis is associated with clients having autoimmune and/or inflammatory diseases, allergies, asthma, previous mononucleosis infection, and chronic fatigue and/or fibromyalgia (Shafrir et al., 2021).

Most clients with endometriosis are in their 30s and nulliparous. Many experience infertility issues. Signs and symptoms of endometriosis usually regress after menopause except when the client takes estrogen supplementation.

Signs and Symptoms

The two major problems associated with endometriosis are cyclic pain and infertility. Endometriosis should be considered in a client seeking infertility treatment even in cases where there are no complaints of pain. Endometriosis pain is deep, unilateral or bilateral, and either sharp or dull. It is constant, as opposed to the spasmodic or colicky pain of primary dysmenorrhea. **Dyspareunia** (painful intercourse) may occur, usually with deep penetration. Rectal pain may occur during defecation. Diarrhea, constipation, and sensations of rectal pressure or urgency are other symptoms of endometriosis.

Management

Treatment may be either medical or surgical. When choosing treatment options, the client must often weigh the need for pain relief and the desire to maintain fertility against potential side effects. The amount of growth and shedding of displaced endometrial tissue is dependent on production of ovarian hormones during the menstrual cycle. Other factors include symptom severity, desire for future fertility, client age, and the effect of endometriosis on nearby organs including urinary and gastrointestinal (GI) tract obstruction. Treatment may include over-the-counter pain relievers such as NSAIDs, ibuprofen (Advil, Motrin IB, others), or naproxen sodium (Aleve) to help ease painful menstrual cramps. For clients not trying to achieve fertility, hormone therapy in combination with pain relievers may be recommended (Mayo Clinic, 2019b).

Continuous oral contraceptives for 6 to 12 months suppress endometrial tissue proliferation, particularly in a client desiring pregnancy after medical treatment. Both the testosterone derivative danazol and gonadotropin-releasing hormone (GnRH) agonists such as leuprolide acetate (Lupron) and nafarelin (Synarel) interfere with hormones needed for ovulation and the menstrual cycle, creating a "pseudomenopause." The client may experience hot flashes, vaginal dryness, insomnia, decreased libido, and reduced bone density. In addition, danazol may produce masculinizing effects, such as deepening of the voice, facial and body hair, and weight gain. The client will take the drug often between 3 and 6 months, depending on the drug and the degree of endometriosis. There are several different surgical treatment options for endometriosis depending on the size, number, and location of lesions, client age, and whether or not it is affecting fertility. **Laparoscopy** (insertion of an illuminated tube into the abdominal cavity) may be performed for lysis of adhesions and laser vaporization of the lesions of endometriosis. This procedure is often used for endometriosis contributing to infertility. For clients with severe pain who no longer wish to have children, a hysterectomy (sometimes including removal of one or both ovaries and fallopian tubes) to remove all lesions is an option. The appendix is a common site of endometriosis and is usually removed at the time of hysterectomy. Removal of both ovaries causes loss of their hormone production and results in early menopause.

Nursing Considerations

Dysmenorrhea varies from mild "menstrual awareness" to incapacitating pain affecting the quality of life for several days each month. An important nursing action is to acknowledge the pain and to encourage the client to verbalize pain relief measures. Suggestions should include nonpharmacologic pain-relief measures such as frequent rest periods, application of heat to the lower abdomen, moderate exercise, and a well-balanced diet. The client should avoid stressful situations during the menstrual period if possible. The nurse should educate the client about expected effects of over-the-counter or prescribed medications and adverse effects. The nurse should address client concerns regarding treatment regimen and provide emotional support.

KNOWLEDGE CHECK

19. What causes primary dysmenorrhea, and how may it be treated?
20. How does endometriosis cause dysmenorrhea, and how can it be treated?
21. What are the major side effects of danazol? Of the GnRH agonists?

Premenstrual Syndrome

PMS is a psychotic neuroendocrine disorder with biologic, psychological, and social parameters. Symptoms are divided into two categories: physical and psychological. PMS is considered a periodic recurrence of a combination of disruptive, physical, psychological, and behavioral changes during the luteal phase of the menstrual cycle. These changes range from mild to severe (Rad et al., 2018). PMS, also called *premenstrual dysphoric disorder* (PMDD), affects about 5% to 10% of clients severely enough to cause significant disruption with their daily lives. Although PMDD is the official diagnostic name for the diagnostic criteria, PMS is now a term ingrained in lay culture and will be used in this chapter. After exclusion of other diagnoses, the following criteria must be met for the condition to be diagnosed as PMS (Rad et al., 2018):

- The signs and symptoms must be cyclic and recur in the luteal phase (after ovulation) of the menstrual cycle.
- The client should be nonsymptomatic during the follicular phase (before ovulation) of the menstrual cycle, and the cycle must include 7 symptom-free days.
- Symptoms must be severe enough to have an impact on employment, lifestyle, and relationships.
- Diagnosis should be based on the client's *prospective* symptom recording or charting of symptoms as they occur rather than recall of symptoms that occurred in the past.

Numerous symptoms have been ascribed to PMS, but a relatively small number make up most complaints. They are divided into physical and psychological symptoms. Box 28.5 lists those that are most common. Occupational or personal stress may worsen PMS. Several PMS diaries with varied amounts of detail are available for the client to record the symptoms and their severity, lifestyle impact, and medications.

Etiology

Although the cause of PMS is unknown, a common theory is that normal fluctuations in gonadal hormones during a cycle, chiefly estrogen and progesterone, trigger central biochemical responses, specifically serotonin. The premenstrual fall in serotonin levels occurs in many clients, but those having PMS may become symptomatic as the estrogen, progesterone, and serotonin levels fall during the luteal phase. Most clients describe a rapid postmenstrual return to a feeling of well-being.

Sociocultural influences may play a factor in PMS. There have been varied symptoms according to geographic location, marital status, education, occupation, and parity. Clients from Western cultures have learned to expect uncomfortable symptoms leading to menstruation. A relationship of PMS has been seen between mothers, daughters, and sisters suggestive of a learned behavior.

CLIENT EDUCATION

Relieving Symptoms of Premenstrual Syndrome

Diet

Decrease consumption of caffeine (coffee, tea, colas, chocolate), which can increase irritability, insomnia, anxiety, and nervousness.

Avoid simple sugars (cookies, cake, candy) to maintain blood glucose levels.

Decrease intake of salty foods (chips, pickles) to reduce fluid retention.

Drink at least 2000 mL (2 quarts) of *water* daily. Do not include other beverages in this total.

Eat six small meals daily to prevent hypoglycemia. Meals should be well balanced, with emphasis on fresh fruits and vegetables, complex carbohydrates, and nonfat milk products.

Avoid alcohol, which can aggravate depression.

Physical Activity

Increase physical activity to relieve tension and decrease depression.

Stress Management

Acknowledge the effect of PMS on daily life and actively plan to avoid stressful situations during the premenstrual period when symptoms are acute.

Use guided imagery, conscious relaxation techniques, warm baths, and massage to reduce stress.

Sleep and Rest

Reduce fatigue and insomnia:

Adhere to a regular schedule for sleep.

Drink a glass of milk (high in tryptophan and known to promote sleep) before bedtime.

Schedule physical activity for mornings or early afternoon.

Engage in relaxing activities such as reading before bedtime.

Management

Treatment of PMS is individualized based on client's symptoms. It is important prior to treatment to eliminate other diagnoses including mental health issues. Supportive therapy including measures to reduce anxiety should be included as part of the treatment plan. Relaxation therapy, physical activity, and dietary modifications to relieve symptoms are also beneficial to overall health and should be included. Small and frequent meals can positively impact mood swings.

Clinical trials have shown supplementation with calcium (1200 mg/day) has some effectiveness, and magnesium supplementation (200 to 400 mg/day) is minimally effective. Carbohydrate-rich foods and beverages may improve the mood and reduce food cravings in some clients. Reducing caffeine intake and taking vitamin E (400 international units [IU]/day) during the luteal phase of the cycle may reduce breast pain (mastalgia) in some clients. A study by Kartal (2019) determined participants preferred complementary and alternative medicine (CAM) methods such as yoga and meditation more than medical treatment to manage PMS symptoms. See Box 28.6

BOX 28.5 Symptoms of Premenstrual Syndrome

Physical Symptoms
Headaches, dizziness
Abdominal bloating or swelling; swelling of the extremities
Breast tenderness
Hot flashes
Abdominal cramps
Generalized muscle and joint pain
Fatigue
Appetite changes: binge eating, cravings
Sleep changes: excessive sleep or insomnia
Decreased libido

Psychological Symptoms
Depression
Feelings of hopelessness
Anxiety
Confusion, forgetfulness, poor concentration
Accident proneness
Irritability and anger
Emotional lability: Tearfulness or readiness to cry, loneliness, mood instability
Reduced interest in activities of living
Social avoidance
Lethargy or high energy

BOX 28.6 Complementary and Alternative Medicine Therapy for Premenstrual Syndrome

Complementary and alternative medicine (CAM) may help some clients with symptoms of premenstrual syndrome (PMS). Measures include acupuncture, massage, homeopathy, hypnosis, yoga, relaxation techniques, osteopathy, movement therapies, and mind–body interventions.

for CAM therapies. Clients with physical, emotional, and cognitive symptoms may be prescribed antidepressant medications, oral contraceptives, or a combination of the two. Estrogen therapy may relieve premenstrual migraines. Bromocriptine (Parlodel) and low doses of danazol may relieve breast pain. Selective serotonin reuptake inhibitors (SSRIs) taken at lower doses than those used to treat depression—such as fluoxetine (Sarafem), sertraline (Zoloft), or paroxetine (Paxil)— are effective for many clients experiencing PMS symptoms.

Nursing Considerations

Nursing considerations include completion of a detailed history and physical examination to eliminate other potential diagnoses. Client education should include lifestyle modifications such as diet and physical activity, expected cyclic changes, and family, if possible, to foster a spirit of support and encouragement.

ABORTION

Abortion is the spontaneous or induced termination of pregnancy before fetal viability. Spontaneous abortion is commonly referred to as miscarriage. Therapeutic abortion occurs when a pregnancy is terminated for medical reasons. In cases of rape or incest, many clients consider termination. Currently the most frequent indication is to prevent birth of a fetus with a significant anatomic, metabolic, or mental deformity. The term elective abortion or voluntary abortion describes the interruption of pregnancy before viability at the request of the client but not for medical reasons. Most abortions done today are elective. Therapeutic and elective abortions involve many social, ethical and legal issues (see Chapter 2).

Methods of Induced Abortion

Methods of induced abortion vary according to gestational period. Termination of pregnancy with medications are performed within 7 weeks of the client's last menstrual period. Medication-induced uterine contractions to end pregnancy provides client privacy, does not require anesthesia, and eliminates risks such as uterine trauma or perforation.

Medications used in induced abortions up to 9 weeks' gestation include the following:

- Mifepristone (Mifeprex, or RU-486) an antiprogesterone drug is followed by misoprostol (Cytotec), a prostaglandin drug commonly used to reduce gastric acid secretion. Oral or vaginal use of misoprostol in therapeutic abortion is unlabeled by the manufacturer.
- Methotrexate (Folex, Mexate) is an antimetabolite also used to treat certain types of cancer. Misoprostol may be prescribed to enhance expulsion of uterine contents.

Surgical abortion procedures are required if the client is more than 7 weeks pregnant or if a medical abortion fails to terminate pregnancy. Up to 12 weeks of gestation, vacuum aspiration with curettage is the most popular method of termination. The cervix is dilated following a local anesthetic and a plastic cannula is inserted into the uterine cavity. Contents are aspirated with negative pressure and the uterine cavity scraped to ensure the uterus is empty. Cramping may last 20 to 30 minutes after the procedure is completed. Complications may include uterine perforation, hemorrhage, cervical lacerations, and adverse reactions to the anesthetic agent.

For second-trimester abortions, cervical dilation with removal of the fetus and placenta is generally performed. The procedure is similar to vacuum curettage but requires greater cervical dilation and a larger aspirator because the products of conception have grown in size and should be removed gradually. Dilation begins with insertion of laminaria—rounded, cone-shaped materials that absorb water—into the cervix 24 hours before the procedure. Other osmotic dilators include Dilapan and Lamicel. The laminaria draw fluid from the cervical canal and expand, causing the cervix to dilate slowly and with minimal trauma. If needed, before aspiration and removal of the products of pregnancy, additional cervical dilation is done.

Induced abortion methods exist for clients in their second trimester and involve the labor process. Laminaria are inserted about 12 hours before the procedure to start cervical dilation. Prostaglandin E_2, which stimulates contractions, may be given via vaginal suppository or intraamniotic infusion. Oxytocin is not effective at inducing labor but it may shorten labor after being established by other methods.

CLIENT EDUCATION

Guidelines for Self-Care after Abortion

Avoid strenuous work or physical activity for a few days.

Bleeding or cramping may occur for 1 to 2 weeks. If severe, seek medical care. Light "spotting" may occur for about a month.

Sanitary pads should be used instead of tampons for the first week to avoid possible infection.

Avoid sex for 1 week to allow the uterine lining to heal and prevent infection.

Contraception should be used if sex is resumed before menstrual period begins. Menstrual periods usually resumes in 4 to 6 weeks.

Temperature should be taken twice each day to detect possible infection; a temperature above 37.8°C (100°F) should be reported to the health care provider.

Follow-up appointment in 2 weeks or as recommended.

Nursing Considerations

It is important for the nurse to provide physical and emotional support. History taking and collection of laboratory data depend on the routine of the health care setting in which the nurse is functioning. Counseling and lending emotional support are nursing responsibilities although a designated counselor also may perform these services.

Nurses should provide client education that relates to self-care after an induced abortion. Spontaneous abortion self-care is similar and includes observation for excessive bleeding or signs of infection (temperature greater than 37.8°C [100°F], foul-smelling vaginal drainage). Nurses also provide information about follow-up visits and contraception. The Rh-negative client should receive Rho(D) immune globulin (RhoGAM).

? KNOWLEDGE CHECK

22. What are the criteria for diagnosing PMS?
23. What should the nurse teach the client and family regarding lifestyle changes that may reduce the symptoms of PMS or increase client and family coping?
24. What drugs may be used in an early induced termination of pregnancy?
25. What discharge teaching is appropriate after termination of pregnancy?

MENOPAUSE

Menopause marks the end of menstrual periods. However, the term is often used to include the endocrine, somatic, and psychological changes that occur at the end of the reproductive period. The process of menopause is termed *climacteric*. *Premenopause* refers to the early part of the climacteric, before menstrual periods cease but after the client experiences symptoms such as irregular menstrual periods. Perimenopause includes premenopause, menopause, and 1 year after menopause. *Postmenopause* refers to the phase after menopause when menstrual periods have ceased.

Unexpected postmenopausal vaginal bleeding should be evaluated in a timely manner because it is suggestive of uterine cancer. Other causes of postmenopausal vaginal bleeding include cancer of the cervix or vagina, endometrial or vaginal atrophy, uterine fibroids or polyps, infection of the uterine lining (endometritis), medications such as hormone therapy and tamoxifen, pelvic trauma, or endometrial hyperplasia.

Age of Menopause

The average age for natural menopause is 51 (North American Menopause Society [NAMS], 2021). The natural climacteric takes place over a 3- to 5-year period. Menopause can be induced or created artificially at any age. Surgical removal of the ovaries or destruction of the ovaries by radiation or chemotherapy causes abrupt, permanent cessation of ovarian function, including the production of estrogen. The most common reason for performing these procedures is treatment of cancer or endometriosis. Younger clients experiencing artificial menopause often have more symptoms than those who experience natural menopause.

Clients may live another 30 years or more after natural menopause. This is often a time in their lives fraught with physiologic, psychological, and social changes that may require a reevaluation of primary roles and restructuring of personal goals.

Physiologic Changes

During the normal reproductive cycle, the ovaries respond to gonadotropins (follicle-stimulating hormone and luteinizing hormone) in a predictable pattern: (1) A follicle matures, (2) the ovary secretes estrogen, (3) ovulation occurs, and (4) the corpus luteum produces progesterone. During the premenopausal period, however, the ovaries are less responsive to gonadotropins, and, although increased amounts of follicle-stimulating hormone are secreted, ovulation is sporadic, and menstrual periods are irregular. With progressive aging, the ovaries become unresponsive, even to high levels of gonadotropins, and ovulation, menstruation, and the secretion of ovarian hormones (estrogen and progesterone) cease.

Estrogen is responsible for the secondary sex characteristics of clients. When estrogen levels decline, the organs of reproduction undergo regression. The labia become thin and pale. The vaginal mucosa atrophies, and vaginal tissue loses its lubrication and therefore is easily traumatized. Dyspareunia is common, and bacterial invasion of the epithelium may occur and lead to frequent vaginal infections. This entire process is referred to as **atrophic vaginitis**. Breasts become smaller, and atrophy of the uterus and ovaries occur. However, a concurrent benefit is that uterine myomas (fibroids) and endometriosis lesions also atrophy. Estrogen deficit can result in atrophic changes in the bladder and urethra that may cause loss of urethral tone and frequent atrophic cystitis.

In addition, absence of estrogen is associated with an adverse change in serum lipids. Serum levels of low-density lipoproteins (LDLs), which carry cholesterol to blood vessels, increase. At the same time, levels of high-density lipoproteins (HDLs), which are known to carry cholesterol to the liver and protect against the development of CAD, decrease.

Many menopausal clients experience hot flashes or flushes, which are the result of vasomotor instability. The cause of vasomotor instability is not known, but it is closely associated with increased secretion of gonadotropins. Hot flashes are characterized by a sudden feeling of heat or burning of the skin, followed by perspiration. They occur more frequently during the night contributing to interrupted sleep and fatigue.

Psychological Responses

Often referred to as the "change of life" individual client responses vary widely. Many clients are relieved their childbearing and child-rearing tasks are ending and perceive this chapter as an exciting time when personal development becomes a priority. Other clients grieve the possibility of childbearing has ended, particularly those who have never given birth.

Depression, mood swings, irritability, and agitation are common climacteric symptoms along with insomnia and fatigue. For some clients, physiologic and psychological symptoms are mild and infrequent while others experience severe, debilitating symptoms.

Therapy for Menopause

Although many clients comfortably experience the changes menopause brings, others seek relief from symptoms. Benefits of hormone replacement therapy (HRT) include decreased incidence of CVD, colorectal cancer, breast cancer, and osteoporosis.

The combination of estrogen and progesterone replacement is usually called *hormone replacement therapy (HRT),* whereas the estrogen-only replacement therapy may be called *estrogen replacement therapy* (ERT). It is common to see HRT used for either or both therapies, however.

Although once routinely prescribed to decrease menopausal symptoms, HRT has associated risks for some clients (Box 28.7). In addition, CAM often is beneficial for clients having mild menopausal symptoms (Box 28.8).

Nursing Considerations

Nursing care should focus on client education regarding the physical and psychological changes that may occur during perimenopause. For clients considering HRT, the nurse should review associated risks and benefits. It is important for the nurse to provide information about Kegel exercises to increase muscle tone around the vagina and urinary meatus and counteract the effects of genital atrophy. The nurse should encourage the client to drink at least eight glasses of water daily to decrease the concentration of urine, flush urine from the bladder, and reduce bacterial growth, thereby preventing atrophic cystitis. The nurse should instruct the client to wipe from front to back after urination and defecation to reduce the transfer of bacteria from the anus to the urinary meatus and help prevent cystitis.

CLIENT EDUCATION

Hormone Replacement Therapy

HRT is individualized because of possible risks specific to the client. Clients may use estrogen-only HRT or estrogen–progesterone HRT for significant discomforts unrelieved by other measures or for beneficial effects. Client education should include both benefits and risks of HRT to ensure that an informed decision is reached. Other topics to include in client education include the following:

Take the medication with meals to reduce nausea.

If a dose is missed, take the medication as soon as you remember, but not immediately before the next scheduled dose. *Do not take double doses.*

If uterus is present, expect withdrawal bleeding when estrogen and progestin are temporarily discontinued.

Report unexpected vaginal bleeding to health care provider.

Stop smoking to reduce the risk for thromboembolism.

Use sunscreen and protective clothing to prevent increased pigmentation.

Continue follow-up physical examinations, including blood pressure measurements, Pap tests, and examinations of breasts, abdomen, and pelvis.

? KNOWLEDGE CHECK

26. What are the effects of estrogen depletion at menopause (either natural or artificial) on the body?
27. What are the major psychological symptoms associated with menopause?
28. What conditions are associated with increased risks with HRT?

BOX 28.7   High-Risk Clients for Hormone Replacement Therapy

Previous episode of breast or ovarian cancer or other estrogen-dependent tumor

Close family history of breast cancer (first-degree relative)

Uterine cancer

Active thromboembolic disease or prior thromboembolic disorder when taking estrogen

Risk for cardiovascular disease

Stroke

Acute or chronic liver disease

Undiagnosed abnormal vaginal bleeding

Gallbladder or pancreatic disease

Diabetes mellitus

Conditions aggravated by fluid retention, such as migraine, epilepsy, cardiac or renal dysfunction, depression

Osteoporosis

Osteoporosis is characterized by decreased bone density, leaving the bones porous, fragile, and susceptible to fractures.

BOX 28.8 Complementary and Alternative Medicine for Menopause

Mind–Body Interventions
Hypnosis
Cognitive behavioral therapy
Biofeedback and relaxation training
Mindfulness-based stress reduction
Yoga
Aromatherapy

Herbal Products, Vitamins, and Supplements
Black cohosh (*Cimicifuga racemosa*)
Wild yam (*Dioscorea*)
Dong quai (*Angelica sinensis*)
Maca (*Lepidium meyenii*)
Pollen extract
Evening primrose oil (*Oenothera biennis*)
Phytoestrogens
Vitamin E

Whole System Alternative Medicine Approaches
Reflexology
Homeopathy
Acupuncture
Traditional Chinese and East Asian medicine

From Johnson, A., Roberts, L., & Elkins, G. (2019). Complementary and alternative medicine for menopause. *Journal of Evidence-Based Integrative Medicine*, 24, 1-14. https://doi.org/10.1177/2515690X19829380.

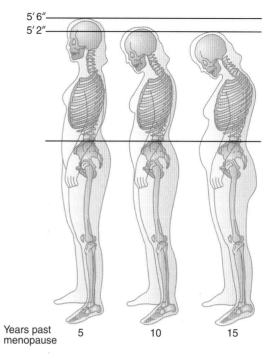

FIG. 28.3 With progression of osteoporosis, the vertebral column collapses, causing loss of height and back pain. *Dowager's hump* is the term used for this curvature of the upper back.

Signs and Symptoms

Osteoporosis has been called the "silent thief" because bone mass is lost over many years with no signs or symptoms. The first noticeable evidence is loss of height and back pain that occurs when the vertebrae collapse. Later signs include the "dowager's hump," which occurs when the vertebrae can no longer support the upper body in an upright position. Secondary to this, the waistline diminishes and the abdomen protrudes as the rib cage moves closer to the pelvis. Depending on the number of fractures, several inches of height may be lost. Fig. 28.3 illustrates progressive changes in posture associated with osteoporosis.

Diagnosis of osteoporosis requires a thorough history, physical examination, and bone mineral analysis. Dual-energy x-ray absorptiometry (DEXA or DXA) is a highly accurate, fast, and relatively inexpensive method for measuring bone mineral density and involves low exposure to radiation. Results can be evaluated with risk factors to direct management. Bone density examination can not only confirm the presence of osteoporosis but also detect low density before a fracture and predict the risk for fracture. Repeating bone density imaging helps determine the rate of bone loss and monitor treatment effectiveness.

Prevention and Medical Management

The major goal of treatment is to prevent or slow osteoporosis and stabilize remaining bone mass. Although research has upheld estrogen therapy to reduce osteoporosis by inhibition of bone resorption, fewer clients are choosing hormone therapy because of its potential adverse effects. In addition,

The vertebrae, wrists, and hips are the most common sites of fractures, with forearms, feet, and toes also susceptible. More than 53 million people in the United States today either have osteoporosis or are at high risk because of low bone mass. Osteoporosis can occur at any age, although the risk for developing the disease increases with age. Osteoporosis is most common in non-Hispanic White biologic females, but the disease affects many older Americans of any race or gender. Hip fractures increase the risk for reduced mobility and death in elderly clients (National Institute of Arthritis and Musculoskeletal and Skin Diseases [NIAMS], 2019).

Risk Factors

The combination of peak bone density and the rate of bone loss influences the severity of osteoporosis. Small-boned, fair-skinned White clients of Northern European descent and Asian clients are at greatest risk for osteoporosis, but African American and Hispanic clients also are at risk. Other risk factors may include a family history of the disease, late menarche, early menopause, and a sedentary lifestyle. Medication therapy such as corticosteroids, some anticonvulsants, or aromatase inhibitors for breast cancer may reduce bone density. Inadequate lifetime intake of calcium or vitamin D is a risk factor. Clients usually reach their peak bone mass between 18 and 25 years. Bone loss usually accelerates with menopause. Osteoporosis occurs when a client loses too much bone, makes too little bone, or both (National Osteoporosis Foundation [NOF], 2021).

many breast cancer survivors take medications such as aromatase inhibitors that suppress or block estrogen because of its effects on tumor cells.

Drug Therapy. Drug categories to reduce osteoporosis include the following:

- Calcitonin (Calcimar, Miacalcin, Fortical), a synthetic hormone, is usually prescribed as a daily nasal spray to reduce factors that cause loss of calcium and increase reabsorption of calcium in the GI tract.
- Bisphosphonates inhibit osteoclasts, reducing bone turnover. Alendronate (Fosamax), risedronate (Actonel), and ibandronate (Boniva) are used to prevent and treat postmenopausal osteoporosis. Oral bisphosphonates may be contraindicated for clients with ulcers or an inflammatory GI disease such as dysphagia or esophagitis. Alendronate and risedronate are also approved to treat bone loss that results from glucocorticoids and to treat biologic male clients with osteoporosis. Zoledronic acid (Reclast) is approved for treatment of postmenopausal osteoporosis and is given by IV infusion yearly. Headache or flu-like pain in muscles or joints may occur for 2 or 3 days after zoledronic acid infusion.
- Raloxifene (Evista), a selective estrogen receptor modulator (SERM), binds to estrogen receptors to reduce bone loss. Because of the combined estrogen agonist and estrogen antagonist effects of SERMs, raloxifene is being studied to see if its effects also improve cardiac health without raising breast or uterine cancer incidence.
- Teriparatide (Forteo) is an injectable parathyroid hormone approved for postmenopausal clients and biologic male clients at high risk for fracture. Current approved duration of use is a maximum of 24 months. Teriparatide stimulates new bone formation, reducing the risk for both vertebral and nonvertebral fractures. Nausea, dizziness, and leg cramps are side effects.
- Denosumab (Prolia) is a gamma-receptor activator of nuclear factor-kappa β (RANK) ligand (RANKL) inhibitor that inhibits osteoclasts. Increased RANKL in postmenopausal clients results in greater bone resorption with the osteoclasts. Denosumab reduces bone loss by inhibiting osteoclasts produced by higher RANKL levels.

Calcium and Vitamin D. Although calcium does not prevent bone loss, other therapies cannot be effective if calcium is deficient. A client 50 years of age and younger needs 1000 mg of calcium daily, and a client 51 years or older needs 1200 mg/day. Daily calcium supplements are recommended because it is difficult to ingest these quantities through food intake only. Vitamin D is necessary for calcium to be absorbed from the intestine. Supplemental vitamin D, 400 to 800 units, is often recommended for clients under 50 years of age; 800 to 1000 units is recommended for those 50 years of age or older (NOF, 2020)

Physical Activity. Weight-bearing and resistance exercise has been shown to be beneficial in slowing loss of bone mass to maintain density if there is adequate calcium and vitamin D intake. Most of the bone mass is acquired by age 18, but muscle-strengthening exercise may continue to build bone into the 30s. High-impact exercise improves bone mineral density but should be avoided in a person who already has fragile vertebrae from osteoporosis. At least 30 minutes of daily therapeutic exercise is needed. Other exercises, such as swimming or water-based exercises, often improve cardiovascular and respiratory fitness while managing weight, although their primary use is not to limit bone loss.

Nursing Considerations

Nurses should counsel clients about lifestyle factors that contribute to bone loss, such as cigarette smoking or excessive alcohol or caffeine intake, and the importance of following the recommended medical regimen. Adolescents and young clients should also be educated about factors that impair, as well as promote their ideal amount of peak bone density. Nurses should include injury prevention information such as fall prevention. Environmental education should include using ample lighting with easily accessible switches, keeping loose cords out of pathway, and using area rugs with nonskid backing. Bathtubs should have nonskid devices, and grab bars should be installed near toilets and tubs. Stairways should have handrail. Consultation with an occupational or physical therapist may be needed if the client has mobility problems.

❓ KNOWLEDGE CHECK

29. Why is osteoporosis called the "silent thief"?
30. How can osteoporosis be prevented?
31. What osteoporosis-related client education topics should the nurse include regarding injury prevention?

PELVIC FLOOR DYSFUNCTION

Pelvic floor dysfunction occurs when muscles, ligaments, and fascia that support the pelvic organs are damaged or weakened. This relaxation of pelvic support allows the pelvic organs to prolapse into, and sometimes out of, the vagina. Pelvic disorders generally occur in the perimenopausal period and may be the delayed result of traumatic childbirth or the effects of aging. Pelvic floor dysfunction may occur in a client who had a hysterectomy.

Vaginal Wall Prolapse

The vagina may prolapse at either the anterior or the posterior wall. Anterior wall prolapse involves the bladder and urethra and is called **cystocele**. Prolapse of the posterior wall produces enterocele or **rectocele**.

Cystocele

When the weakened upper anterior wall of the vagina is no longer able to support the weight of urine in the bladder, cystocele develops. The bladder protrudes downward into the vagina, resulting in incomplete emptying of the bladder. Cystitis is likely to occur because of the stagnant urine. Urethral displacement, formerly termed *urethrocele,* may occur when the urethra bulges into the lower anterior vaginal wall, producing stress urinary incontinence (Fig. 28.4A).

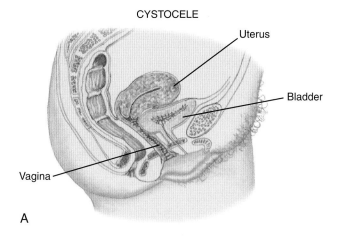

A

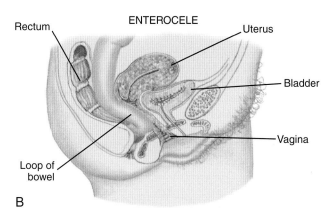

B

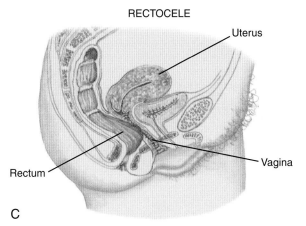

C

FIG. 28.4 Three Types of Vaginal Wall Prolapse. (A) Cystocele: Note bulging of bladder into the vagina. (B) Enterocele: Note loop of bowel between rectum and uterus. (C) Rectocele: Note bulging of rectum into vagina.

Stress incontinence is the loss of urine that occurs with a sudden increase in intraabdominal pressure, such as that generated by sneezing, coughing, laughing, lifting, or sudden jarring motions. The two most common causes of stress incontinence are damage to the normal supports of the bladder neck and urethra that occurs during pregnancy and childbirth and tissue atrophy that occurs after menopause.

Enterocele

Enterocele is prolapse of the upper posterior vaginal wall between the vagina and rectum. This is almost always associated with herniation of the pouch of Douglas (a fold of peritoneum that dips down between the rectum and the uterus) and may contain loops of bowel. Enterocele often accompanies uterine prolapse (Fig. 28.4B).

Rectocele

Rectocele occurs when the posterior wall of the vagina becomes weakened and thin. Each time the client strains at defecation, feces are pushed against the thinned wall, causing further stretching, until finally the rectum protrudes into the vagina. Many rectoceles are small and produce few symptoms. If the rectocele is large, the client may have difficulty emptying the rectum. Some clients facilitate bowel elimination by applying digital pressure along the posterior vaginal wall to keep the rectocele from protruding during a bowel movement (Fig. 28.4C).

Uterine Prolapse

Uterine prolapse occurs when the cardinal ligaments, which support the uterus and vagina, are unduly stretched during pregnancy and do not return to normal after childbirth. This allows the uterus to sag backward and downward into the vagina. Uterine prolapse is less common than in the past, largely because of a reduction in traumatic vaginal deliveries. The condition continues to exist, however, particularly when the client has experienced multiple vaginal deliveries or when the infants were large.

Symptoms

Symptoms of pelvic floor dysfunction often occur during the menopausal period as estrogen diminishes resulting in atrophic changes in the supporting structures. The most common symptoms of vaginal wall prolapse are feelings of pelvic fullness, a dragging sensation, pelvic pressure, and fatigue. Low backache and a sensation of organs "falling out" are sometimes described. Sexual problems related to arousal, orgasm, and painful vaginal intercourse may occur with pelvic floor dysfunction.

Symptoms relate to the structures involved and the level at which support has decreased. For instance, urinary frequency and urgency and urinary incontinence are seen in clients with cystocele because support of the urethra and lower vaginal wall has decreased. Constipation, flatulence, and difficulty defecating are major symptoms of rectocele. Regardless of the location or structure involved, symptoms become worse after prolonged standing and are relieved by lying down.

Symptoms of uterine prolapse are produced by the weight of the descending structures and may include sensations of pelvic pressure, backache, and fatigue. Cervical ulceration and bleeding occur if the cervix protrudes from the vaginal introitus.

Management

Treatment of disorders related to pelvic floor dysfunction depends on the client's age, physical condition, sexual activity, and degree of prolapse. Surgical procedures are usually indicated for clients in severe discomfort. The most common procedures are the anterior and posterior colporrhaphy, often called an A&P repair. The anterior colporrhaphy involves suturing the pubocervical fascia to support the bladder and urethra when a cystocele exists. If a rectocele exists, a posterior colporrhaphy (suturing the fascia and perineal muscles that support the perineum and rectum) is performed. Vaginal hysterectomy may be combined with anterior and posterior repair.

If surgery is contraindicated, a pessary (a device to support pelvic structures) may be inserted into the vagina. The pessary should be inspected and changed frequently by a physician or nurse practitioner to prevent vaginal ulceration, fistula formation, stool impaction, and infection. Vaginal estrogen cream may improve the client's tolerance of the pessary. Topical or systemic estrogen treatment may be indicated.

Nursing Considerations

Pelvic Exercises. Pelvic floor muscle training is directed toward strengthening the levator ani and pubococcygeal muscles that affect urethral closure and pelvic floor support. Kegel exercises are isometric, and one possible application is for the client to consciously contract and relax these muscles slowly 8 to 12 times for a count of 6 to 8 seconds each and repeat this series for three sets. Before pelvic floor muscle training is conducted it is important to determine whether the client can contract the muscles. This is performed by having the client sit with legs apart while urinating and squeezing the muscles to stop the urinary stream. If accomplished then the client should be able to perform pelvic floor muscle training. The client should be instructed to exhale and keep the mouth open to avoid bearing down when contracting their pelvic muscles and then gradually relax the muscle contraction. Variations exist about how frequently to repeat pelvic muscle contractions each day. The client should be informed that in order to maintain muscle tone these exercises should be considered a lifelong therapy.

Measures to help reduce the symptoms of pelvic relaxation may prove helpful. These include lying down with the legs elevated for a few minutes several times a day. Some clients experienced relief by assuming a knee–chest position for a few minutes.

Urinary Incontinence. Evaluation of the characteristics of a client's urinary incontinence guides treatment. The following are three major patterns (National Institute of Diabetes and Digestive and Kidney Diseases [NIDDKD], 2018a):

- Stress incontinence is characterized by urine leakage occurring when intra-abdominal pressure increases. Examples include coughing, sneezing, laughter, or physical exertion.
- Urge incontinence is characterized by urine leakage that accompanies the client's strong desire to empty the bladder.
- Mixed incontinence is characterized by urine leakage associated with both stress and urge incontinence patterns.

Overactive bladder (OAB) may occur with both urge and mixed incontinence. OAB is characterized by frequent sensations of urgency and nocturia and may accompany neurologic, anatomic, or structural disorders.

Research indicates that urinary continence can be improved by teaching the client pelvic floor exercises and bladder training which involves adhering to a prescribed schedule for emptying the bladder (NIDDKD, 2018b). Clients often benefit from information related to commercial incontinence products that protect the skin and prevent odor. These products are made of material trapping urine and prevent constant contact with the skin. Clients often restrict fluids believing this will decrease urinary incontinence. Restricting fluids can make the condition worse because the bladder does not fill to its normal capacity. Furthermore, decreased fluid intake can lead to concentrated urine and can irritate bladder mucous membranes, therefore increasing the urge to void. Alcohol and caffeine also can irritate the bladder and worsen incontinence. Obesity is associated with urinary incontinence. Drug treatment may enhance bladder control. Drugs that may be prescribed include (NIDDKD, 2018b) the following:

- Vaginal estrogen using a cream, tablet, or vaginal ring to reduce atrophy of the urinary and vaginal areas.
- Anticholinergic drugs, including their long-acting versions, such as oxybutynin (Ditropan) or tolterodine (Detrol).
- Other drugs are being studied for possible use in improving bladder control.

❓ KNOWLEDGE CHECK

32. How does cystocele differ from rectocele in terms of location? Symptoms?
33. What causes uterine prolapse, and how is it treated?
34. What are nursing actions to alleviate problems associated with pelvic floor relaxation? Urinary incontinence?

DISORDERS OF THE REPRODUCTIVE TRACT

Benign Disorders

The most common benign conditions of the reproductive tract include cervical polyps, uterine leiomyomas (fibroids), and ovarian cysts.

Cervical Polyps

Polyps are small tumors, usually only a few millimeters in diameter, that are generally on a pedicle (a stalk or stem-like structure). They are caused by proliferation of cervical mucosa and often cause intermittent vaginal bleeding. Cervical polyps are surgically removed in an outpatient setting, and the specimen is sent for pathologic examination to rule out malignancy.

Uterine Leiomyomas

Leiomyomas, also called *fibroids,* are one of the most common gynecologic conditions encountered. Although the cause is unknown, they develop from uterine smooth muscle cells and are estrogen-dependent. As a result, they grow rapidly during

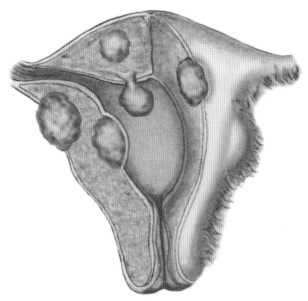

FIG. 28.5 Sites within the uterus where fibroids commonly occur.

the childbearing years, when estrogen is abundant, but shrink during menopause unless growth is maintained by HRT for menopausal symptoms. Fibroids may occur throughout the muscular layer of the uterus and may be prominent near the end of pregnancy as the estrogen levels are high and the uterus is large (Fig. 28.5).

Uterine fibroids do not often cause symptoms. Uterine size is sometimes increased, and excessive menstrual bleeding may occur. Excessive bleeding may result in anemia, weakness, and fatigue. Infertility may be related to uterine fibroids. Additional symptoms include feelings of pelvic pressure, bloating, and urinary frequency that occur when the tumor applies pressure on the bladder. Pressure on the ureter may cause hydroureter (dilation of the ureter). Many symptoms of fibroids depend on the location of the benign uterine tumors.

Treatment depends on multiple factors, including the size, number, and location of the fibroids; the symptoms experienced; whether future childbearing is desired; and how near the client is to natural menopause. In the absence of symptoms, treatment may consist of observation only. If abnormal bleeding is a problem, surgical intervention may be necessary. Hysterectomy may be appropriate for a client who does not desire future childbearing. Myomectomy, or removal of the fibroid from uterine muscle, may be an option for a client desiring future childbearing. Uterine artery embolization (UAE) is a procedure focused on reducing the fibroid size by introducing obstruction in the arteries that supply the fibroid.

Medical treatment with progesterone-only or combination estrogen–progesterone oral contraceptives may reduce excess menstrual flow. Short courses of GnRH agonists may be effective in reducing the size of myomas and lessen symptoms before surgical removal. GnRH agonists cause hot flashes, vaginal dryness, and other discomforts similar to those of menopause and therefore are not tolerated well by some clients. Loss of bone mineral density is an adverse effect of long-term therapy.

Ovarian Cysts

An ovarian cyst may be either follicular or luteal. If the ovarian follicle fails to rupture during ovulation, a follicular cyst may develop. These cysts are usually asymptomatic and may be an incidental finding on an ultrasound. They generally regress during the subsequent menstrual cycle. A lutein cyst may develop if the corpus luteum becomes cystic and fails to regress. A lutein cyst is more likely to cause pain and delay in the next menstrual cycle. Occasionally, an ovarian cyst can rupture or twist on its pedicle and become infarcted, causing pelvic pain and tenderness.

Treatment depends on differentiating a cyst from a solid ovarian tumor that is more likely to indicate cancer. If the client is of childbearing age the provider may opt to wait until after the next menstrual cycle and reexamine the client. Transvaginal ultrasound examination is useful to determine whether it is a fluid-filled cyst or a solid tumor. Laparoscopy may be helpful in ruling out endometriosis. **Laparotomy** (visualization of abdominal or pelvic organs through incision) may be necessary to remove the cyst from the ovary for examination by a pathologist.

Malignant Disorders

The primary sites for cancer in the female reproductive organs are the uterus, ovaries, and cervix. Cancer of the vagina, vulva, and fallopian tubes is relatively uncommon. Although cancer can occur at any age, the incidence increases with age.

CRITICAL TO REMEMBER
Symptoms Requiring Medical Evaluation

Irregular vaginal bleeding
Unexplained perimenopausal or postmenopausal bleeding
Unusual vaginal discharge
Dyspareunia
Persistent vulvar or vaginal itching
Elevated or discolored lesions of the vulva
Persistent abdominal bloating or constipation
Persistent anorexia or vomiting
Blood in stools

Signs and Symptoms

Cancer of the reproductive organs may not be diagnosed until it is advanced because few symptoms are experienced in the early stages. When symptoms occur, they are often nonspecific and could be caused by infection or other benign conditions. Cancer of the ovaries is particularly difficult to diagnose because it may remain "silent" until far advanced, when the chance of long-term survival is greatly reduced.

Risk Factors

Risk factors vary according to the site of the cancer. Risk factors for cervical cancer include a history of STIs, particularly **condyloma acuminatum**, also known as genital warts, caused by the HPV. Prolonged use of unopposed ERT (estrogen-only) predisposes to overgrowth (hyperplasia) of endometrial tissue and is a significant risk factor for uterine cancer. See Box 28.9 for a summary of risk factors for cancer of the reproductive organs.

BOX 28.9 Risk Factors for Cancer of the Reproductive Organs

Uterus
African Americans: higher risk for leiomyosarcoma
Obesity
Nulliparity
Middle aged and older adults
Late menopause (>52 years old)
Diabetes mellitus
Breast, colon, or ovarian cancer
Estrogen replacement therapy

Cervix
Human papillomavirus (HPV) infection
Sexual risks: young age at start of intercourse (<20 years), multiple sexual partners, uncircumcised male partners
Multiple pregnancies
Obesity
Diet low in fruits and vegetables
Smoking
Lower socioeconomic status (may be related to infrequent gynecologic examinations)
History of sexually transmitted infections, such as chlamydia or human immunodeficiency virus (HIV) infection

Ovaries
Menses started at younger than 12 years of age
No child or first child after 30 years of age
Late menopause (>55 years old)
Infertility, infertility drugs
Family history of ovarian, breast, or colorectal cancer
Personal history of breast cancer

Diagnosis

Early diagnosis is strongly associated with long-term survival. Many screening and diagnostic tests are useful. Screening tests include periodic pelvic examinations, Pap tests, ultrasonography, and serum tests for tumor markers such as CA-125, which may be increased with ovarian or other cancers. Genes linked to other cancers, such as *BRCA1* or *BRCA2* mutations, may lead to more diagnostic procedures than if the genetic risk is not apparent. Significant family history of specific cancers of the reproductive organs or linked cancers such as breast and ovarian cancers may alter the risk for a client's development of cancer. Diagnostic procedures such as endometrial biopsy for endometrial cancer and **colposcopy** (examination with a colposcope to magnify cells) can identify patterns of abnormality near the cervical os, where most cancers of the cervix develop. Specific strains of HPV infection are a significant risk factor for cervical cancer even if the original infection has healed.

Management

Treatment of cancer of the reproductive organs is based on the location and extent of the disease and the age and desire of the client to have children. The extent of surgical treatment for these cancers varies with the tumor size, degree of malignancy, and extent of spread beyond the primary tumor site.

Chemotherapy and radiation oncology therapy supplement surgical treatment for many invasive cancers.

Treatment of one type of cancer may be based on previous cancer treatment in the same or related organs. For instance, treatment of previous breast cancer with the chemotherapy drug Adriamycin often means that the client has reached the maximum lifetime amount that can be taken due to the drug's effects on the heart. Drugs such as anastrozole (Arimidex) and exemestane (Aromasin), aromatase inhibitors, may reduce estrogen secretion that increases cancer growth in most breast and reproductive organs.

Cervical Cancer. Testing for HPV often reveals the cervical infection that contributes to cancer. A biopsy of the suspicious area and an endocervical curettage are done for diagnosis if the client is not pregnant. A lesion of early cervical cancer is usually a squamous intraepithelial lesion (SIL). Early treatment of cervical cancer may consist of cryosurgery, destruction of abnormal tissue by laser, loop electrosurgical excision procedure (LEEP), or surgical conization to remove the central cervix. Regular surveillance after cervical cancer therapy is recommended to identify recurrence, particularly in the client who had a high-grade SIL, whose risk for repeated cervical cancer is greater.

Treatment for advanced cervical cancer usually consists of a total abdominal hysterectomy and bilateral salpingo-oophorectomy. Removal of the uterus and ovaries and **sentinel lymph node (SLN) biopsy** may be done via laparoscopy. Adjuvant therapy with radiation and chemotherapy is likely.

Endometrial Cancer. Abnormal vaginal bleeding, usually near or after menopause, is the most common presentation for endometrial cancer. Cancer of the endometrium is the most common cancer of the female reproductive organs. In 2020 the ACS (2020b) estimated about 65,620 new cases of cancer of the uterine corpus will be diagnosed. More than 90% of cases occur in the endometrium (lining of the uterus). About 12,590 clients in the United States will die of cancer of the uterine corpus. Endometrial cancer in the older client is likely to be more advanced. Many clients undergo surgical procedures (hysterectomy and salpingo-oophorectomy) followed by adjuvant chemotherapy and/or radiation therapy.

Ovarian Cancer. Clients with ovarian cancer may be asymptomatic, or they may seek care for abdominal or pelvic pain, increased abdominal girth, and sometimes abnormal bleeding. Total abdominal hysterectomy, bilateral salpingo-oophorectomy, and removal of ovarian tissue in the pelvis may be curative for the earliest stages of ovarian cancer. Surgery for more advanced ovarian cancer improves diagnostic information, allows more accurate staging, and permits surgical reduction of the cancer. Ovarian cancer is usually treated by surgery followed by chemotherapy. However, it may be treated by chemotherapy to reduce the tumor's size, followed by hysterectomy and bilateral salpingo-oophorectomy. A second surgery may be done to determine whether more surgical or adjuvant treatment is needed. Chemotherapy is required after surgery for all but the very early cancers.

KNOWLEDGE CHECK

35. What are the signs and symptoms of leiomyomas (uterine fibroids), and how are they treated?
36. Why is ultrasonography used to evaluate ovarian cysts?
37. What signs and symptoms suggest possible cancer of the reproductive organs and should always be investigated?
38. How may cancer of the following reproductive organs be treated: Cervix? Endometrium? Ovary?

INFECTIOUS DISORDERS OF THE REPRODUCTIVE TRACT

Some infectious disorders of the reproductive tract have mild symptoms while others are more severe and can be fatal. Infections may spread silently in the reproductive organs, allowing damage to the organs before the client reports symptoms.

Candidiasis

Candidiasis, also known as *moniliasis* and *yeast infection,* is the most common form of vaginitis. The cause is believed to be related to a change in vaginal pH that allows accelerated growth of *Candida albicans,* a yeast-like fungus commonly found in the digestive tract and on the skin. Some conditions, such as pregnancy, diabetes mellitus, oral contraceptive use, and systemic antibiotic therapy, result in changes in vaginal pH and flora that favor accelerated growth of *C. albicans.* Although not considered a STI, recurrent candidiasis in sexually active clients may occur. A small number of biologic male partners may have erythema and itching of the glans penis (balanitis).

The main symptoms for candidiasis are vaginal and perineal itching. Vulvar and vaginal tissues are inflamed, causing burning on urination. Vaginal discharge is white with a typical "cottage cheese" appearance. Diagnosis is made by identifying the spores of *C. albicans.*

Treatment may consist of nonprescription or prescription medications. Medications available without prescription include butoconazole, miconazole, clotrimazole, terconazole, and tioconazole by vaginal application. The duration for most of the nonprescription medications for candidiasis ranges from 3 to 7 days, depending on the specific medication. Clients should seek medical attention with the first infection or if the infection persists or recurs frequently. Oral fluconazole is a prescription medication for treatment of candidiasis with a single dose. Clients with more severe candidiasis may need another dose of fluconazole in 4 days. Recurrent yeast infections that resist treatment are associated with diabetes mellitus or HIV infection.

Sexually Transmitted Infections

Many reproductive infections can be transmitted through sexual activity. For some, such as syphilis, gonorrhea, and chlamydial infection, sexual activity is almost the only method of transmission. For others, such as bacterial vaginosis, sexual activity may or may not be the mode of transmission.

Incidence

STIs are most frequent among adolescents and young adults. Biologic females are twice as likely as biologic males to develop infections because microscopic tears from intercourse occur in vaginal mucosa, creating favorable conditions for infections to develop. Many infected clients are asymptomatic. Although the age of the first sexual experience has been declining steadily, sexual activity remains high among adolescents and young adults. The immature vaginal mucosa of the adolescent is more easily injured during sexual activity.

Methods of contraception have a significant impact on the risk for STIs. Barrier methods, such as condoms and female condoms, offer the best protection from infection. Diaphragms, cervical caps, and spermicidal foams and jellies do not offer the same protection as condoms, although they can decrease the risk for cervical and upper genital tract infections. When counseling youth, nurses should emphasize that oral contraceptives can prevent pregnancy but do nothing to prevent exposure to STIs.

Major concerns include the following:
- The vulnerability of clients, especially teenagers, to STIs
- The resistance of some organisms to antibiotics
- The relationship between HIV infection and other STIs
- Asymptomatic clients and failure to seek treatment

Clients should be advised to avoid using alcohol during treatment with metronidazole and for 24 hours after treatment is complete. Sexual partners should refrain from intercourse until a cure is established. Reinfection may result when the client's partner is not treated.

Bacterial Vaginosis. This infection, previously referred to as *nonspecific vaginitis,* is associated with organisms that replace normal lactobacilli with *Gardnerella vaginalis* or *Mycoplasma hominis* or with anaerobic bacteria, such as *Prevotella* or *Mobiluncus.* Causes of the bacterial proliferation are not known, although tissue trauma and vaginal intercourse have been identified as contributing factors. Multiple partners, douching, and lack of vaginal lactobacilli are associated with bacterial vaginosis.

Chief signs and symptoms are a thin, grayish–white vaginal discharge that typically exudes a fishy odor. The diagnosis is made by preparing a saline wet mount and identifying characteristic clue cells (epithelial cells with numerous bacilli clinging to their surface).

Treatment for bacterial vaginosis is directed toward reestablishing the balance of flora in the vagina. Metronidazole has been shown to relieve symptoms and improve vaginal flora. Clindamycin is an alternative treatment. The client should refrain from sexual intercourse until cured or the partner should use a condom.

Chlamydial Infection. The most common STI in Western countries is caused by the Gram-negative bacterium *C. trachomatis.* The incidence is particularly high in sexually active teenagers and young adults. Chlamydial infection is often asymptomatic in biologic females, which makes diagnosis and control of the disease difficult. It should be suspected when the biologic male sexual partner is treated for nongonococcal urethritis and when the culture results for gonorrhea are negative, yet the biologic female exhibits symptoms similar to those of gonorrhea, such as a yellowish vaginal discharge and painful urination. Gonorrhea and chlamydial infections often coexist.

Diagnosis of chlamydial infection can be made by isolating the bacterium in tissue culture, by enzyme-linked immunosorbent assay (ELISA) or by direct fluorescent monoclonal antibody. Tissue culture of the organism is most accurate but requires more time.

Untreated, chlamydial infection ascends from the cervix to involve the fallopian tubes and is one of the chief causes of tubal scarring that results in pelvic inflammatory disease (PID), infertility, or ectopic pregnancy. Treatment is usually directed to eradicate both chlamydia and gonorrhea because the two often coexist. Treatment options include azithromycin (Zithromax), doxycycline (Vibramycin), ofloxacin (Floxin), levofloxacin (Levaquin), and erythromycin. Treatment of all sexual partners is essential to prevent recurrence and further spread. Use of condoms until a cure is established is essential as well.

Gonorrhea. Gonorrhea is an infection of the genitourinary tract that is caused by the gonococcus *Neisseria gonorrhoeae.* Gonorrhea may be asymptomatic in biologic females, but when symptoms do occur, they usually include purulent discharge, **dysuria** (or painful urination), and dyspareunia. Diagnosis is based on a positive culture for the gonococcus. Gonorrhea is associated with PID (which increases the risk for tubal scarring and can result in infertility or ectopic pregnancy), as is chlamydial infection.

Dual treatment of gonorrhea and chlamydial infections is often routine. Additional drugs to those previously discussed for chlamydia with gonorrhea infections include cefixime (Suprax), ceftriaxone (Rocephin), and ciprofloxacin (Cipro). All sexual partners should be treated simultaneously, and intercourse should be avoided or the biologic male should use a condom until a cure is confirmed.

Syphilis. Syphilis is caused by the spirochete *Treponema pallidum,* and it is divided into primary, secondary, and tertiary stages. The first sign of primary syphilis is a painless chancre that develops on the genitalia, anus, or lips or in the oral cavity. At this time, diagnosis is made by identifying the spirochete on dark-field microscopy in material scraped from the base of the chancre. Serologic test results are generally negative in the primary stage. If untreated, the chancre heals in about 6 weeks. The disease is highly infectious at the primary stage.

Although the chancre disappears, the spirochete lives and is carried by the blood to all parts of the body. About 2 months after the initial infection, infected people exhibit symptoms of secondary syphilis, including enlargement of the spleen and liver, headache, anorexia, and a generalized maculopapular skin rash. Skin eruptions, called *condylomata lata,* may develop on the vulva during this time. Condylomata lata resemble warts; they contain numerous spirochetes and are highly contagious. Serologic test results are generally positive at this time.

If untreated, the disease enters a latent phase that may last for several years. Tertiary syphilis, which follows the latent phase, may involve the heart, blood vessels, and central nervous system. General paralysis and psychosis may result.

In addition to identification of the spirochete in material scraped from a chancre, diagnosis is also made by serology. The usual screening test is the Venereal Disease Research Laboratory (VDRL) serum test, which is based on the presence of antibodies produced in response to the infection. The rapid plasma reagin (RPR) and fluorescent treponemal antibody absorption (FTA-ABS) tests are more specific and are often done to confirm a positive VDRL test.

The best treatment for syphilis is parenteral penicillin G. A client allergic to penicillin can be admitted to the hospital for desensitization to penicillin followed by administration of the drug.

Herpes Genitalis. Herpes genitalis is an STI caused by the herpes simplex virus (HSV). Two types of HSV have been identified: type 1 and type 2. HSV-2 usually causes genital lesions, and HSV-1 usually causes oropharyngeal infection. However, either organism may infect the less-frequent location. Transmission occurs through direct contact with an infected person. A person infected with HSV-1 develops antibodies that may reduce the severity of the first HSV-2 infection. A primary HSV-2 infection is one in which the client had no preceding HSV-1 infection and therefore has no antibodies. Transmission may occur from a partner who is infected but has no visible lesions or symptomatic viral shedding.

Within 2 to 12 days after the primary infection, vesicles (blisters) appear in a characteristic cluster on the vulva, perineum, or perianal area. The initial lesions may cause severe vulvar pain and tenderness, as well as dyspareunia. Lesions also may occur on the cervix or in the vagina. With primary infection, the client may experience flu-like symptoms, including fever, general malaise, and enlarged lymph nodes. The vesicles rupture within 1 to 7 days and form ulcers that take an average of 7 to 10 days to heal.

When symptoms abate, the virus remains dormant in the nerve ganglia and periodically reactivates, particularly in times of stress, fever, and menses. Recurrent episodes are seldom as extensive or painful as the initial episode, but they are just as contagious. Diagnosis is often based on clinical signs and symptoms and confirmed by viral culture of fluid from the vesicle.

No cure exists, but antiviral drugs reduce or suppress symptoms, shedding, and recurrent episodes. Antiviral drugs include acyclovir (Zovirax), famciclovir (Famvir), and valacyclovir (Valtrex). Clients should be advised to abstain from sexual contact while the lesions are present to avoid transmission to their partner. If it is an initial infection, clients should abstain until culture-negative, because prolonged viral shedding may occur in such cases.

Human Papillomavirus. Condylomata acuminata, also known as venereal or genital warts, are caused by HPV. The dry, wart-like growths may be small and discrete, or they may cluster and resemble cauliflower (Fig. 28.6). Common sites include the vagina, labia, cervix, and perineal area.

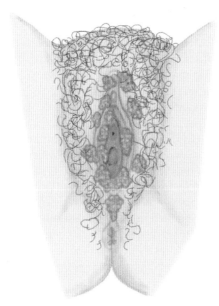

FIG. 28.6 Condylomata acuminata, also called *venereal* or *genital warts,* are caused by the human papillomavirus (HPV).

Condylomata acuminata are of particular concern because of the association of HPV with cervical cancer. Colposcopy, examination by a magnifying instrument called the colposcope, is generally recommended to evaluate abnormal cervical tissue and to identify HPV. Clients having condylomata acuminata should have Pap tests more frequently to detect cervical **dysplasia** (abnormal tissue development).

The goal of treatment is to remove the warts, which easily transmit the HPV between sexual partners. Treatment is determined by the site and extent of the warts and the client's preference. Topical treatment options include podophyllin, trichloroacetic acid (TCA), and bichloracetic acid (BCA). More extensive warts or those that do not respond to topical therapy may require removal by **cryotherapy** (extreme cold), laser vaporization, LEEP, or conization. Interferon, an antineoplastic drug, is sometimes used to treat condylomata acuminata in clients older than 18 years of age who have not responded to conventional therapy.

The client should understand that none of these treatments eradicate the virus and there may be recurrences. Furthermore, all sexual partners must be treated. Sexual contact should be avoided until all lesions are healed, and the use of condoms is recommended to reduce transmission. HPV vaccine is discussed earlier in this chapter.

Acquired Immunodeficiency Syndrome. Acquired immunodeficiency syndrome (AIDS), caused by HIV, remains the most devastating STI in the world today, although new treatments have improved clients' length and quality of life. HIV is found

CLIENT EDUCATION

Sexually Transmitted Infections

What are the most common signs and symptoms of STIs?

Unexpected nonbloody vaginal discharge (increased amount, unusual color, or odor) or vaginal bleeding.

Vulvar itching or swelling.

Pelvic pain, including painful intercourse, painful urination, and abdominal tenderness.

Skin eruptions or changes (rashes, ulcers, warts, blisters).

Flu-like symptoms (fever, swollen or painful lymph glands, loss of appetite, nausea or vomiting).

Presence of symptoms in a sexual partner, even if symptoms are absent in the client.

What are the common methods of diagnosis?

Culture (vaginal discharge, cervix, lesions) to identify organism.

Blood test (serology) to determine whether antibodies for specific diseases are present.

VDRL, RPR, or FTA-ABS test for syphilis; HIV test for human immunodeficiency virus.

How can STIs be prevented?

Establish monogamous relationship with uninfected partner.

Limit number of sexual partners.

Use mechanical and chemical barriers such as a latex condom with every act of intercourse.

Remember that one episode of a STI offers no protection from future infection.

Make sure partner is simultaneously treated to prevent reinfection.

What are the most important things to know about the treatment?

The entire course of medication should be completed even if symptoms subside.

Comply with follow-up evaluation as recommended by the health care provider.

Curtail sexual intercourse until free of infection.

Partner should be examined and treated and a follow-up evaluation done before sexual intercourse is resumed.

Side effects of medications, such as skin rashes, difficulty breathing, or headaches, should be reported.

Not all STIs can be cured (herpes, AIDS, venereal warts); treatment is aimed at slowing the disease and preventing complications.

Are there measures that provide comfort and prevent secondary infections?

Keep the vulva clean but avoid strong soaps, creams, and ointments unless prescribed by the health care provider.

Keep the vulva dry; using a hair dryer on low heat is helpful.

Wear absorbent cotton underwear and avoid pantyhose and tight pants as much as possible.

Take analgesics (aspirin or acetaminophen) as directed by the health care provider.

Cool or tepid sitz baths may provide relief from itching.

Wipe vulva from front to back after urination or defecation, and then carefully wash hands.

in blood, semen, vaginal secretions, urine, saliva, tears, cerebrospinal fluid, amniotic fluid, and breast milk. The primary modes of transmission are intimate contact with infected bodily secretions, exposure to infected blood and blood products, and perinatal transmission from client to infant.

HIV testing is routine for all pregnant clients so treatment can be started if needed, possibly avoiding transmission to the fetus. A client's risk for infection through a heterosexual relationship has surpassed the risk that the HIV infection stems from injectable drug use. Diagnosis of another STI is an indication for HIV testing and requires ongoing testing. Written consent for HIV testing should be incorporated into the client plan of care. No medications have been shown to cure HIV and AIDS. Ongoing research continues to be priority. Updated 2020 guidelines for HIV and AIDS treatment in the pediatric, adult, and perinatal groups may be found at the HIV.gov website: https://www.hiv.gov/hiv-basics/overview/about-hiv-and-aids/what-are-hiv-and-aids.

Nursing Considerations

Nurses have a major role in controlling the spread of STIs and providing information related to treating infections. Clients should be encouraged to exercise preventive measures to avoid infection even when partners do not want to use barrier methods of contraception. Other nursing considerations include the following:

- Educate client regarding signs and symptoms that require medical attention.
- Explain diagnostic or screening tests and follow-up testing requirements.
- Educate about preventive measures and follow-up care.
- Provide client with referrals to support groups.

KNOWLEDGE CHECK

39. What conditions may change the normal flora of the vagina and result in *C. albicans* vaginitis?
40. What are the symptoms of vaginal candidiasis?
41. Why are barrier-type contraceptives recommended to prevent STIs?
42. How do primary and secondary syphilis differ in terms of signs and symptoms and potential for transmitting the disease?
43. How are condylomata acuminata associated with cervical cancer?

Pelvic Inflammatory Disease

PID is an infection of the upper genital tract. The estimated prevalence of self-reported lifetime PID was 4.4% in sexually experienced clients of reproductive age (18 to 44 years), which equates to an estimated 2.5 million clients in the United States with a reported lifetime history of PID diagnosis. The prevalence was highest in clients at increased risk, such as those with previous STIs (CDC, 2020b). Clients who are under 25 years of age are more likely to develop PID because the cervix is not fully matured, increasing their susceptibility to

infectious organisms that ascend into the uterus, fallopian tubes, ovaries, and other pelvic organs. Exposure to multiple sexual partners increases the risk for acquiring an infection that causes PID. Douching increases the risk for PID because it changes the natural vaginal flora that helps resist infection and pushes infectious organisms toward the uterine cavity.

Etiology

Most PID cases are caused by *C. trachomatis* and *N. gonorrhoeae* infections. The remainder are caused by a variety of aerobic and anaerobic organisms such as *Escherichia coli, G. vaginalis, Streptococcus*, group B *Streptococcus, Peptostreptococcus, Peptococcus, Bacteroides* species, *Prevotella, Mycoplasma genitalium, Ureaplasma*, and cytomegalovirus (CMV). These organisms invade the endocervical canal causing cervicitis. Microorganisms ascend and infect the endometrium, fallopian tubes, and pelvic cavity. The chronic inflammatory response results in tubal scarring and peritubal adhesions, which interfere with conception or with transport of the fertilized ovum through the obstructed fallopian tubes to the uterus. Inadequate treatment of a vaginal infection increases the risk that the organisms will ascend into the uterus, infecting deeper reproductive structures and causing PID.

Symptoms

Signs and symptoms of PID vary widely. Some clients are asymptomatic or have subtle symptoms, whereas others experience pelvic pain, fever, purulent vaginal discharge, nausea, anorexia, and irregular vaginal bleeding. Findings during physical examination may include abdominal or **adnexal** (accessory organs) tenderness and tenderness of the uterus and cervix when they are moved during bimanual examination (cervical motion tenderness). Laboratory evaluation may reveal a marked leukocytosis and increased sedimentation rate. A urinalysis is needed to rule out UTI. Cultures for *N. gonorrhoeae, C. trachomatis,* or other suspected infectious organisms help diagnose and best treat PID.

Management

Clients experiencing a severe infection often manifested by fever, abdominal pain, and leukocytosis may require hospitalization. They are most often treated with IV administration of broad-spectrum antibiotics such as ceftriaxone plus azithromycin or doxycycline or cefixime plus azithromycin or doxycycline. IV antibiotic treatment usually can be changed to oral treatment after 48 hours, and the total duration of antibiotic therapy should be 14 days. Laparoscopy may be required to rule out surgical emergencies such as appendicitis or ectopic pregnancy, which have similar signs and symptoms, and to obtain specimens for culture. Pelvic abscess often requires surgical treatment. Outpatient treatment is appropriate for some clients who are not severely ill (CDC, 2020b).

Nursing Considerations

Nurses should educate clients to prevent PID. Preventative measures are either primary or secondary. Primary prevention involves avoiding exposure to these diseases or preventing acquisition of infection during exposure. Primary preventive measures include limiting the number of sexual partners and avoiding intercourse with those who have had multiple partners or other high-risk behaviors such as injectable drug use, which is associated with HIV infection. Barrier methods (latex condoms) used consistently and correctly during all sexual activity help prevent STIs.

Secondary prevention involves keeping a lower genital tract infection from ascending to the upper genital tract or from being further transmitted within the community. This involves seeking medical attention promptly after having unprotected sex with someone who is suspected of having a STI and when vaginal discharge or genital lesions are apparent. Periodic medical assessment is necessary if a client is not in a mutually monogamous relationship even if asymptomatic. Additional measures include taking medication as prescribed and returning for follow-up evaluation.

Toxic Shock Syndrome

Although **toxic shock syndrome (TSS)** is rare, it is a potentially fatal condition caused by toxin-producing strains of *Staphylococcus aureus*. The toxin alters capillary permeability, which allows intravascular fluid to leak from the blood vessels, leading to hypovolemia, hypotension, and shock. The toxin also causes direct tissue damage to organs and precipitates serious defects in coagulation.

If toxin-producing strains of *S. aureus* inhabit the vagina, certain factors increase the risk that the toxin will gain entry into the bloodstream. These include the use of high-absorbency tampons during menstruation and barrier methods of contraception (cervical cap or diaphragm), both of which may trap and hold bacteria if left in place for a prolonged time. Clients having had nasal surgery or previous *S. aureus* wound infections are at greater risk of developing TSS.

Symptoms of TSS include a sudden spiking fever (38.9°C [102°F]) and flu-like symptoms (headache, sore throat, vomiting, diarrhea), hypotension, a generalized rash resembling sunburn, and skin peeling from the palms of the hands and the soles of the feet 1 and 2 weeks after the onset of the illness.

Treatment consists of fluid replacement, administration of vasopressor drugs, and antimicrobial therapy. Corticosteroids may be used to treat skin changes.

Nurses are responsible for educating clients about measures to prevent TSS and should instruct them to do the following:
- Tampon use
  - Wash the hands thoroughly to remove bacteria before inserting tampons.
  - Change tampons at least every 4 hours to prevent excessive bacterial growth on a tampon that is left in place for a longer time.
  - Do not use superabsorbent tampons at any time because they may be left in the vagina for a prolonged period, allowing bacteria to proliferate.
  - Use pads rather than tampons during hours of sleep, which usually exceeds 4-hour segments of tampon use.

- Diaphragm or cervical cap use
  - Wash hands thoroughly before inserting a diaphragm or cervical cap.
  - Do not use a diaphragm or cervical cap during menstrual periods.
  - Remove a diaphragm or cervical cap within the time recommended by the health care provider.

KNOWLEDGE CHECK

44. What organisms cause PID?
45. How can the risk of toxic shock syndrome be reduced?

APPLICATION OF THE NURSING PROCESS: PROMOTING REPRODUCTIVE SYSTEM HEALTH

Case Study

Consider nursing actions as they apply to the case study.

Assessment

Consider a 36-year-old client who arrives for an annual well-being examination. The client is overweight and states, "I eat too much and I eat the kind of food that is bad for you." When answering questions during the history, the client states that many family members have diabetes and says, "I don't want to be sick all the time like most of my family. Can I change anything?"

A single parent, the client also describes her 6- and 10-year-old children as "sitting around too much" and says that they too are overweight. The client reveals the desire to see their children more physically active and is aware that this will help prevent excessive weight gain.

The client works at a fast food restaurant for varying hours per week where health insurance is offered but premiums are too expensive to purchase. The client qualifies for Medicaid, which is the client's major source of funding for medical care.

Identification of Client Health Risks

Although the client has some obvious health problems including financial limitations, there is a personal desire to improve self-health and health of the children. Personal statements indicate an awareness to "do better but not sure where to start." This provides an opportunity for client education to take place targeted toward taking charge of health and influence the health of the children simultaneously.

Planning: Expected Outcomes

Expected outcomes for this brief clinic visit are that the client will do the following:
- Describe affordable food preferences that are healthy and promote weight loss.
- Explore measures to increase activity level including the children.

Interventions

Reinforce the Client's Desire for Change

Ask questions that allow the client to express desired life-style changes that can be accomplished over time. Encourage the client to improve self-health and health of the children. Acknowledge with the client that setbacks may occur, and offer support to help maintain the desire to make positive changes.

Identify Food Preferences

Determining typical food choices and preferences can help the nurse identify beneficial aspects of the current diet and changes that might benefit the client's desire for better health. Ask the client to complete a 24-hour dietary recall including the frequency and timing of meals. Determine what food choices are available when the client is at work. Identify which fruits and vegetables are eaten and whether they are fresh, canned, or cooked. Analyze and share findings of positives associated with current dietary intake. Help clients identify positive dietary changes that could help achieve the desired lifestyle changes. Encourage the client to eat a healthy break-fast daily and to provide a healthy breakfast for the children. Remind the client that eating breakfast will make overeating, or eating unhealthy snacks throughout the day, less likely.

Drinking fewer soft drinks or bottled water might reduce an expense that the client has not considered. Refer the client to a nutritionist.

Financial Assistance

Ask whether the client receives any public assistance such as the Supplemental Nutrition Assistance Program (SNAP) (https://www.nutrition.gov), formerly the food stamps program. Refer to the appropriate source for information about qualifications and application if the client does not receive public assistance. Referral to a social worker may identify other sources for food such as a free lunch program for the children on school days or church or neighborhood groups that have food pantries.

Physical Activity

Explain that daily physical activity helps burn calories and can improve energy level. Explore ways to increase activity such as walking to work, the grocery store, or the post office. Help the client determine whether it is realistic for the children to walk to school with adult supervision. Encourage family playtime at a nearby park.

Evaluation

Although this clinical visit was brief it provides the nurse with an opportunity to encourage the client to pursue lifestyle changes that will improve overall self-health and of the children. Determining measures to improve physical activity level and improve nutrition may motivate the client in the pursuit of change.

SUMMARY CONCEPTS

- The Women's Health Initiative was a 15-year national study to address the best prevention and treatment for three major diseases that affect clients as they age: cardiovascular disease, breast cancer, and osteoporosis.
- Healthy People 2030 goals are health targets for the United States.
- Many clients do not have a primary health care provider, such as a family physician or family nurse practitioner, and depend on their reproductive health provider for their regular health checks.
- A health history helps identify health concerns and risks for specific diseases, actions that can be taken to promote health, and other measures needed to further improve health.
- A complete physical assessment can identify general health problems and guide further testing that should be done.
- Major preventable problems that can create other problems are overweight and obesity, physical inactivity, and smoking.
- Screening procedures may prevent problems and/or identify a problem early, when it is most curable. Some screenings are monthly or annually, some age-based, and others risk-based procedures.
- Disorders of the breast may be benign, such as fibrocystic changes that occur in relation to the menstrual cycle, or malignant. The discovery of breast disorder can create anxiety. Nurses should provide education regarding diagnostic procedures, such as mammogram, ultrasound, fine-needle aspiration biopsy, core needle biopsy, and surgical biopsy.

- One in eight biologic females in the United States develop breast cancer. Besides gender, the greatest risk factors are advancing age, a prior history of breast cancer, and genetic mutations in the *BRCA1, BRCA2,* and *p53* genes. Additional factors include family history (mother, sister, daughter) of breast cancer and previous uterine, ovarian, or colon cancer. Lifestyle factors such as a high intake of dietary fat, smoking, and consumption of alcohol are also suspected to increase risk.
- Management of breast cancer includes surgical removal of the tumor plus varying amounts of surrounding tissue and lymph glands. Adjuvant therapy includes radiation, chemotherapy, hormone therapy, and immunotherapy.
- Breast reconstruction is an integral part of the surgical management of breast cancer. Methods include tissue expansion and autogenous grafts. Reconstruction at the time of surgical tumor removal or a later reconstruction are options for many clients.
- Nursing care for clients with breast cancer focuses on providing emotional support and accurate information.
- Cardiovascular disease kills more clients than breast cancer. Preventive measures include modifying risk factors, such as maintaining a normal weight and stopping smoking. Added preventive measures include controlling hypertension, diet, and glucose level; increasing activity; and, for some clients, taking a low-dose aspirin on a daily basis.
- Pap tests can identify early changes in cervical tissue that may lead to cervical cancer.

- Human papillomavirus vaccine is designed to prevent infection with four strains of human papillomavirus that can result in genital warts or cervical cancer. The best time for immunization is prior to becoming sexually active although it can be started after sexual activity.
- Fecal occult blood testing is a yearly test that may identify colon or rectal cancer early.
- Menstrual cycle disorders include amenorrhea, abnormal uterine bleeding, cyclic pelvic pain, and premenstrual syndrome. Some of the disorders, such as premenstrual syndrome, may respond to lifestyle alterations including changes in diet, exercise habits, and stress management.
- Elective termination of pregnancy may be performed by medical or surgical methods, and each method is associated with social and ethical conflicts.
- Menopause is the final menstrual period, although most people use the term interchangeably with *climacteric*. The climacteric is a combination of endocrine, somatic, and psychic changes that occur at the end of the reproductive cycle. Client responses vary widely but all are in a permanent state of estrogen deficit after menopause that can result in bone loss (osteoporosis), increased risk for coronary artery disease, and atrophic vaginitis.
- Hormone replacement therapy may be prescribed to manage the symptoms of estrogen deficit, such as hot flashes and atrophic vaginitis, and to decrease bone mineral loss that results in osteoporosis. Clients should discuss with health care providers whether hormone replacement therapy is beneficial.

- Hormone replacement therapy has risks and benefits and is contraindicated for clients who have thromboembolic disease, undiagnosed vaginal bleeding, previous episodes of breast cancer or untreated uterine cancer, or chronic liver disease. For these clients, alternative measures are needed to control the symptoms of menopause.
- Relaxation of pelvic support structures occurs as a delayed result of traumatic childbirth and becomes troublesome when a deficiency in estrogen hastens genital atrophy as menopause nears.
- Many infections of the reproductive tract are transmitted by sexual contact. The incidence of sexually transmitted infections is reduced by barrier methods of contraception, particularly the condom, which prevents contact between infected skin or mucosal surfaces and prevents potentially infected ejaculate from entering the lower genital tract.
- Pelvic inflammatory disease is often a complication of untreated sexually transmitted infections, and a large number of cases are caused by chlamydial or gonorrheal infections. Pelvic inflammatory disease can cause infertility or ectopic pregnancy because of scarring of fallopian tubes resulting from inflammatory processes in the pelvic cavity.
- Toxic shock syndrome is a life-threatening condition resulting from infection with toxin-producing strains of *Staphylococcus aureus*. Some infections may be related to use of high-absorbency tampons that trap and hold bacteria in nutrient-rich menstrual blood for an extended time. Tampons and other items that trap bacteria, such as cervical caps and diaphragms, should be removed as directed by the health care provider.

Clinical Judgment and Next-Generation NCLEX® Examination-Style Questions

1. A nurse working in a women's health clinic is caring for a 48-year-old Black female complaining of frequent fatigue, loss of appetite and nausea and/or vomiting, occasional jaw pain, and frequent palpitations. The client states her last menstrual period was "3 years ago." She is 5 feet, 9 inches and weighs 260 lb and denies use of alcohol, tobacco, or illicit drugs. The client is employed as the chief executive officer of a large company and states she is "too busy working to go to the doctor or exercise." She is married with two children ages 23 and 18. Her husband is recently unemployed and provides additional support in maintaining their home, as she is the primary source of family income. The client's father passed away at age 45 from a myocardial infarction, and her mother passed away at the age of 60 from a cerebral vascular accident. **Based on this information, which of the following orders does the nurse anticipate? (Choose all that apply).**
   A. Referral for genetic counseling
   B. Teach the client about aspirin therapy
   C. Assess BUN and creatinine levels
   D. Referral for pulmonology work up
   E. Referral for nutrition counseling
   F. Schedule stress test
   G. Complete lipid profile
   H. Prescribe low-fat, high-sodium diet

   I. Education on when to seek emergency care
   J. Referral to substance abuse counseling
   K. Encourage sedentary lifestyle to conserve energy

2. A nurse is working at a women's health clinic and is caring for a 20-year-old female, G1 T1 A0 L1 who is currently not pregnant. She states she is in a monogamous relationship with the father of her 2-year-old daughter. She is here for her annual examination. **Which of the following question is appropriate to include in obtaining the client's sexual history? (Choose all that apply.)**
   A. At what age did the client become sexually active?
   B. How old is the client's partner?
   C. Has the client ever engaged in homosexual activities?
   D. What form of contraceptive is currently used?
   E. When was the client's last sexual encounter?
   F. Has the client ever been treated for a sexually transmitted infection?
   G. Does the client have a family history of autoimmune diseases?
   H. Has the client ever been treated for a mental health disorder?
   I. How many sexual partners has the client had?
   J. Is the client knowledgeable on how to protect self from sexually transmitted infections?

REFERENCES & READINGS

American Cancer Society (ACS). (2019a). *Breast cancer risk factors you cannot change.* https://www.cancer.org/cancer/breast-cancer/risk-and-prevention/breast-cancer-risk-factors-you-cannot-change.html.

American Cancer Society (ACS). (2019b). *Breast reconstruction options.* https://www.cancer.org/cancer/breast-cancer/reconstruction-surgery/breast-reconstruction-options.html.

American Cancer Society (ACS). (2019c). *Intraductal papillomas of the breast.* https://www.cancer.org/cancer/breast-cancer/non-cancerous-breast-conditions/intraductal-papillomas.html.

American Cancer Society (ACS). (2019d). *Reach to recovery.* www.cancer.org/involved/volunteer/reach-to-recovery.html.

American Cancer Society (ACS). (2020a). *Colorectal cancer screening tests.* https://www.cancer.org/cancer/colon-rectal-cancer/detection-diagnosis-staging/screening-tests-used.html.

American Cancer Society (ACS). (2020b). *Key statistics for uterine sarcoma.* https://www.cancer.org/cancer/uterine-sarcoma/about/key-statistics.html.

American Cancer Society (ACS). (2021a). *Breast cancer risks and prevention.* https://www.cancer.org/cancer/breast-cancer/risk-and-prevention.html.

American Cancer Society (ACS). (2021b). *How common is breast cancer?* https://www.cancer.org/cancer/breast-cancer/about/how-common-is-breast-cancer.html.

American College of Obstetricians and Gynecologists (ACOG). (2021). *Cervical cancer screening. Frequently asked questions.* https://www.acog.org/womens-health/faqs/cervical-cancer-screening.

American Heart Association (AHA). (2020a). *Age-adjusted total CVD mortality rates by race/ethnicity.* https://www.heart.org/en/about-us/2024-health-equity-impact-goal/age-adjusted-total-cvd-mortality-rates-by-race-ethnicity.

American Heart Association (AHA). (2020b). *Prevent CVD.* https://www.yourethecure.org/cvd_prevention.

American Heart Association (AHA). (2020c). *Understanding blood pressure readings.* https://www.heart.org/en/health-topics/high-blood-pressure/understanding-blood-pressure-readings.

American Heart Association. (2021). *Coronary microvascular disease (MVD).* https://www.heart.org/en/health-topics/heart-attack/angina-chest-pain/coronary-microvascular-disease-mvd.

Centers for Disease Control and Prevention (CDC). (2020a). *Overweight and obesity.* https://www.cdc.gov/obesity/index.html.

Centers for Disease Control and Prevention (CDC). (2020b). *Pelvic inflammatory disease (PID)–CDC fact sheet.* https://www.cdc.gov/std/pid/stdfact-pid-detailed.htm.

Centers for Disease Control and Prevention (CDC). (2021). *Vaccines and immunizations.* https://www.cdc.gov/vaccines/index.html.

GARDASIL 9. (2020). *Information about GARDASIL 9.* https://www.gardasil9.com/.

Henry, C., Ekeroma, A., & Filoche, S. (2020). Barriers to seeking consultation for abnormal uterine bleeding: Systematic review of qualitative research. *BMC Women's Health, 20*(123). https://bmcwomenshealth.biomedcentral.com/articles/10.1186/s12905-020-00986-8 (2020).

HIV.gov. (2020). *Overview: About HIV & AIDS: What are HIV and AIDS?* https://www.hiv.gov/hiv-basics/overview/about-hiv-and-aids/what-are-hiv-and-aids.

Johnson, A., Roberts, L., & Elkins, G. (2019). Complementary and alternative medicine for menopause. *Journal of Evidence-Based Integrative Medicine, 24*(25). https://www.ncbi.nlm.nih.gov/pmc/articles/PMC6419242/.

Kartal, Y. A. (2019). Complementary and alternative medicine therapy use of western Turkish students for menstrual symptoms. *International Journal of Caring Sciences, 12*(2). http://www.internationaljournalofcaringsciences.org/docs/56_kartal_original_12_2.pdf.

Klein, D. A., Paradise, S. L., & Reeder, R. M. (2019). Amenorrhea: A systematic approach to diagnosis and management. *American Family Physician, 100*(1), 39–48. https://www.aafp.org/afp/2019/0701/p39.html.

Kour, A., Sharma, S., Sambyal, V., Guleria, K., Singh, N. R., Uppal, M. S., Manjari, M., Sudan, M., & Kukreja, S. (2019). Risk factor analysis for breast cancer in premenopausal and postmenopausal women of Punjab, India. *Asian Pacific Journal of Cancer Prevention, 20*(11), 3299–3304. https://doi.org/10.31557/APJCP.2019.20.11.3299.

Malherbe, K., & Fatima, S. (2021). *Fibrocystic breast disease. StatPearls.* https://www.ncbi.nlm.nih.gov/books/NBK551609/.

Mayo Clinic. (2019a). *DASH diet: Healthy eating to lower your blood pressure.* https://www.mayoclinic.org/healthy-lifestyle/nutrition-and-healthy-eating/in-depth/dash-diet/art-20048456.

Mayo Clinic. (2019b). *Endometriosis.* https://www.mayoclinic.org/diseases-conditions/endometriosis/diagnosis-treatment/drc-20354661.

Mayo Clinic. (2019c). *Fibroadenomas.* https://www.mayoclinic.org/diseases-conditions/fibroadenoma/symptoms-causes/syc-20352752#:~:text=Overview,has%20a%20well%2Ddefined%20shape.

Mayo Clinic. (2019d). *Mammary duct ectasia.* https://www.mayoclinic.org/diseases-conditions/mammary-duct-ectasia/symptoms-causes/syc-20374801.

Mayo Clinic. (2020). *Fibrocystic breasts.* https://www.mayoclinic.org/diseases-conditions/fibrocystic-breasts/symptoms-causes/syc-20350438.

McMullen, E. R., Zoumberos, N. A., & Kleer, C. G. (2019). Metaplastic breast carcinoma: Update on histopathology and molecular alterations. *Archives of Pathology & Laboratory Medicine, 143*(12), 1492–1496. https://doi.org/10.5858/arpa.2019-0396-RA.

National Cancer Institute (NCI) & National Institutes of Health (NIH). (2020). *BRCA gene mutations: Cancer risk and genetic testing.* https://www.cancer.gov/about-cancer/causes-prevention/genetics/brca-fact-sheet.

National Institute of Arthritis, Musculoskeletal, and Skin Diseases (2019). *Osteporosis.* https://www.niams.nih.gov/health-topics/osteporosis.

National Institute of Diabetes and Digestive and Kidney Diseases (NIDDKD). (2018a). *Definition & facts for bladder control problems (urinary incontinence).* https://www.niddk.nih.gov/health-information/urologic-diseases/bladder-control-problems/definition-facts.

National Institute of Diabetes and Digestive and Kidney Diseases (NIDDKD). (2018b). *Treatments for bladder control problems (urinary incontinence).* https://www.niddk.nih.gov/health-information/urologic-diseases/bladder-control-problems/treatment.

National Institutes of Health & National Heart, Lung, and Blood Institute. (n.d.). *Women's Health.* https://www.nhlbi.nih.gov/science/womens-health.

National Osteoporosis Foundation (NOF). (2020). *Calcium and vitamin D.* https://www.nof.org/patients/treatment/calciumvitamin-d/.

National Osteoporosis Foundation (NOF). (2021). *What is osteoporosis and what causes it?* https://www.nof.org/patients/what-is-osteoporosis/.

North American Menopause Society (NAMS). (2021). *Are we there yet? Navigate now with our guided menopause tour.* https://www.menopause.org/for-women/menopauseflashes/menopause-symptoms-and-treatments/are-we-there-yet-navigate-now-with-our-guided-menopause-tour.

Peters, A. T., & Mutharasan, R. K. (2020). Aspirin for prevention of cardiovascular disease. *JAMA, 323*(7). https://jamanetwork.com/journals/jama/fullarticle/2761090.

Rad, M., Sabzevary, M. T., & Dehnavi, Z. M. (2018). Factors associated with premenstrual syndrome in female high school students. *Journal of Education and Health Promotion, 7*(64). https://www.ncbi.nlm.nih.gov/pmc/articles/PMC5963206/#ref1.

RESOLVE. (2021). *Resolve, the national infertility association.* https://resolve.org/support/resolve-support-groups/.

Shafrir, A. L., Palmor, M. C., Fourquet, J., DiVasta, A. D., Farland, L. V., Vitonis, A. F., Harris, H.R., Laufer, M.R., Cramer, D.W., Terry, K.L., & Missmer, S.A. (2021). Co-occurrence of immune-mediated conditions and endometriosis among adolescents and adult women. *American Journal of Reproductive Immunology.* https://doi.org/10.1111/aji.13404.

U.S. Department of Health & Human Services. (2020a). Healthy people 2030. https://health.gov/healthypeople.

U.S. Department of Health & Human Services. (2020b). *Physical activity guidelines.* https://health.gov/our-work/physical-activity/about-physical-activity-guidelines.

World Health Organization (WHO). (2020). Female genital mutilation. Fact sheet published February 2016, updated February 2020. https://www.who.int/news-room/fact-sheets/detail/female-genital-mutilation.

Answers to Knowledge Check

CHAPTER 1

1. Interprofessional education can improve client safety and quality of care by promoting interprofessional team-based client care.
2. A safety bundle is a set of evidence-based practices performed together to improve client outcomes. Maternal safety bundles have been developed for mental health, including depression and anxiety, obstetric hemorrhage, severe hypertension in pregnancy, venous thromboembolism, safe reduction of primary cesarean birth, reduction of peripartum racial/ethnic disparities, support after a severe event, opioid use disorder, prevention of surgical site infections after gynecologic surgery, and enhanced recovery after surgery.
3. The Women's Health Nursing Care Quality Measures include AWHONN's practice standards, which provide standardization and a means to measure the quality of nursing care and practice briefs, which are quick reference guides providing standardized techniques with evidence-based rationales.
4. Birthing centers provide professional care during pregnancy and childbirth in a homelike environment for clients with low-risk pregnancies. They are associated with a nearby hospital to which the client can be transferred in case of unexpected complications. Although the home setting provides comfort and closeness, if transfer to a hospital for unexpected complications is necessary, the time may be an issue. In addition, the client and family must make arrangements for equipment and supplies needed for the birth and care for themselves and their new infant. Labor, delivery, and recovery (LDR) and labor, delivery, recovery, and postpartum (LDRP) rooms offer a comfortable setting that promotes family involvement for birth but within the hospital, where unexpected events and complications can be handled more easily.
5. The purpose of critical thinking is to help nurses make the best clinical judgments based on reason rather than preference or prejudice.
6. Actual client problems reflect health problems that can be validated by the presence of defining characteristics. Risk client problems indicate that risk factors are present that make the person vulnerable to the development of a particular problem that has not yet developed.

7. The terms *goals* and *expected outcomes* (*outcome criteria*) are often used interchangeably to describe desired endpoints of care, but they are different. Broad goals do not have the specific criteria of outcome criteria. Expected outcomes should (1) be stated in terms of the client, (2) be observable and measurable, (3) have a time frame, (4) be realistic, and (5) be worked out with the client and family.
8. Nursing interventions that are not specific and do not identify exactly what is to be done are difficult to implement. Clearly written interventions that provide detailed, objective instructions correct the problem.

CHAPTER 2

1. Characteristics of a functional family include open communication, flexibility in role assignments, agreement of adults on the basic principles of parenting, and resiliency and adaptability.
2. Factors interfering with healthy family functioning include lack of financial resources, absence of adequate family support, birth of an infant who requires specialized care, presence of unhealthy habits such as substance abuse or impaired anger management, and the inability to make mature decisions that are necessary to provide care to an infant.
3. Differing cultures and lack of understanding of cultures (between the nurse and the childbearing family) may create difficulties related to communication style, decision making, eye contact, touch, spirituality and religiosity, and time orientation. Nurses should attempt to reconcile these differences by taking the opportunity to learn about the uniqueness of each client and the cultural beliefs and practices of the family.
4. Integrating harmless traditional cultural practices into the care of the childbearing client demonstrates respect for the culture.
5. Nurses should examine their own cultural values and beliefs to determine ways in which their beliefs may generate conflict with those who hold different cultural beliefs.
6. Cultural negotiation involves providing information while acknowledging that the client may hold views that are different from those of the nurse.
7. Poverty is the underlying factor that causes problems such as inadequate access to health care. The lack of access

to health care includes the inability to pay for it, lack of transportation, lack of care for other children, inaccessible hours for appointments, and language barriers.

8. An important barrier to health care results from the unsympathetic attitude of some health care workers toward those who are unable to pay for prenatal care. Poor families may experience long delays, hurried examinations, rudeness, and arrogance from some members of the health care team. Staff may be overworked and frustrated with the workloads they carry. Clients may wait hours for an examination that lasts only a few minutes. Many never see the same health care provider more than once. These clients may not keep clinic appointments because they do not see the importance of the hurried, impersonal examinations.

9. Poverty is the underlying factor that causes problems such as inadequate access to health care. The lack of access to health care is a major reason for the large number of low-birth-weight infants and the high infant mortality rate.

10. Health care disparities in the United States across racial, geographic, socioeconomic status, age, and gender result in differences in the health outcomes for different groups of people.

11. Battering may start or become worse during pregnancy. The face, abdomen, genitalia, and breasts are frequent sites of injuries. Clients may start prenatal care late and miss appointments. They have an increased risk for uterine rupture, placental abruption, preterm birth, low-birth-weight infant, client and fetal death, sexually transmitted infections (STIs), and postpartum depression.

12. Nurses can examine their own biases to determine whether they accept a common myth that blames the victim. In addition, nurses can consciously practice in ways that empower clients and make it clear that they own their bodies and no one deserves to be beaten.

13. The physically abused person often appears hesitant, embarrassed, or evasive. Eye contact may be avoided, and they may appear ashamed, guilty, or frightened. Signs of present and past injury may be present, such as bruising, swelling, lacerations, burns, scars, and old fractures, as well as genital injuries.

14. Nurses can help establish short-term goals by helping the client acknowledge the abuse, develop a plan for protecting self and children, and identify community resources that provide protection.

15. Victims of human trafficking may have a pattern of "red flags." One red flag may not be indicative of the client being a victim of trafficking in persons (TIP); the nurse should assess for the patterns of possible indicators, which include being accompanied by an individual who insists on answering all questions for the client; reluctance or inability of the victim to reveal their true situation; signs and symptoms of physical and mental abuse; evidence of being controlled; fearfulness; submissiveness; fear of authority figures; lack of identification documents; the client cannot communicate a physical residential address; inconsistencies in stories and/or histories; a client who is foreign or non-English-speaking; homelessness; a history of previous and/or current prostitution charges or sexual abuse; possession of expensive electronics, jewelry, and other luxury items; a history of substance abuse; markings on the body that appear to be branding; and a high number of sex partners relative to age.

16. Ethics examines conduct and distinctions between right and wrong to determine the best course of action. Bioethics applies specifically to the ethics of health care.

17. The deontologic model applies ethical principles to determine what is right. It does not vary the solution according to individual situations. The utilitarian model analyzes the benefits and burdens to determine a course of action that provides the greatest amount of good in a given situation. Belief that every client has basic human rights is the basis for the human rights model.

18. Ethical principles may conflict when the application of one principle violates another.

19. Assessment is used to gather data from all concerned persons. Ethical theories and principles are analyzed to determine whether an ethical dilemma exists. Planning involves identifying as many options as possible and choosing a solution. Interventions must be identified to implement the chosen solution, and the results are evaluated.

20. The belief that abortion is a private choice conflicts with the belief that abortion is taking a life.

21. Punitive approaches are against the ethical principles of autonomy, bodily integrity, and personal freedom. Although the intended plan may be to protect the fetus, such a plan can have unexpected outcomes, causing the client to avoid prenatal care or be dishonest with care providers, causing greater harm to the fetus.

22. Problems involved in the use of advanced reproductive techniques include high cost, low success rate, limitation to the affluent, control of unused embryos, and problem or unexpected pregnancy outcomes.

23. Log off of computer terminals when access is complete. Maintain secret identity codes that access private information. Direct reports to another professional should be done on a "need-to-know" basis rather than reporting to those who do not need to know. Verbal reports should be done in a private area. Care must be taken not to violate client or institutional confidentiality when having any discussion on the internet.

24. State boards of nursing administer the individual states' nurse practice acts, which establish what the nurse is allowed and expected to do when practicing nursing in that state.

25. Standards of care and agency policies influence judgment about malpractice because they describe the level of care that can be expected from practitioners at the time of care.

26. Documentation that provides evidence that the standard of care has been maintained helps defend malpractice claims against nurses. Other actions that help defend malpractice claims include securing informed consent appropriately, acting appropriately as a client advocate in terms of taking a problem through the chain of command, and maintaining expertise.

27. Nurses, concerns about the use of unlicensed assistive personnel include the need to know the capabilities of each UAP and the need to supervise them sufficiently to ensure competence.

28. Short lengths of stay lead to concerns about the client's ability to care for self and infant, potential complications that new parents may not identify, and the fact that parents will not have had time to absorb the necessary teaching. Follow-up phone calls help alleviate some concerns and identify some problems that develop after discharge. In nonmaternity medical situations, many older clients are often discharged early from the hospital. Because the cognitive abilities of a person may decline with advanced age, in these situations it is important to also provide teaching to the client's care provider.

29. Facilities that use phone call follow-up should have regularly reviewed and updated protocols, good documentation forms, and specific instructions to the client about actions to take if further problems develop.

CHAPTER 3

1. Development of the breasts is the first sign of puberty in females. In males, growth of the testes is the first sign, followed by growth of the penis about 1 year later.

2. The female pelvis has a wide, rounded, basin-like shape that favors efficient passage of the fetus during birth. The male pelvis is heavier and narrower and structurally suited for tasks requiring load bearing.

3. Males generally attain a greater adult height than females because they begin their growth spurt about 1 year later than girls and continue growing for a longer period.

4. Female secondary sex characteristics include round hips and breasts, pubic hair, finer skin texture, and a higher-pitched voice. Male secondary sex characteristics include facial and pubic hair, a deeper voice, broader shoulders, and greater muscle mass.

5. The female external reproductive organs are collectively called the *vulva*. The labia majora extend from the mons pubis to the perineum. The labia minora are within and parallel to the labia majora. The clitoris is at the anterior junction of the labia minora. The urinary meatus and vaginal introitus are found within the vestibule (the area enclosed by the labia minora). The hymen partially closes the vaginal opening. The perineum extends from the fourchette (posterior rim of the vaginal opening) to the anus.

6. The three divisions of the uterus are the corpus (body), isthmus (transition zone between corpus and cervix), and cervix (neck). The uterine fundus is the part of the corpus that lies above the entry points of the fallopian tubes.

7. The myometrium is the middle layer of thick uterine muscle between the perimetrium and endometrium. The myometrium includes three types of muscle fibers: (1) longitudinal fibers, mostly in the fundus, to expel the fetus during birth; (2) interlacing figure-eight fibers to compress bleeding blood vessels after birth; and (3) circular fibers to provide constrictions near the fallopian tubes and the internal cervical os, enabling the proper implantation of the fertilized ovum and preventing the reflux of menstrual blood into the fallopian tubes.

8. The fallopian tubes are lined with cells with cilia that beat rhythmically toward the uterine cavity to propel the ovum through the fallopian tube. The fertilized ovum undergoes its early cell divisions in the fallopian tube so that implantation is most likely to occur in the uterine fundus.

9. The two functions of the ovaries are to produce hormones (primarily estrogen and progesterone) and mature an ovum for release during each reproductive cycle.

10. The pelvis is located at the lower end of the spine. The true pelvis is located below the linea terminalis. The true pelvis is most relevant during birth.

11. Pelvic muscles enclose the lower pelvis and support internal reproductive, urinary, and bowel structures. Ligaments maintain internal reproductive organs and their nerve and blood supplies in the proper positions in the pelvis.

12. The ripening follicle secretes estrogen to form new endometrial epithelium and endometrial glands. After ovulation, the follicle (now called the *corpus luteum*) secretes large amounts of both estrogen to continue thickening of the endometrium and progesterone to cause the endometrium to secrete substances to nourish a fertilized ovum.

13. Three ovarian phases of the female reproductive cycle are the follicular (maturation of an ovum), ovulatory (release of the mature ovum), and luteal (secretion of estrogen and progesterone by the corpus luteum). The length of the follicular phase varies more among clients than the other two phases.

14. The endometrial phases are the proliferative, secretory, ischemic, and menstrual phases. The proliferative phase occurs during the first half of the cycle, during which the endometrium thickens in preparation for a fertilized ovum. The secretory phase occurs during the second half of the cycle and is characterized by continued growth of the endometrium, growth of blood vessels and glands, and secretion of substances to nourish a fertilized ovum. If pregnancy does not occur, the endometrium becomes ischemic and necrotic as secretion of estrogen and progesterone from the corpus luteum declines. The old endometrium is shed in the menstrual phase.

15. The cervical mucus becomes thin, clear, and elastic during ovulation to facilitate entrance of sperm from the vagina into the uterus and fallopian tube, thereby enhancing the chances for conception.

16. Montgomery's tubercles secrete a substance during pregnancy and lactation that keeps the nipples soft.

17. Breast size is not related to the amount of milk that can be produced. Breast size is influenced by the amount of fatty tissue in the breast.

18. Milk secretion does not occur during pregnancy because estrogen and progesterone produced by the placenta inhibit its production. Estrogen and progesterone stimulate the growth of the alveoli and ductal system during pregnancy.

19. As a urinary organ, the penis transports urine from the bladder to outside the body during urination. As a reproductive organ, it carries and deposits semen into the vagina during coitus.

20. The two types of erectile tissue in the penis are the corpus spongiosum that surrounds the urethra and the two columns of corpus cavernosum tissue on each side of the penis. The function of erectile tissue is to facilitate entry of the penis into the female's vagina.

21. The scrotum holds the testes away from the body to keep them cooler than the core body temperature, thus facilitating sperm production.

22. The testes function as endocrine glands to produce testosterone and the male gametes (spermatozoa).

CHAPTER 4

1. DNA is the building block of genes. A varying number of genes makes up each chromosome.

2. Genes are too small to be seen under a microscope. They can be studied by analysis of the products they instruct cells to produce, by direct study of the DNA, or through their close association with another gene that can be studied by one of these other methods.

3. Chromosomes can be seen under a microscope when living nucleated cells are dividing. Cell division during the metaphase is a common time for analysis because each chromosome is compact.

4. 46,XY describes the chromosome makeup of a human male. 46,XX describes the chromosomes of a human female. Chromosomal abnormalities are described beginning with the total number of chromosomes, followed by the sex chromosome complement, and followed by the abbreviation that describes the chromosome abnormality.

5. The child of a parent with an autosomal-dominant disorder has a 50% chance of having the same disorder.

6. Blood relationship (consanguinity) of parents increases the likelihood that both share some of the same abnormal autosomal-recessive genes, increasing the chance that their offspring will be affected with a disorder. The closer the parents' blood relationship, the more genes they are likely to share.

7. If both parents carry an abnormal gene for an autosomal-recessive disorder, each child has a 25% chance of receiving both copies of the defective gene and having the disorder. Each child also has a 50% chance of receiving only one copy of the defective gene and being a carrier like each parent. Each child also has a 25% chance of receiving the normal gene from each parent, thereby being neither a carrier nor affected and having no chance of passing the gene to future generations.

8. Males are more likely to have X-linked recessive disorders because they do not have a compensating X chromosome with a normal gene. Each son of a female carrier has a 50% chance of having the trait and a 50% chance of being unaffected. Each daughter of the female carrier has a 50% chance of being a carrier and a 50% chance of being unaffected.

9. A trisomy exists when each body cell contains an extra copy of one chromosome. Down syndrome is the most common trisomy and involves three copies of chromosome 21, for a total of 47 chromosomes in each cell.

10. A monosomy exists when each body cell is missing a chromosome. Turner syndrome (a female with a single X chromosome) is the only monosomy compatible with postnatal life.

11. Genetic material can be lost or duplicated when a chromosome has a structural abnormality. Also, the position of genes on the chromosome may be altered, preventing them from functioning normally.

12. A parent with a balanced chromosomal translocation may have a child with completely normal chromosomes, or the child may have a balanced chromosomal translocation like that of the parent. The offspring may also receive an unbalanced amount of chromosomal material (too much or too little), which often results in spontaneous abortion or birth defects.

13. Multifactorial disorders are typically present and detectable at birth. They are usually isolated defects rather than being present with other unrelated defects. However, sometimes the primary multifactorial defect alters further development and results in other related defects.

14. Factors that may affect the likelihood that a multifactorial disorder will occur or recur include the following: the number of affected close relatives, severity of the defect in those affected, biological sex of the affected person, geographic location, and seasonal variations.

15. The client may be able to prevent exposing the fetus to teratogens by being immunized against infections such as rubella at least 28 days (1 month) before pregnancy, eliminating the use of nontherapeutic drugs such as alcohol and illicit drugs, changing therapeutic drugs to those having a lower risk to the fetus, avoiding deliberate exposure to heat sources such as saunas and hot tubs, and limiting radiation exposure to urgent procedure with lead shielding of the abdomen.

16. A pregnant client with phenylketonuria should follow a low-phenylalanine diet before and during pregnancy to prevent buildup of toxic products that would damage the developing fetus.

17. Adequate folic acid intake of at least 0.4 mg (400 mcg) has been associated with a lower incidence of neural tube defects. Because the neural tube begins closure at 4

weeks of gestation, the client should have adequate intake beginning before conception to ensure the best outcome.

CHAPTER 5

1. Meiosis is a type of cell division that halves the number of chromosomes so that only one of each chromosomal pair goes into each gamete. Meiosis also promotes genetic variation by the process of crossing over, or exchange of chromosomal material between each member of the pair of chromosomes. The union of male and female gametes at conception restores the number of chromosomes to 46 in the offspring.

2. Each oogonium produces one mature ovum after two meiotic divisions. The first meiotic division begins in fetal life and is not completed until shortly before that ovum undergoes ovulation. The second meiotic division begins at ovulation but is not completed unless fertilization occurs.

3. Each spermatogonium undergoes two meiotic divisions to result in four mature spermatozoa. Meiosis begins at puberty, and both meiotic divisions are completed before the sperm mature and are ejaculated.

4. Fertilization usually occurs in the distal third of the fallopian tube (the ampulla), near the ovary.

5. Seminal fluid nourishes and protects the sperm from the acidic environment of the vagina.

6. As sperm approach the ovum, they secrete hyaluronidase to digest a pathway through the corona radiata and zona pellucida. When one spermatozoon finally penetrates the ovum, changes in the zona pellucida prevent other spermatozoa from entering. The cell membranes of the ovum and sperm fuse to allow the sperm to penetrate the ovum. The ovum also completes its second meiotic division.

7. Fertilization is complete and a new human conceived when the nuclei of the ovum and spermatozoon unite.

8. Implantation begins 6 days after conception and is complete by the tenth day.

9. The upper uterus is the ideal location for implantation for three reasons: (1) it has a rich blood supply for fetal gas exchange and nutrition, (2) the thick uterine lining prevents the placenta from attaching too deeply, and (3) the strong interlacing muscle fibers contract to limit blood loss after birth.

10. Nutritive fluids produced in the thick decidua pass to the conceptus by diffusion before a placental circulation is established. Primary chorionic villi, which will form the fetal side of the placenta, extend from the conceptus into the decidua basalis, which will become the maternal side of the placenta, to tap these nutrients.

11. During the first 8 weeks after conception, the embryonic period, all major organ systems develop. The client may be unaware of the pregnancy and may inadvertently expose the embryo to harmful substances. These substances may damage organs that are developing.

12. Gestational age is calculated from the client's last menstrual period and is about 2 weeks longer than fertilization age, which is calculated from conception. Gestational age is most commonly used because the menstrual period provides a specific marker. Ultrasound imaging may further clarify gestational age.

13. At 4 weeks the trachea develops as a bud of the upper digestive tract. After the trachea separates from the upper digestive tract, it branches into the two bronchi, which then divide to form the three lobes of the right lung and the two lobes of the left. Branching continues until terminal air sacs develop.

14. The intestines are contained mostly within the umbilical cord until 10 weeks because they grow more rapidly than the abdominal cavity and the liver and kidneys are relatively large. By 10 weeks after conception, the abdominal cavity has caught up with the growth of its contents and can accommodate them.

15. The fetus usually assumes a head-down position because this position best fits the egg shape of the uterus. Also, the head is heavier and tends to go downward with gravity in the pool of amniotic fluid.

16. Vernix caseosa protects fetal skin from constant exposure to amniotic fluid. Lanugo helps vernix adhere to the skin. Brown fat helps the infant maintain temperature stability in the cooler external environment after birth. Surfactant keeps the lung alveoli from collapsing with each expiration, thus making breathing easier after birth.

17. The placenta gradually takes over the function of the corpus luteum and secretes estrogen and progesterone.

18. Exchange of oxygen, nutrients, and waste products between the client and the fetus takes place in the intervillous spaces of the placenta.

19. The pregnant client's and fetus's blood may be of incompatible blood types and thus should not mix.

20. The fetus can thrive in a relatively low-oxygen environment because of the following:
    a. Fetal hemoglobin carries more oxygen than adult hemoglobin.
    b. The fetus has a higher hemoglobin and hematocrit levels than does the newborn or adult.
    c. Rapid diffusion of carbon dioxide into the blood causes the pregnant client to release oxygen more readily and causes oxygen to combine with fetal blood more readily.

21. Human chorionic gonadotropin (hCG) causes the corpus luteum of the ovary to persist and secrete estrogens and progesterone, which are essential to maintain the uterine lining for implantation. It also facilitates fetal testosterone secretion in the male fetus. Human placental lactogen promotes normal fetal nutrition and growth and client breast development. Estrogens cause enlargement of the uterus and genitalia and enlargement and development of the breasts. Progesterone maintains the secretory endometrium and changes the endometrium into the decidua to nourish the conceptus; progesterone also reduces

uterine contractions to prevent spontaneous abortion. Progesterone facilitates growth and development of the breasts and the cells that will secrete milk. Progesterone may allow immune tolerance of the conceptus.

22. The fetal membranes contain the amniotic fluid that protects the growing fetus and promotes prenatal development by providing a cushion against impacts to the pregnant client's abdomen, maintaining a stable temperature, and allowing symmetric development of the fetus, preventing the membranes from adhering to the developing fetal parts and allowing room and buoyancy for fetal movement.

23. Oxygenated blood enters the fetus through the umbilical vein. Part of the blood goes to the liver, and the rest passes through the ductus venosus to the inferior vena cava. Blood enters the right atrium, where a small amount passes to the right ventricle, and the rest flows through the foramen ovale to the left atrium and then to the left ventricle. Some blood from the right ventricle goes to the lungs to nourish their tissue, and the rest passes through the ductus arteriosus to the aorta, where it joins blood ejected from the left ventricle. Deoxygenated blood returns to the placenta through the two umbilical arteries, which branch off of the internal iliac arteries.

24. Monozygotic twins are conceived when one spermatozoon fertilizes one ovum and the resulting conceptus later divides into two.

25. The placentas and chorions may fuse before birth, making it difficult to determine whether the twins are monozygotic or dizygotic.

26. Dizygotic twins develop from two ova that are each fertilized by a spermatozoon and are like other siblings in a family.

CHAPTER 6

1. The uterine fundus is midway between the symphysis and the umbilicus at 16 weeks, at the level of the umbilicus by 20 weeks, and to the xiphoid process at 36 weeks of gestation.

2. By late pregnancy, blood flow to the uterus and placenta reaches 750 mL/minute, which is 10–15% of total cardiac output at that time. Approximately 90% of this blood goes to the placenta.

3. The cervical mucus plug blocks ascent of bacteria from the vagina into the uterus, thereby providing additional protection of the fetus from possible infection.

4. The major purpose of progesterone in early pregnancy is to stop contractions, help prevent fetal tissue rejection, and, with estrogen, prevent ovulation.

5. During pregnancy the breasts enlarge and become more vascular; the areolae increase in size and become more pigmented; the nipples darken, enlarge, and become more erect; and Montgomery's tubercles become more prominent.

6. Expanded blood volume is needed for the added tissues of pregnancy, to provide blood flow to the placenta, and to allow for loss of blood at childbirth.

7. Physiologic anemia of pregnancy is caused by a greater increase in plasma volume than in red blood cells (RBCs), resulting in a dilution of, but not inadequate, hemoglobin concentration. Iron-deficiency anemia is caused by a true lack of iron that affects hemoglobin levels.

8. In the supine position, the weight of the uterus on the vena cava and aorta impedes blood flow to and from the lower extremities, resulting in decreased cardiac output and supine hypotensive syndrome.

9. During pregnancy, increased circulation through the kidneys is needed to remove metabolic wastes generated by the pregnant client and the fetus. Increased circulation through the skin is necessary to dissipate heat that is generated by accelerated metabolism.

10. Progesterone causes slight hyperventilation and increases sensitivity of the respiratory center to carbon dioxide, leading to a feeling of dyspnea or a heightened awareness of the need to breathe.

11. Flaring of the ribs, widening of the substernal angle, and increased circumference of the chest allow adequate intake of air with each breath.

12. Estrogen causes hyperemia of the gums that may lead to bleeding or gingivitis. Vascular hypertrophy of the gums (epulis) may occur. Excessive salivation (ptyalism) is a problem for some. Progesterone relaxes smooth muscle in the gastrointestinal tract, which slows gastric emptying time and intestinal motility and may lead to heartburn and constipation. Emptying time of the gallbladder is increased, and thicker bile and gallstones may result.

13. Pregnant clients are at increased risk for urinary tract infection because compression of the ureters between the uterus and the pelvic bones and dilation of the ureters and kidney pelvis cause stasis of urine, allowing time for bacteria to multiply and the urine is rich in nutrients due to the excretion of glucose and amino acids.

14. Relaxation of pelvic connective tissue and joints by relaxin and progesterone creates instability and results in a wide stance and "waddling" gait. Lordosis occurs when the large uterus causes the client to lean backward to maintain balance.

15. The hormones follicle-stimulating hormone (FSH) and luteinizing hormone (LH) are suppressed during pregnancy by high levels of estrogen and progesterone to prevent ovulation. Progesterone maintains the endometrium and prevents menstruation.

16. The pregnant client's hormones create increasing resistance of tissues to insulin to provide glucose for the fetus. Normally, the pregnant client produces more insulin to meet the needs.

17. Most, but not all, presumptive signs are subjective. Probable signs are objective. Both can have causes other than pregnancy. Positive indicators of pregnancy have no other possible causes.

18. Many things such as gas, peristalsis, or pseudocyesis (false pregnancy) can be mistaken by the client for fetal movement.

19. Common causes of inaccurate pregnancy test results include a urine specimen that is too dilute or contains protein or blood; ingestion of certain drugs such as some diuretics, anticonvulsants, anti-Parkinson drugs, hypnotics, or tranquilizers; incorrect testing procedure; or testing too early in the pregnancy.

20. The fetus seems vague and unreal during the first trimester. Gradually, physical changes (uterine growth, weight gain, quickening) confirm that a fetus is developing, and the expectant client begins to perceive the fetus as a separate though dependent being.

21. The pregnant client may have increased interest in sex during the first trimester unless nausea or fears of miscarriage are present. Interest is often increased in the second trimester because of pelvic vasocongestion and a general feeling of well-being. The discomforts of the third trimester may decrease sexual responsiveness. Some expectant partners are more interested in sex during pregnancy, but others find the pregnant partner unattractive and fear harming the fetus.

22. The pregnant client explores the role of parent to develop a sense of self in the role and selects behaviors that confirm the idea of fulfilling the role.

23. Pregnancy brings the realization that the parent will have to give up certain aspects of their previous life. This causes a temporary sadness and the need for grief work.

24. Seeking safe passage involves going to a health care provider and following recommendations of the provider and of the culture.

25. Reality boosters include seeing the fetus via ultrasound, hearing the fetal heart, and feeling the fetus move. They are important in making the coming child seem real.

26. Nurses can help partners gain recognition as parents by focusing on the partner as well as the birthing parent, encouraging questions, and including the partner in the plan of care.

27. Information about infant behavior and care is more relevant and therefore more useful after the infant is born.

28. The age of the grandparents, the number and spacing of other grandchildren, and their perceptions of their role help shape the way grandparents respond to an expected grandchild.

29. Toddlers do not understand that a birth is expected and should be told shortly before the expected date. Preschoolers may expect the infant to be a playmate near their age. School-age children may like to be involved and to help prepare for the birth. Adolescents may be embarrassed by evidence of their parents' sexuality, indifferent to the pregnancy, or very involved in preparations.

30. Parents can make any changes in sleeping arrangements several weeks before the infant is born so that other children do not feel displaced by the newborn. They can increase time and attention to older children and reassure them of their love and acceptance.

CHAPTER 7

1. A preconception visit identifies factors that may cause harm to the fetus or the client so that steps can be taken before pregnancy occurs to avoid problems.

2. Medical, surgical, psychological, and obstetric histories are necessary to identify chronic conditions or past difficulties that might affect the outcome of the pregnancy.

3. All caregivers should use the same techniques to measure blood pressure because position and how the blood pressure is taken affect the results. Monitoring changes in blood pressure during pregnancy is an important component of prenatal care.

4. Major risk factors during pregnancy are age under 16 or over 35 years; low socioeconomic status; multiparity; obesity; previous problem pregnancies; preexisting medical disorders or infections; use of substances such as alcohol, tobacco, or illicit drugs; previous fetal or neonatal death; birth of an infant >4000 g; previous preterm birth; and existing medical conditions.

5. The usual schedule of antepartum visits begins in the first trimester and continues every 4 weeks until 28 weeks, then every 2 weeks until 36 weeks, and weekly from 37 weeks to birth.

6. A gradual, predictable increase in uterine size occurs as gestation advances. From approximately 20 weeks until 38 weeks, fundal height in centimeters is nearly equal to gestational age in weeks.

7. In multifetal pregnancies, increased blood volume results in additional work for the heart of the pregnant client. The greatly increased size of the uterus causes greater elevation of the diaphragm and more compression of the large vessels, ureters, and bowel. Nausea and vomiting are more frequent.

8. Relief methods for morning sickness include eating dry carbohydrates (crackers, dry toast, dry cereal) before getting out of bed in the morning. Small, frequent meals and high-protein snacks may help alleviate nausea and vomiting during the day. If necessary, the provider may prescribe vitamin B_6 (pyridoxine), doxylamine, or phenothiazines.

9. Correct posture and body mechanics and exercises such as pelvic rocking can help alleviate backache during pregnancy. Wearing low-heeled shoes and application of heat or acupuncture may also help.

10. The goals of perinatal education are to help pregnant clients and their support persons become knowledgeable consumers; to be active participants in pregnancy and childbirth; and to provide coping techniques for pregnancy, birth, and parenting.

11. Preconception classes generally include information about nutrition before conception, healthy lifestyle, signs of pregnancy, and choosing a caregiver. The emphasis is on the benefits of early and regular prenatal care to reduce risk factors for poor pregnancy outcome. The effects of pregnancy and childbirth on a person's relationships and

career may also be discussed. Early pregnancy (first trimester) classes cover information on adapting to pregnancy and understanding what to expect. Emphasis is on regular prenatal care and avoiding hazards to promote a healthy pregnancy. Second-trimester classes focus on changes occurring during middle pregnancy and what to expect during the third trimester. Teachers discuss childbirth choices and information to help students become more knowledgeable consumers.

12. Childbirth preparation classes during the third trimester focus on self-help measures, what to expect during birth, and how to prepare for the birth of the baby. Specific techniques include pharmacologic and nonpharmacologic pain control.

13. Having a support person during labor increases a client's satisfaction by helping cope with stress, focus on learned techniques, and feel that the experience is being shared.

CHAPTER 8

1. Weight gain during pregnancy helps determine fetal growth. Too little weight gain is associated with preterm birth and low neonatal birth weight; excessive weight gain is associated with large infants.

2. The average client with a normal BMI should gain 11.5 to 16 kg (25 to 35 lb). Underweight clients and those carrying more than one fetus should gain more, and overweight clients should gain less.

3. The average client with a normal BMI should gain approximately 0.5 to 2 kg (1.1 to 4.4 lb) the first trimester and 0.35 to 0.5 kg (0.8 to 1 lb) per week in the second and third trimesters.

4. Although no additional calories are needed during the first trimester, the recommendation for the second and third trimesters is 340 calories and 452 calories.

5. Approximately 71 g of protein per day is recommended during the second half of pregnancy, an increase of 25 g above prepregnancy needs.

6. Fat-soluble vitamins (A, D, E, K) are stored in the fat and are available longer than the water-soluble vitamins (such as B_6, B_{12}, folic acid, thiamine, riboflavin, niacin, C), which are not stored as easily and must be replenished daily. Excessive intake of fat-soluble vitamins is more likely to cause toxicity.

7. Because many pregnancies are not planned and the neural tube forms early in gestation, all female clients of childbearing age should have 400 mcg (0.4 mg) of folic acid daily to prevent birth of infants with neural tube defects from folic acid deficiency. Once pregnancy occurs, 600 mcg (0.6 mg) of folic acid should be taken daily.

8. Iron and folic acid are often below the recommended amounts in the diets of pregnant clients.

9. Excessive intake of vitamins and minerals may be toxic to the fetus and interfere with absorption of other vitamins and minerals.

10. During pregnancy a client should drink approximately 10 cups (or approximately 3 liters) of fluids (mostly water) daily.

11. During pregnancy the client should eat 6 to 8 oz of whole grains, 2½ to 3 cups of vegetables, 2 cups of fruits, 3 cups or the equivalent from the dairy group, and servings equal to 5½ to 6½ oz from the protein group.

12. The nurse should consider traditional foods from the client's culture, the degree to which the traditional diet is followed, and the inclusion of nontraditional foods in the diet.

13. The nurse should assess the client's intake of foods high in vitamins and minerals and the use of vitamin and mineral supplements. It is also important to assess financial resources for food purchase and need for financial assistance for nutritious foods.

14. The vegan can include nonanimal sources of iron; calcium; iodine; omega-3 fatty acids; zinc; riboflavin; and vitamins B_6, B_{12}, and D and combine incomplete protein foods to ensure intake of all essential amino acids. The client may also need to take supplements.

15. Lactose-intolerant clients can choose reduced-lactose dairy products or nondairy calcium-containing foods such as leafy green vegetables, broccoli, peanuts, tofu, salmon, and sardines.

16. Other nutritional risk factors during pregnancy include a history of bariatric surgery, excessive nausea and vomiting, anemia, abnormal prepregnancy weight, eating disorders, food cravings and aversions (including pica), multiparity, closely spaced pregnancies, multifetal pregnancy, and substance abuse.

17. The adolescent may skip meals and vitamin–mineral supplements and eat snacks and fast foods of low nutrient value to be like peers.

18. The lactating person needs more of many nutrients than one who is not pregnant or lactating. Compared to nonpregnant needs, an additional 330 calories is required during the first 6 months of lactation, and 170 calories will be drawn from fat stores. During the second 6 months lactation requires an additional 400 calories compared to nonpregnant needs. The postpartum client who is not breastfeeding can return to their prepregnancy diet, provided it meets recommendations for their age group.

19. The client who is not breastfeeding should decrease calories to the prepregnant level, continue to eat a well-balanced diet including enough protein and vitamin C, and plan to lose extra weight slowly.

CHAPTER 9

1. The three categories of obstetric ultrasound are standard (or basic), limited, and specialized (detailed or targeted). The two routes used for obstetric ultrasound are transvaginal and transabdominal.

2. First-trimester ultrasound is indicated to evaluate the pelvis and pelvic organs such as the uterus, adnexa, and cul-de-sac; to confirm an intrauterine pregnancy, diagnose and assess multiple gestations, gestational

trophoblastic disease, or ectopic pregnancy; evaluate pelvic pain or vaginal bleeding; identify ultrasound markers or severe fetal anomalies and as an adjunct to chorionic villus sampling. During the second and third trimester, ultrasound is used most often to assess fetal anatomy and biometry (the various measurements of the fetus). It may also be used to confirm fetal viability, evaluate structure of the placenta and cord, determine gestational age and assess fetal growth through serial scans, determine fetal presentation, quantify amniotic fluid volume, evaluate components of the biophysical profile, compare fetuses in a multifetal pregnancy, and locate the placenta.

3. During a transabdominal ultrasound, the client is placed in a supine position with the head and knees supported and is tilted to one side by placing a pillow or rolled towel under one hip. The lateral tilt shifts the pregnant uterus off of the vena cava to prevent aortocaval syndrome (supine hypotension), which is caused by decreased blood return to the heart due to compression of the inferior vena cava by the pregnant uterus when the client is supine.

4. In addition to client positioning and comfort during the procedure the role of the nurse related to obstetric ultrasounds may also include assisting with procedures, client teaching, serving as a point of contact for clients and their families, coordination of care by obtaining records, scheduling follow-up appointments, coordinating referrals, and case management of more complex complications. Nurses may also function in expanded roles based on their education, certification, and advanced licensure.

5. Nuchal translucency (NT) is a first-trimester ultrasound measurement of the fluid-filled space measured at the back of the fetal neck. An enlarged NT, often defined as 3.0 mm or greater or above the 99th percentile for gestational age, is associated with trisomy 21 as well as structural abnormalities such as congenital heart defects.

6. Cell-free DNA (cfDNA) screens for fetal trisomy 21, trisomy 18, trisomy 13, sex chromosome anomalies, and selected microdeletions and microduplications.

7. The four serum analytes measured with a second-trimester screening test are human chorionic gonadotropin (hCG), alpha-fetoprotein (AFP), inhibin-A, and unconjugated estriol (uE3).

8. Elevated AFP levels are associated with open neural tube defects (NTDs).

9. Multiple-marker screening, sometimes called a *quad screen,* is the second-trimester screen for four substances (hCG, AFP, uE3, and inhibin A). It is performed to evaluate the risk for trisomy 21, trisomy 18, and NTDs.

10. The major advantage of chorionic villi sampling (CVS) compared with amniocentesis is that it is done in the first trimester (10 to 13 weeks of gestation) and provides faster results. This prevents a long delay between screening and diagnosis and provides results before the client perceives fetal movement. This may ease the pregnancy decision-making process and decrease emotional distress on the client and family.

11. The CVS procedure may be performed transcervically or transabdominally. In both methods, the client will receive genetic counseling about the specific anomaly for which the test is being done as well as information about how the procedure is done and the risk and benefits. An informed consent is obtained. Both methods also use ultrasound guidance before and during the procedure, and the site is aseptically prepared. In the transcervical method, a flexible catheter is inserted through the vagina and cervix to obtain the small specimen of the placenta. In the transabdominal method, an 18- or 20-gauge spinal needle is inserted through the abdominal wall to obtain the specimen. Rh-negative clients should receive RhoGAM following the procedure.

12. Nurses should teach the client about common postprocedure complaints, which include vaginal spotting, beginning as red and transitioning to brown over the first 2 days. Uterine cramping is expected immediately postprocedure but should subside. Other postprocedure teaching should include instructions to rest for 24 hours and avoid exercise, heavy lifting, and sexual intercourse for several days. Symptoms to report are heavy vaginal bleeding, passage of clots or tissue, increasing intensity of uterine cramping, leakage of fluid, or temperature greater than 100.4°F.

13. Second- and third-trimester indications for amniocentesis include prenatal diagnosis of chromosomal, genetic, and metabolic disorders; diagnosis of fetal infection; and therapeutic amniocentesis for amniotic fluid volume disorders such as polyhydramnios.

14. Potential complications associated with amniocentesis are rare but include pregnancy loss (less than 1%), vaginal spotting, or continued leakage of amniotic fluid after the procedure (1% to 2%). Postprocedure client education regarding common complaints and warning signs are similar to that for the CVS—uterine cramping may last several hours, and some clients have low abdominal discomfort for up to 48 hours; a small amount of amniotic fluid leakage on the first day is common. Symptoms to report include increasing intensity of uterine contractions, heavy vaginal bleeding, continued leakage of fluid, or temperature greater than 100.4°F.

15. Surfactant is important for fetal lung maturity because it reduces surface tension on the inner walls of the alveoli, allowing them to stay slightly open during exhalation. Additionally, surfactant stabilizes lung volume, alters lung mechanics, and maintains gas exchange in the lung. Without adequate surfactant, lung walls adhere to one another, making alveoli inflation during inhalation difficult, which in turn increases the amount of pressure required to keep alveoli open. If this situation is not corrected, impaired oxygenation eventually leads to respiratory distress syndrome (RDS) and other neonatal complications, increasing the rates of neonatal morbidity and mortality.

16. The most common indications for PUBS are diagnosis and management of alloimmunization and fetal hydrops. Potential risks include fetal bradycardia and bleeding, umbilical cord lacerations or hematomas, thrombosis, infection, preterm labor resulting in an emergent birth of a compromised fetus, preterm and premature rupture of membranes, and pregnancy loss.

17. The primary goal of antepartum fetal testing (APFT) is identification of fetuses at risk for permanent neurologic injury or stillbirth so timely intervention can be done to decrease perinatal morbidity and mortality rates.

18. The methods used for antepartum surveillance are (1) fetal movement counting (FMC), (2) nonstress test (NST), (3) contraction stress test (CST)/oxytocin challenge test (OCT), (4) biophysical profile (BPP), (5) modified biophysical profile (MBPP), and (6) Doppler flow studies.

19. The primary indications for initiating antepartum fetal testing (APFT) include client, fetal, obstetric and placental indicators (see Table 9.3). Many of these are related to presumed alteration in the maternal-fetal oxygenation pathway.

20. To explain fetal movement counting (FMC), the nurse should tell the client to rest in a quiet location and count distinct fetal movements, such as kicks or rolls. Once 10 movements are perceived, record the number of movements and amount of time on a cell phone app or piece of paper. If you do not feel 10 movements in 1 to 2 hours, or you notice a decrease in the movements, notify your provider.

21. Reactive NSTs contain two or more FHR accelerations within a 20-minute period. Accelerations are defined as visually apparent increases in the FHR that reach a peak of 15 beats per minute (bpm) above the baseline, with the entire acceleration lasting a minimum of 15 seconds but less than 2 minutes ("15 × 15"). Before 32 weeks of gestation, accelerations are defined as visually apparent increases in the FHR that reach a peak of 10 bpm above the baseline with the entire acceleration lasting at least 10 seconds ("10 × 10"). Nonreactive NSTs have less than two accelerations during a 40-minute period.

22. Contraction stress tests (CSTs) determine fetal well-being by monitoring FHR responses to contractions. Healthy, well-oxygenated fetuses can physiologically tolerate the interrupted placental blood flow that occurs during contractions and maintain FHR with normal characteristics such as a stable baseline rate and accelerations. In compromised fetuses, brief interruptions of oxygen transfer during contractions can result in late decelerations.

23. The interpretation criteria for CST are as follows:
    Negative—No late or significant variable decelerations
    Positive—Late decelerations are present with a minimum of 50% of the contractions even when fewer than three contractions occur in 10 minutes
    Equivocal–suspicious—Intermittent late decelerations or significant variable decelerations
    Equivocal—FHR decelerations in the presence of contractions that are more frequent than every 2 minutes or last longer than 90 seconds

Unsatisfactory—Fewer than three contractions in 10 minutes or a tracing that cannot be interpreted
In the event of a positive CST result, the health care team will discuss management options with a client including, but not limited to, further testing or an expedited birth after an evaluation of the entire clinical situation. An equivocal, equivocal suspicious, or unsatisfactory CST result prompts further assessment, including repeat testing within 24 hours, prolonged continuous monitoring, or using adjunct methods of testing unless other clinical factors indicate a need for an expedited birth.

24. The four biophysical characteristics evaluated with ultrasound during a biophysical profile (BPP) are fetal movement, fetal tone, fetal breathing movement, and amniotic fluid amount. Biophysical characteristics are a reflection of the central nervous system (CNS) and provide an indirect means of evaluating fetal oxygenation.

25. Amniotic fluid volume is an important parameter in biophysical profiles (BPPs) and modified biophysical profiles (MBPPs) because decreased amniotic fluid suggests prolonged fetal hypoxia and is a strong indication of fetal compromise.

26. Shunting occurs because the fetus redirects blood from areas not critical to fetal life, such as the kidneys, gastrointestinal tract, and extremities, to the vital organs, which include the heart, brain, and adrenal gland. If changes in oxygenation are prolonged, blood flow to the fetal kidneys ceases. Therefore oligohydramnios in fetuses with normal renal structures and intact amniotic membranes suggests prolonged fetal hypoxia and is a strong indication of fetal compromise.

CHAPTER 10

1. Bleeding is the most common sign of threatened abortion. It may be accompanied by rhythmic cramping, backache, or feelings of pelvic pressure. Gross rupture of membranes and subsequent cervical dilatation and bleeding make the abortion inevitable.

2. Recurrent spontaneous abortions (also called *miscarriages*) most often occur as a result of genetic or chromosomal abnormalities of the embryo or anomalies of the client's reproductive tract.

3. Nurses can facilitate the grief response by being aware that the emotions and the intensity of the emotions experienced with an early loss of the pregnancy vary. Listening and recognizing the meaning of the loss to the client and family is important. Grief often includes feelings of guilt and speculation about whether the client could have done something to prevent the loss. Nurses may help by emphasizing that miscarriages usually occur as the result of factors or abnormalities that cannot be avoided. When nurses demonstrate empathy and unconditional acceptance of the feelings expressed, they support the grief response. Providing information about the grieving and referrals to additional support groups also may be helpful.

4. Scarring of the fallopian tubes is a common factor for the development of ectopic pregnancy in the fallopian tube. Tubal adhesions from a previous tubal infection, appendicitis, or endometriosis increases the risk of an ectopic. A failed tubal ligation, even if performed many years ago, and a history of previous ectopic pregnancy also increase the risk for an ectopic pregnancy in the fallopian tube. Greater incidences of ectopic pregnancies occur in clients who conceived with assisted reproduction, most likely related to the tubal factors that contributed to infertility. Management of tubal pregnancy depends on whether the tube is intact or ruptured. Medical management with methotrexate or surgical management with a linear salpingostomy to remove the pregnancy from the tube may be options for the client with an early ectopic pregnancy if the tube is unruptured. When ectopic pregnancy results in rupture of the fallopian tube, the goal of therapeutic management is to control the bleeding and prevent hypovolemic shock. When the client's cardiovascular status is stable, removal of the effected tube by salpingectomy with ligation of bleeding vessels may be required.

5. Hydatidiform mole is a form of gestational trophoblastic disease that involves abnormal development of the placenta as the fetal part of the pregnancy fails to develop. The first phase of treatment is evacuation of the molar pregnancy from the uterus. The second phase is follow-up to detect malignant changes in remaining trophoblastic tissue.

6. Painless vaginal bleeding in the latter half of pregnancy is the classic sign of placenta previa. Activity limitations, no sexual intercourse, an adult caregiver present at all times, and availability of emergency transportation to the hospital are essential for home care. The client must also be taught to monitor fetal movement and to report a decrease in movement or increase in vaginal bleeding.

7. The classic signs of placental abruption are (a) bleeding, which may be evident vaginally or concealed behind the placenta; (b) uterine pain or tenderness; (c) uterine irritability, with poor relaxation between contractions; (d) abdominal or low back pain; and (e) a high uterine resting tone if an intrauterine pressure catheter is being used. Additional symptoms include a "board-like" abdomen, firm to the touch; port wine–colored amniotic fluid, category II or III fetal heart rate (FHR) pattern and signs of hypovolemic shock.

8. Hemorrhagic shock is the major danger of placental abruption for the pregnant client; anoxia, excessive blood loss, and delivery before maturity are major dangers for the fetus.

9. Hyperemesis gravidarum is believed to be an extreme form of "morning sickness". Morning sickness is self-limiting and causes no serious complications. Hyperemesis is persistent, uncontrollable vomiting that may cause excessive weight loss, dehydration, and electrolyte or acid-base imbalance.

10. Goals of management are to reduce nausea and vomiting, maintain nutrition and fluid balance, and provide emotional support.

11. Fetal complications associated with preeclampsia result from decreased placental perfusion due to the pathologic changes of preeclampsia. The fetus may experience hypoxemia, intolerance to labor, preterm birth, low birth weight, intrauterine growth restriction, or even fetal death.

12. The diagnostic criteria for preeclampsia include hypertension occurring after 20 weeks of gestation usually accompanied by proteinuria. In the absence of proteinuria, hypertension with thrombocytopenia, renal insufficiency, impaired liver function, pulmonary edema, cerebral symptoms or visual changes are also diagnosed as preeclampsia. Nonspecific edema that is severe and generalized is often seen but is no longer considered a classic sign of preeclampsia. Headache, hyperreflexia, visual disturbances, and epigastric pain indicate the disease is worsening. Rest, especially in a lateral position, increases cardiac return and circulatory volume, thus improving perfusion of vital organs and placenta.

13. Vasoconstriction causes rupture of cerebral capillaries and small cerebral hemorrhages. Symptoms of arterial vasospasm include headache and visual disturbances such as blurred vision, "spots" before the eyes, and hyperactive deep tendon reflexes (DTRs).

14. Magnesium sulfate prevents seizures by reducing central nervous system irritability and decreasing vasoconstriction. The primary adverse effect is central nervous system depression, which includes depression of the respiratory center.

15. Pulmonary edema, circulatory or renal failure, aspiration of gastric contents, and cerebral hemorrhage are complications of eclampsia.

16. Assessments for the client with preeclampsia include daily weights, location and degree of edema, vital signs, breath sounds, urinary output, urine for protein, DTRs, and subjective signs such as headache, visual disturbances, and epigastric pain. The fetal heart rate pattern should be assessed. Respiratory rate, oxygen saturation level, consciousness level, and laboratory data such as creatinine, liver enzymes, and magnesium levels should be evaluated. Psychosocial assessment should include the reaction of the client's family and support system. Nursing assessment helps determine whether the condition is responding to medical management, the condition is stable, or the disease is worsening.

17. To prevent seizures, maintain a quiet environment, reduce environmental stimuli, and maintain a therapeutic level of magnesium. Nurses must remain with the client and call for help if a seizure occurs. Attempt to turn the client to a lateral position before the onset of a seizure. Note the sequence and time of the seizure. Insert an airway after the seizure, and suction the client's nose and mouth, administer oxygen, administer medications, and prepare for additional medical interventions.

18. To prevent seizure-related injury, the side rails should be padded and raised. The bed should be in the lowest position with the wheels locked. Oxygen and suction should be readily available. Necessary equipment and medications should be immediately available and checked for proper function at the beginning of each shift.

19. Signs of magnesium toxicity include respiratory rate below 12 breaths per minute, hyporeflexia, chest pain or shortness of breath, altered sensorium (lethargy, drowsiness, disorientation), and serum magnesium level beyond the therapeutic range. If toxicity occurs, discontinue the drug and notify the physician. Calcium gluconate is an antidote for magnesium toxicity and should be immediately available.

20. *H,* Hemolysis; *EL,* elevated liver enzymes; *LP,* low platelets. Major symptoms are pain and tenderness in the right upper quadrant. Additional signs and symptoms may include nausea, vomiting, malaise, headaches, and visual changes. Laboratory data include a low hematocrit level, abnormal liver studies, coagulation abnormalities, and often abnormal renal studies. Palpating the liver could cause trauma, including rupture of a subcapsular hematoma.

21. Preeclampsia occurs only during pregnancy and the early postpartum period. Chronic hypertension is present before pregnancy or before the 20th week of gestation and persists after the postpartum period. Hypertension that remains several weeks postpartum suggests chronic hypertension even if the blood pressure measurements were normal when the client entered care. Treatment may be similar during pregnancy; however, chronic hypertension may be treated with antihypertensive medications before and during pregnancy. Preeclampsia may further complicate chronic hypertension.

22. Administration of Rho(D) immunoglobulin prevents development of anti-Rh antibodies in the client and is recommended after any procedure that includes the possibility of exposure to Rh-positive fetal blood.

23. A client who is sensitized has developed antibodies to the Rh antigen. The pregnant client's anti-Rh antibodies cross the placenta. If the fetus is Rh-positive, the antibodies destroy fetal Rh-positive red blood cells. The fetus becomes anemic, bilirubin concentration increases, and in extreme cases severe neurologic disease can result.

24. Many clients with blood type O have anti-A or anti-B antibodies before they become pregnant, so the first pregnancy can be affected. The effects of ABO incompatibility are milder than Rh sensitization because the primary antibodies of the ABO system are IgM, which do not readily cross the placenta.

25. The hormones of pregnancy cause cellular resistance to insulin, which increases the availability of glucose for the fetus.

26. The pregnant client is at risk for spontaneous abortion (miscarriage); hypertension, especially preeclampsia; urinary tract infections; ketoacidosis; polyhydramnios; premature rupture of the membranes; difficult labor with trauma; cesarean birth; and postpartum hemorrhage. Possible fetal and neonatal effects include congenital malformations; small or large fetal size, depending on the placental vascular supply; fetal hypoxemia; and birth injury. Neonatal effects include hypoglycemia, hypocalcemia, hyperbilirubinemia, and respiratory distress syndrome.

27. Insulin needs decrease during the first trimester and increase sharply during the second and third trimesters (when placental hormones initiate insulin resistance). In the postpartum period, insulin needs decrease as levels of placental hormones decline.

28. Glycosylated hemoglobin gives an accurate evaluation of blood glucose level for the past 2 to 3 months and is not affected by recent intake or restriction of food.

29. Gestational diabetes mellitus (GDM) is first diagnosed during the second or third trimester of pregnancy. Pregestational, type 1 diabetes mellitus usually emerges during childhood or early adulthood and requires insulin for control. Pregestational type 2 diabetes usually occurs in adulthood and is usually managed by diet and/or oral hypoglycemics if not pregnant; during pregnancy, insulin is the preferred treatment. Gestational diabetes is often managed by diet and exercise, although insulin may be needed if fasting or postprandial capillary blood glucose values are persistently high. Due to limited data on the long-term effects of oral hypoglycemics during pregnancy, insulin is the preferred treatment.

30. A glucose challenge test (GCT) is a screening procedure only and requires no fasting before the client drinks a 50-g glucose solution and has a serum glucose drawn 1 hour later. No special client instructions are required. A 3-hour oral glucose tolerance test (OGTT) is performed to diagnose diabetes mellitus, including gestational diabetes. The OGTT requires measurement of a fasting blood glucose level followed by intake of 100 g of glucose solution. Blood glucose levels are determined hourly after the solution is taken at 1, 2, and 3 hours. Prior to the test, the client should be instructed to have 3 days of unrestricted diet and activity followed by an 8 hour fast. They should not eat or smoke throughout the test.

31. The client with GDM has an increased risk for the development of preeclampsia and a cesarean birth. The greatest risk is the increased possibility of development of diabetes later in life. Fetal effects of GDM may include macrosomia, which can result in shoulder dystocia, birth injuries, or cesarean birth but do not include an increased risk for spontaneous abortions (miscarriages), congenital anomalies, or small fetal size due to vascular complications. The newborn is at risk for hypoglycemia and hyperbilirubinemia.

32. The client with obesity should gain 11 to 20 lb during pregnancy.

33. During the intrapartum period, the nurse caring for a client with obesity should assess FHR and uterine activity frequently. In addition, due to the slower rate of labor progress and increased risk for operative vaginal births

and cesarean births, the nurse should assess for signs of dysfunctional labor (abnormal contraction pattern, slow or no cervical change, inadequate fetal descent).

34. Most clients of reproductive age do not have adequate iron stores to meet the demands of pregnancy because of menstrual blood loss and have difficulty meeting the high iron needs of pregnancy with diet alone.

35. The fetal and neonatal effects of iron-deficiency anemia are increased risk for preterm birth, low birth weight, and perinatal mortality. In addition, there may be a negative effect later in life with the mental and psychomotor performance of the child.

36. Pregnancy may worsen sickle cell disease, and the risk of "sickle cell crisis" is increased. These clients also have an increased risk for pyelonephritis, bone infection, heart disease, and hypertensive complications of pregnancy.

37. Frequent measurements of hemoglobin, blood count, serum iron, and iron-binding capacity, as well as folate, are necessary to determine the degree of anemia and iron and folic acid stores. Testing for infections is performed, and noninfected clients who are not immune are immunized as appropriate based on pregnancy status (live vaccines are contraindicated during pregnancy). Both clinical and subclinical UTIs are treated. Frequent fetal surveillance for growth and placental and monitoring for signs of sickle cell crisis are also necessary. The nurse should also be aware that the client's pain could be a pregnancy complication rather than a result of sickle cell crisis.

38. Thalassemia is associated with increased iron absorption and storage, and clients with this disorder are susceptible to iron overload; supplemental iron should not exceed prophylactic dosage unless iron deficiency is documented.

39. The effects of systemic lupus erythematosus in the pregnant client and fetus are increased incidence of hypertensive disorders, including preeclampsia, preterm birth, IUGR, fetal loss, and stillbirth. Congenital heart block, often permanent, is a serious complication for the newborn.

40. Rheumatoid arthritis often markedly improves during pregnancy. However, relapse often occurs within 3 months after childbirth.

41. Hypothyroidism in the pregnant client, most often the result of Hashimoto's thyroiditis, may cause adverse effects on the mental development of the fetus through birth and childhood. A greater risk for miscarriage, preterm birth, and preeclampsia also exists if it is not corrected.

42. Anticonvulsant drugs may be teratogenic. Many have probable or known adverse effects on the fetus. However, generalized seizures may also have adverse fetal effects, so maintaining the anticonvulsant dose as low as possible is important. Newer anticonvulsants, lamotrigine and levetiracetam, have lower rates of structural and cognitive effects and are more often prescribed.

43. The recommended supportive care for clients with Bell's palsy includes eye patching, applying ointment or drops to prevent trauma to the cornea, facial massage, and psychological support. Corticosteroids may be given.

44. Most infants born with CMV are asymptomatic, but 5% to 18% will have symptoms at birth that include jaundice, petechiae, thrombocytopenia, growth restriction, and hydrops. Long-term effects include intellectual and physical disability, seizures, and sensorineural deficits. Congenital CMV is the most common cause of hearing loss in children.

45. The first trimester is the time of organogenesis, when damage can be done to all developing organ systems, and infection may result in loss of the pregnancy or congenital rubella syndrome.

46. A vaccine is available to prevent rubella, but it cannot be given during pregnancy. During pregnancy a client can only avoid situations that pose an increased risk for contraction of rubella. Rubella immunization should be given to the postpartum client before discharge after birth, with instructions that pregnancy should be avoided for 28 days after the immunization.

47. Immunization with varicella-zoster immune globulin is recommended. Because of viral shedding, the infected postpartum client and infant must be isolated from those who are not immune.

48. Vertical transmission of herpesvirus occurs when organisms ascend from active lesions after rupture of membranes and during birth when the fetus comes into contact with infectious tissue and secretions.

49. The fetal and neonatal effects of parvovirus B19 infection are failure of red blood cell production, severe fetal anemia, hydrops, and heart failure often resulting in fetal death. Most infants who survive do very well, although there may be a small risk for developmental delays.

50. Hepatitis B virus is transmitted by contact with infected blood, saliva, vaginal secretions, or semen and readily crosses the placenta. A newborn of a client who is HBsAg-positive should receive hepatitis B immune globulin soon after birth, followed by hepatitis B vaccine. The infant should receive the second and third doses of vaccine at regularly scheduled times.

51. Avoid sexual transmission of HIV by abstinence, decreased number of sex partners (mutual monogamy is best), and using condoms with each sexual act. Intravenous drug users who refuse rehabilitation should be taught to wash the equipment with water, soap, and bleach before each use to reduce transmission of the virus through a soiled needle. Treatment before, during, and after birth can significantly decrease the rate of perinatal transmission.

52. Medical management of the pregnant client with HIV includes the use of multiple antiretroviral drugs from different classes. Ideally, ART is started before conception and continued through the antepartum, intrapartum, postpartum, and neonatal periods. If the client does not seek care, or the infection is not identified until after conception, the medications should be started as soon as possible, even if that is on arrival to the birth facility.

53. The benefits of COVID-19 vaccines for the pregnant client are decreased risk of severe disease during pregnancy and lactation. The evidence is also demonstrating that the vaccines are not only safe for pregnant and lactating clients and their fetuses and newborns but also provide protection to the newborn after birth.

54. Toxoplasmosis can be prevented by cooking meat thoroughly, not touching mucous membranes while handling raw meat, washing kitchen surfaces and hands thoroughly after handling raw meat, avoiding uncooked eggs and unpasteurized milk, washing vegetables and fruit before consumption, and avoiding contact with materials that may be contaminated with cat feces.

55. Intravenous antimicrobial therapy during labor is most effective in preventing neonatal colonization with GBS when the pregnant client is GBS-positive or if the client's GBS status is unknown.

56. Isoniazid and rifampin, with or without ethambutol, are given for 2 months followed by isoniazid and rifampin daily or twice per week for 7 months to treat tuberculosis in the pregnant client. Pyridoxine (vitamin B_6) is added to prevent fetal neurotoxicity. The infant is skin-tested at birth and may be prescribed isoniazid. Isoniazid is usually continued for the infant until the postpartum client's tuberculosis has been inactive for at least 3 months. Infant tuberculosis medication may stop if the postpartum client and family members have received full treatment and show no additional disease. If the skin test result shows conversion to positive, a full course of drug therapy should be given to the infant.

CHAPTER 11

1. Pregnancy interrupts developmental tasks such as the achievement of a stable identity, development of a personal value system, completion of educational goals, and achievement of independence from parents.

2. Teenage clients have an increased chance of perinatal complications, including hypertensive disorders and preterm labor. Their infants are at greater risk for low birth weight and lower 5-minute Apgar scores, which are associated with the need for neonatal intensive care.

3. A variety of teaching methods effective with adolescents include forming small groups with similar concerns, communicating with kindness and respect, using appropriate language understood by teens and conveying empathetic concern with nonverbal communication, using social media and mobile phone applications, and including other family members when appropriate.

4. Prospective teenage parents should be taught early developmental changes to help the young parents understand the normal progression of infant abilities. Explain and demonstrate infant cues, describe the way infants use behaviors to communicate; emphasize eye contact, holding, cuddling, and verbal stimulation are important for the child's development.

5. Mature gravidas often have maturity, problem-solving skills, and emotional and financial resources that may be unavailable to younger parents.

6. The fetus of a mature client is at increased risk for chromosomal anomalies that may be detected by prenatal testing.

7. The older postpartum client may have less energy than younger clients, anticipatory guidance should include measures that will help conserve energy for self and infant care.

8. Neonatal effects of client smoking during pregnancy include risk for low birth weight, increased risk for sudden infant death syndrome (SIDS), and an increased risk of respiratory infections, colic, asthma, bone fractures, and childhood obesity. In addition, tobacco use during pregnancy increases the risk for miscarriage and can cause damage to the fetal brain and lungs.

9. Fetal alcohol syndrome is characterized by slow growth, central nervous system impairment, and cranial and facial anomalies.

10. Effects of cocaine use during pregnancy on the infant include increased risk for miscarriage, IUGR, neonatal abstinence syndrome (NAS), childhood learning difficulties, childhood behavior issues, and vision problems.

11. Pregnant heroin users are placed on methadone or buprenorphine to reduce symptoms of withdrawal and addiction. These drugs can provide a long-acting, steady drug dose to the fetus to avoid the problems of intrauterine overdosage and withdrawal. The dosage is gradually decreased to wean the pregnant client off of the drug.

12. Prenatal behaviors that suggest substance abuse include prenatal care sought late in pregnancy, failure to keep appointments, inconsistent follow-through with recommended regimens, poor grooming, inadequate weight gain, needle punctures, thrombosed veins, signs of cellulitis, defensive or hostile reactions, and severe mood swings.

13. Signs and symptoms of recent cocaine use include profuse sweating, high blood pressure, tachycardia, irregular respirations, lethargic response to labor, dilated pupils, increased body temperature, sudden onset of severely painful uterine contractions, fetal tachycardia, and excessive fetal activity. Emotional signs include anger, caustic or abusive reactions to the caregiver, emotional lability, and paranoia.

14. Interventions are focused on preventing client or fetal injury, maintaining effective communication, providing pain control, and, when the substance is heroin, preventing withdrawal during labor.

15. Parents experience less anxiety when they are gently told about any anomalies of the infant as soon as they are identified and allowed to hold their newborn as soon as possible.

16. Facial, genital, and irreparable defects are likely to affect parenting most.

17. The reaction of parents can be described in terms of a grief response. Initial reactions include shock and disbelief. Denial, anger, and guilt are common.

18. Nurses can promote bonding by handling the infant gently, emphasizing normal traits, helping parents hold and cuddle the infant, and using communication skills to help parents come to terms with their feelings.

19. Discharge planning should include special feeding and other techniques that the infant may require, the follow-up care needed, and referral to agencies and organizations that may be helpful.

20. The way in which the stillborn infant is presented creates memories that the parents will retain. The infant should be washed and taken to the parents while still warm and soft, wrapped in a soft, warm blanket.

21. A memory packet with photographs of the baby, handprints, footprints, a birth identification band, crib card, blanket, cap, and (if possible and parents agree) a lock of hair helps parents grieve.

22. Some birth parents may find a great sense of joy in knowing they could give their child a better life through adoption despite the struggle they have with feelings of guilt, depression, and regret.

23. The nurse should acknowledge the needs and emotions of the adoptive parents. Efforts should be made to give them a private room to process the their emotions and adapt to their new role as parents. Adoptive parents should be taught how to care for an infant and what to expect in terms of growth and development. Demonstrations and return demonstrations may be helpful to assist them in learning to care for their newborn.

24. Nursing responsibilities start with clear and detailed communication with both the surrogate and the intended parents. Care of the surrogate should follow the standard of care for any pregnant client. If the parents do not want the surrogate to breastfeed the infant, instruction should be provided regarding appropriate breast care following birth. The emotional needs of the surrogate should be addressed.

25. Intended parents should receive the infant security bands and their own room. They should be taught how to care for the infant and be incorporated into care and assessments of the infant, as well as be the legal and designated decision makers regarding infant medical decisions. Their emotional needs in adaptation to parenthood should be addressed.

26. The symptoms of postpartum depression differ from those of postpartum "blues" in their intensity and persistence. In postpartum depression, the symptoms are present daily longer than 2 weeks. They include anxiety, feelings of guilt, agitation, fatigue, sleeplessness, feeling unwell, irritability, difficulty concentrating or making decisions, confusion, appetite changes, loss of pleasure in normal activities, crying, sadness, depression, suicidal thoughts, and being less responsive to the infant.

27. Nurses can demonstrate caring, provide anticipatory guidance, help the client verbalize feelings, enhance sensitivity to infant cues, help family members, and explore options and resources.

28. Screening tools include the Edinburgh Postnatal Depression Scale, the Postpartum Depression Checklist, and the Postpartum Depression Predictors Inventory–Revised.

29. Postpartum psychosis usually requires hospitalization, psychotherapy, and appropriate medication.

CHAPTER 12

1. Effacement and dilation of the cervix occur because contractions pull the cervix upward over the fetus and amniotic sac while pushing the fetus and amniotic sac downward against the cervix. The muscle fibers of the upper uterus become shorter to maintain these forces between contractions. The upper two-thirds of the uterus contracts actively to push the fetus down. The lower third of the uterus remains less active, promoting downward passage of the fetus. In addition, the uterus changes shape and becomes more elongated and narrower to maintain pressure of the fetus and amniotic sac against the cervix.

2. The cervix of the nullipara effaces more before it dilates. The cervix of a multipara is usually thicker than that of a nullipara during the entire labor.

3. Changes occurring during labor include the following:
   a. Cardiovascular system—A slight increase in blood pressure and decrease in pulse rate occur as each contraction temporarily stops blood flow to the uterus and shunts 300 to 500 mL of blood into systemic circulation. Supine hypotension may occur if the client lies supine because the heavy uterus compresses the inferior vena cava and reduces blood flow to the heart.
   b. Respiratory system—The depth and rate of respirations increase.
   c. Gastrointestinal system—Gastric motility is reduced during labor, which can result in nausea and vomiting. Controversy exists on whether laboring clients should be allowed to eat or drink during labor. Concerns surround the risk for vomiting and aspiration of undigested foods in the event general anesthesia is required. Evidence supports allowing low-risk laboring clients some form of oral intake. The American Society of Anesthesiologists supports oral intake of clear liquids in low-risk laboring clients.
   d. Urinary system—The sensation of a full bladder is reduced.
   e. Hematopoietic system—Leukocyte counts are as high as 20,000 to 30,000/mm^3, and levels of clotting factors are elevated.

4. Uterine contractions temporarily decrease blood flow to the placenta. If the contractions were sustained, the fetus could not receive freshly oxygenated blood and nutrients and dispose of waste products through the placenta.

5. Labor and vaginal birth primarily benefit the newborn by increasing absorption of fetal lung fluid. They also cause compression of the upper airways, causing some lung fluid to be expelled. These effects reduce the amount of lung fluid remaining in the newborn's respiratory tract

when breathing begins. Labor also stimulates the fetus to secrete catecholamines, which help speed clearance of the lung fluid after birth, stimulate cardiac contraction and breathing, and aid in temperature regulation.

6. The power of labor during the first stage involves uterine contractions. Powers during the second stage include uterine contractions, augmented by the client's voluntary pushing efforts.

7. The three divisions of the true pelvis are the inlet, midpelvis, and outlet.

8. The vertex presentation, in which the fetal head is fully flexed forward, allows the smallest diameter of the fetal head to enter the pelvis. It also more effectively dilates the cervix.

9. ROP: The fetal landmark is the occiput, indicating a vertex presentation. It is located in the pregnant client's right posterior pelvic quadrant. OA: The fetal landmark is the occiput, which is located in the client's anterior pelvis and is not directed toward the left or the right. This is often the presentation just before birth. RSA: The fetal landmark is the sacrum, indicating that the fetus is in a breech presentation. It is located in the client's right anterior pelvis. LMA: The fetal landmark is the mentum, or chin, indicating that the fetus is in a face presentation. The chin is in the client's left anterior pelvis.

10. If the fetus is in the face presentation, the occiput is not accessible to the examiner's fingers during vaginal examination. For this reason the fetal chin (mentum) is used to describe the position (such as RMA [right mentum anterior]).

11. The client may note several changes as labor approaches: increased strength and frequency of Braxton Hicks contractions, lightening, increased vaginal mucus, bloody show, an energy spurt, and a small weight loss.

12. False labor tends to differ from true labor in three major ways. True labor is characterized by contractions that progressively become more frequent, last longer, and are more intense. The discomfort of true labor begins in the lower back and sweeps to the lower abdomen, whereas the discomfort of false labor is more often in the abdomen or groin and is often simply annoying. In true labor, progressive effacement and dilation of the cervix occur, which is the most significant difference from false labor.

13. The transverse diameter of the pelvic inlet is slightly larger than the inlet's anteroposterior diameter. The anteroposterior diameter of the fetal head (in line with the sagittal suture) is slightly larger than the transverse diameter. Therefore the fetal head best fits the pelvis if the sagittal suture is aligned with the pelvic transverse diameter at entry.

14. Because the client's pelvic outlet is usually slightly larger in its anteroposterior diameter than its transverse diameter, the fetal head turns in the mechanism of internal rotation so that the sagittal suture aligns with the anteroposterior diameter as the fetus descends.

15. During the first stage, latent phase, the client is often sociable, excited, and somewhat anxious. During the first stage, active phase, the client becomes less sociable and is inwardly focused. As labor progresses, the client who does not choose epidural analgesia may become irritable and temporarily lose control. During the second stage, the clients energy is usually concentrated on pushing the baby out and rarely interacts with others. A feeling of control and active participation in the birth often accompanies the second stage.

16. Contractions vary among clients, but the general pattern includes increasing frequency, duration, and intensity throughout labor. In the first stage, latent phase, contractions gradually increase until they are about 5 minutes apart, with mild to moderate intensity. In the first stage, active phase, contractions increase from about three contractions in a 10-minute period to five contractions in that same period. Duration of the contractions is steady at 60 to 80 seconds; intensity is moderate to strong. In the second stage, contractions are strong and about 2 to 3 minutes apart and have a duration of about 60 to 80 seconds.

17. Signs that the placenta may have separated include a spherical uterine shape, the rising of the uterus upward in the abdomen, protrusion of the umbilical cord farther outward from the vagina, and a gush of blood.

18. Hemorrhage may occur if the uterus does not remain contracted after birth of the placenta because open blood vessels at the site will not be compressed by the interlacing muscle fibers of the uterus.

CHAPTER 13

1. Childbirth pain differs from other painful experiences because it is part of a normal process, the pain is purposeful and may lead the client to assume different positions that assist in labor progression, the client has time to prepare for it, the pain is intermittent, and it ends with the birth of the baby.

2. Excessive, unrelieved labor pain may result in reduced blood flow to and from the placenta, restricting fetal oxygen supply and waste removal; reduced effectiveness of uterine contractions, which slows labor progress; acid–base imbalance in the pregnant client, and fetal acidosis. Poor pain relief can lessen the joy of childbirth for the client and partner and may have lasting psychological effects. It may also impair interaction with the infant after birth due to exhaustion and trauma.

3. Physical and psychological factors interact to alter the ability to tolerate pain.

4. Four sources of pain present in most labors are cervical dilation, tissue ischemia, pressure and pulling on pelvic structures, and distention of the vagina and perineum.

5. Physical factors that influence pain include the following:
   a. A short, intense labor may be more painful because dilation, effacement, and fetal descent occur rapidly.
   b. A cervix that does not efface or dilate easily is likely to be associated with a longer and more uncomfortable labor.

c. An abnormal fetal position may cause a longer labor as the client's body maneuvers it into a better position. Back pain is especially noticeable if the fetus is in an occiput posterior position.

d. Variations in the client's pelvic size or shape may result in abnormal fetal presentations or positions and in a longer labor because the fetus does not fit through the pelvis easily.

e. Fatigue reduces the client's pain tolerance and ability to use coping skills.

6. Psychosocial factors that influence labor pain include culture, race, anxiety and fear, previous experiences with pain, preparation for childbirth, and the support system.

7. The gate-control theory of pain assumes that a gating mechanism in the dorsal horn of the spinal cord controls the transmission of impulses to the brain for interpretation. Pain impulses are transmitted through small-diameter fibers, whereas other sensations, such as tactile sensations (e.g., massage, heat, cold), are transmitted more quickly through large-diameter fibers. Therefore the impulses transmitted through the large-diameter fibers interfere with, or "close the gate" to, transmission of pain impulses. Impulses from the brain, such as the use of a focal point or breathing techniques, can also impede pain transmission.

8. Nursing actions to promote relaxation include arranging for environmental comfort, maintaining the client's general comfort and dignity, reducing factors that cause anxiety and fear, and using specific relaxation techniques such as helping the client focus on relaxing specific tense muscles.

9. Accurate information and a focus on the normal aspects of childbirth help reduce anxiety and fear. The nurse can empower the birthing couple by providing informed consent and giving them the ability to make choices that feel safe and necessary. Listening to the client's hopes and expectations will help establish trust and lessen fear-driven decision making by the client.

10. Massage increases the release of endorphins, promotes circulation, and reduces muscle tension. Effleurage, light stroking of the abdomen or legs, and rubbing of the back, shoulders, legs, or other areas may be helpful to some clients. Counterpressure applied through sacral pressure, hip squeeze, or knee press may help when the client has back pain with labor. Warmth increases oxytocin release and local blood flow, relaxes muscles, and raises the pain threshold. Cool, damp washcloths placed on the head, throat, or lower abdomen often provides comfort to the laboring client who may be hot.

11. Hyperventilation, which results from rapid, deep breathing, causes excessive loss of carbon dioxide and respiratory alkalosis, vasoconstriction, and, if it persists, can lead to tetany resulting in stiffness of the face and lips and carpopedal spasm.

12. The cleansing breath, or "sigh," helps the client release tension, provides oxygen, and helps the client clear the mind.

13. Lengthy pushing in the second stage has shown greater client fatigue, more operative births, and increased occurrence of category II or III fetal heart rate (FHR) patterns and does not significantly shorten the second stage. Strenuous directed pushing has shown a greater risk for structural and neurogenic injury to a client's pelvic floor. Closed glottis pushing delivers less blood to the placenta, possibly resulting in fetal hypoxia and category II or III fetal heart rate patterns.

14. Drugs taken by the pregnant client can affect the fetus directly, resulting from passage of the medication or its metabolites across the placenta, such as a decrease in fetal heart rate variability after administration of analgesic, or indirectly, secondary to the effect in the client, such as by causing hypotension that reduces placental blood flow and fetal oxygen supply.

15. The major cardiovascular change in pregnancy that effects pharmacologic pain management is aortocaval compression. If the client must be in the supine position, the uterus should be displaced with a wedge under one hip to promote blood return to the heart. Due to respiratory changes of pregnancy, the client is more sensitive to inhaled anesthesia, and the edema of the upper airway may make intubation more difficult. During pregnancy, the stomach is displaced upward by the uterus, peristalsis is slowed, and the tone of the sphincter at the junction of the stomach and esophagus is relaxed. These changes make the client vulnerable to regurgitation and aspiration during general anesthesia. Circulating levels of endorphins and enkephalins are increased during labor; these natural substances have analgesic properties that should reduce the requirements for analgesia and anesthesia. The smaller epidural and subarachnoid spaces, engorged epidural veins, and heightened sensitivity of nerve fibers to local anesthetic agents during pregnancy reduce the amount of analgesics and local anesthetics needed to achieve satisfactory pain management with either an epidural or subarachnoid block.

16. Drugs (prescribed, over-the-counter, or illicit), botanical preparations, and substances such as alcohol may interact with one another. These interactions may be harmful to the client, the fetus, or both and limit pharmacologic pain management options. Knowledge of exactly what drugs the client has used allows the safest choices in pharmacologic pain-relief methods.

17. Neonatal respiratory depression is the primary drawback to the use of opioid analgesia. This effect can be reduced by timing the dose to reduce the amount transferred to the fetus (which varies according to the drug) and by giving the narcotic in small, frequent IV doses at the beginning of the contraction.

18. Airway management (i.e., bag-and-mask ventilation) takes precedence over use of naloxone for the newborn. Naloxone may be used to reverse opioid-induced respiratory depression and to reverse pruritus from epidural opioids in the adult. The respiratory depression may be from systemic or epidural administration of opioids.

19. The two major advantages of regional pain management are that the client can have pain relief and remain alert.

20. Epidural and subarachnoid blocks can cause hypotension. The fall in blood pressure may result in reduced placental blood flow, compromising fetal oxygen supply. Giving the client IV fluids before the block reduces this effect. Other less serious adverse effects are bladder distention, prolonged second stage of labor (epidural), and fever.

21. Epidural or intrathecal opioid analgesics may cause nausea, vomiting, itching, or a combination of these. They may also result in delayed respiratory depression (up to 24 hours), depending on the drug used. Management includes ondansetron or metoclopramide for nausea and vomiting; diphenhydramine, naloxone, or nalbuphine for itching; and pulse oximetry and monitoring of respirations while the opioid is given and up to 24 hours after administration ends, depending on the drug.

22. Failed intubation, client regurgitation with aspiration of acidic gastric contents, and adverse reaction to anesthetic medications are the major potential adverse effects of general anesthesia. If failed intubation occurs, the anesthesia team must manage the airway differently prior to the start of surgery. Additional staff and equipment should be available. The risk for aspiration may be reduced by limiting intake to clear fluids, giving drugs to raise the gastric pH, giving drugs to reduce gastric secretions or speed emptying of the stomach, and using cricoid pressure (Sellick maneuver) to block the esophagus while the endotracheal tube is being inserted. Respiratory depression, primarily in the infant, is minimized by delaying general anesthesia until the surgery team is prepared and by keeping the anesthesia level as light as possible until the umbilical cord is cut. A detailed medical, surgical, and family history may help identify the potential for and adverse reaction to anesthetic medications, but many obstetric clients are young and healthy without significant medical histories, such as surgical interventions with anesthetic agents.

CHAPTER 14

1. Oxygen is carried from the environment to the fetus through a maternal and fetal circulation pathway, which includes the client's lungs, heart, vasculature, uterus, placenta, and umbilical cord. Interruption along this oxygen pathway at one or more points can cause physiologic changes resulting in distinctive fetal heart rate (FHR) characteristics.

2. At term gestation (40 weeks), approximately 500 to 800 mL of the pregnant client's blood perfuses the uterus.

3. The two umbilical arteries carry deoxygenated blood from the fetus to the placenta.

4. Both external and internal electronic fetal monitoring in labor are continuous, providing more data than intermittent assessments and a permanent record on a paper tracing or computer archive system. Common disadvantages are possible limitations to client mobility and a technical atmosphere. Specific to the external ultrasound transducer for monitor FHR and tocotransducer (toco) for uterine activity, additional advantages include that they are easy to apply, may be used during the antepartum and intrapartum periods, and there are no known risks to the client or fetus. There are also telemetry devices that can increase the options for client mobility and position changes. Disadvantages are the need for frequent repositioning of the transducers, the FHR may be doubled or halved in cases of fetal bradycardia or tachycardia, the pregnant client's heart rate may be recorded as fetal data if the ultrasound transducer is placed over the pregnant client's arterial vessels, clients with obesity and preterm or multifetal gestations may be difficult to monitor, and the tocotransducer does not accurately assess the intensity of contractions or resting tone of the uterus between contractions. The toco is location sensitive, poor placement may lead to an absence of or inadequate data, and it is sensitive to client or fetal movement that may be superimposed on the tracing. Internal monitors (fetal scalp electrode [FSE]/intrauterine pressure catheter [IUPC]) are not usually affected by client position changes (although the IUPC needs to be recalibrated with position changes) and do not need to be repositioned to maintain accurate data; the FSE detects FHR between 30 and 240 bpm when clinically required; the IUPC accurately measures all parameters of uterine activity and provides a port that allows amnioinfusion or withdrawal of fluid for testing. However, they are invasive and require cervical dilatation and ruptured fetal membranes. They can cause trauma and infection. There are contraindications such as placenta previa, active infections, and extreme prematurity of the fetus. Telemetry devices are not available; therefore, client mobility is significantly impacted. In cases of intrauterine fetal demise, the FSE may record the pregnant client's heart rate as the FHR, the logic in the software must be turned off to detect fetal arrhythmias, and client position changes may affect the quality of the IUPC data. Nonelectronic fetal monitoring (intermittent auscultation [IA] of FHR and palpation of uterine contractions) promotes the laboring client's mobility and creates a more natural atmosphere. Assessments are possible during ambulation and alternative labor and birthing locations, such as hydrotherapy. The one-to-one nursing care required for this method elevates the level of care, and there is no expensive equipment involved. However, it is not advised for high-risk clients, there is no permanent record or paper tracing, assessment of the fetus is intermittent—significant events may not be detected, periodic and nonperiodic changes in fetal heart rate (FHR) cannot be determined, conditions such as client obesity, hydramnios, client or fetal movement and in some cases, uterine tension during a contraction may reduce the ability to hear the FHR. IA and palpation require a one-to-one nurse-to-client ratio and competency education and ongoing practice for nurses to develop and maintain

the skill. Some clients may be intolerant of the clinician's touch during contractions, conditions such as client obesity may limit the ability to palpate contractions, and contractions cannot be assessed objectively.

5. When palpating uterine contractions, the fingertips are used to indent the uterus at the peak of the contraction. The descriptive terms used are *mild, moderate,* and *firm* or *strong.* A mild contraction can be compared with the tip of the nose—easily indented. A moderate contraction is compared with the chin—it can be slightly indented. A firm or strong contraction is compared with the forehead—unable to indent. The resting tone of the uterus should also be palpated between contractions and the finding recorded. The relaxed uterus is described as *soft.* Increased tone between contractions is abnormal and requires nursing actions.

6. The FHR records on the upper grid of the monitor paper or computer tracing; the uterine activity records on the lower grid.

7. The ultrasound transducer, or external electronic fetal monitor (EFM), detects fetal heart motion to measure fetal heart rate (FHR). A handheld Doppler device uses the same technology. Using a fetoscope or Pinard stethoscope, the listener hears the fetal heart sounds.

8. The accuracy of the uterine activity (UA) data from a tocodynamometer may be affected by the position of the toco on the fundus, the amount of tissue (adipose) between the toco and uterus, and the client's position.

9. Fetal heart rate (FHR) accelerations, whether spontaneous or induced, are predictive of adequate oxygenation and a fetal pH that rules out acidemia.

10. Late decelerations are visually apparent and usually symmetric in shape, with a gradual decrease and return of the fetal heart rate (FHR) to baseline. Late decelerations occur when the onset of the deceleration to the nadir is equal to or greater than 30 seconds, and the onset, nadir, and recovery of the deceleration occurs after the beginning, peak, and end of the contraction. Early decelerations are visually apparent, are symmetric in shape, and have a gradual decrease and return to FHR baseline that mirrors a uterine contraction. The deceleration onset, nadir, and recovery coincide with the beginning, peak, and ending of a contraction. The onset of the deceleration to the nadir is equal to or greater than 30 seconds. Early decelerations are thought to represent a vagal response during fetal head compression. Early decelerations are benign and not associated with an interruption of fetal oxygenation. Variable decelerations are visually apparent, abrupt decreases from onset to nadir of a deceleration. The onset of the deceleration to the nadir is less than 30 seconds. The decrease is at least 15 bpm below the baseline, with the deceleration lasting at least 15 seconds and no longer than 2 minutes from onset to the return to baseline. Deceleration shape, depth, duration, and timing in relationship to contractions may vary. Variable decelerations are suggestive of an interruption of oxygenation at the level of the umbilical cord where cord vessels may be compressed.

11. Frequency is the time (minutes) from the onset of one contraction to the onset of the next contraction. Uterine activity may also be quantified as the number of contractions in a 10-minute window of time, averaged over 30 minutes. Duration is the time (seconds) from the onset of one contraction to the end of the same contraction. Intensity is the strength of the contraction at its peak. It is measured by palpation as mild, moderate, or firm. It is quantified in mmHg with the use of an intrauterine pressure catheter (IUPC). Resting tone is the amount of pressure (tone) in the uterus at rest. Normal resting tone is palpated as soft or relaxed or measured with an IUPC as approximately 10 mmHg. Relaxation time is the amount of time from the end of one contraction to the beginning of the next contraction. During first-stage labor, relaxation time is generally 60 seconds or more; in second-stage labor, it is 45 to 50 seconds or more.

12. Category I FHR is a normal pattern that is strongly predictive of normal fetal acid–base status at the time of observation.

13. The ABCD management approach is a standardized intrapartum FHR management decision model.
    A—Assess oxygen pathway and identify the cause of FHR changes, both maternal and fetal
    B—Begin corrective measures
    C—Clear obstacles to delivery
    D—Determine a delivery plan

14. Conservative corrective measures that may be considered to correct a category II or III fetal heart rate (FHR) pattern include repositioning the client, IV fluid bolus, oxygen supplementation, reducing uterine activity (UA), correcting client blood pressure extremes (hypertension or hypotension), performing amnioinfusion, and modifying second-stage pushing efforts.

15. An IV fluid bolus benefits fetal oxygenation because it maximizes the pregnant client's cardiac output, intravascular volume, and uteroplacental perfusion, resulting in improved fetal oxygenation.

16. Fetal scalp stimulation should elicit an acceleration of the fetal heart rate (FHR). This acceleration is suggestive of adequate fetal oxygenation and a normal fetal acid–base balance at the time of the acceleration.

17. Umbilical cord blood gas sampling is a direct objective method of quantifying fetal acid–base and oxygenation at the time of cord clamping. Blood from the umbilical vein is oxygenated, coming from the placenta to the fetus. Blood from the umbilical arteries is deoxygenated, returning from the fetus to the placenta.

18. Potential obstacles to be considered during the C part of the ABCD approach include the facility (operating room and equipment availability); availability of staff (obstetrician, surgical assistant, anesthesiologist, neonatologist, pediatrician, nursing staff); considerations regarding the client (consent, anesthesia options, laboratory results, need for blood or blood products, need for an IV, urinary catheter and abdominal prep, what is required for a speedy transfer to the operating room

[OR]); considerations regarding the fetus (how many, estimated fetal gestational age and weight, presentation and position, known or anticipated anomalies); and finally, considerations about the monitoring of labor—are adequate data provided to allow appropriately informed management decisions? Measures to overcome these obstacles include preparing the OR; notifying relevant staff; reviewing the client's medical record for consents, laboratory results, and prenatal data; verifying the status of the client's IV; inserting a urinary catheter; and prepping the abdomen for surgery.

CHAPTER 15

1. The nurse should communicate interest, friendliness, caring, and competence when the client and family members enter the birth facility. Determining the their expectations about birth, conveying confidence, assigning a primary nurse, using touch for comfort (if approved by the client), and respecting cultural values are specific strategies that the nurse can use throughout labor. In addition, a nonjudgmental attitude facilitates communication and shows respect to the client as an individual.

2. The nurse should try to identify and incorporate beneficial or neutral cultural practices into care during labor and birth by asking about specific practices that are important during birth and facilitating communication by obtaining a fluent interpreter who is acceptable to the client and family.

3. The nurse should promptly evaluate the client status, the fetal status, and the nearness of birth when a client comes to the hospital or birth center. Prompt assessments should include identification of the client's chief complaint, assessment of the client's vital signs, fetal heart rate and patterns, uterine contractions, progress of labor, client's perception of fetal movement, and evaluation of any high-risk conditions.

4. Grunting sounds, bearing down, sitting on one buttock, and saying, "The baby's coming," suggest imminent birth. In this situation, the nurse notifies the provider promptly, abbreviates the initial assessment, and collects other information after birth.

5. Pregnant clients often bring several people with them to the birthing room and want them to stay during admission. Caution is prudent when asking for sensitive information, such as prior pregnancies, sexually transmitted infections (STIs), and potential abuse, when others are present. The client's partner and other visitors may be unaware of the history. Delay asking intimate information until the client is alone for confidentiality, safety, and accuracy. A victim of domestic violence is unlikely to answer truthfully when others are around.

6. The current status of labor is determined by the assessing the FHR and contraction pattern (frequency, duration, and intensity), status of the amniotic membranes (ruptured or intact), and the vaginal examination (dilation, effacement, and fetal station). The vaginal examination is deferred in cases with active vaginal bleeding and may be deferred or replaced with a sterile speculum exam if the gestation is preterm.

7. Vaginal examinations are limited to minimize the introduction of microorganisms from the perineal area into the uterus, which could lead to infection.

8. The client may specifically request other pain management measures, including epidural analgesia or other medication; express ineffectiveness of current measures; show muscle tension, arching of the back, or panicked activity during contractions; cry or have a tremulous voice; have a tense facial expression; roll in the bed; and express an inability to cope.

9. Frequency of assessment and documentation of FHR depends on the risk status of the client and fetus and the stage of labor. In addition, FHR assessments are recommended before and after procedures or interventions, which might change the intrauterine environment or the relationship of the fetus to its environment.

10. Three major risks associated with AROM and SROM are prolapsed umbilical cord, infection, and placental abruption.

11. Greenish, meconium-stained fluid may be seen in response to transient fetal hypoxia, postterm gestation, or placental insufficiency. Fluid with a foul or strong odor, cloudy appearance, or yellow color suggests chorioamnionitis (inflammation of the amniotic sac, usually caused by bacterial and viral infections).

12. Nurses promote labor progress through client positioning, including frequent position changes; adequate pain management; and teaching the client and support persons.

13. Laboring down, also called delayed pushing, rest and descend, or passive descent is the technique of delaying pushing until the reflex urge to push occurs. This allows uterine contraction to cause most of the fetal internal rotation and descent. Delayed pushing has been shown to result in less client fatigue, decreased pushing time, decreased risk for instrument-assisted and cesarean births, decreased third- and fourth-degree lacerations, decreased injuries to the pelvic floor, and blood loss/rates of hemorrhage equivalent to those of clients who pushed immediately on full cervical dilation.

14. When pushing in a sitting or semi-sitting position, the client's body should be curved around their uterus in a C-shape rather than arching their back. For greatest effectiveness, clients should pull on their knees, handholds, or a squat bar while pushing. Clients should maintain a similar C-shape to their upper body if they push on their side. Sustained pushing while holding a breath (Valsalva maneuver or "purple pushing") or pushing more than four times per contraction reduces blood flow to the placenta, increases intrathoracic pressure, is fatiguing, and should be discouraged.

15. Surfaces that contact the popliteal space behind the knee, such as stirrups, should be padded because pressure on veins and nerves near the surface could lead to thrombus formation or peroneal nerve injury. Also, the client's

upper body should be in the semi-Fowler's or sitting position rather than the supine position.

16. Shortly before birth, the perineum bulges, and the fetal head becomes visible as the pregnant client pushes. At this time birth can occur suddenly.

17. The fetal heart rate (FHR) should be monitored before external version to identify abnormal patterns that would preclude the procedure and to establish a baseline. It should be monitored by Doppler or real-time ultrasound as much as possible during and after external version to detect cord compression that can occur if the umbilical cord becomes entangled during change of the fetal presentation.

18. Uterine activity should be observed after external version for possible onset of labor because this procedure may cause uterine irritability or possible placental abruption; therefore the procedure is done near term.

19. Precautions that promote safe oxytocin induction or augmentation of labor include the following:
    a. Dilution of the oxytocin in an isotonic solution
    b. Piggybacking the oxytocin solution into the port of the primary nonadditive (maintenance) IV line that is nearest the venipuncture site
    c. Starting the oxytocin infusion slowly
    d. Increasing the rate of infusion gradually
    e. Monitoring uterine contractions and fetal heart rate (FHR)

20. Labor may be augmented if it stops or contractions become ineffective. The client whose labor is augmented with oxytocin usually needs less of the drug than the one whose labor is being induced because the uterus is more sensitive to its effects after labor begins.

21. The fetus may have an unfavorable response to oxytocin, manifested by fetal heart rate (FHR) patterns such as tachycardia, bradycardia, decreased variability, and pathologic (late, variable, or prolonged) decelerations.

22. More than five contractions in a 10-minute period, averaged over 30 minutes, contraction durations longer than 120 seconds, increased resting tone of the uterus, and relaxation time of less than 60 seconds between contractions in first-stage labor and 45 to 50 seconds in second-stage labor, and MVUs greater than 250 in first stage and greater than 400 in second stage are signs of increased uterine activity.

23. Administration of oxytocin for a prolonged time may lead to postpartum hemorrhage because the oxytocin receptor sites on the uterine muscle may be saturated and less responsive and the muscle may be fatigued and unable to contract properly to compress bleeding vessels at the placenta site (uterine atony).

24. At least one person, usually an additional nurse, certified to provide neonatal resuscitation should be present at all births. This person's role is dedicated to the assessment and resuscitation of the newborn infant. If the newborn is at risk for complications, there will likely be more than one additional person at the birth.

25. Forceps and vacuum extraction are used to provide traction to assist the client in rotation, expulsion, or both of the fetal head. Special forceps (Piper) can be used to deliver the aftercoming head of the fetus in a breech presentation, but a vacuum extractor can be used only with a cephalic presentation. Forceps may cause fetal injury such as facial bruising and nerve injury. The vacuum extractor may create an artificial caput called a *chignon*. No more than three "pop-offs" should be attempted, and these should not be followed by forceps attempts at vaginal birth.

26. Catheterization before forceps or vacuum extractor eliminates a full bladder, which would reduce available room in the pelvis. Emptying the bladder also reduces the risk of bladder injury.

27. The infant with an asymmetric facial appearance when crying may have facial nerve injury, usually a temporary condition that sometimes occurs when forceps are used to assist birth.

28. The low transverse uterine incision is less likely to rupture during another pregnancy than either of the two vertical incisions. There are, however, valid reasons for the use of vertical incisions.

29. The client expecting a cesarean birth should be taught about the following regarding the operating room and recovery area:
    a. Preoperative procedures, such as skin preparation and insertion of an indwelling catheter and IV.
    b. Description of the operating room, the narrow table, the personnel who will be present, and their functions.
    c. When the partner or support person can come in.
    d. If a regional anesthetic is planned, the client will be awake and feel pulling and pressure sensations but should not expect pain. If a general anesthetic is planned, all preparations will be made before anesthesia is induced, but the surgery will not begin before the client is asleep, and clients will not awaken during the surgery.
    e. In the recovery area, use of oxygen, pulse oximeter, and automatic blood pressure cuff for vital signs; checking of the uterine fundus, incision, lochia, and pain-relief needs.

30. The client who has cesarean birth needs care similar to that of the client who delivers vaginally in terms of vital signs and fundus and lochia assessments. Additional care includes assessment of electrocardiogram pattern, oxygen saturation and respiratory pattern, observation of urine output from the indwelling catheter, observation of the incision or abdominal dressing, functioning of the SCDs, pain management, and respiratory care (turning, coughing, deep breathing). Anesthesia-related care includes level of consciousness (primarily if general anesthesia was used) and return of movement and sensation (primarily if epidural or subarachnoid block was used).

31. REEDA is an acronym used to describe the assessment of a repaired incision or wound such as perineal lacerations, episiotomy or the incision from a cesarean birth. R: redness; E: edema; E: ecchymosis; D: discharge or drainage; A: approximation of edges.

CHAPTER 16

1. Labor dystocia usually occurs during the active phase of first-stage labor (6 cm cervical dilation or more). Uterine contractions become weaker, shorter, and less frequent. It is not painful because the contractions decrease, although the client may become tired. Tachysystole can be either spontaneous or induced and is defined as excessive uterine activity. Tachysystole is more than five contractions in 10 minutes (averaged over 30 minutes). In addition to tachysystole, contractions lasting 2 minutes or longer, contractions with less than 1 minute resting time between, or failure of the uterus to return to resting tone between contractions via palpation, or intraamniotic pressure above 25 mmHg measured by an intrauterine pressure catheter (IUPC) may be of concern. Contractions may be uncoordinated and erratic in their frequency, duration, and intensity. The pregnant client becomes very tired because of nearly constant discomfort.

2. Client position changes encourage the fetus to rotate from an occiput transverse or occiput posterior position to an occiput anterior position; with the client in a hands-and-knees position, the convex surface of the rounded fetal back rotates toward the convex surface of the anterior uterus. The squatting position also increases pelvic diameters and straightens the pelvic curve to facilitate both fetal rotation and descent.

3. A cesarean birth is the usual delivery method of choice for infants in the breech presentation to avoid major complications associated with breech birth, including slow labor, risk for prolapse of the umbilical cord, and the risks associated with possible umbilical cord compression before the head is born.

4. The staff must be prepared for care and possible resuscitation of multiple infants. Duplicate staff and equipment should be ready for every infant expected.

5. Bladder distention during labor can occupy available room in the pelvis, thus impeding labor progress and fetal descent. In addition, it is a potential source of discomfort.

6. Psychological support reduces stress that otherwise can consume energy the uterus needs, inhibit uterine contractions, reduce placental blood supply, impair pushing efforts, and increase pain.

7. Based on Friedman's curve, the average nullipara's cervix dilates about 1.2 cm per hour and expected fetal descent is 1 cm per hour. The average parous client's cervix dilates about 1.5 cm per hour, with minimal descent of 2 cm per hour. Research by Zhang et al. found that labor may take over 6 hours to progress from 4 to 5 cm and over 3 hours to progress from 5 to 6 cm of dilation. Nulliparas and multiparas appeared to progress at a similar pace before 6 cm. They concluded that allowing labor to continue for a longer period before 6 cm of cervical dilation may reduce the rate of cesarean deliveries.

8. Nursing care for the client who has prolonged labor is similar to that for dysfunctional labor. Promoting comfort, energy conservation, emotional support, position changes, and assessments for related complications such as infection should be done. Assessments of the fetus for signs of intrauterine infection and compromised oxygenation are ongoing.

9. Trauma is the primary risk to a client with precipitate labor and may include vaginal wall lacerations and cervical lacerations. Fetal risks may include trauma, such as intracranial hemorrhage or nerve damage, and hypoxia due to intense contractions with a short relaxation period, which reduces the time available for gas exchange in the placenta.

10. Premature rupture of the membranes (PROM) occurs before true labor begins and may occur at any gestational age. Preterm premature rupture of the membranes (PPROM) occurs before 37 weeks of gestation and may be accompanied by contractions. pPROM is more likely to be associated with preterm labor and birth.

11. Infection may be both a cause and a result of premature rupture of the membranes.

12. Labor may be induced if the client is at or near term and it does not begin spontaneously. When the fetus is preterm, the physician must consider multiple factors such as risk for infection (client and fetus/newborn) and risk for complications associated with preterm birth.

13. The nurse should assess the client's vital signs and fetal heart rate (FHR) and teach the client to avoid inserting anything into the vagina, avoid breast stimulation, maintain activity restrictions, and report any uterine contractions or foul odor to vaginal discharge. Temperature should be taken at least four times per day, and report any value greater than 37.8°C (100°F).

14. Symptoms of preterm labor often are vague. They include uterine contractions that may often be painless, the fetus "balling up," menstrual-like cramps, backache, pelvic pressure, changed or increased vaginal discharge, abdominal cramps, and a sense of "feeling bad."

15. Early identification of preterm labor enables management that may delay birth and allow further maturation of the fetus or permit transfer to a facility equipped to care for an immature infant. If preterm birth is likely, emphasis is accelerating fetal lung maturity and providing neonatal neuroprotection.

16. Classifications of drugs to inhibit preterm contractions include magnesium sulfate, calcium agonists, prostaglandin synthesis inhibitors, and beta-adrenergics.

17. To accelerate maturation of the fetal lungs, corticosteroids are given to the pregnant client between 24 and 34 weeks of gestation who is at risk of birth within 7 days. In certain situations, corticosteroids may be administered as early as 22 to 23 weeks and as late as 37 weeks of gestation. The greatest benefits occur if steroids are in the pregnant client's system at least 24 hours before birth. The newborn who is born less than 24 hours after the pregnant

client receives corticosteroids may also benefit; concerns regarding the probability of birth within 24 hours should not prevent administration of corticosteroids.

18. The three potential fetal or newborn risks are reduced placental function and umbilical cord compression before birth and meconium aspiration after birth.

19. If umbilical cord prolapse occurs, the priority of care is to reduce compression and restore normal blood flow through the cord by elevating the presenting part. At the same time, the nurse should summon help to expedite delivery, usually by cesarean birth.

20. Stimulated contractions are potentially more powerful than natural ones and may cause the pressure in the uterus to exceed the uterine wall's ability to withstand that pressure.

21. Shock and hemorrhage are rapidly developing complications of uterine inversion. They are managed by rapid IV fluid and blood replacement. A drug that relaxes the uterus may be given to allow uterine replacement to its proper position, and general anesthesia may be needed. Oxytocin is given after the uterus is returned to the proper position. Hemodynamic monitoring may be required to ensure stabilization.

22. For intrapartum emergencies, nursing considerations include the following: *Prolapsed umbilical cord*—Relieve pressure on the cord to restore adequate blood flow through it until the baby can be delivered. *Uterine rupture*—Attempt its prevention by cautious intrapartum use of uterine stimulants and close monitoring of uterine contractions. *Uterine inversion*—Avoid pressure on the poorly contracted fundus after birth; assess for and correct shock.

CHAPTER 17

1. The three processes involved in involution are contraction of muscle fibers, catabolism, and regeneration of uterine epithelium.

2. The fundus is expected to descend 1 cm (approximately 1 fingerbreadth) per day so that by the fourteenth day after birth it cannot be palpated in the abdomen.

3. A multipara is expected to experience afterpains because repeated stretching of the uterus makes continuous uterine contraction more difficult. Overdistention of the uterus and breastfeeding also cause afterpains. Afterpains are treated with analgesics.

4. Lochia rubra is red, consists mostly of blood, and lasts for 1 to 3 days. Lochia serosa is pink- to brown-tinged and usually lasts from the third to tenth days. Lochia alba is white, cream, or yellowish and may last until 3 to 6 weeks after delivery.

5. Menses will resume in about 6 to 10 weeks for postpartum clients who are formula-feeding. The breastfeeding client may begin menses between 10 weeks and 6 months after childbirth.

6. Breastfeeding delays the return of both ovulation and menstruation.

7. The white blood cell (WBC) count is normally elevated during labor and the immediate postpartum period and may rise to 30,000/mm^3. If the client has a fever or is at increased risk for infection, the nurse should be especially alert for an increase in WBC count and other signs of infection.

8. The postpartum client is at risk for urinary retention because the bladder is less sensitive to fluid pressure, decreasing the urge to void even when the bladder is distended. Trauma of childbirth and lingering effects of regional anesthesia may also make it difficult to void. Urinary tract infection is more likely because stasis of urine allows time for bacteria to multiply. Excessive postpartum bleeding may occur because a full bladder displaces the uterus, causing the uterine muscles to relax.

9. Hyperpigmentation decreases because estrogen, progesterone, and melanocyte-stimulating hormone decrease rapidly after childbirth.

10. Approximately 4.5 to 5.8 kg (10 to 13 lb) are lost during childbirth. An additional 2.3 to 3.6 kg (5 to 8 lb) are lost as a result of diuresis and 0.9 to 1.4 kg (2 to 3 lb) from involution and lochia by the end of the first week.

11. Orthostatic hypotension results from engorgement of visceral blood vessels from decreased intraabdominal pressure after delivery. Signs and symptoms include a 15- to 20-mmHg drop in systolic blood pressure, dizziness, lightheadedness, or faintness when the client moves from lying down to sitting or standing.

12. When tachycardia is noted, assessment of blood pressure (BP), temperature, location and firmness of the fundus, amount of lochia, estimated blood loss at delivery, hemoglobin, hematocrit, temperature, and degree of pain are necessary to help identify the cause. Excitement, pain, anxiety, fatigue, dehydration, anemia, infection, or hypovolemia may cause tachycardia.

13. Uterine massage is necessary when the uterus is not firmly contracted; it is soft or "boggy." The nurse places the nondominant hand above the symphysis pubis to anchor and support the uterus during massage.

14. A cervical or vaginal laceration may cause excessive bleeding even when the uterus is firmly contracted.

15. Assessment of pain, frequent respiratory assessments, auscultation of breath sounds and bowel sounds, inspection of the surgical dressing and wound, and intake and output are necessary for the postcesarean client.

16. Hypostatic pneumonia can be prevented by frequent turning, coughing, breathing deeply, and use of incentive spirometers to help expand the lungs.

17. Early ambulation, tightening and relaxing the abdominal muscles, restriction of carbonated beverages and straws for drinking, pelvic lifts, and simethicone or rectal suppositories as ordered prevent or minimize abdominal distention.

18. Current recommendations include instructing the client to wear a tight bra 24 hours a day until breasts are soft and nontender and express only a small amount of milk if absolutely necessary for pain relief; otherwise, avoid stimulation of the breasts. The client may use cold compresses or gel packs inside the bra for comfort. Cold cabbage leaves also promote comfort. Analgesics may be recommended by the provider.

19. Providing adequate information in a short time is a major problem in preparing parents for discharge.

20. Before discharge, the nurse should be sure that the client has no complications and all assessments and laboratory work are normal, and Rho (D) immune globulin has been administered if appropriate. The client should indicate understanding of self-care instructions, signs of complications and proper responses, and infant care. Postpartum follow-up care should be arranged. Family members or other support persons should be available for support during the early days after discharge.

21. Bonding describes the initial attraction felt by the parents for the infant. Attachment is the development of an enduring, loving relationship between parents and child. It is progressive and requires response from the infant.

22. Maternal touch may progress from fingertipping in the discovery phase to stroking, then enfolding the infant, and then to consoling behaviors.

23. Parents progress from referring to the newborn as "it" to "he" or "she" and then to using the given name. Parents who know the sex of the baby before birth may call the infant by name from before birth.

24. During the taking-in phase, new mothers are focused primarily on their own needs. They are often passive and dependent and repeatedly recount the birth experience. In the taking-hold phase, they become more independent, focus on the infant, and exhibit a heightened readiness to learn.

25. In the letting-go phase, mothers relinquish previous lifestyle patterns to assume the parenting role. Many must give up their idealized expectations of the birth experience, and some must relinquish the infant of their fantasies for the real infant.

26. The anticipatory stage begins during pregnancy as mothers prepare for the birth. The formal stage begins with birth as they become acquainted with the baby. During the informal stage, mothers respond to their infant's unique cues rather than relying on directions from others. The personal stage is attained when mothers feel comfortable with their new role as a parent.

27. Postpartum blues may be related to emotional letdown, discomfort, fatigue, and anxiety about parenting and body image. It is characterized by irritability, fatigue, tearfulness, mood swings, and anxiety. The symptoms are usually unrelated to events, and the condition does not seriously affect the client's ability to care for the infant. With postpartum depression, the depression becomes severe, lasts longer than 2 weeks, or interferes with the client's ability to cope with daily life. Nurses can provide reassurance to the client and teach the family about postpartum blues and warning signs of postpartum depression. Many facilities or providers conduct a screening for depression before discharge.

28. Many partners eagerly look forward to coparenting with their mate. However, they may lack confidence in providing infant care and are sensitive to being left out of instructions and demonstrations of infant care. They may feel others expect them only to provide support to the client.

29. Siblings may feel jealousy and fear that they will be replaced by the newborn in the affection of the parents.

CHAPTER 18

1. The nurse examines previous records to identify factors that would predispose the client to complications such as postpartum hemorrhage.

2. Overdistention of uterine muscles from a twin gestation makes the uterine contraction more difficult and excessive bleeding more likely.

3. The nurse cannot be certain that bleeding is controlled because concealed bleeding can occur in soft tissue and produce a hematoma.

4. Initial management of uterine atony focuses on measures to contract the uterus, such as massaging, expressing clots, and emptying the bladder. Pharmacologic measures include fluid replacement and administration of oxytocin, methylergonovine, or other drugs such as carboprost.

5. Large hematomas may require incision and evacuation of clots, as well as ligation of the bleeding vessel. Small hematomas reabsorb and do not require treatment.

6. The major signs of subinvolution are prolonged lochial discharge, irregular or excessive uterine bleeding, or, occasionally, profuse hemorrhage. Pelvic pain and heaviness, backache, fatigue, and malaise may also be reported.

7. Nurses should teach the client how to palpate the fundus; estimate fundal height; and report abnormalities of lochia, a foul odor, or pelvic pain.

8. Risk factors for thrombus development are venous stasis, hypercoagulability, and injury to the endothelial surface of the blood vessel. Venous stasis increases during pregnancy because of compression of the large vessels by the enlarging uterus. At birth, additional stasis and blood vessel injury may occur, especially if stirrups are used for positioning. Changes in the coagulation and fibrinolytic systems during pregnancy and the postpartum period elevate the factors that favor coagulation and decrease the factors that favor lysis of clots.

9. Heparin remains the long-term treatment of the pregnant client with deep venous thrombosis because warfarin (Coumadin) may be teratogenic and predisposes the fetus to hemorrhage. Heparin is changed to warfarin in the postpartum period.

10. Bed rest is prescribed for the clients with deep vein thrombosis to decrease swelling and to promote venous return from the leg.

11. The nurse assesses clients receiving anticoagulants for unexplained bruising, petechiae, bleeding from the nose or gums, blood in the urine or stools, or increased vaginal bleeding. Signs of hemorrhage, such as tachycardia, falling blood pressure, or other signs of shock, also should be noted.

12. The nurse should assess family structure and function that will need to determine how prepared they are to cope with the client's illness. The nurse should evaluate interactions between the parents and the newborn and determine what support may be needed to facilitate attachment.

13. Cesarean birth or the use of vacuum extraction or forceps may result in trauma that provides a portal of entry for infectious organisms.

14. All parts of the reproductive tract are connected, and organisms can move from the vagina through the cervix, uterus, and fallopian tubes and into the peritoneal cavity. Alkalinity of the vagina during labor, necrosis of the endometrium, and the presence of lochia encourage bacterial growth.

15. When labor is prolonged, organisms have time and opportunity to ascend from the vagina into the uterus, increasing the risk of infection. Also, there may be more vaginal examinations and ruptured membranes for a longer time.

16. Fever, chills, malaise, abdominal pain and cramping, uterine tenderness, purulent foul-smelling lochia, tachycardia, and subinvolution are signs and symptoms of endometritis. It usually is treated by IV administration of antibiotics, antipyretics, and oxytocics to promote involution.

17. Wound infection most often occurs in cesarean incisions, episiotomies, and lacerations.

18. Incisions and lacerations should be inspected for redness, tenderness, edema, and approximation of the edges of the wound, which may pull apart with infection.

19. To prevent urinary tract infection, the client should be advised to drink at least 2500 to 3000 mL of fluid each day and void every 2 to 3 hours during the day. Cystitis and pyelonephritis may be treated with oral antibiotics on an outpatient basis. Severe pyelonephritis or infection may require hospitalization and IV antibiotics.

20. Measures to prevent mastitis include correct positioning of the infant during nursing, frequent emptying of the breasts (feed every 2 to 3 hours), and avoiding nipple trauma and supplemental feedings. In addition, nursing pads should not have a plastic layer, and they should be changed as soon as they are wet; continuous pressure on the breasts caused by tight bras or infant carriers should be avoided.

CHAPTER 19

1. Protective physiologic mechanisms provide compensation to maintain cardiac output and tissue perfusion during hypovolemic states. Circulating blood volume redistributes with preferential shunting of blood to the heart, brain, liver, and lungs and away from nonessential organ systems, including the kidneys and uterus.

2. When shock is suspected or diagnosed, the client's vital signs should be assessed every 5 to 15 minutes and should include the use of a continuous pulse oximeter and electrocardiogram (ECG) monitoring.

3. Massive transfusion protocol (MTF) is indicated if four or more units of blood products within the hour are anticipated and with continued bleeding. MTF includes packed red blood cells, fresh frozen plasma, platelets, and cryoprecipitate.

4. True. Disseminated intravascular coagulation (DIC) is a secondary complication of an underlying condition, not a primary condition.

5. The process of DIC is caused by trauma to tissues, vascular endothelium, and red blood cells.

6. Placental abruption, preeclampsia with severe features/eclampsia, HELLP syndrome, amniotic fluid embolism, sepsis, acute fatty liver disease of pregnancy, retained intrauterine fetal demise, and massive hemorrhage predispose the OB client to DIC.

7. Coagulation laboratories are needed to evaluate coagulopathy. These include fibrinogen, platelet count, prothrombin time (PT), activated partial thromboplastin (APTT), fibrin split products or degradation products, and bleeding time.

8. During the antepartum period, risk factors for sepsis are multiple gestation, ruptured membranes, urinary tract infection, and stillbirth. In the intrapartum and immediate postpartum period, additional risk factors include cesarean or operative vaginal birth, hemorrhage, manual placental extraction or curettage, and retained products of conception.

9. Aggressive fluid resuscitation, lateral positioning of the client, and, if necessary, vasopressor therapy are used to improve hypotension associated with sepsis.

10. Antibiotic therapy should be initiated within the first hour of bundle implementation in a client with suspected sepsis. Whenever possible all necessary cultures should be obtained prior to antibiotic initiation; however, initiation of antibiotics within the first hour is most important.

11. Risk factors related to amniotic fluid embolism (AFE) are not well understood but include advanced client age, multiple gestation, placental abnormalities, preeclampsia/eclampsia, and operative vaginal and cesarean birth.

12. Many clients have a preceding aura, progressive change in mental status, or sense of impending doom prior to an AFE event. These findings should alert the nurse to be suspicious of AFE.

13. Nurses are most likely to recognize and respond when a client experiences an AFE. Initial interventions involve calling for the rapid response team and getting help to the bedside, administering cardiopulmonary support if needed, and placing the client in a left lateral uterine displacement position.

14. Hormonal, metabolic and respiratory changes of pregnancy lead to insulin resistance, an accelerated starvation state, and compensated respiratory alkalosis, which predispose the pregnant client to DKA.

15. Elevated glucose levels, polyuria, polydipsia, nausea/vomiting, fruity ketonic breath, tachycardia, hypotension, dehydration with dry mucus membranes, weakness, altered mental states, and coma are hallmark symptoms of DKA, which may be observed in pregnant clients with this condition.

16. Restore circulating volume, correct hyperglycemia, restore electrolyte balance, and identify and treat the underlying cause are the key principles in management of DKA.

17. Motor vehicle crashes (MVCs), falls, and interpersonal violence are the major causes of trauma-related injuries.

18. The increased blood volume of pregnancy may mask symptoms of blood loss due to trauma.

19. Death of the pregnant client is the most common cause of fetal death resulting from trauma.

20. The primary survey assesses airway, breathing, circulation, disability, and displacement and exposure. This survey focuses on identification of life-threatening injuries and implementing lifesaving interventions. It should be completed within minutes.

21. Hypovolemia (due to hemorrhage, sepsis, preeclampsia), hypoxia (due to respiratory compromise), acidosis (due to hypovolemia or DKA), and pulmonary embolism are the most common causes of cardiac arrest during pregnancy and postpartum.

22. An early key intervention unique to the pregnant cardiac arrest victim is continuous manual displacement of the uterus upward and laterally to optimize circulation and return of blood to the heart.

23. If there is no return to spontaneous circulation and the code has persisted for 4 minutes, it is recommended to proceed with a perimortem cesarean birth if gestational age is greater than 20 weeks.

24. Nurses have significant roles and responsibilities during a code. Some of these are providing reports to additional team members, identifying the team leader and members and roles of each, documenting events, initiating IVs, preparing and administering medications and blood products, performing chest compressions, assisting with airway management, and others.

25. Preeclampsia and sepsis can cause noncardiogenic pulmonary edema. Pneumonia, amniotic fluid embolism, and anaphylaxis are other diseases that can cause noncardiogenic pulmonary edema.

26. Dyspnea, tachypnea, tachycardia, diaphoresis, agitation, anxiety, tightness in the chest, and coughing are symptoms of pulmonary edema. Auscultation of the lungs may or may not reveal crackles, especially early in the disease process.

27. Nursing considerations address the primary goal in the client with pulmonary edema, which is to maintain oxygenation. Interventions include client positioning, administration of supplemental oxygen, limiting client activity, controlling pain and anxiety, and maintaining fluid balance.

28. Cardiovascular disease (CVD) in pregnancy is classified as congenital, acquired, ischemic, and other.

29. The specific cardiac disease or lesion; the client's ability to adapt to physiologic changes in pregnancy, labor, birth, and postpartum; and the development of any pregnancy-related complications affect the perinatal morbidity and mortality associated with CVD.

30. The pregnancy heart team includes maternal-fetal-medicine physicians, obstetricians, cardiologists, anesthesiologists, neonatologists, nurses, social workers, pharmacists, case managers, and other ancillary staff as needed based on the conditions of the pregnant client and fetus.

31. The two most common intrapartum cardiac complications are cardiogenic pulmonary edema and arrhythmias.

CHAPTER 20

1. Hypoxemia, cool air, and handling at birth affect chemoreceptors and sensors that stimulate the respiratory center to cause initiation of respirations at birth.

2. Surfactant reduces surface tension in the alveoli and allows them to remain partially open on expiration, reducing the work of breathing.

3. Fetal lung fluid begins to move into the interstitial spaces shortly before birth and when air enters the lungs at birth. It is absorbed from the interstitial spaces by the lymphatic and vascular systems. A small part of the fluid is squeezed out during birth. After birth, as the infant cries, air moves into the lungs, pushing any remaining fluid into the interstitial spaces where it is absorbed by the pulmonary circulatory and lymphatic systems.

4. The ductus arteriosus closes as a result of increases in blood oxygen and decreased prostaglandins from the placenta. The foramen ovale closes when pressure in the left atrium exceeds that in the right atrium. The ductus venosus closes when the vessels of the cord become occluded (clamped).

5. At birth, increasing oxygen causes the pulmonary blood vessels to dilate. In addition, movement of fetal lung fluid into the interstitial tissues allows more room for expansion of the pulmonary vessels. The ductus arteriosus constricts because of the increased oxygen in the blood when the neonate begins to breathe.

6. Newborns have thinner skin with less subcutaneous fat than older children and adults. They have blood vessels close to the surface and a larger skin surface area. These all contribute to greater loss of heat than in older children or adults.

7. Newborns respond to low temperatures by increasing activity, flexion, vasoconstriction, and nonshivering thermogenesis. Nonshivering thermogenesis (metabolism of brown fat) increases oxygen and glucose consumption, slows production of surfactant, and may cause respiratory distress, hypoglycemia, acidosis, and jaundice.

8. Newborns have higher levels of erythrocytes and hemoglobin than adults. Fetal oxygen exchange in the placenta is less efficient than the lungs. More red blood cells with fetal hemoglobin are needed to adequately oxygenate the cells in the fetus.

9. Stools progress from thick, greenish–black meconium to loose, greenish or yellowish–brown transitional stools to milk stools that are frequent, soft, seedy, and yellow to golden in color if the infant is breastfed and pale yellow or light brown, firmer, malodorous and less frequent if formula-fed.

10. Hypoglycemia is a problem for the newborn because glucose stores are depleted quickly after birth due to stress from birth and the energy needed for respirations, heat production, activity, and transition to extrauterine life. Glucose is the major source of energy in the brain.

11. Infants have an immature liver and more hemolysis of erythrocytes than adults. Trauma at birth, poor early feeding, and an intestinal enzyme that deconjugates bilirubin also increase jaundice.

12. Physiologic jaundice occurs in normal newborns after the first 24 hours of life as a result of hemolysis of unneeded red blood cells and immaturity of the liver. Nonphysiologic jaundice is generally a result of excessive destruction of erythrocytes or problems with bilirubin conjugation, causing bilirubin levels to rise faster and higher than in physiologic jaundice. It begins within the first 24 hours and may necessitate phototherapy. Breastfeeding (early onset) jaundice begins in the first week in breastfed newborns. It is caused by inadequate intake of breast milk. True breast milk jaundice occurs after the first 3 to 5 days of life and lasts longer than physiologic jaundice; it may result from substances in the milk.

13. The newborn's body is composed of a greater percentage of water with more located in the extracellular compartment than in the adult's body. Newborns diurese extracellular fluid in the first week of life, contributing to a weight loss of up to 7% of their birth weight.

14. Newborns receive temporary passive immunity to infections when IgG crosses the placenta in utero. It provides temporary passive immunity to bacteria, bacterial toxins, and viruses to which the pregnant client has immunity. After birth, infants produce IgM as a result of exposure to environmental antigens. It helps protect against Gram-negative bacteria. IgM cannot cross the placenta; its presence in cord blood indicates that the fetus was exposed to the microorganism in utero. IgA does not cross the placenta; the newborn must produce it. IgA helps protect the gastrointestinal and respiratory tracts from infection and is present in breast milk. Therefore breastfed newborns may receive protection.

15. During both periods of reactivity, newborns are active and alert, may be interested in feeding, may have elevated pulse and respiratory rates, and may have transient signs of respiratory distress.

16. In the deep or quiet sleep state, the infant is in a deep sleep with regular, quiet respirations and little response to outside stimuli. In active sleep, infants move about and may have irregular respirations. They are more likely to startle from noise or disturbances and may return to sleep or move to an awake state. The drowsy state is the time between sleep and waking. Eyes may remain closed, or if open, appear glazed and unfocused. In the quiet alert state, the infant is awake and interested in stimuli. This is an excellent time for the parents to interact with the infant. The active alert state is a fussy period that may lead to the crying state if the infant's needs are not met. In the crying state, the cries are continuous and lusty with active body movements and irregular and rapid respirations.

CHAPTER 21

1. Focused assessments of the infant immediately after birth help detect serious abnormalities that need immediate attention. They focus on cardiorespiratory status, thermoregulation, estimation of the gestational age, and the presence of anomalies. A more complete assessment follows when the infant is stable.

2. The cardiovascular assessment includes evaluation of history, airway and breathing, color, heart sounds, and pulses and capillary refill. Blood pressure is assessed if indicated.

3. Taking a rectal temperature is dangerous because it risks perforation of the intestinal wall or other injury to the rectum.

4. Molding of the head is a change in the shape because of normal temporary overriding of cranial bones at the sutures during birth. Caput succedaneum is localized edema from pressure against the cervix, which can cross the suture lines. Cephalhematoma is bleeding between the periosteum and the bone that never crosses suture lines. Molding and caput disappear within a few days, but cephalhematoma may take several months to resolve.

5. Measurements of the infant help determine if in utero growth was adequate for gestational age and if complications are present.

6. Some signs of hypoglycemia are jitteriness, poor muscle tone, respiratory distress (tachypnea, dyspnea, apnea, and cyanosis), high-pitched cry, diaphoresis, low temperature, poor suck, lethargy, irritability, seizures, and coma. Some infants show no signs of hypoglycemia.

7. Using an incorrect site for heel punctures risks injury to the bone (osteomyelitis), nerves, or blood vessels of the heel.

8. Newborn reflexes provide information about the status of the neonate's central nervous system.

9. The first feeding allows the nurse to evaluate the newborn's ability to suck, swallow, and breathe in coordination and assess for signs of esophageal atresia or tracheoesophageal fistula.

10. Infants should void within 12 to 48 hours. Infants void at least one to two times during the first 2 days and at least six times a day by the fourth day.

11. The nurse documents location, size, color, elevation, and texture of marks on the skin; explains marks to parents; and offers emotional support as needed. Subsequent changes from previous descriptions are also documented.

12. The gestational age assessment provides an estimate of the infant's age since conception and alerts the nurse to possible complications related to age and development.

13. The periods of reactivity are important because the infant may need nursing intervention for low temperature, elevated pulse and respirations, and excessive respiratory secretions. During the sleep period, the infant will have relaxed muscle tone and no interest in feeding.

CHAPTER 22

1. Newborns receive vitamin K to prevent vitamin K–dependent bleeding. The eyes are treated with an antibiotic ointment to prevent ophthalmia neonatorum.

2. Nurses can prevent heat loss in newborns by preparing the environment before birth; placing the newborn skin to skin with a parent or under a preheated radiant warmer immediately after birth; keeping them dry, covered, and away from cold objects or surfaces, drafts, and outside windows and walls; and by teaching parents how to prevent heat loss in the newborn.

3. When infants show signs of hypoglycemia, the nurse should follow agency policy and provider orders to check the blood glucose level and temperature, feed the infant colostrum, breast milk or formula, and watch for signs of other complications.

4. Interventions for preventing jaundice include ensuring the infant is feeding well by working with parents and infants having difficulty and teaching parents about jaundice and what observations they should make.

5. Nurses can prevent a baby being given to the wrong parents by always checking the infant's identification and parent's identification every time the two are reunited.

6. Nurses and parents can prevent infant abductions by always being alert for suspicious behavior and stopping anyone who might be taking a baby. Nurses must teach parents how to identify hospital staff and that they should never allow anyone without proper identification to remove their infant from them.

7. Scrupulous handwashing by staff and all who come in contact with newborns (including parents and other family members) is the most important way to prevent infections in newborns. In addition, infant supplies should not be shared, and nurses should be vigilant in assessment for signs of infection.

8. Parents choose circumcision because of the decreased incidence of urinary tract infections, penile cancer, and some sexually transmittable diseases; religious dictates; parental preference; lack of knowledge about care of the foreskin; and a lack of awareness of their choice in the matter. Parents decide against circumcision because it causes pain and carries the risk of hemorrhage, infection, poor cosmetic result, stenosis or fistulas of the urethra, adhesions, necrosis, or other injury to the glans penis. They also question the need for surgery to prevent uncommon conditions.

9. Teach parents to wash the penis daily and when soiled diapers are changed but do not retract the foreskin on an uncircumcised penis until it begins to separate from the glans later in childhood. They can teach the child to retract it to clean after separation occurs. Teach parents of circumcised infants to watch for bleeding and infection and to apply petroleum jelly as instructed unless a PlastiBell was used. Squeeze warm water from a clean washcloth over the penis to wash it. Do not remove the yellow crust or scab that forms over the site; it is part of the healing process and will fall off within 7 to 10 days. If a PlastiBell was used, the ring should fall off in 7 to 10 days.

10. Planning parent teaching includes coordinating teaching to include all topics, setting priorities based on parents' needs, using a variety of teaching techniques, modeling behavior, and teaching intermittently. The nurse should also include other family members and consider culture and language.

11. The first hepatitis B vaccine is given at the birth facility to infants of uninfected clients, as well as to infants of clients who are positive for hepatitis B. Hepatitis B immune globulin is also given to infants of infected clients.

12. Newborn screening tests should be performed after 24 hours of age or as close to discharge as possible, as the blood tests are more sensitive after the first 24 hours. Infants who screen positive for any of the conditions should be retested.

13. Parents obtain information about infant care from friends, family, health care personnel, child care classes, television, books, magazines, and the internet.

14. Nurses may provide follow-up phone calls, home visits, clinic visits, and child care classes.

15. New equipment sold in the United States is generally safe due to government standards for safety. All equipment, especially used or aftermarket equipment, should be checked for safety, and parts should be inspected to ensure that they are strong and functioning properly.

16. Car seats must be chosen according to the size of the infant and must be used correctly to maintain safety. Newborns should be placed in rear-facing car seats in the back seat of the car.

17. Infants are not "spoiled" by prompt attention to their needs. Prompt, consistent response to crying may decrease overall crying later.

18. Nurses can assist parents of crying infants to determine the cause and teach them appropriate techniques for coping with a crying infant. Therapeutic communication techniques can be used to help parents with negative feelings.

19. Diaper rash can be prevented by keeping the area clean and dry and avoiding products to which the infant seems sensitive. If rash occurs, parents should expose the area to air. A thin layer of zinc oxide or petrolatum may speed healing.

20. Infants should not start solid foods until 6 months old.

21. Regurgitation is expulsion of small amounts of milk, often along with a burp. Vomiting involves larger amounts that are expelled with more force.

22. Understanding the infant's changing capabilities helps parents assess situations and the home environment to prevent accidents.

23. Well-baby checkups allow the health care provider to assess the infant's growth and development, observe for abnormalities, provide parent teaching, and give immunizations.

24. Immunizations prevent infants from becoming infected with very serious communicable diseases.

25. Immediate help should be obtained if infants have difficulty breathing, are breathing rapidly, are cyanotic, have extreme pallor, or are hard to arouse from sleep or hard to keep awake.

26. The cause of sudden infant death syndrome (SIDS) remains unknown, but the risk may be increased with sleeping in a prone position or on soft, loose bedding, overheating, parental smoking or drug use during or after pregnancy, and sleeping with another person or on an adult bed or sofa. Infants should sleep alone in a supine position at all times.

CHAPTER 23

1. Infants lose weight as a result of normal excretion of meconium and extracellular fluid during newborn diuresis. Infants should be evaluated for feeding problems if weight loss exceeds 10% of birth weight or if weight loss continues beyond 3 days of age.

2. Colostrum is rich in protein, fat-soluble vitamins, some minerals, and immunoglobulins. Transitional milk has less protein and immunoglobulins but more lactose, fat, and calories than colostrum. Mature milk appears less rich than colostrum and transitional milk, but it supplies all nutrients needed. Properties of mature milk will continue to change as the infant grows, perfectly meeting the infant's nutritional needs.

3. Breast milk is the reference point on which to compare necessary infant nutrition. The nutrients are proportioned for the newborn and change slightly as the infant grows to meet the nutritional needs at that age. Breast milk provides protection against infection and is easily digested, particularly the protein which is digested and absorbed more efficiently than the protein in infant formula. Immunoglobulins, leukocytes, antioxidants, fat-digestive enzymes, and hormones important for growth are present in breast milk but are not available in formula. Commercial formulas contain cow's milk adapted to simulate human milk. Infants may develop allergies to modified cow's milk and may need other types of formula, but they are unlikely to be allergic to human milk. Because of the higher casein to whey proteins in formula compared to breast milk, formula-fed infants will have firmer stools, with a large amount of the protein remaining undigested.

4. Breast milk contains bifidus factor to help establish intestinal flora, leukocytes, lysozymes that are bacteriolytic, lactoferrin to bind iron in bacteria, and immunoglobulins.

5. The two primary (and permanent) contraindications to breastfeeding are (1) infants diagnosed with galactosemia and (2) infants of clients in the United States who have HIV. Some circumstances, such as cancer treatment, herpetic lesions on the nipple, areola or breast, and use of illicit drugs, require temporary cessation in breastfeeding.

6. Support from the clients partner, family and friends, cultural influences, employment demands, and knowledge about each method may influence the choice of feeding method.

7. Suckling causes release of oxytocin, which produces the let-down reflex. Suckling and removal of milk cause the release of prolactin to increase milk production.

8. The level and amount of infant suckling directly affects prolactin release and thus milk production. Therefore, the more the infant breastfeeds, the more milk is produced. Infrequent feedings decrease prolactin output and milk production.

9. Nurses help the client establish breastfeeding during the initial feeding by keeping the newborn in uninterrupted skin-to-skin contact after birth, then help begin breastfeeding when the infant shows feeding cues, ideally within the first hour after birth. Nurses then can help position the infant at the breast and show the parent proper hand positioning. The nurse also can help the infant latch on to the breast, assess the position of the mouth on the breast, check for swallowing, and remove the infant from the breast properly when satisfied.

10. Nurses should teach the parents that breastfeeding is most successful when babies are not on a rigid feeding schedule but are instead allowed to feed as frequently and for as long as they show feeding cues. Parents should be taught to note the quality of a breastfeeding session instead of the length. The infant should suckle vigorously with swallowing noted. When choppy, nonnutritive suckling without the sound of swallowing occurs, the infant should be burped and the feeding completed on the other breast.

11. To wake up a sleepy infant, unwrap the infant's blankets, talk to the infant, change the diaper, rub the infant's back, place the baby skin-to-skin with you, dressed only in a diaper, and express colostrum onto the breast.

12. Sucking from a bottle requires different movements of the mouth and tongue compared to suckling from the breast. The infant who has been fed by bottle may confuse the movements or refuse to breastfeed. Nurses should discourage the use of bottles during the first 2 weeks until the infant learns to breastfeed.

13. To help the client with engorged breasts, the nurse can encourage nursing frequently, applying heat and cold, massaging, and expressing milk to soften the areola.

14. The nurse should advise the client with sore nipples to ensure proper positioning of the infant at the breast, vary the position of the infant, avoid engorgement by frequent feeding, and do not use soap on the nipples. If breast pads are used, remove them when they become wet; avoid pads with plastic lining.

15. The client who plans to work and breastfeed should be taught use of a breast pump and proper storage of milk.

16. There is no one right time for weaning. Breastfeeding for at least 1 year is often recommended. Weaning should be done gradually to help avoid engorgement and help the infant adjust.

17. The parents might ask about the types of formula available, how to prepare it correctly, frequency and amount of feedings, and feeding techniques.

18. Propping bottles risks aspiration of milk. Infants who sleep with a propped bottle have more ear infections, and overfeeding is more likely. In addition, infants need human contact during feeding for security and normal development.

CHAPTER 24

1. Preterm infants appear frail and weak and are small, with limp extremities; poor muscle tone; large head compared to the rest of the body; red, translucent skin; and immature ears, nipples, areolae, and genitals.

2. Factors that increase respiratory problems in preterm infants include lack of surfactant, poor cough reflex, and small air passages.

3. Nursing responsibilities include working with respiratory therapists to manage equipment, monitoring the infant's changing oxygen needs, positioning infants to promote drainage, and suctioning.

4. Nurses wean infants to the open crib by making gradual changes in the environmental temperature; dressing the infant in a shirt, diaper, and hat; and using sleep sacks and double-wrapped blankets in addition to the hat when the infant is out of the incubator.

5. To measure intake and output for infants, all fluids (IV and oral), including medications, are measured. Diapers are weighed to calculate urine output, and drainage, regurgitation, and stools are measured.

6. Preterm infants' kidneys do not concentrate or dilute urine well, and they have large insensible water losses. They lack passive antibodies due to decrease time in utero, have an immature immune system, and are exposed to treatments and situations that may cause infection. Pain causes physiologic and behavioral responses and can have long-term effects; the preterm infant will undergo painful procedures and treatments in the NICU.

7. Nonpharmacologic methods to manage pain in infants include swaddling, facilitated tucking, nonnutritive sucking, sucrose, talking softly, holding, rocking, skin-to-skin positioning, and breastfeeding.

8. The nurse can diminish overstimulation by organizing care, reducing environmental stimuli, promoting rest, promoting motor development, individualizing care, and communicating the infant's needs.

9. Feeding tolerance is assessed by measuring abdominal girth, testing stools for reducing substances and blood, and observing for vomiting or frequent regurgitation. During nipple feedings, the nurse watches for signs of respiratory difficulty, decreased oxygenation, and fatigue.

10. When allowed to set the pace of feedings, infants can stop to rest to conserve energy, regulate breathing, and control the flow of milk.

11. The nurse can help parents who choose to breastfeed their preterm infants by helping them pump and store milk, by teaching breastfeeding techniques adapted to the preterm infant's needs, and by providing support and encouragement.

12. The nurse can help parents feel comfortable with preterm infants by providing warm support; realistic encouragement; and information about the neonatal intensive care unit (NICU) environment, the infant's condition and characteristics, and the equipment and care. This involves making advanced preparations when possible; assisting the parents after birth by facilitating the opportunities to see and touch their infant and allowing the partner to watch the initial NICU care; supporting them with education and physical presence during their visits; facilitating touch, skin-to-skin contact, and interactions with the infant; and preparing for discharge.

13. Beginning early in hospitalization, the nurse should help parents take on gradually increasing responsibility for care of the infant, which will help them prepare for discharge. Helping them prepare their home for the infant is also important.

14. Infants with dysmaturity syndrome may be thin and may have loose skin folds, cracked and peeling skin, minimal vernix, long nails, and meconium staining.

15. Postmature infants may have polycythemia, meconium aspiration, hypoglycemia, and poor temperature regulation.

16. In symmetric growth restriction, all body parts are proportionately small. In asymmetric growth restriction, the head is normal in size but seems large for the body, the weight and abdominal circumference are decreased, and the length is generally normal.

17. Large-for-gestational-age (LGA) infants may have birth injuries such as fractures, nerve injury, cephalhematoma, hypoglycemia, and polycythemia.

CHAPTER 25

1. Effective ventilation is the most important element in resuscitation. Chest compressions and medications are rarely needed. Although most newborns have no difficulty with breathing at birth, up to 10% require some help to begin respirations, and 1% require extensive resuscitative measures.

2. The nurse's role in the care of the infant requiring resuscitation at birth is to begin resuscitation promptly, assist the team, and provide follow-up and parental support.

3. Transient tachypnea of the newborn (TTN) is caused by failure of fetal lung fluid to be absorbed completely in infants who are usually full-term or late preterm. Respiratory distress syndrome occurs in preterm infants as a result of inadequate surfactant (see Chapter 24). TTN

typically resolves faster, causes less alveolar collapse, and results in the need for less supplemental oxygen.

4. Meconium staining is most likely to occur when infants are postterm, small for gestational age (SGA), or compromised before birth by conditions such as placental insufficiency and cord compression.

5. Infants with persistent pulmonary hypertension of the newborn (PPHN) have constriction of the pulmonary blood vessels from inadequate oxygen levels. This increases resistance to blood flow from the heart into the lungs and causes right-to-left shunting of unoxygenated blood through the foramen ovale and patent ductus arteriosus.

6. Kernicterus can be prevented by identifying clients whose infants are at risk for blood incompatibilities, recognizing infants with bilirubin levels that are not normal, and instituting phototherapy when it is needed. Administering Rh immune globulin to pregnant and postpartum clients with Rh-negative blood can prevent Rh blood incompatibilities in future pregnancies, eliminating the risk of hyperbilirubinemia and kernicterus in those newborns.

7. Nurses can help reduce bilirubin in an infant receiving phototherapy by ensuring that the lights or blankets are functioning and positioned properly; exposing as much skin as possible to the light; turning the infant frequently to expose all areas evenly; ensuring adequate milk intake to increase removal of bilirubin by frequent stools; and preventing cold stress or hypoglycemia, which would decrease albumin-binding sites for bilirubin.

8. The role of the nurse in sepsis is to use infection prevention methods, identify infants at risk, watch for early signs, notify the physician, coordinate and administer treatment, observe for change, and support the family.

9. Macrosomia occurs in infants of diabetic mothers (IDMs) because of excessive transfer of glucose, amino acids, and fatty acids from the pregnant client to the fetus. This results in fetal production of insulin and excessive growth in the fetus.

10. Infants of diabetic mothers (IDMs) may develop hypoglycemia after birth because they have high levels of insulin even though they no longer receive glucose from the mother. Infants may need early feeding as a result.

11. The nurse can help the drug-exposed infant rest by minimizing stimulation, swaddling in a flexed position, organizing care to avoid interruptions, and providing a pacifier.

12. The nurse can promote bonding in cases of prenatal drug abuse by helping the parent feel welcome, encouraging participation in infant care, teaching how to respond to the infant's behavior and about the infant's care, and modeling parenting behaviors.

CHAPTER 26

1. Almost all contraceptive methods are used by females, and failure will most affect them.

2. The nurse's role in helping a client with contraception is that of caregiver, counselor, educator, and, at times, health care provider. Providing information to help clients choose contraceptives appropriately and use them correctly is a critical function in each of these roles.

3. Important considerations in choosing contraceptive techniques include safety, protection from sexually transmitted infections (STIs), effectiveness, acceptability, convenience, education needed, benefits, side effects, effect on spontaneity, availability, expense, preference of the client and partner, religious and personal beliefs, and culture.

4. Sterilization and LARC methods may require signed informed consents.

5. Adolescents may have incorrect beliefs, such as that douching will prevent pregnancy, withdrawal (coitus interruptus) is a reliable way to prevent pregnancy, and that their risk of becoming pregnant is low.

6. Adolescents may not seek contraception because they have ambivalent feelings about becoming pregnant, may fear loss of sexual privacy, or may fear pelvic examination.

7. The nurse can teach adolescents effectively by showing sensitivity to their feelings, concerns, needs and different communication styles, being accepting, providing extensive teaching without hurry, and using understandable terms and audiovisual materials.

8. Perimenopausal clients should consider their overall health status when choosing a method of contraception. Those over age 35 and who smoke should not use estrogen-containing contraceptives. Healthy clients in their 40s who do not smoke and are not obese can use combined hormonal contraceptives.

9. Couples choosing sterilization should understand all aspects of the procedure and its permanence.

10. Education for clients choosing intrauterine devices includes information about side effects, including potential change in bleeding patterns, when and how to check the threads, and when to seek medical treatment.

11. Oral contraceptives alter normal hormone changes, preventing ovulation and making the cervical mucus thicker. Progestin-only pills are less effective at inhibiting ovulation than the combined oral contraceptives (COCs), but they also make the endometrial lining unfavorable for implantation while avoiding the side effects and risks associated with estrogen.

12. The most common reason to discontinue use of oral contraceptives is undesired side effects.

13. Clients using oral contraceptives (OCs) need to know when to start the pills, that they must be taken consistently and in the right order every day, what to do if pills are missed, common side effects, and signs that may indicate a problem.

14. Emergency contraception (EC) should be taken as soon as possible after unprotected intercourse or contraceptive failure and is most effective when taken within 72 hours.

15. Barrier methods kill sperm or prevent them from entering the cervix or both.

16. Natural family planning methods avoid drugs, chemicals, and devices, and are acceptable to most religions. Couples need extensive education and high motivation, however, and they risk pregnancy if they make an error.

CHAPTER 27

1. Infertility is strictly defined as the inability to conceive after 1 year of unprotected regular intercourse. A more workable definition that considers the age and other individual factors is the inability of a couple to conceive when desired. Primary infertility is that which occurs in couples who have never conceived. Secondary infertility occurs in those who have conceived before and cannot conceive again.

2. The normal sperm volume should be >1.5 million, total sperm count >39 million, and normal motility >32%. Seminal fluid should liquefy within 30 minutes, allowing motile sperm to move into the uterus without the seminal fluid.

3. Erectile dysfunction, or erection problems, prevent the deposit of seminal fluid with sperm near the female's cervix due to the inability to initiate and maintain an adequate penile erection. Ejaculation abnormalities prevent deposition of the sperm in the upper vagina to achieve pregnancy and may result from retrograde ejaculation, hypospadias, or abnormal ejaculation response (premature, slow, or absent).

4. Abnormalities of the sperm, ejaculation, or the seminal fluid can result from factors such as abnormal hormone stimulation, systemic illness, infections or abnormalities of the reproductive tract, anatomic abnormalities of the reproductive system, exposure to toxins, therapeutic medications, excessive alcohol intake, illicit drug use, elevated scrotal temperature, obstruction, immunologic factors, central nervous system dysfunction, peripheral vascular disease, and psychological disorders.

5. Abnormal ovulation can occur because of hormone disruptions caused by cranial tumors, stress, obesity, eating disorders, systemic disease, and abnormalities in the ovaries or other endocrine glands.

6. Hormone abnormalities associated with ovulation problems interfere with normal buildup and decline of the endometrium. Menstrual periods may be absent, scant, or very heavy.

7. Fallopian tube obstruction may be caused by scarring or adhesions secondary to infections, endometriosis, or pelvic surgery. Congenital anomalies of the reproductive structures also can cause mechanical interference with successful pregnancy.

8. Abnormal cervical mucus can trap sperm and prevent them from entering the uterus and fallopian tube or prevent their preparation (capacitation) for fertilization.

9. Anatomic abnormalities of the uterus or cervix may cause loss of a normal pregnancy by preventing normal implantation. They also may prevent normal placental or fetal growth, or they may increase the risk for miscarriage or previable birth.

10. Endocrine factors associated with repeated pregnancy loss include inadequate progesterone secretion, inadequate endometrial response to progesterone, hypothyroidism and hyperthyroidism, and poorly controlled diabetes in the pregnant client.

11. Immunologic causes of pregnancy loss include an intolerance of the embryo's foreign tissue and systemic lupus erythematosus. Although not always immunologic in origin, thromboembolic disorders may also increase susceptibility to pregnancy loss.

12. Elements included in the history and physical examination include a reproductive history; a medical history; and an examination for undiagnosed endocrine disturbances, tumors, chronic disease, and abnormalities of the reproductive organs. Chromosome analysis is sometimes done. Imaging studies are done if structural abnormalities are suspected.

13. Medications used to induce ovulation include clomiphene citrate, chorionic gonadotropins, gonadotropin-releasing hormone, and human gonadotropins. Clomiphene is a common drug for this purpose. Additional drugs may be given to increase the formation and release of ova and to support a resulting pregnancy.

14. Screening tests related to use of donor sperm include those for blood type and Rh factor, possible genetic abnormalities, and infection. In addition, the male client's history, physical examination, and lifestyle are reviewed for possible problems that might not be revealed by standard tests. Donor sperm are frozen for 6 months to allow identification of infections or other problems that are not evident at the time of collection.

15. In vitro fertilization mixes the male and female gametes outside the body and places embryos back into the uterus. Gamete intrafallopian transfer retrieves ova and then places the ova and sperm into the fallopian tubes, where fertilization occurs. Zygote intrafallopian transfer mixes male and female gametes to allow fertilization and places the fertilized ova into the fallopian tubes. Intracytoplasmic sperm injection (ICSI) is used to retrieve a single sperm and inject it into the cytoplasm of an ovum.

16. Factors that couples consider when seeking infertility help include their age, the length of their attempt to conceive, their desire for a biologic child, and their feelings about adoption or a child-free life.

17. When deciding about infertility evaluations and treatments, the couple considers their personal, social, cultural, and religious values; how difficult treatment may be; the probability of success with treatment; and financial concerns.

18. Psychological reactions to infertility may include guilt, isolation, depression, or stress on the relationship.

19. Parenthood after infertility may be marked by anxiety about the pregnancy, loss of support from infertile couples, or the need for time to accept that their baby is really alive and well.

20. Couples considering adoption must confront their personal preferences, limitations, and prejudices.

21. Couples who lose a pregnancy after a period of infertility often experience grief, but sometimes the grief is mixed with optimism because they were able to achieve pregnancy, even if completion was not possible.

CHAPTER 28

1. Family history is an important part of a health history to assess risk factors that cannot be modified such as heart disease, breast and colon cancers, osteoporosis, and other health problems that should be evaluated further.

2. Important psychosocial assessments include primary and additional languages, reading ability, marital status, employment status and occupation, education level, and evaluation for domestic violence.

3. When taking a sexual history, the nurse should ask about sexual activity, number of partners, age when sexual activity began, method of contraception, history of sexually transmitted infections (STIs) and treatments, and knowledge about and measures used for protection from STIs.

4. Human papillomavirus (HPV) vaccine helps protect individual against cervical, vaginal, and vulvar cancers in females; anal cancer, certain head and neck cancers; and genital warts in both males and females.

5. Vulvar self-examination is recommended to detect signs of precancerous conditions or infections.

6. A Pap test is a cytology specimen of the superficial layers of the cervix and endocervix to detect precancerous and cancerous cells of the cervix.

7. Fecal occult blood testing is important to screen for colon or rectal cancer beginning at age 50.

8. Although biologic female clients may have the "classic" crushing chest pain that is associated with a myocardial infarction, they are more likely to have atypical pain that often is confused with other conditions. These symptoms include fatigue or weakness, upper back pain, nausea and/or vomiting, loss of appetite, dizziness, palpitations, jaw pain, and neck pain. These symptoms may occur at rest or begin during physical activity.

9. Measures to reduce the risk for coronary artery disease include smoking cessation, good nutrition to maintain a normal weight, control high blood pressure and diabetes, exercise, limit alcohol to one drink per day, and, for many, daily low-dose aspirin therapy.

10. Hormonal factors dictate the function, evaluation, and treatment of fibrocystic breast disease. Aspiration of cysts may relieve pain, with follow-up needed only if the cyst recurs or fluid aspirated is suspicious. Specific symptom relief for fibrocystic breast disease has not proved beneficial, but some methods that may be worth trying include wearing a supportive bra to reduce pain from large breasts that stretch ligaments and reducing the intake of caffeine and other stimulants. Other medications that may be tried include oral contraceptives during the second half of the menstrual cycle. Danazol, bromocriptine, and tamoxifen are other possibilities, but their use is temporary.

11. Ultrasound examination, fine-needle aspiration biopsy, core biopsy, or surgical biopsy is used to determine whether a breast disorder is benign or malignant.

12. Staging of breast cancer is important to determine the extent of the breast cancer and to develop a treatment plan.

13. Adjuvant therapy is supportive or additional therapy recommended after surgery to improve the chance of long-term survival. Adjuvant therapy may include radiation therapy, chemotherapy, hormonal therapy, and immunotherapy.

14. The discussion with the client about breast reconstruction options should occur before surgical treatment. Two major methods are the tissue expansion method and autogenous grafts from another area of the client's body. Tissue grafting cannot be done in every client.

15. Preoperative teaching should include the length of the hospital stay and what will happen during that time, dressings, drainage tubes, appearance of incisions for the expected procedures (lumpectomy, mastectomy, reconstruction), and specific exercises to promote flexibility in surgical areas. Lymphedema may occur in the immediate postoperative period, but it usually does not appear until well after discharge.

16. Discharge planning after breast cancer treatment should emphasize the need for continued care and treatment, methods to reduce the risk of wound care of the arm on the affected side, postoperative and adjuvant medications, care of drains, and signs and symptoms that should be reported to the provider. Referral to local support groups also may be helpful.

17. Primary amenorrhea is menstruation that fails to occur by age 15 or within 3 years of breast development. Secondary amenorrhea occurs when the client has not had a menstrual period for 3 months or has had irregular periods for 6 months.

18. Possible causes of abnormal uterine bleeding (AUB) include complications of an unrecognized pregnancy; benign or malignant lesions of the vagina, cervix, or uterus; drug-induced bleeding; systemic diseases, which require prompt treatment; and failure to ovulate. Because clients could have an unrecognized pregnancy, could become anemic, and because malignancy should be ruled out, AUB should not be ignored.

19. Primary dysmenorrhea has no identified pathology. High levels of endometrial prostaglandin diffuse into endometrial tissue, causing spasmodic or colicky pain often called *cramps*. Effective treatment includes rest, application of warmth, oral contraceptives, and prostaglandin inhibitors.

20. Endometriosis lesions grow and proliferate during the follicular and luteal phases of the menstrual cycle and then slough during menstruation. The menstruation from endometriosis lesions occurs in deeper tissue,

causing pressure or pain. Treatment varies with the client's age, whether the client is nearing menopause, the desire for children, the willingness to take the drugs that inhibit excessive tissue growth, and the problems caused to nearby organs by endometriosis. In addition to delaying pregnancy, drug therapy may induce menopausal symptoms. Medical options include NSAIDs, continuous oral contraceptives for 6 to 12 months, danazol, and gonadotropin-releasing hormone (GnRH) agonists. Surgical options include laparoscopy with lysis of adhesions and laser vaporization of the lesions and hysterectomy with removal of one or both ovaries and fallopian tubes and the appendix.

21. The most common side effects of gonadotropin-releasing hormone (GnRH) agonists are hot flashes, vaginal dryness, insomnia, decreased libido, and loss of bone mineral density. Danazol may also cause masculinizing effects and weight gain.

22. Symptoms of premenstrual syndrome (PMS) must be cyclic and recur in the luteal phase of the menstrual cycle; the client should be symptom-free during the follicular phase and the cycle must include seven symptom-free days; symptoms must be severe enough to have an impact on work, lifestyle, and relationships; and the diagnosis must be based on the client's charting of symptoms in a diary as they occur rather than by recall.

23. Common client and family education includes lifestyle modifications such as diet and physical activity, expected cyclic changes, and teaching the family to foster a spirit of support and encouragement.

24. Mifepristone, methotrexate, and misoprostol are drugs that may be used for induced termination of pregnancy up to 9 weeks of gestation.

25. The nurse should teach self-care measures, similar to self-care after spontaneous abortion or miscarriage: observation for excessive bleeding or signs of infection, information about follow-up visits, and contraception information. The client with Rh-negative blood should receive Rho(D) immune globulin.

26. Without estrogen, the reproductive organs begin to atrophy, and the vagina and labia are thinner and more fragile. Vaginal mucosa atrophies and loses its lubrication, making it easily traumatized. The breasts become smaller and atrophy. Bladder changes associated with atrophy make the client more vulnerable to cystitis. Levels of total cholesterol and low-density lipoproteins ("bad" cholesterol) increase, whereas levels of high-density lipoproteins ("good" cholesterol) decrease, increasing the risk for coronary artery disease. Hot flashes occur because of vasomotor instability. Bone mineral loss accelerates in the first few years of the climacteric.

27. Depression, mood swings, and irritability are common psychological symptoms of menopause along with insomnia and fatigue. A client may also greet menopause as freedom from earlier obligations in life as the client shifts responsibility to adult children.

28. A history of breast, ovarian, or uterine cancer; first-degree relative with a history of breast cancer; active or prior thromboembolic disorder; risk for CVD, stroke, or liver disease; undiagnosed abnormal vaginal bleeding; gallbladder or pancreatic disease; diabetes; and conditions aggravated by fluid retention are associated with increased risk of HRT.

29. Osteoporosis is called the *silent thief* because bone mass is lost over many years with no signs or symptoms until the vertebrae collapse or fractures occur.

30. Osteoporosis can be prevented by medications to enhance calcium absorption and inhibit calcium loss (such as calcium and vitamin D supplementation) and by weight-bearing exercises that strengthen muscles and increase bone mass. Prescription medications are also available.

31. Nurses can help clients with osteoporosis prevent fractures by teaching them how to avoid falls by making their environment as safe as possible and to strengthen their bones with medication compliance and load-bearing exercise programs. Adolescents and young clients can also be taught the value of exercise in maintaining long-term bone health.

32. With a cystocele, the weakened upper anterior wall of the vagina cannot support the weight of urine, and the bladder protrudes downward into the vagina, resulting in incomplete emptying of the bladder and consequent cystitis and stress incontinence. With a rectocele, the rectum protrudes into the vagina as the upper posterior wall of the vagina becomes weakened, which may result in difficulty emptying the rectum.

33. Uterine prolapse is caused when the cardinal ligaments are stretched excessively, often with pregnancy, and do not return to normal. This condition is usually treated surgically according to severity and coexisting pelvic floor disorders.

34. Pelvic exercises and bladder training may alleviate symptoms of pelvic floor relaxation and urinary incontinence. Additional measures include teaching about the need to maintain hydration and restrict alcohol and caffeine intake, adherence to weight control programs to reach optimal weight, and use of commercial products to protect the skin and prevent odor. Teaching about any prescribed medications may be indicated.

35. Although leiomyomas do not often cause symptoms, those that do may be associated with increased uterine size and excessive vaginal bleeding, which often results in anemia. Other symptoms are pelvic pressure, bloating, and urinary frequency, depending on the size and location of the fibroids. Treatment depends on size, symptoms, and whether the client desires more children. Surgical treatment options include removal of the fibroids (myomectomy) or hysterectomy. Uterine artery embolization may be an option for the client who does not want surgery. Medical treatment may include oral contraceptives to reduce menstrual flow or short courses

of GnRH agonists to reduce the size and lessen symptoms before surgical removal.

36. Ultrasound is used to distinguish a fluid-filled ovarian cyst from a solid tumor, which requires additional evaluation to determine if the solid tumor is malignant.

37. Signs and symptoms that may indicate cancer of the reproductive organs are irregular vaginal bleeding, unexplained postmenopausal bleeding, unusual vaginal discharge, dyspareunia, persistent vaginal itching, elevated or discolored lesions of the vulva, abdominal bloating, persistent constipation, blood in stools, anorexia, or nausea. Reproductive organ cancers such as ovarian cancer may have no symptoms in the early stages.

38. Cervical cancer may be treated by cryosurgery, destruction of tissue by laser, loop electrosurgical excision procedure (LEEP), electrocoagulation surgical conization, or hysterectomy with chemotherapy for more advanced cases. Endometrial cancer is treated with hysterectomy and bilateral salpingo-oophorectomy plus adjuvant chemotherapy and/or radiation therapy. Ovarian cancer is usually treated by surgery followed by chemotherapy; however, chemotherapy to reduce tumor size followed by surgery to remove malignancy may also be done. A second surgery may be performed to determine if more treatment is needed.

39. Pregnancy, diabetes mellitus, oral contraceptive use, and antibiotic therapy may result in vaginitis caused by *Candida albicans*.

40. Candidiasis causes vaginal and perineal itching, inflamed vulva and vaginal tissue resulting in burning on urination and a thick, white discharge, often with "cottage-cheese" characteristics.

41. Barrier methods of contraception (particularly condoms) protect against the spread of STIs. Condoms offer the best protection, but diaphragms, cervical caps, and spermicidal foams and jellies may decrease the risk for cervical and upper genital tract infection.

42. The major symptom of primary syphilis is a painless chancre that disappears in about 6 weeks; the disease is highly infectious during the primary stage. Symptoms of secondary syphilis are enlargement of the liver and spleen, headache, anorexia, and skin rash. *Condylomata lata* that contain numerous spirochetes and are highly contagious may develop on the vulva.

43. *Condylomata acuminata* (genital warts) are caused by human papillomavirus (HPV), which is associated with cervical cancer.

44. *Chlamydia trachomatis* and *Neisseria gonorrhoeae* cause most cases of pelvic inflammatory disease (PID). Other pathogens, including *Escherichia coli, Gardnerella vaginalis, Streptococcus, Peptostreptococcus, Bacteroides, Prevotella, Mycoplasma, Ureaplasma,* and cytomegalovirus, may cause PID. Other aerobic and anaerobic microorganisms may also cause PID.

45. The risk of toxic shock syndrome can be reduced by thorough hand washing before changing tampons, changing tampons at least every 4 hours, avoiding use of superabsorbent tampons, and using pads rather than tampons during hours of sleep. Wash hands thoroughly before inserting a diaphragm or cervical cap, do not use the diaphragm or cervical cap during menstruation, and the device should be removed within the time limits recommended.

Answers to Next-Generation NCLEX® Examination-Style Questions

CHAPTER 5

1. Oxygenated blood from the placenta enters the fetal circulation through the **1. one** umbilical **2. vein**. About one-third of the blood is directed away from the liver into the **3. ductus venous**, which connects to the inferior vena cava. As blood flows into the right atrium, a flap valve in the septum between the right and left atria called the **4. foramen ovale** directs the highly oxygenated blood into the left atria. Blood from the superior vena cava and the less oxygenated blood from the inferior vena cava flow into the right atrium, to the right ventricle, and into the pulmonary artery. Most of this blood bypasses the fetal lungs and is shunted into the descending aorta through the **5. ductus arteriosus**. The **6. two** umbilical **7. arteries** return the deoxygenated blood to the placenta for oxygenation.

Rationale: A single umbilical vein carries oxygenated blood from the placenta to the fetus. After entering the fetal body, this blood is shunted through the ductus venosus, bypassing the liver, into the inferior vena cava for delivery to the right atrium of the fetal heart. This highly oxygenated blood is directed through the foramen ovale, a flap valve in the atrial septum, into the left atrium, bypassing the fetal lungs. This blood is then pumped into the left ventricle and out of the heart through the aorta to the fetal body.

At the same time, deoxygenated blood enters the right atrium from the superior vena cava and is directed into the right ventricle. It is pumped out of the right ventricle into the pulmonary artery. The ductus arteriosus (DA) connects the pulmonary artery to the descending aorta. The blood is shunted through the DA, bypassing the lungs. In the descending aorta, the deoxygenated blood from the DA mixes with the highly oxygenated blood from the left ventricle and circulates to the lower part of the fetal body.

CHAPTER 6

1. During pregnancy, the uterine fundus reaches the umbilicus at approximately **1. 20** weeks' gestation. After that time, the fundal height is measured from the **2. symphysis pubis** to the top of the fundus in **3. centimeters**. That measurement is approximately equal to the weeks' gestation until **4. 36** weeks, at which time the fetus drops into the pelvis, an occurrence know as **5. lightening**.

Rationale: During pregnancy, the uterus grows at a predictable rate. At approximately 12 weeks' gestation, the fundus (top) of the uterus can be palpated just above the symphysis pubis, at 14 weeks it is between the symphysis and the umbilicus, and by 20 weeks it should be near or at the umbilicus. After 20 weeks, the distance from the symphysis to the fundus is measured in cm and is approximately the same as the weeks' gestation (i.e., at 30 weeks' gestation, the distance from the symphysis to the fundus should be approximately 30 cm). Variations from this growth pattern indicate a need for follow-up. Near 36 weeks' gestation, the fetus drops into the pelvis in preparation for labor and birth. This results in easier lung expansion for the pregnant client and is frequently known as lightening.

2.

Symptom	Presumptive	Probable	Positive
Amenorrhea	X		
Fetal heart rate detected by Doppler or ultrasound			X
Goodell's sign		X	
Positive pregnancy test		X	
Quickening	X		
Fetal movements palpated by examiner			X

Rationale: Presumptive signs of pregnancy are usually subjective changes experienced by the pregnant client. They are the least reliable indicators of pregnancy because they may be the result of conditions other than pregnancy. Amenorrhea, nausea, and vomiting, fatigue, urinary frequency, breast and skin changes, vaginal and cervical color changes (Chadwick's sign), and the client's perception of fetal movement are presumptive signs.

Probable signs of pregnancy are objective findings by an examiner. Although they are more reliable than presumptive signs, they may also be caused by other conditions. Probable signs include abdominal enlargement, cervical softening (Goodell's sign), softening of the isthmus (neck) of the cervix (Hegar's sign), ballottement, Braxton Hicks contractions, and pregnancy tests.

Positive signs of pregnancy can only be caused by pregnancy. They are auscultation of the fetal heart sounds by an examiner, palpation of fetal movement by an examiner, and visualization of the embryo/fetus on sonogram.

3.

	Expected	Requires Follow Up
Darkening of a mole	X	
Decreased frequency of urination		X
Spotting of bright red blood after intercourse	X	
Diarrhea		X
Dizziness when supine	X	
Temperature of 100.8°F		X
Severe backache with flank pain		X

Rationale: Normal physiologic changes of pregnancy result in darkening of moles, spotting after intercourse, and dizziness when supine. Hormonal changes result in the increased pigmentation of the skin including darkening of freckles, moles, and areolae of the breasts. During pregnancy, the cervix becomes hyperemic (increased blood supply) and softens. This friability may result in vaginal spotting following intercourse or a vaginal examination by the provider. When the pregnant client is in the supine position, the weight of the pregnant uterus compresses the vena cava, decreasing blood return to the heart resulting in a drop in blood pressure as well as decreased perfusion of the uterus and placenta. This "aortocaval compression" syndrome causes dizziness, sweating, and feeling faint.

Normal changes of pregnancy result in an increased frequency of urination, especially in the first and third trimesters. Decreased urination could be an indication of dehydration or other issues and requires follow-up. Diarrhea, fever, and severe backache with flank pain are abnormal and require follow-up.

CHAPTER 7

1. The client is a gravida **1.** **5**, para **2.** **3**. The number of term births is **3.** **2**, the number of preterm births is **4.** **1**, the number of abortions is **5.** **1**, and the number of living children is **6.** **3**. The estimated due date for this pregnancy is **7.** **May 19, 2023**.

Rationale: Gravida is the number of times a person has been pregnant, including a current pregnancy. This client is currently pregnant and had 4 previous pregnancies (2013, 2015, 2017 and 2018). Although the 2018 pregnancy resulted in the birth of twins, it was one pregnancy so is only counted once in gravida.

Para is the number of pregnancies a person has carried to 20 weeks gestation or more, regardless of the outcome of the the pregnancy (alive or still birth). A current pregnancy is not counted in para until after the birth. This client had 3 pregnancies which ended after 20 weeks gestation (2013, 2015, 2018). The 2017 pregnancy ended in a miscarriage (spontaneous abortion) before 20 weeks gestation, therefore it is not included in para. Although the 2018 pregnancy resulted in the birth of twins, it was one pregnancy therefore one para.

A term birth is a birth between 37^0 and 41^6 weeks' gestation, so the 2013 and 2015 pregnancies resulted in term births. A preterm birth is a birth between 20^0 and 36^6 weeks' gestation, so the 2018 birth is preterm. Even though twins were born, it is still one birth. An abortion is a pregnancy that ends before 20 weeks' gestation and can be spontaneous (miscarriage) or induced (termination). The 2017 pregnancy was a spontaneous abortion, or miscarriage. This client has 3 living children, the one born in 2013, one born in 2015 and one of the twins born in 2018.

The due date is calculated by using Nagele's rule: LMP - 3 months + 7 days + 1 year. Aug - 3 months = May; 12 days + 7 days - 19; 2022 + 1 year = 2023.

2. B, E

Rationale: D(Rh)-negative and rubella nonimmune laboratory results require follow-up by the nurse. Rh-negative blood type places the client at risk for Rh sensitization if exposed to Rh-positive blood. Rho(D) immune globin (RhoGAM) should be ordered and administered at 28 weeks' gestation, after any invasive procedure or abdominal trauma, and following birth. Nonimmune rubella status places the client and fetus at risk if exposed to rubella during the pregnancy. The client should be notified and taught to avoid situations that could increase the risk of exposure as well as the need for vaccination after the birth of the baby. Rubella vaccine is a live, teratogenic vaccine. Therefore, vaccination during pregnancy is contraindicated. A blood type of "O" may increase the neonate's risk of ABO incompatibility at birth, but no further action is needed at this time. The negative antibody screen indicates that the client is not currently sensitized, and RhoGAM should be administered as indicated. Hematocrit of 34 and hemoglobin of 12 are within the normal range during the first trimester of pregnancy. Nonreactive VDRL indicates that the client does not have a syphilis infection; negative chlamydia indicates no vaginal infection with chlamydia.

3. A, C, E, F

Rationale: Relief measures for nausea and morning sickness include eating a dry carbohydrate before getting out of bed, taking prenatal vitamins at night to avoid stomach upset, eating small frequent meals to avoid an empty or overdistended stomach, choosing a healthy diet that limits fats especially fried foods, using acupressure bands, and drinking peppermint or ginger tea. Although the client should consume plenty of water, it is best to drink separately from meals to avoid overdistention of the stomach.

CHAPTER 8

1. Single, 17-year-old female, heart rate (HR) 106, urine pregnancy test, weight, nausea

Rationale: The client is underweight, BMI 17.79 (106.7 lb), and a teenager with a positive pregnancy test. The client is most likely anxious (HR 106, which should be reassessed during the office visit). The patient is getting adequate rest and most likely is feeling tired from normal pregnancy changes. Morning sickness is the most likely cause of the nausea, and teaching is needed to reassure the client and to provide information on potential relief measures. It is important that the client has a social support system (lives with parents, but client does not want parents to know of pregnancy status). Contraception at this point is irrelevant; it is positive that the client does not use alcohol, tobacco, or drugs. The fetal assessment is normal for 11 weeks.

2.

Nursing Action	Indicated	Contraindicated	Nonessential
Educate client about the relation of nutrition and fetal growth.	X		
Provide education regarding foods that contain iron, calcium, folic acid, and protein.	X		
Ask patient to complete a food diary for 7 days.			X
Suggest vitamin supplementations such as vitamin D, iron, folate, and calcium.	X		
Refer client to a registered dietitian to answer questions and provide further education.	X		
Discuss the need for fluid intake during pregnancy including water, diet sodas, electrolyte enhanced sports drinks, iced tea, and coffee.		X	
Encourage food intake including age-appropriate foods such as hamburgers, fries, chicken nuggets, fried vegetables, and cheese sticks.		X	
Encourage client to eat three healthy meals a day to increase nutrition and avoid snacking.		X	
Provide a scale for home weight monitoring and encourage daily weights for the pregnant client.			X

Rationale: Because the client is a teenager, single, and underweight, it would be essential to teach about nutritional needs during pregnancy. Prenatal vitamins containing folic acid, iron, vitamin D, and calcium intake should be discussed since all are essential minerals or nutrients needed for cellular development of the fetus. Since the client is high risk for nutritional deficits, a consult with a dietitian should be made available. A 7-day food journal or daily weights in early pregnancy are not necessary. One-day food journals or 24-hour recall histories are usually sufficient to determine dietary needs of the pregnancy client.

Due to the patient's morning sickness, high-fat foods should be avoided. Five to six small meals or small meals with snacks are more easily digested and can help with nausea experienced during the day by maintaining a stable blood glucose. A high-protein snack in the evening before bedtime can also help maintain blood glucose levels during the night, thus decreasing morning nausea. Fluid intake should be discussed, but clients should be counseled to avoid excessive caffeine, sugary, or high sodium content drinks. Water should be encouraged. Providing a scale for weight monitoring is not required at this time. Weight assessment will occur in the clinic with follow-up as needed.

3.

Nurse's Responses	Client Questions	Appropriate Nurse's Response for Each Client Question
1. "Normal weight gain during pregnancy is 25–35 lb. You are currently underweight so you should plan on gaining around 30–35 lb to help you have a healthy baby."	"I don't like taking any medicines; why do I need to take these prenatal vitamins?"	5
2. "Protein is important to help your baby grow. You should be eating foods high in protein since you need about 25 grams of protein in your diet every day more than you did before you were pregnant."	"How am I supposed to eat a healthy diet when I feel sick all the time?"	4
3. "Fried foods like chicken nuggets, fries, and fried cheese sticks are high in fat and calories. Candy, sugary soda, and cookies are high in sugar and calories. Foods high in fat can make your nausea worse."	"What foods do I need to avoid?"	3

Continued

Nurse's Responses	Client Questions	Appropriate Nurse's Response for Each Client Question
4. "Morning sickness is a temporary condition that usually goes away after the first trimester of pregnancy. It may be relieved with ginger or peppermint tea. Eating small frequent meals help maintain your blood sugar level and may make eating more tolerable. A nighttime high-protein snack may help maintain your glucose level during the night. Try eating crackers or other carbohydrate before you get out of bed in the morning, that may help with nausea in the morning."	"I don't want to gain weight. How can I keep from gaining weight while I am pregnant?"	1
5. "Folic acid is needed to help your baby develop. Folic acid is available in your diet, but many people do not eat enough foods high in folate."		
6. "Reading food labels will be helpful to identify foods high in protein, carbohydrates, sugars, or fats. Selecting foods low in fat and sugar content provide nutrients you need to help your baby grow and helps you avoid high calorie foods that are not as nutritious."		
7. "Oats, whole grains, fruits, and vegetables are high in fiber to help prevent constipation."		

Rationale: While foods high in fiber, low in fats and sugars, and high in protein are important during pregnancy, these choices do not directly relate to the questions from the client. Folic acid is one supplement included in prenatal vitamins and is not easily obtained in the diet of teenage

clients. Folic acid is necessary in cellular development of the infant and RBC production in the mother. Morning sickness is common and temporary, usually limited to the first trimester. Helping the client understand and utilize methods to reduce nausea can make life easier and pregnancy more enjoyable for the client. This client needs to understand the normal weight gain needed for healthy pregnancies, and since this client is underweight, weight gain should be on the upper edge of the normal range. Reassure the client that the normal maternal body changes and fetal growth necessitate gaining weight. Avoiding fatty foods can help with nausea. Empty calories found in high-sugar foods are nonnutritive calories that are not necessary for fetal development.

4. Laboratory results, parent present at visit, 24-hour food history, supplement use, weight, constipation

Rationale: Maternal vital signs and fetal heart rate are normal. The student does not like taking medications or supplements, but the client is anemic (Hgb 9.8 g/dL) so the iron in the prenatal vitamin and potentially additional iron is necessary. The parent with the client appears to be supportive but also needs encouragement regarding a diet split between small meals and snacks. The client has only gained 0.3 kgs in 6 weeks. Weight gain needs to be discussed with the client with eating goals. The 24-hour food recall indicates the client has needs for additional protein, vegetables, water, and less sugar and potentially caffeine. The nurse should encourage the client to consume three light meals with snacks and complement the wise choices (fruit, peanut butter, cheese, etc.). Constipation can be caused by multiple factors, such as low fiber, decreased fluid intake, and the supplemental iron in the prenatal vitamins. A stool softener may assist the client to have easier bowel movements, but dietary and fluid intake should be included in the client teaching.

5.

Client Response	Effective	Ineffective	Unrelated
"I need to add calcium to my diet. Dairy products, salmon, and calcium-fortified juice will help me add calcium to my diet."	X		
"I should take my iron in the morning with milk to help prevent me from being nauseated when I take it."		X	
"Because the prenatal vitamins make me feel sick, I should not take vitamin supplementation."		X	
"I can consume plain milk, yogurt, cheese, beef, nuts, tofu and green leafy vegetables to increase my protein, iron, and calcium."	X		
"Oats, whole grains, watermelon, prunes, vegetables are high in fiber that can help with constipation."	X		

Client Response	Effective	Ineffective	Unrelated
"Fruit juice, coffee, iced tea, and soda will help me increase my fluids during my pregnancy."		X	
"Since I like sandwiches, ham and turkey lunchmeat should be a staple in my refrigerator."		X	
"If I develop nausea, I need to write down what I ate so I can make a list of foods to avoid."			X
"I need to ensure I take my prenatal vitamin with orange juice because it enhances the amount of iron I get from the medication."	X		

Rationale: The client indicates understanding of food sources for calcium, iron, protein, and fiber. They also understood that iron absorption can be enhanced when taking it with citrus but lacked understanding of iron absorption with dairy products. Client does not understand the need for taking prenatal vitamins and that moving the dose from morning to night can help combat nausea since the client would be sleeping as the prenatal vitamin absorption is occurring. While the client understands the need to increase fluids during pregnancy, the choices of fluids are high in sugar and caffeine, which should be limited during pregnancy. Soda is also high in sodium. Client needs to increase water intake during pregnancy. Juices with reduced sugar content or sugar substitute are acceptable. Decaffeinated iced or hot tea would be acceptable as well. Keeping a food journal for intermittent nausea is not necessary as multiple factors can cause nausea especially during the first trimester of pregnancy.

CHAPTER 9

1. The nurse performing the NST knows there must be **1. two 15 x 15 accelerations (peaks at least 15 bpm above baseline and lasts for at least 15 seconds)** in a **2. 20**-minute period in order for the nonstress test to be reactive

Rationale: Nonstress tests are interpreted as reactive or nonreactive. A reactive NST contains two or more FHR accelerations within a 20-minute period. FHR accelerations indicate an intact CNS and normal autonomic regulation of the FHR, as well as being predictive of the absence of fetal metabolic acidemia at the time of observation. After 32 weeks' gestation the fetus is physiologically mature enough to generate accelerations of 15 x 15 (peaks at least 15 bpm above baseline and lasts for at least 15 seconds); therefore the correct answer is two 15 x 15 accelerations in a 20-minute period.

2. Fetal movement counts serve as an indicator of fetal **1. well-being** based on the premise that the fetus will **2. move** when oxygenating appropriately. Fetal movement **3. increases** at night; therefore fetal movement counts should

occur at the same time every day to give an accurate assessment.

Rationale: Well-being. As a fetus becomes more hypoxic related to interruptions in the oxygenation pathway, activity is reduced to conserve oxygen consumption and maintain energy supplies.

Move. Movement generally reflects an intact and functioning central nervous system and adequate oxygenation.

Increases. Time of the day can potentially influence FMC results. Fetal movement generally peaks between 9:00 PM and 1:00 AM. In this scenario, clients may need to select a different time of day to perform counting.

3.

Client Response	Effective	Ineffective	Unrelated
"It does not matter what time of day I do my fetal movement counts, just as long as I complete them every day."		X	
"If I smoke right before I complete my fetal movement counts, my baby may not move as much."	X		
"I need to complete fetal movement counts at the same time every night."	X		
"If my baby does not move at least 10 times in 1 hour, then I need to call my doctor."	X		
"It does not matter how many times my baby moves, just as long as I feel movement occur daily."		X	
"If I take my prenatal vitamin regularly, it will help my baby move more."			X

Rationale: Fetal movement is an indicator of fetal life. The absence of movement could potentially indicate an adverse perinatal outcome. As the fetus becomes more hypoxic related to interruptions in the oxygenation pathway, activity is reduced to conserve and maintain energy supplies. Teaching clients about the proper way to assess fetal movement is important. Fetal movement peaks at night; therefore consistency in the timing of performing fetal movement counts will provide a more accurate assessment. While the exact number of movements and duration for counting is not established by professional guidelines, typical guidelines include counting for a certain number of movements over a certain time frame. For example, counting 10 movements over a 1 to 2-hour period. Once those 10 movements are achieved, then the counting stops. If the client does not feel 10 movements, then they need to call their provider. Some medications and substances, like cigarettes and alcohol, can alter fetal movement. Smoking causes decreased fetal movement. While prenatal vitamins support a healthy pregnancy, they do not have a direct impact on fetal movement.

CHAPTER 10

Case 1

1.

Lab Results or Other Symptoms	Requires Nursing Follow-Up	Expected Finding
Platelets 90,000/µL	X	
Urine protein-to-creatinine ratio (UPCR) 0.2 mg		X
Headache or visual disturbances (blurred vision, seeing spots)	X	
Bilateral breath sounds clear to auscultation		X
Deep tendon reflexes 4+ in lower extremities	X	
Right-sided epigastric pain	X	
Bilateral lower extremity edema 1+	X	
Hemoglobin 8 g/dL	X	

Rationale: Preeclampsia is a multisystem organ disease process that occurs after 20 weeks of pregnancy. Not one laboratory result or one symptom is definitive for diagnosis of this disease process. Typically it is the whole clinical picture, elevated blood pressure, then possibly increased proteinuria or in the absence of elevated protein, one or more of these diagnostic values: thrombocytopenia (platelets less than 100,000/µL), renal insufficiency (serum creatinine greater than 1.1 mg/dL or a doubling of serum creatinine in the absence of renal disease or a UPCR greater than or equal to 0.3 mg), impaired liver function (elevated liver transaminases 2x normal concentration values, presenting as right-sided epigastric pain), pulmonary edema (adventitious lung sounds), or cerebral or visual symptoms (increased DTRs 3+ or 4+, headache, blurred vision, spots before eyes, double vision, etc.). Although edema is a nonspecific finding and may occur in clients with or without preeclampsia, its presence with other symptoms of preeclampsia warrants follow-up by the nurse. Laboratory studies may identify hepatic, renal, hematologic, or cerebral dysfunction when preeclampsia is severe.

2. Magnesium sulfate is an anticonvulsant that **1. depresses** irritability in the **2. central nervous system** and relaxes smooth muscle. Magnesium is administered either **3. intravenously** or **4. intramuscularly**.

Rationale: While the only known cure for preeclampsia is delivery, medical management includes antihypertensives if blood pressure values meet sustained, severe values (systolic greater than or equal to 160 and/or diastolic greater than or equal to 110) and administration of magnesium sulfate to decrease seizure risk by depression of central nervous system irritability. Preferred administration is intravenously (IV), but intramuscular (IM) is acceptable. While other medications may be used for seizure prevention, magnesium sulfate remains the most commonly used medication. Certain conditions, such as myasthenia gravis or significant cardiac or pulmonary dysfunction, are contraindications for magnesium usage. In those situations, medications such as Dilantin, Ativan, Versed, or Keppra may be used. While magnesium is not an antihypertensive medication, it does cause systemic relaxation of smooth muscle, reducing vasoconstriction and possibly reducing blood pressure.

3. Complaint of shortness of breath, blood pressure = 167/115 mm Hg, heart rate = 138 beats/minute, respirations = 32 breaths/minute, oxygen saturation = 90% (room air), mild wheezing noted to bilateral lower lung fields, magnesium sulfate infusing at 2 g/hour per IV pump

Rationale: Shortness of breath requires immediate attention. The adventitious lung sounds are likely what is causing the client to feel short of breath. One of the adverse effects seen with preeclampsia treated with magnesium sulfate is pulmonary edema (fluid in the lungs). The initial wheezing noted is an early sign of fluid in the pleural space. The abnormal vital signs (VS) noted (hypertension, tachycardia, tachypnea, and low oxygen saturation) all warrant follow-up. The BP shows signs of worsening preeclampsia that needs to be treated with antihypertensives. The HR and RR may be due to the client being anxious due to the shortness of breath, it may be due to ineffective heart function that is allowing fluid to back up into the lungs, or it may be due to an accumulation of magnesium sulfate, nearing toxicity, within the client's system. The SpO_2 lower limit is 92% on room air; therefore this value requires treatment with supplemental oxygen. The last concerning aspect of this assessment is that the magnesium, which may be the potential cause of the abnormal VS and shortness of breath, is still currently infusing. This medication may need to be discontinued and a different seizure prophylactic started. While a nurse can discontinue magnesium in a situation in which they are concerned for the safety of the client, they cannot initiate an additional seizure preventing medication.

Case 2

4.

Nursing Action	Appropriate	Contraindicated	Nonessential
Assess fetal heart rate	X		
Perform vaginal examination to assess for cervical change		X	
Initiate IV	X		
Monitor output	X		
Assess DTRs			X
Access or request prenatal record	X		

Rationale: The client is likely experiencing significant bleeding from a placenta previa. Appropriate nursing actions include assessment of the fetal heart rate to evaluate fetal status and access or request prenatal record to review the results of any sonograms performed. The sonogram report would identify the location of the placenta. Start an IV (based on standing orders or protocols) to ensure IV access for fluid, medication, and possible blood administration, and monitor output as a way to evaluate hydration status and organ perfusion. Urinary output should be at least 30 mL/hour. A vaginal exam is contraindicated because it would potentially rupture the placenta, which covers the cervix in a placenta previa. The placental location should be verified by sonogram prior to anyone performing a vaginal examination. The assessment of DTRs are not essential for this client at this time.

Case 3

5. The nurse teaches the client that preexisting diabetes increases the risk for 1. **miscarriage**, 2. **ketoacidosis**, 3. **birth trauma** and 4. **preeclampsia** in the pregnant client, 5. **congenital anomalies**, 6. **macrosomia (large body)** and 7. **birth injury** in the fetus and 8. **hypoglycemia**, 9. **hypocalecmia**, 10. **hyperbilirubinemia** and 11. **respiratory distress syndrome** in the neonate. In addition, during the first trimester of pregnancy, insulin requirements usually 12. **decreases**, while in the second and third trimesters, the insulin need 13. **increases**.

Rationale: Preexisting diabetes increases the risk to the pregnant client, fetus, and neonate. For the pregnant client, the hormonal changes are different in the first trimester than in the second and third trimesters of pregnancy. During the first trimester, insulin release accelerates, storing glucose in the cells for use later in pregnancy. This increases the risk for hypoglycemia in the first trimester. However, in the second and third trimesters, the sharp rise in hormones results in a state of insulin resistance, which provides ample glucose for the growing fetus but increases the risk for hyperglycemia with ketoacidosis in the pregnant client. The risk for miscarriage is increased, especially if glucose levels are not controlled. The risk for a large baby (macrosomia) increases the risk for birth trauma at delivery, and diabetes is a risk factor for the development of preeclampsia.

For the fetus, there is an increased risk for congenital anomalies (birth defects), especially if glucose levels in the pregnant client are not well controlled in the first trimester. Macrosomia occurs because the high glucose levels from the pregnant client cross the placenta and stimulate fetal production of insulin. The hyperinsulinemia is a growth factor and causes the fetus to grow more than expected. This also increases the risk for trauma at birth. However, if the pregnant client has significant vasculopathy from the effects of diabetes, the placenta may not be supplied with enough blood flow, and the fetus could exhibit intrauterine growth restriction (IUGR).

For the newborn, the glucose from the pregnant client stops when the umbilical cord is clamped and cut. However, the newborn's pancreas continues to release insulin for a short time. This places the baby at risk for hypoglycemia. Hyperbilirubinemia is the result of the breakdown of the extra red blood cells, which form in utero to improve oxygen delivery to the fetal tissues. Neonatal hypocalcemia may be caused by a relative hyperparathyroidism in the pregnant client during gestation or by changes in the magnesium-calcium balance, asphyxia, or preterm birth. These newborns are at risk for respiratory distress first because they are more likely to be born early, either because of preterm labor or a medically indicated preterm birth due to increasing risks of the pregnancy. Secondly, the hyperinsulinemia in the fetus slows the production of cortisol, which is necessary for the synthesis of surfactant.

Because of the hormonal changes described above, the insulin requirement typically decreases during the first trimester and increases during the second and third trimesters.

CHAPTER 11

Case 1

1. Single female, crying, lives alone, sleep pattern, medications, family support, return to work

Rationale: Risk factors for postpartum depression include history of depression (client was on Lexapro prior to pregnancy, and studies indicate that some antidepression medications can be continued during pregnancy with less risk than depression itself); single status, financial concerns, fatigue, lack of sleep, lack of social support, unwanted pregnancy, or complications of pregnancy impacting the mother or infant. The client is single, lives alone, has a history of depression, is financially needy, is not sleeping, and has family support that needs to be refocused to be client-centered. The client has a church community indicating faith most likely is important.

Uncontrollable crying, inability to sleep, unrealistic family comments/expectations, and need for antidepression medication should prompt intervention from the nurse as client is exhibiting signs of postpartum depression versus baby blues (16 days postdelivery is too far out for baby blues—emotional instability is escalating—2 to 8 weeks is the common time for postpartum depression to begin; however, symptoms could be exhibited as far as 1 year from delivery). Medical treatment is indicated for postpartum depression.

2.

Nursing Action	Indicated	Contraindicated	Nonessential
Educate client regarding diet for breastfeeding mothers.			X
Discuss outside support resources such as WIC, La Leche League, church community.	X		
Encourage client to spend time alone to foster a restful environment.		X	

Continued

Nursing Action	Indicated	Contraindicated	Nonessential
Teach family ways to support client at this stage of her postpartum period.	X		
Encourage resting when infant sleeps.	X		
Discuss routine C-section, newborn care, and follow-up.			X
Congratulate client on breastfeeding success thus far and provide formula supplementation information as requested.	X		
Contact health care provider to discuss current assessment of client.	X		
Obtain a consult for lactation consultant to assist client.			X

Rationale: At this time the client's immediate needs are related psychological, emotional, and medical care to treat postpartum depression. The client would not be able to take in routine teaching related to diet, C-section, or newborn care. At this time, priority should be given to helping the client find outside resources for emotional, social, financial, and spiritual support. The health care provider must be notified of the client's emotional well-being given the history of depression (use of Lexapro prior to pregnancy) as this patient needs immediate follow-up and care. The family is physically present daily and most likely needs teaching about how to recognize and support their family member during this depression period. Specific warning signs of postpartum depression and need for immediate interventions need to be understood by the family support system to help identify and/or deter harmful actions to the client or infant. The client should not be alone without the ability to cope. Support is needed to help provide care for infant and client as self-care is ineffective at this point. The client needs encouragement about all the positive influences related to being a new parent. The baby is successfully breastfeeding, normal weight gain, stool, and urine output but is experiencing a normal growth spurt. Relating to the client how well breastfeeding has been thus far and praising the efforts is important to build self-confidence. Encouraging rest while the baby rests is important; however, sleep disturbances are also indicators of postpartum depression. Providing requested information to a client is the responsibility of the nurse and can help the client in decision making.

3.

Client Response	Effective	Ineffective	Unrelated
"Going for a walk with my baby each day will help me get out of the house and get some fresh air."	X		
"So, crying all the time is a sign I might need some extra help, letting my health care provider know I feel overwhelmed is important."	X		
"Because of this condition, I should limit my visitors so my baby and I can get to know each other better."		X	
"I need to rest when my baby rests and let my family help with laundry, cooking, and even baby care if it helps me get some sleep."	X		
"I should discuss with my health care provider restarting my Lexapro since it was so effective before I was pregnant."	X		
"I cannot take Lexapro or any medications like these while I am breastfeeding."		X	
"Baby blues will go away, waiting it out is the best thing to do."		X	
"If I develop any drainage or redness from my C-section scar, I will clean it with peroxide and tell my doctor when I go back to the office in 6 weeks."			X

Rationale: Helping a client recognize the need for exercise, fresh air, positive interactions with infant, and allowing support from family and friends is important to maintaining mental health. It is important that the client and/or family know to contact the health care provider when signs/symptoms of postpartum depression are present or are increasing. Isolation is a negative factor for clients suffering from postpartum depression. Understanding the need to return to antidepression medication and the safety of use during pregnancy and breastfeeding is important to the mental health of the postpartum client. Understanding the difference between baby blues and postpartum depression is important for both clients and families as the family may be the source of recognition of problems and the ones to seek assistance for the postpartum client. Waiting for 6 weeks to follow up with the health care provider for a potential wound infection indicates lack of understanding of need to seek medical care for postoperative infections but is unrelated to teaching the client about postpartum depression.

Case 2

1. Heart rate 132, oxygen saturation 92%, 35 weeks' gestation, rupture of membranes, contractions, pupils, agitation, fetal monitoring, medications, APGARs, infant HR 206, infant oxygen saturation 89%, maternal laboratories

Rationale: The nurse should be suspicious of drug use with multiple factors for this client. The client is overly aggressive and agitated for normal labor, pupils are pinpoint, and partner reports use of marijuana. Pinpoint pupils and preterm precipitous delivery would be more indicative of cocaine utilization and thus more negative impact on the neonate. The client's tachycardia may be due to pain but could also be related to the use of marijuana, cocaine or other drugs. The O_2 saturation of 92% requires supplemental oxygen for fetal oxygenation, and infant is showing signs of distress by fetal monitoring (predelivery) and APGARs, tachycardia, and poor oxygenation postdelivery. Additional maternal and infant laboratory assessment for drug detection is indicated.

2.

Nursing Action	Indicated	Contraindicated	Nonessential
Obtain orders for additional lab work beyond routine admission screen.	X		
Provide immediate postpartum care for client in multibed recovery room.		X	
Encourage skin-to-skin contact with client and infant.		X	
Transfer infant to the NICU.	X		
Encourage labor partner to stay with patient during recovery period.			X
Explain procedures and prepare patient for transfer to the postpartum unit.	X		
Congratulate client on delivery and birth of infant.	X		
Assess infant for irritability, signs of drug withdrawal.	X		
Provide quiet environment with low stimulation for infant in NICU.	X		

Rationale: The clients and infant's immediate needs should be addressed. The infant is in distress, therefore skin-to-skin contact is inappropriate, the infant needs neonatal care, low-stimulus environment, and observation for drug withdrawal due to client's history of marijuana use, behavior in labor, and precipitous preterm delivery. The client should have additional laboratories including drug screening due to behavior, pinpoint pupils, precipitous preterm delivery, partner's report of drug use and potential indications of cocaine use noted. A quiet, low-stimulus environment should be provided for the client immediately postdelivery due to effects of drugs, and the labor partner should be given the option of staying with client or going to the NICU with the infant. It is not necessary for the partner to remain with the client and may be better to decrease external stimuli without visitors present. All procedures should be explained, and the nurse should encourage and congratulate the client regarding the birth.

CHAPTER 12

1. When palpating the fetal head to determine position during an admission vaginal exam, the nurse identifies a "Y" shaped juncture of three bones with a small soft area that is triangle shaped, known as the **1. posterior fontanel**. From this landmark, the nurse follows the **2. sagittal suture** to a larger, diamond-shaped soft area known as the **3. anterior fontanel**.

Rationale: When palpating the fetal head, the juncture of the V-shaped lambdoid suture with the sagittal suture forms a Y with the triangular posterior fontanel at the center. The sagittal suture can be followed to the larger, diamond-shaped anterior fontanel at the junction of the sagittal suture with the coronal suture.

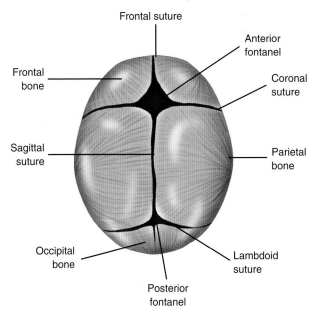

2. The nurse understands the presenting part of the fetus is located **1. 1 cm above the ischial spines**, and the cervix is dilated (opened) **2. 3 cm** and effaced (thinned out) **3. 80%**.

Rationale: The dilation of the cervix is estimated in centimeters by how far apart the examiner can spread their fingers inside the cervix. Completely dilated is 10 cm, when the examiner cannot palpate any of the cervix. Effacement is the thickness or length of the cervix and is estimated in percentage. A completely effaced cervix is paper thin. The fetal station is the relationship of the presenting part of the fetus to the client's ischial spines and is estimated as centimeters above (expressed as a negative number, such as -1) or below (expressed as a positive number, such as +1).

CHAPTER 13

1. A, C, E, F.
Rationale: The experience of pain is personal, and caregivers should not make assumptions about how a client will behave during labor. The unique nature of childbirth pain and the diverse responses to it make nursing management complex. The nurse can miss important cues if the client is either stoic or outspoken about their pain. With either extreme, the nurse may not readily identify critical information such as impending birth or symptoms of a complication. The description of the client's stiffening and minimal interactions are cues that additional pain management strategies should be explored.
2. B, C, D, E, G, I.
Rationale: The client is demonstrating signs of possible epidural catheter migration and requires interventions to stop the medication from adversely affecting the client further. When the medication reaches the bloodstream, an immediate elevation in the client's heart rate is noted. An increase of 20 beats per minute within 45 seconds indicates the epidural is intravascular. However, increased heart rates may also be in relation to experiencing an excessive amount of pain. Other signs of an intravascular injection include numbness of the tongue and lips, a metallic taste in their mouth, lightheadedness, dizziness, tinnitus, or a feeling of impending doom, and they may occur with intravascular injection, although these symptoms usually only occur if a large volume of local anesthesia reaches the client's bloodstream. This anesthetic emergency requires notification of the anesthesia provider and application of the pulse oximeter, and respiratory assessment gives insight into respiratory difficulties that may be present due to the increased level of medication. Increasing the head of the bed and turning off the epidural pump may help to keep the medication level from increasing to a higher level. The effect of the occurrence on the fetus is evaluated by continuous FHR monitoring.
3. I'm feeling lightheaded; vital signs: BP 90/44, pulse rate 124; repeat blood pressures taken every 5 minutes 88/50, 90/48, and 89/50, minimal variability, and recurrent late decelerations.
Rationale: Feeling lightheaded, decreased BP, tachycardia and abnormal or indeterminate FHR changes are symptoms of vasodilation resulting in an interruption of the oxygen pathway to the fetus due to decreased placental perfusion.
4. Increase maintenance IV fluid infusion rate. Administer intravenous phenylephrine, reposition the client to a lateral position, continue blood pressure assessments every 5 minutes.
Rationale: The client was demonstrating symptoms of low blood pressure. A hypotensive episode is a common occurrence following epidural placement due to vasodilation effects of the medication. In this hypotensive instance, the decreased blood flow adversely impacted the fetus causing late decelerations. Correcting the blood pressure will improve blood flow to the intervillous space, correcting the late decelerations and minimal variability. It will also decrease the lightheadedness felt by the client. The anesthesia provider should be notified after independent nursing interventions and those included in protocols or standing orders have been implemented. The report would include assessment findings, interventions provided and the client's response.

Assessment Finding	Effective	Ineffective	Unrelated
FHR BL rate 135 bpm	X		
Blood pressure 118/78 and 122/76	X		
Cervical examination 7 cm/60%/0 station			X
Moderate variability	X		
FHR accelerations	X		

Rationale: The normal FHR baseline, moderate variability, and accelerations are all signs the intervillous space of the placenta is being perfused appropriately and the fetus is adequately oxygenating. The BP increased back to the client's normal range indicating appropriate perfusion postepidural.

CHAPTER 14

1. The nurse recognizes that the fetal heart rate (FHR) baseline (BL) is **1. normal range**. The FHR pattern is reflective of a **2. category I**, which is predictive of **3. normal fetal acid-base status at the time of observation**.
Rationale: The FHR BL is 135 beats per min (bpm), which is within the normal range of 110 to 160 bpm. BL variability is moderate (between 6 and 25 bpm) and there are no variable or late decelerations. Therefore, this is a category I pattern, indicating fetal oxygenation and normal fetal acid-base status at the time of observation.
2. The nurse interprets the FHR pattern as having a FHR BL of 155 beats per minute (bpm) with **1. moderate** variability and **2. recurrent variable decelerations**, which is a periodic pattern. This qualifies as a **3. category II** in the three-tiered categorization system.
Rationale: The FHR BL variability is moderate, between 6 and 25 beats per minute (bpm). The decelerations reach the lowest point less than 30 seconds after they begin and are therefore variable decelerations. An FHR pattern with recurrent variable decelerations and moderate BL variability indicates an interruption of oxygen transfer from the environment to the fetus. However, at the time of observation, the fetus is not experiencing hypoxic injury. This is a category II, or indeterminate pattern.

3. Increase maintenance IV fluid infusion rate, prepare for a potential amnioinfusion, perform a cervical examination, reposition the client to a lateral position, decrease oxytocin infusion.

Rationale: A category II FHR pattern with recurrent variable decelerations and moderate BL variability indicates an interruption of oxygen transfer from the environment to the fetus most likely due to umbilical cord compression. However, at the time of observation, the fetus is not experiencing hypoxic injury. Interventions should relieve cord compression and maximize oxygen delivery to the fetus. Cervical examination is performed to rule out a prolapsed umbilical cord. Amnioinfusion may restore fluid volume to near normal levels and alleviate cord compression. Position changes may alter the relationship of the location of the cord, uterine wall and fetal body parts to relieve the compression. Lateral positions and IV fluid administration maximize cardiac output, placental perfusion and oxygen delivery to the fetus. Decreasing the oxytocin infusion will decrease uterine activity which increases placental perfusion and fetal oxygenation.

CHAPTER 15

1. A, D, E, G, H.

Rationale: The priority for the focused assessment is to determine the current condition of the client (client VS, medical, and obstetric histories), fetus (status of amniotic membranes, client perception of recent fetal movement, FHR), and labor (contraction frequency, intensity, and duration). Information about preparation for labor and birth, last oral intake, spiritual beliefs, and presence of advanced directives can be gathered after the need for immediate interventions is ruled out.

2. C, E, and F.

Rationale: The client should be instructed to return to the birth facility for regular contractions for an hour, occurring approximately every 5 minutes, lasting 1 minute; rupture of amniotic membranes (trickle or gush of fluid from the vagina), and signs of possible complications (decreased fetal movement, vaginal bleeding requiring a pad). Loss of the mucus plug may occur several days or even weeks before true labor begins. The current contraction pattern is irregular and is most likely Braxton Hicks contractions. A return to the birth facility is not necessary until the contractions are regular for about an hour. A bloody show or spotting is likely to occur due to the vaginal examination to determine cervical dilation. The client should be warned that this would be considered normal. Heavy bleeding that requires a sanitary pad may indicate a pregnancy complication and would be an indication to return to the birth facility for further evaluation.

3. The client is at highest risk for **1. infection** because of **2. ruptured membranes, 3. primipara**, and **4. not in active labor**.

Rationale: Once the amniotic membranes rupture, the risk for intrauterine infection increases. The longer the time between rupture of membranes to birth, the greater the risk. Primiparous clients have slower labors than multiparous clients due to the fact that the client is currently 1 cm dilated with irregular contractions, suggesting that the induction of

labor will be a slow process. Precipitous labor is a fast labor (less than 3 hours).

Nursing Action	Indicated	Contraindicated	Nonessential
Position the client supine for better EFM tracing quality		X	
Position the client in a lateral position	X		
Stop the oxytocin infusion	X		
Decrease the oxytocin to half of the current rate		X	
Notify the provider	X		
Consider oxygen administration	X		
Prepare for an emergency cesarean birth		X	
Adjust the EFM to improve the tracing quality			X

Rationale: The client has uterine tachysystole with an abnormal (Category III) fetal heart rate pattern. Essential nursing actions include stop the oxytocin infusion, position the client laterally, consider oxygen administration at 10 L/min via non-rebreather face mask, IV fluid bolus of 500 mL, and notify the provider. Positioning the client in the supine position is contraindicated because it will cause aortocaval compression and decrease placental perfusion, which will further decrease oxygen available to the fetus. Preparing for an emergency cesarean birth is contraindicated at this time. If the uterine activity can be decreased, the fetus may be able to recover. Evaluation of nonsurgical actions will determine the next steps. Adjusting the EFM is not necessary at this time. There is no information in the scenario that indicates an issue with the quality of the EFM tracing.

CHAPTER 16

1. The client states she is cramping and bleeding for the last 2 hours, had an ultrasound once and they said her due date was a couple months from now; laboratories were drawn on her first visit, but she does not know the results; contractions palpate mild, q 7 minutes x 60 seconds, watery bloody fluid

Rationale: Follow-up is required for unknown due date and initial laboratory results. The nurse should attempt to locate those records. Some facilities utilize a common electronic health record, and those results can be shared within their health care system and with outside facilities. Due date is "a couple of months from now" and she is contracting regularly with watery, bloody fluid on her underwear. Contractions increase the risk of possible preterm delivery and loss of fluid increases the client's infection risk. If membranes are ruptured, then hospitalization may be required for the entirety of the pregnancy; therefore confirmation of membrane rupture needs to occur.

2. Answers: A, C, D, E, G.

Rationale: Laboratory results will assist in identifying abnormal values and help develop a treatment plan. OB ultrasound will help identify fetal gestational age. If preterm, a different plan of care is required than for a term fetus. Validation of rupture of membranes assists in identification of risk status for developing infection. Fetal monitoring provides insight into fetal well-being. NPO status is set until the plan of care is determined. An IV or administration of medications (steroids, tocolytic, or magnesium sulfate) may all be required if preterm gestation and risk of preterm delivery is identified. These interventions are based on completing the initial assessment pieces first.

3.

Assessment Finding	Expected	Requires Follow-Up
Contractions decrease to irregular		X
Normal labs	X	
Blood sugar 182		X
Positive AmniSure		X
Cervical exam—appears to not be dilated (closed)	X	

Rationale: While decreasing contractions is good, continual assessment is indicated. Additional follow-up is needed for elevated blood sugar and positive AmniSure (rupture of membranes). The other laboratories and cervical examination are as expected.

4. Preterm birth, infection, umbilical cord prolapse, and anxiety are the priority problems for prevention.

Rationale: The client is estimated at 28 weeks gestation with PPROM and contractions and is therefore at risk for preterm birth and intrauterine infection. In addition, with PPROM and a breech fetal position, there is an increased risk for the umbilical cord to prolapse into the cervix and vagina. This would require immediate birth, which would be preterm. Due to the risks to self and to the fetus/newborn, the client is at increased risk for anxiety. Although bedrest may be prescribed, placing the client at risk for immobility and venous thromboembolism, those potential problems should be addressed after the client is stabilized. Pain may be a problem at some point, but there is no evidence to suggest that it is a current problem.

5. Complains of not feeling well and aching, P 110, T 100.6°F, white blood cell count is 21,000. Contractions are increasing, and she is becoming more restless.

Rationale: Fever, complaints of feeling ill and restlessness, uterine contractions increasing, increased pulse and respirations, and elevated white count are symptoms of an intrauterine infection.

CHAPTER 17

1.

Assessment Finding	Important	Nonessential
BP 129/72		X
HR 102	X	
RR 19		X
Temp 100.5°F	X	
Fundus firm, midline at umbilicus		X
Moderate lochia rubra		X
Cramping while breastfeeding		X
Headache	X	
1+ pedal edema bilaterally		X
Night sweats		X
Hgb 11.1		X
Hct 30		X
WBC 20,000		X

Rationale:

A. BP should be compared to baseline to help determine any deviations. As this patient had recorded BP readings in the 110 to 120/60 to 70, this would not be considered an important finding.

B. HR is tachycardiac (greater than 100) and warrants follow-up. Cause could be associated with pain, dehydration, infection, and excitement. The client denied more than mild cramping; therefore it likely is not pain related. The client also recently had the IV discontinued; therefore it likely is not related to dehydration. While the client could be experiencing excitement, it is unlikely to cause such a drastic increase in heart rate. Further evaluation for infection needs to occur.

C. RR is within normal limits and therefore not concerning.

D. Temperature is elevated and needs to be reported to the provider. While it is common for the temperature to rise in the first 24 hours after childbirth, and can get up to 100.4°F, elevations higher than this would need to be reported. This finding would not be expected.

E. Within 12 hours after delivery. the fundus will be approximately at the umbilicus and will decent 1 cm per day. This finding would be expected.

F. Lochia rubra is expected postpartum days 1 to 3 and may be scant to moderate. This finding would be expected.

G. Afterpains while breastfeeding are due to the release of oxytocin. Analgesics may be used to lessen the discomfort while breastfeeding, but this is not something that requires immediate follow-up.

H. Headache requires immediate and careful assessment to determine the cause. Headaches may be due to changes in fluid and electrolyte balance, anesthesia, or preeclampsia.

I. HCT is low due to increase in plasma volume. This finding would not be considered important unless the patient was demonstrating other symptoms of hypovolemic shock.

J. WBC can increase in the postpartum period up to 30,000/mm³. This finding would not be considered important unless there is an increase of over 30% within 6 hours.

K. Until excess fluid is eliminated, pedal and pretibial edema may be present. This finding would be expected.

L. Diaphoresis aids the elimination of excess plasma volume. This finding would be expected.

2. (1) Explain procedure and rationale. (2) Have Taylor empty bladder. (3) Place Taylor in a supine position with knees flexed. (4) Put on clean gloves and lower perineal pad. (5) Place nondominant hand above symphysis pubis. (6) Palpate using flat fingers of dominant hand starting at umbilicus.

Rationale: Nursing Procedure 17.1 Assessing the Uterine Fundus

3. The nurse needs to include **1. dry the perineum front to back** in the discharge teaching. Should **2. foul odor of lochia** occur after discharge, Taylor should notify the health care provider. The nurse knows the client understands the discharge follow-up instructions when Taylor states **3. "I should contact my provider within the first three weeks."** during teach-back.

Rationale: (1) Drying the perineum front to back prevents contamination from the anal area. All other options are incorrect. (2) Foul odor of the lochia should be reported as it can be an indication of infection. All other options are expected. (3) It is recommended for postpartum clients to have contact with their provider in the first 3 weeks with a comprehensive visit within 4 to 12 weeks. All other options are incorrect.

CHAPTER 18

1.

Nursing Action	Indicated	Contraindicated	Nonessential
Assist the client to the bathroom to empty bladder		X	
Continue to massage the fundus	X		
Raise head of bed 90 degrees		X	
Call for help; notify provider	X		
Increase IV fluids per protocol	X		
Dispose of linens as they become saturated with blood		X	

Rationale: The client has early postpartum hemorrhage. Risk factors include gravida (5), large baby (8 lb 6 oz), long and difficult labor with Pitocin augmentation and epidural anesthesia, vacuum extracted birth, and perineal trauma. Total blood loss before admission to the mother-baby unit was 550 mL (400 at birth and 150 during recovery). Current assessment findings suggest uterine atony. Appropriate nursing actions include continuing uterine massage while assessing for a distended bladder. If the bladder is distended, offer the client a bedpan or insert a urinary catheter. It is unsafe for the client to ambulate to the restroom at this time due excessive blood loss. To increase blood return to the heart, the nurse should raise the foot of the client's bed 10 to 30 degrees, keep the trunk horizontal and slightly raise the head of the bed. The nurse should call for help, asking for the postpartum hemorrhage cart and notify the provider of PPH. IV fluids and medications should be administered according to the facility's PPH protocol. All pads, linens, or other items with blood should be weighed for quantification of blood loss, then saved for the provider to assess as needed.

2.

Assessment	Expected/Normal	Unexpected/Follow-Up Required
Breasts lumps palpated	X	
Temperature 101.3°F		X
Strong, foul odor to lochia		X
Abdominal pain, not relieved with prescribed medications.		X
Uterine fundus at the umbilicus, midline, boggy but responds to uterine massage.		X
Lochia rubra scant	X	

Rationale: The client is at risk for endometritis due to birth by cesarean following a 16-hour labor with membranes ruptured for 14 hours. Temperature of 101.3°F, strong, foul-smelling lochia, abdominal pain not relieved with prescribed medications, subinvolution as evidenced by the uterine fundus at the level of the umbilicus, and boggy are symptoms of endometritis. (The uterus should be approximately 2 cm below the umbilicus and firm.) Other symptoms of endometritis include tachycardia, chills, malaise, and uterine tenderness. These findings require follow-up. As the client's milk comes in, the breasts begin to fill, causing a lumpy feeling when they are palpated. This is a normal finding for a breastfeeding client 2 days after birth. Lochia rubra is a normal finding for the first 3 days after birth and may be scant to moderate in amount.

CHAPTER 19

1.
BP: 146/94
Pulse 114 beats/min
R: 26 breaths/min
Oxygen saturation: 91% (on room air)
Skin: cool and clammy
Lungs: Wheezes noted lower lung bases bilaterally

Uterus: Occasional contractions every 7 to 10 minutes, palpate moderate with relaxation

Twin B: baseline FHTs 155, minimal variability, late decelerations

Rationale: Tachypnea, tachycardia and downward trending pulse oximetry values less than 95% are symptoms of pulmonary edema. Cool clammy skin and adventitious lung sounds on auscultation are additional symptoms. Other symptoms would include dyspnea, anxiety or agitation, coughing, chest discomfort, and air hunger. An elevated systolic blood pressure greater than 140 mmHg or diastolic greater than 90 mmHg requires further investigation. Hypertension in a pregnant client after 20 weeks gestation is suspicious for preeclampsia, which is a risk factor for pulmonary edema. The uterus may contract as the uteroplacental blood flow is decreased with hypoxemia. The fetuses are at risk for compromise due to decreased oxygen availability. Twin B is showing symptoms of an interrupted oxygenation pathway (late decelerations).

2.

Nursing Action	Emergent	Nonemergent
Place oxygen at 8–10 L per nonrebreather FM	X	
Insert a peripheral intravenous line	X	
Monitor vitals signs every 30 minutes		X
Administer morphine sulphate 1–2 mg SIVP	X	
Instruct the patient of radiology coming to perform a bedside CXR		X
Obtain admission lab work: CBC, CMP, type, and screen	X	
Insert Foley catheter		X

Rationale: The immediate goal in management of pulmonary edema is adequate oxygenation of the client. Administration of 8 to 10 L/min of oxygen per nonrebreather face mask is the least invasive, but most effective method. A pulse oximeter value of 95% or greater indicates adequate oxygenation in the pregnant client. Morphine sulfate is administered in small doses to control pain and decrease anxiety, which improves oxygenation. A peripheral IV should be inserted and placed on an infusion pump for the administration of IV medications during a respiratory compromise; fluid intake should be closely monitored. Vital signs should be assessed every 5 to 15 minutes until the client is stable, then every 30 minutes to an hour. Admission lab work, including CBC and CMP will assist the provider with the medical diagnosis.

Instructing the patient that radiology is coming to obtain an CXR is necessary but is not emergent at this time. Urinary output should be closely monitored. Insertion of a Foley catheter is desired, but is not urgent as output can still be measured until it is placed.

3.

Assessment Finding	Effective	Ineffective	Unrelated
Oxygen saturation 95%	X		
Heart Rate: 110 BPM		X	
Respirations 20 breaths per minute	X		
Blood pressure: 136/78			X
Temperature: 98.2°F			X
Uterus: Irritability noted; mild to palpation		X	
Fetus: Twin B: FHTs 150; moderate variability; no decelerations	X		
Lying semi-Fowler's wedged to the right side			X
Intermittent wheezing in the lower lobes bilaterally		X	

Rationale: Initial stabilization of the client's respiratory status including an oxygen saturation of 95% and greater, normalization of respiratory rate, and Category I fetal heart rate pattern indicate gas exchange is improving. Uterine irritability and intermittent wheezing indicate the pregnant client has some continued impaired gas exchange; the nurse should continue to monitor. Changes in blood pressure, temperature, position change are not relevant to evaluating respiratory status.

CHAPTER 20

1. The nurse recognizes that **1. preterm gestation, 2. maternal/newborn blood incompatibilities** and **3. vacuum assisted birth** increase the risk of nonphysiologic (pathologic) jaundice.

Rationale: Hyperbilirubinemia risk factors include prematurity, low birth weight; cephalohematoma/assisted vaginal delivery/trauma, East Asian or American Indian ethnicity, sibling with history of hyperbilirubinemia, breastfed infants/poor intake/delayed meconium passage, infants of diabetic mothers, or ABO incompatibility.

2.

	Indicated	Contraindicated	Nonessential
Place skin-to-skin with parents	X		
Keep infant, clothing, and linens dry	X		
Place bassinet next to window		X	
Prewarm objects before they touch the newborn	X		

	Indicated	Contraindicated	Nonessential
Leave the door to the room open with the bassinet in sight so nursing staff can see the newborn as they pass by.		X	

Rationale: The newborn is at risk for heat loss through conduction, evaporation, convection, and radiation. Placing the infant skin-to-skin with the parent transfers heat from the parent to the newborn through conduction. Keeping the infant and the surroundings dry prevents heat loss through evaporation, and prewarming objects (including hands) before they touch the infant prevents heat loss through conduction. Placing the infant in the bassinet near an open doorway allows heat loss through convection due to the air currents (and it places the infant at risk for abduction!). Placing the bassinet near the window allows heat loss through radiation.

CHAPTER 21

1.

Assessment Finding	Expected/ Normal	Common Variation	Unexpected/ Abnormal
Acrocyanosis	X		
Substernal retraction			X
Faint audible murmur		X	
Respiratory rate 48	X		
Apical heart rate 134	X		
Jitteriness			X
Nasal flaring			X
Large bluish pigmented areas on buttocks		X	
Small white cyst on the face		X	

Rationale: At birth, blood is shunted toward vital organs, such as the brain, heart, and lungs, resulting in blue hands or feet the first few days of life, called acrocyanosis. Intercostal or substernal retractions, tachypnea, nasal flaring, or use of accessory muscles with respirations are abnormal signs of respiratory distress. Normal respiratory rate in the newborn is 30 to 60 breaths/min. Normal heart rate is 120 to 160 beats/min. The ductus arteriosus which allows blood to bypass the lungs during intrauterine life constricts at birth. In some newborns, this process results in a mild murmur, which may resolve spontaneously with in the first few days of

life. However, other signs of cardiovascular status should be assessed and the provider notified. Jitteriness in the newborn is often associated with blood sugar instability and requires follow-up nursing actions. Mongolian spots are large bluish pigmented areas on the buttocks and lower back in many newborns of dark complexions. They usually lighten or disappear by 3 to 5 years of age. Small white cysts on the newborn's face are called milia. They are a normal variation and require no follow-up or treatment.

2.

Assessment Finding	Preterm	Term	Postterm
Tightly flexed posture		X	X
Abundant lanugo	X		
Parchment-like skin with deep cracking			X
Flat areola with no breast tissue palpable	X		
Plantar creases on anterior two-thirds of sole of foot		X	

Rationale: A tightly flexed posture in a newborn is associated with a term or postterm gestational age. Lanugo is abundant in the preterm, bald areas or mostly bald in the term, and completely bald in the postterm newborn. The skin of a preterm newborn is thin, transparent, and gelatinous; by term it is drying, may have superficial peeling or some cracks, rare veins visible; postterm is parchment-like with deep cracks and no visible vessels, it may even be leathery. Breast tissue is nonpalpable in preterm infants and increases with the gestational age; by term there is palpable breast tissue and a visible nipple. Deep creases on the sole of the feet (plantar creases) also increase with gestational age. The preterm infant will not have any creases or will only have them on the anterior one-third of the foot, the term baby has creases on the anterior two-thirds, and the postterm baby has them over the entire foot.

CHAPTER 22

1. A term newborn is rapidly born by spontaneous vaginal delivery and placed directly on the mother's abdomen. This practice is known as **1. skin to skin contact.** This intervention benefits the newborn by promoting: **2. temperature regulation, 3. blood glucose regulation**, and **4. breastfeeding**.
Rationale: Skin-to-skin or kangaroo care is placing a newborn directly on the parent's chest or skin. This has the proven benefit of helping the newborn with thermoregulation, stabilizing glucose levels, and initiating early breastfeeding. It has not been shown to have a direct effect on sensory development, iron stores, or passage of meconium.
2. A, E.
Rationale: With the exception of the baby's temperature, all findings are expected. To warm a cold baby, the nurse should remove all clothing except the diaper, place the infant directly on the skin of the parent (usually the chest),

and cover both with prewarmed blankets. The parent's body temperature will increase until the baby is warmed. Alternately, the baby may be placed on a preheated radiant warmer in the postpartum client's room but does not need to be removed from the room. The admission assessment can be performed with the baby skin-to-skin on the parent's chest. Acrocyanosis (blue extremities) is normal in a newborn due to the immaturity of the circulatory system. Slight crackles on auscultation of the lungs are a common finding in newborns delivered by cesarean. It is due to residual lung fluid, which was not absorbed during labor or expelled during a vaginal birth. In the absence of signs of respiratory complications such as grunting, retractions, nasal flaring, or central cyanosis, no actions are required at this time. The fluid will be absorbed by the lungs with normal respirations. A head-down position, suctioning, and oxygen are not required. It is normal for the newborn to need assistance with latching on. The lactation consultant is not required at this time. Notification of the provider is not required at this time. Independent nursing actions should be implemented to address the newborn's temperature.

3. Parent teaching to decrease the risk of infant abduction includes 1. **matching ID bands are required for staff to give the newborn to an adult, 2. place the baby's bassinet away from the door to the room, preferably on the opposite side of the client's bed**, and 3. **Do not allow anyone without the appropriate picture ID to take the baby out of the room.** Promotion of newborn thermal regulation includes teaching the parents 4. **change the baby's clothing or linens if they become wet, 5. swaddle the baby or place in a sleeping sac when not skin to skin with the parent** and 6. **safe skin to skin positioning requires that the baby's face is visible and the nose and mouth are uncovered.** 7. **If the baby spits up, turn the baby to the side, wipe the face and mouth with a clean cloth and suction gently with a bulb syringe if needed** and 8. **when using the bulb syringe, suction the mouth first, then the nose** are included in parent teaching to decrease the risk of newborn airway obstruction.

Rationale: Parent teaching to decrease the risk of infant abduction includes explaining the use of the ID bands. Each newborn will have two ID bands with a unique number and the parent's information. An identical ID band is placed on the parent at birth. An additional band is available for one other adult. The facility staff should not leave the infant with anyone if they are not wearing the matching band. Facility staff should always transport the baby from the parent's room in the bassinet. The parents should be told not to allow anyone to carry the baby out of the room. The bassinet should be placed away from the doorway to the room to decrease the opportunity for removal from the room without the parent's permission. The baby should never be left unattended. If no one is in the room when the client showers, nursing staff should be notified so that the baby is held in the nursery or at the nurses' station. All hospital staff working with new families should have a picture ID. Parents are taught to verify the picture and the person taking the baby from the room.

Parent instructions to help prevent heat loss include keeping the baby's clothing and linens dry, keeping the stockinette cap on the baby and using skin-to-skin contact with a parent, swaddling, or a sleep sac for warmth. When using skin-to-skin contact, it is important that the baby's face is visible and the nose and mouth are not covered.

To decrease the risk of airway obstruction in the newborn, the parents are taught to wipe the face and mouth with a clean cloth if the baby spits up and gently use a bulb syringe if necessary. Correct use of the bulb syringe includes suction of the mouth first, then the nares. Many newborns will gasp when the nares are suctioned; suctioning the mouth first decreases the risk of inhalation of pharyngeal secretions at this time. All newborns should be placed on their back for sleeping to decrease the risk of sudden infant death syndrome (SIDS).

4. A, C, E, G, H

Rationale: Newborn discharge instructions include when to notify the provider. All facilities will have specific instructions, which are reviewed with the parents and provided in written form. Topics to be included are fever or low temperature (greater than 100.4°F or less than 97.7°F taken axillary). Changes in temperature are sometimes the only symptom of infections in the newborn. Diarrhea, two or more green or watery stools, is also an indication to notify the provider. A gastrointestinal anomaly or infection may be to blame. The newborn can become dehydrated with electrolyte abnormalities when they have diarrhea. The newborn should not sleep more than 6 hours without waking. This is a sign of lethargy, which could indicate illness. Redness around the umbilical cord or stump or yellow drainage from the area indicate an infection at the site and require medical treatment. A yellow coloration in the baby's skin or eyes (jaundice) may indicate hyperbilirubinemia and requires evaluation. Spitting up a small amount after feeding is normal in newborns. Six to eight wet diapers per day indicate that the baby is well hydrated and has adequate intake. It is normal for a few drops of blood to be associated with the umbilical cord falling off. However, if there is active bleeding, the provider should be notified.

CHAPTER 23

1. Weight: 6 lb, 10 oz (3.005 kg); right nipple with slight crack and redness; left nipple with slight redness. Client positions the baby slightly tilted toward the infant's back with the chin pointed downward and the hand supporting the posterior upper part of the head. Latch assessment: L = 1, A = 1, T = 2, C = 0, H = 0. Total score = 4.

Rationale: Weight loss is over 5% at 2 days of age; 10% weight loss is concerning. Reevaluation is warranted. The presence of nipple redness and cracking suggests a latch problem. The Latch assessment is under 7, indicating further evaluation is necessary. Client is positioning baby on its back and holding the head in a position that could restrict the ability to suck and swallow correctly.

2.

Infant Behavior	Positive Hunger Cues	Unrelated to Feeding Cues
Jitteriness		X
Lip smacking	X	
Hand-to-mouth movements	X	
Increased activity	X	
Moro reflex		X
Sucking on hands	X	

Rationale: Lip smacking, hand-to-mouth movements, increased general activity, and sucking on hands are all considered early signs of hunger in newborns. Jitteriness may be a sign of low blood sugar but is not considered a hunger cue. Moro reflex is a normal newborn reflex unrelated to feeding.

3. B
Rationale: 3.118 kg × 110 kcal/day requirement for age 0 to 3 mo = 342.98 cals/24 hours
C
Rationale: 342.98/20 cal/oz = 17.149 divided by six feedings per day = 2.858 oz/feeding. Round to 2.86 oz.

4.

Nurse's Action or Response	Client Question	Appropriate Nurse's Action or Response for Each Client Question
1. "Your baby's stomach is very small so your colostrum is sufficient for the first few days. During the first few days, infants often fall asleep at the breast, but try to feed at least eight times in a 24-hour period and watch for audible swallowing and at least three to four wet diapers by day 3."	"How do I keep my baby awake during a feeding?"	3
2. "Vary the position of the baby every other feeding, avoid using soap on the nipples, and ensure the baby has a wide open latch as if it were taking a bite out of an apple."	"How do I tell if my baby is getting enough from my breast?"	1
3. "Unwrap the baby and feed skin-to-skin. You can also remove the baby and rub the back."	"What can I do about my nipples being sore?"	2
4. "Longer feedings of 45 minutes or more indicate the baby is very hungry."	"After I go home, how do I know how long to feed my baby?"	5
5. "Feedings will vary in length, but generally your baby will slow the suckling pattern greatly and his/her hands will be completely open and relaxed."		
6. "If you baby nurses at least 5 minutes and falls asleep, they should be getting enough milk."		
7. "Use tea bags on the nipples and apply Vaseline or olive oil every few hours to the breast and nipple area."		

Rationale: Newborns should nurse 8 to 12 times a day by day 2 to 3 and should have at least three to four wet diapers daily, increasing to six wet diapers by day 4. Infants often will fall asleep at the breast in the first 48 hours of life and can be awakened by stroking their backs or large muscles and nursing with no clothes or blanket (skin-to-skin). Feedings extending over 45 minutes in length often mean the baby is not transferring milk efficiently and are correlated with poor weight gain. Management of sore nipples includes position changes to put stress on the nipple in different angles and correcting a poor latch. Oils and tea bags have not been shown to help sore nipples and could be unsafe for the infant to ingest.

CHAPTER 24

1.

Client's Response	Effective	Ineffective	Unrelated
"My daughter is being fed every 3 hours, day and night."	X		
"We are keeping the home very quiet."		X	
"I have help from family and friends."	X		
"I am keeping the home warm and the baby wrapped in blankets to prevent getting cold."		X	

Continued

Client's Response	Effective	Ineffective	Unrelated
"We hold the baby four to five times a day."			X
"Developmentally, my baby will crawl at a later time that normal."	X		

Rationale: Many infants needs feedings every 3 hours day and night, to help them gain weight adequately. Infants are accustomed to noises of a nursery 24 hours a day and may not sleep well at first in a quiet home environment. The parents should dress the baby comfortable like each person in the home. It is good to hold the baby and continue to provide skin to skin-in-the home. There is not a length of time to hold the baby. Parents should base their expectations on the infant's corrected age rather than the chronological age.

2.

Nursing Action	Indicated	Contraindicated	Nonessential
"Let the parents know their questions are welcome."	X		
"Continue to instruct the parents not to touch the infant as this could startle the baby and cause the heart rate to increase."		X	
"Use an interpreter as the parents do not understand English."	X		
"Explain the equipment used to care for the infant.	X		
"Teach the parents about skin-to-skin care and touching the baby's hand."	X		

Rationale: An important role of the nurse is providing accurate information to parents. All parents to express concerns before beginning to teach. Encourage them to ask questions about infants care. Show parents how to touch the baby in ways that are appropriate once the baby is stable. Help them hold their baby as soon as possible. The use of an interpreter is recommended in patients who do not speak English. Although language was not discussed in this question, an interpreter should be used as appropriate to the situation. The nurse should explain the use of the equipment used on the baby and the meanings of alarms. As the infant becomes more stable, show parents which forms of touch work best with their infant.

CHAPTER 25

1.

Assessment	Expected	Common Variation	Unexpected
Heart rate 150 bpm	X		
Jittery activity			X
Pink mucous membranes	X		
Yellow tint to skin			X
High-pitched cry			X
Breastfed 10 minutes on both breasts	X		
Fontanels are soft with edema		X	
Total serum bilirubin is 6 mg/dL			X
Dark pink mark on the pack of the neck		X	

Rationale: Normal heart rate for newborns is 120-160, pink mucous membranes suggest adequate oxygenation, breastfeeding for 10 is appropriate. Soft fontanels with edema suggest caput succedaneum which is a common finding following vaginal birth. The dark pin mark on the back of the baby's neck is Nevus Simplex, a common birthmark frequently called angel kisses, stork bites or salmon patches. Jittery activity and a high- pitched cry may be symptoms of hypoglycemia. The nurse should check the capillary glucose with a heel stick per facility protocols. Yellow tint to the skin and total serum bilirubin of 6 mg/dL indicate hyperbilirubinemia (jaundice). The nurse should notify the provider and anticipate an order for phototherapy.

2. The baby's history of 32 weeks' gestation, prolonged rupture of membranes, and maternal history of diabetes puts this baby at risk for developing **1. pathologic** jaundice and **2. hypoglycemia**. Additional assessment and interventions the nurse may include are **3. assess glucose via heelstick**, **4. remove eye patch from eyes during feeding**, **5. turn infant frequently in the warmer**.

Rationale: This infant is at increased risk for pathologic jaundice due to preterm birth. There is also a possibility of infection from prolonged rupture of membranes which is another risk factor for pathologic jaundice. In addition, because the baby's blood is type A-positive and the mother's blood is type O-negative, there is a 'risk for blood incompatibility which further increases this risk. The infant is at increased risk for neonatal hypoglycemia because of the preterm birth and the maternal history of uncontrolled diabetes during pregnancy. Nursing interventions include removing the eye patches after removing the baby from under the bili lights. This will allow bonding to the parents and assessment of the eyes. Additional interventions include turning the infant frequently to allow for the bili lights to reach the entire body of the baby. The nurse should also assess capillary glucose via heelstick per protocol or if the infant becomes symptomatic of hypoglycemia.

CHAPTER 26

1. A, D, F, G, I

Rationale: The acronym *ACHES* can be used to help clients remember warning signs that may indicate complications when using oral contraceptives. Warning signs of possible complications include severe abdominal pain (mesenteric or pelvic vein thrombosis, benign liver tumor, gallbladder disease), chest pain (pulmonary emboli or myocardial infarction, coughing/shortness of breath), severe headache (stroke, migraine), eye problems with complete or partial loss of vision (headache, retinal vein thrombosis, stroke, migraine), and severe leg pain or swelling in the calf or thigh (heat, redness, deep vein thrombosis). Other signs include jaundice, a breast lump, and severe mood swings or depression. The client should contact the health care provider if any of these signs develops.

2. B, D, E, G

Rationale: The patch may be applied to the abdomen, buttock, upper outer arm, or upper torso, excluding the breast. The patch is replaced weekly for 3 weeks, then removed for 7 consecutive days. This will be the time the client will have a period. If the patch falls off, tape should not be used as this will interfere with the contraception.

CHAPTER 27

1.

Client's Statement	Effective	Ineffective	Unrelated
"The timing of ovulation can be affected by many factors."	X		
"Commercial ovulation kits are generally not effective as I am 35 years old."		X	
"When the cervical mucous becomes clear, thin, and slippery, I should be ovulating."	X		
"PCOS can cause anovulation."			X
"Since I am 35 years old, I don't have many eggs left and will stop ovulating."			X
"When using the basal body temperature method, my temperature rises just before ovulation."		X	
"I have a calendar to mark the dates of intercourse."	X		

Rationale: Common prediction methods include commercial ovulation predictor kits and cervical mucous assessment. The accuracy of the commercial kits is not affected by the client's age. Basal body temperature (BBT), or temperature at rest, may be used to identify if ovulation has occurred. The temperature rises slightly with or after ovulation. It is helpful to use a calendar or other method such as a cell phone app to track temperatures and the timing of intercourse in relation to probable ovulation. Women with PCOS may have anovulation or irregular ovulatory cycles, making it difficult to obtain a pregnancy. This is unrelated as the client does not have a history of PCOS and was not discussed by the nurse. As a women reaches the end of her reproductive life, ovulation can become irregular. This is unrelated as the nurse taught how to recognize ovulation.

2.

Medication	Drug action
1. Clomiphene citrate (Clomid)	Stimulates the pituitary gland to produce LH and FSH
hCG	2. Stimulates ovulation when used with gonadotropins. It also stimulates progesterone production
3. Metformin	Given for clients with polycystic ovarian syndrome
Progesterone	4. Luteal phase support; also prepares the uterine lining for implantation

CHAPTER 28

1. B, E, F, G, I

Rationale: Cardiovascular disease (CVD) is the leading global cause of death. Sometimes CVDs may be silent and progress undiagnosed until a client experiences signs or symptoms of a heart attack, a heart failure, an arrhythmia, or a stroke. Whereas some biological female clients have no symptoms, others often experience symptoms with CVD that are atypical of biological male clients: unusual fatigue, upper back pain, nausea and/or vomiting, loss of appetite, dizziness, palpitations, jaw pain, and neck pain. These may occur during rest, begin during physical activity, or be triggered by stress. Major preventable factors include being overweight and obese, physical inactivity, and smoking. A family history of heart disease is especially important when the client is postmenopausal because the level of estrogen, which provides some protection against coronary artery disease (CAD), decreases after menopause, and obesity may increase. If family history, obesity, or other factors increase the client's risk for heart disease, a stress test and analysis of cholesterol and lipid profiles may be ordered and education provided related to aspirin therapy and signs/symptoms that require emergency care or further evaluation. Nutrition counseling for weight loss is also appropriate.

2. A, D, F, I, J

Rationale: The health history identifies risk factors for a variety of conditions, and some topics should be discussed with all clients. These topics include dietary intake, physical activity, habits, and sexual practices. Components of a sexual history include sexual activity (how many partners, age when first sexually active), method of contraception (satisfaction with method, adverse reactions, accuracy of use), previous sexually transmitted infection and treatment, and knowledge or practice of measures to protect self from sexually transmitted diseases, including human immunodeficiency virus (HIV).

GLOSSARY

abortion A spontaneous or elective termination of pregnancy before the 20th week of gestation. Spontaneous abortion is frequently called *miscarriage*.

abruptio placentae See *Placental abruption.*

abstinence syndrome A group of signs and symptoms that occurs when a person who is dependent on a specific drug withdraws or abstains from taking that drug.

acidosis Condition resulting from accumulation of acid (hydrogen ions) or depletion of base (bicarbonate); acid–base balance measured by pH.

acrocyanosis Bluish discoloration of the hands and feet caused by reduced peripheral circulation.

adjuvant therapy Additional treatment that increases or enhances the action of the primary treatment.

adnexa Accessory parts or organs, such as the fallopian tubes and ovaries, associated with the uterus.

afterpains Cramping pain after childbirth caused by alternating relaxation and contraction of uterine muscles.

agonist Substance that causes a physiologic effect.

allele An alternative form of a gene.

alpha-fetoprotein (AFP) Plasma protein produced by the fetus.

ambiguity (ambiguous) Lack of clarity or certainty; having more than one meaning.

ambivalence Simultaneous conflicting emotions, attitudes, ideas, or wishes.

amenorrhea Absence of menstruation. Primary amenorrhea is a delay of the first menstruation, and secondary amenorrhea is cessation of menstruation after its initiation.

amniocentesis Transabdominal puncture of the amniotic sac to obtain a sample of amniotic fluid that contains fetal cells and biochemical substances for laboratory examination.

amnioinfusion Infusion of a sterile isotonic solution into the uterine cavity during labor to reduce umbilical cord compression.

amnion The inner fetal membrane.

amniotic fluid embolism Extremely rare and unpredictable event thought to occur when amniotic fluid enters maternal circulation at or near birth, triggering a sequence of inflammatory immune reactions and coagulopathy. Also referred to as anaphylactoid syndrome of pregnancy.

amniotic fluid index (AFI) An ultrasound examination in which the vertical depth of the largest fluid pocket in each of the four quadrants of the uterus is measured and totaled.

amniotomy AROM—artificial rupture of the fetal membranes (i.e., the amniotic sac).

analgesic Systemic agent that relieves pain without causing loss of consciousness.

anaphylactoid syndrome See *Amniotic fluid embolism.*

anesthesia Loss of sensation, especially to pain, with or without loss of consciousness.

anesthesiologist Physician who specializes in administration of anesthesia.

angina pectoris Myocardial pain usually caused by physical activity or stress; usually called *angina.*

anorexia nervosa Refusal to eat because of a distorted body image and feeling of obesity.

anovulation Menstrual cycles that occur without ovulation.

antagonist Substance that blocks the action of another substance or of body secretions.

antepartum Pertaining to the time during pregnancy before the onset of labor.

apnea A pause in breathing lasting 20 seconds or more or accompanied by cyanosis, pallor, bradycardia, or decreased muscle tone.

apneic spells Cessation of breathing for more than 20 seconds or accompanied by cyanosis, pallor, bradycardia, or hypotonia.

asexual Lack of a sexual attraction or desire for other people.

asphyxia Insufficient oxygen and excess carbon dioxide in blood and tissues.

appropriate for gestational age infant An infant whose size between the 10th and the 90th percentile for gestational age.

aspiration pneumonitis Chemical injury to the lungs that may occur with regurgitation and aspiration of acidic gastric secretions.

assisted reproductive technologies (ART) Medical, surgical, laboratory, and micromanipulation techniques used with ova and sperm to improve chances of conception.

assumptions Beliefs taken for granted without examination.

atony Absence or lack of usual muscle tone.

atrophic vaginitis Inflammation that occurs when the vagina becomes dry and fragile, usually as a result of estrogen deficit after menopause.

attachment Development of strong affectional ties as a result of interaction between an infant and a significant other (e.g., mother, father, parent, sibling, caretaker).

attitude (fetal) Relationship of fetal body parts to one another.

augmentation of labor Artificial stimulation of uterine contractions.

autogenous Tissue that is moved from one part of the body to another part of the same person's body.

autosome Any of the 22 pairs of chromosomes other than the sex chromosomes.

axillary dissection Removal of most of the axillary lymph nodes for staging and treatment of breast cancer.

azoospermia Absence of sperm in semen.

baby blues See *Postpartum blues.*

baroreceptors Cells that are sensitive to blood pressure changes.

basal body temperature Body temperature at rest.

baseline data Information that describes the status of the client before treatment begins.

baseline risk The risk, usually in reference to birth defects or spontaneous abortion, of the general population of pregnant clients who have no identified high-risk factors or invasive procedures.

bias A prejudice that sways the mind.

bicornuate (bicornate) uterus Malformed uterus with two horns.

bilirubin Unusable component of hemolyzed (broken down) erythrocytes.

bilirubin encephalopathy Acute manifestation of bilirubin toxicity occurring in the first weeks after birth.

bisexual Being attracted to people of more than one gender.

bioethics Rules or principles that govern right conduct, specifically those that relate to health care.

biophysical profile (BPP) Method for evaluating fetal status during the antepartum period based on five variables originating with the fetus: fetal heart rate, breathing movements, gross body movements, muscle tone, and amniotic fluid volume.

birth defect An abnormality of structure, function, or body metabolism present at birth that results in physical or mental disability or is fatal.

birth plan A plan describing a couple's preferences for their birth experience. (Also called a *family preference plan.*)

bloody show Mixture of cervical mucus and blood from ruptured capillaries in the cervix; often precedes labor and increases with cervical dilation.

body image Subjective view of one's physical appearance and capabilities; derived from one's own observations and the evaluation of significant others.

bonding Development of a strong emotional tie of a parent to a newborn.

Braxton Hicks contractions Irregular, usually mild uterine contractions that occur throughout pregnancy and become stronger in the last trimester.

breast self-awareness Client's awareness of the normal appearance and feel of their breasts; can include breast self-examination as part of it.

breast self-examination (BSE) Organized monthly evaluation of the breasts by the client; supplements clinical breast examination.

bronchopulmonary dysplasia Chronic pulmonary condition in which damage to the infant's lungs requires prolonged dependence on supplemental oxygen. (Also called *chronic lung disease.*)

brown fat Highly vascular specialized fat that provides more heat than other fat when metabolized.

bulimia Eating disorder characterized by ingestion of large amounts of food followed by induced vomiting, fasting, or use of laxatives or diuretics.

café-au-lait spots Light brown birthmarks.

CAM Abbreviation for complementary and alternative medicine.

caput succedaneum Area of edema over the presenting part of the fetus or newborn resulting from pressure against the cervix; often called *caput*.

carcinoma in situ Malignant neoplasm in surface tissue that has not extended into deeper tissue.

catabolism Destructive process that converts living cells into simpler compounds; process involved in involution of the uterus after childbirth.

caudal regression syndrome A malformation that results when the sacrum, lumbar spine, and lower extremities fail to develop.

cell-free deoxyribonucleic acid (cfDNA) screening A noninvasive prenatal screen for fetal trisomy 21, 18, and 13 as well as sex chromosome anomalies and selected microdeletions and microduplications.

cephalohematoma Bleeding between the periosteum and skull from pressure during birth; does not cross suture lines.

cephalopelvic disproportion Fetal head size that is too large to fit through the maternal pelvis at birth. (Also called *fetopelvic disproportion*.)

cerclage Encircling the cervix with sutures to prevent recurrent spontaneous abortion caused by early cervical dilation.

cervical cap A small cup-like contraceptive device placed over the cervix to prevent sperm from entering.

cervical incompetence or cervical insufficiency An anatomic defect that results in painless dilation of the cervix in the second trimester of pregnancy.

cesarean birth Surgical birth of the fetus through an incision in the abdominal wall and uterus.

Chadwick's sign Bluish–purple discoloration of the cervix, vagina, and labia during pregnancy as a result of increased vascular congestion.

chemical dependence Physical and psychological dependence on a substance such as alcohol, tobacco, or drugs, either legal or illicit.

chemoreceptors Cells that are sensitive to chemical changes in the blood, specifically changes in oxygen and carbon dioxide levels, and changes in acid–base balance.

chignon Newborn scalp edema created by a vacuum extractor.

choanal atresia Abnormality of the nasal septum that obstructs one or both nasal passages.

chordee Ventral curvature of the penis.

chorioamnionitis Inflammation of the amniotic sac (fetal membranes); usually caused by bacterial and viral infections. (Also called *amnionitis* or Triple I-intrauterine infection or inflammation or both.)

chorion The outer fetal membrane.

chorionic villus sampling (CVS) Transcervical or transabdominal procedure to obtain a sample of chorionic villi (projections which develop from the outer fetal membrane and burrow into endometrial tissue during implantation) for analysis of fetal cells.

chromosomes Organization of DNA of specific genes into strings within the cell nucleus.

cilia Hair-like processes on the surface of a cell that beat rhythmically to move the cell or to move fluid or other substances over the cell surface.

cisgender A person who identifies as the sex they were assigned at birth.

climacteric Endocrine, body, and psychic changes occurring at the end of a woman's reproductive period. (Also informally called *menopause*, although this term does not encompass all changes.)

clinical breast examination (CBE) Breast examination by a professional that may identify problems that the client has not identified with breast self-examination (BSE).

clonus Rapidly alternating muscle contraction and relaxation, which may occur when reflexes are hyperactive.

coitus Sexual union between a male and a female.

coitus interruptus Withdrawal of the penis from the vagina before ejaculation.

colostrum Breast fluid secreted during pregnancy and the early days after childbirth.

colposcopy Examination of the vaginal and cervical tissue with a colposcope for magnification of cells.

complementary and alternative medicine (CAM) Nonmainstream or unconventional health care treatments and practices that are generally not used in hospitals and often not reimbursed by insurance companies.

complete protein food Food containing all the essential amino acids.

compliance Stretchability or elasticity of the lungs and thorax that allows distention without resistance during respirations.

conceptus Cells and membranes resulting from fertilization of the ovum at any stage of prenatal development.

condyloma acuminatum A wart-like growth of the skin seen on the external genitalia, in the vagina, on the cervix, or near the anus; may be caused by human papillomavirus (condyloma acuminatum) or by syphilis (condyloma latum).

congenital Present at birth.

congenital anomaly Abnormal intrauterine development of an organ or structure.

congestive heart failure Condition resulting from failure of the heart to maintain adequate circulation; characterized by weakness, dyspnea, and edema in body parts that are lower than the heart.

consanguinity Blood relationship.

containment A method of increasing comfort in infants by swaddling or other means to keep the extremities in a flexed position near the body.

contraception Prevention of pregnancy.

contraction stress test (CST) Method for evaluating fetal status during the antepartum period by observing response of the fetal heart to the stress of uterine contractions that may induce recurrent episodes of fetal hypoxia.

corpus luteum Graafian follicle cells remaining after ovulation that produce estrogen and progesterone.

corrected age Gestational age that a preterm infant would be if still in utero; the chronologic age minus the number of weeks the infant was born prematurely. (May also be called *developmental age*.)

couvade syndrome Pregnancy-related rituals or a cluster of pregnancy-like symptoms experienced by some prospective partners during pregnancy and childbirth.

craniosynostosis Premature closure of the sutures of the infant's head.

crowning Appearance of the fetal scalp or presenting part at the vaginal opening.

cryotherapy Destruction of tissue using extreme cold.

cryptorchidism Failure of one or both testes to descend into the scrotum.

cultural values Principles or standards that guide the thinking, decisions, and actions of a group, particularly during pivotal life events.

culture Sum of values, beliefs, and practices of a group of people that is transmitted from one generation to the next.

cystocele Prolapse of the urinary bladder through the anterior vaginal wall.

decidua Name applied to the endometrium during pregnancy. All except the deepest layer are shed after childbirth.

deontologic model Ethical model stating that the right course of action is the one dictated by ethical principles and moral rules.

developmental task A step in growth and maturation that one must complete before additional growth and maturation are possible.

diabetes mellitus A disorder of carbohydrate metabolism caused by a relative or complete lack of insulin secretion; characterized by glycosuria (glucose in the urine) and hyperglycemia.

diabetogenic Refers to a condition such as pregnancy that produces the effects of diabetes mellitus.

diaphragm A latex dome that covers the cervix and prevents entrance of sperm; must be used with a spermicide to be effective.

diastasis recti Separation of the longitudinal muscles of the abdomen (rectus abdominis) during pregnancy.

dietary reference intakes A label for several terms that estimate nutrient needs; includes recommended dietary allowance, adequate intake, tolerable upper intake level, and estimated average requirement.

dilation Opening.

dilation and curettage (D&C) Stretching of the cervical os to permit suctioning or scraping of the walls of the uterus. The procedure may be performed to obtain samples of endometrial tissue for laboratory examination; or during the postpartum period to remove retained fragments of placenta.

dilation and evacuation (D&E) Wide cervical dilation followed by mechanical destruction and removal of fetal parts from the uterus. After complete removal of the fetus, a vacuum curette is used to remove the placenta and remaining products of conception.

diploid Having a pair of chromosomes that represents one copy of every chromosome from each parent; the number of chromosomes (46 in humans) normally present in body cells other than gametes.

disseminated intravascular coagulation (DIC) Pathologic coagulopathy involving systemic activation of coagulation, clotting, decreased tissue oxygenation and consumption of coagulation factors.

dominant Gene for which a single copy on either the maternal or paternal chromosome can cause the trait to be expressed.

doula A trained labor support person who provides labor or postpartum support or both.

duration Period from the beginning of a uterine contraction to the end of the same contraction.

dyslipidemia Abnormal fat and cholesterol levels.

dysmenorrhea Painful menstruation.

dyspareunia Difficult or painful coitus in the female.

dysplasia Abnormal development of tissue.

dystocia Difficult or prolonged labor; often associated with abnormal uterine activity and cephalopelvic disproportion.

dysuria Painful urination often associated with urinary tract infection.

eclampsia Form of hypertension of pregnancy complicated by generalized (grand mal) seizures.

ectopic pregnancy Implantation of a fertilized ovum in any area other than the uterus; the most common site is the fallopian tube.

EDD Estimated date of delivery; may also be abbreviated EDB (*estimated date of birth*).

effacement Thinning and shortening of the cervix.

effleurage Light stroking or massage of the abdomen or another body part performed during labor contractions.

egocentrism Interest centered on the self rather than on the needs of others.

ejaculation Expulsion of semen from the penis.

emancipated minor An adolescent younger than the age of majority (usually 18 years) who is considered developmentally competent to make certain medical decisions independent of a parent or guardian.

embolus A mass that may be composed of a thrombus (blood clot) or amniotic fluid released into the bloodstream, which may cause obstruction of pulmonary vessels.

embryo The developing baby from the beginning of the third week through the eighth week after conception.

en face Position that allows eye-to-eye contact between the newborn and a parent.

endometrial hyperplasia Excessive proliferation of normal cells of the uterine lining; may be caused by administration of estrogen during the postmenopausal period.

endometriosis Presence of tissue resembling the endometrium outside the uterine cavity.

endometritis Infection of the inner lining of the uterus.

endometrium Lining of the uterus.

endomyometritis Infection of the muscle and inner lining of the uterus.

endoparametritis Infection of the muscle and inner lining of the uterus, as well as the surrounding tissues.

endorphin Substance similar to opioids that occurs naturally in the central nervous system and modifies pain sensations; related to enkephalins.

engagement (fetal) Descent of the widest diameter of the fetal presenting part to at least a zero station (the level of the ischial spines in the maternal pelvis).

engorgement Swelling of the breasts resulting from stasis and distention of the vascular and lymphatic circulations and accumulation of milk as lactation is established.

engrossment Intense fascination and close face-to-face observation between the father and newborn.

enkephalin Substance similar to opioids that occurs naturally in the central nervous system and modifies pain sensations; related to endorphins.

enteral feeding Nutrients supplied to the gastrointestinal tract orally or by feeding tube.

entrainment Newborn movement in rhythm with adult speech, particularly high-pitched tones, which are more easily heard.

epidural space Area outside the dura, between the dura mater and the vertebral canal.

episiotomy Surgical incision of the perineum to enlarge the vaginal opening.

epispadias Abnormal placement of the urinary meatus on the dorsal side of the penis.

erectile dysfunction Consistent inability of a male to achieve or maintain an erection of the penis that is sufficiently rigid to permit successful sexual intercourse. (Also called *impotence.*)

erythema toxicum Benign rash of unknown cause in newborns, with blotchy red areas that have white or yellow papules or vesicles in the center.

erythroblastosis fetalis Agglutination and hemolysis of fetal erythrocytes resulting from incompatibility between maternal and fetal blood. Now known as hemolytic disease of the fetus and newborn (HDFN).

esophageal atresia Condition in which the esophagus is separated from the stomach and ends in a blind pouch.

essential amino acids Amino acids that cannot be synthesized by the body and must be obtained from foods.

ethical dilemma A situation in which no solution seems completely satisfactory.

ethics Rules or principles that govern right conduct and distinctions between right and wrong.

ethnic Pertaining to religious, racial, national, or cultural group characteristics, especially speech patterns, social customs, and physical characteristics.

ethnicity Condition of belonging to a particular ethnic group; also refers to ethnic pride.

ethnocentrism Opinion that the beliefs and customs of one's own ethnic group are superior.

extremely-low-birth-weight infant An infant weighing 2 lb, 3 oz (1000 g) or less at birth.

extremely preterm infant An infant born before 28 weeks' gestation.

extrusion reflex Automatic nervous system response that causes an infant to push anything solid out of the mouth.

familial Presence of a trait or condition in a family more often than would be expected by chance alone.

fantasies Mental images formed to prepare for the birth of a child.

fern test Microscopic appearance of amniotic fluid resembling fern leaves when the fluid is allowed to dry on a microscope slide. (Also called *ferning.*)

fertilization age Prenatal age of the developing baby, calculated from the date of conception. (Also called *postconceptional age.*)

fetal alcohol spectrum disorders All disorders resulting from maternal use of alcohol during pregnancy; includes fetal alcohol syndrome.

fetal alcohol syndrome A group of physical, behavioral, and mental abnormalities that are the most severe effects of fetal alcohol exposure.

fetal growth restriction Failure of a fetus to grow as expected for gestational age (also called *intrauterine growth restriction [IUGR]*).

fetal hydrops See *Hydrops fetalis.*

fetal lie Relationship of the long axis of the fetus to the long axis of the pregnant client.

fetal lung fluid Fluid that fills the fetal lungs, expanding the alveoli and promoting lung development.

fetus The developing baby from 9 weeks after conception until birth.

fingertipping First tactile (touch) experience between the postpartum client and newborn in which the client explores the infant's body, mainly with the fingertips.

first period of reactivity Period beginning at birth in which newborns are active and alert. It ends when the infant first falls asleep.

fontanel Space at the intersection of sutures connecting fetal or infant skull bones.

foremilk First breast milk received in a feeding.

fornix (Pl. fornices) An arch or pouch-like structure at the upper end of the vagina. (Also called a *cul-de-sac.*)

fourth trimester First 12 weeks after birth; a time of transition for parents and siblings.

frequency (of uterine contractions) Period from the beginning of one uterine contraction to the beginning of the next.

gamete Reproductive cell or germ cell; in the female an ovum and in the male a spermatozoon.

gametogenesis Development and maturation of the sperm and ova.

gastroschisis Protrusion of the intestines through a defect in the abdominal wall. The intestines are not covered by a peritoneal sac or skin.

gate-control theory A theory about pain based on the premise that a gating mechanism in the dorsal horn of the spinal cord can open or close a "gate" for transmission of pain impulses to the brain.

gay A person who is emotionally, romantically, or sexually attracted to members of the same gender.

gender expression External appearance of one's gender identity, usually through behavior, clothing, hairstyle, or voice.

gender fluid A person who does not identify with a single fixed gender or has a fluid or unfixed gender identity.

gender identity A person's concept of self as male, female, both, or neither; how they perceive themselves and what the call themselves.

gender incongruence Clinically significant distress caused when a person's gender identity is not consistent with the sex they were assigned at birth.

gene Segment of DNA that directs the production of a specific product needed for body structure or function.

general anesthesia Systemic loss of sensation with loss of consciousness.

genetic Pertaining to the genes or chromosomes.

genetic sex Sex determined at conception by union of two X chromosomes (female) or an X and a Y chromosome (male). (Also called *chromosomal sex.*)

genotype Genetic makeup of an individual.

gestational age Prenatal age of the developing baby (measured in weeks) calculated from the first day of the client's last menstrual period; approximately 2 weeks longer than the fertilization age. (Also called *menstrual age.*)

gestational carrier (or gestational surrogate) A client who carries the embryo of an infertile couple and relinquishes the child to the couple after birth.

gestational trophoblastic disease Spectrum of diseases that includes both benign hydatidiform mole and gestational trophoblastic tumors such as invasive moles and choriocarcinoma.

gluconeogenesis Formation of glycogen by the liver from noncarbohydrate sources such as amino and fatty acids.

glycosuria Glucose in the urine.

gonad Reproductive (sex) gland that produces gametes and sex hormones. The female gonads are ovaries, and the male gonads are testes.

gonadotropic hormones Secretions of the anterior pituitary gland that stimulate the gonads, specifically follicle-stimulating hormone and luteinizing hormone. Chorionic gonadotropin is secreted by the placenta during pregnancy.

Goodell's sign Softening of the cervix during pregnancy.

graafian follicle A small sac within the ovary that contains the maturing ovum.

gravida A pregnant client; also refers to a client's total number of pregnancies, including the one in progress, if applicable.

gynecologic age The number of years since menarche (first menstrual period).

habituation Decreased response to a repeated stimulus.

haploid Having one copy of a chromosome from each pair (23 in humans, or half the diploid number); normal for gametes.

Hegar's sign Softening of the lower uterine segment that allows it to be easily compressed at 6 to 8 weeks of pregnancy.

hematoma Localized collection of blood in a space or tissue.

heme iron Iron obtained from meat, poultry, or fish sources; the form most usable by the body.

heterozygous Having two different alleles for a genetic trait.

hindmilk Breast milk received near the end of a feeding; contains higher fat content than foremilk.

homologous Chromosomes that pair during meiosis, one received from the person's female parent and one from the male parent.

homozygous Having two identical alleles for a genetic trait.

human rights model Ethical model based on the belief that every person has human rights.

hydramnios Excessive volume of amniotic fluid, more than about 2000 mL at term. (Also called *polyhydramnios.*)

hydrops fetalis Heart failure and generalized edema in the fetus secondary to severe anemia resulting from destruction of erythrocytes (hemolytic disease of the fetus and newborn).

hyperbilirubinemia Excessive amount of bilirubin in the blood.

hypercapnia Excess carbon dioxide in the blood, evidenced by an elevated Pco_2.

hyperemia Excess blood in an area of the body.

hypospadias Abnormal placement of the urinary meatus on the ventral side of the penis.

hypovolemia Abnormally decreased volume of circulating fluid in the body.

hypovolemic shock Acute circulatory failure resulting from decreased intravascular volume due to hemorrhage or loss of extracellular fluid.

hypoxemia Reduced oxygenation of the blood, evidenced by a low Po_2.

hypoxia Inadequate availability of oxygen to the body tissues (cells).

iatrogenic Term used to describe an adverse condition resulting from treatment.

impotence See *Erectile dysfunction.*

incomplete protein food Food that does not contain all the essential amino acids.

induction of labor Artificial initiation of labor.

infant mortality rate Number of deaths per 1000 live births that occurs within the first 12 months of life.

infertility Inability of a couple to conceive after 1 year of regular intercourse (two to three times weekly) without using contraception;

also, the involuntary inability to conceive and produce viable offspring when the couple chooses. Primary infertility occurs in a couple who has never conceived; secondary infertility occurs in a couple who has conceived at least once before.

intensity (of uterine contractions) Strength of a uterine contraction at its peak.

intermittent auscultation Using a Delee-Hillis fetoscope, Pinard stethoscope or hand-held Doppler ultrasound to determine the fetal heart rate and regularity at selected intervals based on the client's risk status and unit guidelines and policies.

intrapartum Time of labor and childbirth.

intrauterine device Long-acting contraceptives that are inserted into the uterus to provide continuous pregnancy prevention.

intraventricular hemorrhage Bleeding around and into the ventricles of the brain. (Also called *germinal matrix hemorrhage* and *periventricular–intraventricular hemorrhage.*)

involution Retrogressive changes that return the reproductive organs, particularly the uterus, to their nonpregnant size and condition.

jaundice Yellow discoloration of the skin and sclera caused by excess bilirubin in the blood.

kangaroo care A method of providing skin-to-skin contact between infants and their parents.

karyotype A display of a cell's chromosomes, arranged from largest to smallest pairs, with sex chromosomes displayed as a separate pair.

Kegel exercises Alternate contracting and relaxing of the pelvic floor muscles to strengthen the muscles surrounding the urinary meatus and vagina.

kernicterus Staining of brain tissue caused by accumulation of unconjugated bilirubin in the brain. Bilirubin encephalopathy is the brain damage that results from these deposits.

ketosis Accumulation of ketone bodies (metabolic products) in blood; frequently associated with acidosis.

kilocalorie A unit of heat; used to show the energy value in foods (commonly called *calorie*).

lactation Secretion of milk from the breasts; also describes the period during which a child is breastfed.

lactogenesis The production of milk.

lacto-ovovegetarian A vegetarian whose diet includes milk products and eggs.

lactose intolerance Inability to digest most dairy products because of a deficiency of the enzyme lactase.

lactovegetarian A vegetarian whose diet includes milk products.

lanugo Fine, soft hair that covers the fetus.

laparoscopy Insertion of an illuminated tube into the abdominal cavity to visualize contents, locate bleeding, and perform surgical procedures.

laparotomy Incision through the lower abdominal wall to examine the abdominal or pelvic organs or perform other surgical procedures.

large-for-gestational-age infant An infant whose size is above the 90th percentile for gestational age.

latch Attachment of the infant to the breast.

late preterm infant An infant born between 34 weeks, 0 days and 36 weeks, 6 days of gestation.

lecithin/sphingomyelin ratio (L/S ratio) Ratio of two phospholipids in amniotic fluid used to determine fetal lung maturity; ratio of 2:1 or greater usually indicates fetal lung maturity.

lesbian A woman who is sexually attracted to other women.

let-down reflex See *Milk-ejection reflex*.

letting-go A phase of maternal adaptation that involves relinquishment of previous roles and assumption of a new role as a parent.

libido Sexual desire.

lightening Descent of the fetal head into the pelvic cavity before labor.

linea nigra Pigmented line extending in the midline of the abdomen from the fundus to the symphysis pubis.

linear salpingostomy Incision along the length of a fallopian tube to remove an ectopic pregnancy and preserve the tube.

lipogenic Substance such as insulin that stimulates the production of fat.

lochia Vaginal drainage after birth.

lochia alba White, cream-colored, or light yellow vaginal discharge that follows lochia serosa. Occurs when the amount of blood is decreased and the number of leukocytes is increased.

lochia rubra Reddish or red–brown vaginal discharge that occurs immediately after childbirth; composed mostly of blood.

lochia serosa Pink- or brown-tinged vaginal discharge that follows lochia rubra and precedes lochia alba; composed largely of serous exudate, blood, and leukocytes.

low-birth-weight infant An infant weighing less than 5 lb, 8 oz (2500 g) at birth.

maceration Discoloration and softening of tissues and eventual disintegration of a fetus that is retained in the uterus after its death.

macrosomia Infant birth weight above the 90th percentile for gestational age. Some sources use more than 4000 g (8 lb, 13 oz) or 4500 g (9 lb, 15 oz).

mammogram Study of breast tissue using very-low-dose radiography; primary tool in the diagnosis of breast tumors.

Marfan syndrome A hereditary condition that involves weakness in connective tissue, bones, and muscles; the vascular system is affected, particularly the aorta.

mastitis Infection of the breast.

maternal mortality rate Number of maternal deaths from births and complications of pregnancy, childbirth, and puerperium (the first 42 days after the pregnancy ends) per 100,000 live births.

mature milk Breast milk that replaces transitional milk.

meconium aspiration syndrome Obstruction and air trapping caused by meconium in the infant's lungs, which may lead to severe respiratory distress.

meiosis Reduction cell division in gametes that halves the number of chromosomes in each cell.

melasma Brownish pigmentation of the face during pregnancy. (Also called *chloasma* and *mask of pregnancy*.)

menarche Onset of menstruation, usually between 10 and 16 years of age or within 2 years of the start of breast development.

meningocele Protrusion of the meninges through a defect in the vertebrae; a form of neural tube defect.

menometrorrhagia Uterine bleeding that is irregular in frequency and excessive in amount.

menopause Permanent cessation of menstruation during the climacteric.

menorrhagia Excessive bleeding at the time of menstruation in number of days' duration, amount of blood lost, or both.

methadone A synthetic compound with opiate properties; used as an oral substitute for heroin and morphine in the opiate-dependent person.

metritis Infection of the decidua, myometrium, and parametrial tissues of the uterus.

metrorrhagia Bleeding from the uterus at any time other than during the menstrual period.

milia White cysts, 1 mm in size, on the face.

miliaria (prickly heat) Rash caused by heat.

milk-ejection reflex Release of milk from the alveoli into the ducts. (Also known as the *let-down reflex*.)

mimicry Copying the behaviors of other pregnant clients or mothers as a method of "trying on" the role of advanced pregnancy or motherhood.

mitosis Cell division in body cells other than the gametes.

mittelschmerz Low abdominal pain that occurs at ovulation.

moderately preterm infant An infant born between $28\frac{0}{7}$ to $33\frac{6}{7}$ weeks of gestation

molding Shaping of the fetal head during movement through the birth canal.

Mongolian spots Bruise-like marks that occur mostly in newborns with dark skin tones.

monosomy Presence of only one of a chromosome pair in every body cell.

Montevideo unit Method to quantify intensity of labor contractions with uterine activity monitoring. The baseline intrauterine pressure for each contraction in a 10-minute period is subtracted from the peak pressure.

mortality rate Number of deaths that occur each year by different categories.

morula Fertilized ovum that resembles a mulberry when it contains 12 to 16 cells.

motor block Loss of voluntary movement caused by regional anesthesia.

multifetal pregnancy A pregnancy in which the client is carrying two or more fetuses. (Also called *multiple gestation*.)

multigravida A client who has been pregnant more than once.

multipara A client who has delivered two or more pregnancies at 20 or more weeks of gestation.

multiple-marker testing/screening Sometimes called a quad screen; a maternal blood test for four substances (human chorionic gonadotropin, alpha-fetoprotein, unconjugated estriol, and in the quad screen, inhibin A). It is performed to evaluate a pregnant client's risk for trisomy 21, trisomy 18, and open neural tube defects.

mutation Alteration in DNA sequence in a gene, usually one that adversely affects its function.

myelomeningocele Protrusion of the meninges and spinal cord through a defect in the vertebrae; a form of neural tube defect.

nadir Lowest point, such as the lowest pulse rate in a series.

narcissism Undue preoccupation with oneself.

natural family planning Method of predicting ovulation based on normal changes in a woman's body; also called fertility awareness method.

necrotizing enterocolitis (NEC) Serious inflammatory condition of the intestines, which is often complicated by necrosis of the bowel, perforation, and peritonitis.

neonatal abstinence syndrome A cluster of physical signs exhibited by the newborn exposed in utero to maternal use of substances such as heroin. (See also *Abstinence syndrome*.)

neonatal mortality rate Number of deaths per 1000 live births occurring at birth or within the first 28 days of life.

neural tube defect (NTD) A congenital defect in the closure of the bony encasement of the spinal cord or skull. Includes defects such as anencephaly, spina bifida, meningocele, myelomeningocele, and others.

neutral thermal environment (NTE) Environment in which body temperature is maintained without an increase in metabolic rate or oxygen use.

nevus flammeus Permanent pink to dark reddish–purple birthmark. (Also called *port wine stain*.)

nevus simplex Flat, pink area on the nape of the neck, on the midforehead, or over the eyelids resulting from dilation of the capillaries. (Also called *stork bites*, *salmon patches*, or *telangiectatic nevi*.)

nevus vasculosus Rough, red collection of capillaries with a raised surface that disappears with time. (Also called *strawberry hemangioma*.)

nidation Implantation of the fertilized ovum (zygote) in the uterine endometrium.

nonbinary An adjective describing a person who does not identify exclusively as a man or a woman.

noncompliance Resistance of the lungs and thorax to distention with air during respirations.

nonheme iron Iron obtained from plants and fortified foods.

nonnutritive sucking Sucking during which little or no milk flow is obtained or sucking on an object such as a pacifier or finger.

nonshivering thermogenesis Process of heat production, without shivering, by oxidation of brown fat.

nonstress test (NST) A method for evaluating fetal status during the antepartum period by observing the response of the fetal heart rate to fetal movement.

nuchal cord Umbilical cord around the fetal body, often the neck.

nullipara A client who has never completed a pregnancy beyond 20 weeks' gestation.

nurse anesthetist A registered nurse who has advanced education and certification in administration of anesthetics; also, certified registered nurse anesthetist (CRNA).

nutrient density The quality and quantity of protein, vitamins, and minerals per 100 calories in foods.

nutritive suckling (sucking) Steady, rhythmic suckling at the breast or sucking at a bottle to obtain milk.

occult prolapse See *Prolapsed cord.*

oligohydramnios Abnormally small amount of amniotic fluid, less than about 500 mL at term.

oligospermia A decreased number of sperm in semen, usually considered to be under 20 million per milliliter.

omphalocele Protrusion of the intestines into the base of the umbilical cord.

oogenesis Formation of gametes (ova) in the female.

opiate Any narcotic-containing opium or a derivative of opium.

oral contraceptive Drug that inhibits ovulation; contains progestins alone or in combination with estrogen.

osmotic diuresis Secretion and passage of large amounts of urine as a result of increased osmotic pressure that can result from hyperglycemia.

osteomalacia Softening of bones; precedes osteoporosis.

osteoporosis Increased spaces (porosity) of bone; process usually accelerates after menopause.

ovovegetarian A vegetarian whose diet includes eggs.

ovulation Release of the mature ovum from the ovary.

pain threshold (or pain perception) The lowest level of stimulus one perceives as painful; relatively constant under different conditions.

pain tolerance Maximum pain one is willing to endure. Pain tolerance may increase or decrease under different conditions.

pansexual A person who has the potential for emotional, romantic, or sexual attraction to people of any gender.

Pap test Evaluation of cells taken from the cervix for evaluation of possible cervical cancer.

para A client who has given birth after a pregnancy of at least 20 weeks of gestation; also designates the number of a client's pregnancies that have ended after at least 20 weeks of gestation.

paroxysmal nocturnal dyspnea Respiratory distress occurring when lying down; often associated with congestive heart failure.

peau d'orange Dimpled skin condition in which skin resembles an orange peel; associated with lymphatic edema and often seen over the area of breast cancer.

pedigree A graphic representation of a family's medical and hereditary history and the relationships among the family members. (Also called a *genogram.*)

percutaneous umbilical blood sampling (PUBS) Procedure for obtaining fetal blood through ultrasound-guided puncture of an umbilical cord vessel to detect fetal problems such as inherited blood disorders, acidosis, or infection. (Also called *cordocentesis.*)

perinatologist Physician who specializes in the high-risk pregnancy care of the pregnant client and fetus during the perinatal period (from approximately the 20th week of pregnancy to 4 weeks after childbirth). (Also known as a *maternal-fetal medicine specialist.*)

periodic breathing Cessation of breathing lasting 5 to 10 seconds followed by 10 to 15 seconds of rapid respirations without changes in skin color or heart rate.

persistent pulmonary hypertension Vasoconstriction of the infant's pulmonary vessels after birth; may result in right-to-left shunting of blood flow through the ductus arteriosus, the foramen ovale, or both.

pH test A paper or commercial swab used to test pH; helps determine whether the amniotic sac has ruptured. Nitrazine test.

phenotype The outward expression of a person's genetic makeup; observed characteristics produced by the interaction of genes and environment.

phosphatidylglycerol (PG) A major phospholipid of surfactant whose presence in amniotic fluid indicates fetal lung maturity.

phosphatidylinositol (PI) A phospholipid of surfactant that is produced and secreted in increasing amounts as the fetal lungs mature.

physiologic anemia of pregnancy Decrease in hemoglobin and hematocrit values caused by dilution of erythrocytes from expanded plasma volume rather than by an actual decrease in erythrocytes or hemoglobin.

phytoestrogen Estrogen substance of plant origin.

pica Ingestion of nonnutritive substances such as laundry starch, clay, or ice.

placenta Fetal structure that provides nourishment and removes wastes from the developing baby and secretes hormones necessary for the continuation of pregnancy.

placenta accreta A placenta that is abnormally adherent into the uterine wall. If the condition is more advanced, it is called *placenta increta* (the placenta extends into the uterine muscle) or *placenta percreta* (the placenta perforates through the uterine muscle).

placenta previa Abnormal implantation of the placenta in the lower uterus at or very near the cervical os.

placental abruption Premature separation of a normally implanted placenta. Also called abruptio placentae.

plagiocephaly Flattening or asymmetry of the back of the head.

point of maximum impulse Area of the chest in which the heart sounds are loudest when auscultated.

polycythemia Abnormally high number of erythrocytes.

polydactyly More than 10 digits on the hands or feet.

polydipsia Excessive thirst.

polyhydramnios See *Hydramnios.*

polymerase chain reaction (PCR) A technique to rapidly analyze sequences of genes for in vitro diagnosis of infections; many hereditary characteristics can also be analyzed by the technique.

polymorphism Alternative form of a gene found in the population at a frequency greater than 1%.

polyphagia Excessive ingestion of food.

polyploidy Having additional full sets of chromosomes, such as 69 (triploidy) or 92 (tetraploidy).

polyuria Excessive excretion of urine.

position (fetal) Relation of a fixed reference point on the fetus to the quadrants of the maternal pelvis.

postictal Unresponsive state after a seizure.

postmaturity syndrome Condition in which a postterm infant shows characteristics indicative of poor placental functioning before birth. (Also called *dysmaturity syndrome.*)

postpartum Refers to the first 6 weeks after childbirth.

postpartum blues Temporary, self-limited period of tearfulness experienced by many postpartum clients beginning the first week after childbirth.

postterm infant An infant born after 42 weeks of gestation.

precipitate birth A birth that occurs without a trained attendant present.

precipitate labor An intense, unusually short labor (less than 3 hours).

preeclampsia A hypertensive disorder of pregnancy characterized by new onset of hypertension after 20 weeks' gestation and multisystem involvement.

pregnancy-related mortality rate Death of a client during pregnancy or within 12 months after the end of the pregnancy from any cause related to or worsened by the pregnancy, but not due to accidental or incidental causes.

premature rupture of the membranes Spontaneous rupture of the membranes before the onset of labor (term, preterm, or postterm gestation). Also known as *prelabor rupture of the membranes.*

presentation (fetal) Fetal part that enters the pelvic inlet, or the presenting part.

preterm birth A birth that occurs after the 20th week and before the beginning of the 37th week of gestation.

preterm infant An infant born before the beginning of the 38th week of gestation. (Also called *premature infant.*)

preterm labor Onset of labor after 20 weeks and before the beginning of the 37th week of gestation.

preterm premature rupture of the membranes Rupture of the membranes before the onset of labor in a pregnancy after 20 weeks and before the beginning of the 37th week of gestation. Also known as *preterm prelabor rupture of the membranes.*

primigravida   A client who is pregnant for the first time.

primipara   A client who has given birth after a pregnancy of at least 20 weeks of gestation; also used informally to describe a pregnant client before the birth of the first child.

progestin   Any natural or synthetic form of progesterone.

prolapsed cord   Displacement of the umbilical cord in front of or beside the fetal presenting part. An occult prolapse is one that is suspected on the basis of fetal heart rate patterns; the umbilical cord cannot be palpated or seen.

pseudomenstruation   Vaginal bleeding in the newborn resulting from withdrawal of placental hormones.

psychosis   Mental state in which a person's ability to recognize reality, communicate, and relate to others is impaired.

puberty   Period of sexual maturation accompanied by the development of secondary sex characteristics and the capacity to reproduce.

puerperal infection   A temperature of 38°C (100.4°F) or higher after the first 24 hours and occurring on at least 2 of the first 10 days after childbirth.

puerperium   Period from the end of childbirth until involution of the reproductive organs is complete; approximately 6 weeks.

pulmonary embolus   A potentially fatal complication that occurs when the pulmonary artery is obstructed by a blood clot that was swept into circulation from a vein or by amniotic fluid.

pulse oximetry   Method of determining the level of blood oxygen saturation by sensors attached to the skin.

pulse pressure   The difference between systolic and diastolic blood pressures.

queer   A term used by some people to describe their own fluid gender identity.

quickening   The first movements of the fetus felt by the pregnant client.

recessive   Gene that requires two copies, one from the maternal and one from the paternal chromosome, for the trait to be expressed.

reciprocal attachment behaviors   Repertoire of infant actions that promotes attachment between the parent and newborn.

recommended dietary allowance (RDA)   Level of nutrient intake considered to meet the needs of healthy individuals.

rectocele   Herniation (protrusion) of the rectum through the posterior vaginal wall.

REEDA   Acronym for redness, ecchymosis, edema, discharge, and approximation; useful for assessing wound healing or the presence of inflammation or infection.

reflection   Meditation, attentive consideration.

regional anesthesia   Anesthesia that blocks pain impulses in a localized area without loss of consciousness.

respiratory distress syndrome (RDS)   Condition caused by insufficient production of surfactant in the lungs; results in atelectasis (collapse of the lung alveoli), hypoxia (de-

creased oxygen [O_2] concentration), and hypercapnia (increased carbon dioxide [CO_2] concentration).

retinopathy of prematurity (ROP)   Condition in which injury to blood vessels may cause decreased vision or blindness in preterm infants.

retrograde ejaculation   Discharge of semen into the bladder rather than from the end of the penis.

ripening   Softening of the cervix as labor nears as the result of an increase in water content and the effects of relaxin on the connective tissue of the cervix.

role transition   Changing from one pattern of behavior and one image of self to another.

ruga (Pl. rugae)   Ridge or fold of tissue, as on the male's scrotum and in the female's vagina.

salpingectomy   Surgical removal of a fallopian tube.

seborrheic dermatitis (cradle cap)   Yellowish, crusty area of the scalp.

second period of reactivity   Period of 4 to 6 hours after the first sleep after birth when the newborn may have an elevated pulse rate and respiratory rate and excessive mucus.

secondary sex characteristics   Physical differences between mature males and females that are not directly related to reproduction.

semen   Spermatozoa with their nourishing and protective fluid; discharged at ejaculation.

sensory block   Loss of sensation caused by regional anesthesia.

sentinel lymph node (SLN) biopsy   Technique to remove a minimal number of key lymph nodes to determine spread of the tumor.

sepsis   A systemic infection from bacteria in the bloodstream

seroconversion   Change in a blood test result from negative to positive, indicating the development of antibodies in response to infection or immunization.

servocontrol   Mechanism on a radiant warmer or incubator to regulate the amount of heat produced.

sex chromosome   The X or Y chromosome; females have two X chromosomes, and males have one X and one Y chromosome.

sexual orientation   An inherent or immutable emotional, romantic, or sexual attraction to other people.

short bowel syndrome   A condition caused by a bowel that is shorter than normal.

shoulder dystocia   Delayed or difficult birth of the fetal shoulders after the head is born.

small-for-gestational-age infant   An infant whose size is below the 10th percentile for gestational age.

somatic cells   Body cells other than the gametes, or germ cells.

somatic sex   Gender assignment as male or female on the basis of form and structure of the external genitalia.

spermatogenesis   Formation of male gametes (sperm) in the testes.

spermicide   A chemical that kills sperm.

spina bifida   Defective closure of the bony spine that encloses the spinal cord; a type of neural tube defect.

spinnbarkeit   Clear, slippery, stretchy quality of cervical mucus during ovulation.

standard of care   Level of care that can be expected of a professional as determined by laws, professional organizations, and health care agencies.

station (fetal)   Measurement of fetal descent in relation to the ischial spines of the maternal pelvis. (See also *Engagement.*)

sterility   Total inability to conceive.

strabismus   A turning inward ("crossing") or outward of the eyes caused by poor tone in the muscles that control eye movement.

striae gravidarum   Irregular pink to purple streaks on the pregnant client's abdomen, breasts, or buttocks resulting from tears in connective tissue.

subarachnoid space   Space between the arachnoid mater and the pia mater containing cerebrospinal fluid.

subinvolution   Delayed return of the uterus to its nonpregnant size and consistency.

suckling   Giving or taking nourishment from the breast. Sometimes used interchangeably with *sucking,* which refers only to drawing into the mouth with a partial vacuum, as with a bottle or pacifier.

sudden infant death syndrome (SIDS)   Sudden death of an infant that is unexplained by history, autopsy, or examination of the scene of death.

surfactant   Combination of lipoproteins produced by the lungs of the mature fetus to reduce surface tension in the alveoli, thus promoting lung expansion after birth.

surrogate mother   A fertile woman who is inseminated with the purpose of conceiving and relinquishing a child to an infertile couple.

suspend   To delay or bring to a stop temporarily.

sutures   Narrow areas of flexible tissue that connect fetal skull bones, permitting slight movement during labor.

syndactyly   Webbing between fingers or toes.

tachypnea   Respiratory rate greater than 60 breaths per minute in the newborn after the first hour of life.

taking-hold   Second phase of maternal adaptation during which the client assumes control of care of self and initiates care of the infant.

taking-in   First phase of maternal adaptation during which the client passively accepts care, comfort, and details about the newborn.

teratogen   An environmental agent that can cause defects in a developing baby during pregnancy.

term   Refers to the period of time a pregnancy is expected to last. (Also known as *full term.*)

thermogenesis   Heat production.

thermoregulation   Maintenance of body temperature.

thrombophlebitis   Occurs when the vessel wall develops an inflammatory response to the thrombus. This further occludes the vessel.

thrombus Collection of blood factors, primarily platelets and fibrin, that may cause vascular obstruction.

tocolytic Drug that inhibits uterine contractions.

total parenteral nutrition (TPN) Intravenous infusion of all nutrients known to be needed for metabolism and growth.

toxic shock syndrome Rare, potentially fatal disorder usually caused by a toxin produced by *Staphylococcus aureus*; has been associated with improper use of tampons.

tracheoesophageal fistula Abnormal connection between the esophagus and the trachea.

transcultural nursing Concerned with the provision of nursing care in a manner that is sensitive to the needs of individuals, families, and groups.

transdermal contraceptive patch Adhesive patch containing estrogen and progestin, which are absorbed through the skin to prevent pregnancy.

transducer Device that translates one physical quantity to another, such as fetal heart motion into an electrical signal for rate calculation, generation of sound, or a written record.

transgender A person whose gender identity differs from the sex they were assigned at birth.

transient tachypnea of the newborn Condition of rapid respirations caused by inadequate absorption of fetal lung fluid.

transitional milk Breast milk that appears between secretion of colostrum and mature milk.

translocation Exchange of genetic material between nonhomologous chromosomes.

trimester One of three equal, 13-week parts of a full-term pregnancy.

Triple I Intrauterine infection or inflammation or both. See *Chorioamnionitis.*

trisomy Presence of three copies of a chromosome in each body cell.

tubal sterilization Cutting or mechanically occluding the fallopian tubes to prevent passage of ova or sperm, thus preventing pregnancy. (May also be called *tubal ligation.*)

ultrasound Use of sound waves for visualizing deep structures of the body by recording the reflections (echoes) of high-frequency sound waves directed into the tissue.

uterine atony Lack of tone in the postpartum uterus, which often results in postpartum hemorrhage.

uterine inversion Turning of the uterus inside out after birth of the fetus.

uterine resting tone Degree of uterine muscle tension when the client is not in labor or during the interval between labor contractions.

uterine rupture A tear in the wall of the uterus.

uterine tachysystole More than five contractions in 10 minutes, averaged over 30 minutes

uteroplacental insufficiency Inability of the placenta to exchange oxygen, carbon dioxide, nutrients, and waste products properly between the maternal and fetal circulations.

utilitarian model Ethical model stating that the right course of action is the one that produces the greatest good.

vacuum curettage (vacuum aspiration) Removal of the uterine contents by application of a vacuum through a hollow curette or cannula introduced into the uterus.

vaginal contraceptive ring Flexible ring releasing small amounts of estrogen and progesterone to prevent pregnancy.

validate To make certain that the information collected is accurate.

varicocele Abnormal dilation or varicosity of veins in the spermatic cord.

vasa previa Branching of umbilical cord vessels in the amniotic sac rather than inserting into the placenta.

vasectomy Cutting or occluding the vas deferens to prevent passage of sperm, thus preventing pregnancy.

VBAC Acronym for vaginal birth after cesarean.

vegan A complete vegetarian who does not eat any animal products.

vegetarian An individual whose diet consists wholly or mostly of plant foods and who avoids animal food sources.

vernix caseosa Thick, white substance that protects the skin of the fetus.

version Turning the fetus from one presentation to another before birth, usually from breech to cephalic.

very-low-birth-weight infant An infant weighing 3 lb, 5 oz (1500 g) or less at birth.

vibroacoustic stimulation Use of sound stimulation to elicit fetal movement and acceleration (speeding up) of the fetal heart rate.

well-woman examination Verbal history, physical examination, and screening tests for a woman with no complaints of serious diseases, usually done annually. Often abbreviated WWE.

zygote The developing baby from conception through the first week of prenatal life.

INDEX

Page numbers followed by *f* indicate figures; *t,* tables, *b,* boxes.